# CHEST
# MEDICINE

▼

## ESSENTIALS OF
## PULMONARY AND
## CRITICAL CARE
## MEDICINE

THIRD EDITION

# CHEST MEDICINE
▼

## ESSENTIALS OF PULMONARY AND CRITICAL CARE MEDICINE

### THIRD EDITION

EDITED BY

**RONALD B. GEORGE, M.D.**
Professor and Chairman
Department of Medicine
Louisiana State University School of Medicine
Shreveport, Louisiana

**RICHARD W. LIGHT, M.D.**
Professor of Medicine
University of California, Irvine
Veterans Administration Medical Center
Long Beach, California

**MICHAEL A. MATTHAY, M.D.**
Professor of Medicine and Anesthesia
Associate Director, Intensive Care Unit
Senior Member, Cardiovascular Research Institute
School of Medicine
University of California, San Francisco
San Francisco, California

**RICHARD A. MATTHAY, M.D.**
Boehringer Ingelheim Professor of Medicine
Associate Chairman
Pulmonary and Critical Care Section
Yale University School of Medicine
New Haven, Connecticut

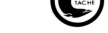

**Williams & Wilkins**
BALTIMORE • PHILADELPHIA • HONG KONG
LONDON • MUNICH • SYDNEY • TOKYO
A WAVERLY COMPANY

*Editor:* David C. Retford
*Managing Editor:* Kathleen Courtney Millet
*Copy Editors:* Thomas Lehr, Anne Schwartz
*Designer:* Ann Feild
*Illustration Planner:* Ray Lowman
*Production Coordinator:* Kimberly S. Nawrozki

Copyright © 1995
Williams & Wilkins
351 West Camden Street
Baltimore, Maryland 21201 USA

Accurate indications, adverse reactions, and dosage schedules for drugs are provided in this book, but it is possible that they may change. The reader is urged to review the package information data of the manufacturers of the medications mentioned.

*Printed in the United States of America*

First Edition 1983, Churchill Livingstone Inc.
Second Edition 1990, Williams & Wilkins

The figures and tables listed below are from George RB, Light RW, Matthay RA (eds): *Chest Medicine,* ed 1. New York, Churchill Livingstone, 1983.
    Figures 1.3–1.5, 1.18, 2.2, 3.1–3.16, 4.1–4.7, 7.1–7.8, 7.11, 7.12, 7.21, 7.22, 8.1–8.13,
              12.2–12.14, 13.2–13.13, 17.6–17.10, 17.14, 18.2–18.11, 22.2–22.5, 22.9,
              22.10
    Tables 4.1, 5.3, 8.2–8.4, 6.1, 13.1–13.5, 13.7–13.11, 17.4, 17.7, 18.2, 22.1, 22.2

**Library of Congress Cataloging-in-Publication Data**

Chest medicine : essentials of pulmonary and critical care medicine /
  edited by Ronald B. George . . . [et al.].—3rd ed.
     p.  cm.
  Includes bibliographical references and index.
  ISBN 0-683-03458-8
  1. Chest—Diseases.  2. Respiratory intensive care.  I. George,
Ronald B.
  [DNLM:  1. Lung Diseases.  2. Lung—physiology.  3. Critical Care.
WF 600 C525 1995]
RC941.C5675  1995
616.2′4—dc20
DNLM/DLC
for Library of Congress                     94-38017
                                    CIP

                                      97 98 99
                           2 3 4 5 6 7 8 9 10

Reprints of chapter(s) may be purchased from Williams & Wilkins in quantities of 100 or more. Call Isabella Wise, Special Sales Department, (800) 358-3583.

# Preface

THE NEED FOR an "essentials" textbook in chest medicine became apparent to the editors in the early 1980s when the specialties of pulmonary disease and critical care medicine exploded with new information and technology. At that time, there were several excellent reference texts available, and there was no need for another large, expensive office reference. Since we published our first edition of *Chest Medicine* in 1983, the concept of "essentials" texts to supplement these large reference works has become extremely popular. The concise editions of the major internal medicine textbooks now outsell the parent texts by a large margin.

With the publication of the third edition of *Chest Medicine*, our original concept of a concise yet comprehensive summary of the field of pulmonary and critical care medicine remains intact. During the 13 years since our first edition appeared, the field has changed and expanded greatly. Critical care has grown into a major area of interest, with multiple textbooks and journals devoted to this field. In response to these changes, we have expanded this section in the current edition from four to seven chapters. Some of the more elementary portions of the earlier edition have been eliminated to limit the size of the textbook. Material readily available elsewhere, such as appendices and basic science chapters, has been replaced with additional clinical chapters. The persistent goal of the editors has been to provide a clinically oriented textbook that can be read from cover to cover during preparation for examinations, or can be easily referred to by the busy clinician.

The material is appropriate for practicing physicians (both primary care and subspecialty), fellows, housestaff, and medical students, as well as for respiratory therapists, physician assistants, and other health care professionals.

As in the Second Edition, we divided the book into four sections: Pulmonary Structure and Function; Diagnostic Studies in Patients with Respiratory Problems; Evaluation and Management of Lung Disease; and The Critically Ill Patient. Every chapter has been extensively rewritten, some by new authors and editors, to ensure the timeliness of the content. New diagnostic procedures are discussed in detail, as are new treatment modalities. The current literature has been reviewed and is referenced.

The editors wish to thank the contributors, whose hard work has brought the text up to date. We also thank the staff of Williams & Wilkins, particularly Dave Retford, Jonathan Pine, Katey Millet, Molly Mullen, Kim Nawrozki, and Tom Lehr. As always, we are grateful to our administrative support staff—Cathy Couvillon, Jill Richardson, and Leslye Stein—who do all the real work and allow us to fulfill our many roles. Most of all we thank our students, housestaff physicians, and fellows, who force us to be current and who make our task a pleasant one. To them, once again, this textbook is dedicated.

Ronald B. George, M.D.
Richard W. Light, M.D.
Michael A. Matthay, M.D.
Richard A. Matthay, M.D.

# Contributors

**Loutfi S. Aboussouan, M.D.**
Clinical Associate
Department of Pulmonary and Critical Care
    Medicine
The Cleveland Clinic Foundation
Cleveland, Ohio

**William McDowell Anderson, M.D.**
Associate Professor
Department of Internal Medicine
University of South Florida College of Medicine
Chief, Pulmonary and Critical Care Medicine
James A. Haley Veterans Affairs Hospital
Tampa, Florida

**Alejandro C. Arroliga, M.D.**
Department of Pulmonary and Critical Care
    Medicine
The Cleveland Clinic Foundation
Cleveland, Ohio

**John R. Balmes, M.D.**
Associate Professor
Department of Medicine
University of California, San Francisco
Chief, Division of Occupational and Environmental
    Medicine
San Francisco General Hospital
San Francisco, California

**Richard B. Berry, M.D.**
Associate Professor of Medicine in Residence
Pulmonary and Critical Care Medicine
University of California, Irvine
Orange, California
Staff Physician, Medical Director of the Sleep
    Laboratory
Veterans Affairs Medical Center
Long Beach, California

**Darryl C. Carter, M.D.**
Professor of Pathology
Yale University School of Medicine
Director, Tissue Retrieval Facility
Comprehensive Cancer Center
New Haven, Connecticut

**Andrew L. Chesson, Jr., M.D.**
Department of Neurology
Louisiana State University School of Medicine
Shreveport, Louisiana

**Steven A. Conrad, M.D., Ph.D., F.A.C.P., F.C.C.M.,
    F.A.C.E.P.**
Associate Professor of Medicine
Section of Pulmonary and Critical Care Medicine
Director, Medical Intensive Care Unit
Louisiana State University Medical Center
Shreveport, Louisiana

**Paul M. Dorinsky, M.D.**
Associate Professor of Medicine
Division of Pulmonary and Critical Care Medicine
The Ohio State University College of Medicine
Director, Medical Intensive Care Unit
Ohio State University Medical Center
Columbus, Ohio

**Jeffrey R. Fineman, M.D.**
Assistant Professor of Pediatrics
Department of Pediatrics
University of California, San Francisco
San Francisco, California

**Ronald B. George, M.D.**
Professor and Chairman
Department of Medicine
Louisiana State University School of Medicine
Shreveport, Louisiana

**Christian Jayr, M.D.**
Anesthesiologist
Institut Gustave Roussy
Villejuif, France

**Mani S. Kavuru, M.D.**
Director, Pulmonary Function Laboratory
Staff Physician
Department of Pulmonary and Critical Care
    Medicine
The Cleveland Clinic Foundation
Cleveland, Ohio

**Françoise Kramer, M.D.**
Assistant Professor of Clinical Medicine
Section of Infectious Diseases
Los Angeles County/University of Southern
  California Medical Center
Los Angeles, California

**Stephanie M. Levine, M.D.**
Assistant Professor of Medicine
Division of Pulmonary Disease/Critical Care
  Medicine
University of Texas Health Science Center at San
  Antonio
San Antonio, Texas

**Richard W. Light, M.D.**
Professor of Medicine
University of California, Irvine
Veterans Affairs Medical Center
Long Beach, California

**C. Kees Mahutte, M.D., Ph.D.**
Associate Professor of Medicine
University of California, Irvine
Irvine, California
Chief, Pulmonary and Critical Care Section
Veterans Affairs Medical Center
Long Beach, California

**Richard A. Matthay, M.D.**
Boehringer Ingelheim Professor of Medicine
Associate Director
Pulmonary and Critical Care Section
Yale University School of Medicine
New Haven, Connecticut

**Michael A. Matthay, M.D.**
Professor of Medicine and Anesthesia
Associate Director, Intensive Care Unit
Senior Member, Cardiovascular Research Institute
University of California, San Francisco School of
  Medicine
San Francisco, California

**Michael S. Niederman, M.D., F.A.C.P., F.C.C.P**
Director, Medical and Respiratory Intensive Care
  Unit
Director, Critical Care Subsection
Pulmonary and Critical Care Medicine
Winthrop-University Hospital
Mineola, New York
Associate Professor
Department of Medicine, State University of New
  York
Stony Brook, New York

**Eric A. Peper, M.D., F.A.C.S.**
Cardiovascular and Thoracic Surgery
Sacramento Cardiovascular Surgeons Medical Group
Sutter Memorial Hospital
Sacramento, California

**Jay I. Peters, M.D.**
Associate Professor of Medicine
Division of Pulmonary Disease/Critical Care
Department of Medicine
University of Texas Health Science Center at San
  Antonio
San Antonio, Texas

**Carrie A. Redlich, M.D., M.P.H.**
Assistant Professor
Department of Internal Medicine
Pulmonary and Critical Care Section
Occupational and Environmental Medicine Program
Yale University School of Medicine
New Haven, Connecticut

**Stephen I. Rennard, M.D.**
Larson Professor of Medicine
Chief, Pulmonary and Critical Care Medicine
University of Nebraska Medical Center
Omaha, Nebraska

**Herbert Y. Reynolds, M.D.**
J. Lloyd Huck Professor of Medicine
Chairman, Department of Medicine
The Milton S. Hershey Medical Center
Pennsylvania State University School of Medicine
Hershey, Pennsylvania

**George A. Sarosi, M.D.**
Chairman
Department of Medicine
Santa Clara Valley Medical Center
San Jose, California
Professor of Medicine
Stanford University School of Medicine
Stanford, California

**Scott A. Sasse, M.D.**
Assistant Professor of Medicine
Section of Pulmonary and Critical Care Medicine
University of California, Irvine
Veterans Affairs Medical Center
Long Beach, California

**H. Dirk Sostman, M.D.**
Professor and Director of Academic Affairs
Department of Radiology
Duke University
Durham, North Carolina

**James K. Stoller, M.D.**
Head, Section of Respiratory Therapy
Department of Pulmonary and Critical Care
    Medicine
The Cleveland Clinic Foundation
Cleveland, Ohio

**Herbert P. Wiedemann, M.D.**
Chairman
Department of Pulmonary and Critical Care
    Medicine
The Cleveland Clinic Foundation
Cleveland, Ohio

# Contents

# PULMONARY

# STRUCTURE

# AND

# FUNCTION

Chapter **1**

# Functional Anatomy of the Respiratory System

**Ronald B. George**
**Andrew L. Chesson, Jr.**
**Stephen I. Rennard**

THE LUNGS PERFORM many important functions, including the filtering of systemic venous blood prior to its entry into the left ventricle and the production and metabolism of vasoactive substances. Their most important function, however, is the exchange of carbon dioxide, a byproduct of cellular metabolism, for oxygen, which is necessary for cellular activity. The respiratory system is ideally designed to perform this vital function 24 hours a day with a minimum amount of work (1).

During a lifetime of breathing the delicate tissues of the lung periphery are constantly exposed to environmental toxins and irritants of varying potency, including viruses, bacteria, and other living organisms as well as cigarette smoke, dust particles, and toxic chemicals. This constant exposure to a hostile environment

TABLE 1.1
RESPIRATORY STRUCTURES AS RELATED TO THEIR FUNCTION

| Function | Structures |
| --- | --- |
| Control of breathing | Respiratory center<br>Peripheral chemoreceptors<br>Afferent and efferent nerves |
| Ventilatory pump | Chest wall and pleura<br>Respiratory muscles |
| Distribution of ventilation | Upper respiratory tract<br>Conducting airways<br>Respiratory bronchioles |
| Distribution of blood | Pulmonary arteries and veins<br>Pulmonary capillaries |
| Gas exchange | Terminal respiratory unit |
| Bronchial clearance | Mucociliary escalator<br>Macrophages |
| Alveolar clearance and defense | Pulmonary lymphatics<br>Alveolar macrophages<br>Humoral mediators<br>Inflammatory cells |

has resulted in the development of an elaborate defense mechanism for the purpose of maintaining the integrity of the lung periphery. Table 1.1 outlines the functional components of respiration and lung defenses and the structures involved. This chapter provides an overview of these structures as they relate to the functions for which they were designed. The pulmonary circulation is discussed in Chapter 2, and the circulatory structures are discussed here only as they relate to the gas exchange units of the lung.

## CONTROL OF BREATHING

Control of respiration in the relaxed, awake human is governed by the interplay of cortical and brainstem respiratory pathways. The automatic respiratory control structures are located in the brainstem, while the voluntary control of respiration is governed primarily by the cerebral cortex.

### BRAINSTEM RESPIRATORY DRIVE

Brainstem transection experiments in animals led to the concept of specific respiratory control centers governing functions such as inspiration, expiration, and pauses during breathing. This concept has gradually been modified toward a consideration of localized regions of respiratory regulation but with a highly interconnected, multilevel feedback system (2–5). The respiratory muscles have no intrinsic automaticity of their own but appear to be regulated in their automatic function by two major regions of respiratory regulation

(Fig. 1.1). The *medullary* center appears to be the generator of respiratory rhythm, while groups of rostral *pontine* respiratory nuclei seem to act to "fine tune" respiratory regulation (5).

In the medullary center two major groups of respiratory neurons are described—the *dorsal respiratory group* (DRG) and a *ventral respiratory group* (VRG) (3). The DRG is located dorsomedially in the medulla. It is primarily composed of inspiratory bulbospinal neurons, which in turn provide input to the spinal inspiratory motor neurons of the phrenic and external intercostal nerves (6). Some cells in the DRG appear to respond to lung inflation stimuli; other cells, to visceral afferent input from the ninth and tenth cranial nerves. These pathways may account for the postulated role of the DRG as an integrator between the input, coming from the pharynx and the lung, and the respiratory motor response. DRG stimuli appear to be transmitted to the VRG for modulation.

The VRG is located ventrolaterally in the medulla. It contains inspiratory and expiratory bulbospinal neurons whose output is to the spinal respiratory motor

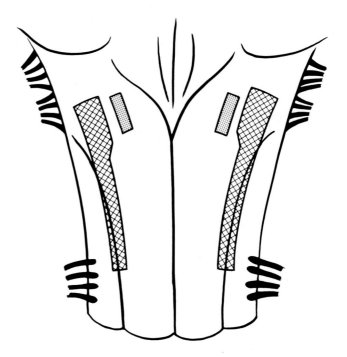

**FIGURE 1.1.** This schematic indicates the location of the dorsomedial (DRG) and ventrolateral (VRG) groupings of respiratory neurons. The *stippled area* represents the dorsomedial group. The *cross-hatched area* represents components of the ventrolateral group. (Adapted, with permission, from Long SE, Duffin J: The medullary respiratory neurons: a review. *Can J Physiol Pharmacol* 62:161–182, 1984.)

neurons for intercostal, abdominal, and phrenic innervation and auxiliary muscles of respiration (7).

### CORTICAL MODULATION

Certain aspects of voluntary respiratory control can override the automatic brainstem respiratory centers. Breath holding and hyperventilation are examples of ways in which cortical modulation can countermand normal respiratory regulation, even to the point where blood gas alterations can be physiologically detrimental. Loss of consciousness (reduction in the state of wakefulness) allows the brainstem regulatory centers to reassert control. Voluntary coughing, singing, speaking, and vital capacity maneuvers are other examples of cortical modulation overriding automatic respiratory efforts. These voluntary pathways originate in cortical neurons with efferent projections, via corticospinal and corticobulbar pathways, to respiratory associated muscles. Afferent impulses during the waking state may activate the reticular formation and modify the respiratory response to chemical or mechanical stimulation. Reduction or absence of wakeful drive responses may play a significant role in the appearance of sleep-related respiratory disorders. During sleep, voluntary control of respiration is no longer active and automatic control and feedback circuits become dominant. This enhances the effect of chemical or metabolic regulatory systems.

### SPINAL PATHWAYS

Integration between voluntary respiration, which is controlled at the cortical level, and automatic respiration, controlled at the brainstem level, occurs via interconnections in the spinal cord. The cortex, DRG, VRG, and other supraspinal brainstem centers descend in the spinal cord to phrenic, intercostal, and abdominal respiratory motor neurons. Cortical fibers descend separately from the involuntary pathways. Integration between these systems occurs at the spinal respiratory motor neurons, where supraspinal active inhibition may occur. This prevents antagonist α motor neuron reflex excitation during the phase of agonist muscle contraction. Ascending sensory input, found in the lateral column of the spinal cord, may further influence respiration (8–10). Special additional input probably comes from pulmonary and chest wall receptors.

### MECHANORECEPTORS IN THE LUNGS AND CHEST WALL

Afferent impulses also arise from the lungs and chest wall. The *chest wall mechanoreceptors* help to measure and modulate forces generated by inspiratory effort (11). The mechanoreceptors include tendon receptors and muscle spindles. *Tendon receptors* inhibit motor activity when the force of contraction reaches potentially injurious levels. *Muscle spindles* in the intercostal muscles and, to a lesser extent, in the diaphragm may help to maintain tidal volume when chest wall movement is impeded (11, 12). The main muscle fibers controlling respiration are supplied by α motor neurons. Spindles, arranged in parallel with the major muscle fibers, are supplied by γ-efferent motor neurons (Fig. 1.2). Stretch of the spindles, seen with inspiration and when chemical drive is increased, increases the motor discharge, via the spindle afferents, to the α motor neuron. This intraspinal connection activates the respiratory muscles to contract until the tension on the spindles is relieved. The muscle spindles provide an immediate feedback system to maintain adequate ventilation in the presence of increased respiratory loads.

### PULMONARY MECHANORECEPTORS

There are at least three kinds of pulmonary parenchymal receptors in the lung that have afferent signals going to the central nervous system (CNS) via the vagus nerve. Irritant receptors, stretch receptors, and juxtacapillary receptors may help modify ventilation by altering the depth and frequency of respiration (13). *Irritant receptors,* located in the airway epithelium, produce hyperpnea and bronchoconstriction and stimulate release of airway secretions when the bronchial tree is exposed to noxious chemical stimuli or sudden mechanical deformation. These receptors are involved in coughing. They also seem to increase ventilatory response to $CO_2$. *Stretch receptors,* located in the airway

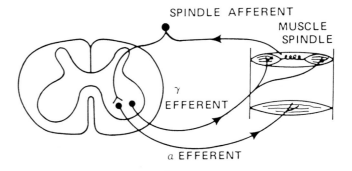

**FIGURE 1.2.** Drawing representing *α*- and *γ*-efferent loops of the muscle spindle. The spindles sense elongation of the monitored respiratory muscle and reflexly assist in control of the strength of contraction. *γ*-Efferents help to maintain adjustment in the efferent loop. (Reprinted with permission from West JB: *Respiratory Physiology—The Essentials.* Baltimore, Williams & Wilkins, 1974, p 126.)

smooth muscle, respond to changes in the lung volume. Apnea may occur (Hering-Breuer reflex) with lung inflation. Irritant and stretch receptors may work to regulate airway diameter during breathing to optimize the relationship between airway resistance and anatomic dead space (13). By exciting stretch receptors, lung inflation may increase the activity of expiratory muscles and restore end-expiratory volume to its usual level. This helps maintain inspiratory muscles at their optimal length and maintain their efficiency. *Juxtacapillary receptors* (J receptors) are within the interstitium of the alveolar wall and are stimulated by distortion of the interstitial space, as with interstitial edema or fibrosis. These receptors may mediate the rapid, shallow breathing that is characteristic of these conditions (12–14).

### CHEMOSENSITIVITY AND CHEMORECEPTORS

A feedback loop exists between changes in arterial blood, $Po_2$, $Pco_2$, or pH and changes in ventilation. This feedback loop facilitates changes in the depth and rate of breathing in response to changes in the metabolic needs of the body.

### EFFECTS OF CHANGES IN $Paco_2$

Carbon dioxide is the most important chemical stimulus in the regulation of respiration in normal individuals. Over a wide range of metabolic activities and varying levels of $CO_2$ production there is normally little variation in $Paco_2$. This is because a slight increase in $Paco_2$ elicits a proportional increase in minute ventilation. Chemoreceptors in the peripheral circulation and central nervous system detect changes and send afferent input to the respiratory centers to effect ventilatory correction. Most of the increase in minute ventilation is in response to changes in the hydrogen ion concentration in the cerebrospinal fluid (CSF) that bathes the medullary chemoreceptors, although chemoreceptors in the carotid and aortic bodies also contribute to the increase in respiration (15, 16).

The body's capacity to store $CO_2$ far exceeds its capacity to store oxygen, and changes in ventilation will cause more rapid and significant changes in $Po_2$ than in $Pco_2$ or pH. Complete cessation of ventilation for 1 minute in a person breathing room air will cause a relatively mild (6 to 10 mm Hg) rise in $Paco_2$, whereas $Pao_2$ will decrease by 40 to 50 mm Hg (17).

### EFFECTS OF CHANGES IN $Pao_2$

The effects of hypoxia on increasing ventilatory effort is by stimulation of the peripheral chemoreceptors

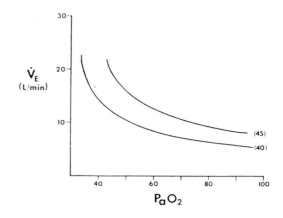

**FIGURE 1.3.** The relationship between arterial $Po_2$ and minute ventilation at different $Paco_2$s (in *parentheses*). The ventilatory response to a hypoxic stimulus is increased by hypercapnia.

located in the carotid and aortic bodies (18). Unlike the central stimulatory effect of hypercapnia, the central effect of hypoxia is respiratory depression (19). In normal individuals at sea level, approximately 10% of the resting respiratory drive is the result of hypoxic stimulation (20). The effect of hypoxia on respiration is not linear. As $Po_2$ falls below 75 mm Hg, respiratory stimulation increases more dramatically, with a marked increase in minute ventilation occurring as levels of 50 to 40 mm Hg are reached (Fig. 1.3). Hypoxia and hypercarbia tend to interact as respiratory stimuli (21), so the ventilatory response to hypoxia is increased in the presence of hypercarbia and vice versa (18).

### pH MODULATION

Hydrogen ions stimulate both the peripheral chemoreceptors in the carotid and aortic bodies and the central chemoreceptors located in the medulla. It is often difficult to separate the influence of hydrogen ion on ventilation from the effect of change in $Pco_2$; however, a low pH at a constant $Paco_2$ can result in increased minute ventilation (22). The ventilatory response to hypercapnia may be either increased by acidosis or decreased by alkalosis at pH levels outside the range of normal.

### VENTILATORY RESPONSES

Since changes in $CO_2$ and $O_2$ have generally consistent effects on respiration in normal individuals, techniques of challenging or stimulating a subject with inhaled gases of different $O_2$ and $CO_2$ mixtures can be used to assess respiratory control or responsiveness.

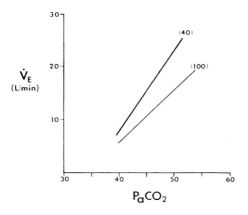

**FIGURE 1.4.** The relationship between arterial $P_{CO_2}$ and minute ventilation at different $Pa_{O_2}$s (in *parentheses*). During hypoxia, the ventilatory response to an increase in $Pa_{CO_2}$ is additionally increased.

Measurement techniques have been derived for testing the relationships between $P_{CO_2}$ and $Pa_{O_2}$ and their effect on respiration in normal and in abnormal persons.

Non–steady-state rebreathing methods for determining ventilatory responses to carbon dioxide have been developed that have simplified measurements of the sensitivity of chemoreceptors (23). When a subject breathes a gas mixture containing 7% $CO_2$, rapid equilibrium of alveolar gas with arterial blood and CNS is achieved. The partial pressures of $P_{CO_2}$ in the breathing circuit, arterial blood, and interstitial fluid of the brain increase at the same rate (4 to 6 mm Hg per minute), so determining alveolar $P_{CO_2}$ with a rapid gas analyzer and comparing it to minute ventilation allows the ventilatory response to $CO_2$ to be determined within a few minutes. The slope of the line relating ventilation to alveolar $P_{CO_2}$ ($\Delta \dot{V}/\Delta P_{CO_2}$) is the ventilatory response to $CO_2$; the normal values range from 0.5 to 8.0 liters/min/mm Hg $P_{CO_2}$ (Fig. 1.4). Responses are generally lower in women, possibly because of their smaller vital capacity.

Ventilatory response to hypoxia can be determined by a similar rebreathing technique with a patient inspiring 7% $CO_2$ in air. Since the hypoxic ventilatory response is influenced by $P_{CO_2}$, a portion of the expired air is diverted through a $CO_2$ absorber. In this manner, a constant arterial $P_{CO_2}$ is maintained while $P_{O_2}$ progressively falls as oxygen is removed from the rebreathing circuit (Fig. 1.3). Either alveolar $P_{O_2}$ can be measured or arterial oxygen saturation may be measured using an ear oximeter. In patients with lung disease, because of their increased alveolar-arterial oxygen gradient, arterial saturation or arterial $P_{O_2}$ must be measured directly.

## VENTILATORY PUMP

The ventilatory pump consists of the chest wall, the respiratory muscles, and the pleural space, which connects the lungs to the chest wall. The chest wall acts as a rigid cylinder within which the lungs are expanded and deflated by the action of the respiratory muscles. The diaphragm, the principal muscle of quiet breathing, moves like a piston within the cylinder, and the movement of this wide-bore piston over relatively short distances represents an efficient method of moving large volumes of air with minimum work. Air moves into and out of the lungs in a to-and-fro manner like the tides of the ocean; thus it is called *tidal* flow.

### CHEST WALL

The bony thorax consists of the spine, the ribs, and the sternum. The basic shape of the thorax is that of a truncated cone (Fig. 1.5). Both the superior and inferior ends of the cone are inclined anteriorly so that the posterior portion of the cone, the spine, is longer than the anterior portion, the sternum. These structures are innervated and may be a source of chest pain. The ribs are hinged on the spine by ligaments and cartilage in such a way that the ribs move upward and outward during inspiration and downward and inward during expiration. This hinging movement results in a change in thoracic volume. In addition, the connective tissue components of the chest wall function as a spring storing mechanical energy. This elastic property of the chest wall is a function both of the geometry of chest

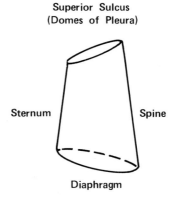

**FIGURE 1.5.** Simplified diagram of the cone-shaped thorax (lateral view). There is anterior-posterior compression, so the thorax is widened laterally; the anterior wall is shorter than the posterior wall, and the superior and inferior planes are inclined anteriorly.

wall structures and of their composition. The extracellular matrix components that determine the mechanical properties of the chest include both the calcified bony ribs and the proteoglycans, elastin, and collagen of the cartilaginous ribs.

The expansion of the chest wall driven by respiratory muscles causes a fall in pressure of the air contained within the lungs, which in turn causes the flow of gas into the lungs. Air continues to flow into the lungs until the intrapulmonary gas pressure equals the atmospheric pressure. As the respiratory muscles relax, expiration begins and the elastic recoil of the chest wall and lungs compresses the air contained within the lungs, resulting in a pressure greater than atmospheric. This causes gas to flow out of the lungs. The movement of the chest wall and lungs during inspiration and expiration is shown in Figure 1.6.

### RESPIRATORY MUSCLES

The respiratory muscles are the only skeletal muscles that are essential to life and have been called by Macklem and his associates "the vital pump" (24). Clinical investigation in recent years has shown that weakness or fatigue of the respiratory muscles is a common cause of hypercapnic respiratory failure and difficulty of weaning from mechanical ventilation (25, 26).

Inspiration requires active work, which is provided by the muscles of inspiration. These include the diaphragm, the inspiratory intercostal muscles, and the accessory muscles of inspiration (the scalenes and sternomastoids). Expiration under normal, quiet conditions is passive and requires no work; however, when ventilatory needs increase due to exertion or when the lungs are abnormal, as in asthma or chronic obstructive pulmonary disease (COPD), expiration often becomes an active process. The muscles of expiration include the internal intercostal muscles and the muscles of the abdominal wall (Fig. 1.7). In quadriplegic patients the pectoralis major and serratus anterior muscles may be used during expiration (27).

Like all skeletal muscle, and unlike the smooth muscle that lines airways, the muscles of respiration have

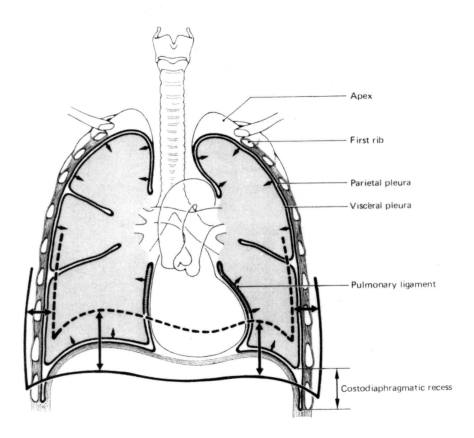

**FIGURE 1.6.**    Frontal section of chest and lung showing pleural space. *Single arrows* indicate retractive force, and *double arrows* show the excursion of the lung bases and periphery between deep inspiration and expiration.

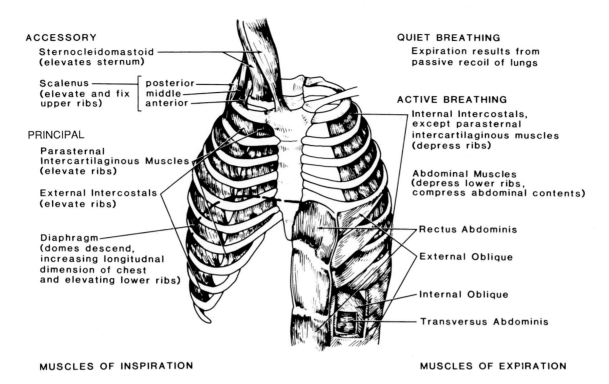

**ACCESSORY**
Sternocleidomastoid
(elevates sternum)

Scalenus
(elevate and fix
upper ribs)
posterior
middle
anterior

**PRINCIPAL**

Parasternal
Intercartilaginous Muscles
(elevate ribs)

External Intercostals
(elevate ribs)

Diaphragm
(domes descend,
increasing longitudnal
dimension of chest
and elevating lower ribs)

**QUIET BREATHING**
Expiration results from
passive recoil of lungs

**ACTIVE BREATHING**
Internal Intercostals,
except parasternal
intercartilaginous muscles
(depress ribs)

Abdominal Muscles
(depress lower ribs,
compress abdominal contents)

Rectus Abdominis

External Oblique

Internal Oblique

Transversus Abdominis

**MUSCLES OF INSPIRATION**                    **MUSCLES OF EXPIRATION**

**FIGURE 1.7.** Diagram of the anatomy of the major respiratory muscles. Left side—inspiratory muscles; right side—expiratory muscles. (Reprinted with permission from Garrity ER, Sharp JT: Respiratory muscles: function and dysfunction. In: *Pulmonary and Critical Care Update*, vol. 2. Park Ridge, IL, American College of Chest Physicians, 1986.)

no basal tone. Release of acetylcholine at the neuromuscular junction is required to initiate the contraction process. Binding of acetylcholine to the N2 nicotinic cholinergic receptor on the target muscle cell initiates a depolarization that in turn releases calcium from the T-tubule system into the cytoplasm. This calcium then activates the ATPase of myosin heavy chain, which converts ATP to ADP, causing the myosin to move along the actin fibers present within the cellular cytoplasm. This movement results in cellular shortening, and in this manner chemical energy is converted from ATP to the mechanical energy needed to drive ventilation. The ATP, in turn, is generated by the mitochondria of the muscle cell by oxidative metabolism or, for brief intervals, from glycolysis. Repolarization of the cell membrane, resequestration of calcium, and cleavage of acetylcholine by acetylcholinesterase results in relaxation of the muscle cell and readies it for another round of contraction.

Resting tidal breathing depends on the diaphragm, which is composed of two distinct portions. The costal and crural diaphragm have separate functions and innervations. The motor innervation to the diaphragm

is via the phrenic nerve, which is derived from the third, fourth, and fifth cervical nerves. Sensory nerves to the crural portion of the diaphragm are also carried in the phrenic nerve; thus, irritation of the center of the diaphragm may cause pain which is referred to the ipsilateral neck or shoulder areas, which are also innervated by the third, fourth, and fifth cervical segments. Sensory innervation of the costal portion of the diaphragm is via the intercostal nerves from the adjacent chest wall, which they also innervate, and pain from the lateral portion of the diaphragm is referred to the chest wall.

With contraction the dome of the diaphragm moves downward, displacing abdominal contents, so that during inspiration the abdomen normally moves outward. Because of the fulcrum effect of the relatively fixed abdominal contents, diaphragm contraction also elevates and increases the diameter of the lower rib cage (Fig. 1.6). The accessory muscles of inspiration become important only during high levels of ventilation and with hyperinflation of the thorax associated with obstructive lung disease. The accessory muscles move the cage upward so that the ribs themselves lie in a more horizontal plane, thus increasing the diameter of the thoracic cage.

Fatigue of the inspiratory muscles occurs when the energy supply is exceeded because of either (a) increased ventilatory demands (vigorous exercise), (b) increased work of breathing (asthma or COPD), or (c) inadequate energy generation by the muscles (hypoxemia, congestive heart failure). Dyspnea is the major complaint when the respiratory muscles become fatigued. The sensation of dyspnea has not been completely explained, but it may be related to a disproportion between the amount of work required and the amount of work the respiratory muscles can perform. Healthy respiratory muscles can increase minute ventilation from a normal resting level of 6 to 7 liters/minute to a maximum of over 100 liters/minute with voluntary effort. However, this maximum level of ventilation cannot be sustained over long periods, and with vigorous exercise minute ventilation is more often maintained at 5 to 6 times the normal resting level. The body adapts to the increased ventilatory demand by increasing the circulation to the muscles of inspiration and by increasing the extraction of oxygen from the diaphragmatic capillaries. Lactate production occurs in normal persons only as a result of breathing against a high resistance leading to fatigue, or breathing low-oxygen mixtures. High levels of blood lactate have been found in patients during severe asthma attacks (28).

Hyperinflation, which occurs in patients with emphysema and during asthma attacks, places the diaphragm at a distinct disadvantage. With hyperinflation the diaphragm is already low and flat so that contraction neither moves the diaphragm downward nor moves the lower rib cage outward. In fact, with severe hyperinflation diaphragm contraction may pull the lower rib cage inward (*Hoover's sign*), causing an expiratory effect on the rib cage (29).

The clinical signs of inspiratory muscle fatigue have been summarized by Macklem's group (24, 25, 30). During early muscle fatigue the ratio of high-frequency to low-frequency electrical activity of the diaphragm as recorded on an electromyogram decreases. This is manifested by an increased respiratory rate; rapid, shallow breathing; and an early fall in the measured arterial $P_{CO_2}$. As muscle fatigue increases, the diaphragm movement diminishes and the accessory muscles assume a greater role. The contraction of accessory muscles produces a negative pressure in the thorax that may actually pull the flaccid diaphragm upward, causing the abdomen to move inward during inspiration; this is called *paradoxical respiration* and indicates significant diaphragm fatigue (25). Respiration may

also shift from predominantly diaphragmatic breathing to predominantly accessory muscle breathing (*respiratory alternans*). In summary, the clinical signs of inspiratory muscle fatigue include rapid, shallow respiration with an initial increase in minute ventilation; an initial fall in $P_{aCO_2}$; often paradoxical respiration and respiratory alternans; and finally a decrease in respiratory rate and minute ventilation leading to hypoventilation and respiratory acidosis.

### PLEURA

As the lungs grow laterally from the mediastinum during fetal development, they grow into a part of the celomic cavity, which is lined with undifferentiated mesenchyme. As the lungs extend into the cavity, they are covered by these mesenchymal cells, which become the parietal pleura. The mesenchymal cells that line the chest wall and mediastinum become the visceral pleura. The visceral and parietal pleura join one another at the lung hila. The parietal pleura contains abundant pain fibers derived from the intercostal nerves, and irritation of this membrane produces a characteristic, well-localized type of chest pain, which is exacerbated by chest wall movement (*pleuritic pain*).

The pleural space is airtight and the two pleural surfaces, parietal and visceral, are separated only by a thin film that contains hyaluronic acid and provides lubrication during lung movement. In the intact system at rest the lung has a natural tendency to become smaller and the chest wall a natural tendency to become larger. They are thus pulling against each other across the pleural space and, since it is airtight and no air can enter, a negative pressure is produced. It is this negative pleural pressure that links the lung to the chest wall and transmits movements of the chest wall to the lung. At rest the average negative intrapleural pressure is about 4 cm $H_2O$. In the upright position this negative pressure is greater at the top of the lungs than at the lung bases because of the effects of gravity on the lungs themselves.

Fluid flows constantly through the pleural space, forming a lubricating film over the surface of the lungs. Recent studies show that approximately 100 ml of pleural fluid is formed each hour, and since this fluid is rapidly absorbed, the pleural space contains a minimal amount of fluid at any given time. Previous theories proposed that pleural fluid was formed from the systemic capillaries adjacent to the parietal pleura and absorbed into the plexus of capillaries under the visceral pleura. Recent studies suggest, however, that the absorption of pleural fluid is more complicated than this and that the parietal pleural lymphatics play a role in the removal of liquid, protein, and other large particles from the pleural cavity (31, 32). The visceral pleural capillaries drain via the pulmonary veins into the left atrium. The pleura and its diseases are discussed further in Chapter 16.

## DISTRIBUTION OF AIR

Before atmospheric air reaches the alveolar-capillary membrane, the air must be conditioned so that it does not injure this delicate surface area. The *upper respiratory tract* is primarily designed to purify, warm, and humidify the air; it consists of the nose, paranasal sinuses, pharynx, and larynx.

### NOSE

The nose contains a layer of epithelial cells overlying a rich capillary plexus, all resting on thin bony plates, the turbinates. The vascular and epithelial structures are responsive to neural and humoral mediators. The nasal tissues can therefore provide for rapid heat exchange, transudation of fluid, or recruitment of inflammatory cells to the nose. The nasal mucosa is normally bathed by thin, watery secretions designed to trap foreign particles and to add moisture to the inspired air. With normal, quiet breathing, inspired air is heated to body temperature and the relative humidity is increased to over 90% during passage through the nose. Resistance to air flow is higher in the nose than in the mouth because of the intricate system of baffles. This is the explanation for mouth breathing during vigorous exercise; in this case the air conditioning function of the nose is lost and dry, cold air may enter the lower airways. In patients with abnormal irritability of the bronchial tree, inspiration of cold air through the mouth during exercise may initiate bronchospasm. Patients with tracheostomy and those being ventilated via endotracheal tubes also lose the function of the nose, and inspired gas must be artificially humidified and warmed to prevent drying and irritation of the lower airways.

### PARANASAL SINUSES

The sinuses are lined by ciliated columnar epithelium and communicate with the nasal passages by narrow openings, which may become occluded when they are inflamed. Cilia within the sinus cavities beat in a pattern that tends to propel secretions toward the opening into the nasal cavity. The function of paranasal sinuses is not completely clear, but they add resonance to voice sounds and may insulate the cranial vault. They also provide lightness to the skull without unduly compromising its protective function. The sinuses

may become inflamed and cause drainage of material into the pharynx (postnasal drip). This material may be aspirated into the lower respiratory tract, especially during sleep, and this may be a source of chronic bronchial irritation.

### PHARYNX

The pharynx is divided by the soft palate into the nasopharynx and the oropharynx. The adenoids, tonsils, and eustachian tubes are located in the nasopharynx. At the base of the tongue is the epiglottis, which protects the laryngeal opening during swallowing. In unconscious patients the base of the tongue may fall posteriorly and obstruct the laryngeal opening. To avoid this the head should be hyperextended and the lower jaw pulled forward. Alternatively, the patient may be placed in a position in which gravity causes the tongue to fall forward. The oropharynx is easily seen through the open mouth and serves as an entryway to both the larynx and the esophagus.

### LARYNX

The larynx contains the vocal cords, which are a vital part of the defense system of the respiratory system since they participate in coughing. Coughing is a major clearance mechanism for material that collects in the larger airways, and it is initiated by irritation of nerves in the walls of the trachea and large bronchi. Coughing is produced by closure of the vocal cords combined with contraction of the respiratory and abdominal muscles, so that high pressures are created in the lower airways. Sudden opening of the vocal cords then allows a rush of air, carrying larger particles of mucus with it. Normally the respiratory tract is free of bacteria below the level of the larynx.

One or both vocal cords may become paralyzed by surgery or injury to the nerves in the neck or thorax. The left recurrent laryngeal nerve descends into the mediastinum and around the arch of the aorta before returning to the larynx. This nerve may become disrupted by cancer involving lymph nodes adjacent to the left hilum, and hoarseness is an ominous sign in patients with carcinoma of the lung. Other diseases such as granulomas, lymphomas, and aortic aneurysms may also interrupt the left recurrent laryngeal nerve in the mediastinum. The right recurrent laryngeal nerve descends only to the level of the subclavian artery, so it is less often affected.

If both vocal cords are paralyzed, they become flaccid near the midline and breathing may be hindered. Large airway obstruction produces a characteristic combination of symptoms, signs, and pulmonary function abnormalities (33). Bilateral vocal cord paralysis causes a variable extrathoracic airway obstruction, which produces inspiratory stridor associated with hoarseness, dyspnea, and anxiety. Tests of ventilatory function, such as a flow-volume loop or a spirogram, may show relatively normal forced expiration, but during inspiration there is a decrease in peak air flow. Carcinoma of the larynx also produces the combination of hoarseness and stridor. However, since this is a fixed obstruction, stridor occurs usually during both inspiration *and* expiration, and pulmonary function tests show both inspiratory and expiratory flow limitation. (For further discussion of upper airway obstruction see Chapter 7.)

The *lower respiratory tract* begins at the junction of the larynx with the trachea and includes the trachea, bronchi, bronchioles, and alveoli. The air conduction system of the lungs is a series of dichotomously branching bronchi and bronchioles, ending blindly in some 300 million alveoli, which collectively form the gas exchange surface (Fig. 1.8). There are normally about 23 generations of airways, of which the first 16 or so are conducting airways, where no gas exchange

occurs, and the last seven or so are respiratory airways, where alveoli appear in progressively larger numbers (34). The average diameter of a daughter branch is smaller than that of its parent branch, but the *total cross-sectional area* of each successive generation *increases* from trachea to alveoli; thus, the total area of the respiratory bronchioles is much greater than that of the trachea (Fig. 1.9).

### TRACHEA

The trachea begins at the base of the neck and extends about 10 to 12 cm to its bifurcation into the right and left main bronchi. It lies immediately anterior to the esophagus and behind the aorta and often lies slightly to the right of the midline after entering the thorax. Its transverse diameter is greater than its anterior-posterior diameter, and it is held open by a series of anterior horseshoe-shaped cartilaginous rings bound posteriorly by fibrous bands. The position of the carina varies according to the position of the neck and the level of inspiration but is normally at about

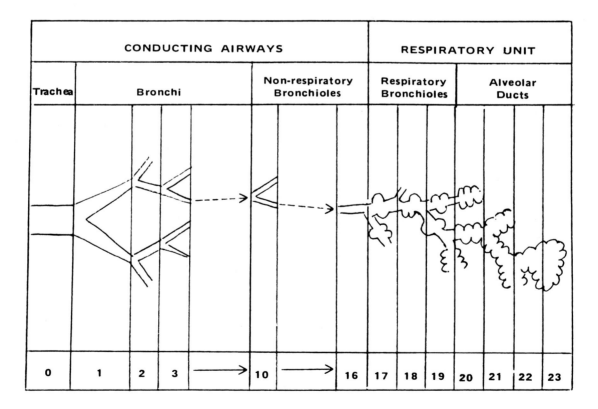

**FIGURE 1.8.** Conducting airways and terminal respiratory unit of the lung. The relative size of the respiratory unit is greatly enlarged. Figures at the bottom indicate the approximate number of generations from trachea to alveoli. (Modified from Weibel ER: *Morphometry of the Human Lung.* Heidelberg, Germany, Springer-Verlag, 1963.)

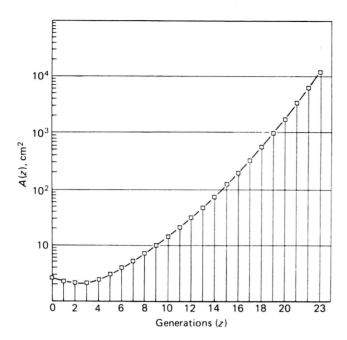

**FIGURE 1.9.** Total cross section of the airways in the human lung by generation. Although each generation of airways is smaller than its parent, the *total* cross-sectional area of each generation is greater than the *total* area of the previous generation. (From Weibel ER: *Morphometry of the Human Lung.* Heidelberg, Germany, Springer-Verlag, 1963.)

the level of the second anterior rib, just below the aortic arch. The angle between the right and left main bronchi is normally acute, varying from 50 to 100.

## BRONCHI

The right main bronchus divides almost immediately into the upper lobe bronchus and the intermediate bronchus. The left main bronchus is considerably longer, extending across the midline approximately 5 cm before it divides into the left upper-lobe and left lower-lobe bronchi. The major bronchi contain large numbers of mucous glands, and their surface is innervated by branches of both the parasympathetic and the sympathetic nervous systems. These nerves are connected to the brain via the vagus nerves. Irritant receptors in large airways initiate the cough reflex, and resultant motor stimuli through the vagi cause bronchoconstriction and mucus secretion. Airway nerves also permit axon-axonal reflexes, so irritation of one site in the airway can lead to bronchoconstriction and/or secretion diffusely. Neuropeptides, including substance P and the neurokinins, are thought

to be important mediators released by these sensory nerves in the airways (35).

The right main bronchus is larger and less deviated from the axis of the trachea than the left; it thus may be considered an extension of the trachea itself. This is an explanation for the more frequent aspiration of foreign material into the right lung. The main bronchi divide into five lobar bronchi, the upper, middle, and lower on the right and the upper and lower on the left. The left upper lobe divides into the apical-posterior and anterior segments and the lingula, which developmentally corresponds to the right middle lobe. The lobes are separated from each other by fissures, which are lined by two layers of visceral pleura.

The lobar bronchi divide into segmental bronchi, 10 on the right and nine on the left (Fig. 1.10). Segments

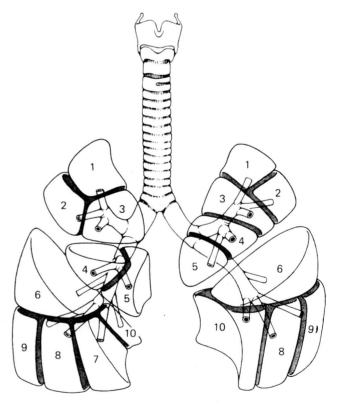

**FIGURE 1.10.** The bronchopulmonary segments. *Upper lobes*: (1) apical, (2) posterior, (3) anterior, (4) superior lingular, and (5) inferior lingular segments. *Middle lobe*: (4) lateral and (5) medial segments. *Lower lobes*: (6) apical (superior), (7) medial basal, (8) anterior basal, (9) lateral basal, and (10) posterior basal segments. The medial basal segment (7) is absent in the left lung. (From Weibel ER: Design and structure of the human lung. In Fishman AP (ed): *Assessment of Pulmonary Function.* New York, McGraw-Hill, 1980.)

are usually separated by delicate connective tissue planes but not by fissures. There is some disagreement concerning the nomenclature of the bronchopulmonary segments; however, the classification of the Thoracic Society of Great Britain, shown in Figure 1.10, is the one most commonly used. A thorough knowledge of the lung segments has become necessary in recent years because of the high incidence of bronchogenic carcinoma, one of the most common neoplasms. These neoplasms commonly occur in lobar and segmental bronchi and produce characteristic patterns, based on their anatomic location, on the chest x-ray film.

The epithelial cells that line the airways change in character from the proximal to the distal airways. In the trachea, the epithelium is pseudostratified with as many as four or five nuclei arranged above each other. Most of the surface area of the basement membrane, however, is covered by basal cells. These small cells with scant cytoplasm have numerous hemidesmosomes, which anchor them to the basement membrane, as well as numerous desmosomes, which provide mechanical anchors for the columnar cells of the epithelium. It is currently thought that all columnar cells extend a slender process that contacts the basement membrane, hence the designation "pseudostratified." These processes may function to regulate the differentiated phenotype of the epithelial cells.

The columnar cells consist predominantly of ciliated cells, with smaller numbers of goblet cells and brush cells. *Ciliated cells* contain motile cilia, which beat in a coordinated manner to move the mucus layer toward the mouth. *Goblet cells*, interspersed among the ciliated epithelial cells, secrete mucus. *Brush cells* contain microvilli resembling those of basal cells in the gut and may function to control fluid balance in the airway lumen. These cells may also represent immature ciliated cells. Following injury, the epithelial cellular components change, and goblet cells or squamous cells, which are usually non-keratinizing and stratified, may replace the population of ciliated cells.

The columnar cells are connected by several types of junctions. Mechanical integrity is thought to depend on desmosomes formed with basal cells and with other columnar cells. Gap junctions between epithelial cells provide for exchange of nutrients and metabolites and may be important in permitting cell-to-cell exchange of mediators that coordinate epithelial functioning. Near the epithelial surface, the epithelial cells are linked by tight junctions. These junctions permit a fusion of the outer leaflet of the lipid bilayer cell membrane of adjacent cells. Since they extend entirely around each cell, these junctions prevent exchange between the apical and basolateral membranes. Tight junctions thus permit the airway epithelium to form a barrier segregating

the airway lumen from the airway parenchyma. In addition, the apical cell surface is segregated from the basolateral cell surface. Many functions, particularly those involved in the regulation of secretion, depend on processes that are localized within the cell membranes.

The epithelium contains numerous glands with ducts that penetrate and empty into the airway lumen. In addition to the trachea, glands are particularly prevalent in the medium-sized bronchi but are sparse in the smaller bronchi. Glands contain two types of secretory cells: *serous cells*, which secrete a variety of peptides including lysozyme, lactoferrin, and the secretory leukoprotease inhibitor as well as ions and water, and *mucous cells*, which secrete mucins. Because the volume of glands is estimated to be forty-fold greater than that of the luminal goblet cells, they are thought to be the major sources of bronchial mucous secretions. Luminal secretory cells and glands, however, may be regulated differently and may make qualitatively different contributions to airways secretions. Hypertrophy of the mucous glands can occur in chronic bronchitis; the *Reid index* (a ratio of the depth of gland penetration to the thickness of the bronchial wall) is a measure of this hypertrophy.

In the proximal airways, the columnar cells are highly elongated, and basal cells are common (Fig. 1.11). In more peripheral airways, the columnar cells gradually become shorter and basal cells become

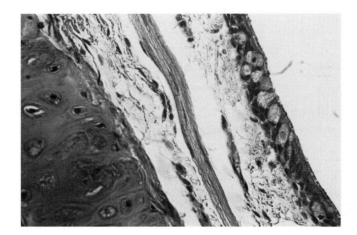

**FIGURE 1.11.** Section through the wall of a large bronchus ($\times 400$). The lumen (right) is lined with pseudostratified columnar epithelial cells containing tiny cilia, which propel mucus toward the trachea. The submucosa is surrounded by a thin layer of smooth muscle. To the left is a part of the cartilage that lends support to the bronchial wall. (Courtesy of Warren D. Grafton, M.D.)

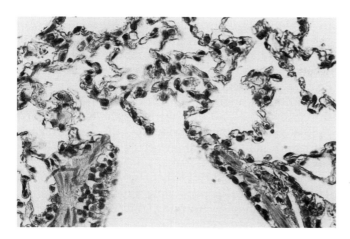

**FIGURE 1.12.** Section through a terminal bronchiole (×400). At the center of the picture the terminal bronchiole is dividing into two respiratory bronchioles, whose walls contain alveoli. The respiratory bronchioles end in alveolar sacs. (Courtesy of Warren D. Grafton, M.D.)

fewer, disappearing in the terminal airways. The total height of the epithelium diminishes as its character changes from pseudostratified to columnar. The walls of the terminal bronchioles are thus quite different from those of the larger airways (Fig. 1.12). Ciliated cells become less numerous and no glands or goblet cells are present. *Clara cells* are often seen scattered between ciliated cells and may project into the airway lumen (36). Recent evidence suggests that these cells contribute, along with the type II alveolar cells, to the surface lining layer of the bronchioles. Clara cells may also function as progenitors for ciliated cells, brush cells, and goblet cells. This may explain why there is a decrease in Clara cells with an increase in epithelial mucous cells in the bronchioles of heavy smokers.

The segmental bronchi bifurcate further until the terminal bronchiole is reached. Each terminal bronchiole has a diameter of about 1 mm, but the total cross-sectional circumference of the terminal bronchioles in human lungs is nearly 2,000 times that of the trachea (Fig. 1.9) (34). Beyond the terminal bronchiole the airways contain progressively larger numbers of alveoli. As shown in Figure 1.8, after approximately three generations of respiratory bronchioles *alveolar ducts* are found. These are totally lined by alveoli.

*Kulchitsky cells* occur most commonly in newborns. These cells appear to be innervated and may produce kinins during the newborn period (37). These cells are the precursors of bronchial carcinoid tumors and probably of small cell carcinomas. Clumps of argyrophilic cells resembling Kulchitsky cells have been discovered

in bronchial, bronchiolar, and alveolar epithelium. The epithelium overlying these structures is modified and consists of nonciliated columnar cells. The capillaries supplying the structure are fenestrated. These *neuroepithelial* bodies are strategically located in such a manner that they may serve to "sniff" the air flowing by them and regulate the caliber of the airways and blood vessels. This would provide a sensitive autoregulatory mechanism for the distribution of inspired air (38).

Ventilation of the conducting airways ceases to be bulk flow at the level of the alveolar ducts. Farther distally, movement of gases is by gaseous diffusion. Ventilation of the gas-exchange surfaces, therefore, depends on how far the gases must travel from the alveolar duct to the alveolar wall. If small peripheral airways become partly or completely occluded, collateral ventilation of alveoli may occur via the *pores of Kohn*, holes in the alveolar walls that connect alveoli directly, or via the *canals of Lambert*, tiny passages from distal airways to adjacent alveoli. This collateral ventilation increases the physiologic dead space and adds to the ventilation-perfusion mismatching seen in diseases that affect the small airways (39). However, it prevents lung segments distal to obstructed airways from becoming atelectatic.

## DISTRIBUTION OF BLOOD

The lungs receive their blood supply from two sources: the bronchial arteries, which contain oxygenated blood from the left ventricle, and the pulmonary arteries, which contain systemic venous blood from the right ventricle. The pulmonary circulation is discussed in detail in Chapter 2. The bronchial arteries supply the walls of the bronchi and bronchioles to the level of the alveoli. There are usually two major bronchial arteries to each lung that originate from the aorta or from the intercostal arteries, although there is a great deal of variation in humans (40). The arteries enter the lungs through the hila and follow the branches of the bronchial tree as far as the terminal bronchioles. The branches form two plexuses, one in the submucosal area of the bronchi and one in the peribronchial area. These two plexuses communicate freely through small arterioles that penetrate the bronchial wall. The bronchial veins from the upper (mainly extrapulmonary) airways join the systemic veins to the right heart. The major portion of blood from the intrapulmonary bronchial circulation anastomoses with the pulmonary circulation in the alveoli, returning to the left atrium via the pulmonary veins. This forms a part of the normal arteriovenous shunting in the lungs (40). The majority of the blood supply to the alveoli is derived from the pulmonary circulation. The walls of the alveoli contain a rich network of pulmonary capillaries, and it is here that the exchange of carbon dioxide for oxygen occurs.

The circulatory pump that supplies systemic venous blood to the gas-exchange units of the lung is the right ventricle. The pulmonary artery emerges from the right ventricle and divides into right and left main pulmonary arteries anterior to the tracheal carina (Fig. 1.13). The left pulmonary artery is slightly higher than the right in most cases, and the right crosses the midline before dividing into an upper and a lower branch. The pulmonary arteries divide into branches corresponding to the divisions of the bronchial tree and supply the terminal arterioles, which enter the center of the terminal respiratory units (TRUs) along with the terminal bronchioles. These in turn break up into pulmonary capillaries, which form networks in the interalveolar septa. The pulmonary circulation is a low-pressure system, and the mean pulmonary artery pressure is normally around 15 mm Hg at rest. The entire cardiac output flows through this low-pressure system, although at rest the capillaries contain only about 100

ml of blood. The blood moves into the capillaries in a pulsatile manner with each heart beat, so that each 100 ml of blood remains in the capillaries for about 0.75 second (with a normal heart rate of 80/minute). This is more than adequate time for gas exchange to occur. Blood flow through the capillaries increases markedly during exercise, and this decreases the time available for gas exchange. In normal humans this is not a problem, since gas equilibration occurs within about 0.25 second (41).

The pulmonary veins form at the periphery of the TRUs and converge separately from the arteries and bronchi, eventually forming the main pulmonary veins, which end in the left atrium. In addition to the alveolar capillaries the pulmonary veins also receive blood from the peripheral bronchial arterial system, accounting for a significant portion of the right-to-left shunt that occurs normally in the lungs. As much as 5% of the cardiac output may be shunted through the lungs in normal humans.

## GAS EXCHANGE AREA

### TERMINAL RESPIRATORY UNIT

In the past, different authors have used various names for the smaller divisions of the lung architecture. To prevent confusion, the *terminal respiratory unit* (TRU) is herein defined as the portion of lung distal to a terminal nonrespiratory bronchiole (42, 43). The TRU has been called the acinus by Lauweryns (44) and the primary lobule by Miller (45). Three to five TRUs together form a *pulmonary lobule* (46), which is separated from its neighboring lobules by an interlobular septum containing lymphatic channels; these interlobular septa may become visible as Kerley's "B" lines on the chest x-ray film when they are distended by fluid or fibrosis.

A stylized version of a TRU is illustrated in Figure 1.14. The unit is designed to perform its basic function of gas exchange efficiently. The terminal bronchiole enters the center of the TRU accompanied by a branch of the pulmonary artery carrying unoxygenated blood from the body tissues. The arteriole divides into a rich network of pulmonary capillaries that cover the alveolar walls and drain into pulmonary venules, which lie in the periphery of the TRU. These venules converge into larger branches situated in the interlobular septa. This arrangement results in the organized perfusion of a lobule from the center to the periphery.

### CELLS OF THE ALVEOLI

Five major cell types have been identified in the alveoli of the lungs (Table 1.2) (47). Type I and type II

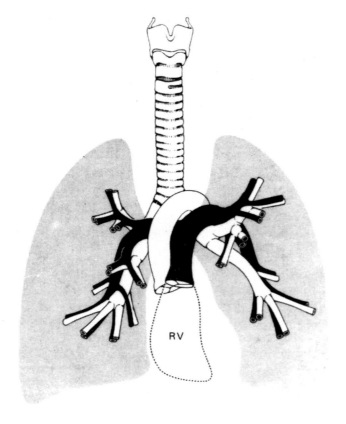

**FIGURE 1.13.** The pulmonary hila, showing the arteries. Note the relationships of the major vessels to the trachea, bronchi, and aorta. (Reprinted from Weibel ER: Design and structure of the human lung. In Fishman AP (ed): *Assessment of Pulmonary Function.* New York, McGraw-Hill, 1980.)

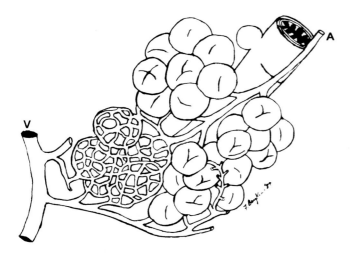

**FIGURE 1.14.** A terminal respiratory unit (TRU), the basic gas-exchanging unit of the lungs. The pulmonary arterial branch (*A*) enters the center of the TRU along with the terminal bronchiole. It anastomoses with the pulmonary venule in the alveolar walls, forming a dense capillary network for gas exchange. Venous drainage is to the periphery of the TRU, where the venous branches (*V*) lie. They coalesce to form the major pulmonary veins, which carry oxygenated blood.

**TABLE 1.2**
**CELLS OF THE ALVEOLAR REGION OF THE HUMAN LUNG**

|  | Cells $n \times 10^9$ | Total % |
|---|---|---|
| Alveolar epithelial cells |  |  |
|    Type I cells | 19 | 8.3 |
|    Type II cells | 37 | 15.9 |
| Endothelial cells | 68 | 30.2 |
| Interstitial cells | 84 | 36.1 |
| Macrophages | 23 | 9.4 |

Reprinted with permission from Crapo JD et al: Cell number and cell characteristics of the normal human lung. *Am Rev Respir Dis* 125:740–745, 1982.

alveolar epithelial cells cover the epithelial surface. Pulmonary endothelial cells, which constitute approximately 30% of the cells in the human lung parenchyma, are discussed in Chapter 2. Interstitial cells provide support for the structures in the alveolar walls. Alveolar macrophages are an important component of the host defense and lung clearance mechanisms.

Most of the alveolar surface is covered by a thin layer of type I *alveolar lining cells* (Fig. 1.15). These epithelial cells have large, thin cytoplasmic extensions that generally extend into several alveoli. They provide a minimal barrier to gas exchange. The alveolar capillary membrane is only 4 to 8 μm thick and consists of the alveolar epithelium, the interstitium containing the basement membranes, and the pulmonary capillary endothelium (Fig. 1.16). The capillaries form a very dense network in the alveolar septa so that the major part of the alveolar surface is covered with capillary blood, providing an ideal arrangement for gas exchange. The alveolar lining cells are highly susceptible to injury by a variety of agents, and they cannot replicate. Thus, the destruction of type I cells is followed by the proliferation of the cuboidal type II *granular pneumocytes*, which rapidly divide and repopulate the alveolar surface. They later differentiate into type I cells, thus allowing for the restoration of the gas-exchanging alveolar surface (48).

The type II granular pneumocytes are found primarily at the junctions of alveolar walls. In addition to being the progenitor cell of the alveolar epithelium, these are the source of alveolar surfactant. Electron micrographs of type II cells demonstrate many lamellar bodies that contain surfactant prior to secretion. Surfactant, defined by its property to lower surface tension, is composed of a mixture of phospholipids and lipid binding apoproteins. The alveolar walls are lined with a thin layer of this surfactant. Lowering surface tension in the alveoli helps to keep the lungs expanded during partial deflation. Surfactant also may have antioxidant and antibacterial properties. The surfactant layer extends proximally into the smaller airways, where Clara cells may contribute to its formation. Surfactant can also coat inhaled particulates and may facilitate their clearance.

Surfactant secretion is increased by both adrenergic and cholinergic stimulation, and by hyperventilation. Ventilation may help to maintain surfactant in a proper monolayer; lack of sighing may contribute to surfactant dysfunction and hence lead to atelectasis. Surfactant lipids appear to be altered in patients with acute lung injury, although the mechanisms for atelectasis and reduced lung compliance that occur in patients with the adult respiratory distress syndrome (ARDS) have not been determined completely; other factors such as altered breathing patterns and fever are also present (48). In vitro studies of Type II alveolar epithelial cells have shown that they can actively transport electrolytes, possibly an important means of maintaining the alveolar subphase liquid composition (49). This capacity for ion transport may also be important in the resolution of alveolar edema (50).

The interstitial cells are thought to be the source of the connective tissue of the alveolar wall. The macromolecules present in the extracellular matrix not only

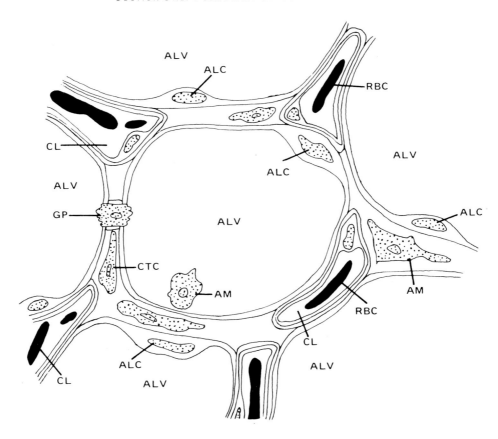

**FIGURE 1.15.** Cells of the alveoli. *ALV,* alveolus; *AM,* alveolar macrophage; *CL,* capillary lumen; *CTC,* connective tissue cell; *RBC,* red blood cell; *ALC,* alveolar lining cell; *GP,* granular pneu-mocyte. (Adapted from Weibel ER: Design and structure of the human lung. In Fishman AP (ed): *Assessment of Pulmonary Function.* New York, McGraw-Hill, 1980.)

help define alveolar architecture, but also contribute to alveolar mechanical properties. Estimates from animal studies suggest that some matrix components, such as collagen, may undergo relatively rapid turnover. Other components, such as elastin, may be exceedingly stable. Destruction of the extracellular matrix, particularly of elastin, is thought to contribute to eventual loss of alveoli. Overproduction of matrix components, in contrast, can lead to alveolar fibrosis, which can also disrupt alveolar gas exchange. In this context, interstitial cells not only produce and degrade matrix macromolecules, but their metabolic activity can be regulated by mediators present in the local milieu. Regulation of interstitial cell activity by local cytokine and cellular networks thus provides a means to maintain alveolar structural integrity despite the numerous stresses the lungs must face.

## LUNG CLEARANCE AND DEFENSES

By virtue of its direct contact with the atmosphere, necessary for gas exchange, the lung is at hazard for injury. Major irritants that invade the respiratory tract include organic agents such as bacteria, fungal spores, and viruses and inorganic agents such as industrial exhaust, dusts, and cigarette smoke. These infectious and noninfectious agents may act together to produce acute or chronic disease. Complicated and effective defense mechanisms have evolved to protect the respiratory tract from these inhaled substances (51).

### PARTICLE DEPOSITION IN THE RESPIRATORY TRACT

The deposition of particles in the lungs depends on their size and density, the distance over which they must travel, and the relative humidity. The method of breathing (i.e., mouth breathing versus nose breathing), the rate of air flow, the minute ventilation, and the depth of breathing also influence the deposition of the aerosol. Defense mechanisms vary depending on where in the respiratory tract particles are deposited as well as on their size and composition. In general, particles larger than 10 $\mu$m in diameter are deposited

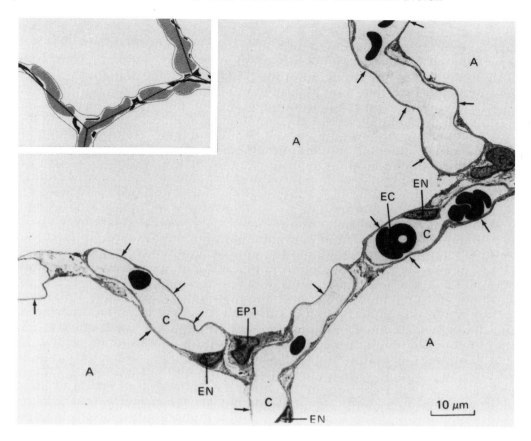

**FIGURE 1.16.** Thin section of alveolar septa from human lung. The major part is occupied by capillaries (*C*), which form the thinnest barrier to air on alternating sides of the septum (*arrows*). Note the distribution of connective tissue fibers (*black spots* on inset). *A*, alveolus; *EN*, endothelium; *EC*, erythrocyte; *EP1*, type I epithelial cell; *F*, fibroblast. (Reprinted from Weibel ER: Design and structure of the human lung. In Fishman AP (ed): *Assessment of Pulmonary Function.* New York, McGraw-Hill, 1980.)

by impaction in the upper respiratory passages. Particles between 2 and 10 μm are carried in the airstream into the lower respiratory tract, where they impact in the bronchial tree. Particles between 0.5 and 3 μm are too small to impact in the airways but are deposited in the gas exchange areas of the lungs (the TRUs). Particles smaller than 0.2 μm are not efficiently deposited in the lung and may be exhaled. Modern nebulizers are capable of generating aerosols containing small particles of controlled size in high concentrations and are thus efficient means of depositing particles in the distal parts of the respiratory tract.

## TRANSPORT SYSTEMS OF THE LUNGS

Three transport systems are available for the removal of inhaled particles from the alveoli: the mucociliary escalator, phagocytes, and the lymphohematogenous drainage system. These systems work together although they operate through different pathways at different rates (51).

## MUCOCILIARY ESCALATOR

The mucociliary escalator functions to transport deposited particles from the level of the terminal bronchioles to the major airways, where they are coughed up and either expectorated or swallowed. The transport rate of this system is about 3 mm/minute and becomes more rapid proximally, where the streams converge. Approximately 90% of the particles directly deposited on the mucus layer are cleared within 2 hours. In the main bronchi, the mucociliary apparatus is formed by the ciliated epithelial cells, the mucus-producing goblet cells, and the mucous glands, which open directly onto the mucosa. In the smaller bronchi and bronchioles mucus is formed from goblet cell secretions. In the smallest peripheral bronchioles, goblet

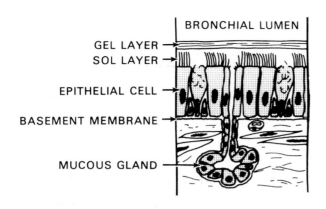

BRONCHIAL LUMEN

GEL LAYER →
SOL LAYER →
EPITHELIAL CELL →
BASEMENT MEMBRANE →
MUCOUS GLAND →

FIGURE 1.17.   The mucociliary escalator. The gel layer of mucus is propelled toward the trachea by the movement of the cilia on the surface of the cells.

cells are not normally seen, and the epithelium is lined by a thin layer of material containing surfactant that is derived from the Clara cells and the type II alveolar cells. This layer flows proximally and is continuous with the mucus layer of the mucociliary escalator.

The mucus, which is the transport medium, is a complex mucopolysaccharide arranged in a double layer on the surface of the epithelium (Fig. 1.17). The external layer is a viscous gel, which acts as a trap to catch and transport deposited particles. The mucus gel is elastic, and the mechanical beating of cilia is therefore able to propel both mucus and any entrapped particulates proximally. Loss of mucus elasticity can impair clearance. The internal sol layer is a thin liquid in which the cilia are able to move easily. The cilia themselves move with a characteristic biphasic rhythm. Beating within the liquid layer and striking the gel layer with their tips, they exhibit a periodic movement, forming wave bands that move the mucus up the bronchial tree toward the larynx. Efficient beating of cilia requires that the sol layer have an appropriate viscosity. In addition, the sol layer must be of the proper thickness so that cilia tips contact the mucus gel on the forward beat, but release on the reverse beat. Effective clearance, therefore, requires a sol layer of appropriate composition and amount.

Many factors can alter clearance. Ciliary motion can be affected by exposure to a variety of substances. Toxic fumes and cigarette smoke, for example, may disrupt normal wave patterns or cause cilia to stop beating completely. Hereditary abnormalities of the cilia alter their movement and result in the "immotile cilia syndrome" (52). This syndrome can result from a variety of cilia defects, several of which can be recognized by electron microscopy of cilia. These hereditary diseases are associated with immotile cilia not only in the lung and upper respiratory tract, but also at other sites where cilia are present such as sperm cells and cells lining the nasal sinuses. Immotile sperm and male infertility, therefore, may be associated with the immotile cilia syndromes. Cilia in the developing embryo are responsible for pushing the developing heart to the left. With immotile cilia, localization is nearly random, and approximately half of individuals will have dextrocardia or situs inversus. The triad of situs inversus associated with bronchiectasis and sinusitis, associated with immotile cilia, is termed Kartagener's syndrome.

Chronic bronchitis, asthma, cystic fibrosis, and acute respiratory infections may cause loss of cilia or abnormal ciliary function. These conditions are also associated with altered mucus secretion. Deoxyribonucleic acid (DNA) derived from inflammatory cells can increase viscosity, and proteolytic enzymes can disrupt mucus elasticity; thus, these disorders are associated with impaired clearance for a number of reasons. It is likely that increased susceptibility to infection in these disorders results, at least in part, from these clearance defects.

The alveolar surface itself is protected to some extent by the normal movement of the surface lining layer into the peripheral bronchi. However, more important to alveolar clearance are two other factors, the alveolar phagocytes and the lymphohematogenous drainage system.

### ALVEOLAR MACROPHAGE

The principal resident phagocyte of the alveoli is the alveolar macrophage. Some replication of these cells may take place in the lung, but they are ultimately derived from precursors in bone marrow which migrate in the peripheral blood as monocytes. Compared to mononuclear phagocytes at other sites (e.g., peritoneal macrophages), alveolar macrophages possess adaptations for the aerobic environment of the lung. Macrophages can phagocytose surfactant and are probably involved in the metabolic turnover of many of the extracellular components of the alveoli. Macrophages also phagocytose both bacteria and nonliving particulates. This process can be augmented by both specific and nonspecific opsonins, which can bind to particulates and subsequently interact with specific macrophage receptors. Following phagocytosis, bacteria may be killed and particles digested by powerful enzymes in the cellular lysosomes. Organic molecules may be further detoxified by oxidases and a variety of transferases.

Macrophages are also able to release a host of cytokines. Through the release of these mediators, macrophages are able to recruit and activate other inflammatory cells. Neutrophils, recruited in response to macrophage-derived chemotactic factors such as leukotriene $B_4$ or interleukin-8 can greatly augment the phagocytic defenses of the lung. Cytokines derived from macrophages can also recruit and activate lymphocytes and pulmonary parenchymal cells. Macrophages are likely, therefore, to play a central role in initiating and maintaining chronic inflammatory processes in the lungs. The ability of macrophages to regulate parenchymal cells, combined with their capability of releasing proteases capable of degrading all components of the extracellular matrix, suggests they may also be crucial regulators of tissue repair and remodeling.

## LYMPHOHEMATOGENOUS DRAINAGE

The third transport system of the lungs is the lymphohematogenous drainage system. The alveolar septum contains connective tissue and is a space that may potentially act as a vehicle for the exit of macrophages from the alveoli. From there macrophages may enter the pulmonary capillaries or the lymphatics of the lung periphery. Inhaled particles probably do not enter lymphatics directly unless inflammation is present, but are carried within phagocytic cells. The speed of transport via the lymphatic system is variable and may take months or years. Collections of macrophages containing large amounts of foreign particles are frequently seen in the lymph nodes of the lungs, where they may remain permanently.

## PULMONARY LYMPHATICS

The lungs and pleura are richly supplied with lymphatics. The purpose of the large flow of lymph from the lungs is twofold. First, it forms a natural mechanism for the removal of excess fluid that moves into the interstitial spaces from the pulmonary capillaries, thus keeping the alveoli relatively free of fluid. Secondly, it forms an important part of the alveolar defense mechanism by transporting macrophages containing inhaled particles from distal areas of the lungs. It is largely because of this rich lymphatic system that bronchogenic carcinoma travels out of the lungs so readily. The lymphatics in the terminal respiratory units converge in the interlobular septa. Movement of lymph is increased by respiratory movements coupled with a series of valves in the lymphatic vessels, which ensures proximal flow. Chronic increased pulmonary capillary pressure, and presumably increased production of pulmonary lymph, can be associated with increased capacity for lymphatic clearance. The lymphatics line the pulmonary arteries and veins as well as the bronchi themselves and converge at the pulmonary

hila, where the hilar lymph nodes are found. From here the thoracic duct drains the left lung, and the right lymphatic duct drains the right. These vessels enter the systemic venous circulation at the junctions of the subclavian and internal jugular veins.

The bronchopulmonary lymph nodes surround the divisions of the lobar bronchi, and hilar glands are clustered at the lung roots. The hilar lymph nodes occur around the upper and lower lobe bronchi and communicate richly via the subcarinal nodes with the opposite side. Paratracheal nodes are found on either side of the trachea and are most prominent on the right. The *azygos* node is found adjacent to the azygos vein at the junction of the right upper lobe bronchus and the right main bronchus. The pulmonary lymphatic system communicates with the lower deep cervical nodes above and with the abdominal lymphatics below. In addition to the hilar and mediastinal lymph nodes there are also lymphatics along the distribution of the internal mammary arteries, near the intercostal arteries adjacent to the posterior ribs, and in the anterior and posterior mediastinum, which receive drainage primarily from the chest wall.

There is some disagreement as to the drainage of the various lobes of the lung, and indeed drainage channels may vary among individuals. In general, the lower lobes drain into the hilar and subcarinal nodes, while the upper lobes more often drain directly to the paratracheal nodes. Thus, cancers arising in lower-lobe bronchi must traverse an extra set of lymph nodes, the hilar group, before reaching the paratracheal chain. The rich system of anastomoses among lymph node groups may account at least in part for the variation in lymphatic drainage of the lobes. Lymphocytes in intrapulmonary and regional nodes may become reactive, and the nodes may enlarge in a variety of inflammatory lung diseases, both infections (e.g., granulomas) and noninfectious (e.g., silicosis).

Lymphocytes accumulate beneath the epithelium of airways, where they are termed bronchus-associated lymphoid tissue (BALT). These airway lymphocytes are thought to participate in the system of mucosal immunity and to be responsible for local responses to antigen with both local and generalized production of immunoglobulin, particularly IgA. Lymphocytes are also present in the pulmonary parenchyma, and their numbers may increase significantly in disease states. While the mechanisms responsible are not fully elucidated, lymphocytes present in the lung are thought to be capable of migrating to regional nodes, circulating in the blood and then relocalizing at specific tissue sites by virtue of the expression of specific "homing receptors."

▼

## REFERENCES

1. Staub NC, Albertine KH: The structure of the lungs relative to their principal function. In Murray JF, Nadel JA (eds): *Textbook of Respiratory Medicine*. Philadelphia, WB Saunders, 1988, pp 12–16.
2. Berger A, Mitchell R, Severinghaus J: Regulation of respiration (part one). *N Engl J Med* 297:92, 1977.
3. Berger A, Mitchell R, Severinghaus J: Regulation of respiration (part two). *N Engl J Med* 297:138, 1977.
4. Berger A, Mitchell R, Severinghaus J: Regulation of respiration (part three). *N Engl J Med* 297:194, 1977.
5. Long S, Duffin J: The medullary respiratory neurons: a review. *Can J Physiol Pharmacol* 62:161, 1984.
6. Merrill EG: Network properties of respiratory neurons. In Feldman JL, Berger DJ (eds): *Proceedings of the International Symposium: Central Neural Production of Periodic Respiratory Movements*. Chicago, Northwestern University, 1982, p 54.
7. Merrill EG: Finding a respiratory function for the medullary respiratory neurons. In Bellairs R, Gray EG (eds): *Essays on the Nervous System*. Oxford, Clarendon Press, 1974, p 451.
8. Remmers JE, Marttila I: Action of intercostal muscle afferents on the respiratory rhythm of anesthetized cats. *Respir Physiol* 24:31, 1975.
9. Remmers JE, Tsiaras WG: Effect of lateral cervical cord lesions on the respiratory rhythm of anaesthetized, decerebrate cats after vagotomy. *J Physiol (Lond)* 233:63, 1973.
10. Remmers JE: Inhibition of inspiratory activity by intercostal muscle afferents. *Respir Physiol* 10:358, 1970.
11. Von Euler C: On the role of proprioceptors in perception and execution of motor acts with special reference to breathing. In Pengelly LD, Rebuck AS, Campbell EJM (eds): *Loaded Breathing*. Don Mills, Ontario, Canada, Longmans, 1974, p 139.
12. Cherniack NS, Fishman AP: Abnormal breathing patterns. *Dis Mon* 7:1, 1975.
13. Widdicombe JG, Fillenz M: Receptors of the lungs and airways. In Neil E (ed): *Handbook of Sensory Physiology, vol 3 pt 1, Enteroceptors*. New York, Springer-Verlag, 1972, p 80.
14. Paintal AS: Vagal sensory receptors and their reflex effects. *Physiol Rev* 53:159, 1973.
15. Leusen I: Regulation of cerebrospinal fluid composition with reference to breathing. *Physiol Rev* 52:1, 1972.
16. Cherniack NS: The regulation of ventilation. In Fishman AP (ed): *Pulmonary Diseases and Disorders*. New York, McGraw-Hill, 1980, p 317.
17. Cherniack NS, Longobardo GS: Oxygen and carbon dioxide gas stores of the body. *Physiol Rev* 50:196, 1970.
18. Biscoe TJ: Carotid body: structure and function. *Physiol Rev* 42:335, 1962.
19. Cherniack NS, Edelman NH, Lahiri S: Hypoxia and hypercapnia as respiratory stimulants and depressants. *Respir Physiol* 11:113, 1970.
20. Stockley RA: The estimation of the resting reflex hypoxic drive to respiration in normal man. *Respir Physiol* 31:217, 1977.
21. Cunningham DJC: The control system regulating breathing in man. *Q Rev Biophys* 6:433, 1974.
22. Biscoe TJ, Purnes MJ, Sampson SR: The frequency of nerve impulses in single carotid body chemoreceptor afferent fibers recorded in vivo with intact circulation. *J Physiol (Lond)* 208:121, 1970.
23. Read DJC: A clinical method for assessing the ventilatory response to $CO_2$. *Australas Ann Med* 16:20, 1967.
24. Macklem PT: Respiratory muscles: The vital pump. *Chest* 78:753–758, 1980.
25. Cohen CA, Zagelbaum G, Gross D, Roussos C, Macklem PT: Clinical manifestations of inspiratory muscle fatigue. *Am J Med* 73:308–316, 1982.
26. Garrity ER Jr, Shart JT: Respiratory muscles: function and dysfunction. *ACCP Pulm Crit Care Update* vol 2, lesson 10, 1986.
27. De Troyer A, Estene M, Heilporn A: Mechanisms of active expiration in tetraplegic patients. *N Engl J Med* 314:740–744, 1986.
28. Roncoroni AJ, Androgue HJA, DeObrutsky CW, Marchisio ML, Herrera MR: Metabolic acidosis in status asthmaticus. *Respiration* 33:85–94, 1976.
29. Minh VD, Dolan GF, Konopka RF, Moser KM: Effect of hyperinflation on inspiratory function of the diaphragm. *J Appl Physiol* 40:67–73, 1976.
30. Roussos C, Macklem PT: The respiratory muscles. *N Engl J Med* 307:786–797, 1982.
31. Weiner-Kronish JP, Albertine KH, Licko V, Staub NC: Protein egress and entry rates in pleural fluid and plasma in sheep. *J Appl Physiol* 56:459–463, 1984.
32. Broaddus VC, Wiener-Kronesh JP, Berthiaume Y, Staub NC: Removal of pleural liquid and protein in lymphatics in awake sheep. *J Appl Physiol* 64:384–390, 1988.
33. Light RW, George RB: Upper airway obstruction (editorial). *Arch Intern Med* 137:281, 1977.
34. Weibel ER: *Morphometry of the Lung*. New York, Academic Press, 1963.
35. Barnes PJ: Airway neuropeptides: roles in fine tuning and in disease? *News Physiol Sci* 4:116–120, 1989.
36. Massaro G: Nonciliated bronchiolar epithelial (Clara) cells. In Massaro D (ed): *Lung Biology in Health and Disease, vol 41, Lung Cell Biology*. New York, Marcel Dekker, 1989, pp 81–114.
37. Lauweryns JM, Peuskens JC, Cokelacre M: Argyrophil, fluorescent and granulated (peptide and amine producing?) AFG cells in human infant bronchial epithelium. Light and electron microscopic studies. *Life Sci* 9:1417, 1970.
38. Lauweryns JM, Peuskens JC: Neuroepithelial bodies (neuroreceptor or secretory organs?) in human infant bronchial and bronchiolar epithelium. *Anat Rec* 172:471, 1972.
39. Terry PB, Traystman RJ, Newball HH, et al: Collateral ventilation in man. *N Engl J Med* 298:10, 1978.
40. Deffebach ME, Charan NB, Lakshminarayan S, Butler J: The bronchial circulation: small, but a vital attribute of the lung. *Am Rev Respir Dis* 135:463–481, 1987.
41. Murray J: *The Normal Lung*, ed 2. Philadelphia, WB Saunders, 1986, p 189.
42. Von Hayek H: *The Human Lung* (trans. Krohl VE). New York, Hafner, 1960.
43. Staub NC: The interdependence of pulmonary structure and function. *Anesthesiology* 24:831, 1963.
44. Lauweryns JM: The blood and lymphatic microcirculation of the lung. In Sommers SC (ed): *Pathology Annual 1971*. New York, Appleton-Century-Crofts, 1971.

45. Miller WS: *The Lung.* Baltimore, Charles C Thomas, 1937.

46. Reid L, Simon G: The peripheral pattern in the normal bronchogram and its relation to peripheral pulmonary anatomy. *Thorax* 13:103, 1958.

47. Crapo JD, Barry BE, Gehr P, et al: Cell number and cell characteristics of the normal human lung. *Am Rev Respir Dis* 125:740–745, 1982.

48. Gail DB, Lenfant CJM: Cells of the lung: biology and clinical implications. *Am Rev Respir Dis* 127:366–387, 1983.

49. Nielson DW, Georke J, Clements JA: Alveolar sub-phase pH in the lungs of anesthetized rabbits. *Proc Natl Acad Sci USA* 78:7119–7123, 1981.

50. Matthay MA, Berthiaume Y, Staub NC: Long-term clearance of liquid and protein from the lungs of unanesthetized sheep. *J Appl Physiol* 59:928–934, 1985.

51. Green GM: In defense of the lung. *Am Rev Respir Dis* 102:691, 1970.

52. Eliasson R, Mossberg B, Camner P, Afzelius BA: The immotile cilia syndrome: a congenital ciliary abnormality as an etiologic function in chronic infection and male sterility. *N Engl J Med* 297:1–6, 1977.

# Chapter 2

# Pulmonary Circulation

**Michael A. Matthay**
**Jeffrey R. Fineman**
**Richard A. Matthay**

THE PRIMARY PURPOSE of this chapter is to discuss the factors that determine blood flow, vascular pressures, and vascular resistance in the normal lung. Also considered is how the structure of the pulmonary circulation influences the distribution of pulmonary blood flow. This review of the normal physiology of the pulmonary circulation provides a foundation for understanding its disorders.

Since the pulmonary circulation has several functions besides gas exchange, a brief discussion of its nonrespiratory functions is included at the end of this chapter. The physiology of transvascular fluid and protein exchange in the microcirculation of the lung is covered in Chapter 22.

## ANATOMY OF THE PULMONARY CIRCULATORY SYSTEM

### THE RIGHT SIDE OF THE HEART

The pulmonary circulation begins at the right ventricle. As illustrated in Figure 2.1, the right ventricle is wrapped approximately halfway around the left ventricle (1). This is due to the difference in pressures developed by the two ventricles during systole. Because the left ventricle contracts with extreme force compared with the right ventricle, it assumes a globular shape, and the septum protrudes into the right heart.

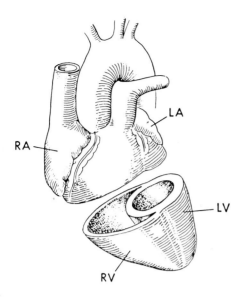

**FIGURE 2.1.** The anatomical relationship of the right ventricle to the left ventricle, showing the globular shape of the left ventricle and the half-moon shape of the right ventricle. *LA*, left atrium; *LV*, left ventricle; *RA*, right atrium; *RV*, right ventricle. (Adapted with permission from Guyton AC: The pulmonary circulation. In *Textbook of Medical Physiology*, ed 7. Philadelphia, WB Saunders, 1986.)

Since both sides of the heart pump essentially the same quantity of blood, the external wall of the right ventricle bulges outward and extends around a large portion of the left ventricle to accommodate this quantity (1).

Owing to the difference in pressures between the two sides of the heart, the right ventricular muscle is slightly more than one-third as thick as that of the left ventricle. In fact, the wall of the right ventricle is only 3 times as thick as the atrial walls, while the left ventricular wall is about 8 times as thick (1).

## THE PULMONARY VESSELS

The lung possesses dual blood supply sources. As part of the systemic circulation, the bronchial circulation provides the nutrition for part of the lung tissue. In contrast, the pulmonary circulation serves the body as a whole, since its primary function is gas exchange (2).

The main pulmonary artery receives the mixed venous blood pumped by the right ventricle. This vessel extends only 4 cm beyond the apex of the right ventricle and then divides into the right and left main branches, which supply blood to the two respective lungs. The main pulmonary artery wall is thin, with a thickness approximately twice that of the vena cava and only one-third that of the aorta (1). The subdivisions of the main pulmonary artery, even the small arteries and arterioles, have much larger diameters than their counterpart systemic arteries. This anatomic arrangement, combined with the fact that the vessel walls are very thin and distensible, makes the pulmonary arterial tree very compliant, averaging 3 ml/mm Hg, which is almost equal to that of the entire systemic arterial tree. This large compliance allows the pulmonary arteries to accommodate the stroke volume output of the right ventricle (1).

The main pulmonary artery branches successively, like the system of airways (see Chapter 1), and the pulmonary arteries accompany the bronchi through the centers of the primary lobules as far as the terminal bronchioles (3). Beyond that point, they form the capillary bed, which lies in the walls of the alveoli. The pulmonary capillaries form a dense network in the alveolar wall, providing an exceedingly efficient arrangement for gas exchange (3). The oxygenated blood leaves the capillary bed in the small pulmonary veins, which run between the lobules and eventually unite to form the four large veins that drain into the left atrium.

Structurally, the interstitial space that surrounds the pulmonary arteries and veins is continuous with the interstitial space around the capillaries in the alveolar septa. Functionally, however, the circulation is surrounded by two different interstitial spaces. As is explained later in this chapter, the alveolar vessels are exposed to different perivascular pressures than the larger, extraalveolar vessels. Consequently, there are important differences in blood flow, vascular resistance, and transvascular fluid flux between alveolar and extraalveolar vessels. Figure 2.2 is a photograph of the extraalveolar interstitial space, which is composed of loose connective tissue, pulmonary arteries, airways, and lymphatics. Lung capillaries, or the alveolar vessels, and the lymphatics are discussed in Chapter 22.

## THE BRONCHIAL VESSELS

The bronchial arteries usually originate from either the proximal portion of the thoracic aorta or one of the first two intercostal arteries. Each lung has at least one bronchial artery. These vessels follow the course of the bronchial tree into the lung parenchyma, where they branch elaborately and rejoin to form plexuses around the bronchi and in the bronchial submucosa (4). The blood flowing in the bronchial arteries is oxygenated blood, in contrast to the partially deoxygenated blood in the pulmonary arteries.

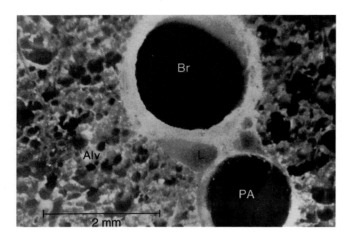

**FIGURE 2.2.**    A photomicrograph from a sheep lung frozen at normal inflation pressure. Note that the bronchus (*Br*), the lymphatic (*L*), and the partially blood-filled pulmonary artery (*PA*) are surrounded by loose connective tissue. This is the extraalveolar interstitial space. Alveolar ducts and alveoli (*Alv*) surround the bronchovascular sheath.

The bronchial arteries supply the lower part of the trachea, the bronchi as far as the respiratory bronchioles, and most of the visceral pleura by anastomoses with numerous other vessels. They also supply the vasa vasorum of the pulmonary artery and vein, the vagi, and the mediastinal structures, particularly the pericardium and the tracheobronchial lymph nodes (3). After bronchial arterial blood has passed through the supporting tissues, most of the blood empties into the pulmonary veins and enters the left atrium rather than passing back to the right atrium (1). An average of 1 to 2% of the total cardiac output takes this route, making the left ventricular output slightly greater than the right ventricular output (1). The anatomic and physiologic aspects of the bronchial circulation are considered in a major review article (4) and a recent text on the bronchial circulation (5).

## PHYSIOLOGY OF THE PULMONARY CIRCULATORY SYSTEM

### PRESSURES IN THE PULMONARY CIRCULATION: METHODS OF MEASUREMENT

In 1941, Cournand and Ranges (6) applied the technique of right atrial catheterization in humans, and in 1946, Bloomfield and associates (7) described pulmonary artery catheterization to measure central circulatory pressures in humans. Normal pressure relationships in the human systemic and pulmonary

circulations are illustrated in Figure 2.3 (3). A direct comparison of intravascular pressures in the pulmonary and systemic circulations in a normal adult man is presented in Table 2.1 (8).

Knowledge of normal pulmonary venous and left atrial pressures is essential to an assessment of the pulmonary circulation. However, it is technically more difficult to measure pressures within the left atrium than within the right heart chambers and pulmonary arterial circulation during cardiac catheterization. This presented a serious practical limitation to studies of the pulmonary circulation until it was learned that "wedge" pressures from an accessible pulmonary artery are almost identical to simultaneously measured end-diastolic pressures from the left atrium (9). To obtain a wedge pressure, blood flow through a branch of the pulmonary artery is occluded by either "wedging" the end of a catheter into the pulmonary artery or inflating a balloon surrounding the catheter in the vessel. Pressures recorded from the tip of the catheter under conditions of "no flow" reflect the pressure downstream within the vascular network at the site of the next freely communicating channels (i.e., pulmonary capillaries or small pulmonary veins), which in turn reflect left atrial pressures (8). The use of bedside pulmonary arterial catheterization has greatly facilitated the determination of pulmonary arterial and wedge pressures. These pressures can now be measured outside the cardiac catheterization laboratory by

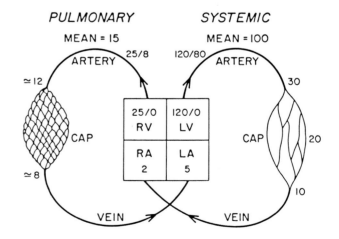

**FIGURE 2.3.**    Comparison of pressure (in mm Hg) in the pulmonary and systemic circulations. Hydrostatic differences modify these. *LA*, left atrium; *LV*, left ventricle; *RA*, right atrium; *RV*, right ventricle. (Reproduced with permission from West JB: *Respiratory Physiology—The Essentials*, ed 4. Baltimore, Williams & Wilkins, 1989.)

**TABLE 2.1**
**COMPARISON OF PULMONARY AND SYSTEMIC HEMODYNAMIC VARIABLES DURING REST AND EXERCISE OF MODERATE SEVERITY IN NORMAL ADULT MAN**

| Condition | Rest (Sitting) | Exercise |
|---|---|---|
| Oxygen consumption, ml/min | 300 | 2,000 |
| Blood flow | | |
|   Cardiac output, liters/min | 6 | 16.2 |
|   Heart rate, beats/min | 70 | 135 |
|   Stroke volume, ml/beat | 90 | 120 |
| Intravascular pressures, mm Hg | | |
|   Pulmonary arterial pressure | 25/8 | 30/11 |
|     Mean | 15 | 20 |
|   Left atrial pressure, mean | 5 | 10 |
|   Brachial arterial pressure | 120/70 | 155/78 |
|     Mean | 88 | 110 |
|   Right atrial pressure, mean | 2 | 1 |
| Resistances, mm Hg/liter/min | | |
|   Pulmonary vascular resistance | 1.67 | 0.62 |
|   Systemic vascular resistance | 13.2 | 6.9 |

Adapted with permission from Murray JF: *The Normal Lung.* Philadelphia, WB Saunders, 1986.

"floating" this catheter through the venous system and right heart into the pulmonary circulation (10, 11). This technique is now applied widely to studies of the pulmonary circulation in healthy subjects and in seriously ill patients. Coupled with indicator dilution approaches to determination of cardiac output, this method renders the once inaccessible human pulmonary circulation readily available for hemodynamic measurements.

There is evidence that pulmonary arterial end-diastolic pressure in normal subjects and in patients without lung disease closely approximates their wedge pressure (12). This correlation occurs because the total pressure difference will be least at the end of diastole, when the blood flow through the pulmonary circulation is lower than at any other point during the cardiac cycle. However, this relationship may not be maintained in the presence of disorders of the pulmonary circulation, and therefore pulmonary arterial end-diastolic pressure should not be assumed to be an accurate measurement of left atrial pressure in patients with any form of lung disease (12–14).

The risks and benefits of the use of bedside pulmonary arterial catheters in critically ill patients have been reviewed in detail (11).

### NORMAL PRESSURES WITHIN THE PULMONARY BLOOD VESSELS

Pressures in the pulmonary circulation are remarkably low (Table 2.1 and Figure 2.3) (4). The mean pressure in the main pulmonary artery is aproximately 15 mm Hg (range, 13 to 18 mm Hg); the systolic and diastolic pressures are about 25 and 8 mm Hg, respectively. In contrast, the mean pressure in the aorta is about 100 mm Hg—5 to 6 times higher than in the pulmonary artery. Pressures in the right and left atria are similar, about 2 and 5 mm Hg, respectively. Thus, pressure differences across the pulmonary and systemic circulations are about 15 − 5 = 10 and 100 − 2 = 98 mm Hg, respectively—a factor of 10 (3).

In keeping with these low pressures, the walls of the pulmonary artery and its branches are remarkably thin and contain relatively little smooth muscle; thus, they are easily mistaken for veins. In contrast, the arteries of the systemic circulation generally have thick walls and the arterioles in particular have abundant smooth muscle (3). The structural differences reflect the different functions of the two circulations. The systemic circulation regulates the supply of blood to various body parts, including those far above the level of the heart (the head or the upstretched arm, for example). In contrast, the lung is required to accept the entire cardiac output at all times. Because the pulmonary circulation is rarely concerned with directing blood from one region to another, its arterial pressures are as low as is consistent with delivering the blood to the top of the lung. This reduces the work of the right heart and maintains it as small as is feasible for efficient gas exchange to occur in the lung (3).

Overall, the distribution of pressures within the pulmonary circulation is more symmetrical than in the systemic circulation, where most of the pressure drop is upstream of the capillaries (Fig. 2.3) (3). Until recently, however, there were no direct measurements of pressure and resistance in the lung microcirculation. Experimental data from direct micropuncture of lung microvessels in adult dogs and adult rabbits have shown that, under normoxic conditions, approximately 50 to 60% of the resistance is in the nonmuscularized microvessels (those with diameters less than 10 to 20 $\mu$m) (15, 16). These vessels may include some small extraalveolar vessels also. However, in newborn animals the majority of the resistance lies in the arterial segment, probably because there is more smooth muscle in the media of the small pulmonary arteries (17, 18).

### PRESSURES AROUND THE PULMONARY BLOOD VESSELS

It is important to distinguish between alveolar and extraalveolar vessels when considering pressures around pulmonary vessels. Alveolar vessels include not only capillaries, but probably small arterioles and venules in the corners of the alveoli (19, 20). Extraalveolar vessels include all of the arteries and veins that course through the lung parenchyma.

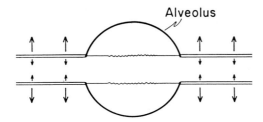

Alveolus

**FIGURE 2.4.** Alveolar and extraalveolar vessels. The first are mainly the capillaries and are exposed to alveolar pressure. The second are pulled open by the expansion of the lung parenchyma, and the effective pressure around them is therefore lower than alveolar pressure. (Adapted with permission from Hughes JMB, Glazier JB, Maloney JE, West JB: *Respir Physiol* 4:58, 1968.)

The caliber of the alveolar vessels is determined by the relationship between alveolar pressure and the pressure within the capillaries. Normally, the pulmonary capillaries are surrounded by gas and hence they derive very little support from the interstitial space and the alveolar epithelium around them. Consequently, the pulmonary capillaries or alveolar vessels will collapse or distend depending on the pressures within and around them. Usually, the effective pressure around the capillaries is alveolar pressure, and when this rises above the pressure inside the capillaries, the capillaries collapse (21).

In contrast, the pressure around the pulmonary arteries and veins, the extraalveolar vessels, can be substantially less than alveolar pressure. As the lung expands, these larger vessels are pulled open by the tension of the surrounding elastic lung parenchyma (Figs. 2.2 and 2.4) (3). Consequently, the effective pressure around these vessels is low; in fact, it is less than the pressure around the whole lung, or intrapleural pressure (22). In fact, micropuncture studies of the lung interstitium in normal and edematous dog lungs have shown that there is a pressure gradient from the alveolar to the extraalveolar and hilar interstitial lung regions that helps to move interstitial liquid to lymphatics and the extraalveolar loose connective tissue. The interstitial pressure at the hilum is $-1.8 \pm 0.2$ cm $H_2O$ relative to pleural pressure (23). This paradox can be explained by the mechanical advantage that develops when a rigid structure such as a blood vessel or a bronchus is surrounded by a rapidly expanding elastic material such as lung parenchyma. In any event, both the arteries and veins increase their caliber as the lung expands (3).

The different interstitial pressures surrounding alveolar and extraalveolar vessels in the lung are impor-

tant factors influencing normal fluid exchange in the lung. This is discussed further in Chapter 22.

## BLOOD VOLUME OF THE LUNGS

The blood volume of the lungs is approximately 12% of the total blood volume of the circulatory system (Fig. 2.5) (1). In the average human being, the two lungs contain approximately 450 ml of blood, of which about 70 to 100 ml is in the capillaries and the remainder is divided up equally between the arteries and the veins.

Under different physiologic and pathologic conditions, the quantity of blood in the lungs can vary considerably. For example, when a person exhales so vigorously that he or she builds up high pressure in the lungs, as when blowing a trumpet, as much as 250 ml of blood can be expelled from the pulmonary circulatory system into the systemic circulation. Also, loss of blood from the systemic circulation by hemorrhage can be partly compensated for by automatic shift of blood from the lung into the systemic vessels (1).

Failure of the left side of the heart because of increased resistance to blood flow through the mitral valve as a result of mitral stenosis causes blood to build up in the pulmonary circulation, greatly increasing the pulmonary blood volume while decreasing the systemic volume. Concurrently, the pressures in the pulmonary circulation increase while the systemic pressures decrease. Exactly the opposite effect takes place when the right side of the heart fails. Because the volume of the systemic circulation is about 7 times that

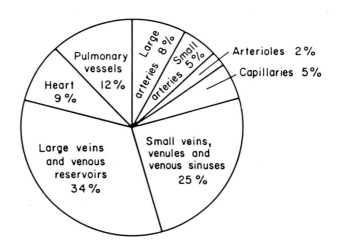

**FIGURE 2.5.** Percentage of the total blood volume in each portion of the circulatory system. (Reproduced with permission from Guyton AC: The pulmonary circulation. In *Textbook of Medical Physiology*, ed 7. Philadelphia, WB Saunders, 1986.)

of the pulmonary system, a shift of blood from one system to the other has a greater effect on the pulmonary than on the systemic circulation (1).

## PULMONARY BLOOD FLOW

Blood flow through the lungs is equal to the cardiac output, except for the 1% that circulates through the bronchial circulation (5). Therefore, the factors that control cardiac output also control pulmonary blood flow. In most conditions, the pulmonary vessels act as passive, distensible tubes that enlarge with increasing pressure and narrow with decreasing pressure. For the blood to be aerated adequately, however, it is important that it be distributed as uniformly as possible to all the different segments of the lung (1).

The volume of blood passing through the lungs each minute ($\dot{Q}$) can be calculated by using the Fick principle. According to this principle, the oxygen ($O_2$) consumption per minute ($\dot{V}O_2$) is equal to the amount of $O_2$ taken up by the blood in the lungs per minute. Since the $O_2$ concentration in the blood entering the lungs is $CvO_2$ and that in the blood leaving the lungs is $CaO_2$,

$$\dot{V}O_2 = \dot{Q}(CaO_2 - CvO_2) \qquad (1)$$

$$\dot{Q} = \frac{\dot{V}O_2}{CaO_2 - CvO_2} \qquad (2)$$

$\dot{V}O_2$ can be measured by collecting the expired gas in a large spirometer and measuring its $O_2$ concentration. Mixed venous blood can be sampled via a catheter in the pulmonary artery and systemic arterial blood by puncture of a systemic artery, usually the brachial or the radial artery. Blood flow ($\dot{Q}$) can then be calculated according to Equation 2.

Pulmonary blood flow also can be measured by the dye dilution technique. With this method, dye is injected into the venous circulation and its concentration in arterial blood is recorded (3, 4). More recently, thermal dilution cardiac output has emerged as a simple and reliable means of determining cardiac output at the bedside (24). A bolus of cold indicator (10 ml 5% dextrose in water) is injected through the right atrial port of a pulmonary arterial catheter, and a thermistor at the tip of the catheter in the pulmonary artery senses a temperature change. The time-temperature curve is then integrated by a bedside computer to give the cardiac output (24). Bedside cardiac output measurements have been very useful in helping to guide therapy for critically ill patients (11, 14).

## DISTRIBUTION OF BLOOD FLOW

Although we have been assuming that all parts of the pulmonary circulation behave identically, considerable inequality of blood flow exists within the human lung (3). This is shown in Figure 2.6.

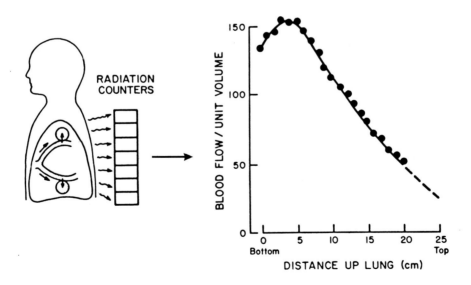

**FIGURE 2.6.** Measurement of the distribution of blood flow in the upright human lung using radioactive xenon. The dissolved xenon is evolved into alveolar gas in the pulmonary capillaries. The units of blood flow are such that if flow were uniform, all values would be 100. Note the small flow at the apex. (Adapted with permission from West JB: *Respiratory Physiology—The Essentials*, ed 4. Baltimore, Williams & Wilkins, 1989.)

The behavior of blood flow in a particular part of the lung depends on the relationship of the intraluminal pressures (arterial, capillary, venous) and the state of contraction of smooth muscle existing in that region.' Since the lung has an appreciable height in erect humans in relation to generally low pressures in the pulmonary vessels, the vessels near the apex must have a lower pressure than those at the bottom of the lung. Thus, it can be predicted that blood flow should vary in different parts of the lung (4).

For measurement of regional blood flow, radioactive xenon ($^{133}$Xe) is dissolved in saline and injected into a peripheral vein. When the solution reaches the pulmonary capillaries, it mixes in alveolar gas because of its low solubility, and the distribution of radioactivity can be measured by counters placed over the chest. In the upright human lung, blood flow decreases almost linearly from the bottom to the top, reaching lowest values at the apex (Fig. 2.6) (3). This distribution is affected by changes in posture and by exercise. When the subject is supine, blood flow in the apical zone increases but flow in the lower lung zone remains virtually unchanged. As a result the distribution from apex to base becomes almost uniform. In this posture, blood flow in the posterior regions of the lungs exceeds flow in the anterior parts. On mild exercise, blood flow in both upper and lower lung zones increases and the regional differences become less (3).

The phenomenon of uneven distribution of blood flow (Fig. 2.6) can be primarily attributed to the hydrostatic pressure differences within the blood vessels. Since the pulmonary arterial system is a continuous

column of blood, the difference in pressure between the top and the bottom of the lung is about 30 cm $H_2O$, or 23 mm Hg (3). This is a large pressure difference for such a low-pressure system as the pulmonary circulation (Fig. 2.3). Thus, the topographic gradient of blood flow is determined by hydrostatic pressure differences in the pulmonary circulation caused by gravity and not, as is the case with the regional distribution of ventilation, by the vertical gradient of intrapleural pressure (8).

The importance of hydrostatic pressure differences on regional blood flow is illustrated in Figure 2.7. This figure demonstrates that at the top of the lung (zone 1) pulmonary arterial pressure falls below alveolar pressure, which is normally close to atmospheric pressure. If this occurs, the capillaries collapse and no flow is possible. Under normal conditions, this does not occur because the pulmonary arterial pressure is just adequate to raise blood to the top of the lung. Zone 1 conditions may be present if the arterial pressure is reduced (e.g., following severe hemorrhage) or if alveolar pressure is raised (e.g., during positive-pressure ventilation). The ventilated but unperfused lung is called alveolar dead space (see also Chapter 4).

Farther down the lung (zone 2), pulmonary arterial pressure rises because of the hydrostatic effect and becomes greater than alveolar pressure. However, venous pressure remains very low and is less than alveolar pressure. Under these conditions, blood flow is determined by the difference between arterial and alveolar pressures, not by the usual arterial-venous pressure difference (3). In fact, venous pressure has

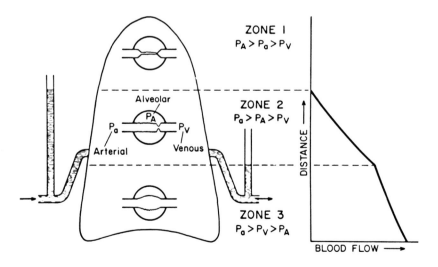

**FIGURE 2.7.** Model to explain the uneven distribution of blood flow in the lung based on the pressures affecting the capillaries. (Adapted with permission from West JB, Dollery CT, Naimark

A: Distribution of blood flow in isolated lung: relation to vascular and alveolar pressure. *J Appl Physiol* 19:713, 1964.)

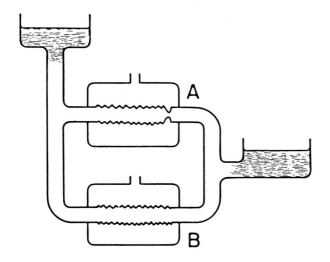

**FIGURE 2.8.** Two Starling resistors, each consisting of a thin rubber tube inside a container. When chamber pressure exceeds downstream pressure as in **A**, flow is independent of downstream pressure. However, when downstream pressure exceeds chamber pressure as in **B**, flow is determined by the upstream-downstream difference. (Adapted with permission from West JB: *Respiratory Physiology—The Essentials*, ed 4. Baltimore, Williams & Wilkins, 1989.)

no influence on flow unless it exceeds alveolar pressure.

West has modeled this situation with a flexible rubber tube inside a glass chamber (Fig. 2.8) (3). When chamber pressure is greater than downstream pressure, the rubber tube collapses at its downstream end, and the pressure in the tube at this point limits flow. The pulmonary capillary bed is really very different from a rubber tube, but the overall behavior is similar and is often called the *Starling resistor, sluice,* or *waterfall* effect. Since arterial pressure increases down the zone but alveolar pressure is the same throughout the lung, the pressure difference is responsible for flow increases. Moreover, increasing recruitment of capillaries occurs down this zone (3).

In zone 3, venous pressure is greater than alveolar pressure, and flow is determined in the usual way by the arterial-venous difference. The increase in blood flow down this region of the lung is associated with distention of the capillaries. Pressure within them (lying between arterial and venous) increases down the zone while the pressure outside (alveolar) remains constant. Thus, the transmural capillary pressure rises and blood flow increases down this zone 3.

Typical patterns of distribution of pulmonary blood

flow are shown in Figure 2.9 (4). The blood flow is less at the apex than at the base of the upright lung (sitting or standing) owing to gravity. Blood flow does not increase uniformly with increasing distance down the lung; it declines again near the bottom. This has been explained by the fact that in tidal breathing, alveoli at the bottom of the lung are relatively less inflated than those at the top. As a result, they exert less of a distending force on the extraalveolar vessels, which therefore are narrower and offer greater resistance so that flow decreases. Thus, maximal inspiration increases the flow of blood to the base of the upright lung, probably because the alveoli at the bottom of the lung expand more during a large inspiration than do those at the top. The extraalveolar vessels subsequently distend, with a resultant fall in resistance so that blood flow at the bottom of the lung increases (4).

When a normal subject lies down, the basal blood flow differences are largely abolished, since the two parts of the lung are nearly at the same hydrostatic level. If a subject lies on his or her side, the dependent lung is better perfused than the contralateral lung (4).

Figure 2.9 also shows the effect of exercise and distribution of blood flow on the lung. The blood flow at the top of the lung increases relatively more than that at the base during exercise, although the perfusion gradient (flow per unit vertical distance) may be nearly the same during exercise as it is at rest.

### PULMONARY VASCULAR RESISTANCE

The resistance of a system of blood vessels may be described by the expression vascular resistance = (input pressure − output pressure)/blood flow. *Pulmonary vascular resistance* (PVR) is determined by the mean inflow pressure in the pulmonary artery ($P_{pa}$), the mean outflow pressure in the pulmonary veins or left atrium ($P_{la}$), and the blood flow through the lungs according to the equation

$$\frac{P_{pa} - P_{la} \text{ (mm Hg)}}{\text{Pulmonary blood flow (liters/min)}} \quad (3)$$
$$= \text{PVR (mm Hg/liter/min)}$$

Determining PVR is a useful way to compare different circulations or the same circulation under different conditions. For instance, the total pressure drop from the pulmonary artery to the left atrium in the pulmonary circulation is only approximately 10 mm Hg, in contrast to a pressure drop of about 100 mm Hg for the systemic circulation (Fig. 2.3). Since the blood flow through these two circulations is virtually identical, PVR is only one-tenth the resistance in the systemic circulation (Table 2.1). Pulmonary blood flow is about 6 liters/minute; hence, in numbers, PVR equals (15 − 5)/6 or about 1.7 mm Hg/liter/minute (3).

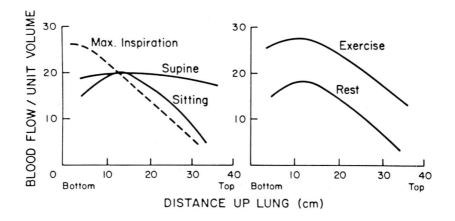

**FIGURE 2.9.** The effect of posture, lung inflation, and exercise on regional pulmonary blood flow. (Adapted with permission from Cherniack RM, Cherniack L, Naimark A: The pulmonary circulation. In *Respiration in Health and Disease,* ed 2. Philadelphia, WB Saunders, 1972, p 63.)

In the systemic circulation, the high resistance is caused largely by the muscular arteries that regulate blood flow to various organs of the body. In contrast, the pulmonary circulation has no such vessels and appears to have as low a resistance as is compatible with distributing the blood in a thin film over a vast area of the alveolar walls (3). Values for a normal PVR at rest and during moderately severe exercise are given in Table 2.1 and are compared with values of systemic vascular resistance (8). Calculation of PVR in a variety of disease states provides a quantitative measurement of the physiologic effect of the clinical disorder.

### Pulmonary Artery and Left Atrial Pressure

The remarkable feature of the normal pulmonary circulation is its ability to accommodate large increases in cardiac output with only a slight increase in pulmonary artery pressure. Thus, although the PVR is extraordinarily low, it has a remarkable facility for becoming even lower as the pressure within the pulmonary circulation rises (3, 8). Experimentally, if pulmonary artery pressure is raised by increasing flow while lung volume and left atrial pressure are held constant, PVR decreases (25). Similarly, if left atrial pressure is raised without allowing pulmonary artery pressure and blood flow to change, then PVR falls (26). Figure 2.10 graphically shows that an increase in either pulmonary arterial or venous pressure causes PVR to decrease. Two mechanisms are probably responsible for this. Under normal conditions, some capillaries are either closed or open but with no blood flow. As the pressure rises, these vessels begin to conduct blood, thus lowering the overall resistance. This is termed *recruitment* and is apparently the chief mechanism for

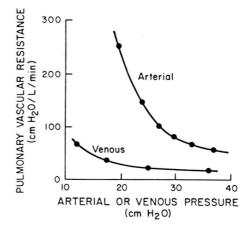

**FIGURE 2.10.** Fall in pulmonary vascular resistance as the pulmonary arterial or venous pressure is raised. When the arterial pressure was changed, the venous pressure was held constant at 12 cm $H_2O$, and when the venous pressure was changed, the arterial pressure was held at 37 cm $H_2O$. Data are from an excised dog preparation. (Adapted with permission from West JB: *Respiratory Physiology—The Essentials,* ed 4. Baltimore, Williams & Wilkins, 1989.)

the fall in PVR that occurs as the pulmonary artery pressure is increased from low levels. The reason some vessels are unperfused at low perfusing pressures is not clear, but this may be caused by random differences in the geometry of the complex network that results in preferential channels for flow. Another possible explanation is that a critical opening pressure must be exceeded in some arteries before they will conduct blood (3). In several clinical disorders that involve the pulmonary circulation, such as restrictive or obstructive lung disease with severe hypoxemia, a rise in pulmonary blood flow (as with exercise) may result in a rise in PVR (see Chapter 10).

### Lung Volume

An additional important determinant of PVR is lung volume. The currently available experimental evidence indicates that changes in lung volume may have opposing effects on vascular resistance in the alveolar and extraalveolar vessels (27, 28). As the lung expands, the extraalveolar vessels are pulled open and their vascular resistance declines. In the case of alveolar vessels, vascular resistance may increase if alveolar pressure rises above the intravascular pressure in the capillaries (i.e., if transmural pressure rises). With inflation to a high lung volume, alveolar pressure can rise with respect to perfusion pressure in the capillaries. These vessels then can be compressed, resulting in an increase in their vascular resistance. In addition, the caliber of the capillaries is reduced at higher lung volumes because of stretching of the alveolar walls (3). Figure 2.11 shows that the resistance offered by alveolar and extraalveolar vessels may change in opposite directions during inflation of the lung from residual volume to total lung capacity (8). The exact magnitude of the changes has not yet been defined.

From the foregoing discussion, it is apparent that PVR can be altered by changes in the caliber of pulmonary vessels, whether the alteration is a mechanical change affecting lung volume or a hemodynamic event affecting pulmonary blood flow and vascular recruitment. A number of other factors can affect pulmonary vascular resistance by dilating or constricting smooth muscle in the walls of pulmonary vessels. Until recently, it was not well established that significant vasomotor control of the pulmonary circulation existed. It is now clear, however, that there is enough smooth muscle in pulmonary arterioles to alter resistance (not much is required in a low-pressure system). Furthermore, this muscle can hypertrophy in a variety of disease states, including congenital heart disease, longstanding mitral stenosis and mitral insufficiency, and some primary lung disorders such as idiopathic primary pulmonary hypertension. In addition, a variety of neurogenic, humoral, and chemical substances can dilate and constrict the pulmonary vascular bed. These factors are discussed in the next section.

### REGULATION OF THE PULMONARY CIRCULATION

This section addresses a number of questions regarding how the pulmonary circulation is regulated:

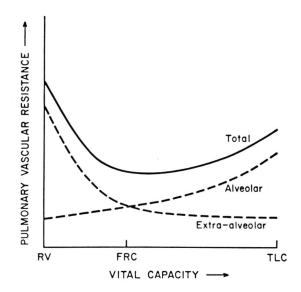

**FIGURE 2.11.** Schematic representation of the effects of changes in vital capacity on total pulmonary vascular resistance and the contributions to the total afforded by alveolar and extraalveolar vessels. During inflation from residual volume (*RV*) to total lung capacity (*TLC*), resistance to blood flow through alveolar vessels increases, whereas resistance through extraalveolar vessels decreases. Thus, changes in total pulmonary vascular resistance form a U-shaped curve during lung inflation, with the nadir at functional residual capacity (*FRC*). (Reproduced with permission from Murray JF: *The Normal Lung.* Philadelphia, WB Saunders, 1986.)

What regulates resting vascular tone in the lung? Do pulmonary vessels respond to autonomic stimuli in the same way as systemic vessels? How does the lung regulate flow in the presence of hypoxia and hypercapnia?

### Resting Vascular Tone

Although pulmonary resistance is about one-tenth the resistance in the systemic circulation, there is some resting vascular tone in the normal pulmonary circulation. It is not certain whether this tone is mediated by very low levels of alpha activity, by low levels of a circulating catecholamine such as norepinephrine, by prostaglandins, or by other factors. The presence of low-grade resting vasoconstriction can be demonstrated by administering vasodilators such as isoproterenol and theophylline, which lower pulmonary artery pressure and pulmonary vascular resistance (29). α-Blockade with phentolamine will also slightly lower pulmonary vascular resistance (30).

### Autonomic Nervous System

There are both α- and β-adrenergic receptors in the pulmonary circulation (31, 32). However, overall the autonomic nervous system exerts minimal control over the pulmonary circulation in the normal human adult (33, 34). In animals, stimulation of sympathetic nerves results in only a slight rise in pulmonary arterial tone, in contrast to the brisk response of the systemic circulation to increased sympathetic activity (35, 36). Moreover, pulmonary vasoconstriction from a variety of stimuli (most importantly, alveolar hypoxia) has been dissociated from the sympathetic nervous system. In the normal human, changes in sympathetic and parasympathetic tone appear to exert their major effect on the pulmonary blood circulation indirectly by changing cardiac output and thereby altering pulmonary blood flow (4). Nevertheless, it may be that sympathetic tone has some secondary effects on pulmonary vascular resistance in certain disease states.

### Catecholamines and Other Agents

Release of large amounts of endogenous catecholamines, such as epinephrine and norepinephrine, can initiate mild vasoconstriction in the lung because of the predominance of $\alpha$ receptors in the pulmonary vessel walls (33). The net effect on pulmonary vascular resistance also depends on their combined $\alpha$ and $\beta$ effects on cardiac output and airway resistance.

There are a variety of other naturally occurring substances with vasoconstrictive properties relative to the pulmonary circulation. These include histamine, angiotensin II, serotonin, and the prostaglandins. Most of these substances have been studied by exogenous administration of pharmacologic doses in experimental animals and in humans. Their function in maintaining normal pulmonary vascular resistance in humans is under investigation. A role has been suggested for each of them in a variety of disease states, but, with a few exceptions, there is little definitive evidence that they mediate clinical disorders of the pulmonary circulation in humans. A brief discussion of their effects on the pulmonary circulation in pharmacologic doses is included here, and a review of their metabolism is provided at the end of this chapter.

Histamine acts principally as a pulmonary vasoconstrictor, probably mediated mostly by $H_1$ receptors (37). In the systemic circulation, however, histamine causes vasodilation. Since histamine is stored in the lung in mast cells and is a potent pulmonary vasoconstrictor, it has been investigated as a mediator of conditions that increase pulmonary vascular resistance (i.e., alveolar hypoxia). However, histamine does not mediate the vasoconstrictor response to alveolar hypoxia (33).

Serotonin (5-hydroxytryptamine) is another agent stored in the mast cells that can cause pulmonary vasoconstriction in experimental animals. Data from direct micropuncture studies show that serotonin produces a rise in pulmonary vascular resistance by increasing both precapillary arterial and postcapillary venous tone (15).

Other substances that can affect pulmonary vascular resistance are agents that are metabolically altered in the lung. These include angiotensin II, bradykinin, and the prostaglandins. In pharmacologic doses, angiotensin II is a potent pulmonary vasoconstrictor. Like histamine, it has been ruled out as a principal mediator of the pulmonary vasoconstriction produced by alveolar hypoxia (38). Bradykinin is a pulmonary vasodilator and, like angiotensin II, has no proven function in the normal pulmonary circulation.

Prostaglandins of different chemical varieties have opposing effects on the pulmonary circulation. Prostaglandins of the F series cause vasoconstriction, while those of the E series cause vasodilation. However, arachidonic acid metabolites (prostaglandins), angiotensin II, and bradykinin have local vascular effects that could be direct or also mediated by a secondary transmitter (39). It is not clear at present how important prostaglandins are in maintaining resting vascular tone in the pulmonary circulation or what role they play in specific disease states (33). However, as discussed in the next section, there is some evidence that lipoxygenase products of arachidonic acid metabolism may play a role in mediating hypoxic pulmonary vasoconstriction and controlling the normal pulmonary circulation, especially in the fetus (40, 41). Also, there is new evidence that several vasodilators stimulate vascular endothelium via a muscarinic receptor to produce a factor (endothelium-derived relaxing factor) that diffuses into adjacent muscle cells and activates a mechanism for relaxation (42) (see below).

### Endothelium-derived Vasoactive Factors

The pulmonary vascular endothelial cells are capable of producing a variety of vasoactive substances that participate in the regulation of normal pulmonary vascular tone. These substances, such as nitric oxide and endothelin-1 (ET-1), are capable of producing vascular relaxation or constriction, modulating the propensity of the blood to clot, and inducing or inhibiting smooth muscle migration and replication (43, 44) (Fig. 2.12).

Nitric oxide is a labile humoral factor produced by nitric oxide synthase from L-arginine in the vascular endothelial cell. Nitric oxide diffuses into the smooth muscle cell and produces vascular relaxation by increasing concentrations of cyclic guanosine 3',5'-monophosphate (cGMP), via the activation of soluble guanylate cyclase. Nitric oxide is released in response to a variety of factors, including shear stress and the binding of certain endothelium-dependent vasodilators

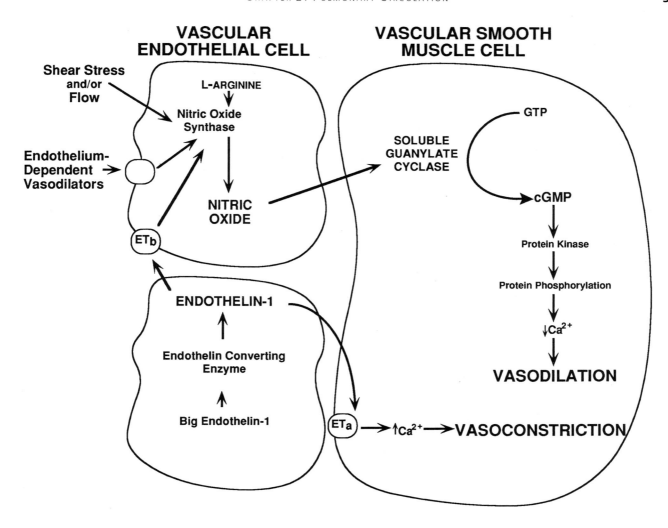

**FIGURE 2.12.** An illustration of the various vasoactive factors produced by pulmonary vascular endothelial cells and their functions. These substances participate in the regulation of pulmonary vascular tone, the clotting of the blood, and also the migration and replication of smooth muscle cells.

(such as acetylcholine, ATP, and bradykinin) to receptors on the endothelial cell. Recent evidence suggests that basal nitric oxide release is an important mediator of resting pulmonary vascular tone in the fetus, newborn, and adult, as well as a mediator of the fall in pulmonary vascular resistance normally occurring at the time of birth (45–48).

Endothelin-1 is a 21–amino acid polypeptide also produced by vascular endothelial cells (49). The vasoactive properties of ET-1 are complex, and studies have shown varying hemodynamic effects on different vascular beds. However, its most striking property is its sustained hypertensive action. In fact ET-1 is the most potent vasoconstricting agent discovered, with a potency 10 times that of angiotensin II. Studies on the

pulmonary circulation have demonstrated that exogenous ET-1 can produce sustained vasoconstriction, transient vasodilation, or a biphasic response of transient vasodilation followed by sustained vasoconstriction. The hemodynamic effects of ET-1 are mediated by at least two distinctive receptor populations, $ET_a$ and $ET_b$. The $ET_a$ receptors are located on vascular smooth muscle cells and mediate vasoconstriction, whereas the $ET_b$ receptors may be located on endothelial cells and mediate both vasodilation and vasoconstriction. The role of endogenous ET-1 in the regulation of normal pulmonary vascular tone is currently unclear (50). Nevertheless, endothelial dysfunction resulting in aberrations of endothelin-1 and nitric oxide has been implicated in a variety of disease states (51).

## Hypoxic Pulmonary Vasoconstriction

One of the most important and striking differences between the pulmonary and systemic circulations is their contrasting responses to hypoxia. In the systemic circulation, hypoxia produces vasodilation, while in the pulmonary circulation hypoxia results in vasoconstriction. The vasoconstriction occurs on the arterial side of the pulmonary circulation when oxygen tension drops to approximately 60 mm Hg or less in the alveoli. A low oxygen tension in the bloodstream does not induce pulmonary vasoconstriction (33, 52). Investigators have speculated that a receptor is present on the adventitial surface of pulmonary arteries that senses alveolar $P_{O_2}$ and initiates vasoconstriction (8, 53). The exact mechanisms that mediate hypoxic pulmonary vasoconstriction, however, have not been precisely determined. Since the response occurs in the isolated lung, neural mechanisms and circulating humoral agents probably are not responsible (52, 53). A number of potential mediators, such as histamine, angiotensin II, and prostaglandins of the F series, have been ruled out as essential factors in hypoxic pulmonary vasoconstriction (33). Recent research efforts have established that the hypoxic vasoconstrictor response may cause pulmonary vessels to constrict by directly affecting smooth muscle membranes, resulting in depolarization, calcium influx, and contraction. For example, verapamil, an agent that blocks cellular calcium influx, can inhibit the hypoxic constrictor response (54). However, the agent responsible for the release of calcium is still unknown (53).

Since the endothelium is necessary for hypoxia-induced contractions of isolated pulmonary arteries, endothelium-derived vasoactive substances have recently been implicated as factors in hypoxic pulmonary vasoconstriction. Although in vitro data suggest that hypoxia impairs nitric oxide activity, in vivo, nitric oxide inhibition potentiates hypoxic pulmonary vasoconstriction. Most likely, nitric oxide is actually released during hypoxia, and the released nitric oxide modulates the pulmonary vasoconstricting response (55, 56, 57). It is unlikely that endothelin-1 mediates acute hypoxic pulmonary vasoconstriction. However, impairment of nitric oxide activity and increased endothelin release may contribute to the pulmonary vasoconstriction and smooth muscle vascular remodeling associated with chronic hypoxia (58, 59).

It has been well established that acidosis potentiates hypoxic pulmonary vasoconstriction (60, 61). In a number of animals, the vasoconstrictor response to an alveolar $P_{O_2}$ of 40 mm Hg doubles when the pH is reduced to 7.20 (Fig. 2.13) (61, 62). In humans, when acidosis has been induced in patients with chronic obstructive

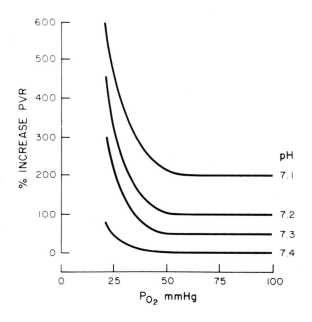

**FIGURE 2.13.** Diagram of the average results from experiments in newborn calves, showing the effect of changes in inspired $P_{O_2}$ on pulmonary vascular resistance (*PVR*) under conditions of different arterial blood pH. As inspired $P_{O_2}$ is decreased, pulmonary resistance increases; this effect becomes exaggerated and occurs at progressively higher $O_2$ values as pH is decreased. (Reproduced from Rudolph AM, Yuan S: Response of the pulmonary vasculature to hypoxia and $H^+$ ion concentration changes. *J Clin Invest* 45:399–411, 1966, by copyright permission of the American Society for Clinical Investigation.)

pulmonary disease, the pulmonary vascular response to hypoxia has been augmented (60).

Considerable attention has been given to the deleterious effects of hypoxic pulmonary vasoconstriction, especially in chronic conditions. Many patients with advanced chronic obstructive lung disease have markedly increased pulmonary resistance that probably predisposes them to cor pulmonale or right heart failure from increased pulmonary artery pressures (13, 63). Therapy with low-flow oxygen can relieve some of the pulmonary hypertension and perhaps prolong life (63).

However, hypoxic pulmonary vasoconstriction also should be regarded as a very useful adaptation, especially in the face of acute respiratory disorders. In patients with pneumonia, pneumothorax, pulmonary edema, or lobar atelectasis, hypoxic pulmonary vasoconstriction decreases blood flow to the poorly ventilated areas of the lung and thereby reduces the degree of venous admixture and arterial hypoxemia. Patients with diffuse lung infiltrates and acute respiratory failure often have mild to moderate pulmonary artery hypertension, part of which may be mediated by local areas of hypoxia and acidosis in poorly ventilated areas of the lung (64). Treatment with agents such as isoproterenol or nitroprusside will increase cardiac output and dilate pulmonary arteries, with a resultant decrease in pulmonary vascular resistance. However, the degree of intrapulmonary right-to-left shunting can also increase with this therapy, and arterial hypoxemia may worsen (65).

## METABOLIC FUNCTION OF THE PULMONARY CIRCULATORY SYSTEM

### METABOLIC NEEDS OF THE NORMAL HUMAN LUNG

The work involved in gas exchange is performed primarily by the respiratory muscles, which provide the mechanical force required for ventilation, and by the heart, which pumps blood through the pulmonary circulation (8). Because gas exchange by diffusion is a passive process that does not require energy, essentially the entire metabolic cost of respiration is supplied by organs other than the lung. Nonetheless, the lung is known to be a metabolically active organ with an oxygen consumption that at times may be appreciable, especially when lung disease is present (8). For instance, six patients with far advanced tuberculosis had pulmonary tissue oxygen consumptions that averaged 12% of the total-body oxygen utilization (66).

The metabolic needs of the normal human lung have never been measured precisely but probably are in the range of 4 to 5% of resting whole-body oxygen consumption. For comparison purposes, the kidney uses about 8% and the brain about 20% of the resting total body $O_2$ consumption (8). Some of the oxygen is used by the lung for processes related to respiration, such as synthesis of surfactant; some is used to satisfy metabolic requirements of about 40 different cell types that make up the lung; and the remainder is used by cells performing nonrespiratory functions such as synthesis, storage, release, activation, and inactivation of a variety of chemical substances (8). Because many of these biochemical activities take place within or on the pulmonary vascular endothelium (67), they are considered in this chapter on pulmonary circulation.

### VASOACTIVE SUBSTANCES

In Table 2.2, the fate of several vasoactive substances during a single passage through the pulmonary circulation is indicated. The extent of removal indicated in Table 2.2 applies only when the concentration of the

**TABLE 2.2**

**SUMMARY OF THE FATE OF CIRCULATING SUBSTANCES DURING A SINGLE PASSAGE THROUGH THE INTACT PULMONARY CIRCULATION**

| Substance | Fate |
| --- | --- |
| Amines | |
| Acetylcholine | Uncertain |
| Serotonin | Almost completely removed |
| Norepinephrine | Up to 30% removed |
| Epinephrine | Not affected |
| Dopamine | Not affected |
| Histamine | Not affected |
| Peptides | |
| Bradykinin | Up to 80% inactivated |
| Angiotensin I | Converted to angiotensin II |
| Angiotensin II | Not affected |
| Vasopressin | Not affected |
| Arachidonic acid metabolites | |
| Prostaglandin $E_2$ | Almost completely removed |
| Prostaglandin $F_{2\alpha}$ | Almost completely removed |
| Prostaglandin $A_2$ | Not affected |
| Prostacyclin (PGI$_2$) | Not affected |
| Thromboxane | Unknown |
| Leukotrienes | Almost completely removed |
| Adenine nucleotides | |
| Adenosine triphosphate | Almost completely removed |
| Adenosine monophosphate | Almost completely removed |

Reproduced with permission from Murray JF: *The Normal Lung.* Philadelphia, WB Saunders, 1986.

substance in the pulmonary arterial blood is low (i.e., in the normal range). In pathologic disturbances, when large amounts of compounds may be released or administered, the capacity of the lung to deal with them may be overwhelmed (8). Moreover, the efficacy of removal may be altered markedly in patients with lung disease (68–71).

### 5-Hydroxytryptamine or Serotonin

5-Hydroxytryptamine (5-HT) may be released from argentaffin cells in the intestine or lungs or from platelets (8). It is now known that the major site for inactivation of 5-HT in the body is the lung, not the liver (71, 72). During a single passage through the lungs 5-HT is rapidly and extensively degraded by monamine oxidase (MAO) to deaminated products, which are released into the circulation (65).

## Histamine

Histamine is present in tissue mast cells and blood basophils and thus is found both within the parenchyma and connective tissue of the lung and within the pulmonary circulation (73). Histamine is thought to be one of the chemical mediators of type I (immediate) hypersensitivity reaction, including atopic asthma. To date, the physiologic significance of the cellular depots of histamine in the lungs of normal humans has not been determined. Furthermore, perfusion studies do not demonstrate removal or inactivation of histamine by the lung (74).

## Bradykinin

Kinins are potent endogenous vasodilator substances that probably play a role in the inflammatory response in hereditary angioneurotic edema and act as a mediator in neonatal circulatory adjustment (8). It has been suggested that bradykinin may have a pathogenic role in some patients with bronchial asthma and anaphylaxis (74). Although the lungs contain relatively large amounts of precursor, bradykinin has not been identified as a secretory product of the lung (8). In fact, the pulmonary circulation of many mammals, including humans, has been shown to inactivate up to 80% of an infused dose, presumably by enzymatic activity (74).

## Angiotensin

Angiotensin I is formed in the bloodstream from an $\alpha_2$-globulin precursor by the action of the enzyme renin. The decapeptide angiotensin I has relatively little vasomotor potency but is rapidly converted to a highly active octapeptide, angiotensin II (8). The transformation from angiotensin I to angiotensin II is caused by angiotensin converting enzyme (ACE), which is located on the luminal surface of the pulmonary endothelium. Although other organs also contain converting enzymes, no physiologically significant conversion of angiotensin I to angiotensin II has been demonstrated in organs other than the lung (74). In addition, the presence of converting activity in the lungs rather than in the blood implies that the renin-angiotensin system has generalized regulatory effects on the circulation rather than just local effects on the afferent glomerular arterioles as proposed previously (8).

## Prostaglandins

Prostaglandins belong to a family of compounds synthesized and released from different organs under varying conditions. Arachidonic acid, an "essential" fatty acid, is rapidly converted by the lung into the primary prostaglandins $PGE_2$ and $PGF_2$, as well as into

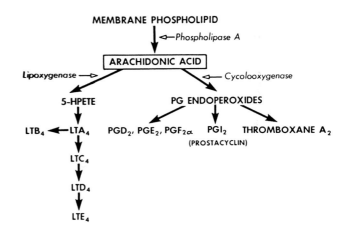

**Figure 2.14.** Pathways of arachidonic acid metabolism. Prostaglandins ($PGD_2$, $PGE_2$, $PGF_{2\alpha}$, and $PGI_2$) and thromboxane $A_2$ are generated via the cyclooxygenase pathway; the leukotrienes ($LTA_4$, $LTB_4$, $LTC_4$, $LTD_4$, and $LTE_4$) are generated via the lipoxygenase pathway. (Adapted with permission from Murray JF: *The Normal Lung.* Philadelphia, WB Saunders, 1986.)

prostacyclin ($PGI_2$), thromboxane $A_2$, and other biologically active products (Fig. 2.14) (75).

The lungs have an important role in both the synthesis and removal of certain prostaglandins (8, 75). Although the normal lung contains detectable quantities of prostaglandins (principally of the F series), these do not appear to be sufficient to cause systemic effects if released (8) (they may, of course, have important local actions). However, in many experimental conditions and presumably in their clinical analogues as well, the synthesis and release of prostaglandins by the lung can be accelerated to a rate at which physiologic consequences result (8). This mechanism may be important in anaphylaxis, mechanical overdistention of the lungs, pulmonary embolism, and pulmonary edema (75). In general, prostaglandins of the F series constrict pulmonary and systemic blood vessels as well as bronchial smooth muscle. In contrast, prostaglandins of the E series dilate systemic vessels, decrease blood pressure, and relax bronchial smooth muscle (75, 76). The prostaglandin endoperoxides, intermediate products in the pathway catalyzed by cyclooxygenase (Fig. 2.14), are unstable but potent constrictors of pulmonary vascular and airway smooth muscle. Thromboxane $A_2$ shares these properties in addition to its ability to aggregate platelets. In contrast, $PGI_2$ is a potent inhibitor of platelet aggregation and a vasodilator (75).

As illustrated in Table 2.2, the lung inactivates nearly all prostaglandins of the E and F series that perfuse it. It does not affect the A and I series. The mechanism of inactivation is related to the presence of an enzyme capable of oxidizing prostaglandin, 15-hydroxyprostaglandin dehydrogenase (74, 75).

### Nitric Oxide

Nitric oxide is produced by the vascular endothelium in both the pulmonary and systemic circulations. Nitric oxide synthase catalyzes the conversion of L-arginine to L-citrulline, which results in the generation of nitric oxide. There is basal production of nitric oxide in the pulmonary circulation as well as stimuli-mediated production. Those stimuli include changes in shear stress, flow, and oxygen tension and the binding of endothelium-dependent vasodilators (such as acetylcholine and adenosine triphosphate) to specific receptors. Production is also induced by cytokines within macrophages. Nitric oxide diffuses across cell membranes and activates soluble guanylate cyclase within the vascular smooth muscle cell, which increases cGMP concentrations. Although its metabolism is complex, nitric oxide is rapidly oxidized and is likely excreted as nitrite and nitrate (43).

### Endothelin-1

Endothelin-1 is also produced by the vascular endothelium in both the pulmonary and systemic circulations. It is synthesized as a prepropeptide containing 203 amino acids, which undergoes cleavage to form the 39–amino acid precursor Big ET-1. Big ET-1 is then cleaved, by an unidentified proteolytic enzyme named endothelin-1 converting enzyme, to the 21–amino acid peptide endothelin-1. Secretion of endothelin-1 is induced by numerous stimuli such as thrombin, calcium, cytokines, and hypoxia. Up to 50% of circulating endothelin-1 is removed during passage through the lungs (50).

### Other Metabolic Functions

The lung is able to secrete immunoglobulins, particularly IgA, in the bronchial mucus, which plays a role in defense against infection. Synthesis of phospholipids that make up pulmonary surfactant is accomplished by alveolar type II epithelial cells. Protein synthesis occurs in the lung, of course, since collagen and elastin form the structural basis of the lung (53). In the future, a better understanding of the mechanisms that control collagen and elastin synthesis will be crucial to determining the factors that result in pathologic rates of collagen and elastin synthesis in various types of acute and chronic lung diseases.

The lung can function as an endocrine organ, and there are several newly discovered metabolic functions of the lung (77).

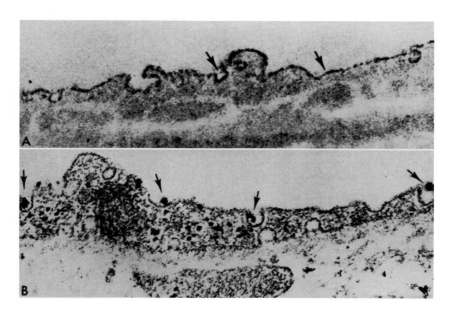

**FIGURE 2.15.** **A**, Section of rat pulmonary capillary endothelium prepared to demonstrate the location of angiotensin converting enzyme. The electron-dense reaction product (*arrows*) is located on the plasma membrane and caveolae intracellulare facing the vascular lumen (original magnification ×76,000). (Reprinted by permission from Ryan US, et al: Localization of angiotensin converting enzyme [Kininase II]. II, Immunocytochemistry and immunofluorescence. *Tissue Cell* 8:125–146, 1976.) **B**, Cytochemical localization of 5′-nucleotidase in blood-free rat product (*arrows*), which does not appear on other membranes or organelles (original magnification ×95,000). (Reprinted by permission from Smith U, Ryan JW: Pinocytotic vesicles of the pulmonary endothelial cell. *Chest* 59:12S7–15S, 1971.)

## LOCUS OF METABOLIC ACTIVITY

Sites at which the various metabolic processes described are carried out have not been identified with certainty. Nonetheless, pieces of evidence suggest that the luminal surface of the pulmonary vascular endothelium is specially endowed to participate in the biochemical transformation of at least some circulating vasoactive substances (8, 78). Electron micrographs have revealed ultrastructural specialization that has been linked with the sites of enzymes that metabolize the adenine nucleotides, angiotensin I, and bradykinin (67). The endothelial surface of pulmonary capillaries has a high density of *caveolae intracellulare* that communicate with the bloodstream through a delicate covering layer (Fig. 2.15). Cytochemical techniques have revealed that adenine nucleotides are metabolized within the caveolae; less direct evidence favors a similar location for the metabolism of angiotensin I and bradykinin (67). These early studies provide an exciting beginning to the structure-function correlations of some of the nonrespiratory activities carried out in the pulmonary circulation (67).

## REFERENCES

1. Guyton AC: The pulmonary circulation. In *Textbook of Medical Physiology*, ed 7. Philadelphia, WB Saunders, 1986.
2. Wagenvoort CA, Wagenvoort N: *Pathology of Pulmonary Hypertension*. New York, John Wiley & Sons, 1977.
3. West JB: *Respiratory Physiology*, ed 4. Baltimore, Williams & Wilkins, 1989.
4. Deffebach ME, Charan NB, Lakshminarayan S, Butler J: The bronchial circulation. *Am Rev Respir Dis* 135:463–481, 1987.
5. Butler J (ed): *The Bronchial Circulation*. Lung Biology in Health and Disease, vol 57. New York, Marcel Dekker, 1992.
6. Cournand A, Ranges HA: Catheterization of the right auricle in man. *Proc Soc Exp Biol Med* 46:462–468, 1941.
7. Bloomfield RA, Lauson HD, Cournand A, et al: Recordings of right heart pressures in normal subjects and in patients with chronic pulmonary disease and various types of cardiocirculatory disease. *J Clin Invest* 25:639–648, 1946.
8. Murray JF: *The Normal Lung*. Philadelphia, WB Saunders, 1986.
9. Hellems HK, Haynes FW, Dexter L: Pulmonary "capillary" pressure in man. *J Appl Physiol* 2:24–29, 1949.
10. Swan HJC, Ganz W, Forrester J, et al: Catheterization of the heart in man with use of a flow-directed balloon-tipped catheter. *N Engl J Med* 283:447–451, 1970.
11. Matthay MA, Chatterjee K: Bedside pulmonary artery catheterization: Risks versus benefits. *Ann Intern Med* 109:826–834, 1988.
12. Jenkins BS, Bradley RD, Branthwaite MA: Evaluation of pulmonary arterial end diastolic pressure as an indirect estimate of left atrial mean pressure. *Circulation* 42:75–78, 1970.
13. Burrows B, Kettel LJ, Niden AH, et al: Patterns of cardiovascular dysfunction in chronic obstructive pulmonary disease. *N Engl J Med* 286:912–918, 1972.
14. Wiedemann H, Matthay MA, Matthay RA: Cardiovascular-pulmonary monitoring in the intensive care unit. *Chest* 85:537–549 (Part I); 85:656–668 (Part II), 1984.
15. Bhattacharya JH, Nanjo S, Staub NC: Micropuncture measurement of lung microvascular pressure during 5-HT infusion. *J Appl Physiol* 52:634–637, 1982.
16. Bhattacharya JH: Pulmonary microcirculation. In Baker CH, Nastuu W (eds): *Microcirculation Technology*. New York, Academic Press, 1986.
17. Raj JU, Chen P, Navazo L: Micropuncture measurements of lung microvascular pressure profile in 3–4 week old rabbits. *Pediatr Res* 20:1103–1111, 1986.
18. Hislop A, Reid L: Pulmonary arterial development during childhood. *Thorax* 28:129–135, 1973.
19. Iliff LD: Extra-alveolar vessels and edema development in excised dog lungs. *Circ Res* 28:524–532, 1971.
20. Gauge A, Nicolaysen G: Alveolar pressure and lung volume as determinants of net transvascular fluid filtration. *J Appl Physiol* 42:476–482, 1971.
21. West JB, Dollery CT, Naimark A: Distribution of blood flow in isolated lung; relation to vascular and alveolar pressures. *J Appl Physiol* 19:173–178, 1964.
22. Goshy M, Lai-Fook SJ, Hyatt RE: Peri-vascular pressure measurements by wick-catheter technique in isolated dog lobes. *J Appl Physiol* 46:950–955, 1971.
23. Bhattachayra J, Gropper MA, Staub NC: Interstitial fluid pressure gradient measured by micropuncture in excised dog lung. *J Appl Physiol* 56:271–277, 1984.
24. Levett JM, Replogle RL: Thermodilution cardiac output: a critical analysis and review of the literature. *J Surg Res* 27:392–404, 1979.
25. Roos A, Thompson LJ Jr, Nagel EL, Prommas DC: Pulmonary vascular resistance as determined by lung inflation and vascular pressures. *J Appl Physiol* 16:77–84, 1961.
26. Borst HG, McGregor M, Whittenberger JL, Berglund E: Influence of pulmonary arterial and left atrial pressures on pulmonary vascular resistance. *Circ Res* 4:393–399, 1956.
27. Howell JGL, Permutt S, Proctor DG, Riley RL: Effect of inflation of the lung on different parts of the pulmonary vascular bed. *J Appl Physiol* 16:71–76, 1961.
28. Mead J, Whittenberger JL: Lung inflation and hemodynamics. In Fenn WO, Rahn H (eds): *Handbook of Physiology*. Washington, DC, American Physiological Society, 1964, vol 1.
29. Bergofsky EH, Bass BG, Ferretti R, Fishman AP: Pulmonary vasoconstriction in response to precapillary hypoxemia. *J Clin Invest* 4:1201–1215, 1963.
30. Porcelli RJ, Bergofsky EH: Adrenergic receptors in pulmonary vasoconstrictor responses to gaseous and humoral agents. *J Appl Physiol* 34:483–488, 1973.
31. Lock JE, Olley PM, Coceani F: Direct pulmonary vascular responses to prostaglandins in the conscious newborn lamb. *Am J Physiol* 238:H631–H638, 1980.
32. Carstairs JR, Nimmo AJ, Barnes PJ: Autoradiographic localization of beta-adrenoreceptors in human lung. *Am Rev Respir Dis* 132:541–547, 1985.
33. Bergofsky EH: Active control of the normal pulmonary

circulation. In Moser KM (ed): *Pulmonary Vascular Disease.* New York, Marcel Dekker, 1979.

34. Widdicombe JG, Sterling G: The autonomic nervous system and breathing. *Ann Intern Med* 126:311, 1970.

35. Ingram RH, Szidon JP, Shalek R, Fishman AP: Effects of sympathetic nerve stimulation on the pulmonary arterial tree of the isolated lobe perfused in situ. *Circ Res* 22:801–815, 1968.

36. Kadowitz PJ, Hyman AL: Effect of sympathetic nerve stimulation on pulmonary vascular resistance in the dog. *Circ Res* 32:221–227, 1973.

37. Tucker A, Weir EK, Reeves JT, Grover RF: Histamine H$_1$ and H$_2$ receptors in the pulmonary and systemic vasculature of the dog. *Am J Physiol* 229:1008–1013, 1975.

38. Hales CA, Kazemi H: Failure of saralasin acetate, a competitive inhibitor of angiotensin II, to diminish alveolar hypoxic vasoconstriction in the dog. *Cardiovasc Res* 11:541–546, 1977.

39. Miller VM, Vanhoutte PM: Endothelium-dependent contractions to arachidonic acid are mediated by products of cyclooxygenase. *Am J Physiol* 248:H432–H437, 1985.

40. Morganroth ML, Reeves JF, Murphy RC, Voelkel NF: Leukotriene synthesis and receptor blockers block hypoxic pulmonary vasoconstriction. *J Appl Physiol* 56:1340–1346, 1984.

41. Soifer S, Loitz RD, Roman C, Heymann MA: Leukotriene end organ antagonists increase pulmonary blood flow in fetal lambs. *Am J Physiol* 249:H5770–H5776, 1985.

42. Furchgott RF: The role of the endothelium in the responses of vascular smooth muscle to drugs. *Annu Rev Pharmacol Toxicol* 24:175–197, 1984.

43. Moncada S, Higgs A: The L-arginine–nitric oxide pathway. *N Engl J Med* 329:2002-2012, 1993.

44. Dinh-Xuan AT: Endothelial modulation of pulmonary vascular tone. *Eur Respir J* 5:757–762, 1992.

45. Palmer RMJ, Ashton DS, Moncada S: Vascular endothelial cells synthesize nitric oxide from L-arginine. *Nature* 333:664–666, 1988.

46. Rubanyi GM, Romero JC, Vanhoutte PM: Flow-induced release of endothelium-derived relaxing factor. *Am J Physiol* 250:H1145–H1149, 1986.

47. Fineman E Jr, Heymann MA, Soifer SJ: N$^w$-nitro-L-arginine attenuates endothelium-dependent pulmonary vasodilation in lambs. *Am J Physiol* 260:H1299–H1306, 1991.

48. Abman SH, Chatfield BA, Hall SL, McMurtry IF: Role of endothelium-derived relaxing factor during transition of pulmonary circulation at birth. *Am J Physiol* 259:H1921–H1927, 1990.

49. Yanagisawa M, Kurihara H, Kimura S, Tomobe Y, Kobayashi M, Mitsui Y, Yazaki Y, Goto K, Masaki T: A novel potent vasoconstrictor peptide produced by vascular endothelial cells. *Nature* 332:411–415, 1988.

50. Rubanyi GM (ed): *Endothelin.* New York, Oxford University Press for the American Physiological Society, 1992.

51. Vane JR, Änggård EE, Botting RM: Regulatory functions of the vascular endothelium. *N Engl J Med* 323:27–36, 1990.

52. Glazier JB, Murray JF: Sites of pulmonary vasomotor reactivity in the dog during alveolar hypoxia and serotonin and histamine infusion. *J Clin Invest* 50:2550–2558, 1971.

53. Cutaia M, Round S: Hypoxic pulmonary vasoconstriction: physiologic significance, mechanism, and clinical relevance. *Chest* 97:706–718, 1990.

54. Tucker A, McMurray IF, Grover RF, Reeves JT: Attenuation of hypoxic pulmonary vasoconstriction by verapamil in intact dogs. *Proc Soc Exp Biol Med* 141:611–616, 1976.

55. Johns RA Jr, Linden JM, Peach MJ: Endothelium-dependent relaxation and cyclic GMP accumulation in rabbit pulmonary artery are selectively impaired by moderate hypoxia. *Circ Res* 65:1508–1515, 1989.

56. Archer SL, Tolins JP, Raij L, Weir K: Hypoxic pulmonary vasoconstriction is enhanced by inhibition of the synthesis of an endothelium derived relaxing factor. *Biochem Biophys Res Commun* 164:1198–1205, 1989.

57. Fineman L Jr, Chang R, Soifer SJ: EDRF inhibition augments pulmonary hypertension in intact newborn lambs. *Am J Physiol* 262:H1365–H1371, 1992.

58. Wong J, Vanderford PA, Winters JW, Chang R, Soifer SJ, Fineman JR: Endothelin-1 does not mediate acute hypoxic pulmonary vasoconstriction in the intact newborn lamb. *J Cardiovasc Pharmacol* 22(Suppl 8):S262–S266, 1993.

59. Adnot S, Raffestin B, Eddahibi S, Braquet P, Chabrier P: Loss of endothelium-dependent relaxant activity in the pulmonary circulation of rats exposed to chronic hypoxia. *J Clin Invest* 87:155–162, 1991.

60. Harvey RM, Enson Y, Betti R, et al: Further observations on the effect of hydrogen ion on the pulmonary circulation. *Circulation* 35:1019–1027, 1967.

61. Rudolph AM, Yuan S: Response of the pulmonary vasculature to hypoxia and H$^+$ ion concentration changes. *J Clin Invest* 45:399–411, 1966.

62. Bergofsky EH, Holtzman S: A study of the mechanism involved in the pulmonary arterial pressor response to hypoxia. *Circ Res* 20:506–519, 1967.

63. Nocturnal Oxygen Therapy Trial Group: Continuous or nocturnal oxygen therapy in hypoxemic chronic obstructive lung disease: a clinical trial. *Ann Intern Med* 93:391–398, 1981.

64. Zapol WM, Snider MT: Pulmonary hypertension in severe acute respiratory failure. *N Engl J Med* 296:476, 1977.

65. Matthay MA, Broaddus VC: Fluid and hemodynamic management in acute lung injury. *Semin Respir Crit Care Med* 15:271–288, 1994.

66. Fritts HW Jr, Richards DW, Cournand A: Oxygen consumption of tissues in the human lung. *Science* 133:1070, 1961.

67. Smith U, Ryan JW: Electron microscopy of the endothelial and epithelial components of the lungs: correlations of structure and function. *Fed Proc* 32:1957–1966, 1973.

68. Gillis CN, Catravas JD: Altered removal of vasoactive substances by the injured lung: detection by lung microvascular injury. *Ann NY Acad Sci* (in press).

69. Carlos WM, Bedrossian MD, Woo J, et al: Decreased ACE in adult respiratory distress syndrome. *Am J Clin Pathol* 70:244–247, 1978.

70. Oparil S, Low J, Koerner TJ: Altered angiotensin I conversion in pulmonary disease. *Clin Sci Mol Med* 51:537–543, 1976.

71. Fisher A, Block ER, Pietra G: Environmental influences on uptake of serotonin and other amines. *Environ Health Perspect* 35:191–198, 1980.

72. Roth RA, Wallace KB, Alper RH; Bailie MD: Effect of paraquat treatment of rats on disposition of 5-hydroxy-tryptamine and angiotensin I by perfused lung. *Biochem Pharmacol* 28:2349–2355, 1979.

73. Gillis CN, Roth JA: Pulmonary disposition of circulating vasoactive hormones. *Biochem Pharmacol* 25:2547–2553, 1976.

74. Vane JR: The release and fate of vaso-active hormones in the circulation. *Br J Pharmacol* 35:202–208, 1969.

75. Said SI: Metabolic functions of the pulmonary circulation. *Circ Res* 50:325–333, 1982.

76. Fanburg BL: Prostaglandins and the lung. *Am Rev Respir Dis* 108:482–489, 1973.

77. Becker KL, Gazdar AF (eds): *The Endocrine Lung in Health and Disease.* Philadelphia, WB Saunders, 1984.

78. Ryan JW, Ryan US: Pulmonary endothelial cells. *Fed Proc* 36:2683–2691, 1977.

# Chapter 3

# Mechanics of Respiration

## Richard W. Light

IN THIS CHAPTER, the factors that determine the volume of the lungs and hemithorax and the movement of air into and out of the lungs are described.

### LUNG VOLUMES—THE DIMENSIONS OF THE RESPIRATORY SYSTEM

Figure 3.1 illustrates the subdivisions of the lungs during various respiratory maneuvers. The *total lung capacity* (TLC) is the total amount of air that is in the lungs after a maximal inspiration. The TLC is dependent on the height, age, and sex of the subject, being larger in taller, younger, and male individuals.

The *vital capacity* (VC) is the maximal amount of air that a subject is able to expire after a maximal inspiration. The *residual volume* (RV) of the lungs is the amount of air that is still in the lungs at the end of a maximal expiration. It is normally approximately 25% of the total lung capacity. The sum of the RV and the VC is equal to the TLC.

The *functional residual capacity* (FRC) is the quantity of air in the lungs and airways at the end of a spontaneous expiration. Therefore it is the resting volume of the lungs. Normally, it is about 40% of the total lung capacity.

The *tidal volume* ($V_T$) is the volume of air that is breathed in during inspiration or out during expiration. It averages about 600 ml in normal subjects under resting conditions. The *minute ventilation* is the total amount of air moved into and out of the lungs during 1 minute. It is equal to the product of the $V_T$ and the respiratory rate.

The *inspiratory capacity* (IC) is the maximal volume of air that can be inspired from the resting level (FRC). The IC is approximately 60% of the TLC. The *inspiratory reserve volume* (IRV) is the IC minus the $V_T$, or the maximal volume of air that can be inspired beyond the $V_T$. The *expiratory reserve volume* (ERV) is the maximal volume of air that can be expired beyond the FRC. The sum of the ERV and the IC is equal to the VC.

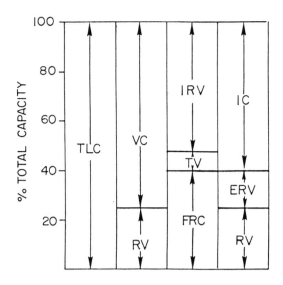

**FIGURE 3.1.** The subdivisions of the lung volume.

## VOLUME-PRESSURE RELATIONS OF THE RESPIRATORY SYSTEM DURING RELAXATION

Everyone who has observed an autopsy realizes that when the chest is opened the lungs collapse and the thorax enlarges. This simple observation illustrates two fundamental static properties of the respiratory system: the lungs tend to recoil inward and the chest wall tends to recoil outward.

The lungs and the chest wall are distensible objects. As with any distensible object, their volume is dependent on their elastic properties and their distending pressure. The distending pressure is the pressure difference between the inner and outer surfaces. In Figure 3.2 the distending pressures for the lungs and the chest are illustrated.

The distending pressure of the lung is termed the *transpulmonary pressure* (PL) and is the alveolar pressure (PA) minus the pleural pressure (Ppl).

$$P_L = P_A - Ppl \qquad (1)$$

The distending pressure for the chest wall (Pw) is the pleural pressure minus the pressure at the body surface (Pbs).

$$P_W = Ppl - Pbs \qquad (2)$$

Note the importance of the pleural pressure in both of these expressions. The distending pressure for the entire respiratory system (Prs) is the sum of the distending pressures for the lung and the chest wall. Since the pleural pressures cancel out, it is the alveolar pressure minus the pressure at the body surface

$$Prs = P_A - Pbs \qquad (3)$$

The elastic properties of a distensible object can be defined by means of a volume-pressure diagram for the object. To construct such a diagram, the volumes of the object at different distending pressures are determined. The relationship between changes in volume and changes in pressure define the *compliance* of the object, which is expressed as follows:

$$\text{Compliance} = \frac{\text{change in volume}}{\text{change in pressure}} \qquad (4)$$

### PRESSURE-VOLUME CURVES FOR THE CHEST WALL, LUNG, AND RESPIRATORY SYSTEM

If the respiratory muscles are completely relaxed and the heart and lungs removed from the thorax, the elastic properties of the thorax can be studied by adding or removing air from the thorax and observing the relationship between the distending pressure and the volume of the thorax. A pressure-volume curve obtained in this manner is depicted in Figure 3.3**A.** Note that the resting volume of the chest wall—that is, the volume at which the distending pressure is zero—is about 50% of the VC.

In a similar manner, if the lungs are removed from the thorax, a pressure-volume curve for them can be obtained. Such a curve is illustrated in Figure 3.3**B.** As the inflating pressure becomes higher, the volume increment with a given pressure increase becomes progressively smaller.

If the subject is relaxed, a pressure-volume curve for the respiratory system can be obtained by increasing or decreasing the alveolar pressures. The curve so obtained for a respiratory system is shown in Figure 3.3**C.** It is the sum of the curves for the chest wall and the lungs. The resting volume of the respiratory system is the volume at which PA is equal to Pbs and the distending pressure is zero. Note that it is the volume at which the distending pressures of the lungs and the chest wall are equal but opposite in sign. This resting volume is the FRC for the patient.

## VOLUME-PRESSURE RELATIONS OF THE RESPIRATORY SYSTEM DURING MUSCULAR EFFORTS

For the volume of the respiratory system to be different than the FRC, muscular effort must be present if the glottis is open and if there is no air flow. In Figure 3.4 the alveolar pressures that can be generated at various lung volumes with maximal inspiratory (Pmax$_{insp}$) and expiratory (Pmax$_{exp}$) efforts are shown. Also shown are the alveolar pressures during relaxation at various lung volumes when there is no flow. The horizontal difference between Pmax$_{insp}$ or Pmax$_{exp}$

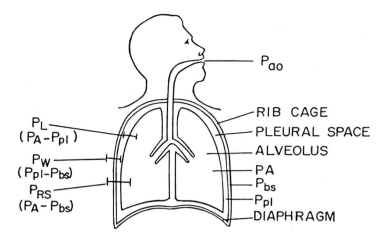

**FIGURE 3.2.** Respiratory pressures influencing ventilation. *Pao,* pressure at the airway opening; *Ppl,* pressure within the pleural space; *PA,* pressure within the alveoli; Pbs, pressure at the body surface; *PL,* pressure difference across the lung; *Pw,* pressure difference across the chest; *PRS,* pressure across the respiratory system.

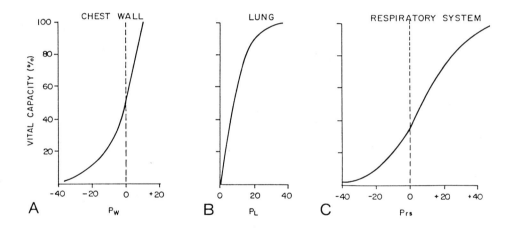

**FIGURE 3.3.** Static pressure-volume relationships for the chest wall (**A**), the lungs (**B**), and the respiratory system (**C**).

and the relaxation pressure gives the net maximal pressure generated by the inspiratory or expiratory muscles, respectively. Note that the higher the lung volumes, the lower the maximal inspiratory pressure and the higher the maximal expiratory pressure. At FRC, the maximal inspiratory pressure is about $-100$ cm $H_2O$, while the maximal expiratory pressure is about $+150$ cm $H_2O$.

From Figure 3.4 it is easy to see that the TLC is the volume at which the maximal negative pressure generated by the inspiratory muscles is equal to the relaxed positive pressure of the respiratory system. Accordingly, the total lung capacity will be reduced if the lung or the chest wall becomes stiffer (less compliant) or if the inspiratory muscles become weaker. Conversely, the TLC will be increased if the lungs or chest wall become more compliant or if the muscles become stronger.

In a similar fashion, the RV is the volume at which the maximal positive expiratory pressure is equal to the relaxed negative pressure of the respiratory system. The RV will increase if there is expiratory muscle weakness or if the pressure-volume curve of the respiratory system is shifted to the left, which can occur with a noncompliant chest wall or a very compliant lung (Fig. 3.3). The RV will decrease if the lower end

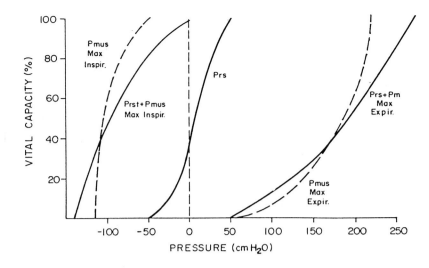

**FIGURE 3.4.** Schematic demonstrating the relationship between the alveolar pressures generated during maximal inspiratory and expiratory efforts. The *dashed lines* indicate the pressure contributed by the muscles.

of the pressure-volume curve for either the lung or the chest wall is shifted to the right.

### MEASUREMENT OF PLEURAL PRESSURE

Since the pleural pressure is the pressure at the inner surface of the chest wall and the outer surface of the lungs, it is an important pressure to measure when studying either normal subjects or patients with pulmonary disease. The pleural pressure can be measured directly by inserting needles, trocars, catheters, or balloons into the pleural space. However, direct measurement of the pleural pressure is not usually done, because of the danger of producing a pneumothorax or an infection of the pleural space. At the present time, pleural pressures are usually measured indirectly, using a balloon positioned in the subject's esophagus. Since the esophagus is located between the two pleural spaces, esophageal pressure measurements provide a close approximation of the pleural pressure at the level of the balloon in the thorax (1). Estimation of pleural pressure by means of an esophageal balloon is not without its pitfalls (1). The volume of air within the balloon must be small so that the balloon is not stretched and the esophageal walls are not displaced; otherwise, falsely elevated pleural pressure measurements will be obtained. Moreover, the balloon must be short and must be placed in the lower part of the esophagus. If care is taken, reliable pressure-volume curves of the lung can be obtained by measuring esophageal pressure at different lung volumes while the subject holds his or her breath with the glottis open

to eliminate the effect of changes in alveolar pressure. Recently it has been demonstrated that reliable measurements of esophageal pressures can be made with micromanometers (2). Use of these devices circumvents some of the problems associated with esophageal balloons.

### PLEURAL PRESSURE GRADIENTS

Although estimation of the pleural pressure via an esophageal balloon gives a value for the pleural pressure, the pleural pressure is not uniform throughout the chest. There is a gradient in pleural pressure between the top and bottom of the lung, with the pleural pressure being lowest or most negative at the top and highest or least negative at the bottom. The main factors responsible for the pleural pressure gradient are probably gravity, mismatching of the shapes of the chest wall and lung, and the weight of the lungs and other intrathoracic structures (3).

The magnitude of the pleural pressure gradient is on the order of 0.50 cm $H_2O$ per centimeter of vertical distance (3). Therefore, in the upright position the difference in the pleural pressure between the apex and the base of the lungs may be 12 cm $H_2O$ or more. Since the alveolar pressure is constant throughout the lungs, the effect of the pleural pressure gradient is that different parts of the lungs have different distending pressures ($P_L$). The transpulmonary pressure is approximately 12 cm $H_2O$ higher in the uppermost than in the lowermost portion of the lungs.

It is thought that the pressure-volume curve is the

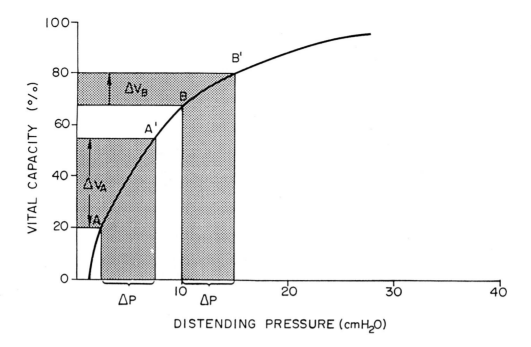

**FIGURE 3.5.** Pressure-volume curve of a normal lung. At functional residual capacity, the alveoli in the lower part of the lung (A) are at a smaller volume than those in the upper part of the lung (B) on account of the pleural pressure gradient. Then, when a given amount of distending pressure ($\Delta P$) is applied to both sets of alveoli, the volume increase of those in the lower parts of the lung ($\Delta V_A$) is much greater than that in the upper parts of the lung ($\Delta V_B$) because of the shape of the pressure-volume curve.

same for different regions of the lung regardless of their location. Therefore, the variation in pleural pressure results in the alveoli in the superior parts of the lung being larger than those in the inferior parts. Moreover, since separate alveoli are at different positions on their pressure-volume curves, a given change in distending pressure causes varying volume changes throughout the lung. For these reasons, at lung volumes above FRC alveoli in the inferior parts expand considerably more than those at the top, as illustrated in Figure 3.5. At low lung volumes, the pleural pressure may become positive in the lower regions of the lung. This positive pressure can compress airways, resulting in alveoli that are not ventilated. This phenomenon is the basis for the closing volume test, which is described in detail in Chapter 8.

## FACTORS HOLDING THE LUNG AGAINST THE CHEST WALL

The pleural pressure throughout most of the thorax is negative at FRC since the lungs and chest wall are, respectively, above and below their resting volumes. Why does the space between the lungs and chest wall (the pleural space) not become filled with either gas or liquid?

Gases move in and out of the pleural space from the capillaries in the visceral and parietal pleura. Since the sum of all the partial pressures in capillary blood ($P_{H_2O}$ = 47, $P_{CO_2}$ = 46, $P_{N_2}$ = 573, and $P_{O_2}$ = 40 mm Hg) averages 706 mm Hg, there should be a net movement of gas into the pleural space only if the pleural pressure is below 706 mm Hg, or below $-54$ mm Hg relative to atmospheric pressure. Since mean pleural pressures this low virtually never occur, the pleural space does not fill up with gas unless there is a communication between the pleural space and either the lungs or the atmosphere or unless there are gas-forming organisms in the pleural space. It is for the same reason that air from a pneumothorax is absorbed.

There is normally a small amount of liquid present in the pleural space. This liquid forms a very thin film of uniform thickness that couples the parietal and visceral pleural surfaces, enabling them to slide over each other with a minimum amount of friction. Normally, a small amount of fluid (~ 0.01 ml/kg/hr) continuously enters the pleural space from either the visceral or parietal pleura (4). All liquid in the pleural space leaves via the lymphatics in the parietal pleura, which have a capacity of about 0.28 ml/kg/hr (5). The movement of fluid into and out of the pleural space is more fully discussed in Chapter 18.

### FACTORS INFLUENCING THE PRESSURE-VOLUME CURVE OF THE LUNG

#### Elastic Recoil of the Lungs

Pressure-volume curves for a lung of a normal individual, a lung from a patient with emphysema, and a lung from a patient with interstitial fibrosis are illustrated in Figure 3.6. As volume is added to the lung, pressure is generated within the system, owing to the tendency of the elastic component to recoil inward. As more volume is added, the pressure increase with each volume increment becomes larger. Eventually, the pressure-volume curve becomes almost flat as the elastic elements reach their limits of distensibility. If more volume is then added, the lungs are liable to rupture because of the very high transpulmonary pressure.

Under static conditions, the pressure generated by the lung is determined solely by its elastic recoil pressure Pst(L). In other words, when the airways are open and there is no air flow, the Pst(L) is equal to PL. If the glottis is open so that the alveolar pressure is zero, the pleural pressure must be equal but opposite in sign to the recoil pressure: Pst(L) = PL = PA − Ppl; but since PA = 0, Pst(L) = −Ppl.

The lungs of patients with emphysema are more distensible than normal lungs because many alveolar walls have been destroyed, resulting in a loss of elastic elements. As illustrated in Figure 3.6, the pressure-volume curve of the patient with emphysema is shifted to the left. The transpulmonary pressure at any given lung volume is less than it is for the normal lung. In contrast, the lungs of patients with interstitial fibrosis are less distensible than normal lungs because the tissue retractive forces are increased. Therefore, the pressure-volume curve of the patient with interstitial fibrosis is shifted to the right. The stiffness of the lung may also be increased when the pulmonary vessels are engorged with blood or when the interstitial spaces are filled with fluid.

#### Origin of Lung Elastic Recoil

The total force causing the inflated lung to recoil inward has two components: the first arises from the elastic properties of the lung tissue itself and the second arises from surface tension. In Figure 3.7 pressure-volume curves are shown for an excised lung when it is inflated with saline and then when it is inflated with air. When a normal excised lung is deflated and then inflated with air, the volume increases very little until a pressure of 8 cm H$_2$O is reached. At pressures above this, the volume increases rapidly until the TLC is approached at about 30 cm H$_2$O. The filling of the lung is uneven, as different areas of the lung are seen to inflate rapidly. Then if the pressure is decreased, the volume of air remaining in the lung remains much greater than at the same pressure during inflation, and the lung deflates evenly. Microscopic observations of subpleural air spaces (6) show that these air spaces are recruited sequentially from largest to smallest during inflation from the gas-free state but that they tend to deflate in parallel without extensive derecruitment. This difference between the inflation and deflation curves and the failure of the lung to return to its original state after deformation is called *hysteresis.* When the lungs are filled with a liquid such as isotonic saline, they begin to expand at a lower pressure, fill uniformly, and require less pressure to fill them completely. When the lung empties after being filled with liquid, very little hysteresis is noted. The differences in the pressure-volume curves with air and saline inflation are due to differences in surface tension.

Surface tension does not represent a true force but arises because any surface has the tendency to decrease to a minimum. The molecules present at the surface of an air-liquid interface are pulled toward the liquid by molecules in the liquid, and this pull is not counterbalanced because the molecules lie on the surface. When one considers a spherical bubble, the surface tension (*T*) in the wall of the bubble tends to contract the bubble

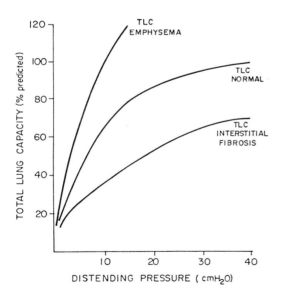

**FIGURE 3.6.** Representative pressure-volume curves from a normal subject, a patient with emphysema, and a patient with interstitial fibrosis.

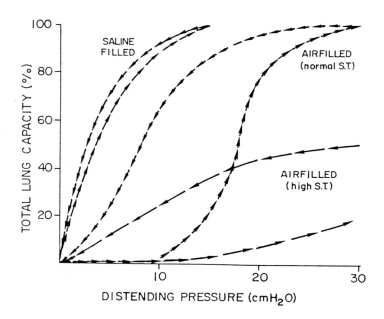

**FIGURE 3.7.** Pressure-volume curves of lungs filled with saline and with air with normal and high surface tension (*S.T.*). The *arrows* indicate whether the lung is being inflated or deflated. When the lung is filled with saline, the effects of surface forces at the air-liquid interfaces are eliminated. The differences be-tween the curves of the saline-filled and air-filled lungs are due to surface forces. The differences between the curve of the lung with normal surface tension and that of the lung with high sur-face tension are due to the reduction of surface forces by surfac-tant.

and the pressure ($P$) due to the gas inside the bubble tends to expand it. At equilibrium,

$$P = \frac{2T}{r} \qquad (5)$$

where $r$ is the radius of the bubble.

From this equation (Laplace's equation) it can be seen that the larger the bubble, the smaller the pressure inside the bubble if $T$ is constant. The lungs are actually two sets of millions of bubbles. Consider what would happen if $T$ were the same throughout the lungs. At any given time, if all the alveoli were not exactly the same size, the pressure in the smaller alveoli would be greater than the pressure in the larger alveoli. Hence, air would flow from the smaller to the larger alveoli. This would exacerbate the pressure differences, and after a short period most alveoli would be collapsed or fully distended, obviously a less than ideal situation.

However, in the normal lung there is no such insta-bility. The reason that the normal lung is stable is a substance called *surfactant* (7). Surfactant is a complex mixture composed of lipids, proteins, and carbohy-drates, secreted by the type II pneumocytes that are present in all alveoli. The major surface-active compo-nent of pulmonary surfactant is the phospholipid di-palmitoyl phosphatidylcholine. Surfactant has two main functions. First, when it is present, the surface tension decreases dramatically as the surface area is decreased. The result of this is that the $T$ in Laplace's equation becomes a variable depending on the radius of the alveoli, such that

$$P = \frac{2T'}{r} = \text{constant} \qquad (6)$$

where $T'$ is the varying surface tension in the presence of surfactant. In this manner surfactant promotes alve-olar stability. Its presence is partly responsible for the hysteresis observed with the inflating lung. It is diffi-cult to open alveoli initially, but once they are inflated, the presence of surfactant allows them to empty evenly in parallel. The second characteristic of surfactant is that it markedly decreases surface tension. It has the lowest surface tension of any biologic substance ever measured and thereby reduces the transpulmonary pressure necessary to achieve a given lung volume. The presence of surfactant also increases the antibacte-rial capabilities of alveolar macrophages and modu-lates lymphocyte responsiveness (7).

The difference between the pressure-volume curves obtained with saline and with air indicate how much of the elastic recoil is due to surface tension (Fig. 3.7). On the inflation part of the curve, much more elastic recoil is due to surface tension than is due to the elastic properties of the lung. For example, to reach a volume of 50% TLC, a total pressure of 18 cm $H_2O$ is necessary with air inflation but only 3 cm $H_2O$ with saline inflation, which indicates that 15 of the 18 cm $H_2O$ of the elastic recoil is due to surface tension. Alternatively, on the deflation limb of the curve with air inflation, a pressure of 8 cm $H_2O$ is necessary for a volume of 50% TLC, and the elastic recoil due to surface tension is only 5 cm $H_2O$.

The importance of surfactant in reducing the surface tension can be appreciated by comparing the pressure-volume curves of isolated lungs with and without surfactant (Fig. 3.7). In the lung with no surfactant and therefore high surface tension, the total lung capacity is not approached even with a distending pressure of 30 cm $H_2O$. Moreover, at 50% TLC, the distending pressure of the deflating lung devoid of surfactant is more than double that of the lung with normal surfactant.

Surfactant is important in several different clinical situations. The infant acute respiratory distress syndrome occurs in infants who are born prematurely, before they have developed sufficient ability to produce surfactant. As a result of the inadequate level of surfactant, their lungs are unstable and have very low compliance. The instability leads to complete atelectasis of many alveoli, which produces a right-to-left shunt and results in profound hypoxemia. The decreased compliance leads to alveolar hypoventilation. Surfactant production can be augmented by administration of corticoids to the mother prenatally. Studies have consistently shown that the administration of exogenous surfactant therapy to premature babies with the infant respiratory distress syndrome results in improved gas exchange and lung mechanics as well as a reduced mortality rate. The administration of exogenous surfactant is now considered to be routine therapy for infants with the respiratory distress syndrome (8).

A lack of surfactant is also thought to play a role in producing the adult respiratory distress syndrome (ARDS) (see Chapter 22). This condition is characterized by diffuse pulmonary infiltrates and marked hypoxia refractory to high inspired concentrations of oxygen. The marked hypoxia is secondary to perfusion of atelectatic alveoli. On account of the atelectatic alveoli, the lungs are very noncompliant, as would be predicted from Figure 3.7. Therapy of the acute respiratory distress syndrome is directed in large part toward increasing lung volume to prevent alveoli from becoming atelectatic (see Chapter 22). Early studies using exogenous surfactant to treat adult patients with ARDS have been promising, but many questions remain to be answered, including the optimal surfactant delivery

technique, the ideal time of surfactant administration, and the optimal exogenous surfactant preparation (7).

## DYNAMICS OF THE RESPIRATORY SYSTEM

In this section, the dynamics of breathing are discussed. First, different types of air flow and resistances to air flow are described. Next, the relationship between alveolar pressures and air flow is reviewed, including the dynamic compression of the airways by positive pleural pressure on forced expiration. Finally, factors influencing the distribution of ventilation and the work of breathing are discussed.

### AIRWAY RESISTANCES

Air moves into and out of the lungs whenever the alveolar pressure differs from the atmospheric pressure (assuming the airways are not obstructed). The *airway resistance* (Raw) is defined as the frictional resistance of the entire system of air passages to air flow from outside the body to within the alveoli. By definition

$$\text{Raw} = \frac{P_A - P_{ao}}{\dot{V}} \quad (7)$$

where $P_A$ is the alveolar pressure, $P_{ao}$ is the pressure at the airway opening, and $\dot{V}$ is the flow rate. This system is analogous to an electrical circuit:

$$R = \frac{V}{I} \quad (8)$$

where $R$ is the electrical resistance, $V$ is the voltage difference, and $I$ is the current.

### Patterns of Air Flow

The resistance to air flow in a tube depends on the type of flow, the dimensions of the tube, and the viscosity and density of the gas. Air flow through tubes can be either *laminar* or *turbulent*. Laminar flow is organized, and the streamlines are everywhere parallel to the sides of the tube and are capable of sliding over one another (Fig. 3.8). The streamlines at the center of the tube move faster than those closest to the walls, producing a flow profile that is parabolic. With laminar flow, the relation between pressure and flow is given by Poiseuille's equation:

$$P = \frac{8\eta l\dot{V}}{\pi r^4} = K_1\dot{V} \quad (9)$$

or

$$\dot{V} = \frac{P\pi r^4}{8\eta l} \quad (10)$$

where $\dot{V}$ is the flow rate, $P$ is the driving pressure (pressure drop between the beginning and end of the tube),

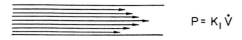

LAMINAR FLOW

$P = K_1 \dot{V}$

TURBULENT FLOW

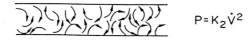

$P = K_2 \dot{V}^2$

TRANSITIONAL FLOW

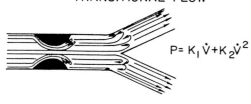

$P = K_1 \dot{V} + K_2 \dot{V}^2$

**FIGURE 3.8.**    Patterns of air flow in tubes.

$r$ and $l$ are the radius and the length of the tube, respectively, and $\eta$ is the viscosity of the gas. Since flow resistance ($R$) is the driving pressure divided by the flow (Equation 7), the resistance with laminar flow is independent of the flow rate:

$$R = \frac{8\eta l}{\pi r^4} = K_1 \qquad (11)$$

Note the critical importance of the tube radius—if the radius of the tube is halved, the airway resistance increases 16-fold. Note also that laminar flow is dependent on the viscosity of a gas but is independent of its density.

Turbulent flow occurs at high flow rates and is characterized by a complete disorganization of the streamlines so that molecules of gas move laterally, collide with one another, and change their velocities (Fig. 3.8). Owing to this disorganization, the pressure drop across the tube is not proportionate to the flow rate as with laminar flow, but rather is proportional to the square of the flow rate:

$$P = K_2\dot{V}^2 \qquad (12)$$

It follows from Equation 7 that the resistance to air flow is proportional to the flow rate:

$$R = K\dot{V} \qquad (13)$$

in contrast with laminar flow. In addition, with turbulent flow the viscosity of the gas becomes unimportant, but an increase in gas density increases the pressure drop for a given flow.

Whether air flow is laminar or turbulent depends to a large extent on a dimensionless quantity called the Reynolds number, Re, which is given by

$$Re = \frac{2rvd}{\eta} \qquad (14)$$

where $r$ is the radius of the tube, $v$ is the average velocity, $d$ is the density of the gas, and $\eta$ is the viscosity of the gas. In straight, smooth, rigid tubes, turbulence occurs when Re exceeds 2000.

In the lung, laminar flow occurs only in the small peripheral airways, where, owing to the large overall cross-sectional area, flow through any given airway is extremely slow. Turbulent flow occurs in the trachea. In the remainder of the lung, owing in large part to the multiple branchings of the tracheobronchial tree, flow is neither laminar nor turbulent, but rather mixed or transitional (Fig. 3.8). With a transitional flow pattern, flow is dependent on both the viscosity and the density of the gas.

### Distribution of Airway Resistance

Toward the periphery in the tracheobronchial tree, the airways become successively narrower. Therefore, from Equation 11 one would anticipate that the major part of the airway resistance would reside in the narrow peripheral airways. However, direct measurements of airway resistance have shown that less than 20% of the total airway resistance is confined to airways with diameters less than 2 mm. The explanation for this apparent paradox is that the progressive branching of the tracheobronchial tree results in an increased average cross-sectional diameter of the peripheral airways, and so resistance does not increase disproportionately (9).

During nasal breathing, the resistance offered by the nose is the largest single component, constituting one-half to two-thirds of the total resistance at low flow rates. The nasal resistance increases disproportionately with increasing flow rates, so during heavy exercise one switches from nasal breathing to mouth breathing. During quiet breathing the mouth, pharynx, larynx, and trachea provide 20 to 30% of the airway resistance. Most of the remainder of the airway resistance is in the bronchi with diameters greater than 2 mm. Less than 20% of the total airway resistance is in the bronchi with diameters less than 2 mm (10).

### Factors Influencing Airway Resistance

Airway resistance depends on the number, length, and cross-sectional area of the conducting airways. Since resistance to air flow in a given airway changes according to the 4th power of its radius, the cross-sectional area within the tracheobronchial tree is by far

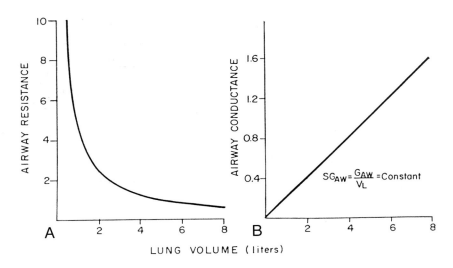

**FIGURE 3.9.** **A**, The relationship between airway resistance and lung volume. **B**, The relationship between airway conductance and lung volume. Note that the relationship between airway resistance and lung volume is not linear, while that between airway conductance and lung volume is linear.

the most important determinant of airway resistance. The airways, like the lung parenchyma, exhibit elasticity and are capable of being compressed or distended. Therefore, the diameter of an airway varies with the transmural pressure applied to that airway; that is, the difference between the pressure within the airway and the pressure surrounding the airway. The pressure surrounding the intrathoracic airways approximates pleural pressure.

As the lung volume increases, the traction applied to the walls of the intrathoracic airways also increases, widening the airways and decreasing their resistance to air flow. The relationship between the lung volume and airway resistance is not linear (Fig. 3.9**A**). However, the relationship between the reciprocal of the airway resistance, the *airway conductance* (Gaw), and lung volume is linear (Fig. 3.9**B**). The *specific airway conductance* (SGaw) is defined as:

$$\text{Specific Gaw} = \frac{\text{Gaw}}{V_L} \qquad (15)$$

where $V_L$ is the volume at which Gaw is measured. Since SGaw is nearly independent of the lung volume in a given patient, it is the index of airway resistance that should be used in the clinical situation. Furthermore, use of this index will reduce the variations in resistance measurements from individual to individual owing to varying body size (11).

Contraction of the bronchial smooth muscles narrows the airways and increases airway resistance. Normally there is a small amount of resting smooth muscle tone in the bronchial smooth muscles. Administration of inhaled bronchodilator drugs to normal subjects leads to a significant decrease in the airway resistance (12). The tone of the bronchial smooth muscle is under the control of the autonomic nervous system. Sympathetic stimulation causes bronchodilation, while parasympathetic stimulation causes bronchoconstriction. Stimulation of the irritant receptors in the tracheobronchial tree induces bronchoconstriction reflexly via the parasympathetic nerve fibers contained in the vagus nerve (13). In patients with lung disease, mucosal edema, hypertrophy and hyperplasia of mucous glands, increased production of mucus, and hypertrophy of the bronchial smooth muscle all tend to decrease airway caliber and contribute to the increased airway resistance.

### PRESSURE-FLOW RELATIONSHIPS

It has been recognized for a long time that there is a limit to the flow rate that can be attained during expiration and that, once this limit is achieved, greater muscular effort does not augment flow. With both laminar flow (Equation 10) and turbulent flow (Equation 12), one would expect higher pressures to be associated with higher flows.

The limitation of flow at different lung volumes is best appreciated from the examination of isovolume pressure-flow curves at different lung volumes. Isovolume pressure-flow curves are constructed by simultaneously measuring the flow, volume, and pleural pressure as a subject inhales and exhales with varying

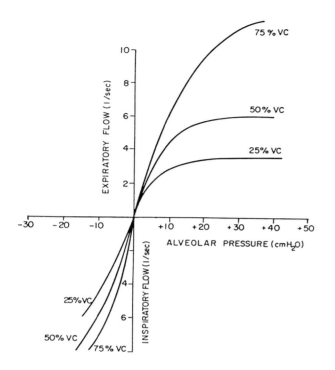

**FIGURE 3.10.** Isovolume pressure-flow curves at 25, 50, and 75% of the vital capacity. Note the limitation of air flow on expiration at alveolar pressures above 20 and 28 cm $H_2O$ at 25 and 50% of the vital capacity, respectively.

amounts of effort that are reflected by changes in pleural pressure. Thus, for any given lung volume there is a set of pleural pressures and flow rates. Since at any given lung volume the elastic recoil pressure of the lung is constant, the pleural pressures can be converted to alveolar pressures by adding the elastic recoil pressure at the lung volume to the pleural pressure.

Figure 3.10 depicts a family of isovolume pressure-flow curves at different lung volumes. Two main characteristics of these curves should be noted. First, for a given alveolar pressure, the higher the lung volume the greater the flow rate during both inspiration (negative alveolar pressure) and expiration (positive alveolar pressure). The explanation for this on inspiration is that the higher the lung volume the lower the airway resistance. The explanation during expiration is not only the lower airway resistance but also the greater elastic recoil of the lung at higher lung volumes, since this latter pressure is important in determining expiratory flow rate (see discussion below).

Second, during expiration at all but the higher lung volumes, as alveolar pressure increases, flow rates increase until a certain alveolar pressure is reached. Then

further increases in alveolar pressure do not result in increased flow. This flow limitation in view of increasing alveolar pressure is surprising, since with both laminar flow (Equation 10) and turbulent flow (Equation 12) one would expect higher pressures to be associated with higher flows. The explanation for this upper limit on expiratory flow is dynamic compression of the airways, which is discussed in the next section. Note that there is no similar limitation of flow on inspiration. Note also that the alveolar pressure necessary to generate the maximum flow is lower at lower lung volumes.

At volumes greater than 75% of the vital capacity, air flow increases progressively with increasing alveolar pressure and is considered *effort dependent.* In contrast, at lung volumes below 75% of the vital capacity, the flow rate reaches a maximum once a given alveolar pressure is reached. At these lung volumes, air flow is considered to be *effort independent,* but the critical alveolar pressure must be reached in order to have maximum flow.

The limitation of flow on expiration, demonstrated in Figure 3.10, is very important to the clinician. The majority of patients with lung disease have obstructive lung disease, which means that it takes them longer than normal to get the air out of their lungs. The two main tests used to diagnose and assess the response of these patients to therapy are the *forced expiratory spirogram* and the *flow-volume loop* (see Chapter 8). With both of these tests, the patient takes a maximal inspiration and then exhales as hard and long as he or she can. From Figure 3.10 it can be seen that at lung volumes below about 75% of the vital capacity these tests are independent of effort after the critical alveolar pressure is reached. Therefore, the tests are reproducible and are invaluable in the management of these patients. Since there is no flow limitation on inspiration, tests dependent on inspiratory flow rates are much less reproducible than are tests dependent on expiratory flow rates.

### Dynamic Compression of the Airways

Limitation of flow on expiration results from dynamic compression of the airways. To illustrate the mechanisms involved in producing flow limitation during a maximal expiratory maneuver, it is useful to consider a model of the lung in which the alveoli are represented by an elastic sac and the intrathoracic airways by a compressible tube, both of which are enclosed within a pleural space (Fig. 3.11).

At a given lung volume when there is no flow (Fig. 3.11**A**), the alveolar pressure is zero. The pleural pressure is subatmospheric and counterbalances the elastic recoil of the lung. To generate expiratory flow, the alveolar pressure must be increased above zero, which is

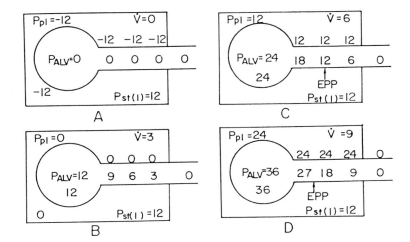

**FIGURE 3.11.** A schematic representation of the equal-pressure point (EPP) concept. In **A** the alveolar pressure is zero, so there is no flow. In **B** the increase in the alveolar pressure is equal to the Pst(L), so the pleural pressure is zero. Here the equal-pressure point is at the airway opening. In **C** the alveolar pressure has increased more, so the pleural pressure must be positive. The pressure drops from the alveolus to different points along the airway are greater because $\dot{V}$ is higher. Accordingly, the EPP moves closer to the alveolus. In **D**, the Ppl has been increased even more and the EPP has moved farther upstream because flow has increased. When flow limitation occurs, the equal-pressure point becomes fixed, and $\dot{V}$max is determined by Equation 18.

accomplished by increasing the pleural pressure. Since the lung volume has not changed, the increase in the alveolar pressure is the same as the increase in the pleural pressure:

$$P_A = Ppl + Pst(L) \qquad (16)$$

The intrabronchial pressure decreases moving downstream (toward the mouth) from the alveolus because of flow resistance. During quiet breathing the pleural pressure does not become positive, and in this situation the intrabronchial pressure is always greater than the pleural pressure (Fig. 3.11**B**). When sufficient expiratory effort is generated, the pleural pressure becomes positive, and in this situation the intrabronchial pressure at some point along the airways is equal to the extrabronchial or pleural pressure (Fig. 3.11**C**). Mead and coworkers (14) designated this point the *equal-pressure point* (EPP). The EPP divides the airways into two components arranged in series: an *upstream segment* from the alveoli to the equal-pressure point, where the distending pressure of the bronchi is positive, and a *downstream segment* from the equal-pressure point to the airway opening, where the distending pressure of the bronchi is negative intrathoracically. It is these downstream segments of the airways that are dynamically compressed during forced expiration.

**Location of Equal-Pressure Point**

When the pleural pressure is subatmospheric, there is no EPP (Fig. 3.11**A**). When the pleural pressure becomes atmospheric, the EPP is at the airway opening (Fig. 3.11**B**). As the pleural pressure becomes more positive, the EPP moves upstream (Fig. 3.11**C** and **D**)—but how far? When flow in the upstream segment is considered, the pressure drop from the alveolus to the EPP is the alveolar pressure minus the pleural pressure, which is the elastic recoil pressure of the lung. The resistance of the upstream segment is designated Rus. Therefore, it follows from Equation 7 that

$$\dot{V} = \frac{Pst(L)}{Rus} \qquad (17)$$

At a constant lung volume Pst(L) is constant. Therefore, the only way that $\dot{V}$ can be increased is for Rus to decrease, which can be accomplished only by having the EPP move upstream. With more and more effort, the EPP moves upstream (Fig. 3.11**B**–**D**) until the pleural pressure reaches a level at which further increases in it do not lead to further increases in $\dot{V}$. The $\dot{V}$ at this pleural pressure is called $\dot{V}$max and corresponds to the flat top at the isovolume pressure-flow curve.

Note by this analysis

$$\dot{V}max = \frac{Pst(L)}{Rus} \qquad (18)$$

and therefore $\dot{V}$max is dependent on two factors: (*a*) the resistance of the upstream segment and (*b*) the recoil pressure of the lung. In other words, a decreased elastic recoil of the lung is just as important in reducing $\dot{V}$max as is increased airway resistance.

Pride and coworkers (15) developed a different analysis of the mechanisms of forced expiration. Their analysis is similar to that of Mead but also takes into account the resistance to collapse of the intrathoracic airways. The analysis has not been publicized as much as the equal-pressure point analysis of Mead, but it better explains the mechanics of forced expiration.

In the model of Pride and coworkers (Fig. 3.12) the airways are divided into two rigid tubes connected in series by a short segment of a collapsible tube. They divided the airways into an upstream segment between the alveoli and the distal end of the collapsible segment and a downstream segment from the end of the collapsible segment to the airway opening. Moreover, they defined the critical closing pressure of the collapsible segment (Ptm′) as the transmural pressure

(Ptm) at which the segment collapsed. As with any distensible object, the transmural pressure is the pressure inside the wall minus the pressure outside the wall. Therefore, the value for Ptm′ indicates the distending pressure that must be maintained to keep the collapsible segment patent. They further assumed that the short, collapsible segment was fully open whenever its distending pressure exceeded Ptm′ and fully collapsed whenever Ptm fell below Ptm′.

The transmural pressure in the collapsible segment is given by the following equation:

$$Ptm = P_A - (\dot{V} \times Rs) - Ppl \qquad (19)$$

where Rs is the resistance of the segment upstream from the collapsible segment. (Note the distinction from Rus, which is the resistance of the segment up-

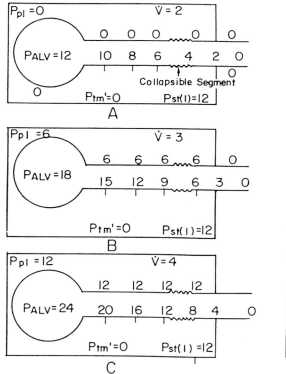

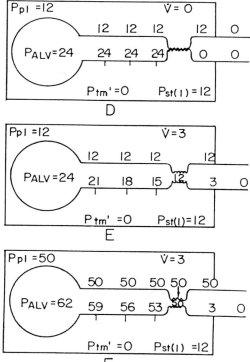

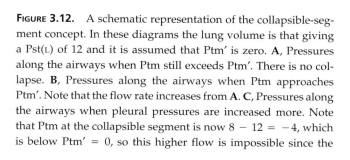

**Figure 3.12.** A schematic representation of the collapsible-segment concept. In these diagrams the lung volume is that giving a Pst(L) of 12 and it is assumed that Ptm′ is zero. **A,** Pressures along the airways when Ptm still exceeds Ptm′. There is no collapse. **B,** Pressures along the airways when Ptm approaches Ptm′. Note that the flow rate increases from **A. C,** Pressures along the airways when pleural pressures are increased more. Note that Ptm at the collapsible segment is now 8 − 12 = −4, which is below Ptm′ = 0, so this higher flow is impossible since the collapsible segment must collapse. **D,** Pressures along the airways when there is no flow. Now Ptm is 24 − 12 = 12, so the airways must open. **E,** Pressure along the airways when the collapsible segment is partially collapsed such that Ptm = Ptm′. **F,** Pressures along the airways when the alveolar pressure is raised much higher. Note that the collapsible segment is more collapsed than in **E** and that the flows in **B, E,** and **F** are also identical. The airway pressures downstream from the collapsible segment in **B, E,** and **F** are also identical.

stream from the EPP in the analysis of Mead et al.)
Since

$$PA = Pst(L) + Ppl \qquad (20)$$

then

$$Ptm = Pst(L) - (\dot{V} \times Rs) \qquad (21)$$

Therefore, as $\dot{V}$ increases, Ptm decreases. When $\dot{V}$ increases to a critical level ($\dot{V}max$), Ptm drops to Ptm'. This is illustrated in Figure 3.12**B**, where Ptm = 6 − 6 = 0 and it is assumed that Ptm' = 0. If flow rates increase more, as illustrated in Figure 3.12**C**, the Ptm would fall below Ptm' (in the illustration Ptm = −4), but by our assumptions, the collapsible segment would be collapsed completely and there would be no flow (Fig. 3.12**D**). However, as soon as flow ceases, the intrabronchial pressure becomes the same as the alveolar pressure, and again Ptm exceeds Ptm' and flow resumes. If the collapsible segment opens all the way, $\dot{V}$ again exceeds $\dot{V}max$, Ptm falls below Ptm', and air flow ceases. Therefore, it is postulated that the collapsible segment acts as a variable resistor, as illustrated in Figure 3.12**E** and **F**. Once the pleural pressure is reached at which dynamic compression of the airways occurs, the collapsible segment partially collapses; as a result the pressure drop between the alveoli and the collapsible segment is such that the Ptm is equal to the Ptm'. As pleural pressures increase more and more (Fig. 3.12**F**), there is a larger and larger pressure drop across the collapsible segment. Note that by this analysis flow and intrabronchial pressures downstream from the collapsible segment do not change once flow limitation is achieved (Fig. 3.12**B, E, F**). From Equation 21, flow limitation occurs when Ptm = Ptm'. Therefore, when Ptm' is substituted for Ptm in Equation 21,

$$Ptm' = Pst(L) - \dot{V}max \times Rs \qquad (22)$$

which can be rewritten as follows:

$$\dot{V}max = \frac{Pst(L) - Ptm'}{Rs} \qquad (23)$$

Note that this analysis of respiratory mechanics is conceptually analogous to a waterfall. The height of the waterfall (i.e., the pressure drop across the collapsible segment) does not affect flow either above or below the waterfall. The flow above the waterfall is given by Equation 23 regardless of the height of the waterfall. The flow below the waterfall is determined by the flow above the waterfall. Since the resistance to flow below the waterfall is fixed, the pressure immediately downstream from the collapsible segment is equal to the product of $\dot{V}max$ and the resistance of the downstream segment.

When Equation 23 is analyzed, it is seen that $\dot{V}max$ depends on three different factors: (*a*) the elastic recoil of the lung (Pst(L)), (*b*) the tendency of the airways to collapse (Ptm'), and (*c*) the resistance of the upstream segment (Rs). Emphysema, chronic bronchitis, and asthma are the three main diseases that cause reduced flow rates on expiration. Analysis of Equation 23 reveals that the predominant mechanism causing reduced flow rates is different with each of these three diseases. With emphysema, the main abnormality is decreased elastic recoil of the lungs; with chronic bronchitis, the predominant abnormality is increased resistance of the upstream segment (Rs), while with asthma the constriction of the bronchial smooth muscles greatly increases the tendency of the airways to collapse (Ptm') and thereby reduces flow rates by this mechanism. Of course with all three diseases, all the factors interact to some extent to produce reduced expiratory flow rates. An explanation for air trapping is also given by Equation 23. Air trapping will occur when the Pst(L) is less than Ptm', for when this condition is met $\dot{V}max$ is zero. Therefore, the lungs cannot empty at lung volumes below which Ptm' exceeds Pst(L).

Experimental evidence supporting this analysis of flow limitation has been provided by Smaldone and Bergofsky [16]. They monitored intrabronchial pressures in excised lungs and demonstrated that the flow-limiting segment consisted of well-demarcated short lengths of the trachea at large lung volumes but of lobar or segmental bronchi at low lung volumes. There was a large pressure drop across the collapsible segment, which at any given lung volume was closely related to the driving pressure. Leaver and coworkers [17] investigated the contribution of the three factors in Equation 23 in producing decreased expiratory flow rates in 17 patients with chronic bronchitis and emphysema. They found that all three factors contributed to reduction in maximal flow. In three of their 17 patients, the reduction in expiratory flow rates could be entirely accounted for by loss of lung elastic recoil and enhanced airway collapsibility.

Although dynamic compression of the airways produces limitation of flow on expiration, it is not without value because it does improve the effectiveness of coughing. In the collapsible segment, the linear velocity of air flow is markedly increased owing to the smaller cross-sectional area. This increased linear velocity leads to a greater shearing force that serves to dislodge secretions and particles from the walls of airways. The shift of the collapsible segment from the trachea to the segmental bronchi as lung volumes get smaller increases the ease with which coughing can remove secretions from most of the larger airways.

### DENSITY DEPENDENCE OF MAXIMAL AIR FLOW

In the normal lung during forced expiration, flow in the peripheral airways is laminar, flow in the medium-sized airways is transitional, and flow in the large airways is turbulent. Only laminar flow is independent of gas *density*. Therefore, if maximal expiratory flow rates are measured with the patient breathing gases of varying densities, the flow rates should remain stable only if there is laminar flow in the flow-limiting segment. If there is either turbulent flow or transitional flow in this segment, breathing a gas with a lower density should result in increased flow rates at a given lung volume. In contrast, laminar flow is dependent on gas *viscosity*.

A mixture of 80% helium and 20% oxygen (He-O$_2$) has a viscosity very similar to that of air but a density that is approximately one-third that of air (18). Since the viscosity of He-O$_2$ is similar to that of air but the density of He-O$_2$ is much lower, one would expect higher maximal flows with the He-O$_2$ only if the flow in the flow-limiting segment were turbulent or transitional. Flow-volume loops from a normal subject obtained while breathing air and with He-O$_2$ are illustrated on the left in Figure 3.13. At all lung volumes above 15% of the vital capacity, the maximum flow rate with He-O$_2$ is greater than that with air. At 50% of the vital capacity the flow rate with He-O$_2$ is 50% higher than it is with air. The percent increase in flow rates with He-O$_2$ at 50% VC is termed the $\Delta\dot{V}max_{50}$. The point at which the flow rates with He-O$_2$ and with air become identical is termed the *isoflow volume* (Viso $\dot{v}$). The normal $\Delta\dot{V}max_{50}$ is 47.3 ± 27.4% (two standard deviations) and does not change with age. The normal

Viso $\dot{v}$ at age 40 is 16.5 ± 13.8% and increases 0.3% for each additional year (19).

In normal subjects, flow at low lung volumes is density independent because the collapsible segment is more peripheral and flow rates are lower. Owing to the much smaller flow rates, the Reynolds number (Equation 14) dictates that the flow will be laminar. Flow-volume loops for a smoker obtained with room air and with He-O$_2$ are illustrated on the right in Figure 3.13. Although the flow-volume loops with room air for the normal person and the smoker are virtually identical, the increases in the flow rates with He-O$_2$ are much less for the smoker. The $\Delta\dot{V}max_{50}$ for the smoker is only 15%, compared with 50% for the nonsmoker, and the Viso $\dot{v}$ is 30% compared with 15% for the nonsmoker.

The use of He-O$_2$ flow-volume loops has its greatest utility in detecting disease of the small peripheral airways. Since the small airways usually contribute a minor portion to the total airway resistance, changes in these airways may not be detectable by measurements of airway resistance. Increased resistance in the small airways should reduce maximal flow, but because of the great variability of flow-volume curves in normal individuals flows may not be reduced below the normal range. However, disease in the peripheral airways should decrease the relative contribution of density-dependent flow to the total pressure drop between the alveoli and the collapsible segment.

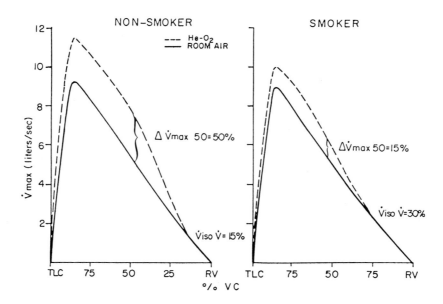

**Figure 3.13.** Flow-volume loops obtained with room air and He-O$_2$ on a normal nonsmoker and an asymptomatic smoker. Although the flow-volume loops on room air are identical, there is a substantially greater improvement in the flow rates with He-O$_2$ in the normal person than in the smoking individual.

Dosman and coworkers (19) obtained flow-volume loops with air and He-$O_2$ for 66 nonsmokers and 48 smokers whose forced expiratory volume in 1 second divided by the forced vital capacity ($FEV_1/FVC\%$) ratios exceeded 70%. With air, only 12% of the smokers had a $\dot{V}max_{50}$ and only 2% had a $\dot{V}max_{25}$ that were more than two standard deviations below those of the nonsmokers. In contrast, with He-$O_2$ 40% of the smokers had a $\varDelta\dot{V}max_{50}$ that was more than two standard deviations below that of the nonsmokers and 52% had a Viso $\dot{v}$ that exceeded those of the nonsmokers by more than two standard deviations. These results show that use of He-$O_2$ during a forced expiratory maneuver allows the detection of functional abnormalities in smokers at a stage when their $\dot{V}max$ is still within the normal range while they are breathing room air. However, the significance of these functional abnormalities in terms of the patient eventually developing chronic obstructive pulmonary disease (COPD) remains to be proved.

Despite the theoretical considerations described above, there has not been widespread utilization of the He-$O_2$ flow-volume loops in clinical pulmonary disease. This is because they have proved difficult to use in healthy subjects and patients because of large intrasubject and intersubject variability and variability in interpretation of the same series of curves by different observers (20).

### DISTRIBUTION OF VENTILATION

The regional distribution of ventilation depends on the distensibility of the peripheral gas exchange units and the resistance of the airways leading to them. The emptying of an elastic reservoir such as the lung through a resistive conduit resembles the discharge of a capacitor through a resistor. If the volume $V$ remaining in the reservoir as a fraction of the initial volume $V_0$ is plotted against time $t$, an exponential curve is obtained whose equation is

$$\frac{V}{V_0} = e^{-t/RC} \qquad (24)$$

where $R$ is the resistance and $C$ is the compliance of the system. When $t$ is equal to $RC$, the exponent has a value of unity and $V/V_0 = e^{-1} = 0.37$. The product $RC$ is the time that it takes the system to reach 37% of its original volume, and this product is termed the *time constant* of the respiratory unit.

When two or more parallel units are subjected to the same inflation or deflation pressure, they will each fill or empty at a rate determined by their individual time constants. If their time constants are equal, the units will fill and empty uniformly. If their time constants are unequal, the units will fill or empty nonuniformly. From Equation 24 it can be seen that an increase in either the resistance or the compliance of a respiratory unit will increase the time that it takes the unit to empty or fill.

### Frequency Dependence of Compliance

Since the time constants of the respiratory units are relatively small (0.01 second), during quiet breathing equilibration between alveolar and mouth pressures occurs at both the end of expiration and the end of inspiration. Therefore, the dynamic compliance of the respiratory system (the change in volume divided by the change in pleural pressure) during quiet breathing is the same as the static compliance. In the normal lung, increases in the breathing frequency up to rates of 80/minute do not affect the measured compliance, because the time constants are small and equilibration between alveolar and mouth pressure still occurs. However, in patients with peripheral airway disease, the time constants of at least some of the respiratory units are increased so that with more rapid breathing, equilibration between alveolar and mouth pressure does not occur at either end-inspiration or end-expiration. Accordingly, the volume change with a given pleural pressure change falls with increasing respiratory rate, and the compliance is said to be *frequency dependent* (21).

In patients with relatively normal expiratory flow rates, the decrease in dynamic compliance with increasing respiratory rates may be marked. Woolcock and coworkers (21) found that the dynamic compliance of mild asthmatics breathing at a respiratory frequency of around 80/minute was less than 50% of the static compliance. A large proportion of the decrease in dynamic compliance is due to the fact that at times of zero flow at the mouth, air is flowing within the lung from one region to another (*pendelluft*). The mechanism for this is illustrated in Figure 3.14. During inspiration alveolus 1 will fill more rapidly than alveolus 2 because of the increased airway resistance of the airways leading to alveolus 2 and hence its larger time constant. If the inspiratory time is short, alveolus 2 will never become completely filled. Then on expiration, the pressure in alveolus 1 will be higher than the pressure in alveolus 2 on account of its larger volume, so flow will go not only from alveolus 1 to the mouth but also from alveolus 1 to alveolus 2. The higher the frequency, the lower the tidal volume to the abnormal region.

Tests of dynamic compliance are sensitive indicators of peripheral airway disease. The time constants of the lung units distal to airways 2 mm in diameter are on

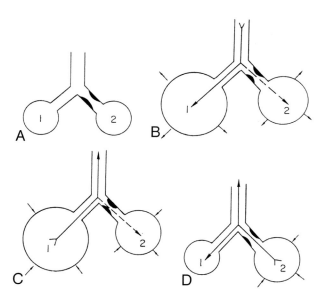

**FIGURE 3.14.** Effects of uneven time constants on ventilation. The airway leading to unit *2* is partially obstructed and therefore unit *2* has a longer time constant. After a slow expiration (**A**), the units have the same size. With a rapid inspiration (**B**), unit *1* fills more than unit *2* because it has a faster time constant. Shortly after the start of a rapid expiration (**C**), air moves not only from unit *1* to the airway opening but also from unit *1* to unit *2* because the pressure in unit *2* is less than the pressure in unit *1*. During the latter phases of expiration (**D**), flow moves from unit *2* to unit *1*. As the respiratory rate is progressively increased, the tidal volume of the abnormal region becomes smaller and smaller.

the order of 0.01 second. Fourfold increases in some time constants are necessary to cause dynamic compliance to become frequency dependent. However, measurements of frequency dependence of compliance are not done in most pulmonary function laboratories because they are time consuming and technically difficult and require the patient to swallow an esophageal balloon.

From the preceding discussion it can be readily appreciated that the time constants of the respiratory units markedly influence the distribution of ventilation. A second factor that is influential is the regional differences in pleural pressures, as discussed earlier in this chapter. Owing to the regional difference in pleural pressure, dependent parts of the lung are ventilated better. Other factors that influence the distribution of ventilation are the *interdependence* that exists between adjacent lung units and the presence of *collateral pathways* for ventilation.

### Interdependence

The lung has a connective tissue framework containing elastic elements. Because contiguous units are attached to each other, they are not free to move independently, but rather the behavior of one unit is influenced by the behavior of its neighbors. This dependence of one respiratory unit on the movements of its neighbors is termed *tissue interdependence*. Another factor that influences interdependence is the relationship between the lung and the adjacent chest wall. If on an inspiratory effort any part of the lung lags in its filling, the shape of the chest wall will be distorted. The local distortion of the chest wall will produce a local decrease in pleural pressure over the slowly filling lung. This local decrease in pleural pressure will be transmitted to the alveoli, thereby producing a greater pressure differential between the mouth and the alveoli. This in turn augments the flow to the area that was lagging and promotes uniformity of ventilation. It has been shown that this interaction between the lung and the chest wall is more important for the preservation of homogeneous ventilation than is lung tissue interdependence (22).

### Collateral Ventilation

*Collateral ventilation* is ventilation of the alveolar structures through passages that bypass the normal airways (23). Without collateral ventilation, alveoli distal to obstructed airways would become atelectatic. The possible pathways for collateral ventilation include interalveolar communications (pores of Kohn), bronchiole-alveolar communications (canals of Lambert), and the interbronchiolar communications of Martin. The relative contributions of these three different types of communications to collateral ventilation is unknown. In a normal human lung, the resistance to collateral ventilation is high and ventilation via collateral channels takes a long time in relation to the time taken for inspiration. However, in patients with emphysema the overall resistance to collateral ventilation is less than the airway resistance (24). Therefore, collateral ventilation may be very important in preserving the uniformity of ventilation in patients with emphysema and other lung diseases. In normal humans there is very little collateral ventilation between different lobes or different segments (25).

### WORK OF BREATHING

During breathing, the respiratory muscles must work to overcome the elastic, flow-resistive, and inertial forces of the lung and chest wall. In the respiratory system, work is expressed as the product of pressure and volume change according to the following equation:

$$Work = \int P \times \Delta V \qquad (25)$$

Therefore, to measure the mechanical work that is done during breathing it is necessary to obtain simultaneous measurements of both the volume change and the pressure that is exerted across the respiratory system.

At the present there is no method available for measuring the total amount of work being done on the lung, the respired gases, the chest wall, the diaphragm, and the abdominal contents because no technique has been developed for determination of the nonelastic resistance of the chest wall. However, the mechanical work performed on the lungs during a breathing cycle can be estimated by simultaneously measuring the changes in the intrathoracic pressures and the volume of the lungs throughout a respiratory cycle.

Figure 3.15 illustrates the information concerning work on the lungs available from such measurements. In the figure the line *ABC* is the static inflation-deflation curve of the lung. The mechanical work necessary to overcome the elastic resistance of the lung is the trapezoidal area *OABCD*. The mechanical work required to overcome the nonelastic resistance is the area of the loop *AECF*. The portion of the loop that falls to the right of line *ABC* (*AECB*) represents the mechanical work necessary to overcome the nonelastic resistance during inspiration. The portion of the loop that falls to the left of line *ABC* (*ABCF*) represents the mechanical work required to overcome the nonelastic resistance during expiration. Note that in Figure 3.15**A**, this area (*ABCF*) lies entirely within area *OABCD*, which represents the elastic energy stored in the system during inspiration. The fact that the area *ABCF* lies within *OABCD* indicates that this stored energy is sufficient to overcome the flow-resistive forces of expiration and no work is required from the expiratory muscles.

When lung disease is present, the work of breathing can increase substantially. The mechanical work done on a lung in which the compliance is reduced by 50% is shown in Figure 3.15**B**. Note that the trapezoidal area *OABCD* is nearly doubled, and hence the work necessary to overcome the elastic resistance is nearly double that for the normal lung. The mechanical work necessary to overcome nonelastic resistance has not changed. In Figure 3.15**C** is shown the mechanical work done on a lung in which the airway resistance is markedly increased. Owing to the increased airway resistance, more-negative pleural pressures must be generated to achieve the same inspiratory flow rates. Therefore, the distance between lines *ABC* and *AEC* is markedly increased and the inspiratory work (*OAECD*) is increased. Also on account of the increased airway resistance, positive pleural pressure occurs

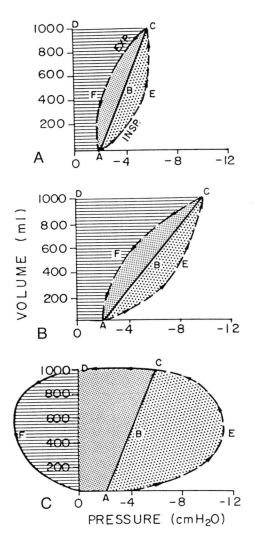

**FIGURE 3.15.** The mechanical work done during a respiratory cycle on a normal lung (**A**), a lung with reduced compliance (**B**), and a lung with increased airway resistance (**C**). See text for explanation.

during expiration, indicating that muscular work is performed. No longer is the stored elastic energy sufficient. The net work during expiration is the area *DFO*. Therefore, the total work during the respiratory cycle is the inspiratory work (*OECD*) plus the expiratory work (*DFO*), and this is increased substantially over the total work in Figure 3.15**A**.

### Relationship between Mechanical Work and Alveolar Ventilation

The work of breathing at any given level of alveolar ventilation is dependent on the pattern of breathing. Large tidal volumes increase the elastic work of breathing, whereas rapid breathing frequencies increase the

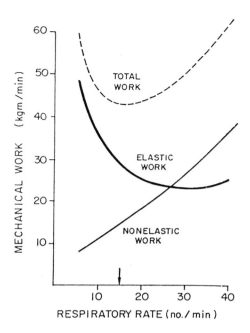

**FIGURE 3.16.** The effect of respiratory rate on the elastic, nonelastic, and total mechanical work of breathing at a given level of alveolar ventilation. Subjects tend to adopt the respiratory rate at which the total work of breathing is minimal (*arrow*).

work against flow-resistive forces (Fig. 3.16). With small tidal volumes a higher total ventilation is required because more ventilation is wasted. Several studies have shown that both normal individuals and patients adopt the respiratory pattern at which work is minimal (Fig. 3.16). The respiratory rate at which the minimum work occurs increases progressively with increased alveolar ventilation. Individuals with pulmonary fibrosis, which is characterized by increased elastic work of breathing, tend to breathe rapidly and shallowly. Individuals with airway obstruction, which is characterized by increased nonelastic work of breathing, usually breathe more deeply and slowly.

### Oxygen Cost of Breathing

To perform the mechanical work necessary for breathing, the respiratory muscles require oxygen. The *oxygen cost of breathing* provides an indirect measure of the work of breathing. The oxygen cost of breathing is measured by determining the total oxygen consumption of the body at rest and at increased levels of ventilation produced by voluntary hyperventilation.

During quiet breathing the total oxygen consumption of the body is between 200 and 300 ml/min. In normal subjects the oxygen cost of breathing is on the

order of 0.5 to 1.0 ml per liter of ventilation and therefore accounts for 3 to 5% of the total oxygen consumption. When an individual exercises, the increase in the oxygen cost of breathing parallels the increase in the oxygen consumption and remains about 4% of the oxygen consumption (26). The oxygen cost of breathing is much greater in patients with lung disease. In one report the oxygen cost of breathing in patients with chronic obstructive pulmonary disease who were ready for weaning was 17% of the total oxygen consumption (27). It is not clear whether or not there is a linear relationship between the oxygen cost of breathing and the level of ventilation in patients with lung disease.

▼

### REFERENCES

1. Milic-Emili J, Mead J, Turner JM, et al: Improved technique for estimating pleural pressure from esophageal balloons. *J Appl Physiol* 19:207–211, 1964.
2. Chartrand DA, Jodoin C, Couture J: Measurement of pleural pressure with esophageal catheter-tip micromanometer in anaesthetized humans. *Can J Anaesth* 38:518–521, 1991.
3. Lai-Fook SJ, Rodarte JR: Pleural pressure distribution and its relationship to lung volume and interstitial pressure. *J Appl Physiol* 70:967–978,1991.
4. Wiener-Kronish JP, Albertine KH, Licko V, Staub NC: Protein egress and entry rates in pleural fluid and plasma in sheep. *J Appl Physiol* 56:459–463, 1984.
5. Broaddus VC, Wiener-Kronish JP, Berthiaume Y, Staub NC: Removal of pleural liquid and protein by lymphatics in awake sheep. *J Appl Physiol* 64:384–390, 1988.
6. Radford EP Jr: Mechanical factors determining alveolar configuration. *Am Rev Respir Dis* 81:743–744, 1960.
7. Lewis JF, Jobe AH: Surfactant and the adult respiratory distress syndrome. *Am Rev Respir Dis* 1993; 147:218–233.
8. Jobe AH: Pulmonary surfactant therapy. *N Engl J Med* 328:861–868, 1993.
9. Hogg JC, Macklem PT, Thurlbeck WM: Site and nature of airway obstruction in chronic obstructive lung disease. *N Engl J Med* 278:1355–1360, 1968.
10. Ferris BG Jr, Mead J, Opie LH: Partitioning of respiratory flow resistance in man. *J Appl Physiol* 19:653–658, 1964.
11. Briscoe WA, Dubois AB: The relationship between airway resistance, airway conductance and lung volume in subjects of different age and body size. *J Clin Invest* 37:1279–1285, 1958.
12. Skinner C, Palmer KNV: Changes in specific airways conductance and forced expiratory volume in one second after a bronchodilator in normal subjects and patients with airways obstruction. *Thorax* 29:574–577, 1974.
13. Nadel JA: Autonomic control of airway smooth muscle and airway secretions. *Am Rev Respir Dis* 115(Suppl):117–126, 1977.
14. Mead J, Turner JM, Macklem PT, et al: Significance of the relationship between lung recoil and maximum expiratory flow. *J Appl Physiol* 22:95–105, 1967.

15. Pride NB, Permutt S, Riley RL, et al: Determinants of maximal expiratory flow from the lungs. *J Appl Physiol* 23:646–662, 1967.

16. Smaldone GC, Bergofsky EH: Delineation of flow-limiting segment and predicted airway resistance by movable catheter. *J Appl Physiol* 40:943–952, 1976.

17. Leaver DG, Tattersfield AE, Pride NB: Contributions of loss of lung recoil and of enhanced airways collapsibility to the airflow obstruction of chronic bronchitis and emphysema. *J Clin Invest* 52:2117–2128, 1973.

18. Drazen JM, Loring SH, Ingram RH Jr: Distribution of pulmonary resistance: effects of gas density, viscosity, and flow rate. *J Appl Physiol* 41:388–395, 1976.

19. Dosman J, Bode F, Urbanetti J, et al: The use of a helium-oxygen mixture during maximum expiratory flow to demonstrate obstruction in small airways in smokers. *J Clin Invest* 55:1089–1090, 1975.

20. Lam S, Abboud RT, Chan-Yeung M, Tan F: Use of maximal expiratory flow-volume curves with air and helium-oxygen in the detection of ventilatory abnormalities in population survey. *Am Rev Respir Dis* 123;234–237, 1981.

21. Woolcock AJ, Vincent NJ, Macklem PT: Frequency dependence of compliance as a test for obstruction in the small airways. *J Clin Invest* 48:1097–1106, 1969.

22. Zidulka A, Sylvester JT, Nadler S, Anthonisen NR: Lung interdependence and lung–chest wall interaction of sublobar and lobar units in pigs. *J Appl Physiol* 46:8–13, 1979.

23. Menkes HA, Traystman RJ: Collateral ventilation. *Am Rev Respir Dis* 116:287–309, 1977.

24. Terry PB, Traystman RJ, Newball HH, et al: Collateral ventilation in man. *N Engl J Med* 298:10–14, 1978.

25. Morrell NW, Roberts CM, Biggs T, Seed WA: Collateral ventilation and gas exchange during airway occlusion in the normal human lung. *Am Rev Respir Dis* 147:535–539, 1993.

26. Coast JR, Rasmussen SA, Krause KM, O'Kroy JA, Loy RA, Rhodes J: Ventilatory work and oxygen consumption during exercise and hyperventilation. *J Appl Physiol* 74:793–798, 1993.

27. Annat GJ, Viale JP, Dereymez CP, Bouffard YM, Delafosse BX, Motin JP: Oxygen cost of breathing and diaphragmatic pressure-time index. *Chest* 98:411–414, 1990.

# Chapter 4

# Ventilation, Gas Exchange, and Oxygen Delivery

## Ronald B. George

## INTRODUCTION

THE UNIQUE AND most important function of the respiratory system is to provide gas exchange between the body and the environment. Oxygen is required for energy generation via oxidative phosphorylation, as well as for support of various metabolic processes. Carbon dioxide ($CO_2$) is produced as the end point of the metabolism of ingested food. The body is limited in its ability to store oxygen and $CO_2$, and thus there must be a continuous exchange of these gases with the environment to prevent hypoxemia and respiratory acidosis.

Gas exchange occurs by passive diffusion across a thin alveolar-capillary membrane, the functional unit of the lungs, which separates pulmonary capillaries from alveolar air spaces. The respiratory muscles bring in fresh air to the alveoli, creating an atmosphere of relatively high oxygen and low $CO_2$. The heart and the pulmonary circulation deliver mixed venous blood from the tissues, which has low oxygen and relatively high $CO_2$ tensions. The gradients thus produced result in the passive transfer of $CO_2$ out of the blood and of oxygen into the blood.

One can determine if alveolar-capillary gas exchange is adequate by measuring arterial blood $P_{O_2}$

and $Pco_2$; if these gas tensions are normal, the gas exchange apparatus is functioning adequately. However, much more can be learned about gas exchange by using a few simple formulas that allow an estimation of the efficiency of ventilation and perfusion. Information about the delivery of oxygen to the tissues where it is required can be gained by the careful use of additional tests, including the analysis of expired gas and mixed venous blood. This chapter demonstrates how this information can be used to assess the efficiency of gas exchange in the lungs and oxygen transport from the lungs to the tissues.

### Normal Blood Gas Tensions and Alveolar-Arterial Differences

In normal subjects at sea level, the arterial $Pco_2$ is 35 to 45 mm Hg and the arterial $Po_2$ is 80 to 100 mm Hg. Normal arterial pH is 7.35 to 7.45. Average normal gas pressures at sea level for alveoli, arterial blood, and mixed venous blood are shown in Table 4.1. Note that there is a difference between alveolar and arterial $Po_2$. This is the result of the normal anatomic shunts, through which 1 to 3% of mixed venous blood flows directly into the systemic circulation without perfusing the alveolar capillaries. This occurs mainly through the bronchial, mediastinal, and left thebesian veins. In normal subjects 21 to 30 years of age, the average alveolar-arterial difference is 5 to 10 mm Hg (1). With the normal aging process, there are gradually more and more lung units with uneven ventilation and perfusion. Thus, in a group of normal adults 61 to 75 years of age, the average alveolar-arterial oxygen difference ($PAo_2 - Pao_2$) was 16 mm Hg (1), and the gradient may go up to 30 mm Hg in normal subjects over age 70.

In a resting adult, cardiac output, and thus pulmonary blood flow, is approximately 6 liters/minute. Alveolar ventilation is normally about 4.5 liters/minute, and the overall *ventilation-perfusion ratio* is approximately 0.8. Normal oxygen consumption ($\dot{V}o_2$) is approximately 250 to 300 ml/minute and normal $CO_2$

production ($\dot{V}co_2$) is approximately 200 to 250 ml/minute, so the average *respiratory exchange ratio* ($\dot{V}co_2/\dot{V}o_2$) is also about 0.8. With a normal hemoglobin concentration of 15 g/dl, and a normal ratio of cardiac output to oxygen consumption, the mixed venous blood contains approximately 5 ml/dl less oxygen than the arterial blood under "steady-state" conditions.

### ALVEOLAR VENTILATION

Of a resting tidal volume of 500 ml, approximately 150 ml (one-third) is required to fill the large airways in which no gas exchange occurs. Since this air is not involved in gas exchange, it is considered wasted and is a part of the physiologic dead space. This portion of the "wasted ventilation" is called the *anatomic dead space* and is present in all individuals. It is approximately equal to the body weight in pounds. Thus, at a resting minute ventilation of 7 liters, if the tidal volume is 500 ml, the respiratory rate is 14/minute, and the physiologic dead space is composed of only the conducting airways (150 ml), the effective alveolar ventilation per minute will be 4.9 liters. In normal young subjects the physiologic dead space is similar to the anatomic dead space. However, in the presence of aging or disease, the physiologic dead space is greatly increased by the presence of underperfused alveoli (*alveolar dead space*).

### HYPOVENTILATION

Overall hypoventilation of the lungs causes a decreased flow of inspired air relative to the venous blood perfusing the lungs. This results in a predictable fall in $Po_2$ and a rise in $Pco_2$ in alveolar gas and capillary blood. While arterial $Po_2$ is dependent on several factors that affect gas exchange, arterial $Pco_2$ is dependent solely on the relationship of $CO_2$ production to alveolar ventilation. Thus, at a given level of $CO_2$ production ($\dot{V}co_2$), the volume of alveolar ventilation ($\dot{V}_A$) per minute may be calculated by using the *alveolar ventilation equation*:

$$\dot{V}_A = \frac{\dot{V}co_2 \times 0.863}{Paco_2} \tag{1}$$

$\dot{V}co_2$ is the $CO_2$ production per minute and may be measured by collecting an expired gas sample. The factor 0.863 corrects for differences in measurement units and conversion from body temperature to standard temperature (BTPS to STPD). In practice, arterial pressure ($Paco_2$) may be substituted for alveolar pressure ($PAco_2$), since they are essentially equal.

The alveolar ventilation equation provides a means for relating inflow of fresh air ($\dot{V}_A$) to the rate of $CO_2$

**TABLE 4.1**
**NORMAL GAS TENSIONS IN ALVEOLI AND ARTERIAL AND MIXED VENOUS BLOOD AT SEA LEVEL**

|               | Alveoli | Arterial Blood | Mixed Venous Blood |
|---------------|---------|----------------|--------------------|
| $Po_2$        | 100     | 95             | 40                 |
| $Pco_2$       | 40      | 40             | 46                 |
| $PH_2O$       | 47      | 47             | 47                 |
| $PN_2$        | 573     | 573            | 573                |
| $PTOTAL$      | 760     | 755            | 706                |

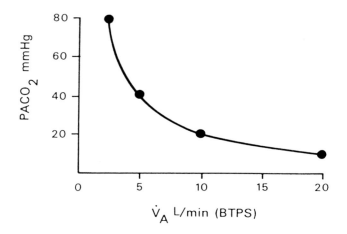

**FIGURE 4.1.** The relationship of alveolar ventilation ($\dot{V}_A$) to alveolar $CO_2$ ($P_{ACO_2}$) at a given $CO_2$ production ($\dot{V}_{CO_2}$) of 200 ml/minute. Increased $CO_2$ production, as with exercise, would shift the curve to the right.

production ($\dot{V}_{CO_2}$). In practice, it is seldom necessary to measure expired $CO_2$, and for practical purposes the equation may be simplified to express the inverse relationship between alveolar (and arterial) $P_{CO_2}$ and alveolar ventilation:

$$P_{ACO_2} \approx \frac{1}{\dot{V}_A} \qquad (2)$$

The inverse relationship of alveolar and arterial $P_{CO_2}$ to alveolar ventilation is shown in Figure 4.1. With a steady $CO_2$ output of 200 ml/minute, halving the alveolar ventilation from 5 liters/minute to 2.5 liters/minute will double the $P_{ACO_2}$ to 80 mm Hg, and doubling alveolar ventilation to 10 liters/minute will halve the $P_{ACO_2}$ to 20 mm Hg. From the shape of this curve, it may be evident that relatively small increases in alveolar ventilation are associated with impressive reductions in $P_{ACO_2}$ when the patient is hypercapnic. $P_{ACO_2}$ can also rise quickly when alveolar ventilation changes by only a small amount in this setting. Conversely, in the setting of hypocapnia, relatively large changes are required to decrease $P_{ACO_2}$ further. It is not uncommon to observe rather large fluctuations in $P_{ACO_2}$ in hypercapnic patients responding to minor changes in ventilation. In response to metabolic acidosis, large changes in ventilation and work of breathing result in only modest changes in acid-base status. Obviously, if $\dot{V}_{CO_2}$ should change owing to increased metabolic activity, as with exercise, a new curve would be derived to the right of the one shown in Figure 4.1.

## THE BOHR EQUATION

While the arterial $P_{CO_2}$ provides a simple method of estimating effective alveolar ventilation, it is also useful in estimating the amount of dead space or "wasted ventilation." This tells us how efficient a patient's breathing pattern is (i.e., how much of each breath is useful and how much is "wasted"). Figure 4.2 illustrates the variables used in calculating dead space ventilation. Note that *partial pressures* are used rather than *concentrations* of gases. The total minute ventilation ($\dot{V}_E$) and expired carbon dioxide ($P_{ECO_2}$) are composed of the effective alveolar ventilation ($\dot{V}_A$), which contains alveolar levels of $CO_2$ ($P_{ACO_2}$), and the dead space ventilation ($\dot{V}_D$), which contains inspired levels of $CO_2$ ($P_{ICO_2}$). This sentence may be written in the form of an equation:

$$\dot{V}_E \times P_{ECO_2} = (\dot{V}_A \times P_{ACO_2}) + (\dot{V}_D \times P_{ICO_2}) \qquad (3)$$

Rearranging and solving for $\dot{V}_D/\dot{V}_E$ (the portion of $\dot{V}_E$ that is wasted), we have the *Bohr equation*:

$$\frac{\dot{V}_D}{\dot{V}_E} = \frac{P_{ACO_2} - P_{ECO_2}}{P_{ACO_2} - P_{ICO_2}} \qquad (4)$$

Furthermore, since $P_{ICO_2}$ breathing room is zero, this factor can be eliminated and arterial $CO_2$ ($P_{aCO_2}$) can be substituted for alveolar $CO_2$ as follows:

$$\frac{\dot{V}_D}{\dot{V}_E} = \frac{P_{aCO_2} - P_{ECO_2}}{P_{aCO_2}} \qquad (5)$$

Arterial $P_{CO_2}$ can be substituted for alveolar $P_{CO_2}$ because they are assumed to be in complete equilibrium (and therefore identical) in the ideal alveolus. The $CO_2$ dissociation curve is relatively flat in the physiologic range (Figure 4.3). Furthermore, the difference between the mixed venous and arterial $P_{CO_2}$ is only about 6 mm Hg, and while venous admixture significantly affects $P_{aO_2}$, it has relatively little effect on $P_{aCO_2}$.

If you collect expired gas for a minute or two, mix it, and determine the partial pressure of $CO_2$, the normal value will be approximately 25 to 30 mm Hg. With a normal arterial $P_{CO_2}$ of 40 and a $P_{ECO_2}$ of 25 mm Hg, the dead space would be calculated as follows:

$$\dot{V}_D/\dot{V}_E = \frac{40 - 25}{40}$$
$$= \frac{15}{40}$$
$$= 0.37 \text{ or } 37\%$$

In patients with lung disease the difference between expired $P_{CO_2}$ and arterial $P_{CO_2}$ increases as the physiologic dead space increases. Comparison of expired $P_{CO_2}$ with the arterial $P_{CO_2}$ will give an estimate of the percentage of wasted ventilation (Equation 5).

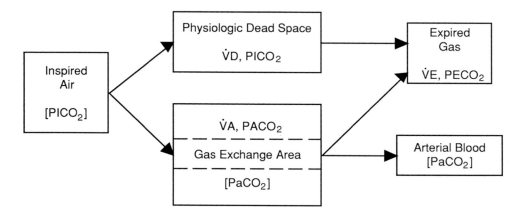

**FIGURE 4.2.** A gas exchange diagram, showing the variables that are measured for the Bohr equation. $P_{ICO_2}$, partial pressure of inspired $CO_2$ (normally zero); $P_{ACO_2}$, partial pressure of $CO_2$ in alveolar air (equal to arterial $P_{CO_2}$); $P_{aCO_2}$, partial pressure of $CO_2$ in arterial blood; $P_{ECO_2}$, partial pressure of $CO_2$ in expired gas; $\dot{V}_D$, dead space ventilation; $\dot{V}_E$, total minute ventilation; $\dot{V}_A$, effective alveolar ventilation.

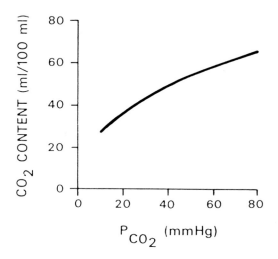

**FIGURE 4.3.** $CO_2$ dissociation curve for a subject with a normal level of saturated hemoglobin. The curve shifts to the right with polycythemia and to the left with anemia. Oxygenation shifts the curve to the right and hypoxemia shifts it to the left (Haldane effect).

## THE ALVEOLAR AIR EQUATION

By comparing *arterial* blood gas values with *alveolar* gas values, one may estimate the impedance to gas transfer across the alveolar capillary membrane. End-expired alveolar gas may be sampled directly; however, the analysis of this expired gas sample includes both functional and nonfunctional alveoli (those that are perfused and those that are not perfused). While there is variation among alveoli depending on their relative ventilation and perfusion, the *average* alveolar $P_{CO_2}$ so nearly equals arterial $P_{CO_2}$ that $P_{aCO_2}$ may substitute for $P_{ACO_2}$ in the alveolar ventilation equation (Equation 1). Thus, $P_{ACO_2} - P_{aCO_2}$ differences are not sensitive indicators of problems with gas exchange. On the other hand, large differences exist between mean alveolar *oxygen* tension and measured arterial oxygen tension, and the *alveolar-arterial oxygen difference* ($P_{AO_2} - P_{aO_2}$) is a practical and relatively sensitive test for assessment of gas exchange. Fortunately, mean alveolar oxygen tension can be calculated with reasonable accuracy by using the *simplified alveolar air equation*:

$$P_{AO_2} = \frac{P_{IO_2} - P_{aCO_2}}{R} \qquad (6)$$

where $P_{AO_2}$ is the calculated alveolar $P_{O_2}$, $P_{IO_2}$ is the partial pressure of inspired oxygen, arterial $P_{CO_2}$ is substituted for alveolar $P_{CO_2}$, and R is the respiratory exchange ratio.

This is a modification of the actual alveolar air equation. In practice, a respiratory exchange ratio of 0.8 is used in Equation 6. Begin and Renzetti (2) have shown that these modifications using an R of 0.8 yield calculated values of $P_{AO_2}$ that are accurate enough for clinical purposes. For example, a subject breathing room air at sea level has an arterial $P_{CO_2}$ of 40 and an arterial $P_{O_2}$ of 90. What are his calculated alveolar $P_{O_2}$ and alveolar-arterial oxygen difference?

We must first calculate $P_{AO_2}$. With the patient breathing room air (21% $O_2$) at sea level (barometric pressure 760 mm Hg and body temperature 37 C), water vapor pressure is 47 mm Hg. Equation 6 becomes:

$$P_{AO_2} = 0.21\,(760 - 47) - \frac{40}{0.8} = 0.21\,(713) - 50$$
$$= 150 - 50$$
$$= 100 \text{ mm Hg}$$

This gives an estimate of the mean alveolar oxygen tension. The difference between alveolar and arterial oxygen tensions can then be calculated by subtracting the measured $Pa_{O_2}$ (90 mm Hg) from the calculated $P_{AO_2}$ (100 mm Hg) to give an alveolar-arterial oxygen difference of 10 mm Hg. As stated above, the normal $P_{AO_2} - Pa_{O_2}$ in young adults averages about 8 mm Hg, and this increases gradually to a mean of 16 mm Hg in the 61 to 75 age group of healthy adults (1). Values significantly above this level indicate the presence of a lung abnormality causing a defect in gas transfer, and this may be assessed whether or not alveolar hypoventilation is present. The simplified alveolar air equation is extremely useful in clinical practice and should be committed to memory.

## Alveolar Perfusion

As noted above, even in normal lungs a small portion of the mixed venous blood bypasses the gas exchange areas and is added to the arterial blood. This is called *venous admixture, shunt, or wasted perfusion*. In older subjects and in patients with respiratory diseases, the venous admixture is increased by a varying extent by the presence of areas with relative underperfusion. With defects in gas exchange, blood is shunted through poorly functional or nonfunctional alveoli into the arterial blood. This section first describes how to calculate *total* perfusion or *cardiac output*, then how to quantify defects in the *distribution* of capillary perfusion.

### Cardiac Output

In the previous discussion it was pointed out that in normal adults alveolar ventilation is about 4.5 liters/minute. Normally, the cardiac output (the total amount of blood perfusing the lungs) is slightly more than this, about 6 liters/minute. Cardiac output is commonly estimated by using Fick's principle, which states that the rate at which oxygen enters the blood during its passage through the lungs is a product of the blood flow and the difference between the oxygen contained in the mixed venous blood and that contained in the arterial blood:

$$\dot{V}_{O_2} = \dot{Q}t\,(Ca_{O_2} - C\bar{v}_{O_2}) \qquad (7)$$

where $\dot{Q}t$ is the total blood flow from the right ventricle (i.e., the cardiac output). Solving for $\dot{Q}t$, we can rewrite this equation as follows:

$$\dot{Q}t = \frac{\dot{V}_{O_2}}{Ca_{O_2} - C\bar{v}_{O_2}} \qquad (8)$$

It should be emphasized that we are now dealing with oxygen *content* in arterial and mixed venous blood rather than with oxygen *tension*, and thus blood hemoglobin levels and the shape of the oxyhemoglobin dissociation curve must be considered. Because hemoglobin is the major oxygen carrier in the blood and because of the sigmoid shape of the oxyhemoglobin dissociation curve, we must calculate oxygen content from $Pa_{O_2}$ using the dissociation curve and measured levels of hemoglobin.

At this point it is reasonable to review the oxyhemoglobin dissociation curve. A few numbers are worth keeping in mind (Figure 4.4). At a normal pH of 7.4 and a normal $Pa_{O_2}$ of 100 mm Hg, the hemoglobin will be approximately 97% saturated. At the shoulder of the oxyhemoglobin dissociation curve, with a $Pa_{O_2}$ of 60 and pH of 7.4, the hemoglobin is about 90% saturated. From here saturation drops quickly, and at a $Pa_{O_2}$ of 40 (the normal mixed venous oxygen tension) the hemoglobin is only about 75% saturated.

The vast majority of the oxygen contained in blood is carried on the hemoglobin molecule. One gram of hemoglobin fully saturated will carry 1.34 ml (3). For example, with a hemoglobin content of 15 g/dl and a saturation of 97%, the oxygen content of arterial blood that is attached to hemoglobin would be:

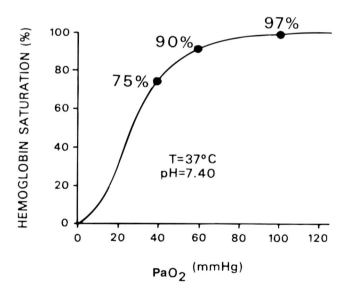

**Figure 4.4.** The normal oxyhemoglobin dissociation curve at pH 7.4 and temperature 37 C. Saturations at three key points are marked. Hyperthermia shifts the curve to the right and hypothermia shifts it to the left. Acidemia shifts it to the right and alkalemia to the left (Bohr effect.)

$$15 \text{ g/dl} \times 0.97 \times 1.34 \text{ ml/g} = 19.5 \text{ ml/dl}$$

In addition to the oxygen attached to hemoglobin, a small quantity is dissolved in arterial plasma, according to the solubility of oxygen in plasma (0.003 ml/dl per mm Hg $P_{O_2}$). At a normal $Pa_{O_2}$ of 100 mm Hg, the dissolved content would be:

$$100 \times 0.003 = 0.3 \text{ ml/dl}$$

The oxygen content of arterial blood for the normal patient in this example would be 19.8 (or about 20) ml/dl. In the normal range of $Pa_{O_2}$, the amount of dissolved oxygen is relatively minute and can be ignored; however, in situations where the $F_{IO_2}$ is high, the amount of dissolved oxygen may become significant.

The blood normally loses about 25% of its oxygen content as it passes through the tissues. With a hemoglobin content of 15 g/dl the arterial blood carries about 20 ml of oxygen per deciliter. With a normal $P\bar{v}_{O_2}$ of 40 mm Hg and a mixed venous saturation of 75%, this same blood carries 15 ml of oxygen per deciliter. Thus, the normal *a-$\bar{v}$ oxygen difference* is 5 ml/dl, and this difference may increase as tissue demands increase in relation to oxygen delivery. With an increase in metabolic demand, the a-$\bar{v}$ oxygen difference increases at the same time the cardiac output increases, thus increasing oxygen delivery simultaneously by two mechanisms.

If cardiac output is insufficient to meet the body's needs, there is a drop in the $P\bar{v}_{O_2}$, since more oxygen must be extracted from the same amount of hemoglobin. In certain situations (e.g., sepsis syndrome), mixed venous oxygen content may increase in the face of low oxygen delivery, due to inability of the tissues to utilize oxygen adequately. Thus, the measurement of mixed venous oxygen (saturation or tension) by indwelling catheters must be interpreted with caution in patients with gas exchange problems. In general, serial measurements are more useful for comparison than are single measurements.

### THE SHUNT EQUATION

While calculation of the alveolar-arterial oxygen gradient ($PA_{O_2} - Pa_{O_2}$) yields an assessment of gas transfer and therefore tells us whether there is wasted perfusion, the actual *percent* of the cardiac output that is shunted through the lungs and unavailable for gas transport may be estimated by using the *shunt equation*:

$$\frac{\dot{Q}s}{\dot{Q}t} = \frac{Cc'_{O_2} - Ca_{O_2}}{Cc'_{O_2} - C\bar{v}_{O_2}} \qquad (9)$$

where $\dot{Q}s/\dot{Q}t$ is the shunt fraction or venous admixture and $Cc'_{O_2}$, $Ca_{O_2}$, and $C\bar{v}_{O_2}$ are the oxygen contents of end-capillary, arterial, and mixed venous blood, respectively. The $Cc'_{O_2}$ is estimated by assuming that end-capillary $P_{O_2}$ is the same as $PA_{O_2}$ (calculated from the alveolar air equation). $Ca_{O_2}$ is calculated from the measured arterial $P_{O_2}$ and the oxyhemoglobin dissociation curve. The $C\bar{v}_{O_2}$ may be estimated by assuming a normal a-$\bar{v}$ oxygen content difference of 5 ml/dl. This estimate of $C\bar{v}_{O_2}$ is not valid unless the cardiac output is adequate and stable, and tissue utilization is intact. If left ventricular function fails to meet the oxygen needs of the tissues, the a-$\bar{v}$ difference is widened; conversely, if tissue utilization is impaired, the a-$\bar{v}$ difference may be narrowed.

At a normal $PA_{O_2}$ of 100 mm Hg and a hemoglobin of 15 g, the hemoglobin is 97% saturated and $Cc'_{O_2}$ is 19.5 ml/dl. If the measured $Pa_{O_2}$ is 80 mm Hg, the hemoglobin is 96% saturated and the $Ca_{O_2}$ is 19.3 ml/dl. Assuming a normal cardiac output, and therefore an a-$\bar{v}$ oxygen content difference of 5 ml/dl, we can calculate the shunt fraction as follows:

$$\begin{aligned}\frac{\dot{Q}s}{\dot{Q}t} &= \frac{Cc'_{O_2} - Ca_{O_2}}{Cc'_{O_2} - C\bar{v}_{O_2}} \\ &= \frac{19.5 - 19.3}{19.5 - 14.5} \\ &= \frac{0.2}{5.0} = 0.04 \text{ or } 4\%\end{aligned} \qquad (10)$$

This relatively small percentage of the cardiac output that represents the normal shunting of blood in healthy people is made up of two components: blood that is perfusing relatively underventilated alveoli, and true shunts that perfuse areas that are not ventilated at all. True shunts in normal people occur because blood from bronchial veins, the veins of the mediastinum, and the thebesian vessels of the left ventricular myocardium empty directly into the systemic arterial circulation.

### VENTILATION-PERFUSION RELATIONSHIPS

In the ideal gas exchange unit, ventilation and perfusion are equally matched and gas exchange is optimum. In real life, however, the situation is much more complex, and a *gradation* occurs from well-ventilated but underperfused areas, to equally ventilated and perfused areas, to areas that are well perfused but underventilated. In diseases that affect the lungs, the areas of equal matching are relatively small, and areas of mismatching of ventilation and perfusion are more important.

Using radioactive xenon scans, West and his colleagues demonstrated that normally, in the upright position, blood flow increases progressively from the top to the bottom of the lungs, and blood flow per unit of lung area is increased approximately 10-fold from apex to base (4). Because of the movement of the diaphragm and larger pressure changes with inspiration around the lower lobe, *ventilation* also increases from top to bottom but not as much as perfusion. The bases are ventilated approximately three times as well as the apices. Thus, there is normally a gradient of both ventilation and perfusion from the top to the bottom of the lungs.

Since blood flow increases relatively more from apex to lung base than does ventilation, there is a decreasing *ratio* of ventilation to perfusion on descending from the apex to the base of the lungs. This is illustrated by the $O_2$-$CO_2$ diagram in Figure 4.5, which is taken from West's monograph. Using the figures from the $O_2$-$CO_2$ diagram, West has estimated that in normal resting humans in the upright position, the $\dot{V}/\dot{Q}$ ratio in the lung apices is about 3.3, while that near the lung bases is only about 0.63. For this reason, oxygen tension in the alveoli at the apex is around 130 mm Hg, while in those at the lung base it is only about 90 mm Hg.

Note that according to the principles outlined above, the majority of the blood flows to the lung bases. Thus, areas at the apices, which are relatively well ventilated and have high $\dot{V}/\dot{Q}$ ratios, are poorly perfused, thus contributing relatively little to the measured $Pa_{O_2}$ in the systemic arterial blood. The gas exchange units near the lung bases, where perfusion is relatively high and $\dot{V}/\dot{Q}$ ratios relatively low, contribute much more to the arterial blood, and since their effects predominate, arterial $P_{O_2}$ primarily reflects areas with relatively low $\dot{V}/\dot{Q}$ relationships. This is a major reason why in normal humans arterial $P_{O_2}$ is slightly less than alveolar $P_{O_2}$. The remainder of the normal $PA_{O_2} - Pa_{O_2}$ gradient is explained by the normal anatomic shunts discussed above. Note in Figure 4.5 that the $P_{CO_2}$ also varies normally from lung apices to lung bases. Because of relative hyperventilation, the $P_{CO_2}$ at the top of the lungs is about 30 mm Hg, while that at the lung bases is around 40 mm Hg.

The $\dot{V}/\dot{Q}$ mismatching discussed above is that which occurs normally in the upright position. Patients with abnormal lungs have much more severe mismatching of ventilation to perfusion. Moreover, at the same horizontal level a lung lobule may contain terminal respiratory units that are adequately ventilated adjacent to underventilated terminal lung units whose bronchioles are completely occluded. Collateral ventilation may occur from a well-ventilated to a poorly ventilated pulmonary lobule, thus increasing the distance that the air must travel and increasing the dead space. The mismatching of ventilation to perfusion in disease occurs throughout the lungs and is difficult to measure with such gross tests of ventilation and perfusion as lung scans and arteriograms. In clinical practice, the amount of $\dot{V}/\dot{Q}$ mismatch is estimated from the amount of hypoxemia that remains after the effects of hypoventilation and true shunting are removed. The effects of hypoventilation are determined from the arterial $P_{CO_2}$ (Equation 1), and the effects of true shunts are estimated by measuring the $Pa_{O_2}$ while the patient breathes 100% oxygen.

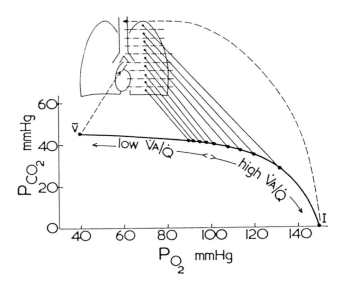

**FIGURE 4.5.** The $O_2$-$CO_2$ diagram showing normal ventilation-perfusion ratios in upright humans, from the top of the lungs to the bottom. The high $\dot{V}/\dot{Q}$ ratio at the apex results in a high $P_{O_2}$ and low $P_{CO_2}$ there. A low $P_{O_2}$ and a high $P_{CO_2}$ are found at the lung base. (Reprinted from West JB: *Ventilation/Blood Flow and Gas Exchange*, ed 4. Oxford, Blackwell Scientific Publications, 1985. With permission of the author and publisher.)

## EFFECTS OF BREATHING 100% OXYGEN

The portion of venous admixture caused by true right-to-left shunts can be separated from that due to poorly ventilated lung units by having the subject breathe 100% oxygen for at least 15 minutes and then calculating the resultant change in shunt fraction (Equation 9). It is important that the patient take deep breaths during this procedure so that even poorly ventilated alveoli receive oxygen. The principle of this maneuver is that breathing 100% oxygen ultimately replaces the nitrogen in all functional lung units, even those that are poorly ventilated. Thus, the hemoglobin in the perfusing capillaries becomes completely saturated. These poorly ventilated alveoli then function as normal lung units as far as oxygen exchange is concerned. Alveolar oxygen tension is calculated from the alveolar air equation (using a respiratory exchange ratio of 1.0), and from that, capillary oxygen content is estimated. Arterial and mixed venous oxygen tensions are measured and oxygen contents are then calculated. Since defects in gas transfer due to $\dot{V}/\dot{Q}$ inequality are eliminated by breathing 100% oxygen, the remaining $\dot{Q}$s is due solely to true right-to-left shunting. Subtracting the true shunt fraction from the total venous admixture (measured while breathing room air) yields an estimate of the contribution of $\dot{V}/\dot{Q}$ mismatching to arterial hypoxemia.

It should be noted that the alveolar-arterial oxygen tension difference normally increases as the $F_{IO_2}$ is increased because the effects of poorly oxygenated blood from the normal right-to-left shunts on the $Pa_{O_2}$ become more pronounced. It is also common for the breathing of pure oxygen to cause absorption atelectasis. This phenomenon occurs when nitrogen from poorly ventilated alveoli is replaced by oxygen, which is subsequently absorbed into the pulmonary capillary blood.

## GAS TRANSFER (DIFFUSION)

Gas transfer across the alveolar-capillary membrane occurs by passive diffusion, which is related to the partial pressures of these gases in the alveoli and in the pulmonary capillaries. The difference in oxygen and $CO_2$ tensions across the membrane represents the driving pressure for diffusion of each gas. It is impossible to measure diffusing capacity for oxygen because the capillary tension cannot be measured. In practice, carbon monoxide diffusion ($D_{CO}$) is measured, since the trace amounts of CO inhaled do not increase the $P_{CO}$ in capillary blood. Diffusing capacity for oxygen ($D_{O_2}$) is about 1.23 times the $D_{CO}$, or about 40 ml/minute/mm Hg (6). During exercise, $D_{O_2}$ may increase by more than three times through pulmonary capillary recruitment and an increase in capillary blood volume.

In the normal human capillary, equilibrium between alveolar and arterial $P_{O_2}$ occurs in less than 0.25 second. Under normal resting conditions, blood spends about 0.75 second in the capillaries. Since it takes only a third of this time for equilibration to occur, a wide safety margin exists, and even a large decrease in diffusion fails to affect gas exchange. The $D_{CO}$ must fall to about 10% of the predicted value before any change in arterial oxygen at rest will occur.

The diffusion process may be affected by an abnormal resistance to diffusion, as in a thickened alveolar-capillary membrane; a decrease in the partial pressure gradient for oxygen across the membrane; or a shortened time for equilibration. At least two of these must

coexist before arterial oxygen is affected. Thus, diffusion may become a factor in gas exchange during exercise (shortened equilibrium time) in a patient with interstitial fibrosis (thickened membrane) or at high altitude (decreased gradient).

For practical purposes, abnormal diffusion plays only a minor role in the hypoxemia seen in patients with lung diseases. This role is of even less importance, since it can be corrected by small increases in the inspired oxygen.

## ARTERIAL HYPOXEMIA

The potential causes of arterial hypoxemia are listed in Table 4.2. In patients who are seen for evaluation of lung disease, arterial hypoxemia is usually the result of a defect in gas transfer, and the causes of hypoxemia not related to abnormal gas transfer (low inspired oxygen concentration, alveolar hypoventilation, and low $P\bar{v}_{O_2}$) are usually readily identifiable. This discussion addresses the differential diagnosis of arterial hypoxemia using a few simple observations and calculations to differentiate among the causes listed in Table 4.2. However, it should be noted that several causes often coexist in the same patient. For instance, the patient who is admitted with an acute exacerbation of COPD may have a combination of alveolar hypoventilation and a defect in gas transfer due to mismatching of ventilation to perfusion. The relative contribution to the arterial hypoxemia should be determined for each of the factors when possible.

### LOW INSPIRED OXYGEN CONCENTRATION

A review of the simplified alveolar air equation emphasizes the importance of $F_{IO_2}$ and barometric pressure on the partial pressure of alveolar oxygen. In the example given above, the barometric pressure at sea level (760 mm Hg) was used; however, people frequently live at higher altitudes and are able to adapt quite well to living at altitudes as high as 2500 m (8200 ft). Nearly 30 million people live at altitudes even

**TABLE 4.2**
**POTENTIAL CAUSES OF ARTERIAL HYPOXEMIA**

| |
|---|
| Low $F_{IO_2}$ |
| Hypoventilation |
| Diffusion defect |
| Ventilation-perfusion mismatch |
| Right-to-left shunt |
| Low mixed venous oxygen tension |

higher, in the Rocky Mountains of North America, the Andes of South America, the Himalayas of Asia, and elsewhere (7). At 8000 ft barometric pressure is approximately 565 mm Hg, the inspired $P_{O_2}$ is about 120 mm Hg, and the alveolar oxygen is approximately 80 mm Hg. In subjects with normal lungs the $Pa_{O_2}$ remains high enough to achieve nearly complete hemoglobin saturation so that oxygen content is not severely affected.

In people living at altitudes above 2500 m, compensation occurs with increased hemoglobin levels and a shift in the oxygen-hemoglobin dissociation curve to the left so that oxygen is unloaded more efficiently to the tissues. Cardiac output increases in response to hypoxemia; however, this decrease in red cell transit time through the pulmonary capillaries in addition to a decrease in mixed venous $P_{O_2}$ tends to emphasize existing $\dot{V}/\dot{Q}$ inequalities. Furthermore, pulmonary hypertension occurs at very high altitudes, and this is associated with an alteration in ventilation-perfusion relationships, which may result in further arterial hemoglobin desaturation. For a further discussion of altitude physiology and adaptation to high altitudes, the reader is referred to the work of West, Hackett, and their associates (8).

Patients undergoing mechanical ventilation because of diffuse lung disease with severe defects in gas exchange (e.g., pneumonia, pulmonary edema, and adult respiratory distress syndrome) may suffer rapid worsening of hypoxemia if the delivered $F_{I_{O_2}}$ falls due to ventilator malfunction or manipulation of the ventilator controls. Such patients are often maintained at the lowest $F_{I_{O_2}}$ that results in nearly complete saturation of the arterial hemoglobin. At levels of $Pa_{O_2}$ below 60 mm Hg a small decrease in $F_{I_{O_2}}$ results in a severe decline in $Sa_{O_2}$ and arterial oxygen content, due to the steep slope of the oxyhemoglobin dissociation curve. Constant monitoring of $Sa_{O_2}$ with pulse oximetry will alert the clinician to such sudden and potentially dangerous decreases in oxygen content.

## HYPOVENTILATION

As noted above, alveolar $P_{CO_2}$ is inversely related to alveolar ventilation; thus, if alveolar ventilation is halved, alveolar and arterial $P_{CO_2}$ values double. The hallmark of alveolar hypoventilation as a cause of arterial hypoxemia is an increase in $Pa_{CO_2}$. Alveolar hypoventilation decreases alveolar $P_{O_2}$ because as $CO_2$ accumulates in the alveoli it displaces oxygen, and so the displaced oxygen is not available for gas exchange. If the arterial $P_{CO_2}$ is normal or low, hypoxemia cannot be explained by alveolar hypoventilation.

In normal patients, alveolar ventilation ($\dot{V}_A$) is a fixed proportion of minute ventilation ($\dot{V}_E$), since dead space ventilation is limited mainly to the anatomic dead space (conducting airways). Thus, we can consider the $\dot{V}_E$ and $Pa_{CO_2}$ to be inversely proportional (see Equation 2). In patients with respiratory problems, the ventilatory pattern may change so that breathing becomes rapid and shallow; thus, a greater part of each breath is composed of dead space ventilation. In such patients, $\dot{V}_A$ may decrease and $Pa_{CO_2}$ may rise without a change in measured minute ventilation ($\dot{V}_E$). A change to slow, deep breaths will result in hyperventilation (low $Pa_{CO_2}$) without a change in $\dot{V}_E$. In patients with chronic lung disease, minute ventilation may be increased although $Pa_{CO_2}$ is elevated, due to an increase in the alveolar dead space and $\dot{V}/\dot{Q}$ mismatching.

Hypoventilation causes hypoxemia due to its effects on the alveolar $P_{O_2}$, a relationship described in the *alveolar air equation* (Equation 6). Any rise in $Pa_{CO_2}$ causes a drop in the alveolar and thus the arterial $P_{O_2}$. Thus, with moderate degrees of alveolar hypoventilation, the $PA_{O_2} - Pa_{O_2}$ remains normal. Recently, it has been shown that marked hypercapnia will reduce the increased $PA_{O_2} - Pa_{O_2}$ that might otherwise exist due to abnormalities in gas exchange (9).

In patients who are hypoxemic and retaining $CO_2$, the relative contribution to the hypoxemia of alveolar hypoventilation can be determined by calculating $PA_{O_2} - Pa_{O_2}$. If this is normal, one can assume that the observed hypoxemia can be corrected by achieving adequate alveolar ventilation. If, however, the $PA_{O_2} - Pa_{O_2}$ is elevated, there is a defect in gas transfer (usually a $\dot{V}/\dot{Q}$ mismatch) in addition to the hypoventilation. In comatose patients who have no associated lung disease, the $PA_{O_2} - Pa_{O_2}$ is within normal limits and the hypoxemia should be corrected completely with adequate ventilation. If, however, the $PA_{O_2} - Pa_{O_2}$ is elevated in the presence of a high $Pa_{CO_2}$, there is an additional defect in gas transfer, and an increased $F_{I_{O_2}}$ or the addition of positive end-expiratory pressure (PEEP) may be necessary.

## DIFFUSION DEFECT

A defect in gas transfer due to diffusion limitation does not occur in normal humans at sea level because even at high cardiac outputs the blood remains in the capillaries long enough for adequate equilibrium. However, during exercise at high altitudes the driving pressure ($PA_{O_2}$) of oxygen in the alveoli may be low enough and the transit time of blood in the capillaries so short that a limitation of diffusion of oxygen into the blood may become a factor in the development of hypoxemia (10). As noted above, three factors may decrease oxygen diffusion and cause hypoxemia: a defect in the lung diffusion capacity of oxygen; a decrease in the oxygen gradient between alveoli and capillary blood; and a decrease in equilibration time. Two or more of these abnormalities must occur for diffusion defects to become a factor in hypoxemia; however, defects in diffusion play a role in certain situations. Diffusion defects are easily corrected by increasing the $FIO_2$.

### VENTILATION-PERFUSION MISMATCH

Ventilation-perfusion mismatching is the most common cause of hypoxemia in patients with lung disease. Marked $\dot{V}/\dot{Q}$ mismatching is manifested by hypoxemia in the presence of a normal, low, or high $Paco_2$. By definition, wasted ventilation ($\dot{V}D/\dot{V}T$) and wasted perfusion ($\dot{Q}s/\dot{Q}t$) are both increased. Measurement of $\dot{V}D/\dot{V}T$ yields an estimate of the amount of wasted ventilation, while calculating the shunt fraction indicates the amount of wasted perfusion.

The $PAO_2 - PaO_2$ is a useful index of the degree of $\dot{V}/\dot{Q}$ inequality in the lungs. Since the distribution of lung abnormalities is not uniform in the presence of disease, various units of the lungs are affected to different degrees. Thus, some areas have relatively high $\dot{V}/\dot{Q}$ ratios and others relatively low ratios. Arterial blood reflects areas with relatively high blood flow, and thus areas with relatively low $\dot{V}/\dot{Q}$ ratios. The majority of diffuse lung diseases, including those affecting the airways such as chronic bronchitis and asthma and those affecting the alveoli such as emphysema and interstitial fibrosis, all result in increased $PAO_2 - PaO_2$ due to $\dot{V}/\dot{Q}$ mismatching. Furthermore, therapeutic measures such as administration of bronchodilators may actually hinder the physiologic attenuation of perfusion to areas of localized hypoxemia, resulting in more severe shunting and a further drop in $PAO_2 - PaO_2$ (11).

The greater the degree of $\dot{V}/\dot{Q}$ inequality present, the higher the $\dot{V}E$ must be to maintain a normal or reduced $Paco_2$. An elevated $\dot{V}E$ with a normal $Paco_2$ is evidence for the presence of a $\dot{V}/\dot{Q}$ abnormality. This is due to an increase in the dead space ventilation. The overventilation of normal lung units required to compensate for low $\dot{V}/\dot{Q}$ units results in an increased gradient between the expired $Pco_2$ and the $Paco_2$, and thus an increase in the $\dot{V}D/\dot{V}T$.

At some point, the work of increasing $\dot{V}E$ becomes too great to sustain, and any further increase in $\dot{V}/\dot{Q}$ mismatch results in a rise in $Paco_2$. This may be slow, as in COPD, or rapid, as in acute asthma attacks. The respiratory center and the respiratory muscles determine the point at which $Paco_2$ begins to rise. The increased $Paco_2$ that occurs is a method of boosting the efficiency of a compromised ventilatory system. The higher the concentration of $CO_2$ in the alveolar gas, and thus in each expired breath, the lower the $\dot{V}E$ required to remove a specific amount of $CO_2$. The effect of the rise in $Paco_2$ on blood pH and central nervous system function limits the extent of this compensatory mechanism. However, with renal compensation, chronic elevations of $Paco_2$ are well tolerated.

During acute hypercapnic exacerbations of COPD, oxygen therapy almost always leads to a further rise in the $Paco_2$. While this has been thought to be due to further depression of the respiratory drive, Aubier et al showed that $Paco_2$ may rise without a significant reduction in $\dot{V}E$ (12). Other investigators have disputed their findings; at any rate, other factors seem to be active in causing the further rise in $Paco_2$ associated with oxygen administration. There is a further increase in $\dot{V}/\dot{Q}$ mismatching due to vasodilation and increased perfusion of poorly ventilated lung units; and the hemoglobin affinity for $CO_2$ is reduced as oxygen saturation increases (Haldane effect). Since the increase in $Paco_2$ is not entirely due to respiratory center depression, progressively worsening hypercapnia is not inevitable.

A moderate increase in $Paco_2$ without mental changes requires no intervention. If hypercapnia progresses and $CO_2$ narcosis ensues, mechanical ventilation may be required. A common practice is to decrease the $FIO_2$ slightly, to "stimulate the respiratory center." This is a gross mistake, as it may result in severe hypoxemia. Progressive hypercapnia rarely kills a patient; severe hypoxemia often does. A reasonable approach is to increase the $FIO_2$ in small increments, while monitoring with a pulse oximeter, using only that $FIO_2$ necessary to achieve a hemoglobin saturation of 90%.

### RIGHT-TO-LEFT SHUNT

The other potential cause of arterial hypoxemia is a true right-to-left shunt. Shunting may occur in conjunction with $\dot{V}/\dot{Q}$ mismatching or hypoventilation, in which case it adds to the severity of the hypoxemia. The contribution of shunting in patients with arterial hypoxemia may be assessed by calculating the shunt fraction with the patient breathing 100% oxygen, as outlined above. The $\dot{Q}s/\dot{Q}t$ that remains after breathing oxygen (correcting that portion caused by $\dot{V}/\dot{Q}$ mismatching) is the percentage of the cardiac output that is actually shunted through unventilated areas.

When breathing mixtures high in oxygen, the amount of oxygen dissolved in the plasma must be included in the estimation of $Cc'O_2$, $CaO_2$, and $C\bar{v}O_2$. This is calculated by multiplying the $PaO_2$ by the solubility coefficient of oxygen in plasma at body temperature, which is 0.003 ml/dl/mm Hg. On breathing 100%

oxygen at sea level, about 2 ml oxygen is dissolved in each 100 ml plasma. It should also be noted that the calculation of $P_{AO_2} - P_{aO_2}$ while breathing 100% oxygen does not require the usual correction for R, since only oxygen and carbon dioxide are left in the alveoli, the nitrogen having been washed out.

Acute lung injuries, such as the adult respiratory distress syndrome (ARDS), cause severe hypoxemia mostly as a result of shunting. Serial changes in gas transfer cannot be determined using the $P_{AO_2} - P_{aO_2}$ gradient, since the increased $F_{IO_2}$ required to treat the hypoxemia is associated with a variable effect on the calculated gradient. An estimate of serial changes in gas transfer can be obtained by comparing the ratio of $P_{aO_2}$ to the $F_{IO_2}$ (13). A $P_{aO_2}/F_{IO_2}$ of 250 or greater is indicative of a relatively mild defect in gas transfer in patients with ARDS; a ratio of 100 or less is a grave prognostic sign, indicating severe lung damage.

### PEEP, MEAN AIRWAY PRESSURE, AND ARTERIAL OXYGENATION

Positive end-expiratory pressure increases end-expiratory lung volume and tends to improve arterial oxygenation by at least three mechanisms: recruitment of atelectatic lung tissue, redistribution of lung water, and reduction of flow to shunt vessels. Similar mechanisms are likely to operate in all techniques that elevate mean airway pressure.

Under passive conditions, mean airway pressure can be raised by increasing minute ventilation, by extending inspiratory time, or by raising end-expiratory alveolar pressure. Such increases of average lung volume generally improve oxygen exchange, especially in lungs that are affected by atelectasis and edema. Conversely, a decrease in mean airway pressure (e.g., by removal of PEEP or a reduction in minute ventilation) can result in a fall in $P_{aO_2}$.

### LOW MIXED VENOUS OXYGEN TENSION

A reduction in $P_{\bar{v}O_2}$ may result in worsening arterial hypoxemia in patients with $\dot{V}/\dot{Q}$ mismatching, right-to-left shunts, or low hemoglobin levels (14). The drop in $P_{\bar{v}O_2}$ may result from a decrease in cardiac output or from an increase in oxygen uptake by the tissues. The lower $P_{\bar{v}O_2}$ increases the effects of right-to-left shunts on arterial $P_{O_2}$ (depending on the intensity of hypoxemic vasoconstriction), further limiting oxygen delivery. In patients with limited cardiac output, factors such as fever, anxiety, and increased work of breathing may be corrected by such measures as lowering the temperature, administering sedation, or adjusting the ventilator. Decreasing oxygen uptake will then result in an increased $P_{\bar{v}O_2}$ (assuming oxygen delivery is unchanged); and this in turn will increase arterial oxygen.

## OXYGEN TRANSPORT

In a normal adult approximately 300 ml of oxygen is used per minute at rest. During exercise, oxygen delivery is related linearly to oxygen uptake, as shown in Figure 4.6. *Systemic oxygen transport*, or the amount of oxygen delivered to the tissues and metabolized per minute, can be calculated by multiplying the arterial blood oxygen content ($C_{aO_2}$) by the cardiac output ($\dot{Q}$). The arterial oxygen content depends on the concentration of functional hemoglobin in arterial blood and the saturation of that hemoglobin with oxygen. The saturation of hemoglobin is dependent on the partial pressure of oxygen in the arterial blood. Thus, systemic oxygen transport depends on the interaction of the *circulatory system* (delivery of arterial blood), *erythropoietic system* (hemoglobin in red blood cells), and *respiratory system* (gas exchange area) according to the following equation:

Systemic oxygen transport (ml/min)
$$= \dot{Q} \text{ (liter/min)} \times C_{aO_2} \text{ (ml/liter)} \qquad (11)$$
$$= \dot{Q} \times \text{(grams hemoglobin} \times 1.34) \times S_{aO_2}$$

| circulatory | erythropoietic | respiratory |
| system | system | system |

where $\dot{Q}$ is the cardiac output and $S_{aO_2}$ is the percent saturation of the hemoglobin. The respiratory system provides the oxygen tension in the pulmonary capillaries, which in turn determines hemoglobin saturation. The above equation does not include the (normally inconsequential) volume of oxygen that is dissolved in the blood.

### THE CIRCULATORY SYSTEM

With a normal resting cardiac output ($\dot{Q}$) of about 6 liters/minute, since each 100 ml of arterial blood contains about 20 ml oxygen, the total amount of oxygen delivered per minute to the tissues at rest is about 1200 ml. The cells use only about 300 ml of this oxygen, which means that about 900 ml remains in the mixed venous blood. The percent of oxygen remaining in the mixed venous blood represents the *average* extraction of oxygen from blood by all the tissues. It is important to understand that while the average oxygen extraction is about 25% of the oxygen present in the arterial blood, oxygen use differs markedly from one organ system to another. For instance, the heart uses essentially all the oxygen it receives, while the kidneys use only a small percentage. It is physiologically appropriate to

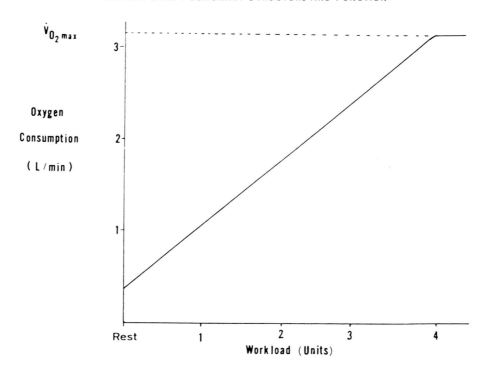

**FIGURE 4.6.** Relationship of oxygen uptake in liters per minute to work intensity, graded in arbitrary units, in a normal subject. In this case the resting oxygen consumption is 350 ml/minute. For a given increase in work load there is a proportional increase in oxygen uptake up to the subject's aerobic capacity ($\dot{V}_{O_2}$max), which is the limit of the oxygen transport capacity. (Courtesy of G. Kinasewitz, M.D.)

have a surplus of oxygen available in case sudden changes in availability or use occur. Thus, the oxygen remaining in the mixed venous blood represents a reservoir for the tissues to call upon should the normal adjustments to demand be temporarily inadequate.

The oxygen extracted from the blood during its passage through the tissues determines the arterial–mixed venous difference in oxygen tension ($Pa_{O_2} - P\bar{v}_{O_2}$). The $P\bar{v}_{O_2}$ is normally about 40 mm Hg, so that with a normal arterial $P_{O_2}$ of 90 mm Hg and an adequate delivery of blood to the tissues, the a-$\bar{v}$ oxygen difference is about 50 mm Hg. A fall in mixed venous $P_{O_2}$ with an increase in the a-$\bar{v}$ oxygen tension difference occurs during exercise, and whenever the oxygen delivery system is stressed. When an abnormal a-$\bar{v}$ difference occurs in the absence of normal stress mechanisms, it is evidence for failure of adequate oxygen delivery. Factors that may alter the validity of this measurement in estimating the adequacy of oxygen delivery are discussed below.

### THE ERYTHROPOIETIC SYSTEM

Each 100 ml of blood normally contains about 15 g of hemoglobin. It is this hemoglobin content that allows for the remarkable oxygen-carrying ability of the blood, normally about 20 ml/dl. This is possible because 1 g of hemoglobin when fully saturated carries 1.34 ml of oxygen. At a normal $Pa_{O_2}$ of over 80 mm Hg, the hemoglobin molecule is almost completely saturated, while at a mixed venous $P_{O_2}$ of 40 mm Hg, the hemoglobin is only about 75% saturated. The ability of hemoglobin to bind oxygen at normal values of arterial $P_{O_2}$ and to give it up at lower values of $P_{O_2}$ is described by the oxyhemoglobin dissociation curve (Fig. 4.4).

To calculate arterial oxygen content, the percent saturation of the hemoglobin ($Sa_{O_2}$) must be determined. The $Sa_{O_2}$ may be estimated from the oxyhemoglobin dissociation curve, provided the $Pa_{O_2}$ and pH are known and the hemoglobin is normal. This is the procedure used in most blood gas laboratories, where $Sa_{O_2}$ is calculated rather than measured. Alternatively, $Sa_{O_2}$ may be measured by using a cooximeter for in vitro measurement or a pulse oximeter for in vivo measurement. Actual measurement is necessary if the shape or position of the oxyhemoglobin dissociation curve is abnormal.

Normally, the relationship of $Sa_{O_2}$ to $P_{O_2}$ is not static but changes with differing conditions, usually to the benefit of the individual. A decrease in blood pH is

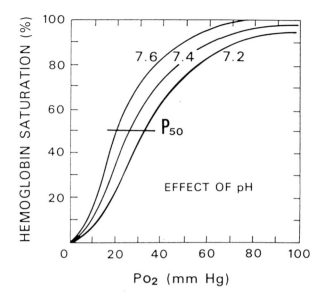

**FIGURE 4.7.** The oxyhemoglobin dissociation curve. The effects of shifts in pH on the affinity of hemoglobin for oxygen (the Bohr effect) are shown. Acidosis shifts the curve toward the right and thus increases oxygen delivery at the tissue level. The affinity of hemoglobin for oxygen is expressed as the $P_{50}$ (the $PaO_2$ at which the hemoglobin is 50% saturated).

associated with a shift in the curve toward the right, as shown in Figure 4.7; thus at the higher pH levels found in the lungs, oxygen is bound more easily, while at lower pH levels found in the tissues, oxygen is freed more easily (the Bohr effect). Lower temperatures shift the curve to the left, while higher temperatures shift the curve to the right.

The binding capacity for oxygen is also affected by an increase or decrease in the 2,3-diphosphoglycerate (2,3-DPG) content of the red cells. Since the 2,3-DPG competes with oxygen for sites on the hemoglobin molecule, increased levels of 2,3-DPG shift the curve to the right and allow for improved oxygen delivery. Carbon monoxide (CO) binds extremely readily with hemoglobin to form carboxyhemoglobin. This decreases the ability of the hemoglobin to carry oxygen. Some inherited abnormal types of hemoglobin are associated with marked changes in the oxyhemoglobin dissociation curve, with either an increased or a decreased affinity of hemoglobin for oxygen.

While almost all the oxygen in arterial blood is carried on the hemoglobin molecule, a small amount is also carried in the plasma as dissolved oxygen. Since the solubility of oxygen in plasma is very low, this portion of the oxygen content is insignificant except in unusual situations, such as in the breathing of high concentrations of oxygen. In patients with carbon monoxide poisoning, CO replaces oxygen on the hemoglobin molecule because its affinity for hemoglobin is greater, producing tissue hypoxia in the presence of a normal hemoglobin level and a normal $PO_2$. In such cases, ventilation with high-oxygen mixtures may prevent hypoxic tissue damage and will augment the elimination of CO.

The affinity of hemoglobin for oxygen and its ability to give up oxygen at the tissue level are commonly assessed by calculating the $P_{50}$, the partial pressure of oxygen at which the hemoglobin is 50% saturated. The $P_{50}$ can be calculated by equilibrating the patient's blood in a tonometer at various $PO_2$ levels and then measuring the saturation of the hemoglobin and plotting a dissociation curve. The normal $P_{50}$ of human blood is 26.6 mm Hg, with a fairly large variability around this level in the presence of disease. The $P_{50}$ may be estimated from a random venous blood sample according to a formula proposed by Lichtman and co-workers (15). In a group of 38 healthy subjects, the mean $P_{50}$ calculated by using this technique was $26 \pm 1.3$ mm Hg. It is important to note that most values of $SaO_2$ reported from the blood gas laboratory are calculated from a nomogram that assumes a normal hemoglobin dissociation curve. For estimation of $P_{50}$, saturation of the venous hemoglobin must be measured directly, for obvious reasons.

## THE RESPIRATORY SYSTEM

The respiratory system is assessed by measurement of $PaO_2$ while breathing room air. If the arterial blood is not adequately oxygenated, there is a defect in gas transfer at the pulmonary capillary level. This may be due to precapillary shunting within the lungs, to mismatching of ventilation with perfusion in the gas transfer units of the lungs, or to hypoventilation. Frequently, several of these factors are abnormal in the same patient. Factors outside the lungs can also affect $PaO_2$. These include extrapulmonary right-to-left shunts, in which case blood never gets to the lungs to be oxygenated, and a decrease in mixed venous $PO_2$.

Inadequate oxygen delivery affects arterial oxygen content by decreasing the mixed venous $PO_2$. In patients with intrapulmonary shunts, since the mixed venous blood is added directly to the arterial blood, there is a dramatic fall in $PaO_2$ secondary to the decrease in $P\bar{v}O_2$ (16). Thus, when the $PaO_2$ deteriorates in a patient with multiple organ system failure, factors other than those directly related to abnormal gas exchange in the lungs must be considered.

## RESPONSES TO INCREASED OXYGEN DEMAND

The need for oxygen by the cells varies depending on the body's level of metabolism. The need for oxygen may increase acutely, as with exercise, or chronically, as in patients with hyperthyroidism. Responses of the three components of the oxygen transport system vary depending on whether the increase is sudden or gradual. In general, responses to chronic increases in demand are more efficient, since the body has more time to adjust.

Acute increases in oxygen demand are common, and the most common of these is physical exercise (Fig. 4.6). Oxygen demand also increases with fever or after the ingestion of food. The earliest and most efficient response to this increased oxygen demand in normal persons is a rise in the cardiac output. The cardiac output may increase to 3 to 4 times its resting value, and by this mechanism oxygen delivery may increase to 3 to 4 liters/minute. In fact, it is the cardiac output that normally defines maximum oxygen uptake and delivery.

Ventilation also increases rapidly with exercise, and a fall in the $Pa_{CO_2}$ is the normal response to exercise above the anaerobic threshold, in response to metabolic acidosis. Moreover, some improvement in $\dot{V}/\dot{Q}$ relationships often occurs during exercise so that $Pa_{O_2}$ rises. However, in health, this improvement in gas exchange does little to increase the amount of oxygen per liter of arterial blood, since the capillary hemoglobin is already essentially saturated. The ventilatory system must, however, be able to keep up with increases in oxygen demand and $CO_2$ production or else the alveolar oxygen concentration will decrease.

The hematocrit actually rises slightly during severe exercise in healthy subjects owing to a reduction in circulating plasma volume. This probably contributes little to the efficiency of oxygen delivery. However, there is also an extracellular metabolic acidosis during heavy exertion, and this results in a shift of the hemoglobin dissociation curve toward the right (Fig. 4.7). In general, a shift of the hemoglobin dissociation curve to the right is a useful defense mechanism, provided the $Pa_{O_2}$ is normal.

A *chronic* increase in oxygen consumption does not occur in health, but increased oxygen demand is characteristic of such diseases as thyrotoxicosis, acromegaly, and some malignancies. In patients with hyperthyroidism or acromegaly, the chronic increase in oxygen demand is met by increases in cardiac output (circulatory system) and blood volume (erythropoietic system). Moreover, a shift in the hemoglobin dissociation curve to the right, which enhances oxygen delivery at the tissue level, may also occur in some diseases, associated with an increase in the $PA_{O_2} - Pa_{O_2}$ gradient. Increased ventilation occurs as a response to an increase in cardiac output.

## RESPONSES TO DEFICIENCIES OF THE OXYGEN TRANSPORT SYSTEM

If oxygen delivery is reduced because of a decrease in cardiac output, hemoglobin concentration, or gas exchange, the tissues respond by extracting additional oxygen from the capillary blood (17). When the $P\bar{v}_{O_2}$ drops below about 30 mm Hg, the cells switch from aerobic to anaerobic metabolism to supply their energy needs. With acute reduction in $P\bar{v}_{O_2}$, there is excess lactic acid production with progressively severe metabolic acidosis (18). Adaptation of the body to deficient oxygen transport therefore involves attempts to improve that transport itself rather than to find alternative metabolic mechanisms.

The circulatory, erythropoietic, and respiratory systems normally function together to ensure adequate oxygen delivery, both at rest and during periods of increased metabolic demand. However, at times any combination of these three systems may fail. In severe multiple organ system failure such as that which occurs with sepsis and the adult respiratory distress syndrome, all three systems may be affected at the same time, resulting in a very high mortality (19).

### FAILURE OF THE CIRCULATORY SYSTEM

Oxygen delivery is markedly affected by a reduction in cardiac output. The immediate compensatory mechanism for a low cardiac output is increased extraction of oxygen from the blood that perfuses the tissues, facilitated by an increase in red cell 2,3-DPG, which displaces oxygen on the hemoglobin molecule and allows more oxygen to be extracted. If this fails to meet tissue demands, anaerobic metabolism occurs and lactate is produced, causing a drop in pH and a further shift to the right of the oxyhemoglobin dissociation curve. The increased extraction of oxygen from capillary blood results in a fall in mixed venous oxygen tension and increased a-$\bar{v}$ oxygen difference.

The balloon-directed pulmonary artery catheter allows sampling of pulmonary artery blood for determination of mixed venous oxygen (20). To measure $P\bar{v}_{O_2}$ accurately, the catheter must be placed proximally in the pulmonary artery and blood should be withdrawn slowly so that admixture with oxygenated postcapillary blood does not occur (21). Insertion of the catheter allows serial measurements of $P\bar{v}_{O_2}$ and mixed venous oxygen saturation ($S\bar{v}O_2$), and calculation of $PaO_2 - P\bar{v}O_2$. It also permits measurement of pulmonary artery and capillary wedge pressures and cardiac output, allowing for an estimate of left ventricular function. Fiberoptic oxygen saturation sensors are now available, allowing for constant monitoring of $S\bar{v}O_2$.

While the mixed venous oxygen tension and a-$\bar{v}$ oxygen difference provide a guide to total oxygen delivery in normal subjects, problems occur when using this measurement in patients with multiple organ failure. In acutely ill patients with ARDS, oxygen use by tissues has been shown to be dependent on the amount of oxygen delivered to those tissues (22). Furthermore, a normal or even high $P\bar{v}O_2$ may be seen with septic shock, intracardiac or arteriovenous right-to-left shunts, or with the use of inotropic drugs to support cardiac function (17). When measured $P\bar{v}O_2$ values are at variance with the clinical appearance it is useful to measure cardiac output directly and to use clinical findings such as mental function and urine output to assess the adequacy of perfusion to vital organs (13), since at present there is no widely accepted method of measuring tissue oxygenation. Gastric tonometry of pH via a nasogastric tube is currently under investigation as a method of estimating tissue oxygenation. This may prove clinically helpful if clinical trials document its reliability.

### Failure of the Erythropoietic System

The normal hematocrit of 40 to 50% is optimum for achieving maximum systemic oxygen delivery. An increase in the hematocrit will increase the oxygen-carrying capacity of the blood within certain limits; however, as the hematocrit rises above 55%, cardiac output falls and the polycythemia becomes a self-defeating mechanism.

The most common abnormality of the erythropoietic system is *blood loss*, either acute or chronic. Acute blood loss stresses the oxygen transport mechanism because it causes not only a drop in hematocrit but also a fall in blood volume. In acute blood loss, it is the loss of circulating blood volume and resultant decrease in cardiac output that is the most critical problem. Oxygen delivery is improved by replacing blood volume even though the hematocrit may remain low. Carbon monoxide poisoning also causes an acute failure of the erythropoietic system by decreasing $SaO_2$. Victims die of tissue hypoxia because the hemoglobin is not available for oxygen transport. In this case cardiac output increases as a response to tissue needs, but this does not correct the defect. The problem remains until the CO is eliminated, a process that takes several hours if

the patient breathes room air but may be shortened if $FIO_2$ is increased.

The principal response to a chronic decrease in circulating red cells (anemia) is an increased heart rate and pulse pressure with a resultant rise in cardiac output. Moreover, with chronic anemia there is an increase in red cell 2,3-DPG with an accompanying shift of the oxyhemoglobin dissociation curve to the right, which decreases hemoglobin-oxygen affinity and makes oxygen more available to the tissues.

### Failure of the Respiratory System

In health, chronic arterial hypoxemia is found only among persons living at high altitudes. In these subjects, polycythemia occurs as a normal defense mechanism. An increase in circulating hemoglobin results in more oxygen being carried per liter of blood at the same $PaO_2$. Cardiac output increases as $PaO_2$ falls, and red blood cell 2,3-DPG rises to allow more efficient unloading of oxygen to the tissues.

In the presence of respiratory diseases that result in arterial hypoxemia, polycythemia and an increase in red blood cell 2,3-DPG are of limited usefulness. The secondary polycythemia that occurs in pulmonary disease is not as effective as that which occurs in normal humans at high altitude; the reasons for this are not entirely clear (23).

In patients with acute respiratory failure it is sometimes possible to aid the compensatory mechanisms by therapeutic interventions. For instance, cardiac output may be improved by maintaining adequate intravascular fluid volumes, while oxygen delivery in the presence of a limited cardiac output may be improved by increasing hemoglobin levels. Oxygen use by the tissues can often be decreased by reducing fever or by administering muscle relaxants to decrease agitation and muscle activity.

*Acknowledgment*

The author wishes to express his sincere appreciation to David R. Dantzker, M.D., and John J. Marini, M.D., who assisted in the revision of this chapter. The ideas and opinions of these experts are evident throughout the text.

▼

### References

1. Mellemgaard K: The alveolar-arterial oxygen difference; its size and components in normal man. *Acta Physiol Scand* 67:10–20, 1966.
2. Begin R, Renzetti AD: Alveolar-arterial oxygen pressure gradient. Comparison between an assumed and actual

respiratory quotient in stable chronic pulmonary disease. *Respir Care* 22:491–500, 1977.

3. Comroe JH Jr, Forster RE, Dubois AB, et al: The lung. In *Clinical Physiology and Pulmonary Function Tests*, ed 2. Chicago, Year Book, 1962.
4. Hughes JMB, Glazier JB, Maloney JE, West JB: Effect of lung volume on the distribution of pulmonary blood flow in man. *Respir Physiol* 4:58–72, 1968.
5. West JB: *Ventilation/Blood Flow and Gas Exchange*, ed 4. Oxford, Blackwell Scientific Publications, 1985.
6. Dantzker DR: Pulmonary gas exchange. In Bone RE et al, (eds). *Pulmonary and Critical Care Medicine*. St Louis, CV Mosby, 1993, pp B-1–13.
7. Baker PT: The adaptive fitness of high altitude populations. In Baker PT (ed): *The Biology of High Altitude Peoples*. Cambridge, Cambridge University Press, 1978, pp 317–346.
8. West JB, Hackett PH, Maret KH, et al: Pulmonary gas exchange on the summit of Mount Everest. *J Appl Physiol* 55:678–687, 1983.
9. Gray BA, Blalock JM: Interpretation of the alveolar-arterial oxygen difference in patients with hypercapnia. *Am Rev Respir Dis* 143:4–8, 1991.
10. West JB, Lahiri S, Gill MB, et al: Arterial oxygen saturation during exercise at high altitude. *J Appl Physiol* 17:617–621, 1962.
11. Tai E, Reid J: Response of blood gas tensions to aminophylline and isoprenaline in patients with asthma. *Thorax* 22:543–549, 1967.
12. Aubier M, Marviano D, Millic-Emili J, et al: Effects of the administration of $O_2$ on ventilation and blood gases in patients with chronic obstructive pulmonary disease during acute respiratory failure. *Am Rev Respir Dis* 122:747–754, 1980.
13. Murray JF, Matthay MA, Luce JM, Flick MR: An expanded definition of the adult respiratory distress syndrome. *Am Rev Respir Dis* 138:720–723, 1988.
14. Dantzker DR: The influence of cardiovascular function on gas exchange. *Clin Chest Med* 4:149–159, 1983.
15. Lichtman MS, Murphy MS, Adamson JW: Detection of mutant hemoglobins with altered affinity for oxygen: a simplified technique. *Ann Intern Med* 84:517–520, 1976.
16. Dantzker DR: The influence of cardiovascular function on gas exchange. *Clin Chest Med* 4:149–159, 1983.
17. Kandel G, Aberman A: Mixed venous oxygen saturation. Its role in the assessment of the critically ill patient. *Arch Intern Med* 143:1400–1402, 1983.
18. Kasnitz P, Druger GL, Yorra F, Simmons DH: Mixed venous oxygen tension and hyperlactatemia. *JAMA* 236:570–574, 1976.
19. Bell RC, Coalson JJ, Smith JD, Johanson WG Jr: Multiple organ system failure and infection in adult respiratory distress syndrome. *Ann Intern Med* 99:293–298, 1983.
20. Swan HJC, Ganz W, Forrester J, et al: Catheterization of the heart in man with use of a flow directed balloon tipped catheter. *N Engl J Med* 283:447–451, 1970.
21. Suter PM, Lindauer JM, Fairley HB, Schlobohm RM: Errors in data derived from pulmonary artery blood gas values. *Crit Care Med* 3:175–181, 1975.
22. Danek SJ, Lynch JP, Weg EG, Dantzker DR: The dependence of oxygen uptake on oxygen delivery in the adult respiratory distress syndrome. *Am Rev Respir Dis* 122:387–395, 1980.
23. Murray JF: *The Normal Lung*, ed 2. Philadelphia, WB Saunders, 1986.

### SUGGESTED READINGS

1. Jones NL: *Blood Gases and Acid-Base Physiology*. Philadelphia, Brian C Decker, 1980.
2. West JB: Assessing pulmonary gas exchange. *N Engl J Med* 316:1336–1338, 1987.
3. West JB: *Respiratory Physiology—The Essentials*, ed 4. Baltimore, Williams & Wilkins, 1989.
4. West JB: Ventilation-perfusion relationships. *Am Rev Respir Dis* 116:919–943, 1977.

# SECTION TWO

▼

# DIAGNOSTIC STUDIES IN PATIENTS WITH RESPIRATORY PROBLEMS

# Chapter 5

# History and Physical Examination

## Ronald B. George

THE PROCESS OF obtaining a meaningful history, performing a good physical examination, and putting the information together to form an initial impression is an art that must be learned by experience. The history and physical examination should lead to a reasonable list of differential diagnoses. This list of impressions, in turn, forms the basis for a diagnostic plan, whereby the number of possible diagnoses is gradually decreased by the results of selected laboratory tests, radiographs, and specialized procedures. This chapter includes some guidelines for this important task.

## OBTAINING A USEFUL HISTORY

The interview is designed to identify the important symptoms and determine their duration. To do this without being led into blind areas of discussion is an important step toward identifying the problem. The interviewer must lead the discussion, avoiding lengthy digressions; on the other hand, the patient must have the freedom to mention items that may prove important as the history unfolds. The patient should not be badgered, but should be made to feel that the interviewer is truly interested in his or her problems. The interviewer should not yawn or act bored, but should instead appear interested in the patient's story.

The chief complaint—the symptom that caused the patient to seek help—and its duration should be identified. Frequently the patient will say that he or she was referred because of an abnormal finding on a chest film or some other laboratory test. However, it is important to determine why that test was made and, if it was part of a routine examination, what changes from previous films resulted in referral.

Once the major complaint and its duration are identified, the development of the patient's symptoms should be investigated chronologically, beginning at the time that the patient first noted a departure from feeling well. The patient should be questioned concerning current and past medications, any allergic reactions or intolerance to foods or drugs, or exposure to contagious illnesses. It is important to determine if other members of the household or coworkers have similar symptoms. It is also useful to obtain information from previous examinations or diagnostic tests. For instance, a previously negative tuberculin skin test is important if tuberculosis is suspected. Elements of the personal, occupational, and social history should be included in the present illness if they are directly pertinent to the patient's current symptoms.

A systematic review of the symptoms of respiratory illnesses and their character and duration should be reported. Nonrespiratory symptoms should also be reviewed, since they may be related to the respiratory disease. Patients with carcinoma of the lung may present with complaints of headaches or seizures related to cerebral metastases; ankle swelling or a history of injury to the lower extremities is important if the patient has a suspected pulmonary embolism. Ascites and edema of the legs may be secondary to heart failure, cor pulmonale, or liver disease, all of which may cause abnormalities on the chest film, while joint pain may be caused by hypertrophic pulmonary osteoarthropathy. It is important to determine if a patient's complaints are seasonal, especially in patients with hay fever, sinusitis, postnasal drip, or asthma.

Previous illnesses and operations should be recorded, since they may be related to the present illness. For instance, childhood measles or pertussis may be the origin of bronchiectasis, and asthma during childhood that disappeared at puberty may return at a later age. Patients with reinfection tuberculosis often relate a history of household contact during their childhood years. Previous operations and biopsies may be the source of pathologic specimens that might be useful for reexamination. If previous chest films are available, they should be obtained for comparison with recent ones.

## Occupational and Exposure History

Cigarette smoking is the most common preventable cause of death in the United States today (1). A smoking history is especially important in patients with respiratory complaints. Passive exposure to cigarette smoke in the home or the workplace is an increasingly recognized cause of respiratory symptoms in children whose parents smoke, and passive smoking has been shown to increase the incidence of respiratory infections (2).

The occupational history is especially important in patients with lung problems, since the lungs are constantly in contact with the environment. The patient should be encouraged to relate his or her job history in chronologic order. Occupational exposure may have occurred many years ago; exposure to asbestos may result in the development of a pleural mesothelioma 25 years or more after the exposure has ceased. It is important to ask the patient if he or she was advised to wear a mask at work or whether his or her fellow workers did so. The type of mask worn and the air source should be identified. Construction workers who are not directly involved in hazardous activities may work in closed areas containing toxic materials; for instance, carpenters, plumbers, and welders often work

in areas where sandblasting is occurring. While the sandblaster may have extensive protection, the workers nearby may be exposed.

Some symptoms of toxic reactions are not related to the lungs. Patients working with galvanized metal (zinc fumes) may complain of nausea, vomiting, and other systemic symptoms. Allergic alveolitis due to thermophilic actinomycetes in workers exposed to moldy hay (farmer's lung) or sugar cane residue (bagassosis) is associated with fever, malaise, and headache in addition to nonproductive cough. The patient should be questioned about particularly irritating odors or upper respiratory symptoms, since toxic fumes usually affect the eyes, nose, and throat and this serves as an early sign of chemical exposure. Upper respiratory symptoms are common in toxic smoke inhalation.

Workers may not be aware of exposures to toxic materials. For instance, office workers have developed allergic alveolitis from air conditioners and humidifiers that were contaminated with fungal spores (3).

The family history is often useful. Cystic fibrosis and the immotile cilia syndromes are inherited, as are the hemoglobinopathies and $\alpha_1$-antitrypsin deficiency. Patients with asthma often have a family history of allergic rhinitis, asthma, or other allergic symptoms. In addition, family members may have similar exposure. Tuberculosis is often spread by household contact, and viral respiratory diseases often affect several family members. Families may be exposed to the oxides of nitrogen (silo filler's disease) or moldy hay while working together on a farm.

## Symptoms of Respiratory Diseases

### Upper Respiratory Tract Symptoms

Rhinorrhea, conjunctivitis, and sneezing are common in patients with allergic rhinitis (hay fever), who may also have asthma; the two syndromes often coincide. Postnasal drip occurs in patients with upper respiratory disease and is manifested during the daytime by frequent clearing of the throat rather than by actual coughing. A postnasal drip is often a problem at night, and eventually may produce a "morning cough" due to chronic irritation of the upper airways.

Nosebleeds (epistaxis) may be a symptom of sinusitis or may be produced by trauma, foreign bodies, or tumors of the nose and nasopharynx. Systemic diseases such as hypertension, polycythemia, and bleeding disorders can also lead to bouts of epistaxis. Wegener's granulomatosis causes necrotizing granulomas of the upper respiratory tract as well as of the lungs. Blood from the nose and nasopharynx sometimes accumulates in the oropharynx and is "coughed up," so the patient thinks that it is coming from the lungs. A history of epistaxis and the finding of blood clots in the nose or nasopharynx are clues that the expectorated blood may be coming from the upper respiratory tract. Hoarseness may result from lesions of the recurrent laryngeal nerve (surgical trauma, mediastinal tumors, or infections) or from diseases of the larynx (tuberculosis, tumors, or allergy).

Patients who present with anaerobic infections of the lungs and pleura (lung abscess, empyema) often have upper respiratory abnormalities leading to aspiration of oral secretions. The patient should be questioned concerning recent mouth or dental surgery, anesthesia, aspiration of a foreign body, neurologic abnormalities, periods of unconsciousness, and seizures.

## CHEST PAIN

Thoracic pain is an alarming symptom, since most people are aware of its association with cardiac disease, lung tumors, and other serious life-threatening diseases. There are two basic types of chest pain: that which arises in the chest wall structures and is conducted through the intercostal and phrenic nerves (lateral or chest wall pain) and that which arises in the internal organs and is conducted through the afferent fibers of the vagus nerve (central or visceral pain). These two types of chest pain will be discussed separately.

*Visceral chest pain* occurs with neoplasms of the major bronchi or mediastinum; abnormalities of the heart, aorta, and pericardium; or diseases that cause esophageal pain, especially reflux esophagitis or tumors. Pain associated with acute bronchitis is usually central and is often accentuated by coughing.

Pain in the substernal area may indicate disease of the heart, pericardium, aorta, or esophagus. Angina pectoris is usually an effort-induced pain that is relieved by rest and vasodilators. It is often referred to the neck, shoulder, or arm. Pericardial pain is sometimes relieved by sitting up or leaning forward. Pain associated with a dissecting aortic aneurysm is frequently reported as severe and deep, and may be referred to the interscapular area of the back. Esophageal pain may mimic angina pectoris and may be relieved by sublingual nitroglycerine, which relaxes esophageal spasm. It is often related to meals and relieved with antacids. Patients with significant esophageal reflux are subject to aspiration, especially at night, and may

present with recurrent bouts of acute bronchospasm and cough, mimicking asthma attacks.

*Chest wall pain* is sharp, often well localized, and is increased by deep breathing or coughing (pleuritic pain or pleurisy). Pleuritic pain is associated with any disease that causes inflammation of the parietal pleura such as infections (pneumonia, empyema, tuberculosis), trauma (pneumothorax, hemothorax, rib fracture), or tumors (cancer, lymphoma, mesothelioma). Older patients may suffer rib fractures following minor trauma or even severe coughing bouts. These fractures may not be visible on the initial chest film, but later callus formation around the fracture may make it apparent in retrospect. Irritation of the intercostal nerves (herpes zoster, spinal nerve root disease) may also lead to localized chest wall pain. Costochondritis of the second to fourth costosternal articulations (Tietze's syndrome) is common and may mimic the pain of myocardial ischemia or other serious diseases. The pain is clearly localized to the costal cartilage, and there is tenderness to pressure and often a palpable enlargement of the costosternal junction.

The peripheral innervation of the diaphragm is from the local intercostal nerves, and irritation of the peripheral diaphragm is referred to the adjacent chest wall. The central diaphragmatic pain fibers are conducted through the phrenic nerves, and pain in the central diaphragm is often felt in the ipsilateral trapezius region at the base of the neck and the shoulder, an area also supplied by the phrenic nerve.

## BREATHLESSNESS

Breathlessness (dyspnea) is the sensation of difficulty in breathing, sometimes interpreted as the inability to take a deep breath. It is one of the most common reasons that patients with chest diseases consult a physician. Breathlessness is difficult to quantitate, since it is subjective and in certain situations (e.g., during and following exercise and at high altitudes) it is normal. While exercise normally produces dyspnea, a rapid increase in breathlessness or a decrease in exercise tolerance is an important symptom. Breathlessness may occur intermittently, as with attacks of asthma, or it may be persistent, as with chronic obstructive pulmonary disease (COPD). It may be influenced by position, as in patients with left heart failure, who complain of orthopnea (dyspnea when lying flat). Orthopnea may also be seen in patients with asthma or chronic airway obstruction.

There are three basic causes of the sensation of breathlessness: an increased awareness of normal breathing, an increase in the work of breathing, and an abnormality of the ventilatory system itself. Increased awareness of normal breathing is usually a result of anxiety, and in this situation the common complaint is that the patient cannot take a satisfactorily deep breath. The breathing pattern is often irregular, with frequent sighs. Severe psychogenic breathlessness is associated with rapid breathing, tingling of the hands and feet, circumoral numbness, respiratory alkalosis, and occasionally tetanic seizures. This *hyperventilation syndrome* is diagnosed only after organic causes, both respiratory and nonrespiratory, have been excluded and the respiratory mechanics and blood oxygen level have been determined to be normal.

The second cause of breathlessness is an increase in the work of breathing. This may be due either to airways obstruction, in which case greater pressures are required to move air into and out of the lungs, or restriction of lung volumes and loss of compliance, in which case greater effort is required to expand the lungs and chest wall.

The third cause of breathlessness is an abnormality of the ventilatory apparatus. This involves dysfunction of the nerves, the respiratory muscles, or the thoracic cage itself. Neurologic abnormalities producing breathlessness include spinal cord injury, ascending polyneuritis, myasthenia gravis, amyotrophic lateral sclerosis, poliomyelitis, and exposure to paralytic agents or neurotoxins. Primary diseases of the respiratory muscles include polymyositis and muscular dystrophy, while examples of chest wall abnormalities include extreme obesity, kyphoscoliosis, large pleural effusions, and space-occupying lesions of the thorax.

## COUGH

Cough receptors are located in the large bronchi, trachea, and larynx and respond to respiratory secretions in the large airways. Irritation of the cough receptors may occur in the absence of abnormal secretions as with inhalation of toxic fumes or a mild asthma attack. In such cases the nonproductive cough serves no useful purpose and may cause mechanical trauma, leading to more coughing. A nonproductive cough may also be a manifestation of anxiety. In such instances it may be useful to suppress the cough, but in most cases coughing aids in airway clearance and suppression is not indicated.

A change in the character or frequency of cough is a common complaint in patients with pulmonary diseases. Most acute and self-limiting coughs are secondary to a viral respiratory infection (4), while chronic and persistent coughs are most often secondary to chronic bronchitis or postnasal drip. Patients who smoke cigarettes have a characteristic "smoker's cough," a manifestation of chronic bronchitis, most noticeable in the morning on awakening. This cough may be productive of mucoid sputum and is often ignored by the chronic cigarette smoker.

Cough may be the sole complaint in patients with mild asthma (5). In such patients the cough may be relieved by a bronchodilator or the avoidance of inhaled allergens. If bronchospasm is not present at the time of examination, reversible airway obstruction may be demonstrated with the use of a nonspecific bronchial challenge such as methacholine (6). Cough with or without bronchospasm may occur as a side effect of $\beta$-adrenergic antagonists as well as the angiotensin converting enzyme (ACE) inhibiting drugs (7).

### SPUTUM EXPECTORATION

If the patient has a productive cough, the duration of sputum expectoration, the character of the sputum, and the presence or absence of blood should be determined. Cigarette smokers with chronic bronchitis have mucoid or occasionally purulent sputum without much change for months or years and without hemoptysis. The sputum is the result of chronic stimulation and hypertrophy of the bronchial glands as a defense mechanism (8).

In patients with COPD and chronic sputum production, it is important to examine grossly the character of an expectorated sputum sample (color, opacity, and consistency). The patient should be asked about any changes in the quantity, color, or opacity, which may indicate an acute infectious exacerbation requiring antibiotic therapy. It is useful to look at an unstained wet preparation of purulent-appearing sputum to identify neutrophils or eosinophils as the cause of the purulence, since therapy is with antibiotics in the case of neutrophils, and with anti-inflammatory agents in the case of eosinophils (9). It is not usually necessary to obtain a Gram stain in cases of chronic bronchitis with acute exacerbation, and the results usually indicate a mixed flora with both Gram-positive and Gram-negative organisms. Likewise, a sputum culture and sensitivity are rarely indicated; antibiotic therapy is empiric, based on the usual causes of such exacerbations.

Viral infections of the lower respiratory tract are associated at first with scant mucoid sputum, which may contain a few streaks of blood. Later the sputum may become copious and purulent with or without bacterial superinfection. Patients recovering from influenza who begin to produce large volumes of purulent sputum associated with a febrile relapse most likely have a bacterial superinfection. Viral and mycoplasmal pneumonias are associated with relatively scant sputum production initially.

Patients with acute lower respiratory tract infections usually produce sputum containing neutrophils. A Gram stain of grossly purulent sputum may help to identify a predominant bacterial organism. In pneumococcal lobar pneumonia the sputum produced early is usually scanty and composed of mucus tinged with blood ("rusty"); later, sputum may become purulent. As opposed to the scant mucoid sputum in early lobar pneumonia, the sputum in patients with bronchopneumonia (frequently a complication of chronic bronchitis) is usually copious and purulent. The chronic production of purulent sputum with episodes of blood streaking is suggestive of severe bronchitis, bronchiectasis, a bronchogenic tumor, or the presence of an aspirated foreign body. Suppurative lung diseases, including bronchiectasis, lung abscess, or bronchopleural fistula with empyema, are associated with expectoration of large volumes of yellow or green sputum. The color is produced by pigments released from degenerating neutrophils. Approximately 60% of patients with lung abscess will have foul-smelling sputum associated with bad breath, anorexia, and weight loss (10).

Asthmatics who are recovering from an acute attack usually produce sputum that is thick and tenacious and contains bronchial mucus plugs. The sputum may be purulent but, when examined, is found to contain predominantly eosinophils rather than neutrophils. A simple wet preparation or a Wright stain allows ready determination of the predominant cell type (9).

Lung tumors and tuberculosis are associated most often with the chronic production of mucoid sputum that may be associated with blood streaking. Hemoptysis is an important symptom in such patients, and it is the appearance of bloody sputum that often brings the patient to the physician.

### Sputum Induction

If the patient is unable to produce sputum, inhalation of a nebulized solution of 3 or 4 ml distilled water or 10% sodium chloride results in the induction of an adequate specimen for examination in over 90% of cases. Any type of nebulizer may be used; however, ultrasonic nebulizers, which produce a concentrated mist, are preferred. The patient should be placed in a private room or isolation booth if he or she is suspected of having a contagious disease. The patient inhales the nebulizer mist deeply and is encouraged to cough frequently, saving all material produced. Chest percussion and/or postural drainage may be used. The procedure is terminated when an adequate specimen is obtained, the nebulizer solution is exhausted, or after a maximum of 15 to 20 minutes. The procedure is most often used for patients suspected of having tuberculosis or a lung malignancy, and to search for *Pneumocystis*

*carinii* infection in patients with the acquired immunodeficiency syndrome (AIDS).

### Gastric Lavage

Aspiration of stomach contents may be used to obtain specimens for mycobacteria or fungi, especially in children who will not produce coughed sputum specimens. The usefulness of gastric washings is based on the fact that most coughed secretions are swallowed rather than expectorated. The procedure is performed immediately upon awakening, before the stomach has emptied. The material must be processed immediately to avoid destruction of the organisms by gastric acidity and enzymes. The presence of acid-fast bacilli in gastric washings is not diagnostic of mycobacterial disease, because saprophytic mycobacteria are often present in the stomach. The procedure has been largely replaced by sputum induction, since sputum induction results in higher yield and less patient discomfort (11).

### HEMOPTYSIS

The term hemoptysis means simply the coughing of blood, and to say that a patient has hemoptysis is not enough. It is important to determine the duration of the hemoptysis and to note whether there is gross blood, blood-tinged sputum, or blood-streaked sputum. An attempt should be made to determine the amount of blood produced and to record whether it is bright red or dark and whether or not it contains blood clots.

Hematemesis, or vomiting of blood, may be confused with hemoptysis; however, hemoptysis tends to produce bloody sputum that is at least partly frothy, while hematemesis does not. Hematemesis more often produces dark red blood that is usually acid, while hemoptysis is alkaline. With hematemesis blood streaking of sputum is unusual, while with hemoptysis it is common. Vomited blood frequently contains food particles, while this is rare with hemoptysis.

The common causes of hemoptysis are shown in Table 5.1. While the majority of episodes in earlier

**TABLE 5.1**
**INCIDENCE OF CAUSES OF HEMOPTYSIS**

| Cause | Percent of Cases |
| --- | --- |
| Bronchogenic carcinoma | 13 |
| Chronic bronchitis | 53 |
| Bronchiectasis | 1 |
| Tuberculosis | 3 |
| Other | 30 |
| Total cases | 320 |

Data compiled from two published series (12, 13).

years were due to bronchiectasis, tuberculosis, or unknown causes, in more recent reports (following the appearance of fiberoptic bronchoscopy), the most common causes are bronchitis and carcinoma (12, 13). One-third of cases are still due to unknown causes. Grossly bloody sputum is often seen in patients with tuberculosis, pulmonary infarction, bronchial adenoma, mitral stenosis, and lung abscess. A ruptured aortic aneurysm communicating with a bronchus usually results in exsanguination. Recurrent episodes of hemoptysis, sometimes massive, may occur in mycetomas that invade air spaces caused by inactive tuberculosis or sarcoidosis.

Bleeding may occur with tumors of the larynx, and in this case hoarseness is frequently present. Problems in the nasopharynx and oropharynx are usually associated with obvious abnormalities of these areas on physical examination. Bleeding dyscrasias often cause hemoptysis, in which case there is usually evidence of hemorrhage elsewhere, for example, in the skin or gastrointestinal tract.

## PHYSICAL EXAMINATION

As in recording the medical history, it is important to develop an organized, systematic approach to examining the patient. Initially, the patient's general condition should be observed and his or her body habitus and state of nutrition noted. The presence of acute distress, such as pain, dyspnea, or mental confusion, should be recorded. Evidence of chronic illness, such as weight loss or debilitation, should also be noted. The patient's psychological attitude, awareness and appreciation of events, handicaps, and use of prosthetic devices should be noted. If the patient is receiving oxygen the amount and method of administration should be recorded.

### INSPECTION AND PALPATION

During the inspection and palpation of the head, neck, and chest, it is useful to have the chest radiograph handy. This is true during the entire examination of the chest because it allows correlation of physical and radiographic findings. In examining the chest, it is useful to recall the normal location of the five lobes of the lungs and their areas of contact with the chest wall (Fig. 5.1).

The nose, throat, and ears should be examined carefully, since lower respiratory diseases are often associated with upper respiratory tract abnormalities. Rhinorrhea and the presence of pale, edematous nasal mucosa occur with allergic rhinitis. Nasal polyps occur with respiratory allergies and may cause epistaxis. The

frontal, ethmoid, and maxillary sinuses are often tender in the presence of sinusitis, which may produce postnasal drip or bleeding. A red, edematous throat may be due to infection, toxic fume exposure, or chronic postnasal drip. Patients with pneumonia often have inflamed mucous membranes due to associated viral or bacterial upper respiratory infections. Oropharyngeal candidiasis (thrush) may be associated with inhaled steroids or antibiotic therapy and is also common in immunosuppressed patients. Tumors, strictures, or inflammation of the oropharynx can cause upper airway obstruction leading to extreme breathlessness, and sleep-related disorders of breathing may occur in the presence of lesions that obstruct the upper airway. Patients with lung abscess or empyema frequently have poor dental hygiene and foul-smelling breath, and may have problems with swallowing.

Sarcoidosis may involve the salivary and lacrimal glands, with dryness of the oral mucosa and conjunctivae; involvement of the parotid gland may be associated with paralysis of the facial nerve (Bell's palsy). Inflammation of the uveal tract in sarcoidosis is detected by slit lamp examination. Drying of the oral mucous membranes may also be associated with anticholinergic drug therapy or with rheumatoid disease (keratoconjunctivitis sicca), which may affect the lungs also.

The position and mobility of the trachea should be determined, since shift of the mediastinum is associated with shift of the trachea, while fixation of the mediastinum by carcinoma or mediastinal fibrosis is associated with decreased tracheal mobility. The position of the trachea is easily ascertained from the front by comparing the distance from the trachea to each clavicular head. Nodes and masses in the neck and supraclavicular areas are usually best palpated from the rear.

An examination of the neck veins is important in patients with lung diseases. Right heart failure and severe obstructive airway disease are associated with neck vein distention. With airway obstruction the veins usually collapse during inspiration unless elevated venous pressure is also present. With obstruction of the superior vena cava there is marked distention of neck veins, sometimes associated with edema of the neck, eyelids, and hands, and dilation of veins over the anterior chest wall.

The presence of tenderness, discoloration, bruises, or scars over the chest wall should be noted. If there is a history of recent trauma and if chest pain is present, an attempt should be made to palpate the chest wall for crepitus indicating the presence of a rib fracture or subcutaneous emphysema. If scars from previous surgery are noted, the patient should be questioned about this. Examination of the spine for kyphoscoliosis

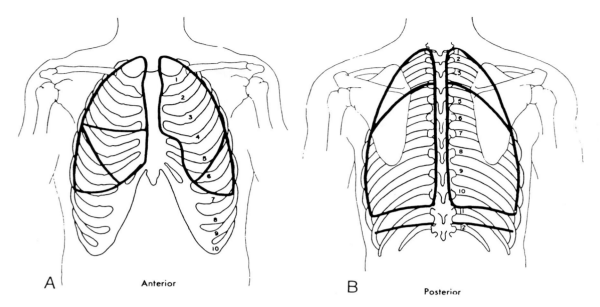

A     Anterior

B     Posterior

**FIGURE 5.1.** **A,** Normal relationship of the lungs to the anterior chest wall. The upper part of the chest overlies the upper lobes. The middle lobe lies under the fourth and fifth interspaces to the right of the heart. The lower lateral chest wall lies over the anterior and lateral basal segments of the lower lobes. **B,** Normal relationship of the lungs to the posterior chest wall. The upper lobe areas are covered by the bones and muscles of the shoulder girdle and are therefore not readily accessible to percussion and auscultation. Most of the posterior chest wall overlies the lower lobes. Diaphragm positions at inspiration and expiration are shown. (Modified from Prior JA, Silberstein JS, Stang JM: *Physical Diagnosis, the History and Examination of the Patient,* ed 6. St. Louis, CV Mosby, 1981.)

may reveal the cause in patients with restrictive lung disease. Expansion of the chest wall should be evaluated both by inspection and by palpation. In patients with severe hyperinflation of the chest due to COPD or asthma, the chest is rounded and "barrel shaped," and because the diaphragm is low and flat there may be inward deflection of the lower chest with inspiration (Hoover's sign). In each step of the physical examination, advantage should be taken of the fact that the chest is a bilaterally symmetrical structure, and each side should be compared with the other as a control. For example, tension pneumothorax produces an ipsilateral hyperinflation of the chest, with hyperresonance and decreased breath sounds.

In patients with significant emphysema and air trapping, pneumothorax may occur spontaneously or with minor trauma, such as chest physical therapy. The presence of a pneumothorax may be difficult to detect on physical examination in such patients, because the findings are similar to those of the underlying COPD (increased thoracic diameter, hyperresonance, decreased breath sounds, decreased fremitus) (14). The pneumothorax may not be evident on inspiratory chest films, because of the pulmonary hyperinflation; an expiratory film is useful in such cases.

## PERCUSSION

Percussion of the chest is useful because the chest contains structures of both air and fluid density, and in the presence of disease their relationships may vary. With pleural effusions, consolidation, large intrathoracic masses, or atelectasis, the chest is dull to percussion. With pneumothorax or hyperinflation, the chest is hyperresonant. The generalized hyperresonance in patients with emphysema may cause the examiner to miss a small pneumothorax; in such patients, mediastinal shift may be limited due to air trapping on the opposite side (14).

Percussion over the area of the diaphragm during maximal inspiration and expiration allows the examiner to estimate the extent of diaphragm motion. This is one of the few objective measurements for assessing diaphragm movement. With emphysema, the diaphragm is low and flat and movement is minimal.

## AUSCULTATION

The examiner should become familiar with the character of normal breath sounds. In the average resting person, inspiration involves approximately one-third

**TABLE 5.2**
**LUNG SOUND NOMENCLATURE**

| Description | Term | Time Expanded Waveform |
|---|---|---|
| Discontinuous | | |
|     Fine (high pitch, low amplitude, short duration) | Fine crackles | ⎯⎯⎯ᴸ⎯⎯ |
|     Coarse (low pitch, high amplitude, long duration) | Coarse crackles | ⎯⎯⎯√⎯⎯ |
| Continuous | | |
|     High-pitched | Wheezes | ∿∿∿∿ |
|     Low-pitched | Rhonchus | ∿∿∿ |

of the respiratory cycle and expiration the remaining two-thirds. Breath sounds vary according to the site of auscultation. Over the trachea, bronchial breath sounds are a normal finding.

Transmission of voice-generated sounds to the chest wall can be evaluated by either palpation or auscultation. Again, it is important to compare the two sides when listening for the conduction of voice sounds. A localized increase in the clarity of whispered or spoken sounds is associated with bronchial breathing and occurs with consolidation around open airways. Several words have been devised to describe this increased conduction of sound through fluid; these include bronchophony, egophony, and whispered pectoriloquy. Decreased conduction of whispered or spoken sounds occurs in the presence of obstructed bronchi, pneumothorax, or large collections of fluid or tissue between the lung and the chest wall.

The terminology of adventitious sounds in the chest has been confusing in the past, and there are still differences in terminology in different countries. In an attempt to unify the terminology a series of symposia have been held in several countries. The recommendations of the International Lung Sounds Association are those used in this chapter (Table 5.2) (15).

### Discontinuous Sounds

The word "rale" was originally devised by Laennec to signify a variety of abnormal chest sounds. Because of the confusion associated with this term, Robertson and Coope introduced the term "crackles" to describe the series of tiny explosions heard over the chest wall during inspiration (16). A number of qualifying adjectives have been used, such as crepitant, subcrepitant, dry, and wet. To avoid confusion only the terms coarse and fine should be used.

A careful analysis of chest physical findings with

**TABLE 5.3**
**CLINICAL CONDITIONS AND TIMING OF CRACKLES**

| Early Crackles | Late Crackles |
|---|---|
| Chronic bronchitis | Diffuse interstitial fibrosis |
| Asthma | Airspace pneumonia |
| Emphysema | Pulmonary congestion and |
| "Atelectatic crackles" |    edema |
| Bronchopneumonia | Sarcoidosis |
| | Scleroderma |
| | Rheumatoid lung |
| | Asbestosis |

waveform analysis has revealed that the *timing* of crackles is important. Those that begin early in inspiration are likely to be associated with airway obstruction (Table 5.3). Early, fine crackles are usually caused by small airway closure at end-expiration and disappear after a few deep breaths. Coarse, early inspiratory crackles are usually associated with bronchitis or bronchopneumonia. Fine, superficial crackles that occur late in inspiration ("Velcro") are usually associated with diseases that cause a restrictive ventilatory defect, such as idiopathic diffuse interstitial fibrosis, asbestosis, and sarcoidosis.

### Continuous Sounds

These sounds have a longer duration than crackles, usually lasting more than 250 msec. They have a musical quality that crackles do not have. Continuous breath sounds are either wheezes, which are high-pitched and arise in small airways, or rhonchi, which are low-pitched and occur in large airways (17). Wheezes generally occur in the presence of bronchospasm and are an important finding in asthma. Occasionally, a wheeze may begin with an audible pop as a small airway opens during inspiration. This crackle, followed by a high-pitched wheeze, has been called a "sibilant crackle" and has the same significance as a wheeze.

The word rhonchus means snore; rhonchi are common in severely ill patients whose secretions have collected in proximal airways. They occur in the presence of large-airway disease (stricture, foreign body, tumor, or mucus secretions), and those that clear with coughing are associated with sputum in larger airways. The presence of a localized wheeze or rhonchus that does not clear with coughing and does not change from one examination to another suggests an intrinsic defect in a large airway, such as a bronchogenic neoplasm. Because of the constricting nature of these lesions, the rhonchus usually occurs during both inspiration and expiration.

### Other Adventitious Sounds

In the presence of air in the pericardium or mediastinum, a coarse, crackling sound called a "mediastinal crunch" may be heard that is synchronous with systole. This sound may be associated with a pericardial friction rub.

A pleural friction rub is a grating sound associated with breathing. Rapid tape recordings have demonstrated that pleural friction rubs are actually a series of tiny explosions, just as crackles are (17). Pleural friction rubs are generally loud and sound as if they are immediately under the stethoscope. They occur during both inspiration and expiration, generally at the end of inspiration and the beginning of expiration. If a patient has pleuritic chest pain, it is useful to ask him or her to point to the location of the pain and to listen over that area, since the rub will be loudest there. The rub will often occur simultaneously with the patient's chest pain.

Pericardial friction rubs are similar to pleural rubs except that they occur with atrial and ventricular systole and diastole. They are best heard at the left sternal border at about the third interspace. It is useful to have the patient stop breathing, at which time the pericardial friction rub should persist. Pericardial and pleural friction rubs may occur simultaneously.

### EXTRAPULMONARY SIGNS

A wide variety of physical findings outside the thorax may occur in patients with pulmonary diseases. Hypoxemia is associated with cyanosis if 5 g/dl or more of reduced hemoglobin is present in the capillary blood. Central cyanosis implies involvement of gas transfer in the lungs and affects the tongue as well as the extremities. Peripheral cyanosis without central cyanosis implies a circulatory problem such as vascular spasm or shock.

Clubbing of the digits may or may not be associated

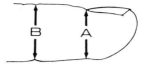

**FIGURE 5.2.** Clubbing of the fingers is best assessed by determining the ratio of the diameter at the base of the nail (**A**) to the diameter at the distal interphalangeal joint (**B**). This ratio is normally less than 1.

with cyanosis. It is seen with many chest diseases, including neoplasms, bronchiectasis, and lung abscess. It may be inherited as a familial trait or may occur with diseases of other organs such as the liver. The most reliable evidence of digital clubbing is an increase in the ratio of the diameter of the digit at the base of the nail to the diameter of the distal interphalangeal joint (Fig. 5.2). This ratio is always less than unity unless clubbing is present.

Patients who have pulmonary neoplasms may have one of several paraneoplastic syndromes, which are usually related to the production of hormones by tumor cells (see Chapter 17). Horner's syndrome occurs when apical lung tumors invade outside the pleura and into the superior cervical ganglion. There is ipsilateral enophthalmos, loss of sweating, and meiosis. Invasion of the brachial plexus nerves by these tumors may produce pain, atrophy, and loss of function in the ipsilateral arm.

## BEDSIDE ASSESSMENT OF CRITICALLY ILL PATIENTS

The development of the modern intensive care unit (ICU) has allowed us to monitor the physiologic processes electronically in severely ill patients. Too often, electronic monitors replace clinical examination. A number of factors interfere with the clinical examination in the ICU, including the condition of the patient, the ICU environment, and the equipment surrounding the patient (Table 5.4). It is a mistake to rely solely on information from sophisticated monitoring devices and laboratory flow sheets, since errors may occur if the data derived are not interpreted in the light of clinical findings. A rapid but careful examination of the patient remains an important diagnostic tool, and should be a part of daily rounds.

Several scoring systems, including APACHE (18) and SAPS (19), have been devised to give baseline information regarding the severity of illness. While there is some debate regarding their prognostic value, it is helpful to have some initial scoring system in order to follow serial changes in the patient's condition.

Reproduced with permission from Fidone JW, George RB. *J Crit Illness* 8:929–936, 1993.

**Table 5.4**

**Problems Encountered in the Physical Examination of Critically Ill Patients**

Environmental interference, such as ambient light and noise, lack of privacy

Reduced cooperation from the patient resulting from impaired consciousness, altered mental state, pain, drug effects

Difficulties in positioning the patient caused by orthopedic traction, abrasion, burns

The presence of therapeutic devices, such as the ventilator, drains, dressings, plaster casts, peritoneal dialysis machines, intra-aortic balloon pump, stomas, catheters, splints

The presence of monitoring devices, including arterial and venous lines, pulse oximeters, spectrometers, blood pressure cuff, electrocardiographic leads

Time limitations caused by nursing procedures, personal hygiene regimens (such as bathing and turning, during which the physician is unable to observe the patient), dressing changes, position changes, physiotherapy, electrocardiograms, bedside procedures, surgical evaluation, visits from friends and family

Visual assessment of the overall status is important. Is the patient awake or comatose? Is he or she receiving mechanical ventilation? What types of tubes are connected to the patient? Is the patient pallid, cyanotic, or jaundiced? Are there rashes or signs of trauma? Cool, cyanotic extremities indicate a low cardiac output (20), but also are found in the presence of peripheral vascular disease and in patients receiving vasopressor therapy. Muscle wasting indicates protein-calorie malnutrition; purpura and bruising suggest a coagulopathy; axillary petechiae suggest fat embolism.

A simple assessment of the patient's level of consciousness, including orientation and response to commands, can yield vital diagnostic and prognostic information. The neurologic status may be assessed using the Glasgow coma scale (Table 5.5) (21). This scale, originally proposed for use in victims of head trauma, is helpful for detecting and quantifying serial changes in the neurologic status. Coma scale scores range from 3 to 15 points; scores below 5 are associated with a very poor prognosis (21).

The vital signs often change rapidly in ICU patients. Palpate the peripheral pulse while watching the ECG monitor to check for a pulse deficit. Check all distal pulses in cannulated arteries. A weak, thready pulse indicates a low cardiac stroke volume, as is seen in cardiogenic or hypovolemic shock. A bounding pulse is common in sepsis associated with a low vascular

resistance and a high cardiac output. Pulsus alternans (every other pulse is weak) is associated with severely depressed left ventricular function. Pulsus paradoxus (a decline in systolic arterial pressure greater than 10 mm Hg with normal inspiration) is present in patients with severe airways obstruction (as in status asthmaticus), as well as in those with pericardial tamponade. High airway pressures during mechanical ventilation may produce pulsus paradoxus.

The rate and depth of respiration should be noted in spontaneously breathing patients. Rapid, shallow breathing is an early and reliable sign of respiratory muscle fatigue. A respiratory rate above 30 per minute suggests that mechanical ventilation should be considered, especially in the presence of abnormal arterial blood gases (22). Evidence of inspiratory muscle fatigue includes use of accessory respiratory muscles, respiratory alternans, and paradoxical abdominal motion. Respiratory alternans, a shift back and forth from chest wall to abdominal breathing, is likely a method of periodically resting certain muscle groups (23). Paradoxical abdominal motion consists of a movement inward rather than outward of the abdomen during inspiration, due to failure of the diaphragm to contract.

Pupils should be checked for size, equality, and reaction to light. Pupil size may be affected by drugs such as opiates that cause constriction, or those that cause dilatation such as catecholamines. Dilated, unreactive pupils are a late sign of brain stem herniation. They may also occur after local trauma, use of mydri-

**Table 5.5**

**The Glasgow Coma Scale**

| | |
|---|---|
| Verbal response (choose one) | |
| Oriented | 5 |
| Confused | 4 |
| Inappropriate words | 3 |
| Incomprehensible | 2 |
| None | 1 |
| Eye opening (choose one) | |
| Spontaneously | 4 |
| To speech | 3 |
| To pain | 2 |
| None | 1 |
| Motor response (choose one) | |
| Obeys commands | 6 |
| Localizes pain | 5 |
| Withdraws | 4 |
| Abnormal flexion | 3 |
| Abnormal extension | 2 |
| None | 1 |
| Total | 3–15 |

Adapted from Teasdale G, Jennett B: Assessment of coma and impaired consciousness: a practical scale. *Lancet* 2:81–84, 1974.

atic agents, third nerve lesions, seizures, or cerebral hypoxia.

Eye reflexes should be noted serially in comatose patients. The pupillary light reflex and corneal touch reflex may be absent initially after a cardiac arrest, but should return within 1 hour. Absence of these reflexes 6 or more hours after cardiac arrest is a very poor prognostic indicator for cerebral recovery. Rapidly rotating the head from side to side stimulates both the vestibular apparatus and proprioceptors in the neck, resulting in the **oculocephalic** or "doll's eye" reflex. The presence of a doll's eye reflex (movement of the eyes in the direction opposite that of head rotation) indicates that brain stem function is intact.

Clinicians should become familiar with the normal ventilator sounds and should be aware of any alarms, auditory or visual. Check the mode of ventilation, the airway pressure, and the exhaled volume indicator. Several of the current ventilators monitor both peak and plateau airway pressures and can quantify the patient's spontaneous efforts versus ventilator-delivered breaths. About 40% of functional ventilator problems occur in the external circuitry. Be alert for leaking humidifiers, disconnections, valve failures, and leaking tubing. Bubbling or gurgling sounds at the mouth indicate a leaking cuff or migration of the cuff outside the larynx. Make sure the alarms have not been manually deactivated.

Migration of the endotracheal tube into a bronchus is a common problem in the ICU. Asymmetric chest expansion and diminished breath sounds over the left hemithorax are characteristic of right main bronchus intubation, which is more common than left main bronchus intubation, due to the architecture of the bronchial tree. The normal tendency of endotracheal tubes is to migrate toward the carina.

When examining the limbs, observe the response to painful stimuli, assess muscle tone and range of joint movement, and check tendon reflexes. Many patients are hypotonic due to metabolic or toxic encephalopathy, drug overdose, anesthesia, or the use of sedatives or neuromuscular blocking drugs. Increased muscle tone is the classic finding in upper motor neuron lesions.

▼

## References

1. U.S. Public Health Service: The health consequences of smoking—cardiovascular disease—A report of the Surgeon General. Washington, DC, U.S. Government Printing Office, 1983.
2. Wall M, Brooks J, Holsclaw D, Redding G: Health effects of smoking on children. ATS Statement. *Am Rev Respir Dis* 132:1137, 1985.
3. Banaszak EF, Thiede WH, Fink JN: Hypersensitivity pneumonitis due to contamination of an air conditioner. *N Engl J Med* 283:271, 1970.
4. Irwin RS, Rosen MJ, Braman SS: Cough, a comprehensive review. *Arch Intern Med* 137:1186, 1977.
5. Corrao WM, Braman SS, Irwin RS: Chronic cough as the sole presenting manifestation of bronchial asthma. *N Engl J Med* 300, 1979.
6. Pratter MR, Irwin RS: The clinical value of pharmacologic bronchoprovocation challenge. *Chest* 85:260, 1984.
7. Bucknall CE, Neilly JB, Carter R, Stevenson RD, Semple PF: Bronchial hyperreactivity in patients who cough after receiving angiotensin converting enzyme inhibitors. *Br Med J* 296:86–88, 1988.
8. Reid L: Measurement of the bronchial mucous gland layer: a diagnostic yardstick in chronic bronchitis. *Thorax* 15:132, 1960.
9. Epstein RL: Constituents of sputum: a simple method. *Ann Intern Med* 77:259–265, 1972.
10. Bartlett JG: Anaerobic infections of the lung. *Chest* 91:901, 1987.
11. Elliott RC, Reichel J: The efficacy of sputum specimens obtained by nebulizer versus gastric aspirates in the bacteriologic diagnosis of pulmonary tuberculosis. *Am Rev Respir Dis* 88:223–227, 1963.
12. Soll B, Selecky PA, Chang R, et al: The use of the fiberoptic bronchoscope in the evaluation of hemoptysis. *AARD* 15:165, 1978.
13. Corey R, Hla KM: Major and massive hemoptysis: reassessment of conservative management. *Am J Med Sci* 294:301–309, 1987.
14. George RB, Herbert SJ, Shames JM, Ellithorpe DB, Weill H, Ziskind MM: Pneumothorax complicating pulmonary emphysema. *JAMA* 234:389–393, 1975.
15. Mikami R, Murao M, Cugell DW, et al: International symposium on lung sounds: synopsis of proceedings. *Chest* 92:342, 1987.
16. Robertson AJ, Coope R: Rales, rhonchi, and Laennec. *Lancet* 2:417, 1957.
17. Forgacs P: Crackles and wheezes. *Lancet* 2:203, 1967.
18. Knaus WA: Prognosis with mechanical ventilation: the influence of disease, severity of disease, age and chronic health status on survival from an acute illness. *Am Rev Respir Dis* 140:S8–13, 1989.
19. LeGall JR, Loriat P, Alperovich A, Glaser P, Granthil C, Mathieu D, et al: Simplified acute physiological score for intensive care patients. *Lancet* 2:741, 1983.
20. Joly HR, Weil MH: Temperature of the great toe as an indication of the severity of shock. *Circulation* 39:131, 1969.
21. Teasdale G, Jennett B: Assessment of coma and impaired consciousness: a practical scale. *Lancet* 2:81–84, 1974.
22. Pardu NE, Winterbauer RH, Allen JD: Bedside evaluation of respiratory distress. *Chest* 85:203–206, 1984.
23. Rochester DF, Arora NS: Respiratory muscle fatigue. *Med Clin North Am* 67:573–579, 1983.

Chapter **6**

# Invasive Diagnostic Procedures

**William McDowell Anderson**
**Richard W. Light**

THE MAJORITY of chest diseases can be diagnosed on the basis of the history, physical findings, pulmonary function tests, and chest radiographs. When these basic procedures are not adequate to define a patient's illness, additional studies are available that allow the physician to define lung abnormalities with precision. These invasive tests, including the various biopsy procedures, not only carry increased risks, but are costly. In this time of fiscal responsibility the clinician must choose, from a battery of increasingly specialized diagnostic procedures, those that are most likely to yield the desired results while having the least risk and cost to the patient. This chapter discusses some of these specialized techniques: thoracentesis, pleural biopsy, bronchoscopy with specialized procedures including bronchoalveolar lavage, protected specimen brushing and transbronchial needle aspiration, transthoracic needle aspiration and biopsy, open lung biopsy, thoracoscopy, and mediastinoscopy. Other tests—such as arterial blood gases and oximetry, capnography, metabolic and nutritional evaluation, and various invasive and noninvasive tests for venous thrombosis—are discussed in the chapters devoted to the diseases for which they are most often used.

## PLEURAL FLUID EXAMINATION

Pleural involvement often accompanies diseases of the lung parenchyma and is usually associated with abnormal amounts of fluid in the pleural space. The amount of pleural fluid present can be estimated by obtaining a lateral decubitus chest radiograph with the suspected side down and measuring the thickness of the fluid between the inner border of the ribs and the lower part of the lung (Fig. 6.1). If the thickness of the fluid is greater than 10 mm, a sample of fluid can usually be obtained for diagnostic thoracentesis.

### THORACENTESIS

The site for insertion of the needle should be determined with care. It is best to make the insertion in the

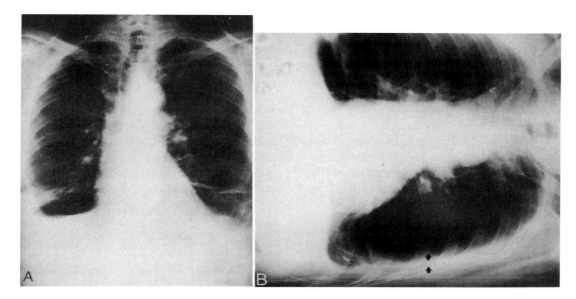

**FIGURE 6.1.** Lateral decubitus radiograph demonstrating pleural effusion. On the erect posteroanterior radiograph (**A**), both costophrenic angles are blunted. In the left lateral decubitus position (**B**), there is a definite fluid line between the outer part of the lung and the inside of the chest wall. Since the distance between the *arrows* was greater than 10 mm, a diagnostic thoracentesis was performed.

posterior region, where the ribs are easily palpable and to where the fluid gravitates. With the patient in the sitting position, the level is identified at which tactile fremitus is lost and the light percussion note becomes dull. Thoracentesis should be attempted first in the interspace below this level.

The handling of the pleural fluid for the different tests is outlined in Table 6.1. For bacterial cultures, 5 ml of pleural fluid should be put into both aerobic and anaerobic culture media. For determination of pleural fluid pH, the sample should be sent to the laboratory on ice in the original syringe.

### PLEURAL FLUID APPEARANCE

The gross appearance of pleural fluid yields useful diagnostic information, and so the color, turbidity, viscosity, and odor of the pleural fluid should be recorded (1). Most transudative and many exudative effusions are clear, straw-colored, nonviscid, and odorless. A white milky appearance indicates chylothorax, a chyliform pleural effusion, or empyema. Pus in the pleural fluid can be distinguished from chylothorax and chyliform effusion, because after centrifugation there is a clear, yellowish supernatant fluid in purulent effusions. A foul odor may be present if empyema is caused by anaerobic organisms.

It requires only 5,000 to 10,000 red blood cells per cubic millimeter to impart a red color to a pleural effusion. Thus, 1 ml of blood in a moderately sized effusion will result in blood-tinged pleural fluid. The diagnostic value of blood-tinged fluid is limited, since over 15% of transudates and over 40% of exudates are blood tinged (2). Grossly bloody effusions have red cell counts above $100,000/mm^3$. This finding is suggestive of one of three disease processes: trauma, malignancy (including malignant mesothelioma and metastatic

**TABLE 6.1**

**DISTRIBUTION OF PLEURAL FLUID OBTAINED WITH DIAGNOSTIC THORACENTESIS**

| Laboratory | Amount (ml) | Tests Ordered |
|---|---|---|
| Bacteriology | 10 | Aerobic and anaerobic cultures<br>Gram stain |
| Tuberculosis and mycology | 5 | Tuberculosis and fungal cultures |
| Cytology | 10 | Cytology |
| Hematology | 5 | Red cell count<br>White cell count<br>Wright stain |
| Chemistry | 5 | Glucose<br>Amylase<br>Lactic dehydrogenase<br>Protein |
| Blood gas | 5 | pH |

neoplasms), or, less commonly, pulmonary embolism (2). A hematocrit should be obtained on grossly bloody pleural fluids to determine whether or not a hemothorax is present. If the pleural fluid hematocrit is more than 50% that of the peripheral blood, a hemothorax is present (see Chapter 18).

### Separation of Transudates from Exudates

The first question that must be answered when a pleural effusion is discovered is whether the effusion is a transudate or an exudate. Transudates by definition are pleural effusions that result from imbalances of the hydrostatic and osmotic forces in the pleural or pulmonary capillaries. Exudates are pleural effusions that result from increased permeability of the pleural or pulmonary capillaries (3). If the effusion is a transudate, no further diagnostic procedures are necessary, and therapy is directed toward the underlying congestive heart failure, cirrhosis, or nephrosis. Alternatively, if the effusion proves to be an exudate, more extensive diagnostic procedures are needed to delineate the cause of the pleural disease.

Exudative pleural effusions can be separated effectively from transudative pleural effusions with the simultaneous use of protein and lactic acid dehydrogenase (LDH) levels in the pleural fluid and serum. Exudates meet at least *one* of the following three criteria, while transudates meet none (4).

1. The pleural fluid protein divided by the serum protein is greater than 0.5;
2. The pleural fluid LDH divided by the serum LDH is greater than 0.6;
3. The pleural fluid LDH is greater than two-thirds of the upper limit of normal for the serum LDH.

In the past decade several other tests—including the pleural fluid bilirubin level, the ratio of pleural fluid to serum bilirubin, the pleural fluid cholesterol, the pleural fluid/serum cholesterol ratio, and the pleural fluid serum albumin gradient—have been suggested as being useful in the separation of transudates from exudates (1). However, it appears that use of the protein and the LDH are as effective as any of the newer criteria in making this differentiation (5). If it is strongly suspected that the patient has a transudative pleural effusion, the most cost-effective use of the laboratory is to order only protein and LDH levels on the pleural fluid. Then, only if these tests demonstrate an exudate are additional tests ordered (1).

### Pleural Fluid Cell Count and Differential

The pleural fluid white blood cell count is of limited value, since it depends on the ratio between the amount of fluid present and the number of cells entering the pleural space. In general, a white cell count of $1,000/mm^3$ or greater suggests an exudate. Parapneumonic effusions usually contain white cell counts above $10,000/mm^3$; however, this is also seen in effusions due to pancreatitis, pulmonary infarction, collagen vascular diseases, malignancy, and tuberculosis (2, 6).

The differential white cell count is a very useful test and should be performed in all cases in which exudates are present. Mesothelial cells normally line the pleural cavity and have a relatively large, round nucleus with light blue cytoplasm. They are occasionally confused with malignant cells, especially in the presence of inflammation, and this may lead to a false diagnosis. They are rarely seen in tuberculous effusions.

If the pleural fluid contains more than 50% lymphocytes, likely diagnoses include granulomatous disease (particularly tuberculosis) and malignancy. Since these are the two types of disease that can be diagnosed with pleural biopsy, the finding of a lymphocytosis in an exudative effusion is an indication for pleural biopsy unless a diagnosis is obtained from the pleural fluid. The presence of neutrophils suggests an acute inflammatory response. Pleural fluid neutrophilia is seen in effusions associated with pneumonia, pancreatitis, pulmonary embolism, and peritonitis. Occasionally, very early tuberculous effusions will have a predominance of neutrophils. The presence of pleural fluid eosinophilia is of little use in the differential diagnosis (1). Most effusions with eosinophil counts greater than 10% are either bloody or associated with a pneumothorax. Other possibilities include a drug reaction, paragonimiasis, asbestos exposure, the Churg-Strauss syndrome, or a resolving parapneumonic effusion.

### Pleural Fluid Chemistries

Pleural fluid protein and LDH levels may be useful in the differential diagnosis of exudates, since a very high LDH level with only moderate protein elevations suggests a malignancy (4). Since the pleural fluid LDH provides an accurate index of the degree of pleural inflammation, it should be measured each time a thoracentesis is performed to reflect whether the process causing the pleural effusion is getting better or worse. A pleural fluid protein level above 6.0 g/dl suggests tuberculosis or a parapneumonic effusion.

The pleural fluid glucose level of transudates and most exudates parallels that of the serum. However, there are seven types of effusions in which the glucose in the pleural fluid is often below 60 mg/dl. These are effusions due to pneumonia, tuberculosis, malignancy, rheumatoid disease, hemothorax, paragonimiasis, and the Churg-Strauss syndrome (1).

The pleural fluid amylase is elevated in pancreatic pleural effusions, in esophageal rupture (in which the markedly elevated amylase is salivary rather than pancreatic), and malignancy (usually adenocarcinoma, associated with elevated salivary amylase). Patients with chronic pancreatic pleural effusions may have only chest symptoms, and, if the pleural fluid amylase level is not measured, the diagnosis of this disease (which is curable surgically) can easily be missed. If there is doubt as to whether the patient has malignancy or pancreatic disease, isoenzymes of amylase should be determined, because the high amylase with malignancy is of the salivary rather than the pancreatic type (7).

The determination of pleural fluid pH is most useful in patients with parapneumonic effusions. A pleural fluid pH below 7.00 in this situation suggests a complicated effusion, that is, one associated with loculation that may go on to develop into an empyema. It has been recommended that a pleural fluid pH below 7.20 is an indication for placement of a chest tube, since progression to empyema is extremely likely (8). Pleural fluid glucose levels are usually decreased concomitantly with pH in patients with parapneumonic effusions. The value of the pH is that it is generally available within a few minutes (whereas the glucose level may take several hours), and the decision for chest tube placement can therefore be made more rapidly. It is extremely important that the fluid be handled anaerobically and sent immediately to the blood gas laboratory for pH determination to ensure its accuracy. In addition to parapneumonic effusions, rheumatoid effusions and effusions associated with malignancy or tuberculosis may have pH levels below 7.20.

## PLEURAL FLUID BACTERIOLOGY AND CYTOLOGY

When a diagnostic thoracentesis is performed, the fluid should be cultured for both aerobic and anaerobic organisms. Mycobacterial and fungal cultures should also be obtained if there is a possibility of tuberculosis or fungal infection. A Gram stain of the fluid should be examined to rule out the presence of bacteria.

A pleural fluid cytologic examination should be ordered if malignancy is suspected; the first pleural fluid cytologic examination will be positive for malignant cells in about 60% of malignant pleural effusions (1). If three separate specimens are submitted, up to 90% of malignant effusions will be positive for malignant cells on cytopathologic examination. Care must be taken that mesothelial cells that have undergone change in response to inflammation are not misinterpreted as malignant cells. Also, pleural effusions in patients with malignancies may be caused by other mechanisms besides direct involvement of the pleura,

including atelectasis or lymphatic obstruction. Pleural fluid cytologic examination and pleural biopsy are additive in their yields, and when a pleural biopsy is performed the fluid obtained during the procedure should always be sent for analysis.

## OTHER TESTS

In special situations useful information may be obtained with additional tests on the pleural fluid. If systemic lupus erythematosus is suspected, a pleural fluid antinuclear antibody (ANA) titer should be obtained, since a titer of 1:160 or above is very supportive of this diagnosis (9). If pleural tuberculosis is suspected, the pleural fluid adenosine deaminase (ADA) and the pleural fluid interferon gamma are useful tests. A pleural fluid ADA level above 70 U/liter virtually establishes the diagnosis of tuberculous pleuritis, while a level below 40 U/liter virtually excludes the diagnosis. A pleural fluid interferon gamma level above 200 pg/ml is nearly diagnostic, while a level below 100 nearly excludes the diagnosis of tuberculous pleuritis (10). Immunohistochemical methods with monoclonal antibodies can be useful in establishing the diagnosis of malignancy and separating mesotheliomas from adenocarcinomas. A recent report suggested that the use of anti-CEA, EMA, and B72.3 was sufficient in over 95% of cases to make these differentiations (11).

Pleural fluid that remains milky or opalescent after centrifugation is either a chylous or a chyliform pleural effusion. A chylous effusion arises when the thoracic duct is severed or obstructed, most often by a tumor involving the mediastinum. A pleural fluid triglyceride level above 110 mg/dl is virtually diagnostic of a chylous pleural effusion.

A chyliform or cholesterol pleural effusion develops when a pleural effusion has been present for a long time. In such cases, for unknown reasons, cholesterol accumulates in the fluid and causes a milky opalescent appearance. Pleural fluid lipid analysis in this case reveals elevated cholesterol and normal triglycerides.

## PLEURAL BIOPSY

Pleural biopsies are obtained rather easily in patients with significant pleural effusions. The biopsy is performed with either the Cope or the Abrams pleural biopsy needle (6). Pleural biopsy is useful in diagnosing granulomatous disease or malignancy of the pleura, and should be performed only if these two diseases are suspected and thus primarily in patients with exudates of relatively long duration.

Prior to performing the biopsy, a thoracentesis should be performed to determine the location for biopsy and to ensure that fluid is present. Bleeding and clotting times should be determined to ensure that there is no bleeding diathesis. In loculated pleural effusions, if localization is difficult, the patient may be examined with ultrasound to determine the best site for biopsy. For patients with large nonloculated effusions, a site in the lower posterior chest approximately two rib interspaces below the tip of the scapula is preferred.

The yield of pleural biopsy depends on patient selection, the technique used, and the number of biopsies performed. In patients with chronic exudates, the pleura is thicker and thus easier to examine. Experience of the person performing the biopsy is correlated with increased yield. If adequate pleura is obtained from three separate biopsies performed on different occasions, tuberculosis can be diagnosed in over 80% and malignancy in over 50% of cases. A pleural specimen should always be sent for mycobacterial and fungal cultures. In patients with tuberculous or fungal effusions, the pleural biopsy cultures may be positive when pleural fluid cultures are not.

## BRONCHOSCOPY

The bronchoscope has become the leading invasive tool of the physician evaluating and treating patients with a wide spectrum of pulmonary disorders and diseases. Direct airway visualization was described by Justav Killian, who reported the use of a laryngoscope to evaluate the lower trachea and main stem bronchi in 1902 (12). By 1928, bronchoscopy was predominantly performed using a rigid bronchoscope for the inspection of large airways, with limited use for extraction of foreign bodies (13). With the introduction of the fiberoptic bronchoscope by Ikeda in the early 1970s, the examination of the airways became more widespread with expanded diagnostic and therapeutic use of the instrument. More recent introduction of video bronchoscopic techniques, combined with computer imaging, can now allow more accurate staging of endobronchial lesions, especially in the management of bronchogenic carcinoma.

The survey of bronchoscopy sponsored by the American College of Chest Physicians (ACCP) reported a mean of 115 procedures performed per physician, among the 466 physicians who reported bronchoscopic procedures (14, 15). A total of over 50,000 procedures were performed in 1989 by this group at costs of $300 to $750. In view of the significant cost of the procedure, and marked therapeutic and diagnostic benefits, this section will review the indications and complications of the procedure, as well as special techniques of bronchial lavage, transbronchial biopsy, and transtracheal needle aspiration and biopsy.

## INDICATIONS

The American Thoracic Society has published guidelines that present the indications for fiberoptic bronchoscopy (16) (Table 6.2). When asked to list the five most common indications for bronchoscopy in their clinical practice, the respondents to the ACCP survey most commonly listed hemoptysis, pneumonia/infection, diffuse pulmonary processes, and other therapeutic reasons. (Interesting findings included the fact that nearly one-fourth of the physicians mentioned cough as one of the five indications.) As with previous surveys, these results suggest that the major indication for fiberoptic bronchoscopy is a suspected lung neoplasm. Characteristics associated with a high risk of carcinoma include an age greater than 40 years and a history of cigarette smoking or other chronic toxic exposure.

Hemoptysis is a common finding of patients with bronchogenic carcinoma and therefore is frequently an indication for diagnostic bronchoscopy. In the series of Weaver and coworkers (17), all patients with carcinoma had (a) age greater than 40 years, (b) an abnormal

**TABLE 6.2**
**INDICATIONS FOR BRONCHOSCOPY**

| Diagnostic | Therapeutic |
|---|---|
| Suspected lung cancer | Remove secretions not |
|   Abnormality on chest |   mobilized by other |
|     radiograph of unknown |   techniques |
|     etiology | Remove foreign bodies |
|   Hemoptysis | Remove abnormal |
|   Unexplained cough |   endobronchial tissue |
|   Localized wheeze | Difficult endotracheal |
|   Positive sputum cytology |   tube intubation |
|   Phrenic or recurrent | Lung lavage for |
|     laryngeal nerve paralysis |   alveolar proteinosis |
|   Superior vena cava | Endobronchial stent |
|     syndrome |   placement |
| Chylothorax | Brachytherapy |
| Unexplained pleural effusion | |
| Lung abscess unresponsive to | |
|   therapy | |
| Endotracheal tube placement | |
|   and complications | |
| Staging of lung cancer | |
| Obtain culture material | |
| Airway trauma | |
| Tracheoesophageal fistula | |
| Assessment of injury from | |
|   noxious fumes or gastric | |
|   content aspiration | |
| Bronchography | |
| Diffuse lung disease | |

chest radiograph, and (c) persistent hemoptysis for longer than 1 week. Other factors that should be considered include the presence of anemia, weight loss, persistent cough, a history of smoking, and male sex. Carcinoma is less of a consideration if the chest radiograph reveals diffuse or nonlocalized abnormalities (2.5% incidence of carcinoma) (18). The prognosis for patients with hemoptysis of undetermined origin (cryptogenic) with a negative bronchoscopy is generally good, usually with resolution of bleeding within 6 months of evaluation (19). Positive results for fiberoptic bronchoscopy and biopsy for endobronchially visible carcinoma are above 90% (20, 21). In nonvisible lesions, the yield is much less and is dependent on the position of the tumor on the chest radiograph. This yield is 94% for hilar abnormalities, 76% for perihilar abnormalities, and 36% for peripheral abnormalities, when a combination of bronchial biopsies, brushings, and washings are analyzed (22). It is also important to perform bronchoscopy in all patients with substantial hemoptysis (over 300 ml per 24 hours) to identify the source of bleeding in case surgery is necessary.

Peripheral pulmonary nodules (coin lesions) represent a particular diagnostic challenge, and the appropriate choice of procedures is controversial (23). Positioning the patient laterally and using biplane fluoroscopy for biopsy instrument localization both probably increase yield compared with single-plane fluoroscopy (24, 25). Bronchoscopic techniques are more sensitive if brush biopsy is performed prior to forceps biopsy to prevent the brush from becoming coated with blood from previous biopsies. In addition, some investigators recommend use of bronchial alveolar lavage, as opposed to bronchial washings, to acquire adequate cytology specimens (26, 27).

Other techniques currently being developed for the diagnosis of peripheral bronchogenic carcinomas are bronchial curettage, ultra-thin fiberoptic bronchoscopy, transbronchial needle aspiration (TBNA), and needle brush. Transbronchial curettage is used predominantly in Japan and involves passage of a single- or double-hinge curette through the bronchoscope and vigorously scraping the tumor. For lesions less than 2 cm in diameter, the yield is 76% for the single-hinged curette and up to 97% for the double-hinged curette (28). Diagnostic yield may be enhanced using the ultrathin (1.8 to 2.2 mm) fiberoptic bronchoscope passed through the channel of a regular bronchoscope. This allows direct visualization of the tumor, which may lead to success with bronchial biopsies (29). The disadvantage of the technique is that a lesion cannot be aspirated or biopsied through the channel. Combining newer techniques of TBNA with bronchial washing

and brushing can increase diagnostic yields in peripheral carcinoma from 48 to 69%. The size of the lesion under biopsy is important: only 33% of studies showed positive results with TBNA plus washing when the lesion was less than 2 cm in diameter, as opposed to a yield of 76% when the lesion was larger than 2 cm (30, 31). Biopsy results may be further enhanced by using the new needle brush biopsy technique. When this procedure was performed along with a regular cytology brush biopsy, TBNA, and a forceps biopsy, the needle brush technique had a diagnostic yield of approximately 50%, with diagnosis exclusively by this technique in four of the 24 patients studied (32).

Other visualization techniques for peripheral lesions, such as the high-resolution computed tomographic (CT) scan, can improve the accuracy of bronchoscopy. When a "bronchus sign" is seen on a CT scan, there is a 90% chance of accurate diagnosis by transbronchial forceps biopsy. This sign is defined as the finding of a bronchus leading directly to a peripheral pulmonary mass. When it is not present, the diagnostic yield of transbronchial biopsy is decreased by 18 to 30% (33, 34). More recently, the use of diagnostic ultrasound through the bronchoscope has shown promising preliminary results in guiding transbronchial biopsies of peripheral lung lesions (35).

The patient with malignant cells in the sputum but no evidence of a neoplasm on a chest radiograph (so-called 'occult cancer') presents a special diagnostic problem. The prevalence of occult lung cancer may increase with the increased application of newer technology, including the solid-state microscope system used for prescreening of sputum cytology specimens. This technology aids in the identification of normal epithelial cells, growing in the proximity of cancerous growths, that exhibit different DNA distribution patterns than the normal cells of individuals without cancer. This phenomenon is referred to as malignancy-associated changes (MACs) (36). Fiberoptic bronchoscopy permits demonstration of the tumor in most cases (37). However, if no lesion is found, all subsegments of the lung must then be sampled (38). Repeat bronchoscopy is occasionally necessary, and if positive results are obtained with either forceps biopsy or two consecutive brush specimens, the procedure may need to be repeated. If results are positive on two different occasions, surgical intervention is recommended (38). To improve the diagnosis of occult lung cancer, photodynamic techniques have been developed that allow photosensitization of malignant cells by administering compounds such as hematoporphyrin or a derivative, dihematoporphyrin. Fluorescent compounds such as these, when injected intravenously, can accumulate in malignant tissue at higher concentrations than in normal tissue (36). When exposed to light, usually a helium-cadmium laser light source administered through a bronchoscope, abnormal tissues contain a fluorescent material and emit a salmon-red fluorescence.

Using this new technique for the diagnosis of occult cancer, the sensitivity for premalignant lesions and carcinoma in situ can be improved from the current level of 48.4% to a sensitivity of 72.5% with similar specificity of approximately 94% (36, 39). Areas of concern found using these techniques can then be evaluated by repeated bronchoscopy or treated locally with laser or surgical resection or therapy with hematoporphyrin phototherapy (40).

While routine bronchoscopy for lung abscess is not indicated, there are certain situations for which the procedure may be useful. For diagnostic purposes, the procedure may be indicated to rule out underlying carcinoma when patients have: (a) few systemic symptoms of infection; (b) no predisposition for aspiration; (c) relatively low white blood cell count ($<11 \times 10^3$ cells/mm$^3$); (d) low-grade fever ($<100$ F orally); and (e) limited infiltrates or lymphadenopathy on initial chest radiograph (41). A rigid bronchoscopic evaluation may be preferable in cases when drainage of a nonresolving abscess is indicated in order to control the airway. Rupture of a massive abscess, with the contents contaminating the rest of the lung and resulting in respiratory failure, has been reported (42).

In immunologically intact hosts with diffuse lung disease the reported diagnostic yield of fiberoptic bronchoscopy with transbronchial biopsy varies according to patient characteristics (43–46). Transbronchial biopsy specimens provide strong evidence for the specific diagnosis when stains for organisms are positive, malignant cells are identified, or granulomas are present. Thus, non-caseating granulomas can be identified in up to 90% of patients with sarcoidosis when four transbronchial biopsy specimens are obtained, especially in advanced stages of disease (45). In Stage II

disease the addition of from 5 to 10 biopsy specimens increased the yield to approximately 95%, with frequent diagnosis being obtained in patients with radiologically normal lungs. Analysis of helper (CD4) and suppressor (CD8) T lymphocytes may help in distinguishing sarcoidosis from hypersensitivity pneumonitis; in the former, the CD4:CD8 ratio may be as high as 20:1, and in the latter, the ratio is decreased or reversed (47). (The further role of bronchoalveolar lavage in the diagnosis of diffuse lung disease is presented in a subsequent section.) In the absence of pathogenic organisms, malignant cells, or granulomas, definitive diagnosis of the cause of diffuse lung disease requires an open lung biopsy. The comparison of the diagnostic yields and complications in four different biopsy procedures used to diagnose diffuse lung diseases is shown in Table 6.3 (44). In patients with idiopathic pulmonary fibrosis, open lung biopsy is the diagnostic procedure of choice; however, some investigators recommend fiberoptic bronchoscopy in the subset of elderly patients with significant respiratory impairment to rule out granulomatous disease, neoplasm, infection, and specific entities such as histiocytosis and pulmonary alveolar proteinosis (48).

In patients who are suspected of having pulmonary tuberculosis or fungal infections and whose sputum smears and cultures are negative, fiberoptic bronchoscopy with transbronchial biopsy may provide a diagnosis (49–51). In a recent retrospective analysis of 67 HIV-positive and 47 HIV-negative patients, an immediate diagnosis of tuberculosis was obtained in 38% of 66 patients who had had a negative sputum smear examination before bronchoscopy (49). There was no significant difference in the yield between HIV-positive and HIV-negative patients. Of interest in this retrospective study was the finding that 91% of the negative sputum samples from pre-bronchoscopy smears eventually yielded positive culture results. In view of these findings, the use of bronchoscopy to diagnose pulmonary tuberculosis before obtaining sputum culture results remains a matter of debate. The benefits of early

**TABLE 6.3**
**RESULTS OF LUNG BIOPSY PROCEDURES**

| Type of Biopsy | Number of Series | Number of Cases | Mortality (%) | Complications (%) | Diagnostic (%) |
|---|---|---|---|---|---|
| Needle core | 9 (1964–74) | 789 | 1.1 | 42.0 | 63 |
| Drill | 10 (1969–76) | 551 | 0.5 | 44.0 | 72 |
| Transbronchial | 8 (1974–78) | 1,289 | 0.2 | 12.8 | 72 |
| Open | 15 (1949–78) | 2,290 | 1.8 | 7.0 | 94 |

Reprinted from Wall CP, Gaensler EA, Carrington CB, et al: Comparison of transbronchial and open lung biopsies in chronic infiltrative lung diseases. *Am Rev Respir Dis* 123:283, 1981.

diagnosis must be weighed against the risk to the patient of bleeding and pneumothorax, and the risk to the bronchoscopist and technicians from nosocomial transmission of tuberculosis. Some investigators suggest that empiric therapy may be a reasonable alternative in appropriate patients (52).

The indications for fiberoptic bronchoscopy in immunocompromised patients with pulmonary infiltrates appears to be increasing with the prevalence of immunosuppressive therapy, organ transplantations, and the acquired immune deficiency syndrome (AIDS). However, the first step in the evaluation of a patient at risk of pulmonary infection is sputum analysis. This has been shown to be useful in the diagnosis of acute bacterial, *Pneumocystis*, fungal, and mycobacterial pneumonias (53). Special procedures, including liquefaction of induced sputum and immunofluorescent monoclonal antibody techniques, have increased the sensitivity of sputum analysis for *Pneumocystis carinii* pneumonia (PCP) in HIV-infected patients (not receiving inhaled pentamidine) to about 92%, a result similar to that obtained using fiberoptic bronchoscopy (54). A variety of techniques are available for the assessment of respiratory disease via fiberoptic bronchoscopy (Table 6.4). The usefulness of fiberoptic bronchoscopy with transbronchial biopsy and bronchoalveolar lavage for specific diseases varies according to disease presentation. With diffuse radiographic infiltrates, the yield for nonbacterial processes such as Pneumocystis pneumonia or pulmonary hemorrhage is 80 to 95% (55). In patients with segmental

or lobar nodular infiltrates, the usefulness of fiberoptic bronchoscopy is more variable (50 to 80%) (55). Specific diagnoses can be obtained in 30 to 55% of cases, with a false-negative rate ranging from 21 to 35% (56). Initial fiberoptic bronchoscopy was shown in a recent series to detect 166 of 173 identifiable pathogens (56). When both BAL and transbronchial lung biopsy were combined, 125 of 127 pathogens were identified (the yield for PCP was 100%). Whether transbronchial lung biopsy adds significantly to the diagnosis of PCP is questionable (57). When bronchoscopic techniques are not productive and localized disease is noticed on the radiograph, needle aspiration biopsy may be an effective procedure in diagnosing pneumonia (57). Open lung biopsy is reserved for (*a*) patients with progressive pulmonary deterioration and a nondiagnostic fiberoptic bronchoscopy; (*b*) patients with an uncorrected coagulopathy in whom BAL cannot be performed or is nondiagnostic; and (*c*) patients receiving mechanical ventilation who have had a nondiagnostic BAL.

Following aspiration of gastric contents, bronchoscopy is not routinely indicated but may be useful if aspiration of food or other solid particles is suspected. Fiberoptic bronchoscopy may be useful diagnostically following gastric acid aspiration, since the mucosa has a typical appearance with erythema and tracheobronchitis (58). Removal of aspirated foreign bodies is possible using the fiberoptic bronchoscope (59), but for most patients, particularly children, rigid bronchoscopy is more efficacious. Following removal of the foreign body, residual granulation tissue may persist for

**TABLE 6.4**

**COMPARISON OF VARIOUS BRONCHOSCOPIC TECHNIQUES TO IDENTIFY INDIVIDUAL ORGANISMS ON A SCALE OF 0 TO 3**

| Organism | Washing | Brushing | Bronchoalveolar Lavage | Biopsy |
|---|---|---|---|---|
| *Pneumocystis carinii* | 2 | 1 | 3 | 3 |
| Viral | | | | |
| Cytomegalovirus | 1 | 1 | 3 | 2 |
| Other viral | 1 | 1 | 2 | 1 |
| Tuberculosis | 3 | 0 | 2 | 3 |
| Fungal | | | | |
| *Candida* | 0 | 0 | 1 | 2 |
| *Aspergillus* | 0 | 0 | 1 | 2 |
| Histoplasmosis | | | | |
| Blastomycosis | | | | |
| Cryptococcosis | | | | |
| Coccidioidomycosis | 2 | 1 | 2 | 1 |
| Bacterial | | | | |
| Routine bacterial | 0 | 3[a] | 2 | 0 |
| *Legionella* | 1 | 1 | 2 | 1 |
| *Nocardia* | 3 | ND[b] | 2 | ND |

Reprinted from Baughman RP: Use of bronchoscopy in the diagnosis of infection in the immunocompromised host. *Thorax* 49:4, 1994.
[a] Protected brush.
[b] ND, not determined.

as long as several months. Even after prolonged periods, this tissue has been shown to regress with the return of patency of the bronchial lumen (59).

For the patient hospitalized in an intensive care unit, bronchoscopy has proved to be both diagnostically and therapeutically important. Olopade reported results of 200 procedures performed between 1985 and 1988. Of these, 87 were done for diagnostic reasons, which included obtaining culture material (82%), evaluating airways (15%), and determining the site of bleeding (3%) (60). Therapeutic indications include treatment for hemoptysis, removal of retained secretions, guided intubation, and removal of foreign bodies. Even in mechanically ventilated patients, foreign bodies can be safely removed with fiberoptic bronchoscopy (61). Acute bronchial tears may also be identified. In the case of more chronic conditions such as bronchopleural fistula, therapy may be instituted to close the fistula with various compounds such as acrylate tissue glue, fibrinogen glue, or gel foam or to insert detachable balloon catheters (62). In many patients the indications for bronchoscopy are both therapeutic and diagnostic.

In patients with suspected bronchiectasis, bronchoscopy may be helpful in obtaining specimens for quantitative culture using the protected specimen brush or bronchoalveolar lavage (see below) (63). Bronchography has often been used to confirm the diagnosis and to assist in planning medical or surgical management (64). The advent of high-resolution computerized tomographic scanning has reduced the need for bronchoscopy to diagnose bronchiectasis (65).

## COMPLICATIONS

Flexible fiberoptic bronchoscopy is generally a well-tolerated procedure with few adverse effects. The commonly recognized complications include hypoxemia, bleeding, fever, cardiac arrhythmias, bronchospasm, pneumonia, and pneumothorax (66–74). Death is rare, occurring during or directly following the procedure, with an incidence of approximately 0.01% (70). Fiberoptic bronchoscopy produces an average decline in $Pa_{O_2}$ of 15 to 20 mm Hg in both intubated and nonintubated patients (66). The resulting hypoxemia may be associated with arrhythmias, myocardial ischemia with associated hypotension, and endogenous catecholamine-induced hypertension (66–70). Proposed mechanisms for these findings include increased airways resistance (in an intubated patient on mechanical ventilation); small airway obstruction from hemorrhage or instilled fluids; or alveolar filling with resulting atelectasis and ventilation/perfusion mismatch (66–68). Patients should be placed on supplemental oxygen via nasal cannula or a specialized face mask. Con-

tinuous monitoring of $Pa_{O_2}$ by transcutaneous oxygen monitor or $Sa_{O_2}$ via pulse oximeter has become essential (66, 67). In the mechanically ventilated patient, peak inspiratory pressure (PIP) must be monitored, as high PIP may lead to pressure-limited decrease in tidal volume ($V_T$) (67). To avoid this complication, monitoring of exhaled $V_T$ and minute ventilation ($V_E$) is helpful and can be done with the monitors on most ventilators. In a recent study of 107 acutely ill ventilated patients with the adult respiratory distress syndrome, fighting the ventilator during the procedure remained the most significant risk factor for associated hypoxemia. This could be adequately relieved with appropriate sedation with a benzodiazepine such as midazolam (15, 78).

Bleeding is one of the most distressing and difficult management problems for the bronchoscopist. Minimal bleeding is defined as 50 ml of blood intermixed with saline lavage, and is not considered to be hazardous. The incidence of clinically significant bleeding varied from a low of 0.5% to a high of 1.3% in one study and appeared to be related to the types of procedures performed at bronchoscopy, including brushing and transbronchial biopsy (71). Risk factors associated with increased bleeding include an immunosuppressed host, platelet dysfunction and coagulopathies, drugs, organ failure, chest malignancy, and uremia (71). Uremia creates a major hazard of bleeding, and approximately 45% of uremic patients have significant hemorrhage after transbronchial biopsy. Pulmonary hypertension is also associated with a high incidence of bleeding and is frequently considered a contraindication to transbronchial biopsy.

Preprocedure evaluation for bleeding includes coagulation parameters as well as a platelet count. While it is occasionally recommended that this be performed in all patients (and is the current practice), the ordering of these studies and other preoperative tests should be based on clinical evaluation (14, 15). A platelet count of 50,000 cells/mm$^3$ has been considered a clinically significant level requiring platelet infusion (71). However, recent reports suggest that fiberoptic bronchoscopy in thrombocytopenic patients is safe, with minor airway bleeding occurring in approximately 8% (72). Patients with dysfunctional platelets as determined by abnormal bleeding time (e.g., in patients with uremia) can be given cryoprecipitate or DDAVP (d-amino-8-D-arginine-vasopressin) (70–72). In addition, the bronchoscope or specialized balloon catheters can be used to tamponade the source of hemorrhage in patients with massive hemoptysis (76, 77). Saline with epinephrine in a 1:20,000 dilution, or either thrombin or a combination of fibrinogen and thrombin may be infused through the bronchoscope or balloon catheter device for the control of hemoptysis (77). Attempts have been made to use fiber glue to treat hemoptysis; however, in patients with massive hemoptysis the continuous stream of blood tends to remove the fiber and glue before a stable clot can form (77). When these measures are not successful, rigid bronchoscopy with direct packing of the bronchus may be indicated. Definitive treatment includes bronchial artery embolization and surgical resection.

Fever is another common complication of bronchoscopy, reported in as many as 16% of patients (73). Pereira et al reported pneumonia in 6% and death from rapidly progressive pneumonia in another 1%. Bacteremia following this procedure has not been demonstrated (73). Careful disinfection, cleaning, and sterilization of scopes is mandatory to prevent this complication (74).

Laryngospasm and bronchospasm are common airway complications, and patients with asthma are at especially high risk (75). The most severe airway obstruction occurs in patients with chronic obstructive pulmonary disease. In these patients, who may have borderline respiratory failure, endotracheal intubation and mechanical ventilation may be necessary during and after the procedure.

## BRONCHOALVEOLAR LAVAGE

The technique of bronchoalveolar lavage (BAL) through the fiberoptic bronchoscope provides an easy and relatively noninvasive means to sample the cellular and soluble components of the lower respiratory tract (79). This procedure has aided in the diagnosis of opportunistic infections and has provided insights into the diagnosis, pathogenesis, and assessment of activity of interstitial and other lung diseases. Most commonly, the procedure involves the insertion and wedging of the bronchoscope into the right middle lobe or lingular lumen: occasionally, a lateral anterior segment of a lower lobe is used. Sterile saline is then instilled in 50- to 60-ml aliquots to a total volume of 100 to 150 ml. With the suction off, the fluid is then either aspirated by hand suction into a syringe or allowed to flow out by gravity into a container. Recovery by this technique yields 60 to 70% of the instilled volume in normal subjects, with smaller amounts in patients (79). Differential cell counts are evaluated on centrifuged preparations containing approximately $4 \times 10^4$ cells/mm$^3$. In a study of patients with interstitial lung disease, the complication rate for BAL procedures was less than 5%. Using the quantity of fluid mentioned above, the investigators found associated minor complications including postbronchoscopy fever (2.5%), pneumonitis

(0.4%), bleeding (0.7%), and bronchospasm (0.7%); none of these complications required therapy (80). BAL is useful in the diagnosis of infection in immunocompromised patients as described above, and is particularly efficacious in patients with AIDS. (56). The isolation of certain organisms is diagnostic of infectious disease. These organisms include *Pneumocystis carinii, Toxoplasma gondii, Strongyloides, Legionella, Histoplasma, Mycobacterium tuberculosis, Mycoplasma,* influenza virus, and respiratory syncytial virus (79). The isolation of cytomegalovirus (CMV) and herpes simplex virus in BAL specimens is not diagnostic by itself, since humans are known to shed these viruses in the respiratory tract in the absence of infection. Stover et al found that lavage had an overall diagnostic sensitivity of 66% and specificity of 100% when evaluated in a group of 92 immunosuppressed patients (81). A new BAL collection system using a transbronchoscopic balloon-tipped catheter (BTC) with a distal ejectable diaphragm is available for collection of distal respiratory secretions (82). Meduri et al found that in nine patients with pneumonia, positive cultures were obtained with the BTC in all nine patients, whereas protective specimen brush cultures were positive in only three (82). Cultures of BAL fluid are considered positive when they contain $10^5$ colony forming units (CFU) of bacteria per milliliter of exudate (79–82). Contamination from injection of lidocaine through the suction channel or from other sources results in concentrations of $10^4$ CFU/ml or less. The argument has been proposed that these studies should not be routinely used because, based on current available data, physicians are not willing to discontinue antibiotic treatment when quantitative bronchoscopic cultures are negative (83).

BAL has gained further diagnostic and therapeutic application in patients with alveolar proteinosis (84). The diagnosis of alveolar proteinosis is considered to be established if the gross appearance of lavage fluid is opaque or murky, and microscopic evaluation reveals (*a*) few alveolar microphages, (*b*) large cellular eosinophilic bodies, and (*c*) appropriate staining of the proteinaceous material (79, 84). Bronchoscopy is also important in the treatment of alveolar proteinosis, as differential lavage of lung segments or a whole lung with either rigid bronchoscopy under general anesthesia or fiberoptic bronchoscopy may be life saving (84). BAL may be useful in the identification of Langerhans' cells in eosinophilic granuloma or histiocytosis (85); hemosiderin-laden macrophages, as seen in pulmonary hemorrhage syndromes (86); and eosinophils in chronic eosinophilic pneumonia and in acute tropical eosinophilia (79). An increase in macrophages and lymphocytes, asbestos bodies, and increased numbers of alveolar macrophages and other inflammatory cells are found in patients with berylliosis, asbestosis, and silicosis, respectively (79). In patients occupationally exposed to silica, as many as 90% of alveolar macrophages obtained by BAL may contain birefringent crystalline particles, compared with fewer than 5% of macrophages containing these particles in persons having only environmental exposure (87). Relative quantitation of the cellular content of BAL fluid is also helpful in the following diagnoses: hypersensitivity pneumonitis, in which there is an increase primarily in suppressor T cells; sarcoidosis, in which there are increased numbers of T helper lymphocytes; and idiopathic pulmonary fibrosis, in which there is an increase in the percentage of neutrophils and eosinophils and possibly an increase in the percentage of T cells (79, 88).

### PROTECTED SPECIMEN BRUSH

The clinical diagnosis of pneumonia, especially in mechanically ventilated patients, may be inaccurate (89). To aid in this diagnosis, Wimberly et al (90) developed a specialized double-catheter brush system with telescoping cannulas and a distal-occluding Carbowax plug. The utility of the culture depends on appropriate technique (91), the absence of concurrent use of antibiotics, and the ability to recover bacteria at a concentration of at least $10^3$ CFU per milliliter of inoculated saline. In nonintubated patients who are not receiving antibiotics, the procedure may have sensitivity as high as 95% (92). Chastre et al (93) performed bronchoscopy in 26 mechanically ventilated patients shortly after death, using the protected specimen brush (PSB) and quantitative culture, followed by quantitative culture of a lung segment removed by thoracotomy. PSB yielded 15 of the 19 bacteria present in the lung and no additional organisms; there were no false negatives; and the false-positive rate in patients receiving antibiotics was 58%, versus 23% in those that were not receiving antibiotics (93). As with quantitative culture of BAL fluid, controversy continues concerning this technique (83). Regardless, in the appropriate patient, these specialized culture techniques provide useful information when specimens are collected and cultured appropriately.

### TRANSBRONCHIAL NEEDLE ASPIRATION

A flexible needle has been developed that can be passed through the bronchoscope channel to penetrate the trachea and bronchi. Transbronchial needle aspiration (TBNA) has been used in the diagnosis and staging of lung cancer (94). TBNA can be useful in the diagnosis of submucosal tumor (erythema, loss of bronchial

markings, or a thickening of the mucosa), a mass extrinsically compressing the bronchial lumen, and necrotic lesions or lesions from which significant bleeding is anticipated (95). When used in combination with other techniques TBNA has a higher yield than forceps biopsy (71 versus 55%). Both are clearly worth doing, since the combined yield is 90% and adding either washing or brushing increases the yield still further to 97% (95). Shure and Fedullo (95, 96) reported 15% of 110 patients with bronchogenic carcinoma diagnosed as positive by transcarinal needle aspiration. There were no false positives, and the aspirate was the only evidence of unresectability in 69% of those in whom it was positive. Only a few false-positive results have been reported with TBNA; these results may be avoided by (*a*) not obtaining a biopsy when a significant amount of secretions cover the mucosa to be biopsied, (*b*) limiting the suction through the bronchoscope prior to the procedure, and (*c*) obtaining the TBNA sample prior to examining the lower airways to prevent contamination.

The complication rate of TBNA is low (94–99). Pneumothorax occurs in only 0.5% of patients who undergo TBNA, and significant bleeding is uncommon even if pulmonary and systemic blood vessels are inadvertently aspirated. Pneumomediastinum and mediastinitis are rare complications. With this low complication rate, TBNA has an important role in the preoperative staging of patients with lung cancer. In spite of these favorable results, the procedure has received criticism by bronchoscopists in the United States (14, 15). This is mostly related to trauma to the scope from the needle when used by inexperienced personnel, as well as poor diagnostic yield. Recent publication of a detailed description of this useful diagnostic technique should help improve its acceptance, as should the increased establishment of onsite cytopathology personnel (97, 98).

### TRANSTHORACIC NEEDLE ASPIRATION AND BIOPSY

Percutaneous needle aspiration and biopsy are useful procedures for patients with lesions of the lung parenchyma and mediastinum (100). Although the majority of these procedures are performed to evaluate solitary or multiple pulmonary nodules in relatively stable patients, these techniques may also be used to diagnose infection, especially in pediatric patients. In a retrospective review of fine-needle (22 gauge) aspiration biopsy at Duke University, 37 (11.7%) of the 316 patients reported were found not to have cancer, with

**TABLE 6.5**
**INCIDENCE OF CHEST DISEASES BIOPSIED WITH FNA AND LNC BIOPSIES OF THE LUNG**[a]

| | Duke University (FNA) | U. of Florida (LNC) |
|---|---|---|
| Primary malignant lung tumors | 501 | 151 |
| Tumors of the pleura | NR[b] | 3 |
| Metastatic malignant tumors | 143 | 8 |
| Lymphoproliferative neoplasms | NR | 8 |
| Inflammatory diseases | | |
|   Nonspecific inflammation | 65 | NR |
|   Fibrosis | NR | 12 |
|   Granuloma | 12 | 3 |
|   Pneumonitis (bacterial) | 5 | 5 |
|   Tuberculosis | NR | 4 |
|   Coccidioidomycosis | NR | 1 |
|   Blastomycosis | 3 | NR |
|   Cryptococcosis | 3 | NR |
|   Candidiasis | 1 | NR |
|   Phycomycosis | 2 | NR |
|   Histoplasmosis | 3 | NR |
|   Aspergillosis | 5 | NR |
|   Abscess | 3 | NR |
|   Infarction of lung | NR | 2 |
|   Others (lipoma, hamartoma, amyloid, sequestration) | NR | 4 |
| Nondiagnostic | 269 | 9 |
| Total | 1,015 | 210 |

Adapted from Johnston WW: Percutaneous fine needle aspiration biopsy of the lung. *Acta Cytol* 28:220, 1984; and Clore F, Virapongse C, Saterfel J: Low risk large-needle biopsy of chest lesions. *Chest* 96:540, 1989.
[a] FNA, fine needle aspiration; LNC, large needle cutting.
[b] NR, not reported.

diagnoses as shown in Table 6.5 (101). This was similar to the results of Clore et al (102), who reported an incidence of inflammatory lesions of 11.9% using large cutting needle (14.5 to 18 gauge) biopsy techniques. As with transbronchial biopsies, onsite review of aspirated material by a cytopathologist enhances the diagnostic yield of the procedure (98).

Complications include pneumothorax, which is most frequent and occurs in 10 to 15% of patients and requires placement of a thoracostomy tube in only 10 to 20% of them. Transient hemoptysis occurs in fewer than 10%, and bacterial contamination of the pleural space is rare. Other complications include allergic anesthetic reactions, vasovagal reflex, soft tissue infection, cancer seeding at the insertion site (from biopsied lesions), and air embolism (less than 0.1%) (100–104).

As with all invasive diagnostic procedures, the risk of percutaneous needle biopsy must be weighed against the potential benefit for the patient. In addition,

the complications of this procedure relative to others—such as transbronchial biopsy and aspiration via fiberoptic bronchoscopy, which has fewer complications—must be considered. Contraindications to the procedure include a bleeding diathesis, bullous lung disease in the area of the biopsy, local cutaneous lesions (e.g., pyoderma or herpes zoster), pulmonary hypertension, or a lesion abutting the mediastinum or hilum. Patients on continuous positive airway pressure (CPAP) or positive-pressure ventilation are at high risk for pneumothorax and should be considered for other ventilatory modes (e.g., jet ventilation) during and after the procedure. Visualization of the lesion for guidance of the procedure may be obtained with computed tomographic scanning, ultrasonography, or fluoroscopy (100–102).

## OPEN LUNG BIOPSY

Open lung biopsy is indicated in the following situations: (*a*) the patient with diffuse pulmonary infiltrates and progressive disease whose diagnosis is not apparent after a careful history, physical examination, sputum analysis, and bronchoscopy with transbronchial biopsy; (*b*) the patient with a progressive localized pulmonary infiltrate whose diagnosis is not apparent after a careful evaluation as described above, including bronchoscopy and transbronchial biopsy; (*c*) the immunocompromised host with pulmonary infiltrates but no specific diagnosis after bronchoscopy with transbronchial biopsy or percutaneous needle aspiration; and (*d*) the patient suspected of having pulmonary malignancy in whom the sputum cytologic examination, bronchoscopy, transbronchial biopsy, and needle aspiration are nondiagnostic (104–108).

Open lung biopsy via limited thoracotomy is a relatively safe procedure with little morbidity (19%) and approximately 0.5 to 0.6% mortality (104–106) (Table 6.6). Biopsy specimens should be taken from at least two sites (an upper-lobe and a lower-lobe site) and should include both abnormal and normal-appearing areas. Obtaining small subpleural samples (especially if pleuritis is present) in dependent segments of the right middle lobe or lingula may yield nonspecific findings. When the procedure is performed and the diagnosis of interstitial infiltrates with suspected fibrosis is found, the pathologist should quantitate both the extent and the severity of the inflammatory or exudative—as well as the fibrotic or reparative—tissue responses noted (105, 106).

In patients with diffuse pulmonary infiltrates and acute respiratory failure, open lung biopsy provided a specific etiologic diagnosis in 66% of patients in one

TABLE 6.6
COMPLICATIONS OF 288 OPEN LUNG BIOPSY PROCEDURES IN
IMMUNOCOMPROMISED PATIENTS

| Complications | No. of Occurrences | % |
|---|---|---|
| Pneumothorax | 22 | 8 |
| Hemothorax | 2 | 0.6 |
| Wound hematoma | 1 | 0.3 |
| Hemoptysis | 1 | 0.3 |
| Wound dehiscence | 1 | 0.3 |
| Incisional neuritis | 1 | 0.3 |
| Tumor recurrence at chest tube site | 1 | 0.3 |
| Death | 2 | 0.6 |
| Totals | 31/288 | 11 |

Reprinted with permission from Matthay RA, Moritz ED: Invasive procedures for diagnosing pulmonary infection. A critical review. *Clin Chest Med* 2:14–15, 1981.

series (105). Diagnosis influenced therapy in 70%; however, only 30% of the patients survived to hospital discharge, and nine patients survived for more than 1 year. This study suggested that open lung biopsy is helpful in yielding an etiologic diagnosis; however, this utility is limited by current shortcomings of therapy (105). In a study (Table 6.7) of 87 consecutive patients reviewed retrospectively by Cheson et al (107), a specific histologic diagnosis was obtained in 62 patients (71%), 33 of whom had infections. Specific therapy was available for 52 patients, and in 33 cases a change in therapy was necessary following the biopsy, for appropriate treatment. Forty-one patients received an adequate course of therapy and 27 (66%) improved clinically, including those with infection, malignancies, and vasculitis. This report suggests that in immunocompromised patients in the pre-AIDS era (from 1971 to 1982) open lung biopsy was safe and accurate in diagnosis, with clinical improvement following biopsy-directed patient management (107).

In contrast, in patients with AIDS, open lung biopsy appears to have a limited role. In 42 patients reported by Fitzgerald and associates (108), 29 patients had a preceding nondiagnostic bronchoscopic procedure and nine had open lung biopsy because of progressive deterioration despite treatment for diseases diagnosed bronchoscopically. Diagnoses of treatable diseases such as cryptococcosis, tuberculosis, and PCP were made in only five of the 42 patients subjected to open lung biopsy in this study, and one of the procedures was a false negative. Based on this and other studies, many investigators suggest that open lung biopsy should be reserved for highly selected patients and that

a second bronchoscopic procedure or thoracoscopy should be considered because of the morbidity associated with open lung biopsy (109).

## THORACOSCOPY

Although thoracoscopy has been a part of thoracic surgical practice for many years, the advent of video-assisted techniques has greatly expanded the indications and uses of this procedure. Where previously thoracoscopy was performed mainly for diagnostic purposes, video-assisted thoracic surgery (VATS) now has assumed a major role in the therapy of chest diseases. Indeed, in some institutions it is now the most commonly used operative approach for some general thoracic surgical practices (110). The primary advantage of VATS is that it produces less morbidity and mortality and shorter hospitalization times than does thoracotomy.

Most VATS procedures are done under general anesthesia, since general anesthesia permits endoscopic surgical manipulation to be done safely and expeditiously (110). After general anesthesia is induced, the thoracoscope is inserted and the ipsilateral lung is collapsed for unimpaired visibility of the intrathoracic structures. Ventilation for the patient is provided via the contralateral lung. At the completion of the VATS procedure, a single chest tube is placed into the pleural space.

### Pleural Effusions

In the diagnosis of pleural disease VATS procedures should be used only when the less invasive diagnostic methods such as thoracentesis and needle biopsy of the pleura have not yielded a diagnosis. In one series of 620 patients with pleural effusions, only 48 (8%) remained without a diagnosis and were subjected to thoracoscopy (111). If the patient has malignancy, thoracoscopy will establish the diagnosis more than 90% of the time. The diagnosis of mesothelioma is probably best made with VATS. However, VATS rarely establishes the diagnosis of benign disease (112). If malignant disease is documented, pleurodesis can be performed at the time of the VATS procedure to control the pleural effusion. VATS procedures may obviate the need for a decortication in patients with complicated parapneumonic effusions (113). In similar manner, thoracoscopy may be useful in breaking down the fibrin membranes that occasionally produce loculations in patients with malignant pleural effusions and, coupled with talc insufflation, may control the process.

**TABLE 6.7**
**REPORTED SERIES OF OPEN LUNG BIOPSY RESULTS IN IMMUNOCOMPROMISED PATIENTS**[a]

| Reference | No. of Patients | Specific Diagnosis (%) | Infection (%) | Change in Therapy (%) | Clinical Improvement (%) | Complications (Mortality) (%) |
|---|---|---|---|---|---|---|
| Greenman et al. (1975) | 48 | 65 | 23 | 73[b] | 69 (70:S) (25:NS) | 8 (0) |
| Rosen et al. (1975) | 47 | >64 | >51 | NR | >34 (>32:S) (7:NS) | 0 (0) |
| Leight et al. (1978) | 42 | 71 | 50 | NR | 65 (S) | |
| Rossiter et al. (1979) | 70 | 55 | 28 | 45 | 75 (74:S) (76:NS) | 10 (0) |
| Singer et al. (1979) | 44 | 61 | 48 | NR | 48 | 34 (0) |
| Toledo-Peyrera et al. (1980) | 13 | 77 | 23 | NR | 84 (80:S) (100:NS) | NR (0) |
| Waltzer et al. (1980) | 22 | 74 | 74 | NR | 77 (75:S) (83:NS) | 9 (0) |
| Jaffe et al. (1981) | 26 | 81 | 50 | NR | 62 | 19 (4) |
| Hiatt et al. (1982) | 68 | 37 | 21 | 28 | 37 (33:NS) (44:S) | 19 (4) |
| Canham et al. (1983) | 20 | 95 | 25 | 29 | <60 | 50 (>10) |

Reprinted from Cheson BD, Samjowski WE, Tang TT, Spruance SL: Value of open-lung biopsy in 87 immunocompromised patients with pulmonary infiltrates. *Cancer* 55:454, 1985.
[a] NS, biopsy specimen was nonspecific; NR, not reported; S, specimen from biopsy revealed a specific diagnosis.
[b] Data limited to 16 hypoxic patients.

## Pneumothorax

Most patients with pneumothorax can be managed satisfactorily with simple aspiration or tube thoracoscopy. However, VATS can eliminate the need for thoracotomy in patients who have a persistent bronchopleural fistula or collapsed lung. At the time of thoracoscopy, bullous disease may be treated with endo-stapling or Nd:YAG laser (114), and attempts at pleurodesis are made with pleural abrasion (115), parietal pleurectomy (114), or the insufflation of talc (116). Which of these three methods is best remains to be determined.

## Interstitial Lung Disease

VATS procedures appear to be particularly useful for obtaining lung biopsies in patients with diffuse interstitial lung disease. Lung biopsy via VATS should not be attempted if the patient requires mechanical ventilation because he or she probably will not be able to tolerate one-lung ventilation. Patients with coagulation disorders or pulmonary hypertension should have an open lung biopsy rather than a VATS procedure. With VATS the visualization of the lung is better than it is with a limited thoracotomy and more areas of the lung can be sampled. Most patients who previously needed an open lung biopsy are currently best managed with VATS procedures (117).

## Pulmonary Nodules

Pulmonary nodules may be safely removed via VATS procedures using the Nd:YAG laser combined with the endoscopic stapling device (110). If the patient is a poor surgical candidate, this wedge resection can serve as the definitive treatment. If the nodule is benign, then no additional procedures need be done. If the patient is a good surgical candidate and has a primary lung cancer, then a lobectomy should probably be performed (110).

## Mediastinal Disease

Some surgeons now prefer VATS procedures to anterior mediastinotomy to approach mediastinal adenopathy located in the aortopulmonary window or the low peri-azygos area. The visibility of the entire mediastinal compartment afforded through the VATS approach is far superior to exploration through an anterior mediastinotomy. VATS procedures can also be used to resect benign posterior mediastinal neoplasms and carefully selected cases of early-stage thymoma (110).

## Miscellaneous Conditions

VATS procedures have also been used for many other thoracic surgical procedures, including ligation of the thoracic duct, creation of a pericardial window,

Zenker's diverticulum, lobectomy, thoracic sympathectomy, benign esophageal tumors, removal of chest wall tumors, and removal of clotted blood with a hemothorax.

## COMPLICATIONS OF THORACOSCOPY

Although there is less morbidity and mortality from VATS procedures than from thoracotomy, there are nonetheless significant complications. Kaiser and Bavaria (118) reviewed the complications of VATS encountered at the Hospital of the University of Pennsylvania between December 1991 and December 1992. They reported that 10% of the VATS procedures were associated with complications. The most common complication was prolonged (longer than 7 days) air leak (3.7%) followed by superficial wound infection (1.9%), and bleeding significant enough to require either transfusion or reoperation (1.9%). In 4.1% of patients, they were unable to successfully complete the intended procedure thoracoscopically and resorted to an open procedure (118).

## MEDIASTINOSCOPY

This endoscopic procedure is used to explore the mediastinum and to obtain biopsies of lymph nodes and other masses. General anesthesia is usually required, although a local anesthetic may be used safely in selected patients in a day surgery setting. All paratracheal nodes and the nodes in the tracheal bronchial angle and proximally along the main bronchi are evaluable, as are the nodes in the anterior compartment of the subcarinal space. Lymph nodes in the aortopulmonary window, as well as the left anterior mediastinum (usually along the phrenic nerve), cannot be reached by conventional mediastinoscopy, nor can the inferior posterior lymph nodes. In addition, nodes along the esophagus and in the inferior pulmonary ligament are not accessible (119).

A modified procedure has recently been developed involving extension of the conventional cervical mediastinoscopy incision using a parasternal approach as an alternative to left anterior mediastinotomy (120). This can aid in the evaluation of lymph nodes in the left hilar or left upper lobe areas. Complications from mediastinoscopy are uncommon, with no operative deaths reported in the series by Luke et al (121) in 1986, from Toronto General Hospital. A complication rate of 2.3% was noted among the 1000 patients described and included hemorrhage, pneumothorax, wound infection, and recurrent laryngeal nerve palsy (121).

Mediastinoscopy is recommended in patients with T2 or T3 primary cancerous lesions, as well as those with T1 lesions in whom the cell type is adenocarcinoma or large-cell carcinoma, even when the computed tomographic studies are negative. If nodes are identified, then cervical mediastinoscopy is performed. Patients with T2 or T3 lesions in the left upper lobe should undergo cervical mediastinoscopy with frozen section; if the other biopsy specimens are negative, a left anterior mediastinotomy through the second intercostal space should be performed (120). These procedures can be performed on an outpatient basis. A recent report of ambulatory mediastinoscopy and anterior mediastinotomy reveals that these procedures permitted a diagnosis to be made in 47 of 158 patients and confirmed unresectable malignant disease in 29 patients, thus barring unnecessary admission to the hospital in 48% of the patients reported (122). Mediastinoscopy may be omitted in patients with T1 squamous cell carcinoma and negative findings on CT. Patients with superior sulcus tumor or significant pleural effusion may be evaluated by mediastinal pleuroscopy on either side (119, 121).

Mediastinoscopy is also used for the diagnosis of other masses in the middle or anterior mediastinum. In one series of 21 such cases (123), definitive diagnoses were obtained in 67%. Since several of these patients had diseases for which the treatment of choice was not surgery, the procedure saved the patient from more extensive exploration. Carlens (124) reported that mediastinoscopy was positive in 96% of 123 cases of sarcoidosis. However, usually the diagnosis of sarcoidosis can be established by less invasive means, such as peripheral lymph node biopsy or transbronchial lung biopsy.

▼

## REFERENCES

1. Light RW: Pleural diseases. *Dis Mon* 28:266–331, 1992.
2. Light RW, Erozan YC, Ball WC Jr: Cells in pleural fluid: their value in differential diagnosis. *Arch Intern Med* 132: 854–860, 1973.
3. Broaddus VC, Light RW: What is the origin of pleural transudates and exudates? (Editorial) *Chest* 102:658, 1992.
4. Light RW, MacGregor MI, Luchsinger PC, et al: Pleural effusions: the diagnostic separation of transudates and exudates. *Ann Intern Med* 77:507–513, 1972.
5. Romero S, Candela A, Martin C, et al: Evaluation of different criteria for the separation of pleural transudates from exudates. *Chest* 104:399–404, 1993.
6. Light RW: *Pleural Diseases.* Philadelphia, Lea & Febiger, 1990.
7. Kramer MR, Ceperao RJ, Pitchenik AE: High amylase in neoplasm-related pleural effusion. *Ann Intern Med* 110:567–569, 1989.

8. Light RW, Girard WM, Jenkinson SG, et al: Parapneumonic effusions. *Am J Med* 69:507–512, 1980.

9. Good JT Jr, King TE, Antony VB, et al: Lupus pleuritis: clinical features and pleural fluid characteristics with special reference to pleural fluid antinuclear antibodies. *Chest* 84:714–718, 1983.

10. Valdes L, San Jose E, Alvarez D, et al: Diagnosis of tuberculous pleurisy using the biologic parameters adenosine deaminase, lysozyme, and interferon gamma. *Chest* 103:458–465, 1993.

11. Frisman DM, McCarthy WF, Schleiff P, et al: Immunocytochemistry in the differential diagnosis of effusions: use of logistic regression to select a panel of antibodies to distinguish adenocarcinomas from mesothelial proliferations. *Mod Pathol* 6:179–184, 1993.

12. Killian G: Direct endoscopy of upper air passages and esophagus: its diagnostic and therapeutic value in search for and removal of foreign body. *J Laryngol Rhinol Otol* 8:461–468, 1902.

13. Ikeda S, Yawai N, Ishikawa S: Flexible bronchofiberscope. *Keio J Med* 17:1–33, 1968.

14. Prakash UBS, Stubbs SE: The Bronchoscopy Survey: some reflexions. *Chest* 100:1660–1667, 1991.

15. Prakash UBS, Offord KP, Stubbs SE: Bronchoscopy in North America: The ACCP Survey. *Chest* 100:1668–1675, 1991.

16. Sokolowski JW, Burgher LW, Jones FL, et al: ATS guidelines for fiberoptic bronchoscopy in adults. *Am Rev Respir Dis* 136:4, 1987.

17. Weaver LJ, Solliday N, Cugell DW: Selection of patients with hemoptysis for fiberoptic bronchoscopy. *Chest* 76:7–10, 1979.

18. O'Neal KM, Lazarus AA: Hemoptysis: indications for bronchoscopy. *Arch Intern Med* 151:171–174, 1991.

19. Adelman M, Haponik EF, Bleecker ER, et al: Cryptogenic hemoptysis. *Ann Intern Med* 102:829–834, 1985.

20. Popovich J Jr, Kvale PA, Eichenhorn MS, et al: Diagnostic accuracy of multiple biopsies from flexible fiberoptic bronchoscopy: a comparison of central versus peripheral carcinoma. *Am Rev Respir Dis* 125:521–523, 1982.

21. Dreisin RB, Albert RK, Talley PA, et al: Flexible fiberoptic bronchoscopy in the teaching hospital: yield and complications. *Chest* 74:144–149, 1978.

22. Cox ID, Bagg LR, Russell NJ, et al: Relationship of radiographic position to the diagnostic yield of fiberoptic bronchoscopy in bronchogenic carcinoma. *Chest* 85:519–522, 1984.

23. Cummings SR, Lillington GH, Richard RJ: Managing solitary pulmonary nodules: the choice of strategy in a close call. *Am Rev Respir Dis* 134:453–460, 1986.

24. Ellis JA: Transbronchial lung biopsy via the fiberoptic bronchoscope. *Chest* 68:524–532, 1975.

25. Kvale PA, Bode FR, Kini S: Diagnostic accuracy in lung cancer: comparison of techniques used in association with flexible fiberoptic bronchoscopy. *Chest* 69:752–757, 1976.

26. Radke JR, Conway WA, Eyler WR, et al: Diagnostic accuracy in peripheral lung lesions. *Chest* 76:176–179, 1979.

27. Pirozynski M: Bronchoalveolar lavage in the diagnosis of peripheral, primary lung cancer. *Chest* 102:372–374, 1992.

28. Ono R, Lake J, Ikeda S: Bronchofiberoscopy with curette biopsy and bronchography in the evaluation of peripheral lung lesions. *Chest* 79:162–166, 1981.

29. Tamaka M, Kohda E, Satoh M, et al: Diagnosis of peripheral lung cancer using a new type of endoscope. *Chest* 97:1231–1234, 1990.

30. Schenk DA, Bryan CL, Bower JH, et al: Transbronchial needle aspiration in the diagnosis of bronchogenic carcinoma. *Chest* 92:83–85, 1987.

31. Shure D, Fedullo PF: Transbronchial needle aspiration of peripheral masses. *Am Rev Respir Dis* 128:1090–1092, 1983.

32. Wang KP, Britt EJ: Needle brush in the diagnosis of lung mass or nodule through flexible bronchoscopy. *Chest* 100:1148–1150, 1991.

33. Gaeta M, Pandolfo I, Volta S, et al: Bronchus sign on CT in peripheral carcinoma of the lung: value in predicting results of transbronchial biopsy. *AJR* 157:1181–1185, 1991.

34. Naidich DP, Sussman R, Kutcher WL, et al: Solitary pulmonary nodules: CT-bronchoscopic correlation. *Chest* 3:595–598, 1988.

35. Goldberg BB, Steiner RM, Liu JB, et al: Ultrasound-assisted bronchoscopy with use of miniature transducer-containing catheters. *Radiology* 190:233–237, 1994.

36. Lam S, MacAulay C, Palcic B: Detection and localization of early lung cancer by imaging techniques. *Chest* 103:12S–14S, 1993.

37. Sanderson DR, Fontana RS, Woolner LB, et al: Bronchoscopic localization of radiographically occult lung cancer. *Chest* 65:608–612, 1974.

38. Marsh BR, Frost JK, Erozan YS, et al: Diagnosis of early bronchogenic carcinoma. *Chest* 73:716S–717S, 1978.

39. Lam S, MacAulay C, Hung J, et al: Detection of dysplasia and carcinoma in situ by a lung imaging fluorescence endoscopy (LIFE). *J Thorac Cardiovasc Surg* 105:1035–1040, 1993.

40. Edell ES, Cortese DA: Bronchoscopic phototherapy with hematoporphyrin derivative for treatment of localized bronchogenic carcinoma. *Mayo Clin Proc* 62:8–14, 1987.

41. Sosenko A, Glassroth J: Fiberoptic bronchoscopy in the evaluation of lung abscesses. *Chest* 87:489–494, 1985.

42. Reider GS, Gracey DR: Aspiration of intrathoracic abscess. *JAMA* 240:1156–1159, 1978.

43. Smith CW, Murray GF, Wilcox BR, et al: The role of transbronchial lung biopsy in diffuse pulmonary disease. *Ann Thorac Surg* 24:54–58, 1977.

44. Wall CP, Gaensler EA, Carrington CB, et al: Comparison of transbronchial and open lung biopsies in chronic infiltrative lung diseases. *Am Rev Respir Dis* 123:280–285, 1981.

45. Gilman MJ, Wang KP: Transbronchial biopsy in sarcoidosis. *Am Rev Respir Dis* 122:721–724, 1980.

46. Roethe RH, Fuller PB, Byrd RB, et al: Transbronchial lung biopsy in sarcoidosis. *Chest* 77:400–402, 1980.

47. Danielle RP, Elias JA, Epstein PE, et al: Bronchoalveolar lavage: role in the pathogenesis, diagnosis, and management of interstitial lung disease. *Ann Intern Med* 102:93–108, 1985.

48. Winterbauer RH: The treatment of idiopathic pulmonary fibrosis. *Chest* 100:233–235, 1991.

49. Kennedy DJ, Lewis WP, Barnes PJ: Yield of bronchoscopy for the diagnosis of tuberculosis in patients with

human immunodeficiency virus infection. *Chest* 102: 1040–1044, 1992.

50. George RB, Jenkinson SG, Light RW: Bronchoscopy in the diagnosis of pulmonary fungal and nocardial infections. *Chest* 73:33–36, 1978.

51. Wallace JM, Deutsch AL, Harrell JH, et al: Bronchoscopy and transbronchial biopsy in evaluation of patients with suspected active tuberculosis. *Am J Med* 70: 1189–1194, 1981.

52. Schluger NW, Rom WN: Current approaches to the diagnosis of active pulmonary tuberculosis. *Am J Respir Crit Care Med* 149:264–267, 1994.

53. Baughman RP: Use of bronchoscopy in the diagnosis of infection in the immunocompromised host. *Thorax* 49: 3–7, 1994.

54. Kovacs JA, Ng VL, Masur H, et al: Diagnosis of *Pneumocystis carinii* pneumonia: improved detection in sputum with use of monoclonal antibodies. *N Engl J Med* 318: 589–593, 1988.

55. Stover DE, Zaman MB, Hajdu SI, et al: Bronchoalveolar lavage in the diagnosis of diffuse pulmonary infiltrates in the immunocompromised host. *Ann Intern Med* 101: 1–7, 1984.

56. Broaddus C, Drake MD, Stulbarg MS, et al: Bronchoalveolar lavage and transbronchial biopsy for the diagnosis of pulmonary infections in the acquired immunodeficiency syndrome. *Ann Intern Med* 102:747–752, 1985.

57. Luce JM, Clement MJ: Pulmonary diagnostic evaluation in patients suspected of having an HIV-related disease. *Semin Respir Infect* 4:93–101, 1989.

58. Wolfe JE, Bone RC, Ruth WE: Diagnosis of gastric aspiration by fiberoptic bronchoscopy. *Chest* 70:458–459, 1979.

59. Lan R, Lee C, Chiang Y, et al: Use of fiberoptic bronchoscopy to retrieve bronchial foreign bodies in adults. *Am Rev Respir Dis* 140:1734–1737, 1989.

60. Olopade CO, Prakash UBS: Bronchoscopy in the critical care unit. *Mayo Clin Proc* 64:1255–1263, 1989.

61. Verea-Hernando H, Garcia-Quijada RC, Ruiz de Galarreta AA: Extraction of foreign bodies with fiberoptic bronchoscopy in mechanically ventilated patients. *Am Rev Respir Dis* 142:258, 1990.

62. McManigle JE, Fletcher GL, Tenholder MF: Bronchoscopy in the management of bronchopleural fistula. *Chest* 97:1235–1238, 1990.

63. Pang JA, Cheng A, Chan HS, et al: The bacteriology of bronchiectasis in Hong Kong investigated by protected catheter brush and bronchoalveolar lavage. *Am Rev Respir Dis* 139:14–17, 1989.

64. Morcos SK, Anderson PB, Baudouin SV, et al: Suitability of and tolerance to Iotrolan 300 in bronchography via the fiberoptic bronchoscope. *Thorax* 45:628–629, 1990.

65. McGuinness G, Naidich DP, Leitman BS, et al: Bronchiectasis: CT evaluation. *AJR* 160:253–259, 1993.

66. Ghows MB, Rosen MJ, Chuang MT, et al: Transcutaneous oxygen monitoring during fiberoptic bronchoscopy. *Chest* 89:543–544, 1986.

67. Dellinger RP: Fiberoptic bronchoscopy in adult airway management. *Crit Care Med* 18:882–887, 1990.

68. Peacock AJ, Benson-Mitchell R, Godfrey R: Effect of fiberoptic bronchoscopy on pulmonary function. *Thorax* 45:38–41, 1990.

69. Trouillet J, Guiguet M. Gibert C, et al: Fiberoptic bronchoscopy in ventilated patients. *Chest* 97:927–930, 1990.

70. Credle WF Jr, Smiddy JF, Elliott RC: Complications of fiberoptic bronchoscopy. *Am Rev Respir Dis* 109:64–72, 1974.

71. Cordasco EM Jr, Mehta AC, Ahmed M: Bronchoscopically induced bleeding. *Chest* 100:1141–1147, 1991.

72. Weiss SM, Hert RC, Gianola FJ, et al: Complications of fiberoptic bronchoscopy in thrombocytopenic patients. *Chest* 104:1025–1028, 1993.

73. Pereira W, Kovnat DM, Kahn MA, et al: Fever and pneumonia after flexible fiberoptic bronchoscopy. *Am Rev Respir Dis* 112:59–64, 1975.

74. Prakash UBS: Does the bronchoscope propagate infection? *Chest* 104:552–559, 1993.

75. Sahn SA, Scoggin C: Fiberoptic bronchoscopy in bronchial asthma. A word of caution. *Chest* 69:39–42, 1976.

76. Saw EC, Gottlieb LS, Yokoyama T, et al: Flexible fiberoptic bronchoscopy and endobronchial tamponade in the management of massive hemoptysis. *Chest* 70: 589–591, 1976.

77. Tsukamoto T, Sasaki H, Nakamura H: Treatment of hemoptysis patients by thrombin and fibrinogen-thrombin infusion therapy using a fiberoptic bronchoscope. *Chest* 96:473–476, 1989.

78. Berger R, McConnell JW, Phillips B, et al: Safety and efficacy of using high-dose topical and nebulized anesthesia to obtain endobronchial cultures. *Chest* 95: 299–303, 1989.

79. Goldstein RA, Rohatgi PK (eds): American Thoracic Society Statement: clinical role of bronchoalveolar lavage in adults with pulmonary disease. *Am Rev Respir Dis* 42:481–486, 1990.

80. Strumpf IJ, Feld MK, Cornelius MJ, et al: Safety of fiberoptic bronchoalveolar lavage in evaluation of interstitial lung disease. *Chest* 80:268–271, 1981.

81. Stover DE, Zaman MB, Hajdu SI, et al: Bronchoalveolar lavage in the diagnosis of diffuse pulmonary infiltrates in the immunosuppressed host. *Ann Intern Med* 101:1–7, 1984.

82. Meduri GU, Wunderink, RG, Leeper UV: Management of bacterial pneumonia in ventilated patients. *Chest* 101: 500–508, 1992.

83. Niederman MS: Diagnosing nosocomia pneumonia: to brush or not to brush. *J Intensive Care Med* 6:151–152, 1991.

84. Martin RJ, Coalson JJ, Rogers RM, et al: Pulmonary alveolar proteinosis: the diagnosis by segmental lavage. *Am Rev Respir Dis* 121:819–825, 1980.

85. Chollet S, Soler P, Dournovo P, et al: Diagnosis of pulmonary histiocytosis X by immunodetection of Langerhans cells in bronchoalveolar lavage fluid. *Am J Pathol* 115:225–232, 1984.

86. Kahn FW, Jones JM, England DM: Diagnosis of pulmonary hemorrhage in the immunocompromised host. *Am Rev Respir Dis* 136:155–160, 1987.

87. Christman JW, Emerson RJ, Graham GB, et al: Mineral dust and cell recovery from bronchoalveolar lavage of healthy Vermont granite workers. *Am Rev Respir Dis* 132:393–399, 1985.

88. Leatherman JW, Michael AF, Schwartz BA, et al: Lung T cells in hypersensitivity pneumonitis. *Ann Intern Med* 100:390–392, 1984.

89. Fagon JY, Chastre J, Hance AJ, et al: Evaluation of clinical judgement in the identification and treatment of nosocomial pneumonia in ventilated patients. *Chest* 103: 547–553, 1993.

90. Wimberly D, Faling LJ, Bartlett JG: A fiberoptic bronchoscopy technique to obtain uncontaminated lower airway secretions for bacterial culture. *Am Rev Respir Dis* 119:337–343, 1979.
91. Meduri GU: Ventilator-associated pneumonia in patients with respiratory failure: a diagnostic approach. *Chest* 97:1208–1219, 1990.
92. Pollack HM, Hawkins EL, Bonner JR, et al: Diagnosis of bacterial pulmonary infections with quantitative protected catheter cultures obtained during bronchoscopy. *J Clin Microbiol* 17:255–259, 1983.
93. Chastre J, Viau F, Brun P, et al: Prospective evaluation of the protected specimen brush for the diagnosis of pulmonary infections in ventilated patients. *Am Rev Respir Dis* 130:924–929, 1984.
94. Wang KP, Terry PB: Transbronchial needle aspiration in the diagnosis and staging of bronchogenic carcinoma. *Am Rev Respir Dis* 127:344–347, 1983.
95. Shure D, Fedullo PF: Transbronchial needle aspiration in the diagnosis of submucosal and peribronchial bronchogenic carcinoma. *Chest* 88:4–51, 1985.
96. Shure D, Fedullo PF: The role of transcarinal needle aspiration in the staging of bronchogenic carcinoma. *Chest* 86:693–696, 1984.
97. Wang KP: How I do it. Transbronchial needle aspiration. *J Bronchol* 1:63–68, 1994.
98. Davenport RD: Rapid on-site evaluation of transbronchial aspirates. *Chest* 98:59–61, 1990.
99. Witte MC, Opal SM, Gilbert JG, et al: Incidence of fever and bacteremia following transbronchial needle aspiration. *Chest* 89:85–87, 1986.
100. Sokolowski JW, Burgher LW, Jones FL Jr, et al: American Thoracic Society Guidelines for percutaneous transthoracic needle biopsy. *Am Rev Respir Dis* 140:255–256, 1989.
101. Johnson WW: Percutaneous fine needle aspiration biopsy of the lung. *Acta Cytol* 28:218–224, 1984.
102. Clore F, Virapongse C, Saterfel J: Low risk large-needle biopsy of chest lesions. *Chest* 96:538–541, 1989.
103. Wallace JM, Batra P, Gong H, et al: Percutaneous needle lung aspiration for diagnosing pneumonitis in the patient with acquired immunodeficiency syndrome (AIDS). *Am Rev Respir Dis* 131:389–392, 1985.
104. Matthay RA, Moritz ED: Invasive procedures for diagnosing pulmonary infection. A critical review. *Clin Chest Med* 2:14–15, 1981.
105. Warner DO, Warner MA, Divertie MB: Open lung biopsy in patients with diffuse pulmonary infiltrates and acute respiratory failure. *Am Rev Respir Dis* 137:90–94, 1988.
106. Gaensler EA, Carrington CB: Open lung biopsy for chronic diffuse infiltrative lung disease: clinical, roentgenographic, and physiological correlations in 502 patients. *Ann Thorac Surg* 30:411–426, 1980.
107. Cheson BD, Samlowski WE, Tang TT, et al: Value of open-lung biopsy in 87 immunocompromised patients with pulmonary infiltrates. *Cancer* 55:453–459, 1985.
108. Fitzgerald W, Bevelagua FA, Garay SM, et al: The role of open lung biopsy in patients with acquired immunodeficiency syndrome. *Chest* 91:659–661, 1987.
109. Murray JF, Mills J: Pulmonary infectious complications of human immunodeficiency virus infection. *Am Rev Respir Dis* 141:1356–1372, 1990.
110. Landreneau RJ, Mack MJ, Hazelrigg SR, et al: The role of thoracoscopy in the management of intrathoracic neoplastic processes. *Semin Thorac Cardiovasc Surg* 5:219–228, 1993.
111. Kendall SW, Bryan AJ, Large SR, Wells FC: Pleural effusions: is thoracoscopy a reliable investigation? A retrospective review. *Respir Med* 86:437–440, 1992.
112. Daniel TM: Diagnostic thoracoscopy for pleural disease. *Ann Thorac Surg* 56:639–640, 1993.
113. Ferguson MK: Thoracoscopy for empyema, bronchopleural fistula, and chylothorax. *Ann Thorac Surg* 56:644–645, 1993.
114. Linder A, Friedel G, Toomes H: Prerequisites, indications, and techniques of video-assisted thoracoscopic surgery. *Thorac Cardiovasc Surg* 41:140–146, 1993.
115. Cannon WB, Vierra MA, Cannon A: Thoracoscopy for spontaneous pneumothorax. *Ann Thorac Surg* 56:686–687, 1993.
116. Milanez JRC, Vargas FS, Filomeno LTB, et al: Intrapleural talc for the prevention of recurrent pneumothorax. *Chest* 106:1162–1165, 1994.
117. Ferson PF, Landreneau RJ, Dowling RD, et al: Comparison of open versus thoracoscopic lung biopsy for diffuse infiltrative pulmonary disease. *J Thorac Cardiovasc Surg* 106:194–199, 1993.
118. Kaiser LR, Bavaria JE: Complications of thoracoscopy. *Ann Thorac Surg* 56:796–798, 1993.
119. Pearson FG: Staging the mediastinum: role of mediastinoscopy and computed tomography. *Chest* 103:346S–348S, 1993.
120. Ginsberg RJ, Rice TW, Goldbert M, et al: Extended cervical mediastinoscopy. *J Thorac Cardiovasc Surg* 94:673–678, 1987.
121. Luke WP, Todd TRJ, Cooper SD: Prospective evaluation of mediastinoscopy for assessment of carcinoma of the lung. *J Thorac Cardiovasc Surg* 91:53–56, 1986.
122. Vallieres E, Page A, Verdent A: Ambulatory mediastinoscopy and anterior mediastinotomy. *Ann Thorac Surg* 52:1122–1126, 1991.
123. Widstrom A, Schnurer L: The value of mediastinoscopy–experience of 374 cases. *J Otolaryngol* 7:103–109, 1978.
124. Carlens E: Mediastinoscopy. *Ann Otol Rhinol Laryngol* 74:1102–1112, 1965.

Chapter **7**

# Chest Imaging

**H. Dirk Sostman**
**Richard A. Matthay**

THE LUNGS ARE composed of a complex of tissues, each of which has a unique function but all of which together perform the act of respiration (1). The morphologist examines each tissue and describes its normal or abnormal characteristics. The radiologist similarly can assess individual components of the lungs through application of special techniques such as bronchography and angiography. The most commonly and generally used examination is the plain chest film (taken without added contrast material) (Figs. 7.1 and 7.2). The plain radiograph is the cornerstone of chest radiographic diagnosis (1). All other radiographic procedures, such as fluoroscopy, tomography, and special contrast studies, are strictly ancillary. With few exceptions, establishing the presence of a disease process by plain radiography of the chest should constitute the first step; if this first examination does not show clearly the nature and extent of the lesion, additional studies can be done to complement the plain chest radiograph.

Accordingly, in this chapter the normal chest radiograph and the normal radiographic anatomy of the airways and the pulmonary vasculature are discussed first; then special chest radiographic views, fluoroscopy, tomography, ultrasound, magnetic resonance imaging, contrast examinations, and ventilation-perfusion scans are reviewed. Radiographic manifestations of diseases of the lungs, mediastinum, diaphragm, chest wall, and pleura are discussed in subsequent chapters.

## CONVENTIONAL CHEST RADIOGRAPHY

### RADIOGRAPHIC TECHNIQUE

The basic principles of radiographic technique are as follows: (*a*) positioning must be such that the x-ray

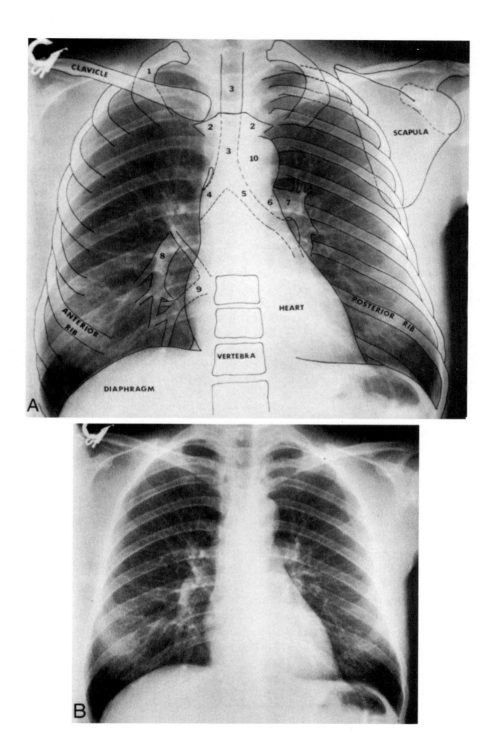

**FIGURE 7.1.** **A**, Posteroanterior (PA) chest radiograph with diagrammatic overlay. Various structures are identified by label or numbers. *1*, first rib; *2*, upper portion of manubrium; *3*, trachea; *4*, right main bronchus; *5*, left main bronchus; *6*, main pulmonary artery; *7*, left pulmonary artery; *8*, right interlobar pulmonary artery; *9*, right pulmonary vein; *10*, aortic arch. **B**, Chest radiograph of the same subject without diagrammatic overlay.

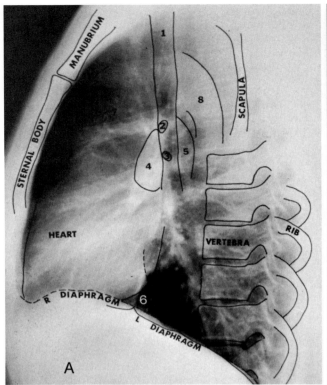 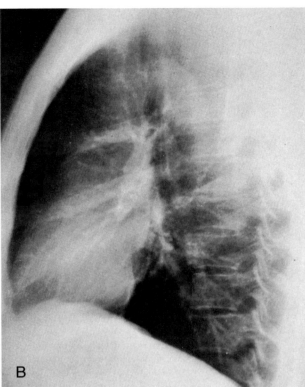

**FIGURE 7.2.** **A**, Lateral chest radiograph of the same patient as in Figure 7.1, with diagrammatic overlay. Structures are identified by labels or numbers. *1*, trachea; *2*, right upper lobe bronchus; *3*, left upper lobe bronchus; *4*, right pulmonary artery; *5*, left pulmonary artery; *6*, inferior vena cava; *7*, ascending aorta; *8*, descending aorta. **B**, Lateral chest radiograph without diagrammatic overlay.

beam is properly centered, the patient's body is not rotated, and the scapulae are rotated sufficiently anteriorly to be projected free of the lungs; (*b*) respiration must be fully suspended, preferably at total lung capacity; (*c*) exposure factors should be such that the resultant radiograph permits faint visualization of the thoracic spine and the intervertebral disks so that lung markings behind the heart are clearly visible (2).

## ROUTINE PROJECTIONS

The normal chest radiograph in the posteroanterior (PA) and lateral projections is shown in Figures 7.1 and 7.2. A diagrammatic overlay shows the normal anatomic structures numbered or labeled in both projections. In young persons or in asymptomatic patients a PA projection alone is generally used as a screening procedure (3). From an analysis of over 100,000 chest radiographs of a hospital-based population, Sagel and coworkers (4) concluded that routine screening examinations, obtained solely because of hospital admission or scheduled surgery, are not warranted in patients under 20, and that the lateral projection can be safely eliminated from routine screening examination in patients 20 to 39 years of age. A lateral film should be obtained whenever chest disease is suspected and in screening examination of patients 40 years of age or older.

For the PA film, the x-ray beam is projected from the back to the front of the patient, with the film cassette against the anterior thorax. Because the heart is in the front of the thorax, there is much less cardiac and mediastinal magnification on a PA than on an anteroposterior (AP) film (5).

The upright position is used because in this position the diaphragms are lower and the lungs are larger since the abdominal viscera do not push the diaphragms up as they do in the supine position. If pleural fluid is present, it is more easily identified on the upright film than on a supine film, since it gravitates to the dependent portion of the thorax, where small spaces such as the costophrenic angles are filled and altered in contour. Ultrasound is more sensitive than the chest radiograph for detecting small to moderate-size pleural effusions. Air-fluid levels, as seen in lung abscess and hydropneumothorax, are clearly visible on the upright chest film. If fluid must be identified and the patient cannot stand or sit upright, a lateral decubitus film should be obtained.

It is not always possible nor is it always advisable to take films upright or in the PA projection. The very sick patient must be recumbent, and infants and young children are usually radiographed in the supine position.

The lateral view adds valuable information about certain areas that are not seen well on the PA view (3). This is particularly true of the anterior part of the lung close to the mediastinum, which may be obscured by the overlying heart and aortic shadows, the mediastinum, and the vertebral column (Figs. 7.1 and 7.2). Moreover, a small pleural effusion is best seen, and often only seen, as blunting of a costophrenic sulcus posteriorly (3).

## PORTABLE CHEST RADIOGRAPHS

Portable radiograph films that are made in the intensive care unit, operating suite, or patient's room are generally of poorer quality than the erect PA radiograph or even recumbent films made in the radiology department. Positioning is difficult in a hospital bed, and consequently the patient's true position is often unknown, which causes difficulty in assessing the pulmonary vascularity or the presence of pleural fluid. The film focal distance is short, with resultant magnification of the heart and aorta and obscuration of part of the lung fields. Further, the x-ray generator used on portable equipment is not as powerful as stationary generators available in the x-ray department. Hence, it is preferable to obtain a film in the radiology department unless the patient absolutely cannot be moved without hazard. If a portable film must be done, an upright portable film is preferable to a supine film. The position and the distance from the beam generator to the film should be recorded on the film.

Recent advances in storage phosphor technology have made it possible to significantly improve the consistency and quality of portable radiographs and to produce them in a digital format so that they may be transmitted easily to video terminals (which might be located, for example, in the intensive care unit).

## OBSERVER ERROR

As Fraser and Paré have emphasized, radiologic diagnosis of chest disease begins with identification of an abnormality on a radiograph; what is not seen cannot be appreciated (1). Many studies of the accuracy of diagnostic procedures (6–9), notably those by Garland and coworkers, have revealed an astonishingly high incidence of both intraobserver and interobserver error among experienced radiologists. For example, in one series (6) the interpreters missed almost one-third of radiographically positive minifilms and overread about 1% of negative films; in another series (7), based only on positive radiographs, interobserver error ranged from 9 to 24% and intraobserver error from 3 to 31%. Since these figures are derived from studies by competent, experienced observers, it is clear that no student of chest radiography should be lulled into a false sense of security concerning his or her competence to detect a lesion.

To minimize observer error, a radiograph can be inspected in two ways, each of which may be employed usefully in different situations. *Directed search* is a method by which a specified order of inspections is carried out, for example thoracic and extrathoracic scans, followed by examination of soft tissues, bony thorax, mediastinum, diaphragm, pleurae, and finally the lungs themselves (1). The lungs usually are analyzed by individual inspection and comparison of the zones of the two lungs from apex to base. Such a method *must* be used by those in training, for it is only through the exercise of this routine that the pattern of the normal chest can be recognized (1).

The alternative method of inspection is *free search*, in which the radiograph is scanned without a preconceived orderly pattern. This is the method employed by the majority of experienced radiologists. However, such free search must be followed by an orderly pattern of inspecting to avoid overlooking less obvious abnormalities.

It is important to view every chest radiograph from a distance of at least 6 to 8 feet or through diminishing lenses (1). There are two reasons: (*a*) the slight nuances of density variation between similar zones of the two lungs can be appreciated better at a distance, and (*b*) the visibility of shadows with ill-defined margins is improved significantly by minification (10).

As a further means of reducing the frequency of "missing" lesions radiographically, the practice of double viewing has been advocated (1, 6, 10). In one study, the dual interpretation by the same observer on two occasions or by two different observers decreased by at least one-third the number of positive films missed (6). Many physicians, particularly chest physicians and surgeons, become highly competent in radiograph interpretation as a result of many years of personal viewing; if their chest radiograph reading is done in consultation with the radiologist, the second look may reveal abnormalities missed on the first interpretation.

## Radiographic Anatomy of the Airways

### The Trachea and Main Bronchi

The trachea is a midline structure; however, a slight deviation to the right after entering the thorax is a normal finding and should not be misinterpreted as evidence of displacement (Fig. 7.1) (1). The walls of the trachea are parallel except on the left side just above the bifurcation, where the aorta commonly impresses a smooth indentation; rarely, the azygos vein causes a smaller indentation at the tracheobronchial angle on the right side (1).

The trachea divides into the two major bronchi at the carina. The angle of bifurcation is varied and is most acute in asthenic persons (1). The course of the right main bronchus distally is more vertical than that of the left.

The transverse diameter of the right main bronchus at total lung capacity is greater than that of the left (average 15.3 mm versus 13.0 mm in adults) (11), although its length before the origin of the upper lobe bronchus as measured at necropsy is shorter (average 2.2 cm compared with 5 cm on the left) (Fig. 7.3) (12, 13).

The air column of the trachea, both major bronchi, and the intermediate bronchus should be visible on well-exposed standard radiographs of the chest in the frontal projection (Fig. 7.1). A thin vertical shadow is usually well visualized on lateral chest radiographs; it is formed by the posterior boundary of the tracheal air column (Fig. 7.2). This thin band is chiefly the posterior tracheal wall and is formed anteriorly by the junction of the tracheal air column and the tracheal wall and posteriorly by the junction of aerated lung in the right retrotracheal space with the external aspect of the tracheal wall and a thin layer of areolar tissue (14).

Pathologic processes within the mediastinum (e.g., carcinoma of the middle third of the esophagus) or in the medial portion of the right upper lobe can lead to deformity or obliteration of the posterior tracheal band, providing evidence for a pathologic process that otherwise might not be readily apparent (1).

### The Lobar Bronchial Segments

The anatomic distribution of the bronchial segments is illustrated in Figure 7.3. Each of the lobes divides into segments, which have been classified by the nomenclature shown in Table 7.1 (1).

Of clinical significance is the fact that several segmental bronchi are located posteriorly, which renders them frequent recipients of aspirated material and likely sites for the development of aspiration pneumonia. The dorsally located segments that are frequent

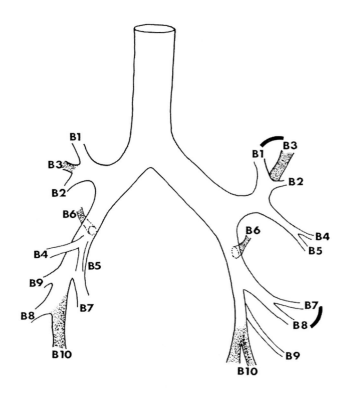

**Figure 7.3.** Diagram of the bronchopulmonary segments, following the Boyden classification. Segments that are relatively more posteriorly located are shaded; these areas are frequent sites of aspiration pneumonia. See Table 7.1 for correspondence of the Boyden system with the more frequently used Jackson-Huber classification. Note that the latter combines the segments connected with bars on the diagram into single segments.

sites for aspiration include the posterior segment of the right upper lobe (B3); the posterior basal and superior segments of the right lower lobe (B10, B6); and the posterior basal and superior segments of the left lower lobe (B10, B6) (Fig. 7.3).

Lobar consolidation of the lung is frequently associated with loss of volume (atelectasis). However, atelectasis of pulmonary segments occurs less often because collapse is prevented by collateral air drift; thus, most radiographic presentations of atelectasis are lobar (3). The patterns of atelectasis of various lobes are illustrated in Figures 7.4 through 7.8. It is important to recognize the patterns of atelectasis, since it is a common manifestation of bronchial obstruction by carcinoma of the lung. Atelectasis is common in the postoperative period, when it is due in part to inadequate clearing of secretions, and it may be seen in other conditions, such as asthma, in which viscid mucus occludes bronchi. It may also occur secondary to aspiration of a foreign body.

**TABLE 7.1**

**NOMENCLATURE OF BRONCHOPULMONARY ANATOMY**

| Jackson-Huber | Boyden |
| --- | --- |
| Right upper lobe | |
|   Apical | B1 |
|   Anterior | B2 |
|   Posterior | B3 |
| Right middle lobe | |
|   Lateral | B4 |
|   Medial | B5 |
| Right lower lobe | |
|   Superior | B6 |
|   Medial basal | B7 |
|   Anterior basal | B8 |
|   Lateral basal | B9 |
|   Posterior basal | B10 |
| Left upper lobe | |
|   Upper division | |
|     Apical-posterior | B1, B3 |
|     Anterior | B2 |
| Lower (lingular) division | |
|   Superior lingular | B4 |
|   Inferior lingular | B5 |
| Left lower lobe | |
|   Superior | B6 |
|   Anteromedial | B7, B8 |
|   Lateral basal | B9 |
|   Posterior basal | B10 |

Adapted from Fraser RG, Paré JAP, Paré PD, et al: *Diagnosis of Diseases of the Chest,* ed 3. Philadelphia, WB Saunders, 1988, vol 1, p 37.

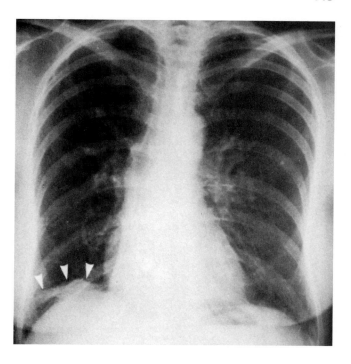

**FIGURE 7.4.** PA chest radiograph showing density in the right lung base behind the right portion of the cardiac silhouette obliterating the medial silhouette of the right hemidiaphragm. This is right lower lobe atelectasis. Note the relative paucity of vascular markings in the aerated portion of the right lung due to compensatory overaeration. Immediately above the right hemidiaphragm there is an area of linear atelectasis as well (*arrowheads*).

## RADIOGRAPHIC ANATOMY OF THE HILA AND PULMONARY VASCULAR SYSTEM

The major vascular structures in the thorax that are visible on the normal chest radiograph are the aorta, pulmonary arteries, and pulmonary veins (15). Each will be discussed individually, but first the normal hila will be described.

The hila are composed of the pulmonary arteries and their main branches, the upper lobe pulmonary veins, the major bronchi, and the lymph nodes. The lower lobe pulmonary veins do not cross the hila and therefore do not contribute to the hilar shadows (15). The bronchi account for little of the hilar opacity, since they are filled with air, and normally lymph nodes are too small to add to the size or density. Therefore, normal hilar shadows consist mostly of the large pulmonary arteries and upper lobe veins (Figs. 7.9 and 7.10) (15).

The main pulmonary artery is 4 to 5 cm in length and about 3 cm in diameter in adults. It lies entirely within the pericardial sac, as does its bifurcation (15). The right pulmonary artery lies posterior to the aorta and the superior vena cava and anterior to the right main bronchus (Figs. 7.9 and 7.11). It remains within the pericardium until it gives off its first branch, and the artery continues as the descending or interlobar division to supply the middle lobe and right lower lobe. It accounts for the lower portion of the right hilum (15).

The left pulmonary artery lies within the pericardium for a short distance before entering the lung. This vessel divides within the left hilum after passing immediately anteriorly and laterally to the lower portion of the left main bronchus (Figs. 7.9 and 7.11) (1).

The component distribution pattern of pulmonary veins (Fig. 7.10) involves two large veins on each side entering the mediastinum slightly below the pulmonary arteries and anterior to them (Fig. 7.11). It may be difficult to distinguish arterial and venous trunks within the lungs owing to superimposition of artery and vein (1), especially in the upper lobes where their course is parallel; in the lower lung fields the veins run more horizontally than the arteries and can often be distinguished.

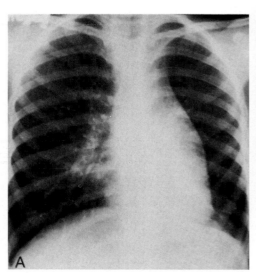
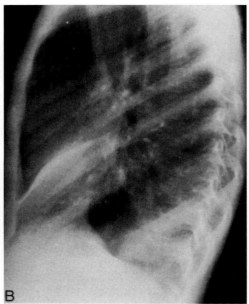

**FIGURE 7.5.** **A,** PA chest radiograph demonstrating middle lobe and left lower lobe atelectasis. The middle lobe atelectasis is seen as a triangular density obliterating the right cardiac silhouette. The left lower lobe atelectasis is demonstrated as a triangular-shaped area of increased density behind the left cardiac silhouette. Note that medial silhouette of the left hemidiaphragm is not visible. **B,** Lateral view of the same patient. The middle lobe atelectasis is more easily visible on this view, seen as a linear area of density overlying the heart silhouette. The left lower lobe atelectasis is seen as an area posteriorly and inferiorly, giving increased density to the vertebral bodies, which it overlies, and obliterating the silhouette of the left hemidiaphragm posteriorly.

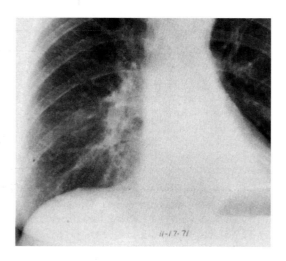

**FIGURE 7.6.** PA chest radiograph of another patient with left lower lobe atelectasis. Note the similarity to Figure 7.5**A**.

The caliber of the hilar pulmonary artery is important and should be assessed carefully. A significant sign is a change in caliber from one examination to another, particularly in relation to the diagnosis of pulmonary hypertension (1). Radiographic measurement of a segment of the pulmonary vascular tree may provide useful information (16). The width of the right descending pulmonary artery has been measured in over 1000 normal adult subjects (16). The upper limit in inspiration was 16 mm in males and 15 mm in females; during expiration it was 1 to 3 mm greater. Pulmonary artery hypertension is generally associated with enlargement of the right descending pulmonary artery.

## SPECIAL CHEST RADIOGRAPHIC VIEWS

### OBLIQUE VIEWS

In addition to the PA and lateral views, other projections serve special purposes. Oblique views may be invaluable in delineating a pulmonary or mediastinal mass or pulmonary infiltrate from structures that overlie it on the PA and lateral view. A pleural effusion or mediastinal mass is often well demonstrated on oblique views (5). Oblique views are also useful for studying lesions that are visible in the PA view but not in the lateral view. They may help in determining the site of origin of an intrathoracic lesion. By observing the rotation of a lesion in relation to a rib or to the heart or aorta, it may be possible to ascertain how close the lesion is to that structure and thereby infer its site and sometimes even its point of origin (5). When there are bilateral lesions on the PA view, it may be difficult to decide from the lateral view which shadow belongs

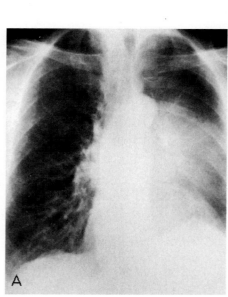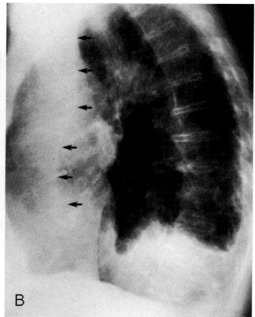

**FIGURE 7.7.** **A,** Chest radiograph of a patient with left upper lobe atelectasis. Note that the upper portion of the left heart border is not visible and there is a hazy density in the left upper lung field. There is evidence of volume loss in the left hemithorax (elevation of the left hemidiaphragm, shift of the heart and medi-astinal structures to the left, and closer spacing of the left ribs than the right ribs). **B,** Lateral view of the same patient. The collapsed left upper lobe forms an anteriorly located density, which is outlined in the figure by *arrows*. This is because the left upper lobe collapsed upward and forward.

to which side. Oblique views usually resolve this dilemma (5). Some reports have emphasized the value of oblique chest radiographs in detecting pleural plaques due to asbestosis. They are also helpful in the differential diagnosis of cardiac and great vessel enlargement, since the border-forming structures of the cardiomediastinal silhouette are different in oblique projections than those in the frontal and lateral views.

Oblique positions are named according to which part of the chest is closest to the cassette: right anterior oblique (RAO) view, with the right front of the patient against the cassette, and left anterior oblique (LAO) view, with the left front of the patient against the cassette. The standard angles relative to the coronal plane are 45 for the RAO and 60 for the LAO (5).

### LATERAL DECUBITUS VIEWS

The lateral decubitus film is useful for demonstrating a small amount of free pleural fluid or pneumothorax, the extent of a cavity or lung abscess, and the mobility of a mediastinal mass with gravity. As little as 25 to 50 ml of pleural fluid can be visualized (17). This view is particularly useful in determining if blunting of a costophrenic sulcus is due to pleural effusion or to pleural thickening (3). Pleural thickening is usually

a scar following organization of an exudate or blood in the pleural space (3). The decubitus film may also be helpful in shifting free fluid out of the way to visualize the underlying lung (2, 3, 5). Bilateral decubitus films are usually necessary if the effusion is moderately sized or large.

A lateral decubitus view is taken with the patient on his or her side, the x-ray beam aimed parallel to the floor, and the area of interest closest to the film. Air rises and fluid falls; so when, for example, right pneumothorax is suspected, the patient should be placed on the left side with the film and x-ray beam centered over the uppermost part of the right chest. For right-sided pleural fluid, on the other hand, the patient should be lying on the right side, with centering over the dependent portion of the right chest (5).

### LORDOTIC VIEW

The original purpose of the lordotic view of the chest was to partially uncover the pulmonary areas from the bony grid created on the PA film by the ribs and clavicles. When the tube is angled upward, the shadows of the clavicles are projected above the thorax and the ribs become more horizontal (Fig. 7.12) (5). The anterior part of each rib is thereby superimposed on its

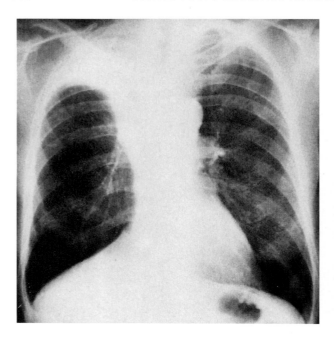

**FIGURE 7.8.** Right upper lobe atelectasis shown on the PA chest radiograph. Note the disparity in vascular markings between the right and left lungs. This is evidence of compensatory hyperinflation of the nonatelectatic portions of the right lung. Note that the right upper lobe collapse does not obliterate the cardiomediastinal silhouette as much as the left upper lobe collapse did. This is partly because the left upper lobe moves forward as well as upward as it collapses (see Fig. 7.7**A** and **B**), while the right upper lobe moves mostly upward, and partly because of differences in the mediastinal contour.

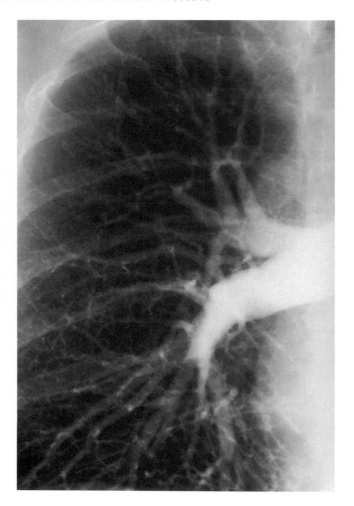

**FIGURE 7.9.** Normal pulmonary artery anatomy is shown on the arterial phase of a normal pulmonary arteriogram, obtained by injecting iodinated contrast material directly into the right main pulmonary artery.

posterior portion, reducing the number of obscuring bony structures. Thus, the lordotic projection enables evaluation of the apical portion of the lungs by displacing shadows of the first rib and the clavicle, which may be confusing on the PA projection (3). The lordotic view is also useful for recognizing collapse of the lingula or middle lobe when these areas become very thin and cast minimal shadows on the PA film (5). Lordotic and reverse lordotic views are often good for determining if a lesion is anterior or posterior. An anterior lesion is projected upward, as are other anterior structures (such as ribs and clavicles). The opposite is true for a posterior lesion. A reverse lordotic film produces exactly the opposite changes.

### EXPIRATION FILM

Although chest radiographs are routinely taken at full inspiration, an expiratory film may be helpful under appropriate circumstances. For example, a small pneumothorax is often difficult or impossible to see on a routine inspiratory PA film. On expiration, the volume of the thorax and of the lungs within it is reduced, but the amount of air in the pleural sac remains essentially unchanged. The pneumothorax then occupies a larger percentage of the area of the thorax and is more easily visible. Also, when a film is taken in expiration, the lungs appear denser, since the blood-containing vessels are crowded into a smaller space. Since the blackness of the pneumothorax does not change, the density gradient between the pneumothorax and the lungs becomes larger and this also makes the pneumothorax easier to see.

Another indication of the expiratory film is to demonstrate air trapping. The bronchi increase in diameter with each inspiration and decrease with each expiration. With a foreign body or tumor in a main bronchus,

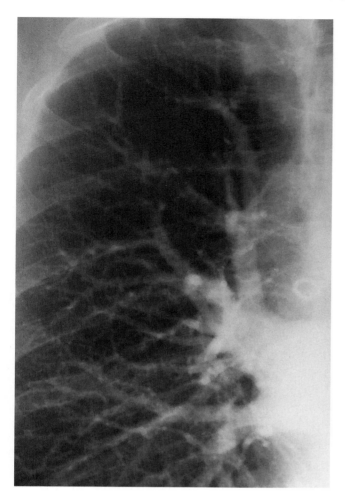

**Figure 7.10.** Levophase (venous and left heart phase) of the same pulmonary arteriogram shown in Figure 7.9. Note the differing course of the pulmonary veins as related to the pulmonary arteries.

a valve action may occur, with air bypassing the obstruction on inspiration and becoming trapped on expiration. With expiration, the normal lung is reduced in volume and becomes less radiolucent. The obstructed portion of the lung retains its air, thereby retaining its radiolucency and forcing the mediastinum to shift toward the contralateral side. If a patient has a unilateral respiratory wheeze, air trapping is likely, and an expiratory film is mandatory (5).

## Other Views

The *overpenetrated grid* radiograph is useful for evaluating densities that lie behind the heart or diaphragm and are seen poorly on routine radiographs. Stereoscopic views can be helpful in localizing any pulmonary lesion and are particularly useful with apical lesions, because they can separate pulmonary lesions from the overlying clavicle and first rib (3).

*Magnification* radiographs are used occasionally in diffuse lung disease to clarify minute details of the pulmonary parenchyma (10). Double-exposed films in inspiration and expiration are sometimes helpful in evaluating motion of the diaphragms.

## Fluoroscopy

Fluoroscopy of the chest is useful for examining the movement of pulmonary and cardiac structures and for localizing a pulmonary lesion that is only visible in one of the two conventional radiographic projections. It is particularly helpful for examining diaphragmatic motion (3, 18). When searching for diaphragmatic paralysis, it is often best to use the lateral projection so that motion of both hemidiaphragms can be observed simultaneously (3). A paralyzed hemidiaphragm moves paradoxically. This paradoxical motion is often difficult to appreciate during quiet breathing but usually becomes readily apparent during a quick, short "sniff" (sniff test). Localized weakness in part of one hemidiaphragm (eventration) is often misinterpreted as diaphragmatic paralysis. This error can be avoided by fluoroscopy in the lateral projection; partial eventration is then manifested by paradoxical motion of one portion of the hemidiaphragm, whereas the other portion moves normally. Eventration of an entire hemidiaphragm is impossible to distinguish from paralysis, since in both instances the entire hemidiaphragm moves paradoxically (3).

Fluoroscopy of the heart is useful for demonstrating calcification in cardiac valves or coronary arteries. Fluoroscopy often helps to identify the nature of a mediastinal lesion. When fluoroscopy is combined with a barium swallow, lesions within the esophagus can be seen. Moreover, the pattern of displacement of the esophagus by a mass in the middle mediastinum helps to determine the nature of the mass (3, 18). Respiratory maneuvers affect the size of large venous structures in the chest, which become smaller during a Valsalva maneuver and larger during a Müller maneuver. These maneuvers do not change the size of solid masses. Pulsation of a mediastinal mass suggests it is vascular. However, pulsation must be interpreted with care: masses that are adjacent to the aorta often transmit its pulsations and appear to be pulsating; in contrast, large aortic aneurysms often pulsate poorly (3).

Chest fluoroscopy also can be useful when trying to determine if a suspected pulmonary nodule on a

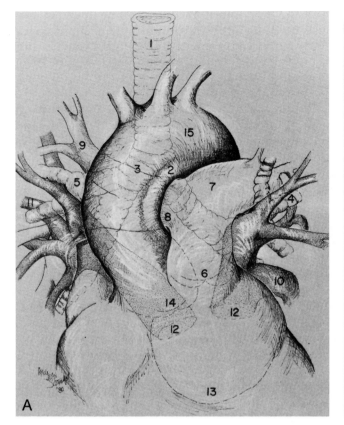
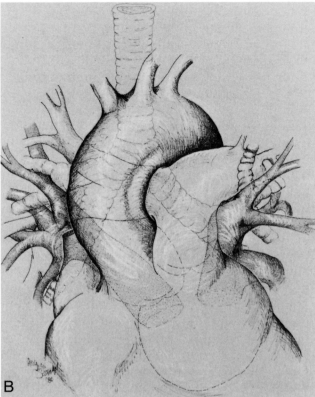

**Figure 7.11.** **A**, Depiction of the bronchial and vascular interrelationships in the mediastinum and hilum. Some of the individual structures are identified by numbers: *1*, trachea; *2*, left main bronchus; *3*, right main bronchus; *4*, segmental left upper lobe bronchus; *5*, right upper lobe bronchus; *6*, pulmonary valve; *7*, left main pulmonary artery; *8*, right main pulmonary artery; *9*, right upper lobe (truncus anterior) pulmonary artery; *10*, left lower lobe pulmonary vein; *11*, right upper lobe pulmonary vein; *12*, entrance of pulmonary vein to left atrium; *13*, left atrium; *14*, aortic valve; *15*, aortic arch. **B**, Depiction of the mediastinal, bronchial, and vascular structures without overlying identifying numbers.

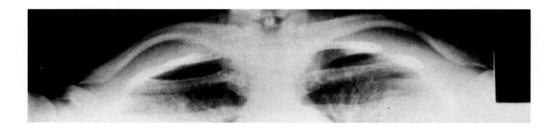

**Figure 7.12.** Normal apical lordotic view of the chest. Compare with Figure 7.1 to appreciate the difference in visualization of the lung apices.

chest radiograph (*a*) is real versus a superimposition of unrelated shadows or (*b*) is intrapulmonary versus extrapulmonary.

In past years, fluoroscopy of the chest was used as a screening procedure for routine chest examination (2, 3). This is no longer acceptable for at least three reasons: (*a*) the patient's exposure to x-rays is much greater during even a short fluoroscopic examination than during standard radiographs; (*b*) small lesions in the lung fields are overlooked at fluoroscopy; and (*c*) usually no permanent record of the fluoroscopic examination is available. However, fluoroscopy of the chest is warranted when specific information is being sought (3) or when it is necessary to monitor "on line" the performance of a special procedure, such as needle aspiration of a pulmonary mass or transbronchial biopsy.

## TOMOGRAPHY

### INDICATIONS FOR TOMOGRAPHY

Tomography is useful when there is a need for precise knowledge of the morphologic characteristics of lesions visible on plain radiographs whose nature is obscured by superimposed images lying superficial or deep to them (2).

Tomography provides clearer visualization of shadows that on plain radiographs are indistinct because of image summation, for example the bronchi or the pulmonary interstitium (2). Tomograms are widely used to determine the presence, size, number, and location of pulmonary nodules. Preoperative tomography is commonly used to detect pulmonary metastases and to determine if an apparently solitary lesion is in fact single. Further, within a solitary nodule, the detection of calcium is an important piece of data that is best obtained by tomography. Calcium usually denotes a benign rather than a neoplastic nodule, especially if there are multiple calcifications or if the calcium is centrally located, laminated, or homogeneous (18).

### CONVENTIONAL TOMOGRAPHY

If the x-ray tube and film are in motion during exposure, the resulting radiograph (called a *tomogram* or *laminagram*) will show a sharply focused plane or "cut" through the body with adjacent planes blurred (18). The thinness of the plane and successful blurring of the other planes are factors that can be controlled to some degree to determine the ultimate appearance of the film. Since the distance of the x-ray tube from the table determines the plane in focus, the films are usually made in a series of cuts so that each level through the lung is visualized sharply (Fig. 7.13), without overlying shadows (18). Posterior oblique tomography at an angle of 55 has been recommended for displaying a clearer outline of the anatomic components of the hila (19). Conventional tomography accurately detects calcification within pulmonary nodules and other thoracic lesions.

In most institutions, conventional tomography has been largely or completely superseded by computerized tomography (CT) in evaluating pulmonary nodules (Fig. 7.14), the hila, the mediastinum, and the lung parenchyma. However, conventional tomography remains an accurate and useful technique.

### COMPUTED TOMOGRAPHY

The development of CT brought diagnostic medical imaging into the modern age. It combined the basic phenomenon upon which the field of radiology was founded (differential x-ray attenuation by tissues) with the basis of subsequent developments (use of non-film x-ray detectors, digital computers, and video displays). Previous methods of forming radiographic images all used direct geometric projection of an x-ray shadowgraph of the patient's body upon a piece of film by a large-area beam of x-ray photons. CT uses a series of planar projections made by a thin beam of x-ray photons. These planar projections are mathematically recombined by the *computer* to form a cross-sectional *tomographic* image of the patient that displays the attenuation values of the many small areas ("picture elements" or "pixels"). CT thus introduced into clinical practice an entirely new approach to diagnostic imaging, aspects of which have subsequently been utilized in digital radiography, fluoroscopy, ultrasound, and magnetic resonance imaging. The diagnostic advantages of CT are due to its transaxial tomographic (slice-like) format and its high sensitivity to differences in electron density (and thus in x-ray attenuation) between different tissues. In addition, since the x-ray attenuation measurements are stored in the computer, the image can be enhanced or manipulated mathematically. For example, the technique of high-resolution CT (HRCT), a valuable method of studying the lung parenchyma, combines very thin slices with mathematical filtering of the computer data to produce increased edge definition in the final image.

Thoracic CT has found widespread use in the assessment of masses and neoplasms, including primary lung cancer (20–24), hilar and mediastinal masses (Fig. 7.15) (25, 26), and pulmonary nodules (Fig. 7.14) (27–33). It is now the standard of care for patients with such conditions who require diagnostic imaging beyond the plain chest radiograph and its simple variants (e.g., fluoroscopy). However, it should be emphasized that many patients with lung cancer or mediastinal and hilar masses do not require imaging beyond the basic chest radiograph. High-resolution CT of the lung parenchyma (Fig. 7.16) has been developed in the last few years and has become widely used for evaluating interstitial lung disease (34–38) and bronchial abnormalities (39–42). CT has application in vascular imaging in the thorax, most notably for suspected aortic dissection (Fig. 7.17) (43, 44) and superior vena cava obstruction. In addition, CT is unsurpassed in the detection and localization of pericardial and pleural fluid collections (Fig. 7.18) (45–48). Finally, CT may be used effectively to guide percutaneous biopsy (49) and drainage (50) of thoracic lesions. The patient is imaged to localize the lesion, and the skin entry site is identified with the aid of the CT scanner's positioning lights. A similar approach can be used to localize fluid collections or pneumothoraces that are not responding to

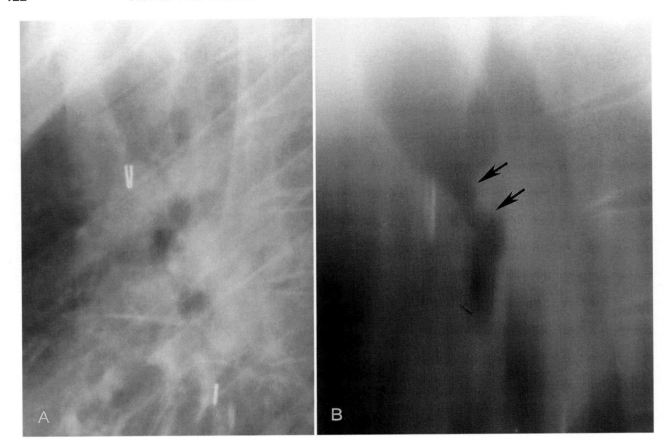

**FIGURE 7.13.** The value of plain tomography in evaluating pathology of the central airways. **A**, Lateral chest radiograph in a patient after resection of esophageal carcinoma who presented with wheezing. The lower portion of the tracheal air column is not well seen, but the presence of a lesion is not clear. **B**, Lateral tomogram through the trachea. Note that the overlying surgical clip that is seen clearly in **A** is blurred on the tomogram. This is the means by which tomography produces clearer visualization of selected planes. The tomogram clearly shows the presence of a constricting tumor recurrence narrowing the lower trachea (*arrows*).

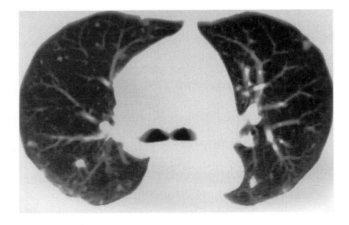

**FIGURE 7.14.** CT is the method of choice for detecting pulmonary metastases (as shown here in a patient with metastatic melanoma) and other kinds of pulmonary nodules.

blindly placed thoracostomy tubes, and then to guide percutaneously placed drains into the refractory collections.

## MAGNETIC RESONANCE

MR imaging (MRI) is based upon magnetization of the patient's tissue, generation of a weak electromagnetic signal by the application of a radiofrequency pulse, and spatially mapping that signal by manipulating its frequency and phase in a location-dependent manner using magnetic field gradients. Unlike CT, MRI does not require mechanical motions of the scanner and therefore can image directly in non-transaxial planes. However, like CT it is a tomographic technique.

Although electromagnetic radiation is involved, the energy levels used in MRI are well below the levels needed to ionize molecules, and MR imaging appears

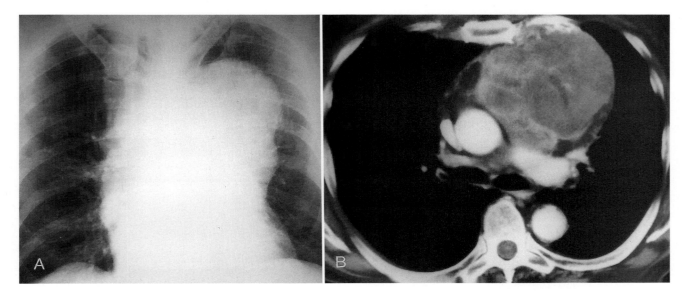

**FIGURE 7.15.** CT is the method of choice for detailed evaluation of most patients with mediastinal masses. **A,** The PA chest radiograph in this patient shows a large mass. **B,** The CT scan clearly delineates the anterior mediastinal location of the mass and separates it from the mediastinal vasculature, facilitating both the differential diagnosis and the surgical planning.

to be remarkably free of significant bioeffects. However, the strong magnetic field is a major safety hazard, since the magnetic forces near a whole-body MR imager are strong enough to cause significant projectile hazards. For example, an oxygen cylinder brought into an MR examination room will fly into the bore of the magnet with a *terminal velocity of about 45 mph*. The possibility of displacements or torques on metallic implants within patients must also be considered. Finally, the magnetic field can operate reed relays in cardiac pacemakers and cause a change in the pacing mode. Accordingly, strict security around MR facilities is essential to prevent patients with certain types of metallic implants from entering the scanner and to prevent medical personnel from carrying into the scan room objects that could become projectiles.

MRI produces extremely high contrast between different types of soft tissue. This soft tissue contrast is based upon intrinsic properties of the tissues and also upon operator-selectable machine parameters. The tissue properties are (*a*) the tissue concentration of protons available to produce an MR signal ("proton density"), (*b*) the presence of motion or blood flow, and (*c*) two tissue properties known as T1 and T2, time constants that describe how quickly an MR signal can be generated (T1) from a tissue and how quickly the MR signal, once generated, decays (T2). In general, pathologic tissues have long T1 times and appear dark on those MR images whose appearance is conditioned primarily by T1 effects ("T1-weighted images"). Usually, pathologic tissues also have long T2 times and appear bright on T2-weighted images. Flowing blood also can appear either bright or dark on MR images, depending on the examination technique that is used.

The usefulness of MRI in thoracic diseases is more limited than that of CT; for most patients who require further imaging beyond the plain chest radiograph, CT is the preferred initial choice because it is more effective, less expensive, and more widely available (49). In certain situations, however, MRI is useful to answer questions that remain after a CT examination has been performed. These situations include indeterminate mediastinal, chest wall, or vascular invasion by lung carcinoma (20, 23, 51) and the evaluation of suspected hilar masses (25, 26). In still other patients, MRI is the initial procedure of choice because the patient is allergic to contrast material that may be deemed necessary for a particular CT examination (52). The most common setting in which this occurs (Fig. 7.19) is suspected aortic dissection (43, 53–55), but an allergy to contrast material can mandate the use of MRI for other vascular imaging problems as well (51). Finally, there are a few conditions in which MRI has a real diagnostic advantage over CT and should be used as the initial procedure of choice. These include upper-extremity deep venous thrombosis (DVT) (56), brachial plexopathies and superior sulcus tumors (Fig. 7.20) (57–59), and cardiac and paracardiac masses (60, 61).

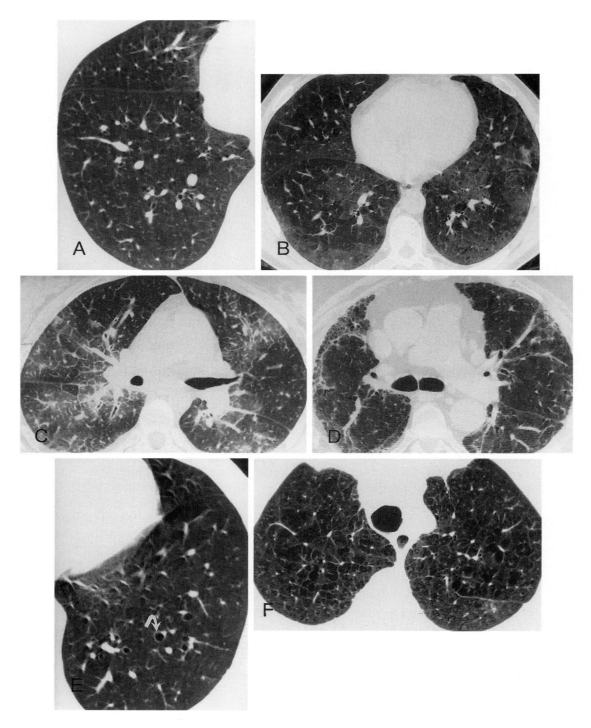

**FIGURE 7.16.** Examples of various common findings on high-resolution CT of the lung parenchyma. **A,** Normal lung. The vessels, bronchi, and fissures are seen clearly. **B,** Patient with alveolitis. There is multifocal faint opacification of the lungs, referred to as "ground-glass opacity." This usually, but not always, indicates the presence of an active, treatable process. **C,** Patient with lymphangitic carcinomatosis. Nodularity, bronchial wall thickening, and interlobular septal (interstitial) thickening are present. **D,** Patient with idiopathic pulmonary fibrosis. Char-acteristically subpleural changes of fibrosis and cyst formation ("honeycombing") are clearly visible on the HRCT image. **E,** Patient with focal bronchiectasis. Note the dilated bronchi compared with **A** and also compared with associated vessels in the same area, forming the so-called "signet-ring" (*arrow*) appearance. **F,** Patient with diffuse emphysema. Areas of destroyed lung tissue are apparent (due to their low density) as dark regions usually without definite walls.

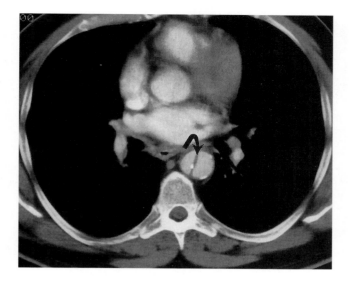

**FIGURE 7.17.** This contrast-enhanced CT section shows a Type B aortic dissection. The intimal flap, containing a fleck of calcium, is well seen (*arrow*).

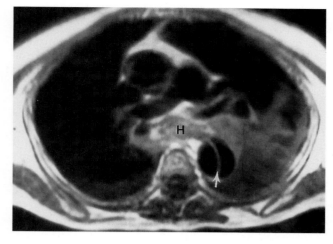

**FIGURE 7.19.** MRI was done in this patient with suspected aortic dissection who had renal dysfunction and thus was a poor candidate for intravenous contrast-enhanced CT. The intimal flap of a type B dissection is visible (*arrow*), and a mediastinal hematoma ("H") was found as well.

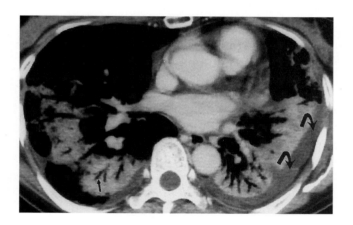

**FIGURE 7.18.** The left pleural effusion (*curved arrows*) is clearly visualized in this patient and easily distinguished from the adjacent lung consolidation. Note, in the consolidated areas of both left and right lungs, the presence of "air bronchograms" (one is indicated in the right lung by a small straight *arrow*).

## ULTRASOUND

Like CT and MRI, ultrasound is a tomographic technique. Ultrasound has limited usefulness in evaluating the lungs, since the sound beam is transmitted poorly by the air-containing alveoli and airways. However, there are two situations in which ultrasound is very useful for evaluating chest diseases. First, ultrasound is widely used to evaluate disorders of the heart and aortic root. Areas in which the heart and mediastinal

structures touch the chest wall without lung intervening are used as "acoustic windows" for transmission of the sound beam into the mediastinum. Ultrasound is the procedure of choice to detect or exclude pericardial effusion. Unique information can also be obtained concerning valvular heart disease such as mitral stenosis, the presence of vegetations or clots in the cardiac chambers, and global or segmental abnormalities of cardiac contraction. The second situation in which ultrasound is useful in the evaluation of chest pathology is in precisely localizing pleural effusions for aspiration or drainage (62, 63). It should be emphasized that ultrasound should not be routinely used for this purpose, because most effusions can be safely and easily aspirated after localization by physical examination.

## CONTRAST EXAMINATIONS

Air is the "natural" contrast material on which the diagnostic value of the plain chest film depends. Supplementary information is gained by introducing extraneous contrast material into different structural compartments of the thorax. "Positive" contrast material, such as barium sulfate suspension, is commonly introduced into the esophagus, while other suitable media are used to visualize cardiac chambers, trachea and bronchi, pulmonary vessels, aorta, bronchial and mediastinal arteries, superior vena cava, and mediastinal veins. Intravenously administered contrast material has become commonly used in many CT and MRI examinations outside of the thorax. For CT iodinated

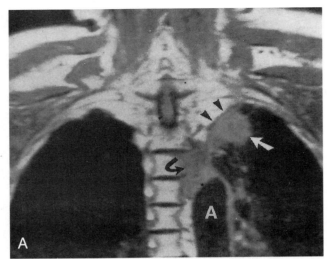

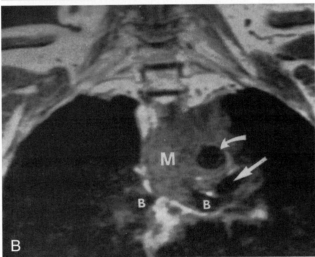

**FIGURE 7.20.** Magnetic resonance (MR) images of a 61-year-old man with a left superior sulcus (Pancoast) tumor, a squamous cell carcinoma. *Top,* Coronal T1-weighted MR scan reveals a mass (*white arrow*) that is confined within the apical pleura. The subpleural fat, which has high signal intensity (*arrowheads*), is preserved. Medially, the mass is infiltrating the mediastinum (*black curved arrow*) and is contiguous with the thoracic aorta (*A*). *Bottom,* Coronal MR scan 20 mm anterior to *top* demonstrates extension of the mass (*M*) into the mediastinum. The relationship of the mass to the aortic arch (*curved arrow*), main pulmonary artery (*straight arrow*), and bronchi (*B*) can be appreciated. (Reproduced with permission from Takasugi JE, Rapaport S, Shaw C: Superior sulcus tumors: the role of imaging. *J Thorac Imaging* 4:41–48, 1989.)

contrast material is used, while for MRI metal chelates are employed. In thoracic imaging with CT and MRI, the use of contrast is more selective and contrast is administered in a minority of examinations. To achieve "negative" contrast, air or other gases can be introduced, although this is no longer done in clinical practice.

### BARIUM SWALLOW

Of all the contrast examinations, the barium swallow, which is usually done under fluoroscopic guidance, is the simplest to perform. The esophageal lumen is outlined by radiopaque barium sulfate. Abnormalities of the esophagus itself, such as tumor or achalasia, can be seen (3). Formerly used to assess mediastinal masses and cardiac enlargement, the barium swallow has been replaced for these purposes by more specific tests, such as CT, MRI, and ultrasound.

### BRONCHOGRAPHY

The trachea and bronchi can be better defined by instillation of radiopaque contrast medium into the lumina of the trachea and bronchial tree (bronchography). It is mostly used for diagnosing bronchiectasis and mapping its location before surgical resection. In the past, prior to development of the flexible bronchoscope, bronchography was used to demonstrate an obstructing lesion that was inaccessible to the rigid bronchoscope. Today, bronchography is rarely done. Bronchiectasis is infrequent and seldom requires surgical treatment (5). When present, it can be visualized accurately with the less hazardous CT examination. The advent of fiberoptic bronchoscopy has rendered fewer lesions inaccessible to direct vision, and bronchoscopic brush or forceps biopsy and transthoracic needle puncture are more precise methods of diagnosing a pulmonary lesion than bronchography. If bronchography is performed, it should be done in conjunction with fiberoptic bronchoscopy.

### PULMONARY ANGIOGRAPHY

Pulmonary angiography (Figs. 7.9 and 7.10) involves the rapid injection of a radiopaque dye into the pulmonary circulation via a catheter into the superior vena cava, right atrium, right ventricle, or main pulmonary artery; or by selective injection into the right or left pulmonary artery or branches of these (2, 3). Direct injection into the pulmonary artery branches invariably produces the clearest opacification of the pulmonary vascular tree, and this superior visualization usually outweighs any disadvantage inherent in the catheterization procedure (2).

Angiography is principally useful for investigating pulmonary thromboembolic disease. In recent years, the popularization of ventilation and perfusion ($\dot{V}/\dot{Q}$) scans of the lung using radioactive isotopes has relegated pulmonary angiography to a secondary role in most cases. The accuracy of $\dot{V}/\dot{Q}$ scans for diagnosing pulmonary thromboemboli has recently been assessed and has been shown to be definitive in some circumstances but inaccurate in others (64). Angiography is almost always indicated when massive pulmonary embolus is suspected as the basis for circulatory collapse and immediate surgical intervention is contemplated. If surgical interruption of the inferior vena cava is planned because of failure of medical therapy or if thrombolytic therapy is planned, pulmonary angiography should usually be done. Angiography is commonly used in a clinical setting in which anticoagulation is considered dangerous or in patients in whom $\dot{V}/\dot{Q}$ scan results are equivocal or the clinical and lung scan evaluations lead to markedly different conclusions.

Less common indications for angiography include (*a*) suspected congenital abnormalities of the arterial system, such as agenesis or hypoplasia of a pulmonary artery; (*b*) suspected congenital abnormalities of the pulmonary venous circulation, such as anomalous pulmonary venous drainage and pulmonary varix; and (*c*) suspected pulmonary A-V malformations. In some instances, noninvasive techniques such as CT, ultrasound, and MRI will provide diagnostic information in these settings.

The decision to perform pulmonary angiography should be made carefully, since the procedure is associated with slight morbidity and rare mortality. However, these risks are not great in experienced hands (65).

Before injection of contrast material into the pulmonary artery, the pulmonary artery pressure should always be measured since it is dangerous to perform angiography in a patient with severe pulmonary arterial hypertension. If physiologic measurements such as wedge pressure or oxygen saturations are needed, they should be obtained before contrast material is injected, since contrast material has numerous physiologic effects that may alter these parameters.

## VENTILATION-PERFUSION LUNG SCANNING

There has been a rapid evolution of imaging devices and radiopharmaceuticals for the study of regional pulmonary function by inhalation and perfusion scintigraphy. Although the number of indications for lung scanning has increased, the major clinical application is in evaluation for pulmonary thromboembolism and

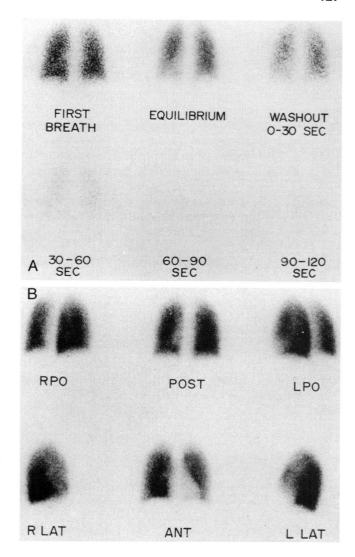

**FIGURE 7.21.** **A,** Ventilation phase of a ventilation-perfusion scan. Note that in the "first-breath" and "equilibrium" images there is homogeneous distribution of the radioactivity in both lungs. Note that in the "wash-out" phase (which is performed by serial imaging when the patient is no longer breathing in radioactive gas, so that the gas already in the lungs is imaged as it exits from the lungs) there is no evidence of abnormal retention of radioactive gas. **B,** Perfusion images of the same patient. It is important to obtain at least six views of the lungs. In this patient the perfusion is normal, with no focal defects seen in the images. The radioactive particles are injected with the patient lying supine. Note on the right and left lateral views that there is more perfusion in the posterior (dependent) portions of the lungs. This is a graphic demonstration of the effect of gravity on the pulmonary perfusion gradient.

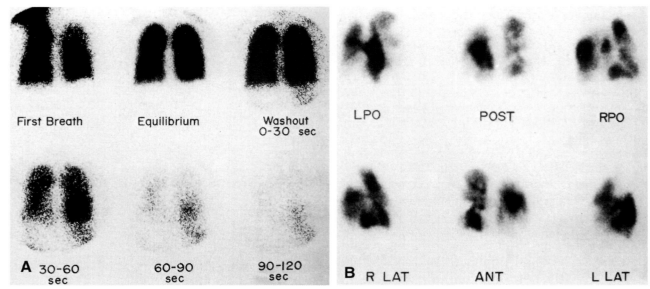

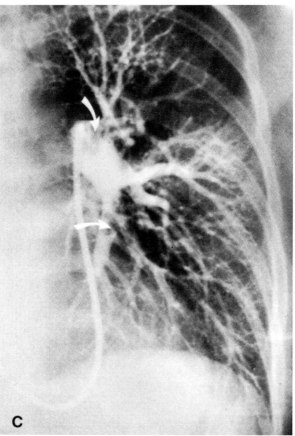

**FIGURE 7.22.** **A**, Ventilation scan in a patient with pulmonary embolism. There is no significant abnormality in ventilation. Focal activity in the later images is due to concentration of xenon in the liver. **B**, Perfusion scan in the same patient. Multiple perfusion defects that are wedge-shaped and bilateral are seen in the perfusion images. This is a classic appearance for pulmonary embolism. **C**, Selective pulmonary arteriogram on the same patient. Multiple filling defects in pulmonary arteries are demonstrated (*arrows*). This is angiographic proof of pulmonary embolism.

performance of preoperative lung function studies (64, 66, 70). It is beyond the scope of this chapter to describe in detail the imaging techniques and methods of interpretation of lung scans. They are only summarized here, and the interested reader is referred to reviews of this subject (66–68).

## INSTRUMENTATION

Lung scans are obtained by measuring $\gamma$-radiation emitted from the chest after radiopharmaceuticals are injected into the bloodstream or inhaled into the air spaces. Ventilation-perfusion scintigraphy is performed with gamma cameras, which permit viewing a large area at once.

Interfacing the gamma camera with a computer allows quantification of pulmonary ventilation and perfusion scans and measurement of regional ventilation and perfusion ratios. Thus, prior to lung resection, the surgeon can discover the contribution to overall pulmonary function of the region of lung to be resected. Perfusion lung scans can be obtained for either particulate or gaseous radionuclides. For the particulate type, a standard quantity of particles (usually macroaggregates of human serum albumin) with a size of 10 to 60 $\mu$m is injected into a peripheral vein. Because the particles are larger than capillaries, they lodge in the first capillary bed encountered (66). Techniques for assessing pulmonary ventilation involve the inhalation of a radioactive gas or a nebulized aerosol of a radioactive material (such as albumin labeled with $^{99m}$Tc). For the latter, the particles must be small enough (less than 1 $\mu$m in diameter) to reach the alveoli.

As stressed previously, the major indication for lung scanning is the investigation of pulmonary thromboembolism. Perfusion studies are diagnostically valuable only when the scan image is normal or can be compared with a current chest radiograph and ventilation scan. The absence of perfusion in an area of lung is nonspecific. It can be due to thromboembolic disease or to primary pulmonary vascular disease such as arteritis; it can be secondary to airway obstruction or other abnormalities of ventilation; or it can result from destruction of lung parenchyma, as in bullous emphysema. Only when the areas of perfusion abnormality correspond to pulmonary segments or subsegments (indicating a distribution comparable with the distribution of the pulmonary arteries) and ventilation in the analogous area is normal can pulmonary vascular disease be diagnosed with confidence. Pulmonary vascular disease is most commonly due to pulmonary embolism, and thus the assumption is made that areas of normal ventilation and abnormal perfusion are due to

pulmonary embolism. The diagnostic scheme for evaluating perfusion defects with and without ventilation and chest radiographic abnormalities is presented in detailed reviews (66–69). A normal lung scan (Fig. 7.21) excludes pulmonary embolism for all practical purposes. Multiple perfusion defects in areas of normal ventilation (Fig. 7.22*A*, *B*) are characteristic of pulmonary embolism. Intermediate patterns are more difficult to interpret. In many of those cases, a pulmonary angiogram (Fig. 7.22*C*) must be done to make the diagnosis accurately.

▼

## REFERENCES

1. Fraser RG, Paré JAP, Paré PD, et al: The normal chest. In Fraser RG, Paré JAP, Paré PD, et al (eds): *Diagnosis of Diseases of the Chest*, ed 3. Philadelphia, WB Saunders, 1988, vol 1, pp 1–291.
2. Fraser RG, Paré JAP, Paré PD, et al: Methods of roentgenologic and pathologic investigation. In Fraser RG, Paré JAP, Paré PD, et al (eds): *Diagnosis of Diseases of the Chest*, ed 3. Philadelphia, WB Saunders, 1988, vol 1, pp 315–387.
3. Miller TW: Radiographic evaluation of the chest. In Fishman AP (ed): *Pulmonary Diseases and Disorders*, ed 2. New York, McGraw-Hill, 1988, vol 1, pp 479–528.
4. Sagel SS, Evans RG, Forrest JV, et al: Efficiency of routine screening and lateral chest radiographs in a hospital based population. *N Engl J Med* 291:1001–1004, 1974.
5. Felson B: The chest roentgenologic work up. *Basics of RD* 81:1–4, 1980.
6. Garland LH: Studies on the accuracy of diagnostic procedures. *AJR* 82:25–38, 1959.
7. Garland LH: On the scientific evaluation of diagnostic procedures. *Radiology* 52:309–327, 1949.
8. Garland LH, Cochrane AL: Results of international test in chest roentgenogram interpretation. *JAMA* 149:631–634, 1952.
9. Felson B, Morgan W, Bristol VC, et al: Observations on the results of multiple readings of chest films on coal miners pneumoconiosis. *Radiology* 109:19–23, 1973.
10. Tuddenham WJ: Problems of perception in chest roentgenology: facts and fallacies. *Radiol Clin North Am* 1: 277–289, 1963.
11. Fraser RG: Measurements of the caliber of human bronchi in three phases of respiration by cinebronchography. *J Can Assoc Radiol* 12:102–112, 1961.
12. Merendino KA, Kirilak LB: Human measurements involved in tracheobronchial resection and reconstruction procedures; report of case of bronchial adenoma. *Surgery* 35:590–597, 1954.
13. Jesseph JE, Merendino KA: The dimensional interrelationships of the major components of the human tracheobronchial tree. *Surg Gynecol Obstet* 105:210–214, 1957.
14. Bachman AL, Teixidor HS: The posterior tracheal band: a reflector of local superior mediastinal abnormality. *Br J Radiol* 48:352–359, 1975.
15. Felson B: *Chest Roentgenology*. Philadelphia, WB Saunders, 1973.
16. Chang CH: The normal roentgenographic measurements

of the right descending pulmonary artery in 1,085 cases. *AJR* 87:929–935, 1962.

17. Hesser I: Roentgen examination of pleural fluid. A study of the localization of free effusions, the potentialities of diagnosing minimal quantities of fluid and its existence under physiological conditions. *Acta Radiol Suppl (Stockh)* 86:1–80, 1951.

18. Scanlon GT: Use of radiology in the diagnosis of lung disease. In Baum GL (ed): *Textbook of Pulmonary Diseases*, ed 2. Boston, Little Brown, 1974, pp 85–102.

19. Favez G, Willa C, Heinzer F: Posterior oblique tomography at an angle of 55 degrees in chest roentgenology. *AJR* 120:907–915, 1974.

20. Webb WR, Gatsonis C, Zerhouni EA, et al: CT and MR imaging in staging non–small cell bronchogenic carcinoma: report of the Radiologic Diagnostic Oncology Group. *Radiology* 178:705–713, 1991.

21. Patterson GA, Ginsberg RJ, Poon PY, et al: A prospective evaluation of magnetic resonance imaging, computed tomography, and mediastinoscopy in the preoperative assessment of mediastinal node status in bronchogenic carcinoma. *J Thorac Cardiovasc Surg* 94:679–684, 1987.

22. Friedman PJ: Lung cancer staging: efficacy of CT. *Radiology* 182:307–309, 1992.

23. Heelan RT, Demas BE, Caravelli JF, et al: Superior sulcus tumors: CT and MR imaging. *Radiology* 170:637–641, 1989.

24. McLoud TC, Bourgouin PM, Greenberg RW, et al: Bronchogenic carcinoma: analysis of staging in the mediastinum with CT by correlative lymph node mapping and sampling. *Radiology* 182:319–323, 1992.

25. Levitt RG, Glazer HS, Roper CL, et al: Magnetic resonance imaging of mediastinal and hilar masses: comparison with CT. *AJR* 145:9–14, 1985.

26. Glazer GM, Gross BH, Aisen AM, et al: Imaging of the pulmonary hilum: a prospective comparative study in patients with lung cancer. *AJR* 145:245–248, 1985.

27. Khan A, Herman PG, Vorwerk P, et al: Solitary pulmonary nodules: comparison of classification with standard, thin-section and reference phantom CT. *Radiology* 179:477–481, 1991.

28. Zwirewich CV, Vedal S, Miller RR, et al: Solitary pulmonary nodule: high resolution CT and radiologic-pathologic correlation. *Radiology* 179:469–476, 1991.

29. Davis SD: CT evaluation for pulmonary metastases in patients with extrathoracic malignancy. *Radiology* 180:1–12, 1991.

30. Chang AE, Schaner EG, Conkle DM, et al: Evaluation of computed tomography in the detection of pulmonary metastases: a prospective study. *Cancer* 43:913–916, 1979.

31. Robertson PL, Boldt DW, DeCampo JF: Paediatric pulmonary nodules: a comparison of computed tomography, thoracotomy findings and histology. *Clin Radiol* 39:607–610, 1988.

32. Costello P, Anderson W, Blume D: Pulmonary nodule: evaluation with spiral volumetric CT. *Radiology* 179:875–876, 1991.

33. Feuerstein IM, Jicha DL, Pass HI et al: Pulmonary metastases: MR imaging with surgical correlation—a prospective study. *Radiology* 182:123–129, 1992.

34. Remy-Jardin M, Remy J, Deffontaines C, et al: Assessment of diffuse infiltrative lung disease: comparison of conventional CT and high-resolution CT. *Radiology* 181:157–162, 1991.

35. Munk PL, Müller NL, Miller RR, et al: Pulmonary lymphangitic carcinomatosis: CT and pathologic findings. *Radiology* 166:705–709, 1988.

36. Mathieson JR, Mayo JR, Staples CA, et al: Chronic diffuse infiltrative lung disease: comparison of diagnostic accuracy of CT and chest radiography. *Radiology* 171:111–116, 1989.

37. Lee JS, Im J-G, Ahn JM, Kim YM, Han MC: Fibrosing alveolitis: prognostic implication of ground-glass attenuation at high-resolution CT. *Radiology* 184:451–454, 1992.

38. Aberle DR, Gamsu G, Ray CS, et al: Asbestos-related pleural and parenchymal fibrosis: detection with high-resolution CT. *Radiology* 166:729–734, 1988.

39. Munro NC, Cooke JC, Currie DC, et al: Comparison of thin section computed tomography with bronchography for identifying bronchiectatic segments in patients with chronic sputum production. *Thorax* 45:135–139, 1990.

40. Silverman PM, Godwin JD: CT/bronchographic correlations in bronchiectasis. *J Comput Assist Tomogr* 11:52–56, 1987.

41. Grenier P, Maurice F, Musset D, et al: Bronchiectasis: assessment by thin-section CT. *Radiology* 161:95–99, 1986.

42. Naidich DP, Funt S, Ettenger NA, et al: Hemoptysis: CT-bronchoscopic correlations in 58 cases. *Radiology* 177:357–362, 1990.

43. Petasnick JP: Radiologic evaluation of aortic dissection. *Radiology* 180:297–305, 1991.

44. Godwin JD: Conventional CT of the aorta. *J Thorac Imaging* 5(4):18–31, 1990.

45. McLoud TC, Flower CDR: Imaging the pleura: sonography, CT, and MR imaging. *AJR* 156:1145–1153, 1991.

46. Waite RJ, Carbonneau RJ, Balikian JP, et al: Parietal pleural changes in empyema: appearances at CT. *Radiology* 175:145–150, 1990.

47. Aberle DR, Balmes JR: Computed tomography of asbestos-related pulmonary parenchymal and pleural diseases. *Clin Chest Med* 12:115–131, 1991.

48. Friedman AC, Fiel SB, Fisher MS, et al: Asbestos-related pleural disease and asbestosis: A comparison of CT and chest radiography. *AJR* 150:268–275, 1988.

49. Fink I, Gamsu G, Harter LP: CT-guided aspiration biopsy of the thorax. *J Comput Assist Tomogr* 6:958–962, 1982.

50. Lee KS, Im J-G, Kim YH, et al: Treatment of multiloculated empyemas with intracavitary urokinase: a prospective study. *Radiology* 179:771–775, 1991.

51. Webb WR, Sostman HD: MR imaging of thoracic disease: clinical uses. *Radiology* 182:621–630, 1992.

52. Katayama H, Yamaguchi K, Kozuka T, et al: Adverse reactions to ionic and nonionic contrast media. *Radiology* 175:621–628, 1990.

53. White RD, Dooms GC, Higgins CB: Advances in imaging thoracic aortic disease. *Invest Radiol* 21:761–778, 1986.

54. Solomon SL, Brown JJ, Glazer HS, et al: Thoracic aortic dissection: pitfalls and artifacts in MR imaging. *Radiology* 177:223–228, 1990.

55. Kersting-Sommerhoff BA, Higgins CB, White RD, et al: Aortic dissection: sensitivity and specificity of MR imaging. *Radiology* 166:651–655, 1988.

56. Hansen ME, Spritzer CE, Sostman HD: Assessing the patency of mediastinal and thoracic inlet veins: value of MR imaging. *AJR* 155:1177–1182, 1990.

57. Rapoport S, Blair DN, McCarthy SM, et al: Brachial plexus: correlation of MR imaging with CT and pathologic findings. *Radiology* 167:161–165, 1988.

58. Castagno AA, Shuman WP: MR imaging in clinically suspected brachial plexus tumor. *AJR* 149:1219–1222, 1987.

59. Gupta RK, Mehta VS, Banerji AK, et al: MR evaluation of brachial plexus injuries. *Neuroradiology* 31:377–381, 1989.

60. Freedberg RS, Krozon I, Runnancik WM, et al: The contribution of magnetic resonance imaging to the evaluation of intracardiac tumors diagnosed by echo-cardiography. *Circulation* 77:96–103, 1988.

61. Barakos JA, Brown JJ, Higgins CB: MR imaging of secondary cardiac and paracardiac lesions. *AJR* 153:47–50, 1989.

62. Yan PC, Luh KT, Shen JC, et al: Ultrasonography and ultrasound guided aspiration biopsy. *Radiology* 155:451–456, 1985.

63. Ammann AM, Brewer WH, Maull KI, et al: Traumatic rupture of the hemidiaphragm: Real-time sonographic diagnosis. *AJR* 140:915–916, 1983.

64. The PIOPED Investigators: Value of the ventilation-perfusion scan in acute pulmonary embolism: results of the prospective investigation of pulmonary embolism diagnosis. *JAMA* 263:2753–2759, 1990.

65. Nicod P, Peterson K, Levine M, et al: Pulmonary angiography in severe chronic pulmonary hypertension. *Ann Intern Med* 107:565–568, 1987.

66. Anderson PO, Martin EC: Pulmonary embolism: diagnosis with multiple imaging modalities. *Radiology* 164:297–312, 1987.

67. Gottschalk A, Juni J, Sostman HD, et al: Ventilation-perfusion scintigraphy in the PIOPED study. Part I: Data collection and tabulation. *J Nucl Med* 34:1109–1118, 1993.

68. Gottschalk A, Sostman HD, Juni J, et al: Ventilation-perfusion scintigraphy in the PIOPED study. Part II: Evaluation of criteria and interpretations. *J Nucl Med* 34:1119–1126, 1993.

69. Wernly JA, DeMeester TR, Kirchner PT, et al: Clinical value of quantitative ventilation-perfusion lung scans in the surgical management of bronchogenic carcinoma. *J Thorac Cardiovasc Surg* 80:535–543, 1980.

70. Boysen PG, Block AJ, Olsen GN, et al: Prospective evaluation for pneumonectomy using the 99m-technetium quantitative perfusion lung scan. *Chest* 72:422–425, 1977.

# Chapter 8

# Clinical Pulmonary Function Testing, Exercise Testing, and Disability Evaluation

**Richard W. Light**

MEASUREMENTS OF VENTILATORY FUNCTION
    **Measurement of Expiratory Flow Rates**
    **Measurement of Airway**
        **Hyperresponsiveness**
    **Measurement of Lung Volumes**
    **Airway and Pulmonary Tissue**
        **Mechanics**
    **Distribution of Ventilation**
    **Gas Transfer and Exchange**
EXERCISE AND EXERCISE TESTING

**Exercise Physiology and**
    **Pathophysiology**
**Measures of Work Capacity**
**Determinants of Work Capacity**
**Training**
**Aging and Exercise Performance**
**Performance of Exercise Testing**
**Use of Pulmonary Function and**
    **Exercise Tests**

PULMONARY FUNCTION TESTING consists of the performance of a set of maneuvers to detect and quantitate disorders of pulmonary ventilation and gas exchange. These tests provide objective evidence of the presence, type, and degree of abnormality. They allow for assessment of the course of a disease state over time, evaluation of the effectiveness of a therapeutic intervention, and determination of the risk of pulmonary complications of surgical procedures. In general, testing of the pulmonary system requires relatively little invasiveness or risk, enabling one to undergo repeated studies over relatively short intervals.

This chapter provides an overview of clinical pulmonary function testing as it exists today. The tests commonly performed in well-equipped clinical laboratories are discussed. The objective is not to detail the techniques but rather to emphasize the fundamental concepts.

### Nomenclature

The field of pulmonary function testing has acquired a system of nomenclature that may appear confusing to the student but has an underlying structure that is easily mastered. The American College of Chest Physicians and the American Thoracic Society Joint

Committee on Pulmonary Nomenclature has provided a set of recommendations, which are followed in this chapter (1). Where older terminology is commonplace, it is given as well.

## MEASUREMENTS OF VENTILATORY FUNCTION

### MEASUREMENT OF EXPIRATORY FLOW RATES

Measurements of flow rates and cumulative exhaled volumes are the backbone of pulmonary function testing. The reader is referred to a recent monograph by

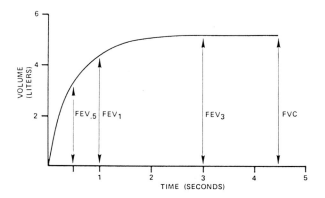

**FIGURE 8.1.** A typical forced expiratory spirogram showing the timed volumes obtained from the graph. $FEV_{0.5}$, $FEV_1$, and $FEV_3$ represent the forced expired volume at 0.5, 1, and 3 seconds, respectively. The forced vital capacity (FVC) is the maximum volume that can be forcefully exhaled.

the American Thoracic Society for guidance in the selection and calibration of equipment for this testing (2).

### Simple Spirometry

With this test, the subject inhales maximally to total lung capacity (TLC) and then exhales as rapidly and forcefully as possible. The cumulative exhaled volume is recorded on the $y$ axis and time on the $x$ axis (Fig. 8.1). From the curve a series of timed volumes and flows are measured. The *forced vital capacity* (FVC) is the total volume exhaled. The $FEV_{0.5}$, $FEV_1$, and $FEV_3$ are the cumulative volumes exhaled after 0.5, 1.0, and 3.0 seconds, respectively. Although the $FEV_{0.5}$, $FEV_1$, and $FEV_3$ are volume measurements, they convey information on obstruction to flow because they are measured over a known period of time. They may be decreased by any process that inhibits expiratory flow, by a decrease in the TLC, or by lack of effort on the part of the subject.

A more sensitive means of evaluating obstruction is to express the forced expired volumes as a percentage of the vital capacity, abbreviated as $FEVt/FVC$, with $t$ representing time of measurement. The ratio is relatively independent of the patient's size. The $FEV_1/FVC$ is a specific measure of airway obstruction with or without associated restriction of lung volumes. Normally it is 75% or greater. The $FEV_3/FVC$ includes flows at relatively low lung volumes when flow rates are decreased relatively early in disease, and thus it may be abnormal in early airway obstruction. It is normally 95% or greater in adults.

Average flows can be graphically measured from

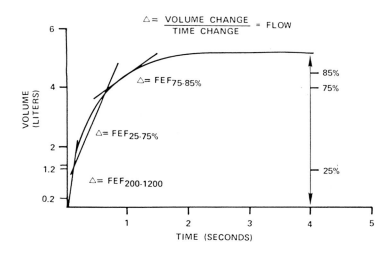

**FIGURE 8.2.** A typical forced expiratory spirogram showing the averaged flows obtained from the graph. The flow between 200 and 1200 ml of expired air ($FEF_{200-1200}$) is taken at high lung volume near TLC. The average flow between 25 and 75% of the

expired vital capacity ($FEF_{25-75\%}$) measures flow in the midportion of the expired volume. The average flow between 75 and 85% of the expired vital capacity ($FEF_{75-85\%}$) measures flow at low lung volumes.

the spirogram. Since flow is the change in volume with time, these *forced expiratory flows* (FEFs) may be determined graphically by dividing the volume change by the time required to make the change. Typically, the average flow between 25 and 75% of the vital capacity ($FEF_{25-75\%}$)—formerly called the maximal midexpiratory flow rate (MMF)—is recorded (Fig. 8.2). Other flows that are frequently reported include the flow between 75 and 85% of the vital capacity ($FEF_{75-85\%}$) and between 200 and 1200 ml of expired air ($FEF_{200-1200}$). These three average flow rates demonstrate marked variability in normal subjects (3). Accordingly, the 95% confidence limits for their normal values are so wide as to limit their utility in detecting disease in an individual subject.

Measures obtained from the FVC maneuver, whether recorded as spirograms or flow-volume loops, require the cooperation of the patient. It is recommended that a minimum of three acceptable FVC maneuvers be performed. If a subject has large variability between expiratory maneuvers, reproducibility criteria may require that up to eight acceptable maneuvers be performed. For the test results to be considered valid, the largest FVC and the second-largest FVC should not vary by more than 5% or 100 ml, whichever is greater. In addition, the largest $FEV_1$ and the second-largest $FEV_1$ should meet the same criteria. These reproducibility criteria are used as a guide to determine whether more than three FVC maneuvers are needed. The largest FVC and the largest $FEV_1$ should be recorded (2).

### Flow-Volume Studies

The development of sophisticated electronic pulmonary function testing equipment has led to the popularity of the flow-volume curve. For this test, the subject makes a forced exhalation from TLC, as with the forced expiratory spirogram, followed by a forced inspiration. The recording device plots volume on the horizontal axis and flow on the vertical axis. Values of FEF are taken at volumes representing 25, 50, and 75% of the exhaled vital capacity and are recorded as $FEF_{x\%}$ ($\dot{V}max_{x\%}$), with $x$ representing the exhaled fraction of the vital capacity (VC).

The flow-volume curve during forced exhalation has a characteristic appearance. The curve shows a rapid ascent to peak flow and a subsequently slow linear descent proportional to volume (Fig. 8.3). The initial portion of the curve depends at least in part on the effort of the patient. As a subject exerts increasing effort during exhalation, higher flow rates are generated. However, the latter two-thirds of the curve is relatively effort independent. For each point on the volume curve, a maximal flow exists that cannot be exceeded

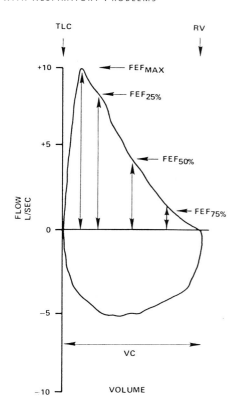

**FIGURE 8.3.** A typical flow-volume loop from a normal subject showing both expiratory (*upper*) and inspiratory (*lower*) portions. Instantaneous flows may be measured after 25% ($FEF_{25\%}$), 50% ($FEF_{50\%}$), and 75% ($FEF_{75\%}$) of the vital capacity has been exhaled. The peak flow is easily measured as the value of the peak of the graph.

regardless of the effort of the patent (see discussion of isovolume pressure-flow curves in Chapter 3). However, it must be emphasized that the maximal flow at a given lung volume will be achieved only if the patient generates sufficient intrathoracic pressure so that flow limitation is reached.

The flow-volume loop carries a great deal of information (4). Early in the development of obstructive airway disease, expiratory flow at low lung volumes is decreased but the volume exhaled is normal. This results in an expiratory curve that declines rapidly until the lung volume gets low, then persists at a low flow rate until the residual volume (RV) is reached (Fig. 8.4**A**). More severe obstructive disease results in an accentuation of upward concavity (5) with a greatly decreased maximal flow (Fig. 8.4**B**). Intrathoracic large airway obstruction, as in the trachea, results in decreased flows at larger lung volumes, while the flows at low volumes are relatively unaffected. The result is a flattening of the flow-volume loop (Fig. 8.4**C**). The

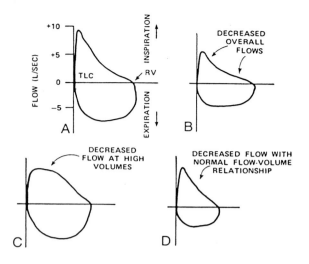

**FIGURE 8.4.** Common examples of abnormal flow-volume loops. **A,** Mild obstructive airway disease characterized by decreased flow at low lung volume when elastic support is reduced. **B,** Significant obstructive airway disease characterized by decreased overall flows with a further decrease at low lung volumes. **C,** Variable intrathoracic large airway obstruction in which peak flow is decreased at higher lung volumes with preservation of normal flow-volume relationship at lower lung volumes. **D,** Restrictive pulmonary disease with decreased vital capacity and flows but preservation of normal flow-volume relationships.

curve for patients with restrictive lung disease is one that has decreased volume and peak flow but a normal relationship between the two (Fig. 8.4**D**).

There have been many studies comparing the flow-volume curves obtained when the subject is breathing air and breathing low-density gas mixtures such as 80% helium and 20% $O_2$. The clinical usefulness of these tests remains to be proved (6). The reader is referred to Chapter 3 for a further discussion of these tests.

**Peak Expiratory Flow Rate**

The peak expiratory flow (PEF) is the highest flow rate that occurs during a forced exhalation from TLC. The PEF occurs very early in expiration, when the flow rates are effort dependent. A low value can result from slightly submaximal effort rather than from airway obstruction. In general, a relatively accurate prediction of the $FEV_1$ can be obtained from the PEF by multiplying the PEF (in liters per minute) by 9 to get the $FEV_1$ in milliliters (7).

The most common situation in which the PEF is used clinically is home monitoring. The availability of inexpensive small, portable devices allows patients to objectively measure their degree of airway obstruction on an ambulatory basis. It seems likely that patients' use of objective measures of airflow obstruction will lead to improvement in the ability of the patients (in cooperation with their physicians) to alter their medication regimen. However, no studies have yet demonstrated that this is indeed the case (8).

**Maximal Voluntary Ventilation**

The maximal voluntary ventilation (MVV) is the volume of air a subject can ventilate with maximal effort over a brief period. With this test, subjects are instructed to breathe rapidly and deeply for 12 to 15 seconds, and the cumulative expired volume is recorded. The results of the test are heavily dependent on subject cooperation and effort. Since the MVV can be predicted relatively accurately ($r = 0.94$) from the $FEV_1$ by multiplying the $FEV_1$ by 40 (9), routine performance of this test is not recommended.

MEASUREMENT OF AIRWAY HYPERRESPONSIVENESS

Individuals with asthma have by definition hyperresponsive airways. At times when they are evaluated in the pulmonary function laboratory, their spirometry may be within normal limits. The diagnosis of asthma can still be established by demonstrating bronchial hyperreactivity to the inhalation of various agents. The two agents most commonly used to provoke bronchial responses are histamine and methacholine. Additional agents that are used at times include distilled water, cold air, and exercise. With the typical procedure, the inhaled dose of the provocative agent is plotted on a logarithmic scale against the change in lung function, expressed as a percentage change from the normal value measured after an initial test dose of normal saline. Then the dose that produces a 20% fall in the $FEV_1$ is determined. Hyperresponsiveness is said to be present when the dose of histamine or methacholine that causes a 20% fall in the $FEV_1$ is 8.0 $\mu$mol or less. The lower the dose that induces the 20% decrease in $FEV_1$, the more hyperresponsive the individual. The primary uses of these tests are to establish the diagnosis of asthma in patients whose spirometry is normal and to quantitate the degree of hyperresponsiveness in known asthmatics (10).

Inhalational challenge tests are becoming more important for the diagnosis and management of patients with obstructive airway disease. One primary use is to exclude the diagnosis of asthma in patients with asthma-type symptoms or cough (10). A positive test in this situation is very suggestive that the patient has asthma, but it should be remembered that 3 to 6% of asymptomatic individuals have airway hyperresponsiveness (11). A second primary use is to diagnose and follow subjects with occupational asthma. A third primary use is to document the severity of asthma and to assess the response to treatment (10). It should be noted that there is a high incidence of airway hyperresponsiveness in smokers with obstructive airway disease. In a recent study of 3700 male and 2200 female smokers with $FEV_1/FVC$ less than 70%, 63% of the men and 87% of the women had a positive response to methacholine (12).

## MEASUREMENT OF LUNG VOLUMES

### Spirometric Volume Determinations

The spirometric volume determinations are relatively simple to perform. The typical testing procedure consists of having a subject breathe several times with a normal, resting tidal pattern while recording the volume continuously. The subject is next instructed to inspire maximally, then exhale as completely as possible, but slowly, and then return to tidal breathing. A forceful expiration may induce air trapping and thus result in a lower volume measurement. A typical graph is given in Figure 8.5, from which the following measurements may be made:

*Tidal volume* (VT): The average of the normal resting ventilatory excursions;

*Inspiratory reserve volume* (IRV): The maximum volume that may be inhaled beyond a normal tidal breath;

*Expiratory reserve volume* (ERV): The maximum volume that may be exhaled from a resting ventilatory level after a normal tidal expiration;

*Vital capacity (slow)* (VC): The total volume of air that may be moved into or out of the lungs, including the inspiratory reserve, tidal, and expiratory reserve volumes;

*Inspiratory capacity* (IC): The maximum volume of air that may be inhaled from a resting level, including the tidal volume and the inspiratory reserve volume.

The main problem with the spirometrically determined lung volumes is that they do not provide any indication of the volume of air remaining after a maximal expiration, which is the *residual volume* (RV). Therefore, alternative methods must be used if one desires to measure the *total lung capacity* (TLC), which is the sum of the RV and VC. These alternative methods include gas dilution methods and body plethysmography.

### Gas Dilution

The *closed-circuit helium dilution* method is performed by having the subject rebreathe a known volume of gas in a closed-circuit spirometer containing

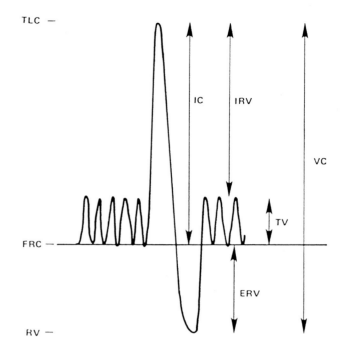

**FIGURE 8.5.** Volume tracing of a spirometer, showing the lung volumes and compartments measured from the tracing. The tracing is obtained by having the patient breathe quietly for a period of time, followed by a deep inspiration, and then a slow, complete expiration. The patient then returns to tidal breathing. The total lung capacity (*TLC*), functional residual capacity (*FRC*), and residual volume (*RV*) are shown for orientation. The measurements include the tidal volume (*TV*), inspiratory reserve volume (*IRV*), expiratory reserve volume (*ERV*), inspiratory capacity (*IC*), and vital capacity (*VC*).

helium as a tracer (13) (Fig. 8.6). Helium is inert and does not readily diffuse across the alveolar-capillary membrane. The helium equilibrates throughout the volume of the entire patient-spirometer system. The carbon dioxide generated is removed and the oxygen lost is replenished with 100% oxygen to maintain a constant volume in the system. If the patient begins and ends the test at the end of a normal expiration, the functional residual capacity is determined. The residual volume is then obtained by subtracting the measured ERV from the calculated FRC. This method is sensitive to errors from leakage of gas and also fails to measure the volume of gas in lung bullae.

A second method is the *open circuit* or *multibreath nitrogen washout* technique (14) (Fig. 8.7). The nitrogen normally present in the lungs is used as the tracer gas. The subject begins breathing 100% oxygen at the end of a normal expiration (FRC). As the nitrogen is "washed out," the expired gas is collected and the concentration

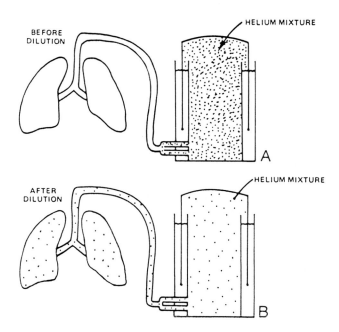

**FIGURE 8.6.** Diagram of the closed-circuit helium method for determination of the functional residual capacity. Prior to equilibration (**A**), the helium tracer is distributed in the spirometer circuit only; after equilibration with the patient's lungs by having him or her rebreathe the gas mixture (**B**), the helium is diluted and distributed throughout the lungs and spirometer. Measurement of the spirometer gas volume and the amount of dilution of the helium tracer enables calculation of the total system volume. The FRC is calculated by subtracting the spirometer volume from the system volume.

of nitrogen is continuously monitored. When the concentration in the expirate falls to a low level, the FRC may be determined by measuring the volume of gas exhaled and the nitrogen concentration of this gas in a manner similar to that used in the helium dilution method. This method has the advantage that it permits a simultaneous assessment of intrapulmonary gas mixing. This method is also sensitive to errors from gas leakage and does not measure the volume of gas in poorly communicating air spaces such as bullae.

Two other measurements of lung volume can be obtained from the dilution of gases used in standard tests of pulmonary function. One involves the measurement of the mean concentration of nitrogen in the air exhaled after an inspiration of 100% oxygen with the single-breath nitrogen washout test. The other involves measuring the change in concentration of helium used as the inert tracer gas in the single-breath measurement of the diffusing capacity. However, since the time for dilution of the tracer gas is relatively short for both

of these methods, the TLC will be underestimated in patients with severe maldistribution of ventilation (15).

From the measurements obtained by spirometry and the gas dilution methods all of the lung volumes may be determined. All three techniques can give faulty results if the test begins and ends at a volume different from that to be measured, which is either the FRC or the RV. With the helium dilution method, gas leaks in the system can cause an overestimation of helium dilution and thus yield falsely elevated values.

## Plethysmographic Volume Determinations

The technique of plethysmography is an alternate method used to measure the volume of the lungs (16). It is important to note that the results of these tests may differ from the results obtained by using gas dilution or washout methods. The gas dilution methods measure *communicating* FRC or RV, while the plethysmographic techniques measure both the *communicating* and *noncommunicating* compartments. Noncommunicating or poorly communicating air spaces are often present as a result of disease in which "air trapping" occurs. A pneumothorax is another example of a noncommunicating space. These gas compartments are compressible and therefore are included in the plethysmographic measurement but are not reflected in the gas dilution determination. The gas volume measured by a plethysmograph is known as the *thoracic gas volume* ($V_{TG}$) and in disease states is frequently higher than the value measured by gas dilution.

The measurement of $V_{TG}$ via plethysmography is based on Boyle's law, which states that the product of the pressure times the volume of the gas in the thorax is constant if the temperature is unchanged. The subject is seated comfortably in the airtight plethysmograph and temperature equilibration is allowed to occur (Fig. 8.8). With the airway occluded, the subject makes inspiratory and expiratory efforts against the occluded airway. The lung volume can then be calculated, since changes in the volume of the thorax are reflected by changes in the pressure in the box and changes in the thoracic pressure are reflected by changes in the pressure recorded at the mouth.

The procedure described above is usually initiated at the end of a normal expiration, so the $V_{TG}$ is equivalent to FRC. By combining this measurement with spirometric measurements, one may determine all the lung volume compartments, as in the gas dilution methods. The volumes determined by plethysmography are subject to error if the test is performed at an inappropriate starting volume. The measurement reflects the actual volume in the thorax at the start and end of the test.

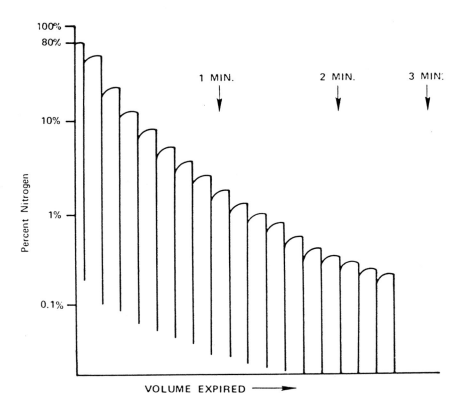

**FIGURE 8.7.** Graph of log nitrogen concentration versus volume exhaled in the multibreath nitrogen washout test used for determination of FRC and intrapulmonary gas mixing. The peak of the curve for each breath represents the end-tidal $N_2$ concentration. Analysis of the curve generated by the peak concentrations enables assessment of the homogeneity of gas distribution. On the log scale, mixing in the presence of ideal gas distribution would result in a curve that is nearly a straight line, with a rapid decrease in the concentration of $N_2$ to below 2.5%. By monitoring the volume exchanged, along with the $N_2$ concentration, the FRC may be calculated.

## AIRWAY AND PULMONARY TISSUE MECHANICS

The tests discussed so far are affected by such extrapulmonary factors as thoracic and abdominal muscle function and the properties of the thoracic cage. It is possible to assess the mechanical properties of the lungs themselves by using tests that require more sophisticated equipment. These tests are discussed briefly in the paragraphs that follow.

### Airway Resistance

Airway resistance (Raw) must be measured during air flow. By definition the airway resistance is the driving pressure divided by the flow that results from the pressure differential. Resistance to flow in the airways may be measured through the use of body plethysmography (17). In measuring total airway resistance, the pressure differential is that between the alveoli and the atmosphere. It is not possible to measure alveolar pressure directly when air is flowing, but a body plethysmograph can be used to measure it indirectly. The flow at the mouth may be measured simultaneously to enable calculation of airway resistance. It is important to measure Raw at low flow rates (less than 0.5 liter/second) so that the measurement does not reflect dynamic compression of the airways (see Chapter 3).

Airway resistance changes with lung volume, so the Raw determination is made at a known volume, usually the FRC. The relationship is inverse: thus an increase in lung volume results in a decreased resistance. The inverse of airway resistance is *airway conductance* (Gaw), or flow per pressure change. Airway conductance is nearly linearly related to lung volume (see Fig. 3.9**B**). The specific airway conductance (Gaw/$V_L$ or SGaw) is therefore independent of the lung volume and is the measurement that should be used in evaluating changes in airway resistance with time in an indi-

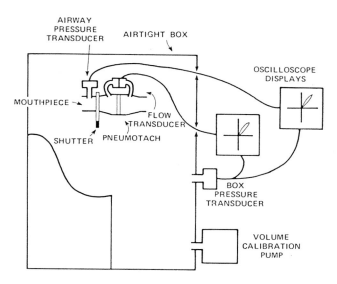

**FIGURE 8.8.** Body plethysmograph for the measurement of thoracic gas volume and airway resistance. The type shown is a pressure plethysmograph, which uses pressure changes in the box to estimate lung volume changes. Pressure transducers are used to monitor the box and mouth pressures. A flow transducer allows simultaneous recording of flow at the mouth. From these measurements, the thoracic gas volume and the airway resistance may be calculated using the techniques outlined in the text.

vidual patient or in comparing a given patient to normal values.

### Lung Compliance

The distensibility of the lungs is assessed by measuring lung compliance, which is determined from the relationship between changes in transpulmonary pressure and changes in lung volume.

The measurement of *static compliance* is performed with a spirometer to measure volume change and with pressure transducers to measure pressures in the airway and esophagus. The pleural pressure is estimated from the pressure within a balloon placed in the esophagus. The subject inspires to TLC and begins a slow expiration. The air flow at the mouth is interrupted at small volume decrements of approximately 500 ml, during which time the volume and pressures are recorded. Since the airway pressure during occlusion of the airway is identical to alveolar pressure, the *transpulmonary pressure* is calculated as the difference between airway and esophageal pressures. The lung volumes and corresponding transpulmonary pressures are plotted to give a static lung compliance curve (Fig. 8.9). The slope of the curve ($\Delta V / \Delta P$) at any given volume represents the *static lung compliance* (CLst) at that

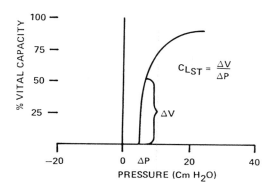

**FIGURE 8.9.** Volume-pressure graph obtained by measuring the pressure during static conditions at various lung volumes with the glottis closed. The test is usually performed by interrupting flow intermittently during an expiration from TLC while recording transpulmonary pressure and volume above FRC. The transpulmonary pressure is the alveolar pressure measured at the mouth minus the pleural pressure measured with an esophageal balloon. The pressure and volume points are plotted as a curve. The static compliance is measured as the slope of the curve at a given point, usually just above FRC.

volume. The portion of the curve 500 to 1000 ml above the FRC is usually chosen for the measurement, since at higher lung volumes the relationship becomes highly nonlinear. The static compliance is often normalized to the absolute lung volume at which the measurement is made and is termed *specific compliance* (CLst/VL). The reason for this is that compliance is directly related to absolute lung volume.

Static lung compliance reflects the elasticity of the lung parenchyma. It increases slightly with advancing age owing to changes in the elastic fibers of the lungs. It also increases in emphysema. A decreased compliance suggests interstitial disease or one with alveolar filling such as pulmonary edema.

During the measurement of static lung compliance, the transthoracic pressure (alveolar minus atmospheric) may be recorded in addition to the transpulmonary pressure to permit calculation of *total lung compliance* (CTst). This measurement includes pulmonary and chest wall factors. The difference between the transthoracic and transpulmonary pressures may be used to calculate the *chest wall compliance* (Cwst).

### DISTRIBUTION OF VENTILATION

Tests of gas distribution are used to give a measure of the homogeneity of the distribution of inspired gas to the alveoli. In the normal lung, gas is transported along all airways and is distributed relatively equally to all areas of the lung, with more distribution to the lower regions of the lung in the upright subject. This is because alveoli in the upper zones are more distended than in the lower zones at FRC and are less able to expand. In certain disease states, especially those with destruction of pulmonary tissue, there is a variable degree of inhomogeneity that alters the intrapulmonary distribution of gas within each region. Several tests are available to detect this type of abnormality.

### Single-Breath Nitrogen Elimination Test

The single-breath $N_2$ test may be used to assess the homogeneity of gas distribution (18). The results of the test give an index that reflects the overall mixing ability of the lungs, but no anatomic indication of areas of poor distribution is possible.

The test is performed with the subject seated after normal breathing of room air for a few moments. The subject exhales to residual volume, and then slowly inhales a breath of 100% oxygen to total lung capacity (TLC). During a slow expiration (under 1 liter/second), the concentration of nitrogen in the exhaled air is recorded continuously as a function of the volume exhaled. The resulting curve consists of four phases, which are depicted in Figure 8.10.

The shape of the curve can be explained on the basis of the underlying physiology. At RV the alveoli in the upper portions of the lungs are larger than those in the lower portions because of the more-negative pleural pressure at the top part of the lung. At TLC all the

alveoli are approximately the same size. Therefore, when an individual takes a breath of 100% $O_2$ from RV, the nitrogen concentration in the alveoli in the upper portion of the lungs will be greater at TLC than that in the lower portion of the lungs. On expiration, the dead-space gas (100% oxygen) is exhaled first and is noted as phase I, in which the nitrogen concentration is zero. The nitrogen concentration rises abruptly (phase II) when alveolar gas with nitrogen begins to be exhaled. Phase III represents alveolar gas exhalation. If gas distribution were perfectly homogeneous, all alveoli would empty at an approximately equal rate and the phase III line would be horizontal. Nonhomogeneous emptying of the lungs results in different rates of nitrogen expiration, and there is normally a slight rise of the phase III line. In conditions of abnormal intrapulmonary mixing, the beginning of phase IV occurs when the small airways in the bases of the lungs begin to close, leaving only the upper zones, which have higher $N_2$ concentration, to empty, causing the abrupt increase in slope (19).

From the curve the following measurements are made:

*Anatomic dead space* (VDanat): The volume of phase I and approximately half of phase II;

*Phase III slope:* The change in nitrogen concentration over 1 liter of the initial portion of phase III;

*Closing volume* (CV): The volume above the RV, at which phase IV begins to occur, reported as percent of VC;

*Closing capacity* (CC): The CV plus the RV, reported as percent of TLC.

The phase III slope is an index of uniformity of gas distribution. Normally there is less than a 2% change in nitrogen concentration per liter during phase III. Increases in its value reflect relatively greater inhomogeneity than normal. Indeed, in one large study of over 2500 adults, the slope of phase III was more strongly associated with mortality than was the $FEV_1$ (20). The CV was proposed as a sensitive indicator of small airway disease (21) and was thought to hold promise as a predictive test for the development of chronic obstructive pulmonary disease. However, subsequent studies designed to prove this contention were disappointing (22). At the present time, this test is rarely used in the clinical situation.

### Multibreath Nitrogen Washout

The use of this test to measure the FRC was described in a previous section (see Figure 8.7). It may also be used to assess the homogeneity of ventilation. The nitrogen concentration after 7 minutes is used as an index of the homogeneity of ventilation. Normally it is less than 2.5%. If uneven gas distribution exists

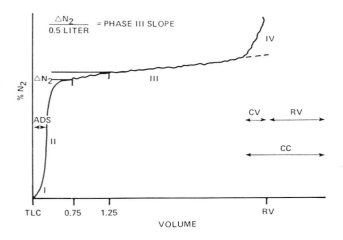

**FIGURE 8.10.** Graph of nitrogen concentration versus volume exhaled in the single-breath nitrogen test. Measurement of $\Delta N_2$ is the change in nitrogen concentration over the curve from 750 to 1250 ml. The phase III slope is the slope of the line over an initial portion of the curve, equal to the change in $N_2$ concentration over a 1-liter portion of the curve. Measurements of closing volume and anatomic dead space are made directly from the graph.

owing to slower emptying of some lung compartments, the washout is prolonged and the nitrogen concentration after 7 minutes is greater than 2.5%. Occasionally, the multibreath nitrogen washout test may be abnormal when the single-breath nitrogen test is normal. This has been attributed to the exchange of gas with bullae or similar compartments, which is too slow to affect the single-breath test but is detectable by the washout method owing to the prolonged tidal breathing.

### Radioactive Xenon Distribution

The two tests of distribution described above provide an index giving some overall indication of the *degree* of inhomogeneity. Visualization of the *distribution* of gas may be performed with the radioactive xenon test, in which the subject breathes a gas mixture containing $^{133}$Xe while his or her chest is scanned with a gamma camera. The $^{133}$Xe isotope may also be dissolved in saline and injected intravenously. Since the gas is poorly soluble in blood, it is almost completely eliminated in one passage through the lungs. Scanning over the chest wall immediately after injection yields an estimate of relative perfusion to various areas, and the rate of clearance from these areas indicates their relative ventilation. These uses of xenon are described in more detail in Chapter 7.

### GAS TRANSFER AND EXCHANGE

The ability of gases to transfer across the alveolar-capillary membrane is assessed by analyzing the concentration of respiratory gases on both sides of the membrane or by assessing the ease with which a foreign gas transfers from the alveoli to the blood. There are several factors that affect the process of gas exchange, including the total surface area available for gas exchange, the diffusion characteristics of the alveolar-capillary membrane, the perfusion of the capillaries with blood, and the matching of ventilation to perfusion. These tests, however, give an overall index of diffusion and do not allow an assessment of each of the factors involved.

### Blood Gas and Acid-Base Analysis

The measurement of the pH and partial pressures of oxygen and carbon dioxide in the arterial and venous blood is fundamental to the diagnosis and management of patients with pulmonary disorders. These measurements not only are valuable in the management of critically ill patients but also enable one to determine a number of clinically useful indexes of cardiopulmonary function, including venous admixture (physiologic shunt fraction) and physiologic dead space fraction. They reflect the overall function of the cardiopulmonary system with respect to gas exchange. Detailed information on the use and interpretation of these measurements is presented in Chapter 4.

### Carbon Monoxide Diffusing Capacity

The diffusing capacity of the lungs ($D_L$) is a measure of the ability of gases to diffuse from the alveoli into the pulmonary capillary blood. Carbon monoxide is the usual test gas since it is not normally present in the lungs or blood and since it is much more soluble in blood than in lung tissues. When the diffusing capacity is measured with carbon monoxide, the test is called the carbon monoxide diffusing capacity ($D_{LCO}$).

To determine $D_{LCO}$, the amount of CO transferred per unit time and the average partial pressure difference of the gas across the alveolar-capillary membrane must be measured. The following equation represents this basic principle:

$$D_{LCO} = \frac{\dot{V}_{CO}}{P_{ACO} - P_{cCO}} \quad (1)$$

where $\dot{V}_{CO}$ is the uptake of carbon monoxide and $P_{ACO}$ and $P_{cCO}$ are the partial pressures of carbon monoxide in the alveolar gas and capillary blood, respectively. The final result for $D_{LCO}$ is expressed as milliliters of carbon monoxide transferred per minute per millimeter of mercury pressure gradient. Since the $D_{LCO}$ is directly related to the alveolar volume, it is frequently normalized to this value ($D_L/V_A$), which allows for its interpretation in the presence of abnormal lung volumes.

*Techniques*

The most common manner by which the diffusing capacity is measured is the *single-breath carbon monoxide test* ($D_{LCO_{SB}}$) (23). With this method, the subject exhales to RV and then inhales a full breath of a gas mixture containing a low concentration of CO and 10% He. The subject holds his or her breath for 10 seconds and then exhales completely (Fig. 8.11). The initial alveolar volume and $P_{ACO}$ are derived from measurements of the helium concentrations in the inspired and expired air and the carbon monoxide concentrations in the inspired gas. The final $P_{ACO}$ is assumed to be the end-expiratory partial pressure of carbon monoxide. It is assumed that the $P_{ACO}$ declines exponentially and that the capillary partial pressure is negligible. The $D_{LCO}$ can then be easily computed from the following equation:

$$D_{LCO} = \frac{V_A \times 60}{(P_{bar} - 47) \times t} \ln \frac{P_{ACO_i}}{P_{ACO_t}} \quad (2)$$

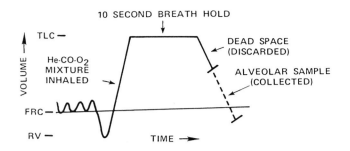

**FIGURE 8.11.** Kymograph tracing during the single-breath $D_{LCO}$ maneuver. The patient first exhales to residual volume, then takes a full breath of a known mixture of oxygen, helium, and carbon monoxide. The breath is held at full inspiration for 10 seconds to allow gas transfer, then the subject exhales. After the initial dead space is exhaled, a sample of alveolar gas is collected and analyzed. The difference in gas concentration between the inhaled gas and the alveolar gas sample allows for calculation of the transfer of carbon monoxide from the lungs.

where $V_A$ is the original lung volume, Pbar is the barometric pressure, $t$ is the time of breath holding, and $P_{ACO}i$ and $P_{ACO}t$ are the initial and final partial alveolar pressures of carbon monoxide. Recommendations for the standard technique for this measurement have been published (24).

A second technique is the *steady-state method* ($D_{LCO_{SS}}$), of which there are several variations. With these methods, the subject rebreathes a gas with a known CO concentration until CO uptake reaches a steady state, at which point several measurements are made for the calculation of the entities in Equation 1. The various methods differ in the way in which the mean $P_{ACO}$ and the capillary $P_{CCO}$ are calculated (25).

A less commonly used technique is the *rebreathing method* ($D_{LCO_{RB}}$) (24), in which a subject rebreathes a CO-He mixture for approximately 1 minute. The gas mixture and the measurement and calculations are nearly identical to those for the single-breath technique.

The choice of the technique used depends on several factors. The single-breath technique is the one most widely used, because it is simple and quick to perform. It is possible, however, that this technique does not give truly physiologic results, since breath holding does not provide proper conditions for complete gas distribution. It is also the method that is most sensitive to ventilation-perfusion abnormalities. It cannot be used for measurements during exercise. The steady-state and rebreathing methods can be applied to exercise testing and are less affected by ventilation-perfusion abnormalities but are more difficult and time-consuming to perform.

*Factors Influencing the Diffusing Capacity*

The resistance to the diffusion of carbon monoxide from the alveoli to the blood is determined primarily by two factors, the state of the alveolar-capillary membrane and the amount of hemoglobin in the pulmonary capillaries available for uptake of carbon monoxide (26). Mathematically, the following formula expresses this relationship:

$$\frac{1}{D_L} = \frac{1}{D_M} + \frac{1}{\theta V_c} \qquad (3)$$

where $D_L$ is the diffusing capacity of the lung, $D_M$ represents the membrane component, $V_c$ is the capillary blood volume, and the coefficient $\theta$ is the rate at which CO binds to intracellular oxyhemoglobin. Normally the two components on the right side of Equation 3 contribute approximately equally to the measured $D_{LCO}$ (27).

Both quantitative and qualitative abnormalities in the alveolar-capillary membrane may alter the measured $D_{LCO}$. The measured $D_{LCO}$ will depend on the total surface area available for gas exchange. Therefore, large individuals will have a higher $D_{LCO}$ than small individuals. Also the removal of a portion of the lung will reduce the $D_{LCO}$. In areas of the lung that are poorly ventilated, carbon monoxide will not be transferred and a reduced diffusing capacity will result. In a given patient, a higher $D_{LCO}$ will be obtained with a higher lung volume (28).

The $D_{LCO}$ may also be reduced if there is increased resistance to diffusion across the alveolar membrane. Historically, qualitative abnormalities in the alveolar-capillary membrane have been considered to be primarily due to an increased thickness of the membrane. However, the relative contribution of a "thick" membrane to loss of $D_{LCO}$ appears to have been overestimated. In diseases with interstitial thickening, other factors such as an alteration in the alveolar architecture with loss of surface area for gas exchange appear to play a greater role in producing the low $D_{LCO}$ (26).

The second major factor that influences the diffusing capacity, which is represented by the last term in Equation 3, is the ability of the blood to accept and bind carbon monoxide. Fundamentally, this is dependent on two factors: the pulmonary capillary blood volume and the level of hemoglobin in this capillary blood. The pulmonary capillary blood volume is obviously reduced in areas of the lung that are not perfused. Changes in position and alterations in intrathoracic pressure at the time of measurement can both alter pulmonary capillary blood volume.

Diffusing capacity measurements are usually made to determine the status of the lung. Since anemia can result in a decreased diffusing capacity in the presence of a normal lung, it is recommended that diffusing capacity measurements be corrected for the level of hemoglobin in the blood by using the following equation (24):

Adjusted $D_{LCO}$ = observed $D_{LCO}$

$$[(10.22 + Hb)/1.7 Hb] \qquad (4)$$

## EXERCISE AND EXERCISE TESTING

In recent years exercise pathophysiology and exercise testing have received more and more attention. This is because an individual's capacity to function on a daily basis is more closely related to the maximal performance of his or her pulmonary and cardiovascular systems than to the performance of these organ systems at rest. If an individual is perfectly comfortable at rest but becomes very dyspneic with minimal exercise, he or she will be miserable. Life is a series of exercises that range from grooming oneself to feeding oneself to generating an income through work. Under normal conditions, one's ability to perform exercise depends on the capacity of the circulatory and respiratory systems to increase the transport of oxygen to the exercising muscles and on the status of the local factors that determine whether the increased quantity of oxygen reaches the cell interior, where it is used to produce energy for muscle fiber contraction. If a certain activity requires a greater oxygen consumption than can be generated by the individual, that activity is closed to that individual.

There are in general four reasons to study individuals while they exercise. First, an exercise test can quantitate the degree of functional impairment. The maximal work load tolerated by the individual or the oxygen consumption during maximal exercise ($\dot{V}O_2max$) can be measured and compared with those predicted for individuals of the same age, size, and sex. Second, analysis of the results of the exercise test will help indicate whether the limiting factor is pulmonary, cardiac, or due to lack of conditioning or to poor effort. Third, responses to various therapeutic interventions (e.g., vasodilator therapy for intractable heart failure) can be assessed with serial exercise tests. Fourth, the results of the exercise test will provide the basis for the development of a rational reconditioning program.

This section briefly considers alterations in the respiratory and circulatory systems that occur during exercise. Excellent reviews are available that discuss the physiologic responses to exercise and training in more depth (29–33). In addition, the use of exercise testing in the differential diagnosis of work intolerance and disability evaluation is discussed.

### EXERCISE PHYSIOLOGY AND PATHOPHYSIOLOGY

To exercise, an individual must generate more energy. Adenosine triphosphate (ATP) is the obligatory energetic intermediary in the transduction of ingested food energy into the mechanical energy of muscle contraction and work. ATP is generated primarily through the oxidation of carbohydrate and fat. When insufficient oxygen is present, ATP can also be generated via the anaerobic metabolism of carbohydrates to lactic acid. However, anaerobic metabolism is much less efficient than aerobic metabolism. To generate the same amount of energy with anaerobic as with aerobic metabolism, approximately 18 times as much glucose must be used. Accordingly, to all intents and purposes an individual's ability to exercise is limited by his or her capacity to deliver oxygen to the exercising muscles and use the delivered oxygen (33).

The oxygen required to perform various tasks is shown in Table 8.1. Note that the oxygen requirements vary more than 15-fold, from 200 ml/minute at rest to

**TABLE 8.1**
**ENERGY REQUIREMENTS FOR AN AVERAGE-SIZED ADULT DURING VARIOUS ACTIVITIES**

| Activity | $O_2$ Consumption (ml/min) |
|---|---|
| Rest, supine | 200 |
| Sitting | 240 |
| Standing relaxed | 280 |
| Eating | 280 |
| Conversation | 280 |
| Typing | 360 |
| Dressing, undressing | 460 |
| Propulsion, wheelchair | 480 |
| Driving car | 560 |
| Peeling potatoes | 580 |
| Walking 2.5 mph | 720 |
| Making beds | 780 |
| Bricklaying | 800 |
| Showering | 840 |
| Swimming 20 yd/min | 1000 |
| Golfing | 1000 |
| Walking 3.75 mph | 1120 |
| Tennis | 1420 |
| Ambulation, braces and crutches | 1600 |
| Shoveling | 1700 |
| Ascending stairs, 22-lb load, 54 ft/min | 3240 |

From Gordon EE: Energy costs of activities in health and disease. *Arch Intern Med* 101:702, 1958. Reproduced with permission of the author and publisher.

more than 3200 ml/minute for carrying loads up stairs. Note also that eating and conversing require relatively low levels of oxygen consumption. Therefore, it becomes evident that if a patient is breathless during an interview or during eating, it will be very difficult for that patient to dress himself or herself, take a shower, drive a car, or do any housekeeping. The fact that propulsion of a wheelchair takes much less oxygen than does walking at 2.5 mph suggests that more people with severe exercise limitation might benefit from this device. If physicians keep in mind the oxygen requirements for the activities listed in Table 8.1, they can counsel their patients more rationally in what they should and should not do.

## MEASURES OF WORK CAPACITY

As mentioned earlier, an individual's ability to perform muscular work is dependent on his or her capacity to transport oxygen from the atmosphere to the mitochondria of the cells in the exercising muscles. The best metabolic index of the work capacity in a given individual is the maximum $O_2$ consumption per unit time ($\dot{V}O_2$max) of the individual. Prediction equations for the $\dot{V}O_2$max are given later in this chapter (Equations 8–11). The $\dot{V}O_2$max can be determined by measuring oxygen consumption ($\dot{V}O_2$) at progressively higher work loads (30). Eventually a point is reached at which higher work loads do not result in higher $\dot{V}O_2$, and by definition the highest $\dot{V}O_2$ value attained is $\dot{V}O_2$max. The leveling off of $\dot{V}O_2$ provides objective evidence that the subject has attained maximal aerobic power. The energy for the additional work is provided by anaerobic metabolism. Thus, demonstration that the blood lactate levels are substantial (8 mM/liter or greater) also indicates that the subject has attained maximal aerobic power. However, it is notable that one cannot demonstrate such a plateau in many exercising individuals (34).

Since maximum exercise is at times uncomfortable to the subject, many exercise laboratories attempt to derive the $\dot{V}O_2$max from a $\dot{V}O_2$ measured at a submaximal load. This can be done because in most individuals there is a linear relationship between heart rate and $\dot{V}O_2$ after the $\dot{V}O_2$ reaches a certain level. The maximum heart rate for an individual can be estimated by subtracting the patient's age from 220. Therefore, if $\dot{V}O_2$ is measured at two submaximum exercise levels, $\dot{V}O_2$max can be estimated as demonstrated in Figure 8.12. This method of determining the $\dot{V}O_2$max by derivation from submaximal load is relatively accurate for normal subjects, deconditioned patients, and most patients with heart disease. However, it is usually not applicable to patients with moderate to severe pulmonary disease

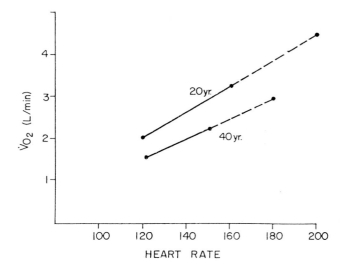

**FIGURE 8.12.** Predicting the $\dot{V}O_2$max from submaximal exercise levels. On the top line, a 20-year-old had a $\dot{V}O_2$ of 2100 at a heart rate of 120 and a $\dot{V}O_2$ of 3250 at a heart rate of 160. By extrapolating to a heart rate of 200 (220 − 20), we find an estimated $\dot{V}O_2$max of 4500. In an analogous manner the 40-year-old represented by the bottom line was found to have an estimated $\dot{V}O_2$max of 3000 ml/minute.

**TABLE 8.2**
**RELATIONSHIP BETWEEN $O_2$ CONSUMPTION AND OTHER MEASURES OF WORK**

| $O_2$ Consumption (ml/min) | kpm/min | watts | METS |
|---|---|---|---|
| 225 | 0 | 0 | 1 |
| 900 | 300 | 50 | 4 |
| 1500 | 600 | 100 | 7 |
| 2100 | 900 | 150 | 10 |
| 2800 | 1200 | 200 | 13 |
| 3500 | 1500 | 250 | 16 |
| 4200 | 1800 | 300 | 19 |
| 5000 | 2100 | 350 | 22 |

because their exercise is limited by their ventilatory abilities and they do not achieve their predicted maximum heart rate. Many patients with left ventricular failure also fall far short of reaching their predicted maximal heart rate (35).

Other indexes of work capacity frequently used are watts, kilopound meters (kpm) per minute, and multiples of resting $O_2$ consumption (metabolic equivalents, or METS). The relationship between these indexes of work capacity and the $\dot{V}O_2$ is shown in Table 8.2. Most bicycle ergometers are calibrated in watts or in kpm per minute, and therefore a reasonable estimate of the $\dot{V}_{O_2}$ for bicycle ergometer exercise can be obtained from Table 8.2. When exercise is performed on a treadmill, the $\dot{V}_{O_2}$ is dependent on the patient's weight, the speed of the treadmill, and the inclination of the treadmill. Nomograms are available (36) for the prediction of an individual's $\dot{V}_{O_2}$ from his or her weight and the speed and inclination of the treadmill. Therefore, relatively accurate estimates of $\dot{V}_{O_2}$ can be obtained without the collection of expired gases. Such estimates do not take into consideration the contribution of anaerobic metabolism to the work performed. Moreover, with repeated testing individuals tend to become more efficient on both the treadmill and the bicycle ergometer. Hence, these indirect estimates of the $\dot{V}_{O_2}$ tend to overestimate actual improvements in the $\dot{V}_{O_2}$.

### DETERMINANTS OF WORK CAPACITY ($\dot{V}_{O_2}$MAX)

The oxygen consumption ($\dot{V}_{O_2}$) of an individual is given by the following equation:

$$\dot{V}_{O_2} = \dot{Q} \times (Ca_{O_2} - C\bar{v}_{O_2}) \qquad (5)$$

where $\dot{Q}$ is the cardiac output, $Ca_{O_2}$ the oxygen content of arterial blood, and $C\bar{v}_{O_2}$ the oxygen content of mixed venous blood. Since almost all the oxygen in the blood is bound to hemoglobin, Equation 5 can be rewritten as follows:

$$\dot{V}_{O_2} = \dot{Q} \times [Hb] \times (Sa_{O_2} - S\bar{v}_{O_2}) \times 1.34 \qquad (6)$$

where Hb is the concentration of hemoglobin in the blood, $Sa_{O_2}$ is the hemoglobin saturation in arterial blood, $S\bar{v}_{O_2}$ is the hemoglobin saturation of mixed venous blood, and 1.34 is the amount of oxygen it takes to fully saturate 1 g of hemoglobin. From Equation 6 one can readily appreciate that the $\dot{V}_{O_2}$max is dependent on the cardiac output, the hemoglobin concentration, the arterial oxygen saturation, and the ability of the exercising muscles to extract oxygen from the blood during maximum exercise as reflected by the $S\bar{v}_{O_2}$. We will discuss exercise physiology by examining the factors that influence the different terms in Equation 6.

### Cardiac Output

The cardiac output is the limiting factor for $\dot{V}_{O_2}$max in normal subjects (30). Attempts to go beyond maximal work capacity are associated with a further increase in ventilation but no further increase in the cardiac output or $\dot{V}_{O_2}$max. The cardiac output during exercise increases linearly with increasing $\dot{V}_{O_2}$. Although an increase in cardiac output can result from an increase in either heart rate or stroke volume or both, most of the increase in cardiac output during exercise is related to increases in the heart rate, and the increases in stroke volume are proportionately smaller.

The cardiac output at a given $\dot{V}_{O_2}$ is essentially identical in trained and untrained subjects during arm and leg exercise and during running, bicycling, and swimming. Therefore, the $\dot{V}_{O_2}$ gives an indirect evaluation of the cardiac output. The cardiac output is approximately 5 liters plus the $\dot{V}_{O_2}$ times 5. Therefore the cardiac output with a $\dot{V}_{O_2}$ of 1 liter/minute is approximately 10 liters/minute, while the cardiac output with a $\dot{V}_{O_2}$ of 3 liters/minute is approximately 20 liters/minute.

The work capacity of patients with heart disease is also limited by their cardiac output. In general, cardiac patients generate the same maximal heart rates as do normal subjects, but since they have much lower stroke volumes than do normal individuals, the cardiac output at a given heart rate is reduced in proportion to the reduction in the stroke volume. In these patients the cardiac output can be improved by surgical correction of valvular defects, improvement of the perfusion of the myocardium by rehabilitative training or surgery, or administration of inotropic agents such as digitalis (35).

### Hemoglobin Concentration

From Equation 6, it is obvious that Hb is a critical factor in determining $\dot{V}_{O_2}$max. Either an abnormally high or a low Hb may be associated with a decreased work capacity. The explanation for the decrease in work capacity with a low Hb is obvious. Support for the relationship between the Hbg and exercise tolerance is provided by a recent study of patients with kidney disease on chronic dialysis. When these patients were given erythropoietin such that their Hbg increased from 7.3 to 10.8 g/dl, their exercise capacity increased from 108 to 130 watts (37).

The detrimental effects of a very high Hb on $\dot{V}_{O_2}$max is not immediately apparent from Equation 6. Nevertheless, too high a hematocrit and Hb can result in increased viscosity of the blood, which in turn can decrease the maximum cardiac output. If the reduction in cardiac output is proportionately greater than the increase in Hb, $\dot{V}_{O_2}$max will be reduced. This appears to be the case for both the experimental animal and the COPD patient with polycythemia. In dogs the systemic oxygen transport during exercise is reduced when the animals are made polycythemic (38). In COPD patients, reduction of the hematocrit from above 60% to below 55% results in a marked improvement in exercise tolerance, which indicates that the increase in cardiac output is proportionately greater than the decrease in Hb (39).

In recent years athletes have attempted to increase

their performance by transfusions; the practice is popularly called "blood doping." It appears that such practices do indeed result in a significant increase in the $\dot{V}O_2$max. One report (40) summarized the results from 30 subjects who participated in four different investigations. These individuals exercised before and within 72 hours of reinfusing two 450-ml blood units. Overall erythrocyte reinfusion led to a mean increase in the $\dot{V}O_2$max of 0.357 liter/minute. In general, for every 1% increase in Hb there was a 1% increase in the $\dot{V}O_2$max, but there was marked interindividual variability in this relationship.

Smoking can affect work capacity by transforming normal hemoglobin into carboxyhemoglobin (CO-Hb), which has no value in terms of $O_2$ transport. Smokers generally have CO-Hb values around 4 to 7%. In normal subjects it has been shown that $\dot{V}O_2$max decreases proportionately to the level of CO-Hb. A CO-Hb of 10% is associated with approximately a 10% decrease in the $\dot{V}O_2$max (41).

### Peripheral $O_2$ Extraction ($S\bar{v}O_2$)

During exercise there is increased $O_2$ extraction by the exercising muscles, which results in a lowered mixed venous saturation ($S\bar{v}O_2$). The contribution of the decreased $S\bar{v}O_2$ to $\dot{V}O_2$ is obvious from Equation 6. Mixed venous blood is a mixture of the venous blood returning to the right heart from exercising muscles and from the remainder of the body. Blood returning from heavily exercising muscles is quite desaturated, with a $P\bar{v}O_2$ of 10 to 15 mm Hg and an $S\bar{v}O_2$ less than 10% (42). In superbly conditioned subjects at exhaustion, the mixed venous saturation averages about 10% (42).

Some authors have proposed that exercise is limited by the diffusion of oxygen from the capillaries to the mitochondria in the exercising muscles (33). In particular, there seems to be a "bottleneck" in the diffusion of oxygen from the capillary to the mitochondria as the oxygen enters the muscle cell before it combines with myoglobin (33). However, most maintain that the oxygen delivery to the muscles is the factor that limits exercise, since the hemoglobin is less than 10% saturated in blood emanating from a highly trained muscle.

During exercise the distribution of the systemic vascular resistance is altered so that a higher percentage of the blood is distributed to the exercising muscles. In unfit people this vasoregulation during exercise is suboptimal. They fail to adjust their regional peripheral vascular resistance, and so their exercising muscles receive less of the cardiac output. Therefore, their $S\bar{v}O_2$ at exhaustion is considerably higher than 25%. It follows from Equation 6 that their $\dot{V}O_2$ at a given level of cardiac output is lower than it is in the conditioned individual, since the $SaO_2 - S\bar{v}O_2$ is smaller (31). Other dysfunctions of the peripheral circulation can also result in a suboptimal distribution of cardiac output and a high $S\bar{v}O_2$ at maximal exercise.

### Arterial Oxygen Saturation ($SaO_2$)

The $SaO_2$ depends on the alveolar $O_2$ tension ($PAO_2$) and the alveolar-arterial $O_2$ gradient ($PAO_2 - PaO_2$). The $PAO_2$ in turn is dependent on the partial pressure of the inspired $O_2$ ($PIO_2$), the $PaCO_2$, and the respiratory exchange ratio (R), as shown by the alveolar air equation:

$$PAO_2 = PIO_2 - PaCO_2 \times [FIO_2 + (1 - FIO_2)/R] \qquad (7)$$

where $FIO_2$ is the fractional concentration of $O_2$ in inspired gas. Note that an elevation of $PaCO_2$ will decrease the $PAO_2$. In normal subjects the $PaCO_2$ tends to remain constant or decrease with increasing levels of exercise to maintain a constant pH (43). Therefore the $PAO_2$ remains constant or increases. However, in some patients with COPD, the ventilatory reserve is insufficient to eliminate the additional $CO_2$ produced with exercise. Accordingly, the $PaCO_2$ increases and the $PAO_2$ decreases (44). For a given level of pulmonary dysfunction, patients in whom the $PaCO_2$ increases during exercise will have higher exercise tolerance, since they do not have to breathe as much to get rid of the same amount of $CO_2$ (44).

The $PAO_2 - PaO_2$ results from venous admixture ($\dot{Q}va/\dot{Q}t$), which is the fraction of the cardiac output that reaches arterial blood and acts as though it had not been exposed to alveolar gas. Venous admixture has three components: (a) that which results from the perfusion of units with low $\dot{V}/\dot{Q}$ ratios; (b) that which results from the failure of the capillary $PO_2$ and the alveolar $PO_2$ to reach equilibrium; and (c) that which results from true right-to-left shunts. In patients with lung disease, the majority of the $PAO_2 - PaO_2$ gradient is due to inadequate ventilation of perfused alveoli. The amount of ventilation required to fully oxygenate the blood in a given alveolus is dependent on both the amount of perfusion and the degree of venous desaturation. West (45) has shown that in a lung unit with a ventilation-perfusion ratio ($\dot{V}/\dot{Q}$) of unity the $PaO_2$ will fall from 100 to 42 mm Hg as $P\bar{v}O_2$ falls from 100 to 10 mm Hg.

The best way to understand this phenomenon is to consider a numerical example. In Table 8.3 are listed the oxygen requirements to achieve full saturation of 100 ml blood at different $S\bar{v}O_2$ levels and the corresponding $PAO_2$ if this much oxygen is extracted from 100 ml of ventilated air. It can be seen that when the $S\bar{v}O_2$ falls below 55%, the resulting $PAO_2$ falls drastically, and accordingly the $PaO_2$ must fall. In the same

## Table 8.3
### Influence of S$\bar{v}$O$_2$ on P$a$O$_2$ Assuming R is 0.8 and Hb 15 g/100 mL

| S$\bar{v}$O$_2$ % | O$_2$ Required for Sa$O_2$ = 100% ml | P$a$O$_2$ if Sa$O_2$ = 100% $\dot{V}/\dot{Q}$ = 1 | $\dot{V}/\dot{Q}$ = 3 |
|---|---|---|---|
| 75 | 5 | 115 | 138 |
| 65 | 7 | 101 | 134 |
| 55 | 9 | 87 | 129 |
| 45 | 11 | 73 | 124 |
| 35 | 13 | 58 | 120 |
| 25 | 15 | 44 | 115 |

example, if the $\dot{V}/\dot{Q}$ ratio had increased to 3, the P$a$O$_2$ when the S$\bar{v}$O$_2$ is 25% would still be over 100 mm Hg.

The above example illustrates that a $\dot{V}/\dot{Q}$ ratio of 1 is not ideal during exercise. If the S$\bar{v}$O$_2$ is substantially decreased, the $\dot{V}/\dot{Q}$ ratio must increase concomitantly or arterial desaturation will result. The cardiac output of a normal subject at rest is about 5 liters/minute and increases fourfold to a level of 20 liters/minute on maximal exercise. The minute ventilation increases from 5 liters/minute at rest to 80 liters/minute during maximal exercise. Thus the overall $\dot{V}/\dot{Q}$ ratio increases from unity at rest to 4 to 1 during maximal exercise, and arterial desaturation does not normally result from the above mechanism.

Another factor that can increase the P$a$O$_2$ − P$a$O$_2$ is a reduced diffusing capacity of the lungs. If, at the end of the capillary, the P$O_2$ of the blood has not reached that of the alveolus, the P$a$O$_2$ − P$a$O$_2$ will be increased. Such an increase is said to be due to a diffusion abnormality. It is generally accepted that in normal individuals, complete equilibrium occurs between alveolar and capillary blood even during heavy exercise except when the individual is breathing low levels of oxygen. However, the Sa$O_2$ is decreased in nearly 50% of elite cyclists and runners. A diffusion limitation is the most likely explanation for the desaturation in these athletes, but ventilation-perfusion imbalances could play a role (46).

It is thought that a reduced diffusing capacity does not contribute to the P$a$O$_2$ − P$a$O$_2$ at rest, even in lung patients with markedly reduced diffusing capacities. However, when a patient with a reduced diffusing capacity exercises, equilibrium between the alveolar and capillary P$O_2$ may not occur, since the venous blood is more desaturated and the capillary transit time is shorter. Shepard (47) in a theoretical analysis demonstrated that a reduced diffusing capacity can cause a

substantial reduction in Sa$O_2$ during exercise. Moreover, once the P$a$O$_2$ − P$a$O$_2$ is increased owing to diffusion limitations, slight increases in $\dot{V}O_2$ lead to dramatic reductions in Sa$O_2$. For example, if the diffusing capacity is 16, the Sa$O_2$ will start to fall when the $\dot{V}O_2$ reaches 1600 and will fall to less than 70% when the $\dot{V}O_2$ reaches 1800 ml/minute, assuming that the S$\bar{v}$O$_2$ was 50%. In general, the higher the cardiac output, the more rapid the transit of blood in the pulmonary capillaries. Once the level is reached at which equilibrium between the alveoli and capillaries does not occur, further increases in the velocity of flow or decreases in S$\bar{v}$O$_2$ lead to large decreases in Sa$O_2$.

The reduction in Sa$O_2$ due to a given fractional shunt ($\dot{Q}s/\dot{Q}t$) depends on the S$\bar{v}$O$_2$. For example, if the $\dot{Q}s/\dot{Q}t$ is 25%, the Sa$O_2$ will be 94% if S$\bar{v}$O$_2$ is 75% but will decrease to 81% if S$\bar{v}$O$_2$ is 25%. In view of the marked reduction in the S$\bar{v}$O$_2$ during strenuous exercise, one might expect that the Sa$O_2$ would decrease substantially in many individuals during heavy exercise and that this reduction would limit their exercise capabilities. However, Sa$O_2$ does not change in normal subjects even during exhaustive physical work. Most patients with lung disease have an increased P$a$O$_2$ − P$a$O$_2$ at rest, and the majority of this increase is due to perfusion of units with low $\dot{V}/\dot{Q}$ ratios. As mentioned previously, patients with COPD increase their ventilation more than their cardiac output during exercise so that their P$a$O$_2$ does not decrease. This increase in total ventilation tends to improve the ventilation of units with low $\dot{V}/\dot{Q}$ ratios and decreases the fraction of the $\dot{Q}s/\dot{Q}t$ that is due to perfusion of poorly ventilated alveoli. The net effect of exercise on Sa$O_2$ depends on whether the $\dot{Q}s/\dot{Q}t$ decreases enough to compensate for the decreased S$\bar{v}$O$_2$.

### Ventilatory Limitation

As mentioned earlier, the cardiac output is the factor limiting exercise in normal subjects. At maximal exercise they have ventilatory reserve as manifested by their ability to increase their ventilation voluntarily. However, the exercise capacity of most individuals with moderate or severe lung disease is limited by their ventilatory abilities. Normal individuals are unable to maintain minute ventilations above 60% of their maximal voluntary ventilation (MVV). Patients with lung disease are also unable to sustain minute ventilations much above 60% of their MVV without developing dyspnea and respiratory muscle fatigue (48). Therefore, their exercise capabilities are limited by their ventilation even though their arterial blood gases frequently remain unchanged at exhaustion.

In addition to their reduced ventilatory reserves, patients with lung disease have increased ventilatory requirements for a given level of exercise. The ventilatory requirement is determined by the $CO_2$ production ($\dot{V}CO_2$), the $PaCO_2$, and the wasted ventilation fraction of each breath ($V_D/V_T$). In patients with lung disease, the $V_D/V_T$ is much higher at rest (mean 0.45) than it is in normals (mean 0.28). Moreover, during exercise the $V_D/V_T$ on the average does not change in patients with COPD, while it falls below 0.20 in normal individuals (44, 49).

Therefore, the patient with lung disease needs more ventilation for a given work load. The ventilatory equivalent for $CO_2$ ($\dot{V}E/\dot{V}CO_2$) is a measure of the efficiency with which additional $CO_2$ is eliminated. The normal $\dot{V}E/\dot{V}CO_2$ is about 30, but with COPD it can exceed 50 (50).

### Anaerobic Metabolism

Exercise requires an increase in $O_2$ flow to the mitochondria of the exercising muscles. If the increase in $O_2$ flow is insufficient to generate the required ATP, anaerobic metabolism must be used to generate the ATP. The anaerobic threshold is the highest level of work that can be done without inducing a sustained metabolic acidosis. The anaerobic threshold normally occurs at between 50 and 60% of the $\dot{V}O_2$max.

Lactic acid is the end product of anaerobic metabolism. The metabolic acidosis that results from its accumulation produces the subjective feeling of fatigue that precludes extensive periods of anaerobic exercise. When lactic acid is produced it is immediately buffered, predominantly by the bicarbonate system:

$$H^+ lactate^- + Na^+HCO_3^- \rightarrow Na^+lactate^- + CO_2 + H_2O$$

The above reaction causes a reduction in the bicarbonate levels and an increase in the production of carbon dioxide gas. With progressive work loads, the relationship between the work load or the $\dot{V}O_2$ and the $\dot{V}E$ is linear until the anaerobic threshold is reached. Above the anaerobic threshold $\dot{V}E$ increases more than $\dot{V}O_2$ for two reasons: (a) the increased carbon dioxide produced in the buffering of lactate must be eliminated, and (b) the metabolic acidosis produced in the buffering process acts as a respiratory stimulant so that $\dot{V}E$ increases more than $\dot{V}CO_2$ and $PaCO_2$ falls. In general it appears that normal individuals and patients with cardiovascular or pulmonary disease attempt to regulate their ventilation such that the arterial pH remains stable (51).

The anaerobic threshold is best documented by demonstrating an increase in the blood lactate concentration. This is usually accompanied by a decrease in the plasma bicarbonate concentration. One can also try to identify the anaerobic threshold by examining the results of the expired gas analysis. One method is to

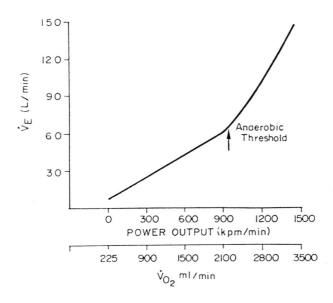

**Figure 8.13.** Determination of anaerobic threshold from plot of $\dot{V}E$ versus work load or $\dot{V}O_2$. The anaerobic threshold is identified as the work load at which the $\dot{V}E$ starts to increase out of proportion to the $\dot{V}O_2$ or the work load.

plot $\dot{V}E$ versus the work load. The anaerobic threshold occurs when $\dot{V}E$ increases out of proportion to the work load (Fig. 8.13). A second method examines plots of the $\dot{V}E/\dot{V}O_2$ and the $\dot{V}E/\dot{V}CO_2$ versus the work load. The anaerobic threshold is the point where $\dot{V}E/\dot{V}O_2$ rises while $\dot{V}E/\dot{V}CO_2$ remains stable when plotted against work rate. A third method examines the relationship between the $\dot{V}O_2$ and the $\dot{V}CO_2$ and identifies the anaerobic threshold as the point where the $\dot{V}CO_2$ increases disproportionately to the $\dot{V}O_2$ (52). Recent studies have shown that noninvasive methods are very inaccurate in identifying the anaerobic threshold in patients with COPD (53). Moreover, the majority of patients with severe lung disease do not reach their anaerobic threshold (53).

### Training

It is widely recognized that it is possible to increase the maximum amount of exercise that a subject can perform by a period of physical training. By the same token, periods of inactivity will decrease the maximum amount of exercise that an individual can perform. In one study (54), $\dot{V}O_2$max was measured in a group of elite Swedish swimmers at the height of their competitive swimming careers and then 4, 6, and 8 years after they had stopped swimming competitively. In these individuals $\dot{V}O_2$max decreased much more rapidly than would be expected from aging alone, and the

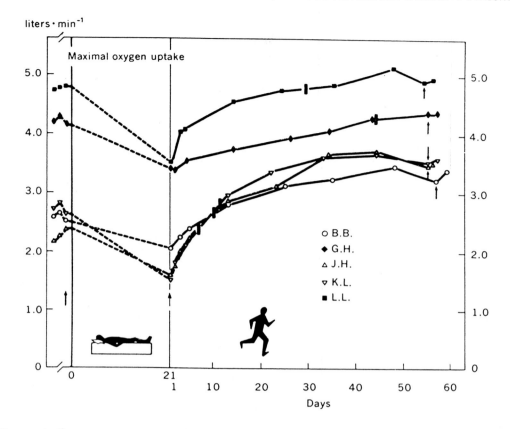

**FIGURE 8.14.** Changes in $\dot{V}O_2$max with bed rest and training. *Heavy bars* mark the time during the training period at which the maximal oxygen uptake had returned to the control value obtained before bed rest. Originally the top two patients were well conditioned, while the bottom three patients were poorly conditioned. (From Saltin B, Blomqvist G, Mitchell JH, et al: Response to exercise after bed rest and after training. A longitudinal study of adaptive changes in oxygen transport and body composition. *Circulation* 38(Suppl 7):1, 1968. By permission of the American Heart Association, Inc.)

rapid decrease persisted even between the 6th and 8th years. In another study (55), five adult males with varying degrees of physical fitness were studied before and after 21 days of bed rest and then periodically during 60 days of intensive reconditioning (Fig. 8.14). During the 21 days of bed rest, $\dot{V}O_2$max fell by over 25% in each of the five individuals. During the reconditioning period, $\dot{V}O_2$max initially increased rapidly, then increased at a slower rate, and then appeared to level off after a mean of about 45 days. The $\dot{V}O_2$max at the end of the training period had increased substantially more in the unfit than in the fit individuals.

In general there are three different factors that should be considered in conditioning programs, namely, the intensity, the duration, and the frequency of the exercise (56). Of the three, the intensity is the most important. To increase $\dot{V}O_2$max, the oxygen transport system must be challenged with exercise demanding at least 50% of the person's $\dot{V}O_2$max. Moreover, the

further above 50% of $\dot{V}O_2$max is the demand of the exercise, the more rapid will be the improvement in $\dot{V}O_2$max and the greater the eventual change. However, training should not be performed much above the anaerobic threshold. One can use the pulse to guide the intensity of exercise in that the anaerobic threshold is usually exceeded when the pulse is greater than 77% of the predicted maximal pulse (57). The exercise program should be performed at least twice a week, but every other day is preferable. The minimal duration of each training session should be 15 minutes, with 45 minutes optimal. The degree of improvement in $\dot{V}O_2$max after 2 months of training is dependent on the initial level of fitness and the intensity of the exercise, as outlined in Table 8.4 (56).

The improvement in physical performance capacity that results from regularly performed, vigorous exercise involves multiple adaptive reactions occurring primarily in the circulatory system. The maximum cardiac

TABLE 8.4
EXPECTED IMPROVEMENT IN $\dot{V}O_2$MAX AFTER TRAINING 3 TIMES A WEEK FOR 45 MINUTES FOR 2 MONTHS

| Initial Status | | Expected Improvement (%) | | |
|---|---|---|---|---|
| Level of Fitness | $\dot{V}O_2$max ml/kg/min | Exercise at 50–70% $\dot{V}O_2$max | Exercise at 70–90% $\dot{V}O_2$max | Exercise at 90–100% $\dot{V}O_2$max |
| Low | 30 | 10 | 25 | 40 |
| Medium | 45 | 3 | 8 | 20 |
| Excellent | 60 | 0 | 0 | 5 |

output increases through an increase in the maximum stroke volume arising from two factors. First, the myocardial function improves, so that with a given peripheral vascular resistance the maximum cardiac output is increased. Second, local adaptive processes in the exercising muscle decrease the vascular resistance of the exercising muscles, so that the total vascular resistance is decreased and a higher fraction of the cardiac output is distributed to the exercising muscles. With conditioning, the improved myocardial function is a generalized process so that if nonconditioned muscles are exercised, the maximum cardiac output will still be increased. In contrast, the redistribution of the cardiac output is specific in that if nonconditioned muscles are exercised, the distribution of the cardiac output to them will not be facilitated.

An important by-product of the redistribution of the cardiac output to the exercising muscles is its effect on $S\bar{v}O_2$. When a larger fraction of the cardiac output goes to the exercising muscles, the $S\bar{v}O_2$ decreases because of the very low $S\bar{v}O_2$ of the larger fraction of the cardiac output returning from the exercising muscles. From Equation 6 it can be readily appreciated that this decrease in $S\bar{v}O_2$ will increase $\dot{V}O_2$max substantially.

Training also leads to changes in the muscle that has undergone training such that it can take up more oxygen (32). In particular there is an increase in the oxidative capacity due to an increase in mitochondrial volume and enhancement of the enzyme systems that promote the use of free fatty acids. These changes lead to a lower $SaO_2$ at the end of the capillary. In addition, an increase in the vascular conductance due to an increase in the capillary density increases oxygen extraction by increasing the surface area for oxygen movement.

It should be noted that the expected improvements outlined in Table 8.4 are those for normal individuals. Even though patients with COPD frequently have a very low $\dot{V}O_2$max at the start of a physical training

program, their $\dot{V}O_2$max usually does not increase by more than 10% (58–60) during a training program. Moreover, endurance training in COPD patients does not result in an increase in mitochondrial enzyme activities as it does in normal subjects (61). In recent years there has been much interest in training the respiratory muscles of patients with lung disease. However, a recent meta-analysis of the results of respiratory muscle training concluded that there was little evidence that patients with COPD clinically benefited from respiratory muscle training (62).

### AGING AND EXERCISE PERFORMANCE

As an individual ages, his or her capacity to exercise decreases. In untrained individuals there is an approximately 10% decrease per decade in the $\dot{V}O_2$max starting at age 25 (31). In trained individuals, the decrease in the $\dot{V}O_2$max is approximately 6% per decade (31). The initial $\dot{V}O_2$max is approximately 50% higher in the trained individual, but the absolute decrease in the $\dot{V}O_2$max is less in the trained individual. In the sedentary individual, most of the decline (72%) in the $\dot{V}O_2$max is due to a decreased cardiac output, while the remaining 28% is due to reduced peripheral oxygen extraction (31). Decreases in the stroke volume are more important than decreases in the heart rate in producing the decrease in the $\dot{V}O_2$max (31). Interestingly, sedentary individuals above the age of 60 who embark upon a vigorous training program can improve their $\dot{V}O_2$max by approximately 25% (63). However, their exercise capabilities still remain far below those of individuals who remained trained throughout their lives (31, 63).

### PERFORMANCE OF EXERCISE TESTING

Although the exercise test must in general be tailored to the individual patient, we believe that most exercise tests should be conducted along the following guidelines: The patient should be studied on a treadmill or bicycle ergometer at increasing work loads. The test should be performed in the presence of a physician and with constant cardiac monitoring. Resuscitation equipment, including a defibrillator, should be immediately at hand. The work load should be increased until the patient becomes physically exhausted.

However, it should be noted that the progressive ergometer test has little relevance to normal activities and may give no insight into the patient's difficulties in coping with daily living. Therefore, self-paced walking tests (55) such as the 12-minute test or 6-minute test have been developed. These tests have the advantage of being a more natural test of exercise capacity. They are reproducible and simple. However, they give information only on overall exercise tolerance and they allow no physiologic measurements during the exercise. Self-paced walking tests have their greatest utility in evaluating the patient's response to a therapeutic intervention. In general, we prefer a 12-minute walking test because there is less variance (64).

The data collected during ergometer or treadmill exercise tests will depend on the information desired from the test. In general, there are four stages of exercise testing (36). In stage 1 exercise testing, the patient is exercised at increasing work load until exhaustion, with monitoring of the heart rate and ventilation. Since the $\dot{V}O_2$ can be estimated from the work load, this test will make it possible to determine if the subject's exercise capabilities are within normal limits. An estimate of the $\dot{V}O_2$ can be obtained from nomograms that relate the power output or the treadmill grade and speed to the $\dot{V}O_2$ (35). Cardiovascular dysfunction is suggested by a stage 1 test demonstrating a heart rate that is high relative to the work load and an early onset of the anaerobic threshold as evidenced by nonlinear increases in ventilation. A ventilatory limitation is suggested when the maximum ventilation reaches 35 times the $FEV_1$ and the anaerobic threshold and the maximum predicted heart rates are not achieved.

In stage 2 exercise testing, mixed expired gases are also collected and analyzed. The additional information provided includes the $\dot{V}O_2$, the $\dot{V}CO_2$, the $\dot{V}E/\dot{V}O_2$, and the $\dot{V}E/\dot{V}CO_2$. Therefore, the aerobic capacity ($\dot{V}O_2max$) can be accurately determined. In addition, cardiac outputs and stroke volumes can be estimated if a rebreathing procedure is used to obtain the mixed venous $PCO_2$. These measurements are useful in further defining the factors limiting exercise but are unnecessary if the exercise capacity is normal.

In stage 3 exercise testing, arterial blood gases are also collected. The additional data permit detection of hypoxemia, hypercapnia, and respiratory or metabolic acidosis during exercise. In addition, the $V_D/V_T$ can be calculated. If the only reason for the measurement of arterial blood gases is to detect hypoxemia, a pulse oximeter is a possible noninvasive alternative. However, it should be noted that some pulse oximeters consistently overestimate the $SaO_2$ during hypoxemia while exercising. With the Biox-Ohmeda pulse oximeter the mean bias in one study was 6.1% (65).

In stage 4 exercise testing, a Swan-Ganz catheter is inserted into the pulmonary artery. The additional information provided includes the pressures in the lesser circulation, the mixed venous blood gases, and the cardiac output as calculated by the Fick method.

## Predicted Values for $\dot{V}O_2max$

The following equations provide predicted values for the $\dot{V}O_2max$ (66, 67).

*Males*

$\dot{V}O_2max$ (liters/minute)
$$= 4.2 - 0.032 \times age\ (SD \pm 0.4) \quad (8)$$

$$\dot{V}O_2max\ (ml/kg/minute) = 60 - 0.55 \times age\ (SD \pm 7.5) \quad (9)$$

*Over the Age of 55*

$$\dot{V}O_2max\ (liters/minute) = 2.43\ (SD \pm 0.44) \quad (10)$$

$$Work\ load\ (watts) = 179\ (SD \pm 36) \quad (11)$$

*Females*

$\dot{V}O_2max$ (liters/minute)
$$= 2.6 - 0.014 \times age\ (SD \pm 0.4) \quad (12)$$

$\dot{V}O_2max$ (ml/kg/minute)
$$= 48 - 0.37 \times age\ (SD \pm 7.0) \quad (13)$$

*Over the Age of 55*

$$\dot{V}O_2max\ (liters/minute) = 1.49\ (SD \pm 0.31) \quad (14)$$

$$Work\ load\ (watts) = 104\ (SD \pm 25) \quad (15)$$

### USE OF PULMONARY FUNCTION AND EXERCISE TESTS

Pulmonary function tests and exercise tests can be used to answer many different questions. This section is organized according to the various questions that might be asked.

### Does the Patient Have Lung Disease?

This is the question that is most frequently asked. The answer to this question is obtained primarily by comparing the results from a given individual to those obtained from a normal population. The predicted value of a test for a given patient represents the mean value of a group of normal individuals with similar characteristics. The characteristics involved depend on the test but usually include height, age, and sex. The predicted value is calculated from a prediction equation, usually an algebraic equation derived from multiple linear regression. Associated with each predicted value is a range representing the expected variation in the group of normal individuals. Conventionally this range has been defined as a somewhat arbitrary percentage of the predicted value. A better approach, which is gaining acceptance, is to use a range based on the *standard error of the estimate* obtained in the analysis of the normal group. In this manner, the range that includes 95% of the normal individuals can be calculated. A test result is labeled as abnormal only if it falls outside the range in which 95% of normals lie. This method takes into account intersubject variability. For specific equations, a number of references are available (68–74).

When a patient is initially evaluated, it is recommended that only spirometry be obtained. If the FVC, $FEV_1$, and $FEV_1/FVC$ are all within normal limits, then one can assume that the patient does not have significant obstructive or restrictive ventilatory dysfunction. At times a diffusing capacity can be obtained in addition to the spirometry since patients with lung disease, especially pulmonary vascular disease, may have normal spirometry but an abnormal diffusing capacity. Usually there is no reason to obtain lung volume measurements or spirometry after the administration of bronchodilators in patients who have normal spirometry.

Inhalation challenge tests are useful at times in patients with normal spirometry. Asthma is an episodic disease and many patients will have normal spirometry at least part of the time. Inhalational challenge tests can demonstrate airway hyperresponsiveness in such patients and suggest the diagnosis. In a similar manner, cough in some patients is due to airway hyperresponsiveness, and an inhalational challenge test may be necessary to demonstrate the airway hyperresponsiveness if the spirometry is within normal limits (10). It should be remembered that 3 to 6% of asymptomatic individuals do have airway hyperresponsiveness.

It should also be pointed out that the maximal exercise test is sometimes abnormal in patients with mild lung disease when the spirometry and diffusing capacity are normal. In a recent study of asymptomatic patients with serological evidence of beryllium disease, results from the maximal exercise tests were more sensitive than were spirometry or the diffusing capacity in identifying abnormalities. A rise in the $V_D/V_T$ during exercise was the most common abnormality (75).

## What Type of Lung Disease Does My Patient Have?

Once a patient has been found to have abnormal pulmonary function, the type and degree of dysfunction are sought. In general, abnormalities in pulmonary function can be classified as obstructive ventilatory dysfunction, restrictive ventilatory dysfunction, and mixed ventilatory dysfunction.

### Obstructive Ventilatory Dysfunction

By definition, obstructive ventilatory dysfunction occurs when there are reduced expiratory flow rates

**TABLE 8.5**
**CRITERIA FOR QUANTITATING DEGREE OF OBSTRUCTION**

| Grade | $FEV_1/FVC$ | $FEV_1$ (ml) |
|---|---|---|
| Very severe | <0.30 | <600 |
| Severe | 0.3–0.4 | 600–1000 |
| Moderate | 0.4–0.6 | 1000–2000 |
| Mild | 0.6–0.7 | 2000–3000 |
| Very mild | 0.7–pred. value | >3000 |

with maximal effort due to increased expiratory resistance. As discussed in Chapter 3, the increased expiratory resistance can be due to either increased airway resistance or decreased elastic recoil of the lung.

In determining whether airway obstruction is present, one should look at the $FEV_1/FVC$ and the $FEV_3/FVC$. In general, if the $FEV_1/FVC$ is above 0.75 and the $FEV_3/FVC$ is above 0.95 the patient does not have significant obstructive ventilatory dysfunction. These ratios will be reduced if the patient has obstructive ventilatory dysfunction. The forced vital capacity is often reduced with moderate to severe airway obstruction as a result of air trapping. The peak expiratory flow and the forced expiratory flows at different lung volumes are also reduced.

The degree of obstructive ventilatory dysfunction can be quantitated as outlined in Table 8.5. The absolute value of the $FEV_1$ should be used only if it has been demonstrated that the patient does not have restrictive ventilatory dysfunction. This can be done either with lung volume determinations or by the demonstration of lung hyperinflation on a chest radiograph. The patient is classified according to the most severe criterion that he or she meets. For example, if the $FEV_1/FVC$ is 0.35 and the $FEV_1$ is 1800 ml, the individual is classified as having severe obstructive ventilatory dysfunction.

### Restrictive Ventilatory Dysfunction

By definition, restrictive pulmonary dysfunction indicates that the TLC is reduced. Most volume compartments are affected, which results in decreases in VC, RV, and FRC as well as the total lung capacity. Frequently the residual volume is not reduced by as great a percentage as the other lung volumes. A diagnosis of restrictive impairment is made when the vital capacity falls below the predicted normal range and is associated with reductions in the other volume compartments. If the patient has no obstructive ventilatory dysfunction, restrictive ventilatory dysfunction can be established from spirometry. However, if the patient has obstructive ventilatory dysfunction the FVC can be reduced due to the obstruction, and therefore the diagnosis of restrictive ventilatory dysfunction can

TABLE 8.6
## TABLE 8.6
### CRITERIA FOR QUANTITATING DEGREE OF RESTRICTION

| Grade | VC % Predicted | TLC % Predicted |
|-------|----------------|-----------------|
| Very mild | >80 | >90 |
| Mild | 60–80 | 70–90 |
| Moderate | 30–60 | 50–70 |
| Severe | <30 | <50 |

only be established if lung volumes, including RV, are measured. When both the $FEV_1$ and the FVC are reduced with spirometry, one can get some idea whether the individual has predominantly obstructive or restrictive ventilatory dysfunction by comparing the value for the $FEV_1$ and the FVC expressed as a percentage of the predicted value. If the individual has predominantly restrictive dysfunction, the FVC will be reduced proportionately more than the $FEV_1$. Alternatively, if the individual has predominantly obstructive dysfunction, the $FEV_1$ will be reduced proportionately more than the FVC.

The degree of restrictive ventilatory dysfunction can be quantitated as outlined in Table 8.6. Results of other ventilatory function tests—such as time forced expiratory volumes, expiratory flows, and MVV—are either normal or slightly reduced with restrictive impairment. Although the $FEV_1$ and $FEV_3$ expressed as a percentage of the predicted value are reduced in individuals with restrictive ventilatory dysfunction, the $FEV_1$/FVC and the $FEV_3$/FVC are normal or greater than predicted, which indicates an absence of airway obstruction.

### Mixed Ventilatory Dysfunction

Some patients have both obstructive and restrictive ventilatory dysfunction. Lung volume measurements, including a determination of the residual volume, are necessary in such cases to quantitate the degree of dysfunction. Since the $FEV_1$ is reduced from the restrictive dysfunction, only the $FEV_1$/FVC should be used in quantitating the obstruction.

## Does My Patient Have Predominantly Asthma, Chronic Bronchitis, or Emphysema?

The three main diseases that produce obstructive ventilatory dysfunction are asthma, chronic bronchitis, and emphysema. Some indication as to the pathogenesis of the obstruction can be obtained from the pulmonary function laboratory. However, it must be noted that in the older smoker the obstructive ventilatory dysfunction is usually due to a combination of all three diseases.

Measures of airway resistance are useful in separating the three entities. With pure emphysema, airway resistance is normal and the expiratory flow limitation is due to loss of lung elastic recoil. Therefore, an increased airway resistance indicates that the airways are abnormal and that the patient has a component of asthma or bronchitis. Emphysema results in destruction of pulmonary parenchyma and therefore loss of surface area for gas exchange. Accordingly, the DLco is reduced with emphysema, while it is normal with asthma or chronic bronchitis.

### Bronchodilator Testing

By definition the obstructive ventilatory dysfunction with asthma is reversible. Therefore, many laboratories perform spirometry before and after administration of bronchodilators to distinguish asthma from chronic bronchitis and emphysema. A positive response is usually said to be present if the $FEV_1$ improves by at least 15% *and* 200 ml above baseline. However, it should be noted that most patients who appear to have chronic bronchitis or emphysema will have an improvement of 15% or more in their $FEV_1$ if they are repeatedly tested (76). It appears that responses to bronchodilators are useful in predicting responses to oral corticosteroids in patients with COPD. Nisar and coworkers (77) administered 5 mg albuterol and 500 $\mu$g ipratropium bromide acutely to 100 patients with COPD (mean age 62 and mean $FEV_1$ ~1000 ml). They reported that 33 responded to neither, 16 responded to albuterol only, 17 responded to ipratropium only, and 34 responded to both. Twenty-two patients improved after oral corticosteroid administration for 2 weeks, including 10 who improved after acute administration of both albuterol and ipratropium, five who improved only after acute administration of albuterol, two who improved only after acute administration of ipratropium, and three who did not improve after acute administration of either drug (77). Other studies have failed to demonstrate a relationship between the short-term response to bronchodilators and the long-term improvement with bronchodilators (78).

### Large Airway Obstruction

A relatively uncommon cause of obstructive ventilatory dysfunction is upper or large airway obstruction. However, it is important not to overlook this possibility, because its presence is life threatening. Upper airway obstruction is manifested as a reduction in peak flow in early expiration and normal flows during the latter part of the expiration (see Fig. 8.4C). If the obstruction in the large airway is variable, its site inside or outside the thoracic inlet determines its effects on flow rates. Variable intrathoracic obstruction primarily affects forced expiratory flows, since positive pleural pressures cause further decrease in the size of the large airway. Variable extrathoracic obstruction affects forced inspiration, since the intratracheal negative pressure on inspiration tends to make the trachea collapse more. These changes are best demonstrated with the flow-volume loop as described above. The ratio of the $FEV_1$ to the $FEV_{0.5}$ is almost always greater than 1.5 except when obstruction of the large airways is present (79).

### Is My Patient Going to Develop Lung Disease?

In the natural history of COPD, disease first develops in the small peripheral airways. Since only 10 to 20% of the total airway resistance is in these airways, the usual tests for obstructive ventilatory dysfunction such as the $FEV_1/FVC$ are normal when significant disease is present (80). Accordingly, many different tests have been proposed, including the closing volume, the slope of phase III on the single-breath nitrogen washout test, comparison of flow-volume loops obtained with room air and a mixture of helium and oxygen, and sophisticated analyses of the forced expiratory spirogram. However, none of these have been shown to be very useful in predicting the development of significant COPD (22), and they are not recommended. A more cost-effective alternative is to ask the patient if he or she smokes. If the answer is affirmative, efforts should be expended to get him or her to stop smoking. Another test that may prove useful in predicting the development of disease is airway hyperresponsiveness as documented by inhalational challenge. In one study, airway hyperresponsiveness to methacholine was quite useful in predicting which nonsmoking men would develop wheezing (81).

### Is My Patient Responding to Therapy?

Once the diagnosis of pulmonary dysfunction is confirmed and therapy is undertaken, how should the response of the patient to therapy be monitored? The simplest way is to ask the patient how he or she feels. However, patients with lung disease are notoriously poor at assessing their pulmonary function. In one study of 82 asthmatics, more than 20% had an $FEV_1$ less than 70% of predicted when they were symptom free, and many did not become symptomatic when the $FEV_1$ fell to less than 50% of predicted after the inhalation of methacholine (82). Likewise, the physical examination of patients with COPD is less than ideal in quantitating the response to therapy. It has been shown that there is only a very poor correlation between the auscultatory findings and the pulmonary function test results in patients with COPD (83).

Therefore, to evaluate the response to therapy, serial tests of pulmonary function should be obtained. Usually spirometry is sufficient, and it is recommended that spirometry be performed each time a patient with pulmonary dysfunction is seen. The best indices for following patients with obstructive lung disease are the absolute values of the $FEV_1$ and the FVC, and not the $FEV_1/FVC$ ratio, since the latter is very dependent on the duration of expiration. However, it should be noted that spirometry is not perfect for assessing the response to therapy. For the patient the most important consideration is whether his or her functional capabilities improve. However, significant improvements in spirometric results are not necessarily associated with increased exercise tolerance (84). Nevertheless, it is impractical to perform repeated exercise tests on most patients with pulmonary dysfunction.

Recent theories concerning the pathogenesis of chronic airway obstruction have focused on airway inflammation and airway hyperresponsiveness (10). Accordingly, serial inhalational challenge tests are being used more and more frequently to assess a patient's response to a therapeutic regimen. For example, a recent study documented that when aerosolized steroids were given to 16 mild asthmatics for 1 year, the hyperresponsiveness improved in 15 of the 16, and in five individuals the methacholine test became normal (85). Although at the present time such tests are used primarily in research situations, their use in the clinical setting will probably become more widespread in the future.

### Why is My Patient Short of Breath on Exertion?

Many patients complain of exercise intolerance. An explanation for the exercise intolerance is frequently lacking even after a careful history, physical examination, chest roentgenogram, electrocardiogram, and routine tests of pulmonary function. The performance of an exercise test will frequently permit identification of the factor producing limitation in an individual patient. The characteristic profiles of exercise tests in patients limited by obstructive ventilatory dysfunction, exercise-induced asthma, restrictive ventilatory dysfunction, pulmonary hypertension, cardiovascular dysfunction, poor physical condition, and poor effort are described below.

#### Obstructive Ventilatory Dysfunction

The exercise capacity of most patients with COPD is limited by their respiratory system. In general, this limitation is due to the facts that their ventilatory capacity is limited by their lung disease and that their ventilatory requirement for a given work load is increased since their wasted ventilation ($V_D/V_T$) is increased. The cardiovascular response to exercise in patients with COPD appears to be relatively normal, since the cardiac output for a given $\dot{V}O_2$ is relatively normal (86).

The typical results of an exercise test of a patient with ventilatory limitation are as follows: (a) the patient stops exercising due to shortness of breath rather than leg fatigue (although even among those with $FEV_1$ below 40% of predicted, a sizable percentage stop on account of leg fatigue) (87); (b) the $\dot{V}O_2$max is reduced, and $\dot{V}E$ at exhaustion is at least 35 times the $FEV_1$ or 70% of the MVV (87); (c) the $VD/VT$ at rest is usually elevated and does not decrease with exercise, and the $\dot{V}CO_2/\dot{V}E$ is above 30; (d) for a given $\dot{V}O_2$ the heart rate is higher than normal, but the maximum heart rate is reduced because the $\dot{V}O_2$max is so low (72); (e) the anaerobic threshold is frequently not reached owing to the ventilatory limitation; (f) arterial blood gases during exercise may be unchanged from rest or may reveal an increased $PaCO_2$ or a decreased $PaO_2$.

### Exercise-Induced Asthma

Exercise can precipitate bronchospasm in some individuals. If exercise-induced asthma is suspected, spirometry should be obtained before the exercise test and at 5-minute intervals after completion of the exercise test. The exercise should be for 6 to 8 minutes at an intensity of 85 to 90% of the predicted maximal heart rate. The diagnosis is established if the $FEV_1$ falls more than 10% after performance of the exercise test. Having the patient inhale dry air such as from a meteorologic balloon filled from a cylinder of compressed room air will enhance the chances of inducing asthma (88).

### Restrictive Ventilatory Dysfunction

Many patients with interstitial diseases such as pulmonary fibrosis, sarcoidosis, or pneumoconiosis have subnormal exercise tolerance. The exercise capacity in most of these patients is limited by a reduced ventilatory capacity (89–91). The reduced FVC results in a relatively low maximal tidal volume, which necessitates a very high respiratory rate. This limitation, coupled with a decreased efficiency of gas exchange (increased $VD/VT$), leads to decreased exercise tolerance. Arterial blood gases during exercise usually reveal hypoxemia, and endurance exercise can be prolonged with supplemental oxygen (89).

### Pulmonary Hypertension

The exercise tolerance as reflected by the $\dot{V}O_2$max of patients with primary pulmonary hypertension is markedly reduced. The exercise capacity of these patients appears to be limited by a low cardiac output. The anaerobic threshold occurs at a relatively low work load, and the oxygen pulse is much lower than normal. The $PaO_2$ also tends to decrease in these patients with exercise. Although the ventilation at any given work load is higher in these patients than in normals (due

to the increased $VD/VT$ and the early onset of anaerobic metabolism), there is no evidence that these patients are ventilatory limited (92).

### Cardiovascular Dysfunction

The exercise capacity of patients with cardiovascular dysfunction is limited by their cardiac output, as is that of normals. The main abnormality in such patients is a decreased stroke volume. Accordingly, their cardiac output at a given heart rate is less than normal. The maximum heart rate often is normal but sometimes is markedly reduced (35).

The typical results of an exercise test in a patient with cardiac dysfunction are as follows (50): (a) the $\dot{V}O_2$max is reduced but the $\dot{V}E$ is less than 35 times the $FEV_1$ and less than 70% of the MVV; (b) the $VD/VT$ is near normal and the $\dot{V}CO_2/\dot{V}E$ is below 30; (c) the heart rate is elevated relative to the $\dot{V}O_2$ (owing to the low stroke volume) and the anaerobic threshold is reached at a low $\dot{V}O_2$; (d) arterial blood gases reveal a normal $PaO_2$ but a reduced $PaCO_2$ and a metabolic acidosis.

### Lack of Fitness

The results of exercise tests in an unfit individual are similar to those in a patient with cardiovascular disease. The anaerobic threshold will be reached at a low $\dot{V}O_2$ because of the poor distribution of the cardiac output. The maximum heart rate is normal and the $\dot{V}E$ is below 35 times the $FEV_1$. Arterial blood gases are similar to those of patients with cardiovascular dysfunction.

### Malingering

Some individuals complain of exercise intolerance when their initial evaluation reveals no abnormalities that can explain such intolerance. Frequently the question arises as to whether they are actually impaired, particularly when litigation or disability compensation is involved. When subjected to a maximal exercise test, such individuals may not give maximum effort. Therefore, they will have decreased $\dot{V}O_2$max. However, aside from this decrease, there will be no evidence that they are limited by any of the above mechanisms. More specifically, their $\dot{V}E$ will be less than 35 times their $FEV_1$; their maximal heart rate will be reduced, but the $\dot{V}O_2$ for a given heart rate will be normal; they will fail to reach their anaerobic threshold and their blood lactate levels will be less than 8 mM/liter; and arterial blood gases will not demonstrate hypercapnia, hypoxia, or a metabolic acidosis.

If an individual appears not to give a maximum effort, a good approximation of their actual $\dot{V}O_2$max can be obtained by extrapolating the results of their exercise test to the maximal predicted heart rate as shown in Figure 8.12. If their ventilatory reserve at exhaustion is less than their cardiac reserve percentagewise, then the extrapolation should be made with the ventilation rather than with the heart rate.

### Is My Patient Physically Impaired from His or Her Lung Disease?

New and revised social legislation entitles an increasing number of Americans to compensation for disability. As a result, physicians are being asked more and more frequently to quantify impairment of health. The term *impairment* implies a physiologic, anatomic, or mental functional deficit, whereas the term *disability* implies an inability to perform or a limitation in the performance of tasks within a social environment. Rating of impairment falls within the sphere of the physician's expertise. In contrast, adjudication of disability requires consideration of additional factors, such as educational or cultural level and availability of suitable work, and is generally an administrative function outside the realm of the physician's practice. The following discussion concerns itself only with quantifying the degree of impairment. The recommendations are those of the American Thoracic Society (93, 94).

*Tests of Pulmonary Function*

In the evaluation of respiratory impairment, the first step is to obtain pulmonary function testing. It is recommended that the first step include both forced spirometry measurements and testing for single-breath diffusing capacity. The results of these tests will allow the majority of subjects to be appropriately categorized as to their degree of impairment as follows:

*Normal.* FVC  80% of predicted, *and* $FEV_1$  80% of predicted, *and* $FEV_1/FVC$  0.75, and $D_{LCO}$  80% of predicted.

*Mildly impaired* (usually not correlated with diminished ability to perform most jobs). FVC 60 to 79% predicted, *or* $FEV_1$ 60 to 79% predicted, *or* $FEV_1/FVC$ 0.60 to 0.74, *or* $D_{LCO}$ 60 to 79% of predicted.

*Moderately impaired* (progressively lower levels of lung function correlated with diminishing ability to meet the physical demands of many jobs). FVC 51 to 59% of predicted, *or* $FEV_1$ 41 to 59% of predicted, *or* $FEV_1/FVC$ 0.41 to 0.59, *or* $D_{LCO}$ 41 to 59% of predicted.

*Severely impaired* (unable to meet the physical demands of most jobs, including travel to work). FVC 50% or less of predicted, *or* $FEV_1$ 40% or less of predicted, *or* $FEV_1/FVC$ less than 0.40, *or* $D_{LCO}$ 40% or less of predicted.

*Exercise Testing*

Subjects found to have no impairment or mild impairment on the basis of their pulmonary function tests are usually able to perform all but the most unusually physically demanding of jobs. Patients with severe impairment usually are unable to perform almost all jobs, if for no other reason than they are frequently unable to travel back and forth to their place of work.

Patients with mild or moderate impairment who complain of shortness of breath while working should be considered as possible candidates for exercise testing. Exercise testing is useful because there is not a close relationship between tests of pulmonary function and $\dot{V}O_2$max (Fig. 8.15). In such cases the exercise testing is performed for two reasons. First, to determine

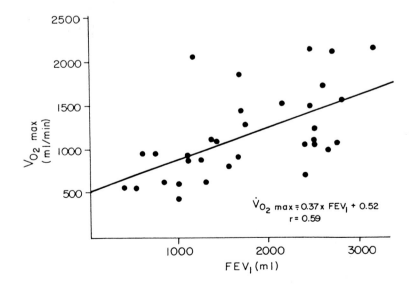

**FIGURE 8.15.**   Relationship between the $\dot{V}O_2$max and the $FEV_1$. Note how poorly the $\dot{V}O_2$max correlates with the $FEV_1$. (Data courtesy Dr. V. D. Minh.)

whether an individual is significantly impaired, and second, to determine whether the impairment is due to pulmonary dysfunction or some other cause. At a minimum, the testing should include measurement of ventilation ($\dot{V}E$), tidal volume, and frequency of breathing. Most testing should be done in laboratories that can also measure the composition of expired gas and arterial oxygen saturation.

The following rating of impairment is recommended:

1. If the $\dot{V}O_2max$ is greater than 25 ml/kg/minute, the subject will be capable of continuous heavy exertion throughout an 8-hour shift and of all but the most physically demanding of jobs.
2. If the $\dot{V}O_2$ is between 15 and 25 ml/kg/minute, and 40% of the observed $\dot{V}O_2max$ is greater than the average metabolic work requirement of the subject's job, then the subject should be able to perform that job comfortably.
3. If the $\dot{V}O_2max$ is less than 15 ml/kg/minute, the subject will be unable to perform most jobs because he or she would be uncomfortable in traveling back and forth to the place of employment.

*Impairment with Asthma*

The determination of impairment in patients with asthma differs from that with other respiratory diseases because of the following factors: (*a*) in asthmatics the condition is much more variable; (*b*) the condition is associated with hyperresponsiveness to various agents such as dusts, fumes, and gases that the patient may encounter while working; (*c*) environmental or occupational exposures may increase airway inflammation, which on repeated exposures can become chronic and irreversible.

The American Thoracic Society has recently developed guidelines for the evaluation of impairment in patients with asthma (95). In summary, these guidelines suggest the following three factors be considered in determining the level of impairment: (*a*) the post-bronchodilator $FEV_1$; (*b*) the reversibility of the $FEV_1$ or the degree of airway hyperresponsiveness; and (*c*) the minimal amount of medication required by the patient. An asthmatic is severely impaired if the $FEV_1$ is less than 50% of predicted while taking at least 20 mg prednisone orally. The reader is referred to the recent ATS statement for further details about impairment in the asthmatic (95).

▼

## REFERENCES

1. Pulmonary terms and symbols: a report of the ACCP-ATS Joint Committee on Pulmonary Nomenclature. *Chest* 67:583–593, 1975.
2. Official statement of the American Thoracic Society: standardization of spirometry—1987 update. *Am Rev Respir Dis* 136:1285–1298, 1987.
3. Cochrane GM, Prieto F, Clark TJ: Intrasubject variability of maximal expiratory flow volume curve. *Thorax* 32:171–176, 1977.
4. Hyatt RE, Black LF: The flow volume curve: a current perspective. *Am Rev Respir Dis* 107:191–199, 1973.
5. Kapp MC, Schachter EN, Beck GJ, et al: The shape of the maximum expiratory flow volume curve. *Chest* 94:799–806, 1988.
6. Meadows JA III, Rodarte JR, Hyatt RE: Density dependence of maximal expiratory flow in chronic obstructive pulmonary disease. *Am Rev Respir Dis* 121:47–53, 1980.
7. Heaf PJD, Gillam PMS: Peak flow rates in normal and asthmatic children. *Br Med J* 1:1595–1596, 1962.
8. Clark NM, Evans D, Mellins RB: Patient use of peak flow monitoring. *Am Rev Respir Dis* 145:722–725, 1992.
9. Campbell SC: A comparison of the maximum voluntary ventilation with the forced expiratory volume in one second: an assessment of subject cooperation. *J Occup Med* 24:531–533, 1982.
10. Cockcroft DW, Hargreave FE: Airway hyperresponsiveness. Relevance of random population data to clinical usefulness. *Am Rev Respir Dis* 142:497–500, 1990.
11. Rijcken B, Schouten JP, Mensinga TT, Weiss ST, De Vries K, Der Lende RV: Factors associated with bronchial responsiveness to histamine in a population sample of adults. *Am Rev Respir Dis* 147:1447–1453, 1993.
12. Buist AS, Connett JE, Miller RD, Kanner RE, Owens GR, Woelker HT: Chronic obstructive pulmonary disease early intervention trial (Lung Health Study). Baseline characteristics of randomized participants. *Chest* 103:1863–1872, 1993.
13. Meneely GR, Ball CO, Kory RC, et al: A simplified closed circuit helium dilution method for the determination of the residual volume of the lungs. *Am J Med* 28:824–831, 1960.
14. Darling RC, Cournand A, Richards DW: Studies on the intrapulmonary mixing of gases. II. An open circuit method for measuring residual air. *J Clin Invest* 19:609–618, 1940.
15. Burns CB, Scheinhorn DJ: Evaluation of single-breath helium dilution total lung capacity in obstructive lung disease. *Am Rev Respir Dis* 130:580–583, 1984.
16. Dubois AB, Botelho SY, Bedell GN, et al: A rapid plethysmographic method for measuring thoracic gas volume: a comparison with a nitrogen washout method for measuring functional residual capacity in normal subjects. *J Clin Invest* 35:322–326, 1956.
17. Dubois AB, Botelho SY, Comroe JH Jr: A new method for measuring airway resistance in man using a body plethysmograph: values in normal subjects and in patients with respiratory disease. *J Clin Invest* 35:327–335, 1956.
18. Comroe JH, Fowler WS: Lung function studies. IV. Detection of uneven alveolar ventilation during a single breath of oxygen: a new test of pulmonary disease. *Am J Med* 10:408–413, 1951.
19. Buist AS, Ross BR: Quantitative analysis of the alveolar plateau in the diagnosis of early airway obstruction. *Am Rev Respir Dis* 108:1078–1087, 1973.
20. Menkes HA, Beaty TH, Cohen BH, Weinmann G: Nitrogen washout and mortality. *Am Rev Respir Dis* 132:115–119, 1985.

21. McCarthy DS, Spencer R, Greene R, Milic-Emili J: Measurements of "closing volume" as a simple and sensitive test for early detection of small airway disease. *Am J Med* 52:747–753, 1972.

22. Buist AS, Vollmer WM, Johnson LR, McCamant LE: Does the single-breath $N_2$ test identify the smoker who will develop chronic airflow limitation? *Am Rev Respir Dis* 127:293–301, 1988.

23. Ogilvie CM, Forster RE, Blakemore WS, Morton JW: A standardized breath holding technique for the clinical measurement of the diffusing capacity of the lung for carbon monoxide. *J Clin Invest* 36:1–17, 1957.

24. Official statement of the American Thoracic Society: single breath carbon monoxide diffusing capacity (transfer factor). Recommendations for a standard technique. *Am Rev Respir Dis* 136:1299–1307, 1987.

25. Lewis BM, Lin TH, Noe FE, Hayford-Wesling EJ: The measurement of pulmonary diffusing capacity for carbon monoxide by a rebreathing method. *J Clin Invest* 38:2073–2086, 1959.

26. Weinberger SE, Johnson TS, Weiss ST: Use and interpretation of the single breath diffusing capacity. *Chest* 78:483–488, 1980.

27. Bates DV, Varvis CJ, Donevan RE, Christie RV: Variations in the pulmonary capillary blood volume and membrane diffusion component in health and disease. *J Clin Invest* 39:1401–1412, 1960.

28. Ferris BG (ed): Epidemiology standardization project: recommended standardized procedures for pulmonary function testing. *Am Rev Respir Dis* 118 (pt 2):62–72, 1978.

29. Wasserman K, Hansen JE, Sue DY, Whipp BJ: *Principles of Exercise Testing and Interpretation.* Philadelphia, Lea & Febiger, 1986.

30. Sutton JR: Limitations to maximal oxygen uptake. *Sports Med* 13:127–133, 1992.

31. Ogawa T, Spina RJ, Martin WH III, Kohrt WM, Schechtman KB, Holoszy JO, Ehsani AA: Effects of aging, sex and physical training on cardiovascular responses to exercise. *Circulation* 86:494–503, 1992.

32. Crawford MH: Physiologic consequences of systematic training. *Cardiol Clin* 10:209–221, 1992.

33. Honig CR, Connett RJ, Gayeski TEJ: $O_2$ transport and its interaction with metabolism; a systems view of aerobic capacity. *Med Sci Sports Exerc* 24:47–53, 1992.

34. Myers J, Walsh D, Buchanan N, Froelicher VF: Can maximal cardiopulmonary capacity be recognized by a plateau in oxygen uptake? *Chest* 96:1312–1316, 1989.

35. Arnold SB, Byrd RC, Meister W, et al: Long-term digitalis therapy improves left ventricular function in heart failure. *N Engl J Med* 303:1443–1448, 1980.

36. Jones NL, Campbell EJM: *Clinical Exercise Testing,* ed 2. Philadelphia, WB Saunders, 1981.

37. Barany P, Freyschuss U, Pettersson E, Bergstrom J: Treatment of anaemia in haemodialysis patients with erythropoietin: long-term effects on exercise capacity. *Clin Sci* 84:441–447, 1993.

38. Weiss AB, Calton FM, Kuida H, Hecht HH: Hemodynamic effects of normovolemic polycythemia in dogs at rest and during exercise. *Am J Physiol* 207:1361–1366, 1964.

39. Chetty KG, Light RW, Stansbury DW, Milne N: Exercise performance of polycythemic chronic obstructive pulmonary disease patients. Effect of phlebotomies. *Chest* 98:1073–1077, 1990.

40. Sawka MN, Young AJ, Muza SR, et al: Erythrocytes reinfusion and maximal aerobic power. *JAMA* 257:1496–1499, 1987.

41. Horvath SM, Raven PB, Dahms TE, et al: Maximal aerobic capacity at different levels of carboxyhemoglobin. *J Appl Physiol* 38:300–303, 1975.

42. Astrand PO, Rodahl K: *Textbook of Work Physiology,* ed 2. New York, McGraw-Hill, 1977.

43. Oren A, Wasserman K, Davis JA, Whipp BJ: Effect of $CO_2$ set point on ventilatory response to exercise. *J Appl Physiol* 51:185–189, 1981.

44. Light RW, Mahutte CK, Brown SE: Etiology of $CO_2$ retention at rest and during exercise in chronic airflow obstruction. *Chest* 94:61–67, 1988.

45. West JB: Ventilation-perfusion relationships. *Am Rev Respir Dis* 116:919–943, 1977.

46. Powers SK, Martin D, Dodd S: Exercise-induced hypoxaemia in elite endurance athletes. Incidence, causes and impact on $Vo_2max$. *Sports Med* 16:14–22, 1993.

47. Shepard RH: Effect of pulmonary diffusion capacity on exercise tolerance. *J Appl Physiol* 12:487–488, 1958.

48. Belman MJ, Mittman C: Ventilatory muscle training improves exercise capacity in chronic obstructive pulmonary disease patients. *Am Rev Respir Dis* 121:273–280, 1981.

49. Jones NL: Normal values for pulmonary gas exchange during exercise. *Am Rev Respir Dis* 129(Suppl):S44–S46, 1984.

50. Brown HV, Wasserman K: Exercise performance in chronic obstructive pulmonary diseases. *Med Clin North Am* 65:525–547, 1981.

51. Koike A, Hiroe M, Taniguchi K, Marumo F: Respiratory control during exercise in patients with cardiovascular disease. *Am Rev Respir Dis* 147:425–429, 1993.

52. Beaver WL, Wasserman K, Whipp BJ: A new method for detecting anaerobic threshold by gas exchange. *J Appl Physiol* 60:2020–2027, 1986.

53. Belman MJ, Epstein LJ, Doornbos D, Elashoff JD, Koerner SK, Mohsenifar Z: Noninvasive determinations of the anaerobic threshold. Reliability and validity in patients with COPD. *Chest* 102:1028–1034, 1992.

54. Eriksson BO, Engstrom I, Karlberg P, et al: A physiological analysis of former girl swimmers. *Acta Paediatr Scand* 217(Suppl):68–72, 1971.

55. Saltin B, Blomqvist G, Mitchell JH, et al: Response to exercise after bed rest and after training. A longitudinal study of adaptive changes in oxygen transport and body composition. *Circulation* 38(Suppl 7):1–78, 1968.

56. Knuttgen HG: Development of muscular strength and endurance. In Knuttgen HG (ed): Neuromuscular mechanisms for therapeutic and conditioning exercise. Baltimore, University Park Press, 1976, p 97.

57. Goldberg L, Elliot DL, Kuehl KS: Assessment of exercise intensity formulas by use of ventilatory threshold. *Chest* 94:95–98, 1988.

58. Degre S, Sergysels R, Messin R, et al: Hemodynamic responses to physical training in patients with chronic lung disease. *Am Rev Respir Dis* 110:395–402, 1974.

59. Cockcroft AE, Saunders MJ, Berry G: Randomized controlled trial of rehabilitation in chronic respiratory disability. *Thorax* 36:200–203, 1981.

60. Holle RHO, Williams DV, Vandree JC, Starts GL, Schoene RB: Increased muscle efficiency and sustained

benefits in an outpatient community hospital-based pulmonary rehabilitation program. *Chest* 94:1161–1168, 1988.

61. Belman MJ, Kendregan BA: Exercise training fails to increase skeletal muscle enzymes in patients with chronic obstructive pulmonary disease. *Am Rev Respir Dis* 123:256–261, 1981.

62. Smith K, Cook D, Guyatt GH, Madhavan J, Oxman AD: Respiratory muscle training in chronic airflow limitation: a meta-analysis. *Am Rev Respir Dis* 145:533–539, 1992.

63. Kohrt WM, Malley MT, Coggan AR, Spina RJ, Ogawa T, Ehsani AA, Bourey RE, Martin WH III, Holloszy JO: Effects of gender, age, and fitness level on response of VO$_2$max to training in 60 to 71 year olds. *J Appl Physiol* 71:2004–2011, 1991.

64. Bernstein ML, Despars JA, Singh N, Avalos K, Stansbury D, Light RW: Reanalysis of the 12-minute walk test in COPD patients. *Chest* 105:163–167, 1994.

65. Orenstein DM, Curtis SC, Nixon PA, Hartigan ER: Accuracy of three pulse oximeters during exercise and hypoxemia in patients with cystic fibrosis. *Chest* 104:1187–1190, 1993.

66. Blackie SP, Fairbarn MS, McElvaney GN, Morrison NJ, Wilcox PG, Pardy RL: Prediction of maximal oxygen uptake and power during cycle ergometry in subjects older than 55 years of age. *Am Rev Respir Dis* 139:1424–1429, 1989.

67. Jones NL, Makrides L, Hitchcock C, et al: Normal standards for an incremental progressive cycle ergometer test. *Am Rev Respir Dis* 131:700–708, 1985.

68. Morris AH, Kanner RE, Crapo RO, Gardner RM: *Clinical Pulmonary Function Testing: A Manual of Uniform Laboratory Procedures,* ed 2. Salt Lake City, Intermountain Thoracic Society, 1984.

69. Clausen JL, Zarins LP (eds): *Pulmonary Function Testing —Guidelines and Controversies.* New York, Academic Press, 1982.

70. Knudson RJ, Lebowitz MD, Holberg CJ, Burrows B: Changes in the normal maximal expiratory flow-volume curve with growth and aging. *Am Rev Respir Dis* 127:725–734, 1983.

71. Morris JF, Koski A, Temple WP, et al: Fifteen-year interval spirometric evaluation of the Oregon predictive equations. *Chest* 92:123–127, 1988.

72. Withers RT, Bourdon PC, Crockett A: Lung volume standards for healthy male lifetime nonsmokers. *Chest* 92:91–97, 1988.

73. Crapo RO, Morris AH: Standardized single breath normal values for carbon monoxide diffusing capacity. *Am Rev Respir Dis* 123:185–189, 1981.

74. Knudson RJ, Kaltenborn WT, Knudson DE, Burrows B: The single-breath carbon monoxide diffusing capacity. Reference equations derived from a healthy nonsmoking population and effects of hematocrit. *Am Rev Respir Dis* 135:805–811, 1987.

75. Pappas GPP, Newman LS: Early pulmonary physiologic abnormalities in beryllium disease. *Am Rev Respir Dis* 148:661–666, 1993.

76. Curtis JK, Liska AP, Rasmussen HK, et al: The bronchospastic component in patients with chronic bronchitis and emphysema. *JAMA* 197:693–696, 1966.

77. Nisar M, Earis JE, Pearson MG, Calverley PMA: Acute bronchodilator trials in chronic obstructive pulmonary disease. *Am Rev Respir Dis* 146:555–559, 1992.

78. Guyatt GH, Townsend M, Nogradi S, et al: Acute response to bronchodilator. An imperfect guide for bronchodilator therapy in chronic airflow limitation. *Arch Intern Med* 148:1949–1952, 1988.

79. Rotman HH, Liss HP, Weg JG: Diagnosis of upper airway obstruction by pulmonary function testing. *Chest* 68:796–799, 1975.

80. Wright JL, Lawson LM, Pare PD, et al: The detection of small airways disease. *Am Rev Respir Dis* 129:989–994, 1984.

81. Sparrow D, O'Connor GT, Basner RC, Brosner B, Weiss ST: Predictors of the new onset of wheezing among middle-aged and older men. *Am Rev Respir Dis* 147:367–371, 1993.

82. Rubenfeld AR, Pain MC: Perception of asthma. *Lancet* 1:882–884, 1976.

83. Marini JJ, Pierson JD, Hudson LD, et al: The significance of wheezing in chronic airflow obstruction. *Am Rev Respir Dis* 120:1069–1072, 1979.

84. Tobin JM, Hughes JA, Hutchison DC: Effects of ipratropium bromide and fenoterol aerosols on exercise tolerance. *Eur J Respir Dis* 65:441–446, 1984.

85. Juniper EF, Kline PA, Vanzieleghem MA, Ramsdale EH, O'Byrne PM, Hargreave FE: Effect on long-term treatment with an inhaled corticosteroid (budesonide) on airway hyperresponsiveness and clinical asthma in nonsteroid-dependent asthmatics. *Am Rev Respir Dis* 142:832–836, 1990.

86. Light RW, Mintz HM, Linden GS, Brown SE: Hemodynamics of patients with severe chronic obstructive pulmonary disease (COPD) during progressive upright exercise. *Am Rev Respir Dis* 130:391–395, 1984.

87. Killian KJ, Leblanc P, Martin DH, Summers E, Jones NL, Campbell EJM: Exercise capacity and ventilatory, circulatory, and symptom limitation in patients with chronic airflow limitation. *Am Rev Respir Dis* 146:935–940, 1992.

88. Mahler DA: Exercise-induced asthma. *Med Sci Sports Exerc* 25:554–561, 1993.

89. Bye PB, Anderson SD, Woolcock AJ, et al: Bicycle endurance performance of patients with interstitial lung disease breathing air and oxygen. *Am Rev Respir Dis* 126:1005–1012, 1982.

90. Burdon JGW, Killian KJ, Jones NL: Pattern of breathing during exercise in patients with interstitial lung disease. *Thorax* 38:778–784, 1983.

91. Matthews JI, Hooper RG: Exercise testing in pulmonary sarcoidosis. *Chest* 83:75–81, 1983.

92. D'Alonzo GE, Gianotti LA, Pohil RL, et al: Comparison of progressive exercise performance of normal subjects and patients with primary pulmonary hypertension. *Chest* 92:57–62, 1987.

93. Medical Section of the American Lung Association: Evaluation of impairment/disability secondary to respiratory disease. *Am Rev Respir Dis* 126:945–951, 1982.

94. Medical Section of the American Lung Association: Evaluation of impairment/disability secondary to respiratory disease. *Am Rev Respir Dis* 133:1205–1209, 1986.

95. Medical Section of the American Lung Association: Guidelines for the evaluation of impairment/disability in patients with asthma. *Am Rev Respir Dis* 147:1056–1061, 1993.

# SECTION
## THREE
▼

# EVALUATION AND MANAGEMENT OF LUNG DISEASE

# Chapter 9

# Asthma

## Mani S. Kavuru
## Herbert P. Wiedemann

BRONCHIAL ASTHMA affects 3 to 5% of the U.S. population, making it a frequently encountered clinical problem in both the pediatric and adult population. It is a major cause of morbidity in the United States and around the world. During the past decade, despite an increasing understanding of the pathogenesis of asthma, there has been an increase in the morbidity and mortality due to asthma. There are several potential reasons for this trend, although there is no general agreement.

Much new information has implicated airway inflammation in the pathogenesis of airway hyperreactivity and clinical asthma. Asthma is a heterogeneous disease, and multiple mechanisms are likely involved in the pathogenesis, rather than a single unifying mechanism. The development of specific antagonists to the various mediators is accelerating our understanding of this disease. As a product of this understanding, it is to be hoped that additional therapeutic agents will emerge for subgroups of asthmatics. This chapter reviews recent trends in epidemiology, pathogenesis, and management principles of bronchial asthma.

## DEFINITION AND CLASSIFICATION

Despite a number of formal attempts over a 30-year period, a universally accepted definition of asthma is unavailable (1–5). It is likely that asthma is not a specific disease, but a syndrome that derives from multiple precipitating mechanisms and results in a common clinical complex involving reversible airway obstruction (6). Important features of this syndrome include episodic occurrence of dyspnea and wheezing, air flow obstruction with a bronchodilator-reversible component, bronchial hyperresponsiveness to a variety of nonspecific and specific stimuli, and airway inflammation. All of these features need not be present. During the past 5 to 10 years, as a result of bronchoalveolar lavage studies involving asthmatics, airway inflammation has become integral to the definition of asthma. Although there is some overlap in features between asthma and other chronic obstructive air flow disorders such as chronic bronchitis, emphysema, and cystic fibrosis, it is essential to make this distinction. Asthma typically occurs in younger individuals who are nonsmokers. In general, the baseline level of functioning, exercise tolerance, and spirometric parameters in asthmatics are much better preserved between acute exacerbations than in individuals with emphysema or chronic bronchitis. Patients with asthma exhibit a tremendous heterogeneity in the clinical features and the severity of disease. Asthma can range from being a rare and mild nuisance, occurring perhaps only in relation to specific triggers such as pollen or exercise, to being a severe, unrelenting, and occasionally fatal disease without a definable external cause.

Asthma traditionally has been classified as either extrinsic or intrinsic. Patients with extrinsic asthma tend to have a childhood onset, positive skin test reactions to many antigens (atopy), a strong family history of atopy and asthma, and often a predictable seasonal variation of their asthma. Intrinsic asthma is not associated with any known immunologic reactions to external antigens, usually begins in adulthood, and exhibits little seasonal variation. However, this classification system is not particularly useful or relevant to the clinical management or treatment of most asthmatic patients, especially adults.

## EPIDEMIOLOGY

### INCIDENCE, PREVALENCE

The true prevalence of asthma is difficult to ascertain due to the lack of a standard definition and the variations in epidemiologic methodology that have been used. In most surveys, asthma is found to be more common in children than in adults and slightly more frequent in males than in females. In the United States, a national survey by the Public Health Service in 1970 estimated that 3% of the population had asthma (7, 8). In this survey, 60.3% of asthmatic individuals consulted a physician for asthma during the previous year and about 50% were using a medication or treatment for asthma. In a smaller study, using better clinical documentation, performed in the Michigan town of Tecumseh, the 12-month prevalence of asthma was 4.0% in males and 3.4% in females (8, 9). National Health and Nutritional Examination Surveys conducted 5 years apart, in 1975 and 1980, reported a significant increase in the prevalence of asthma from 4.8% to 7.6% among 6- to 11-year-old children (10).

Based on National Health Interviews Survey (NHIS) results from 1980 through 1990, the age-adjusted prevalence rate for self-reported asthma increased 38% from 3100 to 4290 per 100,000 population (from 6.8 million to 10.3 million persons affected) (11). The rate increased 50% for females and 27% percent for males. From 1981 through 1988, the annual prevalence rate of asthma in black females increased from 2750 to 6060 per 100,000; from 1980 through 1989, the rate for white females increased from 2960 to 4700 per 100,000.

Skobeloff and coworkers conducted a retrospective review of all asthma admissions from southeastern Pennsylvania to define the role of age and sex as risk factors for asthma hospital admission. There were 33,269 patients admitted for asthma treatment over a 4-year period that included 67 hospitals in five counties (12). In the 0- to 10-year-old age group, males were admitted nearly twice as often as age-identical females. In the 11- to 20-year-old age group, admissions for males and females were nearly identical. Between 20 and 50 years of age, the female-to-male ratio was nearly 3:1. Length of stay increased proportionally as the patient age increased, and the length of stay was greater for females than for males. Overall, the authors concluded that adult females are more severely affected by asthma.

Recent data suggest alarming upward trends in both the morbidity and mortality due to asthma. In 1990, the cost of illness related to asthma was estimated to be $6.2 billion, or nearly 1% of all U.S. health-care costs (13). Inpatient hospital services represented the largest single direct medical expenditure for asthma, approaching $1.6 billion. Forty-three percent of the economic impact of asthma was associated with emergency room use, hospitalization, and death. Nearly two-thirds of the visits for ambulatory care were to physicians in primary care specialties, including pediatrics, family medicine, general practice, and internal medicine.

### TRENDS IN ASTHMA-RELATED MORTALITY

Data from the National Center for Health Statistics disclosed gradual decreases in the number of deaths from asthma each year in the United States to a low of 1,674 in 1977 (11). From 1980 through 1989, however, the age-adjusted death rate for asthma as the underlying cause of death increased 46% from 1.3 per 100,000 population (2,891 deaths) to 1.9 per 100,000 (4,867 deaths). During this period, the death rate increased 54% for females (from 1.3 to 2.0 per 100,000) and 23% for males (from 1.3 to 1.6 per 100,000) (11). The annual asthma death rate was consistently higher for blacks than for whites during this period. For blacks the rate increased 52% (from 2.5 to 3.8 per 100,000), compared with a 45% increase (from 1.1 to 1.6 per 100,000) for whites. The increase in the death rate for black and white females was similar; however, the increase in the death rate for black males was more than twice that for white males. The increase in mortality rates has been even more dramatic in other countries, including

Australia, England-Wales, West Germany, Japan, and Canada (14–17).

A number of recent studies have critically reviewed whether the recent mortality trends are real or an epidemiologic artifact (18–20). Clearly, the accuracy of the statistics depends on the accuracy of physician certification of the cause of death. Two large retrospective studies on the accuracy of certification of death due to asthma from England (21) and New Zealand (22), involving detailed inquiry of relatives, doctors, hospital records, and autopsy results by a medical reviewing panel, accepted 70% of these deaths as being accurately attributed to asthma. The accuracy was highest for persons aged less than 35 and the accuracy declined with increasing age. A recent study of a mortality cohort of 339 asthma-related deaths from the Mayo Clinic found that the death certificate had a sensitivity of 42% and a specificity of 99% compared with an expert review panel (23). Therefore, asthma mortality rates, determined from death certificate data, may underestimate actual asthma-related mortality.

The ninth revision of the International Classification of Diseases (ICD-9), which took effect in 1979, increased assignment of deaths to asthma and decreased assignment to bronchitis and emphysema (18). Since 1979, deaths labeled as asthmatic bronchitis on a death certificate are classified as asthma. In older age groups, the effect of this change increased reported asthma mortality by 35% or more, but in 5- to 34-year-olds the effect was negligible. In 15- to 34-year-old persons in the United States, asthma deaths increased with no reduction in deaths attributed to nonasthmatic disease, suggesting that diagnostic transfer is unlikely. Therefore, the increase in mortality rate in the younger age groups cannot be explained by the code revision alone. Also, the continued increase in reported mortality since 1979 must be due to factors other than the one-time change in death assignment coding. In summary, the recent increases in mortality due to asthma appear to be real and cannot be simply explained by false-positive reporting or a revision in the ICD coding.

There are several potential causes for increased mortality due to asthma, including a change in the prevalence of asthma, change in the severity of disease, inadequate objective assessment of disease severity, toxicity of current therapy, or suboptimal usage of anti-inflammatory therapy.

There are numerous retrospective studies that have examined the circumstances of asthma-related deaths (24–26). Also, there are several case-controlled studies comparing matched survivors to patients who died of asthma (27, 28). Review of these and other studies suggests that asthma deaths are of two types: type 1, slow onset–late arrival; and type 2, sudden onset (29). Consensus from these studies is that there are several risk factors that contribute to type 1 fatal asthma, including prior serious asthma, requiring emergency room visits or mechanical ventilation. Factors that may interfere with compliance and access to medical care include socioeconomic factors, certain psychological features, and racial/cultural factors. Other factors include inadequate objective assessment of asthma severity by pulmonary function testing. Inadequate treatment with either inhaled or systemic corticosteroids is also a frequently described finding. Therefore, undertreatment and underestimation of asthma severity are important contributing factors in type 1 asthma-related fatalities (30).

A number of recent studies have highlighted that some patients die suddenly and unexpectedly with acute asthma (so-called type 2 deaths). Wasserfallen and coworkers analyzed 34 patients intubated and mechanically ventilated for severe asthma and noted three patterns of decompensation in terms of the delay between onset of symptoms and endotracheal intubation (31): group I, rapid decompensation in less than 3 hours; group II, gradual respiratory failure (9.2 ± 7.7 days; and group III, acute deterioration after unstable asthma (4.2 ± 3.6 days). It was noted that the sudden asphyctic group I type was more frequent in young men and was associated with extreme hypercapnia with a higher incidence of respiratory arrest, but the recovery was more rapid with shorter duration of mechanical ventilation. Authors suggested that bronchospasm was a primary mechanism in this group with "hyperacute" deterioration. Kallenbach and colleagues studied 81 patients with acute asthma in whom mechanical ventilation was required (32). Patients with a short attack duration (hyperacute attacks with a period from onset of attack to mechanical ventilation less than 3 hours) were significantly associated with near fatality. Also, patients with a shorter attack duration had a more rapid bronchodilator response and the duration of mechanical ventilation was shorter. Sur et al studied the histologic differences in the airways of three patients who died from sudden-onset asthma (type 2) and four patients of the more common slow-onset asthma (type 1) (33). In the sudden-onset fatal asthma group, neutrophils exceeded eosinophils in the airway submucosa. These authors concluded that sudden-onset fatal asthma is immunohistologically distinct from slow-onset fatal asthma.

In summary, it appears that there is a relatively small subset of patients with status asthmaticus who have a predominantly hyperacute, bronchospastic component (34, 35). Whether the fundamental mechanism in this subset is based on bronchospasm, smooth muscle contraction, neural mechanisms, or yet-unknown inflammatory mechanisms remains to be established (36). Certainly, any patient with status asthmaticus should be maximally treated with inhaled β agonists in addition to systemic anti-inflammatory therapy.

## THE β-AGONIST CONTROVERSY

There has been much controversy surrounding the potential role of β-agonist preparations in the increasing asthma mortality (37–39). The hypothesis is that excessive or regular use of β-adrenergic bronchodilators can actually worsen asthma, perhaps contributing to morbidity and mortality. Several studies from New Zealand suggested that the use of inhaled β agonists increases the risk of death in severe asthma (17, 40, 41). More recently, Sears et al conducted a placebo-controlled, crossover study in patients with mild stable asthma to evaluate the effects of regular versus on-demand inhaled fenoterol therapy for 24 weeks (42). In the 57 patients who did better with one of the two regimens, only 30% had better asthma control when receiving regularly administered bronchodilators, whereas 70% had better asthma control when they employed the bronchodilators only as needed. This study has been widely criticized for several reasons (39): (a) patients had mild asthma requiring only 2.9 actuations of the metered dose inhaler (MDI) per day (subjects were excluded if they required more than 8 actuations per day); (b) the β agonist employed was fenoterol, which has significantly greater β-adrenergic stimulating ability and an intrinsically shorter duration of action than the β agonists used in the United States; (c) subjects were not permitted to use any other bronchodilators; and (d) data presented in the study were qualitative, with no indication of the magnitude of the differences or means of assessing possible clinical significance.

In a second well-publicized study, Spitzer et al conducted a matched, case-controlled study using a health insurance database from Saskatchewan, Canada, of a cohort of 12,301 patients for whom asthma medications had been prescribed (43). Data were based on matching 129 case patients who had fatal or nearly fatal asthma with 655 controls. The use of β agonist administered by an MDI was associated with an increased risk of death from asthma, an odds ratio of 5.4 per canister of fenoterol, 2.4 per canister of albuterol, and 1.0 for background risk (i.e., no fenoterol or albuterol). The primary limitation of this study, and indeed case-controlled studies in general, is concern regarding the comparability of the two groups in terms of the severity of the underlying disease. The correlation of severity of illness with both the usage of inhaled β agonist

and increased mortality makes it difficult to judge an independent effect of the inhaled β agonist. All anti-asthma medications were used more by the subjects who died of asthma than by the controls. A subsequent report by the same authors, after adjusting for disease severity between the two groups, maintained that a significant correlation exists between β-agonist use and asthma mortality (44). A recent meta-analysis evaluated the association between β-agonist use and death from asthma from six case-control studies. Statistical integration revealed a significant, although extremely weak, relation between β-agonist use and death from asthma. This relation emerged only when β agonists were administered with a nebulizer, and there was no association between β-agonist use and death when β agonists were administered by MDI (45).

Overall, the exact contribution of β agonists to the recent mortality trend remains unknown. There is sufficient concern regarding fenoterol to avoid its use. (Fenoterol is not available in the United States.) Also, if patients require increasing numbers of puffs of other β-agonist aerosols, this is usually a marker for the need for more effective anti-inflammatory therapy. β-Agonist aerosols remain a critical part of the regimen for acute emergency room management of bronchial asthma. However, for long-term maintenance therapy, whether regular use should be restricted remains unknown. The National Asthma Education Program (NAEP) guidelines recommend as-needed use of inhaled β agonists (4). If a patient exceeds three to four puffs a day of a β agonist, additional therapy should be considered.

## NATURAL HISTORY

The natural history of asthma is complex and not well defined. In general, childhood asthma is frequently self-limited and carries a better prognosis than adult-onset asthma (8). In one large study, one-half of 449 children with onset of asthma before age 13 became symptom free during 20-year follow-up (9, 46). Another one-fourth had only minimal symptoms, which could be prevented by avoiding specific exacerbating factors such as dust or animals. The severity of asthma in childhood correlates with the persistence of asthma into adulthood and the severity of adult asthma in the childhood-onset group (47, 48). It is generally thought that asthma, unlike other chronic obstructive airway disorders, does not inexorably progress from mild to severe disease. However, there are some studies that suggest that asthma alone can cause irreversible air flow obstruction (49–51). Data from Bronnimann and Burroughs suggest that after the second decade, asthmatic subjects show a low rate of remission (52). Adults with a history of childhood asthma have a significant risk of future active asthma. In general, atopy is not useful in predicting remissions or relapses. Despite common belief, allergic rhinitis is not a harbinger of subsequent asthma. Although allergic rhinitis and asthma frequently coexist, if asthma does not occur within 1 year of the onset of allergic rhinitis, then there is only a 5 to 10% risk of asthma developing later (53). About 20% of asthmatics develop disease after age 65 (54).

## PATHOLOGY AND PATHOGENESIS

Early pathologic observations have been made in patients who have succumbed to a severe exacerbation of asthma (55–57), although some information is available from asthmatic patients who died of other causes (58) and patients with symptom-free asthma (59). The pathologic findings in fatal asthma include (a) infiltration with eosinophils, (b) thickening of the basement membrane, (c) hypertrophy of the airway smooth muscle, (d) desquamation of the epithelium, (e) mucosal edema, and (f) mucus plugs containing shed epithelial cells and proteinaceous and cellular components of the inflammatory reaction (55).

More recently, information from experimentally induced asthma as well as studies involving bronchoalveolar lavage (BAL) and endobronchial biopsy of milder, chronic human asthma has contributed to the hypothesis that airway inflammation is a fundamental aspect of asthma (60–62). This concept underlies the growing clinical and investigational interest in the use of various anti-inflammatory agents in the treatment of asthma. The relationship between airway inflammation and bronchial hyperreactivity remains unclear (63, 64).

There are several well-described human models of experimentally induced asthma that form the basis of our current understanding of the pathogenesis of asthma (63, 65). A well-known model involves an allergic asthmatic challenged with an inhaled allergen to which he is sensitive (Fig. 9.1) (66, 67). This challenge results in a biphasic decline in respiratory function, an early asthmatic response (EAR) that occurs within minutes and resolves by 2 hours, and a late asthmatic response (LAR) that usually occurs within 6 to 8 hours and may last for 24 hours or longer (68). The LAR, which appears to occur in 50% of adult asthmatics (69), is associated with increased airway reactivity to nonspecific stimuli (such as methacholine or histamine) and a cellular infiltrate in airway lavage fluid. Pretreatment with β agonists blocks only the EAR, whereas corticosteroids block only the LAR, and cromolyn sodium and nedocromil block both phases. In human

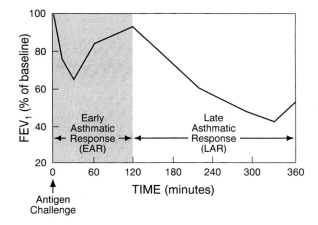

**FIGURE 9.1.** Biphasic decline in lung function, as measured by forced expiratory volume in 1 second ($FEV_1$), in an allergic asthmatic after inhalation of an allergen (see text for details).

studies, exposure to ozone results in LAR and influx of polymorphonuclear neutrophils in BAL (63). In the allergen and western red cedar (plicatic acid) model of asthma there again appears an LAR, but the lavage fluid has an influx of both polymorphonuclear cells and eosinophils. These and other studies suggest that the specificity of the stimulus affects the nature of the inflammatory process after exposure.

These observations in experimentally induced asthma have been extended to chronic stable asthma. Beasley and coworkers studied eight atopic stable asthmatics and four controls (62). Endobronchial biopsies of stable asthmatics showed extensive mucosal inflammation characterized by epithelial sloughing, eosinophil infiltration of the submucosa, and basement membrane thickening. Also, BAL studies in these stable asthmatics showed the presence of a fivefold increase in the shed epithelial cells and mast cells. Martin et al analyzed BAL fluid in a group of asthmatics with nocturnal asthma and compared them to asthmatics without nocturnal asthma. BAL was performed at 4:00 PM and 4:00 AM, which showed a significant increase in neutrophils, eosinophils, and lymphocytes in patients with symptomatic nocturnal asthma at 4:00 AM compared with asthmatics without nocturnal symptoms (70). These studies suggest that airway inflammation plays a significant role in both experimentally induced asthma and stable chronic human asthma. Numerous studies have suggested that the inflammation in asthma differs significantly from the inflammatory response seen in other airway or pulmonary parenchymal diseases by the distinct absence of bronchiolitis, fibrosis, and granulation tissue. The reasons for this remain unclear (38).

Numerous studies have recently advanced the notion that the T lymphocyte plays a pivotal role in the regulation and expression of local eosinophilia and IgE production in both asthma and allergic disease (71–73). Lavage fluid from patients with atopic asthma reveals expression of CD4-positive T helper cells. It appears that T helper cells can be further categorized as $T_{H1}$ or $T_{H2}$ cells based on the profile of cytokines these cells are capable of releasing (74). The $T_{H1}$ cell produces interleukins 2 and 3 (IL-2, IL-3), granulocyte-macrophage colony-stimulating factor (GM-CSF), and interferon gamma (INF-$\gamma$), which leads to delayed hypersensitivity-type inflammatory response. On the other hand, $T_{H2}$ lymphocytes mediate allergic inflammation in atopic asthmatics by a cytokine profile that involves interleukin-4 (which directs B lymphocytes to synthesize IgE), interleukin-5 (which is essential for the maturation of eosinophils), interleukin-3, and GM-CSF. Therefore, preliminary evidence suggests that atopic asthma is regulated by activation of a $T_{H2}$-like T-cell population (75).

The emerging paradigm of the asthma inflammatory cascade involves a complex interaction of resident airway cells, recruited inflammatory cells, a variety of cytokines, and a variety of pro-inflammatory chemical and neurogenic mediators (Fig. 9.2). The critical and rate-limiting steps in this process remain incompletely understood.

## CLINICAL EVALUATION

The history and physical examination are important for several reasons: (*a*) to confirm a diagnosis of bronchial asthma and exclude asthma "mimics" such as upper airway obstruction (UAO), congestive heart failure, etc.; (*b*) to assess the severity of air flow obstruction and the need for hospitalization; (*c*) to identify factors that might place a patient at particular risk for poor outcome, including death; and (*d*) to identify comorbid diseases that may complicate the management of bronchial asthma, such as allergy to avoidable external triggers, sinusitis, or gastroesophageal reflux.

### DIAGNOSIS

In most instances, the diagnosis of asthma is not difficult. The typical patient exhibits dyspnea, and wheezes can be heard throughout the lung fields. It is

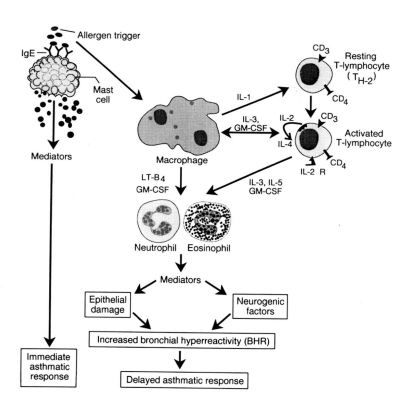

**FIGURE 9.2.** Asthma inflammatory cascade: summary of proposed mechanisms.

essential to specifically inquire about nocturnal symptoms, since this is often missed (76). The clinician needs to remain alert both to possible atypical presentations of asthma and to conditions that may mimic asthma. Some individuals with symptomatic airway hyperresponsiveness exhibit a bothersome nonproductive cough rather than wheezing (77–81). Identification of the "cough variant" asthma syndrome may require the use of a bronchoprovocation test to document the presence of airway hyperreactivity. Such patients often achieve excellent symptomatic relief with the use of inhaled bronchodilator medication (82). However, 29% of Irwin's patients in whom reactive airway disease was diagnosed as a cause of cough, required prednisone to resolve their cough (83). No trials have compared the effectiveness of inhaled $\beta$ agonists with theophylline or inhaled corticosteroids.

The most important asthma mimic is upper-airway obstruction (UAO). Such obstruction can be caused by tumors, laryngeal spasm, aspirated foreign bodies, and tracheal stenosis, to name just a few potential causes. Patients with UAO may present with dyspnea and wheezing (stridor) that might be very difficult to distinguish from asthma on clinical inspection alone (although careful auscultation should reveal that the

wheeze is located over the superior aspect of the thorax or neck). Some patients with chronic UAO have been misdiagnosed and treated for months or even years as "refractory" asthmatics. Failure to diagnose and treat acute life-threatening UAO can have obvious consequences as well. Upper airway obstruction can be detected through analysis of the flow-volume loops (expiratory and inspiratory) and confirmed by bronchoscopy.

The shape of the flow-volume loop may provide insight into the nature and location of airway obstruction. Figure 9.3 depicts several characteristic patterns of the loop that help to localize the site of obstruction and help distinguish asthma from asthma mimics such as UAO. Normally, there is a limitation of air flow at high lung volumes, which produces a sharp peak (peak expiratory flow rate, or PEFR) in the expiratory limb of the flow-volume loop during periods of maximal flow. Both asthma and emphysema are examples of typical obstructive airway disorders characterized by a concavity of the expiratory limb of the flow-volume loop with a fairly well preserved inspiratory limb. With UAO, the shape of the loop is related to the level of the obstruction (above or below the thoracic inlet) and the net effect of pressures acting on the extratho-

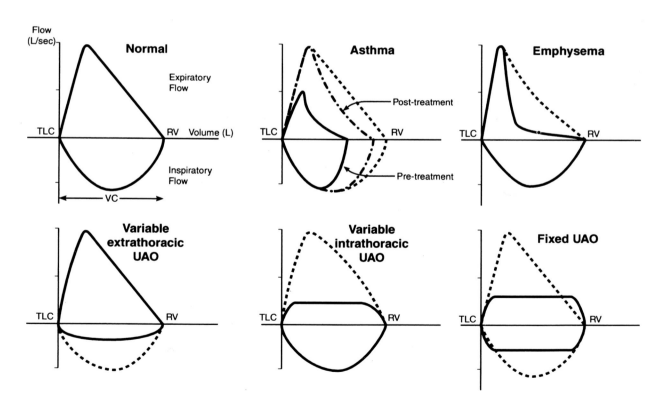

**FIGURE 9.3.** Representative flow-volume loops (see text for details). *TLC*, total lung capacity; *RV*, residual volume; *VC*, vital capacity; *UAO*, upper-airway obstruction.

racic or intrathoracic airway, which include the atmospheric pressure, intraluminal pressure, and intrapleural pressure. The flow-volume loop shows flattening of the inspiratory limb with variable extrathoracic UAO, likely due to a lesion involving the glottic or subglottic area. On the other hand, flattening limited to the expiratory limb of the flow-volume loop occurs with variable intrathoracic UAO, usually on the basis of an obstructing lesion of the mid or distal trachea. "Box-like" flattening of both the inspiratory and expiratory limbs of the flow-volume loop occurs with a fixed UAO due to any etiology.

Over the past decade, several reports have described patients with functional vocal cord disorders that mimic attacks of bronchial asthma ("factitious asthma") (84–87). The typical history involves episodes of wheezing and dyspnea that are refractory to standard therapy for asthma. These individuals may have wheezing that is often loudest over the neck, but the wheezing is often transmitted over both lung fields and may be misdiagnosed as bronchial asthma. During episodes of wheezing, the maximal expiratory and inspiratory flow-volume loop is consistent with variable extrathoracic UAO. The pathophysiology of factitious asthma, as noted by laryngoscopy, appears to be adduction of the true and false vocal cords throughout the respiratory cycle, including the inspiratory phase. During asymptomatic periods, both the flow-volume loop and the laryngoscopic examination are normal. Interestingly, methacholine or histamine provocation testing is usually negative for airway hyperreactivity. Christopher et al described a variety of personality styles and psychiatric diagnoses in these individuals and suggested that factitious asthma is a form of conversion reaction (84). They described a dramatic response to speech therapy and psychotherapy in these patients with factitious vocal cord dysfunction. In general, factitious asthma should be included in the differential diagnosis of difficult-to-control asthma.

## ASSESSING ASTHMA SEVERITY

Assessing the severity of an asthmatic episode is important in determining the therapeutic approach. Although the magnitude of wheezing bears some relationship to the severity of air flow obstruction, use of auscultation alone is unreliable (88). In particular, wheezing may become weak or inaudible as air flow rates become significantly reduced. An early study by McFadden and coworkers evaluated the relationship between clinical and physiologic manifestations of acute bronchial asthma serially during initial therapy in the emergency room (89). Regardless of the initial presentation of the patients, when they became asymptomatic, the overall mechanical function of the lungs was only about 40 to 50% of predicted normal values. When they were without signs of asthma on examination, lung function was only 60 to 70% of predicted values. This study reinforces the need for objective measurement of air flow obstruction during acute asthma.

Patients may have a poor ability to perceive the presence and severity of air flow obstruction until it becomes quite severe (90–93). Some patients have remained asymptomatic even with an $FEV_1$ of 50% of predicted (94). Despite this, patients often have a better appreciation of the severity of air flow limitation than their physician, who is relying on the history and physical examination (95). It is true that physical findings such as pulsus paradoxus (inspiratory decline in systolic blood pressure greater than 12 mm Hg), accessory muscle use including sternocleidomastoid muscle retraction, respiratory rate greater than 30 and heart rate greater than 130 are generally associated with more severe air flow obstruction (96, 97). However, none of these signs alone or in combination are specific or sensitive (98, 99).

The importance of directly and objectively measuring air flow is underscored by the relative insensitivity of either arterial blood gases or subjective assessments for detecting anything less than severe obstruction. The measurements most frequently used for assessing air flow are the forced expiratory volume in 1 second ($FEV_1$) and peak expiratory flow rate (PEFR). Both the $FEV_1$ and PEFR yield comparable results (100–102). Severe air flow obstruction is indicated by a peak flow less than 120 liters/minute or an $FEV_1$ less than 1 liter.

Several attempts have been made to formulate a scoring index for the purpose of grading the severity of acute asthma and predicting the need for hospitalization (Table 9.1) (103–109). Fischl described an index predicting relapse and the need for hospitalization in 205 patients with acute bronchial asthma (109). Of the 205 patients, 120 were successfully treated and discharged from the emergency room, 45 were hospitalized, and 40 were treated and discharged from the emergency room, but had relapses within 10 days. A predictive index based on awarding one point for each of a combination of seven factors on initial presentation, including tachycardia (heart rate above 120/minute), tachypnea (respiratory rate above 30/minute), pulsus paradoxus (18 mm Hg or above) and PEFR (120 liters/minute or less) was developed. Presence of four or more of the seven factors upon presentation to the emergency room (prior to therapy) was 95% accurate in predicting the risk of relapse and 96% accurate in predicting the need for hospitalization. However, two

TABLE 9.1
PROPOSED SPIROMETRIC CRITERIA FOR ADMISSION

| Basis | Indications for Admission | Reference No. |
|---|---|---|
| Initial presentation | • Fischl index 4 | 109 |
| | • Inability to perform spirometry | 104, 105 |
| | • $FEV_1$ <0.61 | 105 |
| Initial flow rate and response to first treatment | • Unresponsive to epinephrine and PEFR <60 liters/min | — |
| | • Unresponsive to bronchodilators and <16% change initial PEFR value | 104, 106 |
| | • <0.15-liter increase in $FEV_1$ after subcutaneous administration of bronchodilator | 105 |
| | • PEFR <100 liters/min initially and <160 liters/min after 0.25 mg terbutaline | 107 |
| | • $FEV_1$ <30% of predicted value; not improving to >40% of predicted value; >4 hours therapy needed | 108 |
| Initial flow rate and response to full treatment | • PEFR <100 liters/min and <300 liters/min after full treatment | 107 |
| | • $FEV_1$ <0.61 and <1.6 liters after full treatment | 105 |
| | • Change in $FEV_1$ <400 ml after bronchodilator administration | 98 |
| Other | • Deterioration of PEFR by 15% after initial good response to bronchodilator therapy | 106 |

Modified from Brenner AS: The acute asthmatic in the emergency department: the decision to admit or discharge. *Am J Emerg Med* 3:74–77, 1985.

subsequent studies failed to support the clinical utility of this method (110, 111). Another early study indicated that the response to initial therapy could be a useful guide (98). Patients whose $FEV_1$ improved by more than 400 ml had an early relapse rate of only 29%, whereas those who failed to demonstrate such an improvement in $FEV_1$ had a 67% relapse rate.

The chest roentgenogram may be helpful to exclude other pathologic conditions (pneumonia, pneumothorax) but does not provide useful information to grade the severity of asthma. In fact, hyperinflation is the most common finding on the chest roentgenogram in patients with acute asthma. Clinical judgment should be used to decide which patients receive a chest roentgenogram (112).

Although life-threatening severe hypoxemia can occur in asthma, it is relatively uncommon and is readily treated with supplemental oxygen. Perhaps of more concern is the evaluation and correct interpretation of the arterial carbon dioxide tension ($Paco_2$) (113–115). Mild and moderate degrees of air flow obstruction in asthma are usually accompanied by a hyperventilation response and a low $Paco_2$. As air flow obstruction becomes more severe, $Paco_2$ rises to about 40 mm Hg. The onset of hypercapnia usually begins when the $FEV_1$ declines below 750 ml or 25% of the predicted value (Fig. 9.4) (113, 116). Thus the finding of a normal $Paco_2$ in a patient with asthma should be viewed with some concern, since mild to moderate degrees of acute air flow obstruction are usually associated with hyperventilation. Any increase in $Paco_2$ above 40 mm Hg

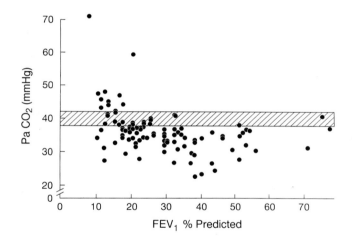

FIGURE 9.4. Correlation of the severity of acute airway obstruction with the arterial carbon dioxide tension in asthma. (From McFadden ER, Lyons HA: Arterial blood gas tension in asthma. Reprinted by permission of the *New England Journal of Medicine,* 278:1027–1032, 1968.)

should be viewed with proportionately increasing alarm, since this heralds severe air flow obstruction and respiratory muscle fatigue. Nowak et al prospectively compared arterial blood gas and pulmonary function measurements in 102 episodes of acute bronchial asthma initially seen in the emergency room (117). The $Pao_2$, $Paco_2$, and pH were unable to distinguish patients requiring admission from those who could be discharged. All patients with $Paco_2$ greater than 42 mm Hg and/or severe hypoxemia ($Pao_2$ less than 60 mm Hg) had a PEFR below 200 liters/minute or an $FEV_1$ below 1.0 liter. In general, in patients with an acute asthma exacerbation, arterial blood gas determination can be limited to patients who have evidence of severe air flow obstruction by a screening air flow measurement.

In the absence of completely reliable objective indicators, clinical judgment is necessary to help decide which patients with acute asthma require hospitalization.

## Comorbid Conditions

### Gastroesophageal Reflux

The relationship between asthma and gastroesophageal reflux (GER) is quite controversial (118, 119). There are several possible associations between asthma and GER: (a) these are two common diseases that coexist independently in some patients; (b) GER either exacerbates or is causally related to the pathogenesis of asthma; or (c) bronchial asthma and/or anti-asthma medications exacerbate or induce gastroesophageal disease (120, 121). It is likely that all three of these possibilities occur in subsets of patients with bronchial asthma. Some degree of reflux appears to be normal or "physiologic," especially for several hours in the postprandial period. The probable mechanisms for GER-induced asthma are (a) acid stimulation of sensory nerve fibers in the lower esophagus, with reflex vagal bronchoconstriction (122), and (b) microaspiration of acid into the trachea (123).

Published literature provides conflicting data as to the role of subclinical or unsuspected GER as a trigger for asthmatic symptoms. Gastroesophageal reflux should be considered in patients with refractory asthma. Patients who have a history of excessive belching, burping, heartburn, and perhaps nocturnal exacerbations should be further assessed or empirically treated for GER. If the history is characteristic of GER, it is reasonable to prescribe empiric medical management for reflux esophagitis by a variety of conservative measures, including administration of $H_2$ blockers (119). If a patient has persistent symptoms of GER and/or refractory asthma despite aggressive medical therapy, then a variety of diagnostic studies are available to evaluate GER. These include upper GI radiography, intraesophageal pH monitoring for 24 hours, esophageal motility studies (manometry), and upper endoscopy with esophageal biopsy (119, 124). These studies may objectively assess the presence of reflux and perhaps identify a correlation with the patient's respiratory symptoms. They may also help to assess the presence of a hiatal hernia or other anatomic abnormalities that may be contributing to aspiration. For the occasional patient who has persistent gastroesophageal symptoms and difficult-to-control asthma, despite a very aggressive medical regimen as described above, a variety of anti-reflux surgical procedures remain an option (125, 126).

### Drug-induced Asthma

A variety of over-the-counter and prescription medications may contribute to acute bronchospasm. The respiratory symptoms may either be an isolated response or be part of a generalized systemic anaphylaxis. The overall magnitude of drug-induced bronchospasm in the United States remains unknown (127). Nonsteroidal anti-inflammatory drugs (NSAIDs) are by far the most common cause of drug-induced asthma. Other agents that have received a lot of attention in the literature include sulfites, $\beta$-adrenergic blocking agents, angiotensin converting enzyme (ACE) inhibitors, tartrazine, and a variety of miscellaneous agents (127–129). The vast majority of cases of drug-induced asthma are the result of an idiopathic pharmacologic reaction to the compound (130). However, other mechanisms include (a) immunologic IgE-requiring mechanism, (b) direct non-IgE related release of mast cell mediators, and (c) induction of an irritative effect by a variety of cellular mechanisms. Drug-induced asthma should be suspected in all patients with difficult-to-control or steroid-dependent asthma. Careful history of all prescribed and over-the-counter medications should be obtained for all patients with asthma.

### Allergic Bronchopulmonary Aspergillosis

The clinical course of an occasional patient with bronchial asthma may be complicated by pulmonary parenchymal infiltrates on the chest radiograph. The differential diagnosis for an infiltrate is extensive. However, specific entities to consider in an asthmatic include (a) typical and atypical infections, (b) allergic bronchopulmonary aspergillosis (ABPA), (c) chronic eosinophilic pneumonia and other pulmonary infiltrate and eosinophilia (PIE) syndromes, and (d) allergic granulomatosis with angiitis (Churg-Strauss disease). Discussion here will be limited only to ABPA.

Allergic bronchopulmonary aspergillosis (ABPA) can be regarded as a complicated or special form of asthma in which immunologic reactions to *Aspergillus* species, usually *Aspergillus fumigatus*, play an important pathogenic role. Clinical syndromes analogous to ABPA have also been described in which noninvasive fungi other than *Aspergillus* appear to be the culprit. These related syndromes have been grouped under the term allergic bronchopulmonary fungoses (ABPF) (131).

*Historical Aspects and Epidemiology*

ABPA was first described in England in 1952 (132). In the United States, the first reported case did not appear until 1968 (133), and for several years ABPA was considered an extremely rare disease in this country. However, the relative paucity of reported cases may in part reflect underdiagnosis of this entity. In 1983, a survey of seven institutions in the United States with a known interest in ABPA identified a total of 352 patients with ABPA diagnosed since the late 1960s (134). The exact prevalence of the disease remains unknown. The vast majority of the reported cases in this country cluster in Illinois, Wisconsin, Minnesota, California, and Michigan (134). This geographic distribution likely reflects the diagnostic interest and knowledge of regional physicians, but a true difference in geographic incidence cannot be excluded as a possible explanation.

*Diagnoses and Clinical Features*

ABPA is an episodic and recurrent disorder with wheezing as an almost universal symptom (135). Mild or early cases resemble simple asthma and may resolve without therapy. More severe or chronic cases exhibit features of bronchiectasis with cough productive of purulent-appearing sputum that sometimes contains brownish sputum "plugs." A characteristic of advanced ABPA is proximal bronchiectasis with normal tapering of distal bronchi (131).

The classic patient with ABPA has asthma, recurrent or fixed pulmonary infiltrates on the chest roentgenogram, proximal bronchiectasis, dual (immediate and late) skin test response to *A. fumigatus,* elevated total serum IgE level (above 1000 ng/ml), peripheral blood eosinophilia (above 1000/mm$^3$), and serum precipitins (specific IgG) to *A. fumigatus* (131, 136). *Aspergillus* species can frequently be identified or cultured from respiratory secretions.

Although recognition of the classic patient with ABPA should not be difficult, it is noteworthy that none of the individual diagnostic features listed in the preceding paragraph are completely specific or sensitive for the diagnosis of ABPA. Therefore, in patients who do not exhibit the full constellation of findings, differentiation of ABPA from other diseases may be difficult. In particular, it may be difficult to distinguish uncomplicated or typical asthma from ABPA. Many patients with asthma have an elevated serum IgE, peripheral eosinophilia, precipitins to *A. fumigatus* (about 10% of asthma patients), or positive skin test reactivity. Furthermore, patients with asthma may at times exhibit an abnormal chest roentgenogram (atelectasis, pneumonia, etc.).

Patterson and colleagues have suggested that an index of elevated IgE and IgG serum antibodies *specific* against *A. fumigatus* is of value in separating ABPA patients from asthma patients who have cutaneous reactivity to *Aspergillus* species (137, 138). Using this method, it was revealed that about 6% of asthma patients with cutaneous reactivity to *Aspergillus* species fulfill criteria for ABPA (139). However, the quantitative assay for specific serum IgE or IgG is not widely available. Furthermore, it remains unclear whether ABPA needs to be rigorously excluded in all patients with chronic asthma, since the treatment for both is likely to include corticosteroids.

In patients with features suggestive of ABPA (asthma, lung infiltrates, elevated serum IgE, peripheral eosinophilia) but lacking evidence of specific immune sensitivity to *Aspergillus* species (absent precipitating antibodies, negative skin tests), the possibility of disease due to a different fungus should be considered. Such allergic bronchopulmonary fungoses (APBF) have been described (syndromes of candidiasis, curvulariosis, dreschleriosis, etc.) (131). In such cases, a diagnostic-therapeutic trial of prednisone may be warranted. If sera are obtained and stored before the initiation of therapy, subsequent assays (search for serum precipitins to specific fungal antigens) may provide insight to the specific cause (131).

It has been proposed that ABPA be described according to a five-stage classification system: acute (stage I), remission (stage II), exacerbation (stage III), corticosteroid-dependent asthma (stage IV), and fibrotic end-stage (stage V) (140). Such a system may provide guidance in both the recognition and management of ABPA, although the natural history of ABPA still remains rather poorly defined and is probably quite variable.

*Treatment*

Prednisone is the drug of choice for treatment of ABPA. Patients who receive other therapy for asthma (cromolyn, inhaled bronchodilators, inhaled corticosteroids) without systemic corticosteroids appear to have an increased number of exacerbations and a greater likelihood of a progressive deterioration of lung function (131, 141). When exacerbations of ABPA are treated with prednisone, it seems that most patients will maintain stable long-term lung function (131, 142–145).

The suggested dosage of prednisone for stages I and III is 0.5 mg/kg daily for 2 weeks (or longer if lung infiltrates are slow to improve), followed by conversion to alternate-day therapy for another 3 months (131). Such therapy usually clears the patient's symptoms and chest roentgenogram. The total serum IgE is usually significantly reduced as well, but may not return to the normal level.

If clinical symptoms recur after cessation of prednisone therapy, resumption of therapy is indicated. However, monitoring of clinical status alone is insufficient, since asymptomatic pulmonary infiltrates can occur, presumably with the potential for progressive asymptomatic lung damage. The need for frequent chest roentgenograms, however, is obviated by the recognition that serum IgE levels are helpful in detecting asymptomatic relapses of ABPA (145).

During the first year off therapy, serum IgE measurements should be obtained frequently (perhaps every 4 to 6 weeks) to determine the patient's baseline value and to detect subsequent relapse. Once a patient's baseline is determined, a subsequent 100% rise in total IgE suggests a relapse. In many cases, the chest roentgenogram will indicate a new infiltrate. According to current concepts, even asymptomatic relapses of ABPA should be treated with a reinstitution of prednisone therapy.

## MANAGEMENT

The National Asthma Education Program (NAEP) expert panel report provides an excellent algorithmic framework for the management of bronchial asthma (4). The general goals of asthma therapy include the following: (a) maintain normal activity levels, including exercise; (b) maintain a nearly "normal" pulmonary function test; (c) prevent chronic and troublesome symptoms and recurrent exacerbations of asthma; and (d) avoid adverse effects from asthma medications. Overall, asthma therapy has four key components according to the expert panel report: (a) patient education; (b) lung function measurement, both initially and during periodic evaluation, including home PEFR monitoring; (c) environmental control with avoidance of asthma triggers; and (d) pharmacologic therapy.

### PATIENT EDUCATION

Asthma self-management education has received increasing attention in the literature recently (146, 147). A number of recent studies have highlighted the beneficial effects as well as the limitations of adult asthma education in clinical practice. At Bellevue Hospital, a randomized crossover trial was conducted to evaluate an outpatient educational program involving 104 adult asthmatics previously requiring multiple hospitalizations for asthma attacks (148). The program involved a combination of widely accepted modalities, including vigorous education about self-management skills, a written crisis plan, easy access to a nurse practitioner,

home PEFR monitoring, and proper MDI technique. The program enrollment resulted in a threefold reduction in readmission rate and a twofold reduction in hospital day use rate. Notably, this study excluded patients with psychiatric disease, who have increased risk of asthma morbidity and mortality (149). Wilson et al conducted a randomized controlled trial with 1-year follow-up in a group of 323 adults with moderate to severe bronchial asthma (requiring three or more physician visits for asthma during a screening year) at a Kaiser Health Plan center (150). Patients were assigned to one of four treatment groups (small-group education, individual education, information workbook control group, or usual control group with no supplemental education). Small-group and individual asthma education programs improved patient understanding, control of asthma symptoms, and MDI technique. The small group was somewhat more effective. Additional controlled studies involving formal asthma education programs have documented their effectiveness in reducing the use of health services (151, 152). Other studies have documented the cost effectiveness of an adult asthma education program (153). However, attendance rates for formal asthma education programs have ranged from 31 to 66% (154, 155). Yoon and colleagues reported that attenders at an asthma education program were more likely to be women, nonsmokers, and patients from a higher socioeconomic status (156).

A recent study of patients with chronic asthma in a general practice setting found that only one in three patients used at least half of the prescribed amount of medication daily (157). Similarly, a number of studies have documented improper MDI technique in the majority of patients (158–160). Several studies have shown that only 40% of physicians correctly performed four or more of the seven steps in the recommended MDI inhalation maneuver (161–163). A provocative study of patients participating in the lung health study described a phenomenon of inhaler "dumping" in patients with chronic obstructive lung disease whose inhaler usage was monitored by self-reporting, canister weighing, and use of electronic recording devices (164). The investigators found that by self-report, 87% of patients stated compliance with prescribed inhaler use (at least twice a day), and 85% compliance was observed if canister weights were used as a measure of compliance. However, only 52% compliance was observed when the measure of compliance was the electronic monitoring device. Nearly 18% of patients who are uninformed about the function of the electronic recording device were found to have dumped their inhaler over a 3-hour time period just prior to appointments.

Aerosol delivery of the $\beta$ agonists can be achieved

through the use of a hand-held MDI in most patients. Proper instruction in the MDI technique is important to ensure effective use (158). It has been shown that increased deposition in the lung occurs when the actuator is held 2 to 4 centimeters from an open mouth position (165). Likewise, beginning inhalation at the end of normal expiration or at functional residual capacity (FRC) is likely to optimize distribution of the inhaled aerosol (165). Optimal use of an MDI delivers only about 10% of the medication dose to the lung, whereas as much as 85% is deposited in the oropharynx (3). The use of a volume reservoir or spacer device is advantageous, especially in patients who are unable to learn or perform the unassisted MDI technique (3, 166). Use of the volume reservoir may improve lung deposition to 15% of the dose and reduce oropharyngeal deposition to 5% (thereby potentially decreasing side effects as well). Powered nebulizers have traditionally been used in patients with significant bronchospasm and in most hospital inpatients. However, recent studies suggest that properly supervised MDI aerosol delivery is as efficacious as powered nebulizer delivery, even in patients with acute or severe air flow obstruction (167–169). Data from non-ICU hospitalized patients suggests that use of MDIs rather than nebulizers results in substantial savings in direct costs (i.e., therapist's time) (170).

## ALLERGEN AVOIDANCE: ENVIRONMENTAL CONTROL MEASURES

A variety of population and clinical studies have strongly suggested that exposure to aeroallergens, in a susceptible host, is associated with allergic sensitization in a subset of patients with both acute and chronic asthma (171–173). It is generally accepted that environmental control measures to reduce exposure to allergens should be considered in most asthmatics and immunotherapy should be reserved for selected patients only (174, 175). Broadly speaking, aeroallergens can be divided into outdoor allergens (pollen and molds) and indoor allergens (house dust mites, animal allergens, cockroach allergen, and indoor molds). Exposure to outdoor allergens is best reduced during the peak pollen season by remaining indoors, in an air-conditioned environment with the windows closed, as much as possible.

Much attention in the literature has recently focused on the composition of house dust and indoor allergens (176). It appears that house dust itself is not an allergen, but there are allergic components within house dust. Fecal pellets from two house dust mites, *Dermatophagoides farinae* and *Dermatophagoides pteronyssinus*, contain several well-characterized allergens (Der f I, Der f II, Der p I, and Der p II) (177). Similarly, allergens from cat dander (Fel d I) and cockroaches (Bla g I, Bla g II) have been well described. Data suggest that certain environmental conditions such as high temperature, high humidity, and perhaps closed urban surroundings can increase allergen burden from these sources. A variety of studies have quantitatively measured these allergens and have recommended "safe" levels (178). Specific recommendations have been published to help reduce indoor allergen burden (178). Overall, it seems clear that indoor allergens contribute to some morbidity related to asthma and that strategies to minimize allergen exposure are warranted in most patients with asthma.

### PHARMACOTHERAPY

Figure 9.5 depicts the overview of therapy as outlined in the 1991 National Asthma Education Program (NAEP) expert panel report (4). The pharmacotherapy for asthma can be classified as symptomatic therapy with bronchodilators ($\beta$ agonists, theophylline) or "disease-modifying" therapy with anti-inflammatory agents (corticosteroids, cromolyn, nedocromil). Medications commonly used in the treatment of asthma, along with possible routes and schedules of administration, are listed in Table 9.2. The NAEP guidelines target therapy based on the severity of asthma (Table 9.3). The NAEP defines mild asthma as intermittent and brief (less than 1 hour) wheezing, cough, dyspnea up to two times weekly, absence of symptoms between exacerbations, and nocturnal symptoms fewer than two times a month. Also, the $FEV_1$ or PEFR are greater than 80% of the patient's personal best PEFR. For mild asthma as defined in this fashion, the guidelines recommend as-needed use of one to two puffs of a $\beta_2$ agonist and/or cromolyn for exposure to various triggers. Moderate asthma is defined as symptoms occurring more than one to two times weekly, exacerbations that affect sleep and activity level, the need for occasional emergency care, and $FEV_1$ or PEFR 60 to 80% of baseline with a 20 to 30% variability when symptomatic. For moderate asthma, the guidelines recommend the addition of inhaled corticosteroids or cromolyn to the as-needed inhaled $\beta_2$ agonist. Alternatively, sustained-release theophylline may be added, especially for nocturnal symptoms. The NAEP defines severe asthma as continuous symptoms with activity limitation, frequent exacerbations, frequent nocturnal symptoms, and occasional hospitalization and emergency treatment. The $FEV_1$ or PEFR are less than 80% of the patient's personal best PEFR. According to the NAEP, severe asthma should be treated with a burst of oral corticosteroids at 40 mg a day for 1 week and then tapered for 1 week, in addition to the inhaled corticosteroids and as-needed inhaled $\beta_2$ agonists.

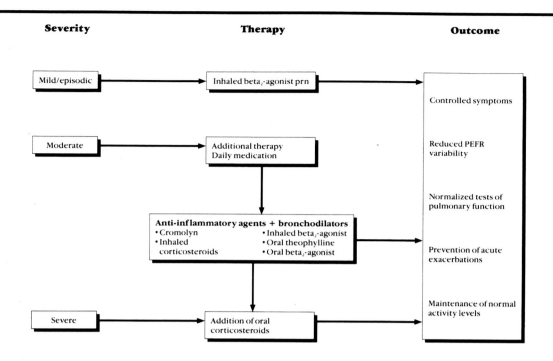

**FIGURE 9.5.** Management of asthma: overview of therapy. (Reproduced from *National Asthma Education Program: Expert Panel Report. Guidelines to the Diagnosis and Management of Asthma.* Bethesda, MD, National Institutes of Health, 1991, p 73.)

### Bronchodilators: $\beta$-Adrenergic Agents

The $\beta$-adrenergic agonist drugs have structural similarities by virtue of a common catechol nucleus. The catecholamines (isoproterenol or isoetharine) are rapid acting, potent, and relatively nonselective $\beta_1$ agonists (179). Resorcinols (metaproterenol, terbutaline, and fenoterol) and saligenins (albuterol and salmeterol) represent a modification of the central catechol nucleus, with resultant longer duration of action and greater $\beta_2$ airway selectivity. Stimulation of the $\beta$ receptors activates adenyl cyclase, causing formation of intracellular cyclic AMP. This in turn provides energy for compartmental shifts in calcium, which results in bronchial smooth muscle relaxation. The major therapeutic actions of $\beta$ stimulation in the treatment of asthma include bronchodilation, facilitation of mucociliary clearance, and inhibition of acute mediator release from mast cells. $\beta$ Agonists do not have an effect on cellular inflammation or the late asthmatic response.

In 1967, Lands and coworkers found that $\beta$ receptors could be subclassified into $\beta_1$ and $\beta_2$ receptors (180). $\beta_2$ Receptors mediate bronchodilation, whereas $\beta_1$ receptors increase heart rate and contractility. In the treatment of air flow obstruction, it is generally advantageous to use agents with a relatively selective $\beta_2$ effect such as metaproterenol, albuterol, terbutaline, and fenoterol to minimize side effects. Nevertheless, undesirable side effects occur even with selective agents, particularly when delivered orally. In particular, muscle tremor may occur due to stimulation of $\beta_1$ receptors in skeletal muscle. Vasodilation of peripheral vessels, another action of $\beta_2$ stimulation, may cause reflex tachycardia and palpitations. At higher doses, the selective agents may also directly stimulate myocardial $\beta_1$ receptors.

Salmeterol xinafoate is a long-acting $\beta_2$ agonist approved for use for asthma in MDIs in the United States in 1994. This agent has a long lipophilic side chain, which confers a long duration of action (8 to 17 hours). In vitro studies suggest that salmeterol is more potent than albuterol and has a slower onset. Short-term clinical trials have shown salmeterol to be better than albuterol with regular doses as well as on-demand, with a similar incidence of adverse reactions. In view of the "$\beta$-agonist controversy" as discussed earlier, the precise role of salmeterol remains unclear. Salmeterol is contraindicated in acute asthma episodes due to its

**TABLE 9.2**

**PHARMACOLOGIC AGENTS FOR THE TREATMENT OF ASTHMA**

| Class | Generic Name | Brand Name (Manufacturer) | Delivery Route/Device | Suggested Dosage (Adults) | Cost[a] | Comments |
|---|---|---|---|---|---|---|
| $\beta$-Adrenergic agents | Albuterol sulfate | Proventil (Schering) | MDI (90 $\mu$g/puff) | Acute: 2–4 puffs q 4–6 hr; max: 16–20 puffs/day Prophylaxis: 2 puffs 15 min before exercise | $18.76/17-g MDI (200 puffs) | Inhaled agents have fewer systemic side effects; $\beta_2$-selective agents are albuterol, bitolterol, metaproterenol, pirbuterol, salmeterol, terbutaline |
| | | | Solution for nebulizer (0.083%, 0.5%) | 2.5–10 mg q 6–8 hr (0.083%) (3 ml) or (0.5%) (0.5 ml) | $35.39/3 ml × 25 (0.83%) $15.52/20 ml (0.5%) | |
| | | | Tablets (2, 4 mg) | 2–4 mg q 6–8 hr; max: 32 mg/day | 2 mg: $34.61/100 4 mg: $51.61/100 | |
| | | | Repetabs (sustained release tablets), 4 mg | 4 mg q 12 hr | $57.98/100 tabs | |
| | | Ventolin (Glaxo) | MDI (90 $\mu$g/puff) | Max: 16–30 puffs/day | $18.76/17-g MDI (200 puffs) | |
| | | | Rotohaler (200 $\mu$g/Rotacap) | 200–400 $\mu$g q 6–8 hr; max dose = 2.4 mg/day | $17.92/Rotohaler & 24 Rotacaps | |
| | | | Solution for nebulizer (0.083%, 0.5%) | 2.5–10 mg q 6–8 hr | $32.40/3 ml × 25 (0.083%) $15.53/20 ml (0.5%) | |
| | | Volmax (Muro) | Sustained-release tablets (4, 8 mg) | 4–8 mg q 12 hr | 4 mg: $33.82/60 tabs | |
| | | Airet (Adams Labs) | Solution (0.083%) | 2.5–10 mg q 6–8 hr | $32.40/3 ml × 25 | |
| | | Albuterol (various generic) | Solution (0.083%, 0.5%) | 2.5–10 mg q 6–8 hr | $8.75–$14.50/20 ml (0.5 ml) | |
| | Metaproterenol sulfate | Alupent (Boehringer) | MDI (650 $\mu$g/puff) | 2–3 puffs q 3–4 hr; max = 12 puffs/day | $18.46/14-g MDI (200 puffs) | |
| | | | Solution (0.4%, 0.6%) | 0.3 ml in 2.5 ml NS q 4–6 hr | $37.43/2.5 ml × 25 | |
| | | | Tablets (10, 20 mg) | 10 mg q 6–8 hr, up to 20 mg | 10 mg: $32.14/100 20 mg: $45.60/100 | |
| | | Metaprel (Sandoz) | MDI (650 $\mu$g/puff) | 2–3 puffs q 3–4 hr; max = 12 puffs/day | $10.20/14-g MDI (200 puffs) | |
| | | | Solution (5%) | 0.3 ml in 2.5 ml NS q 4–6 hr | $7.02/10 ml | |
| | | | Tablets (10, 20 mg) | 10 mg q 6–8 hr, up to 20 mg | 10 mg: $11.46/100 20 mg: $15.30/100 | |
| | Terbutaline sulfate | Brethaire (Geigy) | MDI (200 $\mu$g/puff) | 1–2 puffs q 4–6 hr | $16.75/7.5-ml MDI (300 puffs) | |
| | | | Solution for SC injection or nebulizer (1 mg/ml) | 0.25 mg SC q 15–30 min; max = 0.50 mg/4 hr, 0.75–2.5 mg nebulized with NS | 1-ml ampule (1 ml/ampule): $16.36/10 ml | |
| | | | Tablets (2.5, 5 mg) | 2.5–5 mg tid; max = 15 mg/24 hr | 25 mg: $22.35/100 50 mg: $32.19/100 | |
| | | Bricanyl (Marion Merrell Dow) | MDI (200 $\mu$g/puff) | 1–2 puffs q 4–6 hr | N/A | |
| | | | Tablets (2.5, 5 mg) | 2.4–5 mg tid; max = 15 mg/24 hr | 2.5 mg: $26.58/100 5 mg: $38.10/100 | |
| | Isoetharine HCl | Bronkometer (Sanofi Winthrop) | MDI (340 $\mu$g/puff) | 1–2 puffs q 4 hr | $23.50/15-ml MDI | |
| | | Many | Solutions for inhalation | 0.25–1 ml nebulized with NS | $20.50/15 ml to $26.91/10 ml | |

TABLE **9.2**—*Continued*

| Class | Generic Name | Brand Name (Manufacturer) | Delivery Route/Device | Suggested Dosage (Adults) | Cost[a] | Comments |
|---|---|---|---|---|---|---|
| β-Adrenergic agents (cont'd) | Epinephrine | Medihaler-Epi (3M Pharm) | MDI (300 μg/puff) | 2 puffs qid | $19.50/15-ml MDI | |
| | | Many | Solutions for inhalation (15 ml) | nebulized q 2–3 hr | $91.54/12 | |
| | | Adrenalin chloride (Parke-Davis) | SC injection 1:1000 (1 mg/ml) | 0.2–0.5 mg SC (0.2–0.5 ml SC) q 20 min | $12.07/7 ml | |
| | Isoproternol HCl | Medihaler-ISO (3M Pharm) | MDI (800 μg/puff) | 1–2 puff qid | $21.42/15-ml MDI | |
| | | Isuprel Mistometer (Sanofi Winthrop) | MDI (131 μg/puff) | 1–2 puffs qid | $22.74/16.8-g MDI | |
| | | | Solution (0.5%, 1%, 5%) | 0.5 ml in 2.5 ml NS q 3–4 hr | $111.00/0.5 ml × 100 vials | |
| | | | Tablets (glossets 10, 15 mg) | 10–2 mg q 4 hr | $27.64/50 tablets | |
| | Pirbuterol acetate | Maxair (3M Pharm) | MDI (200 μg/puff) | 1–2 puffs q 4–6 hr; max = 12 puffs/day | $19.56/25.6-g MDI (300 puffs) | |
| | | | AutoHaler | 2 puffs q 6 hr | $26.70/14-g MDI (400 puffs) | |
| | Bitolterol mesylate | Tornalate (Sanofi Winthrop) | MDI (370 μg/puff) | 2 puffs q 6 hr | $26.70/14-g MDI (400 puffs) | |
| | Salmeterol | Serevent (Glaxo) | MDI (50 μg/puff) | 2 puffs q 12 hr | N/A | |
| | Procaterol (investigational) | Pro-Air (Parke-Davis) | MDI (10 μg/puff) | 2 puffs q 8 hr | N/A | |
| Inhaled corticosteroids | Beclomethasone dipropionate | Beclovent (Allen & Hanburys) | MDI (42 μg/puff) | 2 puffs tid-qid; max = 20 puffs/day | $23.41/17-g MDI (200 puffs) | Need more than 400 μg/day to maintain off oral steroids, no adrenal suppression if <800–1200 μg/day |
| | | Vanceril (Schering) | MDI (42 μg/puff) | 2 puffs tid-qid; max = 20 puffs/day | $26.51/16.8-g MDI (200 puffs) | |
| | Flunisolide | Aerobid (Forest) | MDI (250 μg/puff) | 2 puffs bid; max = 8 puffs/day | $34.95/20-g MDI (100 puffs) | |
| | Triamcinolone acetonide | Azmacort (Rhone-Poulenc Rorer) | MDI (100 μg/puff) | 2–4 puffs qid; max = 16 puffs/day | $34.95/20-g MDI (240 puffs) | |
| | Budesonide (investigational) | Pulmicort (Astra) | MDI (50, 200 μg/puff) | 400–1600 μg in divided doses bid-qid | N/A | |
| | Fluticasone dipropionate (investigational) | Flovent (Glaxo) | Diskhaler powder inhaler (50, 100, 250 μg/puff) | 100–800 μg/day | N/A | |
| Systemic corticosteroids | Prednisone | Many | Tablets (1, 5, 10, 20, 50 mg) | 10–50 mg/day | 1 mg: $3.20/100<br>5 mg: $4.15/1000<br>10 mg: $5.99/100<br>20 mg: $11.60/100<br>50 mg: $25.49/100 | Long-term systemic side effects; cataracts, osteopenia, cushingoid features, immune suppression, hypertension |
| | Methylprednisolone sodium succinate | Medrol (Upjohn) | Tablets (2, 4, 8, 16, 24, 32 mg) | 4–48 mg/day | 2 mg: $28.98/100<br>4 mg: $54.70/100<br>8 mg: $19.19/25<br>16 mg: $59.33/50<br>24 mg: $34.98/25<br>32 mg: $42.58/25 | |

**TABLE 9.2—Continued**

| Class | Generic Name | Brand Name (Manufacturer) | Delivery Route/Device | Suggested Dosage (Adults) | Cost[a] | Comments |
|---|---|---|---|---|---|---|
| Systemic corticosteroids (cont'd) | Methylprednisolone sodium succinate (cont'd) | Solu-Medrol (Upjohn) | IV (40, 125, 500, 1000 mg) | 1–2 mg/kg q 4–6 hr | $2.00/40-mg act-o-vial $5.31/125-mg act-o-vial $17.88/500-mg acto-o-vial $32.19/1000-mg act-o-vial | |
| | Hydrocortisone sodium succinate | Solu-Cortef (Upjohn) | IV (100, 250, 500, 1000 mg) | 4 mg/kg q 4–6 hr | $3.34/100-mg act-o-vial $7.56/250-mg act-o-vial $14.71/500 mg act-o-vial $29.29/1000-mg act-o-vial | |
| Cromoglycates | Cromolyn sodium | Intal (Fisons) | Spinhaler (20-mg capsules) | 20 mg qid | $35.44/60 capsules | Contraindicated in acute asthma |
| | | | MDI (800 $\mu$g/puff) | 2 puffs qid | $35.03/8.1-g MDI (112 puffs) | |
| | | | Solution (20 mg/2-ml ampule) | 1 ampule qid | $141.05/2 ml × 100 ampules | |
| | Nedocromil sodium | Tilade (Fisons) | MDI (1.75 mg/puff) | 2 puffs bid-tid-qid | $21.85/16-g MDI (112 puffs) | |
| Methylxanthines | Aminophylline | Various | IV | **Load:** If not on theophylline at home, 5–6 mg/kg over 20 min; if on theophylline, level pending, 3 mg/kg over 20 min; a bolus of 0.5 mg/kg will increase level by 2 in the average adult. **Maintenance:** 0.5–0.9 mg/kg/hr 200–400 mg bid-qid | $16.25/25 20-ml vials | Decreased clearance with cirrhosis, CHF, erythromycin, cimetidine, troleandomycin. Increased clearance with smoking, young age, and phenobarbital. Need to follow serum levels |
| | Theophylline | Anhydrous, immediate release (Slo-Phyllin, Theolair, Quibron, Elixophyllin, etc.) | PO | | $22.62/100 | Normal dose range for an average adult is 300 to 1200 mg/day; immediate release preparations: dose should be given every 6 to 8 hr; sustained-release preparations: dose may be given every 12 to 24 hr; this dose range is an approximate starting point; however, whenever possible, serum levels should be monitored, i.e., 8 hr after a dose, after 5 to 6 consecutive doses |
| Anticholinergics | Atropine sulfate | Many | Solution 0.2% (1 mg/0.5 ml) 0.5% (2.5 mg/0.5 ml) | 0.025 mg/kg diluted with 3–5 ml NS q 6–8 hr (1–2.5 mg) | N/A | Minimal side effects with ipratropium |
| | Ipratropium bromide | Atrovent (Boehringer) | MDI (18 $\mu$g/puff) | 2–4 puffs qid; max = 12 puffs/day | $26.14/14-g MDI (200 puffs) | |
| | | | Solution 0.02% (500-$\mu$g unit dose vial) | 500 $\mu$g tid-qid | | |

[a] Prices are average wholesale price (AWP) estimates for 1993, largely obtained from *1993 Red Book* (Montvale, NJ, Medical Economics Co.). The AWP represents what a retail pharmacist or a dispensing physician might pay for a drug, without discounts. The prices approximate what a consumer might pay, especially in regard to the spread between the high and low prices.

**Table 9.3**
**Grading Clinical Severity of Asthma by National Asthma Education Program (NAEP) Guidelines**

Mild
- Intermittent, brief (<1 hr) symptoms up to two times per week
- Infrequent nocturnal symptoms (<2 times per month)
- Asymptomatic between exacerbations
- Forced expiratory volume ($FEV_1$) or peak expiratory flow rate (PEFR) >80% baseline

Moderate
- Symptoms >1–2 times per week
- Exacerbations may last days, affect sleep, activity
- Need for occasional emergency room care
- $FEV_1$ or PEFR 60–80% baseline

Severe
- Continuous symptoms
- Frequent exacerbations, nocturnal symptoms
- Limited activity level
- Need for occasional hospitalization
- $FEV_1$ or PEFR <60% baseline

slow onset of action. Salmeterol may represent an alternative to theophylline for nocturnal asthma.

For several reasons, the use of oral $\beta$-adrenergic agonists is gradually falling into disfavor (3). Oral delivery of these agents is significantly confounded by patient-to-patient variability in bowel absorption and first-pass hepatic metabolism (3). Aerosol delivery provides a more rapid onset of action, a comparable sustained response, and a significantly decreased incidence of side effects (3, 181). Aerosols have traditionally been administered through MDIs or dry powder inhalers (DPIs) for ambulatory care, while small-volume wet nebulizers have been used in emergency departments, on hospital wards and intensive care units, and in young children (182). Despite the fact that a large number of studies have found comparable bronchodilation for $\beta$ agonists administered by MDI or wet nebulization in patients with acute asthma, (167–169), the National Asthma Education Expert Panel recommends delivery of aerosolized bronchodilators by wet nebulization for management of acute asthma in the emergency room (4). Nebulizer therapy continues to be widely prescribed for a number of reasons: (a) it is widely believed that acutely tachypneic patients are unable to use MDIs optimally, even with a spacer device; (b) patients are usually on MDI therapy at home, and an acute episode requiring emergency care typically represents a failure of home therapy, therefore patients expect alternative therapy; and (c) there is a widespread belief that nebulizer therapy is more effective than MDI usage in treating acute exacerbations of airway obstruction (183).

The environmental impact of chlorofluorocarbons (CFCs) used in pressurized metered dose inhalers has received much recent attention (184–188). Most currently used MDIs contain a blend of CFC propellants including CFC-12 (primary propellant), CFC-11 (primary solvent), and CFC-114 (moderates pressure and density). The CFCs (or Freons) used in MDIs represent 0.5% of the annual worldwide production of these compounds. CFCs are ideal propellants because of their stability and clinical safety.

A number of international conferences have been held that have resulted in an agreement to ban the use of CFCs after 1995, including medical use (187). A number of pharmaceutical companies have responded to this challenge by developing new inhalers that do not use CFCs. One strategy is to utilize a non-CFC propellant such as hydrofluorocarbon-134a. A second strategy is to use breath-actuated dry powder inhalers (DPIs). Examples of DPIs currently available (or under development) are the Spinhaler (Fisons), Rotahaler (Allen and Hanbury), Diskhaler (Allen and Hanbury), Turbuhaler (Astra), and multidisk powder inhaler (Glaxo). In addition to being environmentally safe, the breath-actuated powder devices do not require the exact patient coordination and synchronization typically necessary for MDI use (189, 190). Also, the powder preparations can be inhaled without the need for a spacer extension device. However, these devices do require a minimum inspiratory flow rate from a spontaneously breathing patient, and their use may sometimes cause throat irritation. Further studies demonstrating comparability and safety of these devices need to be conducted.

Much evidence suggests that patients with acute severe air flow obstruction have higher dosage requirements for an aerosolized $\beta$ agonist than do those with less severe, stable airway obstruction. In many hospitals, standard therapy for acutely ill patients involves the administration of a $\beta$ agonist at 20– to 30-minute intervals. A number of studies have suggested that $\beta$ agonists may be effectively and safely administered continuously by a variety of nebulization devices for up to 72 to 96 hours in children with asthma (191, 192). Two studies have extended these findings to adults with acute asthma (193, 194). Colacone and associates randomly assigned 42 patients with acute, severe asthma to receive 5 mg albuterol by intermittent bolus nebulization at times 0 and 60 minutes or 0.2 mg/ml albuterol continuously by a calibrated nebulizer with an output of 25 ml/hour (193). Each patient received 10 mg of albuterol over 2 hours. The authors found that continuous and bolus nebulization were equally effective in the early management of asthma in the emergency room. Both modes of therapy were well tolerated. Interestingly, heart rate was significantly increased at 30 and 90 minutes in the bolus nebulization group. Olshaker and associates performed an open-label, prospective study of 76 adults with acute asthma exacerbation in the emergency room (194). The patients were given three continuous nebulizer treatments over 45 minutes; each dose was 2.5 mg albuterol and 3 ml of normal saline. All patients showed objective and subjective improvement, including an average improvement in baseline peak flow of 150%. This therapy was well tolerated with no significant tachyarrhythmia, despite the fact that the patients had underlying hypertension and coronary artery disease. In a study by Lin and colleagues, seven adults with asthma were given continuously nebulized albuterol at 0.4 mg/kg/hour delivered over 4 hours (195). Patients with a history of coronary artery disease were excluded. The mean patient age was 30.9 years. Patients showed a significant improvement in $FEV_1$. There also was a mean increase in heart rate of 16.3%. One patient withdrew because of supraventricular tachycardia. In six of seven patients, serum albuterol levels at the end of treatment were greater than 25.0 ng/ml. The authors concluded that use of high-dose continuously nebulized albuterol can result in markedly elevated serum albuterol levels and potential cardiac stimulation in some patients with asthma.

Patients with acute air flow obstruction refractory to intermittent, frequently aerosolized $\beta$-agonist therapy may be candidates for continuously nebulized bronchodilator therapy until the effects of anti-inflammatory therapy are achieved (196). Recommended regimens are albuterol, 2.5 to 15 mg/hour, or terbutaline, 2 to 8 mg/hour. A variety of delivery methods for continuous nebulization have been described. Patients should receive continuous nebulization until they have improved enough to tolerate intermittent aerosol treatment every 4 hours. Extensive experience in children and the two reports in adults suggest that this approach is safe, although further studies in adults with underlying coronary artery disease are required.

Subcutaneous injection of $\beta$ agonist is frequently used in the emergency treatment of acute asthma (197). In severe air flow obstruction, aerosol penetration to the bronchial tree may be suboptimal compared to systemically administered medication. Although epinephrine (0.3 to 0.5 ml of 1:1000 aqueous solution) has long been used, terbutaline is available for subcutaneous administration as well. Epinephrine should be used extremely cautiously in patients with cardiac disease (especially if complicated by arrhythmias or severe hypertension) or hyperthyroidism (197). Despite theoretical expectations, subcutaneous terbutaline is not associated with a decreased incidence of cardiac

side effects in comparison with subcutaneous epinephrine (197, 198).

Intravenous administration of $\beta$ agonist has been used in the treatment of severe acute bronchospasm (199). The theoretical rationale for this approach is to overcome problems related to decreased drug penetration and decreased $\beta$-adrenergic receptor responsiveness, and thereby expose $\beta$ receptors to continuous and saturating levels of drugs (200). Most of the experience with this therapy comes from Europe. In the United States, albuterol is not available for intravenous delivery. Albuterol might be preferable to isoproterenol, since the chronotropic effect is far less. However, it is not clear in which patients, if any, intravenous delivery is preferable over aerosol or subcutaneous administration. Available comparisons between intravenous albuterol and aerosol albuterol for the treatment of acute asthma provide conflicting conclusions (199, 201, 202).

A number of mechanisms have been advanced to describe potential side effects related to regular administration of $\beta$ agonists. These include paradoxical bronchoconstriction (203), downregulation of $\beta_2$-agonist receptors, tachyphylaxis as a result of depletion of norepinephrine stores (204), decreased protection against various stimuli (205, 206), and an increase in bronchial hyperreactivity (207). A recent review of adverse reaction reports for inhaled $\beta_2$-adrenergic bronchodilators submitted to the U.S. Food and Drug Administration (FDA) between 1974 and 1988 identified 126 reports of paradoxical bronchoconstriction associated with the use of MDIs and 58 reports associated with nebulization solution (203). The denominator is difficult to ascertain, but approximately 78 million MDI canisters were distributed between 1985 and 1990. A number of mechanisms have been postulated for paradoxical bronchoconstriction, including hypotonicity and acidity of the solution (208, 209), and preservatives such as benzalkonium chloride (210), sorbitan, oleic acid, edetate disodium, sulfites (211, 212) and alcohol. A recent report demonstrated paradoxical bronchoconstriction with nebulized albuterol but not with terbutaline, suggesting that this reaction could be specific to the drug preparation rather than a class effect (213). Overall, paradoxical bronchoconstriction is likely quite rare.

### Bronchodilators: Methylxanthines

The naturally occurring methylxanthines caffeine and theobromine, found in coffee and tea respectively, have been used for hundreds of years in the treatment of bronchospasm (214). Currently, the most frequently prescribed methylxanthines are theophylline (used orally or intravenously) and aminophylline (the ethylenediamine salt of theophylline for intravenous use).

Although the methylxanthines are proven bronchodilators, their mechanism of action remains unknown. Until recently, it was believed that relaxation of bronchial smooth muscle occurred through inhibition of the enzyme phosphodiesterase and the resulting intracellular accumulation of cyclic adenosine monophosphate. However, it is now known that theophylline does not inhibit phosphodiesterase at the therapeutic concentrations used in patients (214). Another proposed mechanism, direct blockage of adenosine receptors, appears untenable since the xanthine derivative enprofylline has negligible adenosine antagonism and yet exhibits more potent bronchodilatory action than does theophylline (214, 215). Several other mechanisms have been proposed, including translocation of intracellular calcium, prostaglandin antagonism, stimulation of endogenous catecholamine release, and direct $\beta$-agonist activity (216). However, in each case, it appears that the activity occurs at theophylline concentrations higher than those used clinically.

Although the mechanisms of action of theophylline are speculative, it is nevertheless clear that theophylline affects many different organs, and its actions are not limited to bronchodilation. For example, several studies suggest that theophylline may improve diaphragm function, especially during fatigue of this muscle (217, 218). Intravenous aminophylline improves right and left ventricular ejection fraction in patients with chronic obstructive lung disease (219). Oral therapy with theophylline produces a similar effect, which can be sustained for at least 4 months (220). Theophylline also stimulates the respiratory response to hypoxia but not hypercapnia (221). It is not clear which of these "alternative" actions of theophylline may play a therapeutic role in patients, but it is noteworthy that theophylline reduces dyspnea in some patients with chronic obstructive lung disease despite the absence of reversible air flow obstruction (222). The role of theophylline as an immunomodulator has recently received attention by the finding that slow-release theophylline increases suppressor T-cell counts in the peripheral blood of antigen-challenged asthmatics (223). Further studies are necessary to define the clinical importance of the nonbronchodilator effects of theophylline.

The role of aminophylline in the treatment of acute, severe asthma remains controversial (149, 224, 225). The expert panel on the diagnosis and management of asthma has not recommended routine use of aminophylline in the treatment of asthma in the emergency department (4). However, both the expert panel and the British Thoracic Society recommend the routine use of oral or intravenous theophylline in patients admitted to the hospital for an acute exacerbation of asthma (4,

226). Early studies suggested that the addition of aminophylline to maximal therapy with inhaled $\beta$ agonists in the emergency room had little effect on pulmonary function parameters during 3 hours' observation (227–229). A recent meta-analysis of 13 controlled trials compared aminophylline therapy with a control regimen consisting of albuterol, epinephrine, or other sympathomimetic bronchodilators (230). Overall, the pooled data found no difference between the aminophylline-treated group and the control groups, with three studies favoring aminophylline, three favoring the control regimen, and seven showing no difference between the two.

More recently, a number of studies have evaluated the role of aminophylline in the treatment of acute exacerbation of asthma when used in addition to inhaled $\beta$ agonists and intravenous corticosteroids both in the emergency room and in the hospital for both adults and children (231–236). In a prospective study of 133 adult patients (232) maximally treated with intravenous corticosteroids and inhaled $\beta$ agonists, administration of aminophylline resulted in a threefold decrease in the hospital admission rate for patients treated with aminophylline (6%) compared with placebo recipients (21%). Surprisingly, the reduction in admissions occurred despite an absence of clinical effect in pulmonary function as measured by spirometry. The admission decision was made by noninvestigator house staff by use of preexisting guidelines for admission. Huang and coworkers, in a placebo-controlled randomized trial of aminophylline infusion in addition to inhaled albuterol and intravenous methylprednisolone, found that the improvement in $FEV_1$ at 3 hours was greater in the aminophylline group (29% ± 23% compared with 10% ± 10%) and that the aminophylline-treated patients required fewer nebulizations of albuterol (234). A concern with this study is whether the patients received maximal inhaled $\beta$-agonist therapy. Also, it is unclear how the decision to administer "as-needed" albuterol therapy was made, since this is one of the end points of the study. In contrast, two recent studies in children did not find intravenous theophylline to add to the management of hospitalized pediatric asthmatics maximally treated with nebulized albuterol and intravenous corticosteroids (235, 236).

During the past decade, with the development of long-acting and potent inhaled $\beta_2$ agonists and inhaled corticosteroids, theophylline has been relegated to a third-line drug for the chronic maintenance therapy of asthma. Theophylline has been supplanted by the other two classes of medication for the following reasons: weak bronchodilating properties, modest and unclear anti-inflammatory properties, and potential side effects (numerous drug interactions, need to monitor serum levels, and the low therapeutic-to-toxicity ratio). Although this medication is generally less effective as a single agent than aerosol $\beta$ agonists, at least some patients will achieve an enhanced benefit from combination therapy. Additionally, therapeutic advantages have been demonstrated when oral theophylline was combined with aerosol metaproterenol (237), aerosol salbutamol (238), inhaled terbutaline (239), and oral terbutaline (240). Maintenance therapy with oral theophylline is also valuable in steroid-dependent asthmatics. In a placebo-controlled, randomized, and double-blind trial of steroid-dependent asthmatics, theophylline reduced the daily corticosteroid requirement (241). The availability of sustained-release formulations provides theophylline with a role in the treatment of nocturnal asthma (242). Particularly useful in this regard are the "once-a-day" formulations (e.g. Theo-24 and Uniphyl) (243–246).

The potentially serious toxicity of theophylline mandates that the clinician be aware of certain pharmacokinetic features of the drug and the implication for dosing regimens. A recent retrospective chart audit evaluated 40 adult inpatients with theophylline toxicity (levels greater than 25 mg/liter) to identify preventable factors (247). The study found that two-thirds (27 of 40 patients) of the inpatients became toxic because of inpatient or emergency department theophylline administration. A set of recurring management errors include a delay in taking action from the time toxic blood levels were drawn, inappropriately high dosing of patients with congestive heart failure, failure to recognize obvious symptoms of toxicity, recurrent toxicity, emergency department treatment of already toxic patients, and overlapping of intravenous and oral therapy. The clearance of theophylline is affected by many different factors (Table 9.4) and exhibits significant variation among adults. The proper maintenance dose of theophylline should be given in accordance with the estimated clearance using guidelines provided (Table 9.5). Aminophylline contains about 80% theophylline. Maintenance doses should be calculated using lean body weight. Serum theophylline levels need to be obtained to confirm the appropriateness of the chosen maintenance dose and to guide adjustments of the dose, if necessary. Prior to initiation of the intravenous maintenance dose, a loading is required. The recommended loading dose of theophylline is 5.6 mg/kg (216). This will yield a serum level of approximately 10 to 12 $\mu$g/ml. The loading dose is not adjusted to account for expected variations in drug clearance, since this consideration affects only the maintenance dose. However, the loading dose recommendation assumes that the patient has an initial blood theophylline level

**TABLE 9.4**
**FACTORS THAT ALTER THEOPHYLLINE CLEARANCE[a]**

| | |
|---|---|
| Decreased clearance | |
|   Severe liver disease | ↓↓↓ |
|   Congestive heart failure | ↓↓↓ |
|   Cimetidine | ↓↓ |
|   Troleandomycin | ↓↓ |
|   Acute illness in ICU | ↓↓ |
|   Fever | ↓ |
|   Erythromycin | ↓ |
|   Oral contraceptives | ↓ |
|   Old age | ↓ |
|   Viral infection | ↓ |
| Increased clearance | |
|   Smoking | |
|   Phenytoin | |
|   Young age | |

Modified from Jenne JW: Theophylline use in asthma. *Clin Chest Med* 4:645–658, 1984.
[a] ↓↓↓, Marked reduction (70–90%)
↓↓, Considerable reduction (~50%)
↓, Mild to moderate reduction (25–50%)

of zero. In patients who are currently taking methylxanthines, an appropriate reduction in the loading dose should be made.

Theophylline has a narrow therapeutic index. In fact, side effects and toxicity are sometimes noted at blood levels considered to be within the therapeutic range (10 to 20 $\mu$g/ml), making it impossible to disassociate adverse effects from therapeutic actions on all patients (214). The so-called minor side effects of theophylline include nausea, anorexia, diarrhea, insomnia, tachycardia, and tremor (216). Although these side effects become increasing prominent at blood levels above the therapeutic range, they are not uncommon at therapeutic or even subtherapeutic levels and may necessitate the cessation of therapy. The major life-threatening side effects are seizures and ventricular arrhythmias. Although major toxicity is relatively rare at blood levels less than 35 $\mu$g/ml, it is important to realize that the major side effects can occur without warning signs. Thus, the absence of minor side effects is not by itself adequate assurance that toxic blood levels are not present. Theophylline-induced seizures are relatively refractory to therapy and are reported to have a mortality of 50% (216, 248). Life-threatening ventricular arrhythmias usually occur at blood levels greater than 35 $\mu$g/ml. Fortunately, such arrhythmias are usually responsive to lidocaine or other therapies (216, 249). Of interest, therapeutic concentrations of theophylline appear to have little, if any, significant adverse effects on cardiac rhythm, even in patients with underlying ventricular ectopy (250, 251). Nevertheless, it is

**TABLE 9.5**
**MAINTENANCE DOSAGES OF INTRAVENOUS AMINOPHYLLINE AND THEOPHYLLINE**

| | Calculated Typical Dose[a] | | | |
|---|---|---|---|---|
| | Aminophylline | | Theophylline | |
| | (mg/kg/hr) | (mg/day) | (mg/kg/hr) | (mg/day) |
| Nonsmokers | 0.50–0.70 | 900 | 0.40–0.60 | 800 |
| Smokers | 0.90 | 1300 | 0.75 | 1100 |
| Cimetidine use | 0.30–0.40 | 600 | 0.25–0.30 | 500 |
| Cor pulmonale | 0.25–0.30 | 500 | 0.20–0.25 | 400 |
| Hepatic insufficiency | 0.20–0.25 | 450 | 0.18–0.20 | 350 |

From American Thoracic Society: Standards for the diagnosis and care of patients with chronic obstructive pulmonary disease (COPD) and asthma. *Am Rev Respir Dis* 136:225–244, 1987.
[a] Calculation should be based on lean body mass.

reasonable to exercise caution in the use of theophylline in patients with cardiac disease or rhythm disorders.

The presence of a dangerously high theophylline blood level (greater than 35 to 40 $\mu$g/ml), especially if accompanied by toxic side effects, requires urgent attention. In such emergent situations, theophylline blood levels can be rapidly lowered by instituting hemoperfusion with activated charcoal (252), or by the oral administration of activated charcoal (253). Of interest, the orally administered charcoal is effective even when toxicity is due to intravenous aminophylline. Thus, using oral activated charcoal should be considered while the hemoperfusion apparatus is being prepared (216). A recent study identified predictors of major toxicity in a series of 249 patients with theophylline intoxication (peak serum level greater than 30 mg/liter) (254). This study found that (*a*) the risk of major toxicity in patients with acute theophylline intoxication is best predicted by the peak serum theophylline concentration; (*b*) patients with chronic theophylline intoxication have a greater risk for major toxicity, at lower serum theophylline concentrations, than those with acute intoxication and that this risk cannot be predicted by the peak serum theophylline concentration. Age above 60 provides the best predictor of major toxicity in cases of chronic theophylline toxicity.

**Anticholinergic Agents**

For more than two centuries, naturally occurring anticholinergic substances (stramonium, found in the *Datura* plant, and atropine) have been used in the treatment of asthma. In general, these agents are less effective than $\beta$ agonists, and the systemic side effects after inhalation are considerable. However, the duration of action of the anticholinergic medications is often considerably longer than the $\beta$ agonists (255). Recently,

the availability of a quaternary derivative of atropine, ipratropium bromide (Atrovent), which is topically active but poorly absorbed (and therefore has minimal side effects), has stimulated renewed interest in using anticholinergic agents for both asthma and chronic obstructive pulmonary disease. Ipratropium bromide is available either in solution for use in a nebulizer or in a metered dose inhaler. When administered via metered dose inhaler, the recommended dose is 2 puffs (40 $\mu$g) four times daily. Of interest, ipratropium bromide, in contrast to atropine, does not reduce mucociliary clearance in normal subjects or in patients with airway disease (256, 257). An unpleasant, bitter taste appears to be the only significant unwanted feature of inhaled ipratropium.

The role of anticholinergic agents such as ipratropium (Atrovent) in the treatment of stable asthma is not yet clearly defined (258). When used as a single agent, ipratropium has been shown in some studies to be almost as effective as isoproterenol (259), albuterol (260), terbutaline (261), and metaproterenol (262). However, other clinical trials have indicated ipratropium to be less effective than either metaproterenol (263) or fenoterol (264). The discrepancy regarding the efficacy of ipratropium may be explained by patient selection; it is probable that there are "responders" and "non-responders" to ipratropium (262). It is difficult to predict which patients might respond to ipratropium, but patients with a "psychogenic" component to their asthma (in which vagal tone may play an important role) constitute a group that might be relatively responsive (265, 266). Several studies indicate that combining ipratropium with a $\beta$-adrenergic agent is more effective in the treatment of chronic asthma than either drug alone (263, 264, 267).

The role of inhaled anticholinergic agents in the

management of acute asthma is quite limited. The usefulness of atropine is limited by systemic side effects (268). Ipratropium is generally inferior to the β agonists as sole therapy for acute asthma. A number of studies have shown that the combination of high-dose ipratropium (500 μg) and a β-adrenergic agent is more effective than either drug used alone (269–271).

## Anti-inflammatory Agents: Corticosteroids

The central role of airway inflammation in the pathogenesis of both acute and chronic asthma (both mild and severe) has been reviewed in detail. It is safe to say that there is a consensus that anti-inflammatory treatment should represent a primary therapeutic approach for acute severe asthma in the emergency room setting (by use of parenteral or oral corticosteroids), in addition to repetitive dosing of inhaled β agonists. For long-term maintenance therapy of patients with chronic asthma, treatment focus has shifted away from use of bronchodilator therapy alone, and toward earlier use of inhaled anti-inflammatory therapy.

Potential mechanisms of corticosteroid action includes effects on leukocytes (T lymphocytes, polymorphonuclear neutrophils), synthesis of regulator proteins, catecholamine receptors or function, eicosanoid synthesis and function, and vascular endothelial integrity (272). Although the precise mechanism of action of glucocorticoids is not known, recent advances in understanding the molecular mechanisms of the glucocorticoid receptor, steroid responsive target gene elements, and cytokine biology have provided new insights (Fig. 9.6) (273–275). There is a single glucocorticoid receptor (GR) that is localized to the cytoplasm of target cells in airway epithelium and endothelium of bronchial vessels. After a glucocorticoid binds to a cytosolic GR, this complex translocates to the nucleus, where it binds to specific glucocorticoid response elements of genes, which either inhibit or stimulate transcription in steroid-responsive target genes. Steroids inhibit the transcription of several cytokines, including interleukin-1 (IL-1), tumor necrosis factor α (TNF-α), granulocyte-macrophage colony stimulating factor (GM-CSF), and interleukins 3, 4, 5, 6, and 8. The well-known eosinopenic effect of corticosteroids is believed to be due to the inhibitory effects on circulating IL-5 and GM-CSF (276). Steroids also increase the synthesis of lipocortin-1, which has an inhibitory effect on phospholipase $A_2$ and therefore inhibits the production of lipid mediators such as leukotrienes, prostaglandins, and platelet activating factor. Additional effects include inhibiting mucus secretion in airways and increasing the expression of β receptors by increasing gene transcription.

The efficacy of systemic corticosteroids (oral or intravenous) in acute severe asthma is quite well established in 15 clinical trials of acute asthma in adults

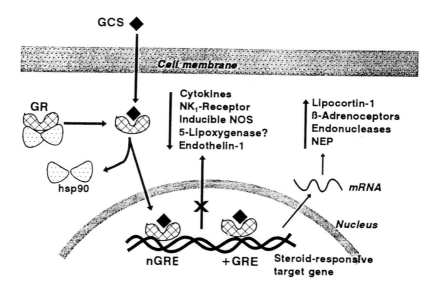

**Figure 9.6.** Molecular mechanism of glucocorticosteroid (*GCS*) action. GCS binds to a cytosolic glucocorticoid receptor (*GR*) that is normally bound to two molecules of heat shock protein (*hsp 90*). The activated GR translocates to the nucleus, where it binds to specific glucocorticoid receptor elements (GREs) in the upstream regulatory region of genes, which either inhibit (*nGRE*) or stimulate (*+GRE*) transcription of steroid-responsive target genes (of which many are likely to be relevant in asthma therapy). (From Barnes PJ, Pedersen S. Efficacy and safety of inhaled corticosteroids in asthma. *Am Rev Respir Dis* 148:S2, 1993.)

(277). Fanta and colleagues demonstrated that in patients with acute severe episodes of asthma refractory to 8 hours of conventional bronchodilator therapy, the subjects given intravenous corticosteroids had significantly greater resolution of airway obstruction by the end of 24 hours (278). Littenberg and Gluck demonstrated that the prompt use of glucocorticoids in the emergency treatment of severe asthma can prevent significant morbidity, reduce the number of hospitalizations, and effect substantial savings in health care costs (279). In contrast, Stein and Cole, in a placebo-controlled trial of 81 adults with acute asthma in the emergency room, failed to show that early administration of intravenous corticosteroids reduces the hospital admission rate (18% for the steroid group and 13% for the control group) (280). However, the admitted patients did begin with lower PEFRs and responded less at 2 hours to inhaled bronchodilators. It is likely that the severity of underlying airway obstruction and inflammation on initial presentation is what determines the need for admission (149). It is clear that the onset of action is delayed at least 6 to 12 hours following systemic administration of corticosteroids (281).

Much has been published about systemic corticosteroid therapy for patients with acute and chronic asthma as to the type of steroid preparation, route of administration (parenteral versus oral), (282), the ideal dosage, (283), and the duration of taper (284). Although several studies have suggested that there are differences in penetration of different corticosteroid preparations in the lung, their clinical relevance is unclear (285, 286). For parenteral use, methylprednisolone is preferred over hydrocortisone because of more potent anti-inflammatory properties and for being less expensive (277). For oral therapy, the available preparations appear to be fairly comparable, although cortisone and prednisone require hydroxylation before they become active. Since bioavailability after oral therapy is quite high for prednisone, some have recommended "noninvasive" therapy by the use of oral steroids in acute asthma exacerbation (287). Although the optimal dosage for systemic steroids has not been established, McFadden's review of the available studies suggests that hydrocortisone equivalent to 14 mg/kg per 24 hours is effective therapy for acutely ill asthmatic adults (277). It is common practice to administer 120 to 180 mg of methylprednisolone per day intravenously, or 150 to 225 mg of prednisone or 600 to 900 mg of hydrocortisone by the oral route (277). Likewise, the optimal schedule of steroid withdrawal following an acute exacerbation is not well established. In one study, Lederle et al suggested that the relapse rate was not different between a steroid taper over 1 week compared to 7 weeks, although the relapse rate was quite high in both groups (284).

Common complications of prolonged systemic corticosteroid therapy include edema, truncal obesity, moon facies, striae, capillary fragility (leading to purpuric skin lesions), muscle wasting, osteoporosis (and vertebral compression fractures), posterior subcapsular cataracts, exacerbation of glucose intolerance, and worsening of hypertension (272, 288). Patients receiving long-term corticosteroid therapy also have an increased susceptibility to infections. Suppression of the hypothalamic-pituitary-adrenal (HPA) axis is a potentially serious complication of ongoing systemic corticosteroid therapy (272). Whereas normal adrenal function usually returns within 24 to 96 hours after a 2- to 4-week course of systemic corticosteroids, significantly prolonged depression of adrenal function may occur if corticosteroids are given for longer than 1 month (273, 289, 290). If adrenal function is suspect, corticosteroids should be tapered gradually rather than abruptly discontinued, and high doses should be given during surgery or other periods of significant stress. It is not clear what is the best method to assess the integrated function of the HPA axis (275). The rapid ACTH (Cortrosyn) stimulation test may prove helpful (289). Others advocate an early-morning plasma cortisol determination; values above the middle part of the normal range indicate an ability to respond to surgical stress without difficulty (291). A low normal value may indicate suppression of the HPA axis.

A number of recent BAL and biopsy studies in patients with bronchial asthma have shown that 3 months' therapy with inhaled corticosteroids reduces inflammatory changes (292–294). Interestingly, a study by Lungren and coworkers showed that even after 10 years of inhaled corticosteroids, the basement membrane thickening persisted (295). Additional studies have shown that inhaled steroids reduce airway responsiveness as measured by methacholine, histamine, or exercise. This reduction in responsiveness (as assessed by an increase in $PC_{20}$ of histamine or methacholine) occurs over several weeks to several months, and usually ranges in the order of one or two doubling dilutions (275, 296, 297). Some have questioned whether these slight changes have clinical significance (38).

Numerous recent studies have shown that inhaled steroid therapy provides effective symptomatic control of chronic asthma (298, 299). Haahtela and colleagues conducted a prospective parallel group trial involving 103 asthmatics over a 2-year period, randomly assigned to receive 600 $\mu$g of inhaled budesonide twice a day or 375 $\mu$g of inhaled terbutaline twice a day (300). Asthma in these patients was newly diagnosed in the previous year and for the most part was mild. The group treated with budesonide showed a significant reduction in symptom scores and in use of rescue $\beta_2$ agonist and an improvement in morning and evening peak expiratory flow rates. This study is limited by the fact that the $\beta$ agonist was only administered on a twice-a-day basis and that a spacer device was not specified for either group. Kertjens et al noted that inhaled beclomethasone at 800 $\mu$g per day improved symptoms and lung function over a 2.5-year period in patients with chronic asthma when given in addition to $\beta$ agonist inhaled therapy (301). Dompeling and coworkers, in a 4-year prospective study, showed that therapy with beclomethasone 400 $\mu$g two times daily slowed the deterioration of lung function of asthmatics, compared to bronchodilator therapy alone (302). A number of studies have shown that higher doses of inhaled steroids reduces the need for maintenance oral steroids (303–307). Barnes has suggested that inhaled steroids are the treatment of choice in the management of nocturnal asthma (308).

Both the binding affinity to GR and the skin

blanching test are in-vitro parameters that are often used to compare relative potency of inhaled glucocorticoids (Table 9.6). Also, the pharmacokinetics of inhaled steroids and the subsequent elimination of these agents determines both the efficacy and the side effects (Table 9.7, Fig. 9.7). Long-term comparative clinical studies are needed before the clinician can rationally choose between the currently available inhaled glucocorticoids (275).

Side effects of inhaled corticosteroids are being increasingly recognized as a potential problem (309). The factors that may contribute to toxicity include the total dose, the dosing schedule, whether or not a spacer device is used, whether mouth rinsing is used, and the sensitivity of the parameter used to assess systemic toxicity (275, 310). The adverse effects of inhaled corticosteroids can be broadly classified as topical or systemic (311). The three main topical side effects are cough, oral candidiasis, and dysphonia. Slow inhalation, use of a spacer device, and gargling reduce the incidence of these side effects (312). The systemic side effects may include suppression of the HPA axis, adverse effects on bone metabolism including osteoporosis, slowing of growth in children and adolescents, linkage to cataract formation, bruising and dermal thinning, and psychological changes (275, 310, 313, 314). Many studies have suggested that doses of inhaled corticosteroids in excess of 800 $\mu$g/day in adults or 400 $\mu$g/day in children appear to result in dose-related suppression of the HPA axis, with substantial interindividual variability and response (310). The HPA axis suppression has been most commonly assessed by morning serum cortisol level and 24-hour urinary cortisol excretion. The clinical significance of these changes over the long duration is not known. In patients who require doses in excess of 800 $\mu$g, use of a spacer device in conjunction with a metered dose inhaler and the use of mouthwashing may reduce suppression of the HPA axis. Twice-a-day dosing appears to have fewer side effects. Some studies suggest

**TABLE 9.6**
**RELATIVE BINDING AFFINITY FOR HUMAN LUNG GLUCOCORTICOID RECEPTOR AND TOPICAL BLANCHING POTENCY IN HUMAN SKIN**

| Glucocorticosteroid | Binding Affinity | Blanching Potency |
|---|---|---|
| Dexamethasone | 1.0 | 1 |
| BDP/BMP[a] | 0.4/13.5 | 600/450 |
| Budesonide | 9.4 | 980 |
| Flunisolide | 1.8 | 330 |
| Triamcinolone acetonide | 3.6 | 330 |
| Fluticasone propionate | 18.0 (Rat tissue) | 1200 |

From Barnes PJ, Pedersen S: Efficacy and safety of inhaled corticosteroids in asthma. *Am Rev Respir Dis* 148:S7, 1993.
[a] BDP, beclomethasone dipropionate; BMP, beclomethasone monopropionate.

**TABLE 9.7**
**PHARMACOKINETICS OF INHALED GLUCOCORTICOSTEROIDS**

| | Plasma Half-life (hr) | Volume of Distribution (liters/kg) | Clearance (liters/min) | First-Pass (%) |
|---|---|---|---|---|
| Triamcinolone acetonide | 1.5 | 2.1 | 1.2 | — |
| Beclomethasone dipropionate | — | — | — | — |
| Flunisolide | 1.6 | 1.8 | 1.0 | 20 |
| Budesonide | 2.8 | 4.3 | 1.4 | 10 |
| Fluticasone dipropionate | 3.1 | 3.7[a] | 0.87 | — |

From Barnes PJ, Pedersen S: Efficacy and safety of inhaled corticosteroids in asthma. *Am Rev Respir Dis* 148:S7, 1993.
[a] Assuming a mean body weight of 70 kg.

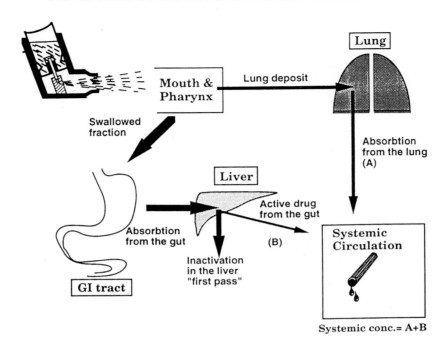

**FIGURE 9.7.** The fate of inhaled steroids. The amount of an inhaled glucocorticosteroid reaching the systemic circulation is the sum of the pulmonary and orally bioavailable fraction. The fraction deposited in the mouth will be swallowed, and the systemic availability will be determined by absorption from the gastrointestinal tract and degree of first-pass metabolism. The fraction deposited in the intrapulmonary airways is likely to be more or less completely absorbed in active form to the systemic circulation, as there is no evidence for any degree of metabolic inactivation in currently used inhaled steroids. The systemic concentration will be reduced by continuous recirculation and inactivation in the liver. (From Barnes PJ, Pedersen S. Efficacy and safety of inhaled corticosteroids in asthma. *Am Rev Respir Dis* 148:S9, 1993.)

that beclomethasone may have a somewhat greater propensity to produce adrenal suppression in comparison with budesonide at higher doses, although the relevance for this is not clear. Inhaled corticosteroids with doses as low as 400 $\mu$g/day have been associated with the development of osteoporosis (314).

### Anti-Inflammatory Agents: Cromolyn Sodium and Nedocromil Sodium

Cromolyn sodium has been available in the United States since 1973 (315, 316). This medication is poorly absorbed orally and therefore is effective only when inhaled. Initially, cromolyn was available only as a 20-mg capsule containing finely powdered cromolyn and lactose particles delivered by a turbo inhaler (Spinhaler). Its usefulness in this form was limited by oral pharyngeal irritation and cough. Subsequently, cromolyn was introduced as a nebulizer solution in 1982 and in a pressurized metered dose inhaler in 1986.

Cromolyn sodium administered prior to allergen exposure blocks both the early and late asthmatic response following antigen inhalation (317). Cromolyn has not demonstrated smooth muscle relaxant properties and therefore is not a bronchodilator. It has long been held that the primary mechanism of action appears to be inhibition of mediator release from mast cells. Although the exact mechanism by which cromolyn inhibits mast cell mediator release is not known, it is believed to inhibit calcium influx by phosphorylation of a membrane protein. Other mechanisms of action of cromolyn include suppression of nonmyelinated vagal sensory nerve endings, inhibition of inflammatory cells other than mast cells, and reduction of airway permeability.

A large number of studies have documented the protective effect exerted by cromolyn against provocative stimuli such as allergen, cold air, $SO_2$, and exercise (317). The drug is most effective when administered before challenge. The protective effects against nonspecific agents such as methacholine and histamine have been less established. A number of studies have evaluated the effect of cromolyn on nonspecific bronchial hyperreactivity. Studies in which cromolyn was administered for longer than 6 weeks suggest an improvement in airway reactivity. Despite initial notions that cromolyn would be more effective in extrinsic than intrinsic asthma, most carefully designed studies do not support this concept. About 60 to 79% of asthmatics show a response to cromolyn. Studies comparing cromolyn and theophylline in the short-term management of chronic asthma suggest that both of these agents are equally effective, with perhaps greater side effects with theophylline. There are some data to show that there is an additive effect between these two agents. Toogood and coworkers did not find any advantage to adding cromolyn to an established regimen of beclomethasone (318).

Nedocromil sodium (Tilade) is structurally different than cromolyn, but it has very similar pharmacologic activities. Nedocromil was approved for use in the United States in MDIs in 1992. The mechanism of action of nedocromil appears to be quite similar to cromolyn. A number of in vitro and in vivo studies suggest that nedocromil blocks both the early and late asthmatic response. Nedocromil has anti-inflammatory properties on a number of cells. There is some suggestion that nedocromil may be more potent in inhibiting bronchial C-fiber nerve endings.

A recent meta-analysis reviewed all known placebo controlled, double-blind, randomized clinical trials involving nedocromil (a total of 4,723 patients from 127 centers) (319). This included both published and unpublished material. The authors compared the treatment effects of nedocromil and placebo using six efficacy variables, including symptom scores, peak flows, $FEV_1$, and inhaled bronchodilator use. The numerous studies were classified by trial design into five groups. Overall, nedocromil is more effective than placebo in treating asthma and is of most benefit to patients who are receiving monotherapy with bronchodilators (320-322). The aggregate data suggested that nedocromil is less potent than inhaled corticosteroids, although some inhaled corticosteroid-sparing effects were noted. A recent nedocromil sodium workshop concluded that nedocromil could represent an alternative to cromolyn, although there was no clear advantage for nedocromil over inhaled steroids, and the costs are higher (323).

Overall, inhaled anti-inflammatory agents should be part of the maintenance therapy for most patients with chronic asthma. Inhaled corticosteroids are preferred in the majority of patients because of proven efficacy, greater potency than cromolyn or nedocromil, and effectiveness when administered twice a day as opposed to four times a day (324). Also, there are more data supporting improvement of inflammation as assessed by BAL and endobronchial biopsy in patients treated with inhaled corticosteroids (325). In patients in whom there is a high concern for toxicity of inhaled corticosteroids (i.e., children, or patients requiring high doses of inhaled corticosteroids), cromolyn or nedocromil represents a rational alternative. Also, for patients who continue to be symptomatic despite very high doses of inhaled corticosteroids, the addition of nedocromil seems reasonable (325–327). Additional studies directly comparing inhaled corticosteroids and nedocromil for newly diagnosed bronchial asthma are required.

## EXPERIMENTAL THERAPY

A minority of patients continue to have troublesome asthma symptoms with frequent exacerbations requiring hospitalization despite maximal conventional therapy. Literature suggests that this is a small subset, perhaps 5 to 20% of all asthmatics (288, 328). The reversible factors that contribute to this subset of "steroid-dependent" asthma include patient noncompliance, poor self-management strategies by the patient, inadequate control of allergen burden at home, inadequate inhaler technique, and suboptimal pharmacotherapy prescription by the physician. Data from the placebo arm of a number of studies have clearly shown that a compulsory traditional management plan, with frequent follow-up in perhaps an asthma center, can reduce the need for oral steroids by 16 to 40% in "steroid-dependent" asthmatics (329, 330).

Carmichael et al described 58 patients with chronic asthma who were clinically resistant to treatment with prednisolone (defined as absence of a 15% increase in $FEV_1$ after a 7-day course of at least 20 mg of prednisolone daily) (331). Dykewicz and colleagues studied the natural history of 40 randomly selected adult asthmatic patients refractory to inhaled beclomethasone and $\beta$ agonists, and dependent on long-term prednisone therapy (mean duration 6.2 $\pm$ 5 years) (332). Over a 3– to 5-year period, 24 patients (60%) had unchanged long-term prednisone requirement, 13 patients (32.5%) improved with a reduction in prednisone requirement, and three patients (7.5%) deteriorated with increased prednisone requirement. Unfortunately, this study did not report the maintenance dose of beclomethasone. Corrigan et al evaluated the possible mechanism of chronic asthmatics with clinical glucocorticoid resistance (333). Patients were defined as having glucocorticoid resistance if there was less than a 30% increase in $FEV_1$ after 2 weeks of daily prednisone, 20 mg for the first week and 40 mg for the second week. Glucocorticoid pharmacokinetics, receptor characteristics, and inhibition of peripheral blood T-cell proliferation by glucocorticoid were assayed. Overall, the investigators noted a relative insensitivity of T lymphocytes to glucocorticoid in patients with clinical glucocorticoid resistance compared to matched glucocorticoid-sensitive asthmatics. They noted that the resistance does not reflect abnormal glucocorticoid clearance. Additional studies by this group suggested that activated T lymphocytes may be the target, and perhaps an anti–T lymphocyte drug such as cyclosporine may be particularly useful in glucocorticoid-resistant asthmatic patients. Overall, the clinical relevance of glucocorticoid resistance in patients with chronic steroid-dependent asthma remains speculative and poorly understood (334).

Barnes classified the new pharmacologic agents for asthma based on (a) improvement of an existing class of drugs or (b) development of novel compounds (335). The literature is replete with numerous studies demonstrating the efficacy of alternative anti-inflammatory therapies that provide a steroid-sparing effect in asthma (336–338). Discussion here will be limited to methotrexate, troleandomycin, cyclosporine, and leukotriene antagonists.

Methotrexate has been evaluated in steroid-dependent asthma in five recent clinical trials (330, 339–342). The rationale for methotrexate trials in asthma is based on the longstanding experience with anti-inflammatory properties of this drug in rheumatoid arthritis and psoriasis. Methotrexate is an inhibitor of dihydrofolate reductase, which appears to inhibit neutrophil-dependent inflammation. Mullarkey et al conducted a placebo-controlled crossover study in 14 steroid-dependent asthmatics (average starting prednisone dose of 26 mg/day, range of 10 to 60 mg) (329). Patients were randomly assigned to 12 weeks of placebo or methotrexate (15 mg p.o. per week) and then switched to the alternate form of therapy. They were seen every 3 weeks in follow-up. On the average, 36.5% less prednisone was required when patients received methotrexate than when they received placebo. The same group published a follow-up experience of 31 cushingoid asthmatics on daily prednisone and inhaled corticosteroids who were treated with low-dose methotrexate for 18 to 28 months (339). They found that the mean prednisone dose was reduced from 26.9 mg/day to 6.3 mg/day in the 25 patients who completed the study; 15 patients discontinued the regular use of prednisone. Similarly, Shiner and coworkers conducted a 24-week placebo-controlled trial of 69 steroid-dependent asthmatics (mean daily prednisolone dose was 14.2 mg/day) and found that during 12 weeks of treatment, steroid doses were tapered by 16% in both the methotrexate and placebo groups (341). However, between 12 and 24 weeks, the prednisolone dose was reduced by a greater portion in the methotrexate than the placebo group (50% versus 14%). Patients were evaluated every 4 weeks in the study. Five of the 38 patients taking

methotrexate had liver function abnormalities. Erzurum et al conducted a double-blind, parallel-group study over 13 weeks in prednisone-dependent asthmatics (average daily dose of 20 mg, range 15 to 30 mg), in which 19 patients received either methotrexate (5 mg intramuscularly every week) or placebo (330). What was unique about this study was that patients were seen on a weekly basis and there was a 1-month baseline period during which conventional therapy was maximized and attempts to reduce the baseline prednisone was made. Overall, both groups reduced their oral prednisone dose by about 40% and the authors concluded that methotrexate did not produce significant benefit in corticosteroid-dependent asthma. A more recent study by Coffey et al evaluated 11 subjects with steroid-dependent asthma (mean of 28 mg/day prednisone) in a placebo-controlled crossover trial for 12-week periods (342). The study found that the placebo group was able to reduce the prednisone dose by about 20% and that methotrexate was not superior to placebo. In summary, based on the available studies, it is difficult to recommend therapy with methotrexate outside the setting of a clinical trial.

Both oral and parenteral gold preparations have been used in the therapy of steroid-dependent asthma (343–346). These studies have generally found that the addition of gold can decrease corticosteroid requirement, can improve symptoms, and perhaps can improve bronchial hyperreactivity as well. In addition to a number of methodologic limitations with these studies, overall patient tolerance has been poor and the incidence of side effects has been as high as 37%, including diarrhea, skin eruptions, and proteinuria. There are no data on long-term side effects or patient compliance with gold therapy for patients with bronchial asthma.

Another steroid-sparing approach in the treatment of chronic asthma has been the use of troleandomycin, a macrolide antibiotic. A number of open-label studies have demonstrated a reduction in corticosteroid dose when troleandomycin is added to the medical regimen of patients with asthma (347–350). The principal effect of troleandomycin is the prolongation of the plasma half-life of corticosteroids through the inhibition of their elimination (methylprednisolone half-life increased from 2.46 hours before troleandomycin to 4.63 hours 1 week after troleandomycin) (348). Published protocols highlight the importance of using methylprednisolone rather than prednisone in conjunction with troleandomycin to have the steroid-sparing effect (350, 351). A recent placebo-controlled parallel group study over a 2-year period was performed in 75 steroid-dependent asthmatics comparing troleandomycin plus methylprednisolone versus methylprednisolone alone (352). Patients in both groups achieved alternate-day steroid therapy, and the reduction in methylprednisolone dose was not significantly different between the treatment groups. However, the patients in the troleandomycin group were observed to have significantly more steroid-related side effects as assessed by serum IgG, blood sugar, cholesterol, and osteoporosis. In summary, this is a well-designed study that strongly supports the notion that the steroid-sparing properties of troleandomycin are a pharmacologic phenomenon and do not translate into fewer long-term steroid-related side effects. Based on this study, further trials with troleandomycin are probably not indicated.

Cyclosporine is an immunosuppressive agent with a number of properties, including inhibition of mediator release from mast cells and basophils and inhibition of the synthesis of lymphokines, with the subsequent downregulation of $CD4^+$ T lymphocytes. Since recent data have implicated the T lymphocyte as playing a critical role in chronic asthma, a number of investigators have evaluated cyclosporine in steroid-dependent asthma (353–355). Most recently, Alexander et al conducted a double-blind, placebo-controlled, crossover trial of cyclosporine (initial dose 5 mg/kg per day) or placebo for 12 weeks with a 2-week washout period (355). In 30 of 33 patients in the cyclosporine group, there was a significant increase in peak expiratory flow rate and $FEV_1$ in addition to a 48% reduction in the frequency of disease exacerbations. Corticosteroid dosage reduction was not attempted in this study. The well-known side effects of cyclosporine include hypertension, hypertrichosis, neurological disturbances, and nephrotoxicity.

The sulfidopeptide or cysteinyl leukotrienes ($LTC_4$, $LTD_4$, and $LTE_4$), formerly the slow-reacting substance of anaphylaxis (SRS-A), are formed by the lipoxygenation of arachidonic acid by the enzyme 5-lipoxygenase (356–358). Much information has accumulated over the past 10 years that suggests that the cysteinyl leukotrienes play a role in spontaneously occurring human asthma (359). These compounds are released by mast cells and eosinophils and they are known to have a variety of potent effects, including bronchoconstriction, increasing permeability, and enhancing airway reactivity. The cysteinyl leukotrienes can be recovered from nasal secretions, bronchoalveolar lavage fluid, and urine of patients with asthma (360, 361).

A number of pharmacologic antagonists have recently been developed that further support the role of leukotrienes in a number of models of human asthma (362, 363). Specifically, potent competitive receptor antagonists to $LTD_4$ inhibit asthmatic responses with challenge involving allergen, exercise, cold dry air, and aspirin (364–367). Zileuton, a 5-lipoxygenase inhibitor, was recently evaluated in the treatment of mild to moderate chronic asthma in a placebo-controlled parallel study over 4 weeks (368). A total of 139 asthmatics with an $FEV_1$ between 40 and 75%, who were not on other therapy, were randomized to zileuton 2.4 g/day or 1.6 g/day or placebo. It was noted that zileuton increased the $FEV_1$ within 1 hour of administration to a level of 14.6% above baseline. In addition, after 4 weeks of zileuton therapy, there was a 13.4% increase in the baseline $FEV_1$ along with a reduction in symptoms and the frequency of $\beta$-agonist use. The cysteinyl leukotriene production, as reflected by recovery of $LTE_4$ in the urine, decreased by 39% at the dose of 2.4 g/day. This study supports the notion that inhibition of leukotriene synthesis at the 5-lipoxgenase level on a chronic basis may produce a clinically relevant benefit. This agent was well tolerated, but long-term studies need to be performed.

## SUMMARY

Much new information has emerged from intensive research in asthma in the past 5 to 10 years. However, as evidenced by a recent consensus conference (369), there are many unresolved questions regarding the fundamental factors involved in the pathogenesis of asthma, the etiology of upward trends in morbidity and mortality of asthma, and the utility of newer therapeutic agents on the long-term management of asthma. The interaction between genetic factors, atopic status, and environmental factors (including allergen exposure, viral infections, and atmospheric pollutants) to produce the familiar symptoms of the airway disease remains unclear. Whether asthma is a single disorder with a unique cause or a syndrome of multiple disorders with several etiologic mechanisms remains unclear. The critical and rate-limiting steps in the asthma inflammatory cascade remain to be established. Also, the natural history of the disease, the significance of airway hyperreactivity in asymptomatic individuals, the impact of long-term anti-inflammatory therapy, and the toxicity of long-term therapy all remain unclear. Future therapeutic strategies will in large part be dependent on the answers to some of these unresolved issues.

▼

## REFERENCES

1. Ciba Foundation Guest Symposium. Terminology, definitions and classification of chronic pulmonary emphysema and related conditions. *Thorax* 14:286, 1959.

2. Scadding JG: The meaning of diagnostic terms in bronchopulmonary disease. *Br Med J* 2:1423, 1963.

3. American Thoracic Society: Standards for the diagnosis and care of patients with chronic obstructive pulmonary disease (COPD) and asthma. *Am Rev Respir Dis* 136:225–244, 1987.

4. National Heart, Lung, and Blood Institute, National Asthma Education Program: *Expert Panel Report. Guidelines for the Diagnosis and Management of Asthma.* Bethesda, MD, National Institutes of Health 1–136, 1991.

5. International consensus report on diagnosis and management of asthma. National Heart, Lung and Blood Institute, National Institutes of Health, Bethesda, MD. *Eur Respir J* 5:601–641, 1992.

6. Snapper JR: Inflammation and airway function: the asthma syndrome (editorial). *Am Rev Respir Dis* 141:531–533, 1990.

7. U.S. Department of Health: *Prevalence of Selected Chronic Respiratory Conditions—United States, 1970.* U.S. Department of Health, Education, and Welfare Series 10, No. 84, 1973.

8. Bonner JR: The epidemiology and natural history of asthma. *Clin Chest Med* 5:557–565, 1984.

9. Broder I, Higgins MW, Mathews KD, et al: Epidemiology of asthma and allergic rhinitis in a total community, Tecumseh, Michigan. *J Allergy Clin Immunol* 53:127–138, 1974.

10. Gergen PJ, Mullally DI, Evans R: National survey of prevalence of asthma among children in the U.S., 1976–1980. *Pediatrics* 81:1–7, 1988.

11. Asthma—United States, 1980–1990. *MMWR* 41:733–735, 1992.

12. Skobeloff EM, Spivey WH, St. Clair SS, et al: The influence of age and sex on asthma admissions. *JAMA* 268:3437–3440, 1992.

13. Weiss KB, Gergen PJ, Hodgson TA: An economic evaluation of asthma in the United States. *N Engl J Med* 326:862–866, 1992.

14. Woolcock AJ: Asthma. In Murray JF, Nadel JA (eds): *Textbook of Respiratory Medicine.* Philadelphia, WB Saunders, 1030–1068, 1988.

15. Jackson RT, Beaglehole R, Rea HH, et al: Mortality from asthma: a new epidemic in New Zealand. *Br Med J* 285:771–774, 1982.

16. Sears MR, Rea HH, Beaglehole R: Asthma mortality: a review of recent experience in New Zealand. *J Allergy Clin Immunol* 80:319–325, 1987.

17. Wilson JD, Sutherland DC, Thomas AC: Has the change to beta-agonists combined with oral theophylline increased cases of total asthma? *Lancet* 1:1235, 1981.

18. Sears MR: Epidemiological trends in bronchial asthma. In Kaliner MA, Barnes PJ, Persson CGA (eds): *Asthma, Its Pathology and Treatment.* New York, Marcel Dekker, 1991, pp 1–49.

19. Sly RM: Mortality from asthma. *J Allergy Clin Immunol* 84:421–434, 1989.

20. Buist AS, Sears MR, Reid LM, et al: Asthma mortality: trends and determinants. *Am Rev Respir Dis* 135:1037–1039, 1987.

21. British Thoracic Association: Death from asthma in two regions of England. *Br Med J* 285:1251–1255, 1982.

22. Sears MR, Rea HH, Beaglehole R, et al: Asthma mortality in New Zealand: a two–year national study. *NZ Med J* 98:271–275, 1985.

23. Hunt LW, Silverstein MD, Reed CE, et al: Accuracy of the death certificate in a population-based study of asthmatic patients. *JAMA* 269:1947–1952, 1993.

24. Rea HH, Sears MR, Beaglehole R, et al: Lessons from the national asthma mortality study: circumstances surrounding death. *NZ Med J* 100:10–13, 1987.

25. Sly RM: Mortality from asthma, 1974–1984. *J Allergy Clin Immunol* 82:705–717, 1988.

26. Benatar SR: Fatal asthma. *N Engl J Med* 314:423–429, 1986.

27. Rea HH, Seragg R, Jackson R, et al: A case-control study of deaths from asthma. *Thorax* 41:833–839, 1986.

28. Barger LW, Vollmer WM, Felt RW, Buist AS: Further investigation into the recent increase in asthma death rates: a review of 41 asthma deaths in Oregon in 1982. *Ann Allergy* 60:31–39, 1988.

29. Strunk RC: Death due to asthma. *Am Rev Respir Dis* 148:550–552, 1993.

30. Weiss KB, Wagener DK: Changing patterns of asthma mortality: identifying target populations at high risk. *JAMA* 264:1683–1687, 1990.

31. Wasserfallen JB, Schaller MD, Feihl F, et al: Sudden asphyxic asthma: a distinct entity? *Am Rev Respir Dis* 142:108–111, 1990.

32. Kallenbach JM, Frankel AH, Lapinsky SE, et al: Determinants of near fatality in acute severe asthma. *Am J Med* 95:265–272, 1993.

33. Sur S, Crotty TB, Kephart GM, et al: Sudden-onset fatal asthma. *Am Rev Respir Dis* 148:713–719, 1993.

34. Molfino NA, Nannini LJ, Rebuck AS, et al: The fatality-prone asthmatic patient. *Chest* 101:621–623, 1992.

35. Barriot P, Riou B: Prevention of fatal asthma. *Chest* 92:460–466, 1987.

36. Reid LM: The presence or absence of bronchial mucous in fatal asthma. *J Allergy Clin Immunol* 80:415–416, 1987.

37. Robin ED, McCauley R: Sudden cardiac death in bronchial asthma and inhaled beta-adrenergic agonists. *Chest* 101:1699–1702, 1992.

38. McFadden ER, Gilbert IA: Medical Progress: Asthma. *N Engl J Med* 327:1928–1937, 1992.

39. Nelson HS, Szeffler SJ, Martin RJ: Regular inhaled beta-adrenergic agonists in the treatment of bronchial asthma: beneficial or detrimental. *Am Rev Respir Dis* 144:249–250, 1991.

40. Grant IWB: Asthma in New Zealand. *Br Med J* 286:364, 1983.

41. Grainger J, Woodsman K, Pearce N, et al: Prescribed fenoterol and death from asthma in New Zealand, 1981–7: a further case-control study. *Thorax* 46:105–111, 1991.

42. Sears MR, Taylor DR, Pring CG, et al: Regular inhaled beta-agonist treatment in bronchial asthma. *Lancet* 336:1391–1396, 1990.

43. Spitzer WO, Suissa S, Ernst P, Horwitz RI, et al: The use of B-agonists and the risk of death and near death from asthma. *N Engl J Med* 326:501–506, 1992.

44. Ernst P, Habbick B, Suissa S, et al: Is the association between inhaled beta-agonist use and life-threatening asthma because of confounding by severity? *Am Rev Respir Dis* 148:75–79, 1993.

45. Mullen ML, Mullen B, Carey M: The association between B-agonist use and death from asthma. *JAMA* 270:1842–1845, 1993.

46. Rackemann FM, Edwards MC: Asthma in children. *N Engl J Med* 246:858–863, 1952.

47. Blair H: Natural history of childhood asthma. *Arch Dis Child* 52:613–619, 1977.

48. Martin AJ, McLennan LA, Landau LI, et al: The natural history of childhood asthma to adult life. *Br Med J* 1:1397–1400, 1980.

49. Brown PJ, Greville HW, Finvcane KE: Asthma and irreversible airflow obstruction. *Thorax* 39:131–136, 1984.

50. Stellman JL, Spicer JE, Cayton RM: Morbidity from chronic asthma. *Thorax* 37:218–221, 1982.

51. Braman SS, Kaemmerlen JT, Davis SM: Asthma in the elderly: a comparison between patients with recently acquired and long-standing disease. *Am Rev Respir Dis* 143:336–340, 1991.

52. Bronnimann S, Burrows B: A prospective study of the natural history of asthma. *Chest* 90:480–484, 1986.

53. Broder I, Barlow PP, Horton RJM: The epidemiology of asthma and hay fever in a total community, Tecumseh, Michigan. *J Allergy* 33:524–531, 1962.

54. Lee HY, Stretton TB: Asthma in the elderly. *Br Med J* 4:93–95, 1972.

55. Hogg JC: The pathology of asthma. *Clin Chest Med* 5:567–571, 1984.

56. Dunnill MS, Massarella GR, Anderson JA: A comparison of the quantitative anatomy of the bronchi in normal subjects, in status asthmaticus, in chronic bronchitis, and in emphysema. *Thorax* 24:176–179, 1969.

57. MacDonald JB, MacDonald ET, Seaton A, et al: Asthma deaths in Cardiff 1963–74: fifty-three deaths in hospital. *Br Med J* 2:721–723, 1976.

58. MacDonald JB, Seaton A, Williams DA: Asthma deaths in Cardiff 1963–74: ninety deaths outside hospital. *Br Med J* 1:1493–1495, 1976.

59. Laitinen LA, Heino M, Laitinen A, et al: Damage of the airway epithelium and bronchial reactivity in patients with asthma. *Am Rev Respir Dis* 131:599–606, 1985.

60. Smith DL, Deshazo RD: State of the art: Bronchoalveolar lavage in asthma: an update and perspective. *Am Rev Respir Dis* 148:523–532, 1993.

61. Djukanovic R, Roche WR, Wilson JW, et al: Mucosal inflammation in asthma. *Am Rev Respir Dis* 142:434–457, 1990.

62. Beasley R, Roche WR, Roberts JA, et al: Cellular events in the bronchi in mild asthma and after bronchial provocation. *Am Rev Respir Dis* 139:806–817, 1989.

63. Sheppard D: Airway hyperresponsiveness: mechanisms in experimental models. *Chest* 96:1165–1168, 1989.

64. O'Bryne PM, Hargreave FE, Kirby JG: Airway inflammation and hyperresponsiveness. *Am Rev Respir Dis* 143:S35–S37, 1991.

65. Bigby TD, Nadel JA: Asthma. In Gallin JI, Goldstein IM, Snyderman R (eds): *Inflammation: Basic Principles and Clinical Correlates*, ed 2. New York, Raven Press, 1992, pp 889–906.

66. Herxheimer H: The late bronchial reaction in induced asthma. *Int Arch Allergy* 3:323–328, 1952.

67. Cartier A, Thomson NC, Frith PA, et al: Allergen-induced increase in bronchial responsiveness to histamine: relationship to the late asthmatic response and change in airway caliber. *J Allergy Clin Immunol* 70:170–177, 1982.

68. O'Bryne PM, Dolovich J, Hargreave FE: Late asthmatic responses. *Am Rev Respir Dis* 136:740–751, 1987.

69. Booij-Noord H, De Vries K, Sluiter HJ, et al: Late bronchial obstructive reaction to experimental inhalation of house dust extract. *Clin Allergy* 2:43–61, 1972.

70. Martin RJ, Cicutto LC, Smith HR, et al: Airway inflammation in nocturnal asthma. *Am Rev Respir Dis* 143:351–357, 1991.

71. Robinson DS, Hamid Q, Ying S, et al: Predominant T$_{H2}$-like bronchoalveolar T-lymphocyte population in atopic asthma. *N Engl J Med* 326:298–304, 1992.

72. Rochester CL, Rankin JA: Is asthma T-cell mediated? *Am Rev Respir Dis* 144:1005–1007, 1992.

73. Kay TB: Helper (CD4) T cells and eosinophils in allergy and asthma. *Am Rev Respir Dis* 14:S22–S26, 1992.

74. Kay AB: Origin of type 2 helper T cells. *N Engl J Med* 330:567–568, 1994.

75. Wilson JW, Djukanovic R, Howarth PH, Holgate ST: Lymphocyte activation in bronchoalveolar lavage and peripheral blood in atopic asthma. *Am Rev Respir Dis* 145:958–960, 1992.

76. Turner-Warwick M: Epidemiology of nocturnal asthma. *Am J Med* 85:6–8, 1988.

77. Glauser FL: Variant asthma. *Ann Allergy* 30:457, 1972.

78. McFadden ER: Exertional dyspnea and cough as preludes to acute attacks of bronchial asthma. *N Engl J Med* 292:555–559, 1975.

79. Corrao WM, Braman SS, Irwin RS: Chronic cough as the sole manifestation of bronchial asthma. *N Engl J Med* 300:633–637, 1979.

80. Hannaway PJ, Hopper GDK: Cough variant asthma in children. *JAMA* 247:206–208, 1982.

81. Johnson D, Osborn LM: Cough variant asthma: a review of the clinical literature. *J Asthma* 28(2):85–90, 1991.

82. Ellul-micallef R: Effect of terbutaline sulphate in chronic "allergic" cough. *Br Med J* 287:940, 1983.

83. Irwin RS, Corrao WM, Pratter MR: Chronic persistent cough in the adult: The spectrum and frequency of causes and successful outcome of specific therapy. *Am Rev Respir Dis* 123:413–417, 1981.

84. Christopher KL, Wood RP, Eckert RC, et al: Vocal-cord dysfunction presenting as asthma. *N Engl J Med* 308:1566–1570, 1983.

85. Downing ET, Braman SS, Fox MJ, et al: Factitious asthma: physiological approach to diagnosis. *JAMA* 248:2878–2881, 1982.

86. Miller RD, Hyatt RE: Evaluation of obstructing lesions of the trachea and larynx by flow-volume loops. *Am Rev Respir Dis* 108:475–481, 1973.

87. Kavuru MS, Eliachar I, Sivak ED: Management of the upper airway in the critically ill patient. In: Sivak ED, Higgins T, Seiver A, eds. *The High Risk Patient: Management of the Critically Ill*. Baltimore, Williams & Wilkins, 1995; pp 189–211.

88. Shim CS, Williams MH Jr: Relationship of wheezing to the severity of obstruction in asthma. *Arch Intern Med* 143:890–893, 1983.

89. McFadden ER, Kiser R, DeGroot WJ: Acute bronchial asthma: relations between clinical and physiologic manifestations. *N Engl J Med* 288:221–225, 1973.

90. FitzGerald JM, Hargreave FE: The assessment and management of acute life-threatening asthma. *Chest* 95:888–894, 1989.

91. Guidelines for the evaluation of impairment/disability

in patients with asthma. *Am Rev Respir Dis* 147: 1056–1061, 1993.

92. Toren K, Brisman J, Jarvholm B: Asthma and asthma-like symptoms in adults assessed by questionnaires: a literature review. *Chest* 104:600–608, 1993.

93. Juniper EF, Guyatt GH, Ferrie PJ, et al: Measuring quality of life in asthma. *Am Rev Respir Dis* 147:832–838, 1993.

94. McFadden ER Jr: Clinical-physiologic correlates in asthma. *J Allergy Clin Immunol* 77:1–5, 1986.

95. Shim CS, William MH: Evaluation of the severity of asthma: patients versus physicians. *Am J Med* 68:11–13, 1980.

96. Knowles GK, Clark TJH: Pulsus paradoxus as a valuable sign indicating severity of asthma. *Lancet* 11:1356–1359, 1973.

97. Rebuck AS, Pergelly LD: Development of pulsus paradoxus in the presence of airways obstruction. *N Engl J Med* 288:66–69, 1973.

98. Kelsen SG, Kelsen DP, Fleegler BF, et al: Emergency room assessment and treatment of patients with acute asthma: adequacy of the conventional approach. *Am J Med* 64:622–628, 1978.

99. Carden DL, Nowak RM, Sarkar D, et al: Vital signs including pulsus paradoxus in the assessment of acute bronchial asthma. *Ann Emerg Med* 12:80–83, 1983.

100. Wright BM, McKerrow CB: Maximum forced expiratory flow rate as a measure of ventilatory capacity: with a description of a new portable instrument for measuring it. *Br Med J* 2:1041–1047, 1959.

101. Berube D, Cartier A, L'Archeveque J, et al: Comparison of peak expiratory flow rate and $FEV_1$ in assessing bronchomotor tone after challenges with occupational sensitizers. *Chest* 99:831–836, 1991.

102. Clark NM, Evans D, Mellins RB: Patient use of peak flow monitoring. *Am Rev Respir Dis* 145:722–725, 1992.

103. Brenner BE: The acute asthmatic in the emergency department: the decision to admit or discharge. *Am J Emerg Med* 3:74–77, 1985.

104. Banner AS, Shah RS, Addington WW: Rapid prediction of need for hospitalization in acute asthma. *JAMA* 235:1337–1338, 1976.

105. Nowak RM, Gordon KR, Wroblewski DA, et al: Spirometric evaluation of acute bronchial asthma. *J Am Coll Emerg Phys* 8:9–12, 1979.

106. Lulla S, Newcomb RW: Emergency management of asthma in children. *Pediatrics* 97:346–350, 1980.

107. Nowak RM, Pensier MI, Sarkar DD, et al: Comparison of peak expiratory flow and $FEV_1$ admission criteria for acute bronchial asthma. *Ann Emerg Med* 11:64–69, 1982.

108. Fanta CH, Rossing TH, McFadden ER Jr: Emergency room treatment of acute asthma: Relationships among therapeutic combinations, severity of obstruction, and time course of response. *Am J Med* 72:416–422, 1982.

109. Fischl MA, Pitchenik A, Gardner LB: An index predicting relapse and need for hospitalization in patients with acute bronchial asthma. *N Engl J Med* 305:783–789, 1981.

110. Rose CC, Murphy JG, Schwartz JS: Performance of an index predicting the response of patients with acute bronchial asthma to intensive emergency department treatment. *N Engl J Med* 310:573–576, 1984.

111. Centor RM, Yarbrough B, Wood JP: Inability to predict relapse in acute asthma. *N Engl J Med* 310:577–580, 1984.

112. Gershel JC, Goldman HS, Stein REK, et al: The usefulness of chest radiographs in first asthma attacks. *N Engl J Med* 309:336–339, 1983.

113. McFadden ER Jr, Lyons HA: Arterial blood gas tension in asthma. *N Engl J Med* 278:1027–1032, 1968.

114. Franklin W: Treatment of severe asthma. *N Engl J Med* 290:1469–1472, 1974.

115. Jackson LK: Functional aspects of asthma. *Clin Chest Med* 5:573–587, 1984.

116. Hopewell PC, Miller RT: Pathophysiology and management of severe asthma. *Clin Chest Med* 5:623–634, 1984.

117. Nowak RM, et al: Arterial blood gases and pulmonary function testing in acute bronchial asthma. *JAMA* 249:2043–2046, 1983.

118. Pack AI: Acid: a nocturnal bronchoconstrictor? *Am Rev Respir Dis* 141:1391–1392, 1990.

119. Pope CE: Acid-reflux disorders. *N Engl J Med* 331:656–660, 1994.

120. Singh V, Jain NK: Asthma as a cause for, rather than a result of, gastroesophageal reflux. *J Asthma* 20:241–243, 1983.

121. Hubert D, Gaudric M, Guerre J, et al: Effect of theophylline on gastroesophageal reflux in patients with asthma. *J Allergy Clin Immunol* 81:1168–1174, 1988.

122. Ing AJ, Ngu MC, Breslin ABX: Pathogenesis of chronic persistent cough associated with gastroesophageal reflux. *Am J Respir Crit Care Med* 149:160–167, 1994.

123. Schan CA, Harding SM, Haile JM, et al: Gastroesophageal reflux-induced bronchoconstriction: an intraesophageal acid infusion study using state-of-the-art technology. *Chest* 106:731–737, 1994.

124. Mattox HE, Richter JE: Prolonged ambulatory esophageal pH monitoring in the evaluation of gastroesophageal reflux disease. *Am J Med* 89:345–356, 1990.

125. Perrin-Fayolle M, Gormand F, Braillon G, et al: Long-term results of surgical treatment of gastroesophageal reflux in asthmatic patients. *Chest* 96:40–45, 1989.

126. Larrain A, Carrasco E, Galleguillos F, et al: Medical and surgical treatment of nonallergic asthma associated with gastroesophageal reflux. *Chest* 99:1330–1335, 1991.

127. Meeker DP, Wiedemann HP: Drug-induced bronchospasm. *Clin Chest Med* 11(1):163–175, 1990.

128. Hannaway PJ, Hopper GDK: Severe anaphylaxis and drug-induced beta-blockade. *N Engl J Med* 308:1536, 1983.

129. Stoller JK, Elghazawi A, Mehta AC: Captopril-induced cough. *Chest* 93:659–661, 1988.

130. Hunt LW, Rosenow EC: Drug-induced asthma. In Weiss EB, Stein M (eds): *Bronchial Asthma: Mechanisms and Therapeutics*, ed 3. Boston, Little, Brown, 1993, pp 1099–1113.

131. Greenberger PA: Allergic bronchopulmonary aspergillosis and fungoses. *Clin Chest Med* 9:599–608, 1988.

132. Hinson KFW, Moon AJ, Plummer NS: Bronchopulmonary aspergillosis. *Thorax* 7:317–333, 1952.

133. Patterson R, Golbert TM: Hypersensitivity disease of the lung. *Univ Mich Med Cent J* 34:8–11, 1968.

134. Akiyama K, Ricketti AJ, Greenberger PA, et al: Identification of allergic bronchopulmonary aspergillosis in the United States. *Immunol Allergy Prac* 5:29–31, 1983.

135. Glimp RA, Bayer AS: Fungal pneumonias. Part 3: allergic bronchopulmonary aspergillosis. *Chest* 80:85–94, 1981.

136. Rosenberg M, Patterson R, Mintzer R, et al: Clinical and

immunologic criteria for the diagnosis of allergic bronchopulmonary aspergillosis. *Ann Intern Med* 80: 405–414, 1977.

137. Patterson R, Greenberger PA, Ricketti AJ, et al: A radioimmunoassay index for allergic bronchopulmonary aspergillosis. *Ann Intern Med* 99:18–22, 1983.

138. Greenberger PA, Patterson R: Application of enzyme-linked immunosorbent assay (ELISA) in diagnosis of allergic bronchopulmonary aspergillosis. *J Lab Clin Med* 99:288–293, 1982.

139. Greenberger PA, Patterson R: Allergic bronchopulmonary aspergillosis and the evaluation of the patient with asthma. *J Allergy Clin Immunol* 81:646–650, 1988.

140. Patterson R, Greenberger PA, Radin RC, et al: Allergic bronchopulmonary aspergillosis: staging as an aid to management. *Ann Intern Med* 96:286–291, 1982.

141. Safirstein BH, D'Souza MF, Simon G, et al: Five-year follow-up of allergic bronchopulmonary aspergillosis. *Am Rev Respir Dis* 108:450–460, 1973.

142. Nichols D, Dopico GA, Braun S, et al: Acute and chronic pulmonary function changes in allergic bronchopulmonary aspergillosis. *Am J Med* 67:631–637, 1979.

143. Patterson R, Greenberger PA, Halwig JM, et al: Allergic bronchopulmonary aspergillosis: natural history and classification of early disease by serologic and radiologic studies. *Arch Intern Med* 146:916–918, 1986.

144. Patterson R, Greenberger PA, Lee TM, et al: Prolonged evaluation of patients with corticosteroid-dependent asthma stage of bronchopulmonary aspergillosis. *J Allergy Clin Immunol* 80:663–668, 1987.

145. Ricketti AJ, Greenberger PA, Patterson R: Serum IgE as an important aid in management of allergic bronchopulmonary aspergillosis. *J Allergy Clin Immunol* 74:68–71, 1984.

146. Clark NM: Asthma self-management education: research and implications for clinical practice. *Chest* 95: 1110–1113, 1989.

147. Parker SR, Mellins RB, Sogn DD: Asthma education: a national strategy. *Am Rev Respir Dis* 140:848–853, 1989.

148. Mayo PH, Richman J, Harris W: Results of a program to reduce admissions for adult asthma. *Ann Intern Med* 112:864–871, 1990.

149. Reed CE, Hunt LW: The emergency visit and management of asthma. *Ann Intern Med* 112:801–802, 1990.

150. Wilson SR, Scamagas P, German DF, et al: A controlled trial of the two forms of self-management education for adults with asthma. *Am J Med* 94:564–576, 1993.

151. Tougaard L, Krone T, Sorknaes A, et al: Economic benefits of teaching patients with chronic obstructive pulmonary disease about their illness. *Lancet* 339:1617–1520, 1992.

152. Bailey WC, Richards JM, Brooks M, et al: A randomized trial to improve self-management practices of adults with asthma. *Arch Intern Med* 150:1664–1668, 1990.

153. Bolton MB, Tilley BC, Kuder J, et al: The cost and effectiveness of an education program for adults who have asthma. *J Gen Intern Med* 6:401–407, 1991.

154. Clark NM, Feldman CH, Evans D, et al: The impact of health education on frequency and cost of health care use by low income children with asthma. *J Allergy Clin Immunol* 78:108–115, 1986.

155. Hilton S, Sibbald B, Anderson HR, et al: Controlled evaluation of the effects of patient education on asthma morbidity in general practice. *Lancet* 1:26–29, 1986.

156. Yoon R, McKenzie DM, Miles DA, et al: Characteristics of attenders and non-attenders at an asthma education program. *Thorax* 46:886–890, 1991.

157. Dekker FW, Dieleman FE, Kaptein AA, et al: Compliance with pulmonary medication in general practice. *Eur Respir J* 6:886–890, 1993.

158. Shim C, Williams MH Jr: The adequacy of inhalation of aerosol from canister nebulizer. *Am J Med* 69:891–894, 1980.

159. Epstein SW, Manning CPR, Ashley MJ, et al: Survey of the clinical use of pressurized aerosol inhalers. *Can Med Assoc J* 120:813–816, 1979.

160. Appel D: Faulty use of canister nebulizers for asthma. *J Fam Pract* 14:1135–1139, 1982.

161. Kelling JS, Strohl KP, Smith RL, et al: Physician knowledge in the use of canister nebulizers. *Chest* 4:612–614, 1983.

162. Guidry CG, Brown WD, Stogner SW, et al: Incorrect use of metered dose inhalers by medical personnel. *Chest* 101:31–33, 1992.

163. Hanania NA, Wittman R, Kesten S, et al: Medical personnel's knowledge of and ability to use inhaling devices. *Chest* 105:111–116, 1994.

164. Tashkin DP, Rand C, Nides M, et al: A nebulizer chronolog to monitor compliance with inhaler use. *Am J Med* 91(Suppl 4A):33S–36S, 1991.

165. Dolovich M, Ruffin RE, Roberts R, et al: Optimal delivery of aerosols from metered dose inhalers. *Chest* 80(Suppl): 911–915, 1981.

166. Sackner MA, Kim CS: Auxillary MDI aerosol delivery systems. *Chest* 99(Suppl):161S–170S, 1985.

167. Shim CS, Williams MH Jr: Effect of bronchodilator administered by canister versus jet nebulizer. *J Allergy Clin Immunol* 73:387–390, 1984.

168. Turner JR, Corkery KJ, Eckman D, et al: Equivalence of continuous flow nebulizer and metered dose inhaler with reservoir bag for treatment of acute air flow obstruction. *Chest* 93:476–481, 1988.

169. Colacone A, Afilado M, Wolkove N, et al: A comparison of albuterol administered by metered dose inhaler (and holding chamber) or wet nebulizer in acute asthma. *Chest* 104:835–841, 1993.

170. Orens DK, Kester L, Fergus LC, et al: Cost impact of metered dose inhalers vs small volume nebulizers in hospitalized patients: The Cleveland Clinic Experience. *Respir Care* 36:1099–1104, 1991.

171. Sporik R, Holgate ST, Platts-Mills TAE, et al: Exposure to house-dust mite allergen (Der pI) and the development of asthma in childhood. *N Engl J Med* 323:502–507, 1990.

172. Call RS, Smith TF, Morris E, et al: Risk factors for asthma in inner city children. *J Pediatr* 121:862–866, 1992.

173. Gelber LE, Seltzer LH, Bouzoukis JK, et al: Sensitization and exposure to indoor allergens as risk factors for asthma among patients presenting to hospital. *Am Rev Respir Dis* 147:573–578, 1993.

174. Creticos PS: Immunotherapy with allergens. *JAMA* 268: 2834–2839, 1992.

175. Platts-Mills TAE: Allergen-specific treatment for asthma. *Am Rev Respir Dis* 148:553–555, 1993.

176. Platts-Mills TAE, de Week AL: Dust mite allergens and asthma—a worldwide problem. *J Allergy Clin Immunol* 83:416–427, 1989.

177. Platts-Mills TAE, Pollart SM, Chapman MD, et al: Role

of allergens in asthma and airway hyperresponsiveness: relevance to immunotherapy and allergen avoidance. In Kaliner MA, Barnes PJ, Persson CGA, (eds): *Asthma: Its Pathology and Treatment*. New York, Marcel Dekker, 1991, pp 595–631.

178. Hamilton RG, Chapman MD, Platts-Mills TAE, et al: House dust aeroallergen measurements in clinical practice: a guide to allergen-free home and work environments. *Immunol Allergy Pract* 14:96–112, 1992.

179. Kaliner M, Lemanske R: Rhinitis and asthma. *JAMA* 268: 2807–2829, 1992.

180. Lands AM, Arnold A, McAuliff JP, et al: Differentiation of receptor systems activated by sympathomimetic amines. *Nature* 214:597–598, 1967.

181. Popa VT: Clinical pharmacology of adrenergic drugs. *J Asthma* 21:183–207, 1984.

182. Newhouse MT: Emergency department management of life-threatening asthma. *Chest* 103:661–663, 1993.

183. Aerosol consensus statement. *Chest* 100:1106–1109, 1991.

184. Newman SP: Metered dose pressurized aerosols and the ozone layer. *Eur Respir J* 3:495–497, 1990.

185. Kerr RA: Ozone destruction worsens [news report]. *Science* 252:204, 1991.

186. Fisher DA, Hales CH, Wang WC, et al: Model calculations of the relative effects of CFCs and their replacement on global warming. *Nature* 344:513–516, 1990.

187. Epstein SW: Is the MDI doomed to extinction? *Chest* 103:1313, 1993.

188. Molina MJ, Rowland FS: Stratospheric risk for chlorofluoromethanes: chlorine atom-catalysed destruction of ozone. *Nature* 249:810–812, 1974.

189. Brown PH, Lenny J, Armstrong S, et al: Breath-actuated inhalers in chronic asthma: comparison of Diskhaler and Turbohaler for delivery of beta-agonists. *Eur Respir J* 5:1143–1145, 1992.

190. Newman SP, Weisz AWB, Talaee N, et al: Improvement of drug delivery with a breath activated pressurized aerosol for patients with poor inhaler technique. *Thorax* 46:712–716, 1991.

191. Moler FW, Hurwitz ME, Custer JR: Improvement in clinical asthma score and PaCO$_2$ in children with severe asthma treated with continuously nebulized terbutaline. *J Allergy Clin Immunol* 81:1101–1109, 1988.

192. Chipps BE, Blackney DA, Black LE, et al: Vortran high output extended aerosol respiratory therapy (HEART) for delivery of continuously nebulized terbutaline for the treatment of acute bronchospasm. *Pediatr Asthma Allergy & Immunol* 4(4):271–277, 1990.

193. Colacone A, Wolkove N, Stern E, et al: Continuous nebulization of albuterol (Salbutamol) in acute asthma. *Chest* 97:693–697, 1990.

194. Olshaker J, Jerrard D, Barish RA, et al: The efficacy and safety of a continuous albuterol protocol for the treatment of acute adult asthma attacks. *Am J Emerg Med* 11: 131–133, 1993.

195. Lin RY, Smith AJ, Hergenroeder P: High serum albuterol levels and tachycardia in adult asthmatics treated with high-dose continuously aerosolized albuterol. *Chest* 103:221–225, 1993.

196. Portnoy J, Nadel G, Amado M, Willsie-Ediger S: Continuous nebulization for status asthmaticus. *Ann Allergy* 69:71–79, 1992.

197. Shim C: Adrenergic agonists and bronchodilator aerosol therapy in asthma. *Clin Chest Med* 5:659–668, 1984.

198. Amory DW, Burham SC, Cheney FW Jr: Comparison of the cardiopulmonary effects of subcutaneously administered epinephrine and terbutaline in patients with reversible airway obstruction. *Chest* 67:279–286, 1975.

199. Jederlinic PJ, Irwin RS: Status asthmaticus. *Intensive Care Med* 4:166–184, 1989.

200. Parry WH, Martorano F, Colton EK: Management of life-threatening asthma with intravenous isoproterenol infusion. *Am J Dis Child* 130:39–42, 1976.

201. Lawford P, Jones BJM, Milledge JS: Comparison of intravenous and nebulized salbutamol in initial treatment of severe asthma. *Br Med J* 1:84, 1978.

202. Williams S, Seaton A: Intravenous or inhaled salbutamol in severe acute asthma? *Thorax* 32:555–558, 1977.

203. Nicklas RA: Paradoxical bronchospasm associated with the use of inhaled beta-agonists. *J Allergy Clin Immunol* 85:959–964, 1990.

204. Galant SP, Durisetti L, Underwood S, et al: Decreased beta-adrenergic receptors on polymorphonuclear leukocytes after adrenergic therapy. *N Engl J Med* 299: 933–936, 1978.

205. Cheung D, Timmers MC, Zwinderman AH, et al: Long-term effects of a long-acting $\beta_2$-adrenoceptor agonist, salmeterol, on airway hyperresponsiveness in patients with mild asthma. *N Engl J Med* 327:1198–1203, 1992.

206. Pearlman DS, Chervinsky P, LaForce C, et al: A comparison of salmeterol with albuterol in the treatment of mild-to-moderate asthma. *N Engl J Med* 327:1420–1425, 1992.

207. van Schayck CP, Graafsma SJ, Visch MB, et al: Increased bronchial hyperresponsiveness after inhaling salbutamol during one year is not caused by subsensitization to salbutamol. *J Allergy Clin Immunol* 86:793–800, 1990.

208. O'Callaghan C, Milner AD, Swarbrick A: Paradoxical deterioration in lung function after nebulized salbutamol in wheezy infants. *Lancet* 2:1424–1425, 1986.

209. Beasley R, Rafferty P, Holgate S: Paradoxical response to nebulized salbutamol in wheezy infants [letter]. *Thorax* 42:702, 1987.

210. Zhang G, Wright WJ, Tam WK, et al: Effect of inhaled preservatives on asthmatic subjects: benzalkonium chloride. *Am Rev Respir Dis* 141:1405–1408, 1990.

211. Koepke JW, Selner JC, Dunhill AL: Presence of sulfur dioxide in commonly used bronchodilator solutions. *J Allergy Clin Immunol* 72:504–508, 1983.

212. Koepke JW, Christopher KL, Chai H, et al: Dose-dependent bronchospasm from sulfites in isoetharine. *JAMA* 251:2982–2983, 1983.

213. Finnerty JP, Howarth PH: Paradoxical bronchoconstriction with nebulized albuterol but not with terbutaline. *Am Rev Respir Dis* 148:512–513, 1993.

214. Rossing TH: Methylxanthines in 1989. *Ann Intern Med* 110:502–504, 1989.

215. Lunell E, Andersson KE, Persson CG, et al: Intravenous enprofylline in asthma patients. *Eur J Respir Dis* 65: 28–34, 1984.

216. Bukowskyj M, Nakatsu K, Munt PW: Theophylline reassessed. *Ann Intern Med* 101:63–73, 1984.

217. Aubier M, DeTroyer A, Sampson M, et al: Aminophylline improves diaphragm contractility. *N Engl J Med* 305: 242–252, 1981.

218. Murciano D, Aubier M, Lecocguic Y, et al: Effects of

theophylline on diaphragmatic strength and fatigue in patients with chronic obstructive pulmonary disease. *N Engl J Med* 311:349–353, 1984.

219. Matthay RA, Berger HJ, Loke J, et al: Effects of aminophylline upon right and left ventricular performance in chronic obstructive pulmonary disease: noninvasive assessment by radionuclide angiocardiography. *Am J Med* 65:903–910, 1978.

220. Matthay RA, Berger HJ, Davis R, et al: Improvement in cardiac performance by oral long-acting theophylline in chronic obstructive pulmonary disease. *Am Heart J* 104: 1022–1026, 1982.

221. Lakshminarayan S, Sahn SA, Weil JV: The effect of aminophylline on ventilatory responses in normal man. *Am Rev Respir Dis* 117:33–38, 1978.

222. Mahler D, Matthay RA, Snyder PE, et al: Sustained-release theophylline reduces dyspnea in nonreversible obstructive airway disease. *Am Rev Respir Dis* 131: 22–25, 1985.

223. Ward AJ, McKenniff M, Evans JM, et al: Theophylline: an immunomodulatory role in asthma? *Am Rev Respir Dis* 147:518–523, 1993.

224. Lam A, Newhouse MT: Management of asthma and chronic airflow limitation: are methylxanthines obsolete. *Chest* 98:44–52, 1990.

225. Milgrom H, Bender B: Current issues in the use of theophylline. *Am Rev Respir Dis* 147:533–539, 1993.

226. British Thoracic Society: Guidelines for management of asthma in adults. *Br Med J* 301:651–653, 1990.

227. Rossing TH, Fanta CH, Goldstein, et al: Emergency therapy of asthma: comparison of the acute effects of parenteral and inhaled sympathomimetics and infused aminophylline. *Am Rev Respir Dis* 122:365–371, 1980.

228. Siegel D, Sheppard D, Gelb A, et al: Aminophylline increases the toxicity but not the efficacy of an inhaled beta-adrenergic agonist in the treatment of acute exacerbations of asthma. *Am Rev Respir Dis* 132:283–286, 1985.

229. Fanta CH, Rossing TH, McFadden ER, Jr: Treatment of acute asthma—is combination therapy with sympathomimetics and methylxanthines indicated? *Am J Med* 80: 5–10, 1986.

230. Littenberg B: Aminophylline treatment in severe, acute asthma: a meta-analysis. *JAMA* 259:1678–1684, 1988.

231. Self TH, Abou-Shala N, Burns R, et al: Inhaler albuterol and oral prednisone therapy in hospitalized adult asthmatics. Does aminophylline add any benefit? *Chest* 98: 1317–1321, 1990.

232. Wrenn K, Slovis CM, Murphy F, Greenberg RS: Aminophylline therapy for acute bronchospastic disease in the emergency room. *Ann Intern Med* 115:241–247, 1991.

233. McFadden ER: Methylxanthines in treatment of asthma: the rise, the fall, and the possible rise again (editorial). *Ann Intern Med* 115:323–324, 1991.

234. Huang D, O'Brien RG, Harman E, et al: Does aminophylline benefit adults admitted to the hospital for an acute exacerbation of asthma? *Ann Intern Med* 119: 1155–1160, 1993.

235. DiGiulio GA, Kercsmar CM, Krug SE, et al: Hospital treatment of asthma: lack of benefit from theophylline given in addition to nebulized albuterol and intravenously administered corticosteroid. *J Pediatr* 122: 464–469, 1993.

236. Carter E, Cruz M, Chesrown S, et al: Efficacy of intravenously administered theophylline in children hospitalized with severe asthma. *J Pediatr* 122:470–476, 1993.

237. Shim C, Williams MH Jr: Comparison of oral aminophylline and aerosol metaproterenol in asthma. *Am J Med* 71:452–455, 1981.

238. Leopold D, Handslip P: Additive interaction of aminophylline and salbutamol in asthma: an in vivo study using dose-response curves. *J Int Med Res* 7(Suppl 1): 52, 1979.

239. Smith JA, Weber RW, Nelson HS: Theophylline and aerosolized terbutaline in the treatment of bronchial asthma: double-blind comparison of optimal doses. *Chest* 78:816–818, 1980.

240. Wolfe JD, Tashkin CP, Calvarese B, et al: Bronchodilator effects of terbutaline and aminophylline alone and in combination in asthmatic patients. *N Engl J Med* 298: 363–367, 1978.

241. Nassif EG, Weinberger M, Thompson R, et al: The value of maintenance theophylline in steroid-dependent asthma. *N Engl J Med* 304:71–75, 1981.

242. Barnes PJ, Greening AP, Neville L, et al: Single-dose slo-release aminophylline at night prevents nocturnal asthma. *Lancet* 1:299–301, 1982.

243. Arkinstall WW, Atkins ME, Harrison D, et al: Once-daily sustained-release theophylline reduces diurnal variation in spirometry and symptomatology in adult asthmatics. *Am Rev Respir Dis* 135:316–321, 1987.

244. Tilles DS, Hales CA: Comparison of 12-hour and 24-hour sustained-release theophylline in outpatient management of asthma. *Chest* 91:370–375, 1987.

245. Mangura BT, Maniatis T, Abdel Rahman MS, et al: Bioavailability of a once daily-administered theophylline preparation: a comparison study. *Chest* 90:566–570, 1986.

246. Helm SG: Diurnal stabilization of asthma with once-daily evening administration of controlled-release theophylline: a multi-investigator study. *Immunol Allergy Pract* 9(11):414–419, 1987.

247. Schiff GD, Hegde HK, LaCloche L, Hryhorczuk DO: Inpatient theophylline toxicity: preventable factors. *Ann Intern Med* 114:748–753, 1991.

248. Zwillich CW, Sutton FD, Neff TA, et al: Theophylline-induced seizures in adults: correlation with serum concentrations. *Ann Intern Med* 82:784–787, 1975.

249. Hendeles L, Bighley L, Richardson RH, et al: Frequent toxicity from IV aminophylline infusions in critically ill patients. *Drug Intell Clin Pharm* 11:12–18, 1977.

250. Dutt AK, DeSoyza ND, Au WY, et al: The effect of aminophylline on cardiac rhythm in advanced chronic obstructive pulmonary disease: correlation with serum theophylline levels. *Eur J Respir Dis* 64:264–270, 1983.

251. Banner AS, Sunderrajan EV, Agarwal MK, et al: Arrhythmogenic effects of orally administered bronchodilators. *Arch Intern Med* 139:434–437, 1979.

252. Fleetham JA, Ginsburg JC, Nakatsu K, et al: Resin hemoperfusion as treatment for theophylline-induced seizures. *Chest* 75:741–742, 1979.

253. Berlinger WG, Spector R, Goldberg MJ, et al: Enhancement of theophylline clearance by oral activated charcoal. *Clin Pharmacol Ther* 33:351–354, 1983.

254. Shannon M: Predictors of major toxicity after theophylline overdose. *Ann Intern Med* 119:1161–1167, 1993.

255. Mann JS, George CF: Anticholinergic drugs in the treatment of airways disease. *Br J Dis Chest* 79:209–228, 1985.

256. Yeates DB, Aspin N, Levison H, et al: Mucociliary tracheal transport rates in man. *J Appl Physiol* 39:487–495, 1975.

257. Pavia D, Bateman JRM, Sheahan NF, et al: Effect of ipratropium bromide on mucociliary clearance and pulmonary function in reversible airways obstruction. *Thorax* 34:501–507, 1979.

258. Johns KA, Busse WW: Anticholinergic drugs: what role in asthma? *J Respir Dis* 10:35–50, 1989.

259. Schleuter DP, Neumann JL: Double blind comparison of bronchial and ventilation perfusion changes to Atrovent and isoproterenol. *Chest* 73:982–983, 1978.

260. Grandordy B, Thomas V, Marsac J: Compared bronchodilation after inhaled salbutamol and ipratropium bromide in asthma (abstract). *Am Rev Respir Dis* 129(part 2):A91, 1984.

261. Jindal SR, Malif SR: Clinical experience with terbutaline sulfate and ipratropium bromide in bronchial asthma. *Indian J Chest Dis Allied Sci* 21:130–133, 1979.

262. Storms WW, Bodman SF, Nathan RA, et al: Use of ipratropium bromide in asthma: results of a multi-clinic study. *Am J Med* 81(Suppl 5A):61–66, 1986.

263. Bruderman I, Cohen-Aronovski R, Smorzik J: A comparative study of various combinations of ipratropium bromide and metaproterenol in allergic asthmatic patients. *Chest* 83:208–210, 1983.

264. Ruffin RE, McIntyre E, Crockett AJ, et al: Combination bronchodilator therapy in asthma. *J Allergy Clin Immunol* 69:60–65, 1982.

265. McFadden ER Jr, Luparello T, Lyons H, et al: The mechanism of action of suggestion in the induction of acute asthma attacks. *Psychosom Med* 31:134–143, 1969.

266. Neild JE, Cameron IR: Bronchoconstriction in response to suggestion: its prevention by an inhaled anticholinergic agent. *Br Med J* 290:674, 1985.

267. Rebuck AS, Gent M, Chapman KR: Anticholinergic and sympathomimetic combination therapy of asthma. *J Allergy Clin Immunol* 71:317–323, 1983.

268. Karpel JP, Appel D, Briedbart D, et al: A comparison of atropine sulfate and metaproterenol sulfate in the emergency treatment of asthma. *Am Rev Respir Dis* 133:727–729, 1986.

269. Bryant DH: Nebulized ipratropium bromide in the treatment of acute asthma. *Chest* 88:24–29, 1985.

270. Ward MJ, McFarlane JT, Davies D, et al: A place for ipratropium bromide in the treatment of severe acute asthma. *Br J Dis Chest* 79:374, 1985.

271. Rebuck AS, Chapman KR, Abboud R, et al: Nebulized anticholinergic and sympathomimetic treatment of asthma and chronic obstructive airways disease in the emergency room. *Am J Med* 82:59–64, 1987.

272. Dunlap NE, Fulmer JD: Corticosteroid therapy in emphysema. *Clin Chest Med* 5:669–683, 1984.

273. Morris HG: Pharmacology of corticosteroids in asthma. In Middleton E, Reed CE, Ellis EF (eds): *Allergy: Principles and Practice*. St. Louis, CV Mosby, 1978.

274. Corticosteroids: their biologic mechanisms and application to the treatment of asthma. *Am Rev Respir Dis* 141(Suppl):1–96, 1990.

275. Barnes PJ, Pederson S: Efficacy and safety of inhaled corticosteroids in asthma. *Am Rev Respir Dis* 148:S1–S26, 1993.

276. Robinson D, Hamid Q, Ying S, et al: Prednisolone treatment in asthma is associated with modulation of bronchoalveolar lavage cell interleukin-4, interleukin-5, and interferon-γ cytokine expression. *Am Rev Respir Dis* 148:401–406, 1993.

277. McFadden ER: Dosages of corticosteroids in asthma. *Am Rev Respir Dis* 147:1306–1310, 1993.

278. Fanta CH, Rossing TH, McFadden ER: Glucocorticoid in acute asthma: a critical controlled trial. *Am J Med* 74:845–851, 1983.

279. Littenberg B, Gluck EH: A controlled trial of methylprednisolone in the emergency treatment of acute asthma. *N Engl J Med* 314:150–152, 1986.

280. Stein LM, Cole RP: Early administration of corticosteroids in emergency room treatment of acute asthma. *Ann Intern Med* 112:822–827, 1990.

281. McFadden ER, Kiser R, deGroot WJ, et al: A controlled study of the effects of single doses of hydrocortisone on the resolution of acute attacks of asthma. *Am J Med* 60:52–59, 1976.

282. Ogirala RG, Aldrich TK, Prezant DF, et al: High-dose intramuscular triamcinolone in severe, chronic, life-threatening asthma. *N Engl J Med* 324:585–589, 1991.

283. Haskell RJ, Wong BM, Hansen JE: A double-blind, randomized clinical trial of methylprednisolone in status asthmaticus. *Arch Intern Med* 143:1324–1327, 1983.

284. Lederle FA, Pluhar RE, Joseph AM, Niewoehner DE: Tapering of corticosteroid therapy following exacerbations of asthma. *Arch Intern Med* 147:2201–2203, 1987.

285. Vichyanond P, Irvin CG, Larsen GL, et al: Penetration of corticosteroids into the lung: evidence for a difference between methylprednisolone and prednisolone. *J Allergy Clin Immunol* 84:867–873, 1989.

286. Greos LS, Vichyanond P, Bloedow DC, et al: Methylprednisolone achieves greater concentrations in the lung than prednisolone. *Am Rev Respir Dis* 144:586–592, 1991.

287. Aelony Y: Non-invasive oral treatment of asthma in the emergency room. *Am J Med* 78:929–936, 1985.

288. Adinoff AD, Hollister JR: Steroid-induced fractures and bone loss in patients with asthma. *N Engl J Med* 309:265–268, 1983.

289. Dixon RB, Christy NP: On the various forms of corticosteroid withdrawal syndrome. *Am J Med* 68:224–230, 1980.

290. Scoggins CH, Petty TL: *Clinical Strategies in Asthma*. Philadelphia, Lea & Febiger, 1982.

291. Plumpton FS, Besser GM: The adrenocortical responses to surgery and insulin-induced hypoglycemia in corticosteroid-treated and normal subjects. *Br J Surg* 56:216–219, 1969.

292. Laitinen LA, Laitinen A, Haahtela T: A comparative study of the effects of an inhaled corticosteroid, budesonide, and a β₂-agonist, terbutaline on airway inflammation in newly diagnosed asthma: a randomized double-blind, parallel-group controlled trial. *J Allergy Clin Immunol* 90:32–42, 1992.

293. Djukanovic R, Wilson JW, Britten YM, et al: Effect of an inhaled corticosteroid on airway inflammation and symptoms of asthma. *Am Rev Respir Dis* 145:699, 1992.

294. Jeffrey PK, Godfrey RW, Adelroth E, et al: Effect of treatment on airway inflammation and thickening of basement membrane reticular collagen in asthma. *Am Rev Respir Dis* 145:890–899, 1992.

295. Lungren R, Soderberg M, Horstedt P, et al: Morphological studies on bronchial mucosal biopsies from asthmatics before and after ten years treatment with inhaled steroids. *Eur Respir J* 1:883–889, 1988.

296. Juniper EF, Kline PA, Vanzieleghem MA, et al: Effect

of long-term treatment with an inhaled corticosteroid (Budesonide) on airway hyperresponsiveness and clinical asthma in non–steroid dependent asthmatics. *Am Rev Respir Dis* 142:832–836, 1990.

297. Juniper EF, Kline PA, van Zieleshem MA, et al: Long-term effects of budesonide on airway responsiveness and clinical asthma severity in inhaled steroid-dependent asthmatics. *Eur Respir J* 3:1122–1127, 1990.

298. Li JTC, Reed CE: Proper use of aerosol corticosteroids to control asthma. *Mayo Clin Proc* 64:205–210, 1989.

299. Geddes DM: Inhaled corticosteroids: benefits and risks. *Thorax* 47:404–407, 1992.

300. Haahtela T, Jarvinen M, Kava T, et al: Comparison of a $\beta_2$-agonist, terbutaline, with an inhaled corticosteroid, budesonide, in newly detected asthma. *N Engl J Med* 325:388–392, 1991.

301. Kertjens HAM, Brand PLP, Hughes MD, et al: A comparison of bronchodilator therapy with or without inhaled corticosteroid therapy for obstructive airways disease. *N Engl J Med* 327:1413–1419, 1992.

302. Dompeling E, van Schayck CP, van Grunsven PM, et al: Slowing the deterioration of asthma and chronic obstructive pulmonary disease observed during bronchodilator therapy by adding inhaled corticosteroids. *Ann Intern Med* 188:770–778, 1993.

303. Meltzer EO, Kemp JP, Orgel A, Izu AE: Flunisolide aerosol for treatment of severe, chronic asthma in steroid-independent children. *Pediatrics* 69:340–345, 1982.

304. Smith MJ, Hodson ME: High-dose beclomethasone inhaler in the treatment of asthma. *Lancet* 1:265–269, 1983.

305. Toogood JH: High dose inhaled steroid therapy for asthma. *J Allergy Clin Immunol* 83:528–536, 1989.

306. Laursen LC, Taudorf E, Weeke B: High-dose inhaled budesonide in treatment of severe steroid-dependent asthma. *Eur J Respir Dis* 68:19–28, 1986.

307. Tarlo SM, Broder I, Davies GM, et al: Six-month double-blind controlled trial of high dose, concentrated beclomethasone dipropionate in the treatment of severe chronic asthma. *Chest* 93:998–1002, 1988.

308. Barnes PJ: Inflammatory mechanisms and nocturnal asthma. *Am J Med* 85 (suppl 1B): 64–70, 1988.

309. Toogood JH: Complications of topical steroid therapy for asthma. *Am Rev Respir Dis* 141:S89–S96, 1990.

310. Lipworth BJ: Clinical pharmacology of corticosteroids in bronchial asthma. *Pharmacol Ther* 58:173–209, 1993.

311. Breslin ABX: New developments in anti-asthma drugs. *Med J Aust* 158:779–782, 1993.

312. Newman SP, Moren F, Pavia D, et al: Deposition of pressurized suspension aerosols inhaled through extension devices. *Am Rev Respir Dis* 124:317–320, 1981.

313. Allen MB, Ray SG, Leitch AG, et al: Steroid aerosols and cataract formation. *Br Med J* 299:432–433, 1989.

314. Luengo M, Picado C, Del Rio L, et al: Vertebral fractures in steroid dependent asthma and involutional osteoporosis: a comparative study. *Thorax* 46:803–806, 1991.

315. Patalano F, Ruggieri F: Sodium cromoglycate: a review. *Eur Respir J* 2:556S–560S, 1989.

316. Kuzemko JA: Twenty years of sodium cromoglycate treatment: a short review. *Respir Med* 83(Suppl):11–16, 1989.

317. Murphy S, Kelly HW: Cromolyn sodium: a review of mechanisms and clinical use in asthma. *Drug Intell Clin Pharm* 21:22–35, 1987.

318. Toogood JH, Jennings B, Lefcol NM: A clinical trial of combined cromolyn/beclomethasone treatment for chronic asthma. *J Pediatr* 67:317–324, 1981.

319. Edwards AM, Stevens MT: The clinical efficacy of inhaled nedocromil sodium (Tilade) in the treatment of asthma. *Eur Respir J* 6:35–41, 1993.

320. Callaghan B, Teo NC, Clancy L: Effects of the addition of nedocromil sodium to maintenance bronchodilator therapy in the management of chronic asthma. *Chest* 101:787–792, 1992.

321. North American Tilade Study Group: A double-blind multicenter group comparative study of the efficacy and safety of nedocromil sodium in the management of asthma. *Chest* 97:1299–1306, 1990.

322. De Jong JW, Teengs JP, Postma DS, et al: Nedocromil sodium versus albuterol in the management of allergic asthma. *Am J Respir Crit Care Med* 149:91–97, 1994.

323. Geddes DM, Turner-Warnick M, Brewis RAL, et al: Nedocromil sodium workshop. *Respir Med* 83:265–267.

324. O'Byrne RM: Is nedocromil sodium effective treatment for asthma? [editorial] *Eur Respir J* 6:5–6, 1993.

325. Bel EH, Timmers MC, Hermans J, et al: The long term effects of nedocromil sodium and beclomethasone dipropionate on bronchial responsiveness to methacholine in nonatopic asthmatic subjects. *Am Rev Respir Dis* 141:21–28, 1990.

326. Svendsen UG, Jorgensen H: Inhaled nedocromil sodium as additional treatment to high dose inhaled corticosteroids in the management of bronchial asthma. *Eur Respir J* 4:992–999, 1991.

327. Wong CS, Cooper S, Britton JR, et al: Steroid sparing effect of nedocromil sodium in asthmatic patients taking high doses of inhaled steroids. *Thorax* 46:768P–769P, 1991.

328. Kemp JP: Approaches to asthma management. *Arch Intern Med* 153:805–828, 1993.

329. Mullarkey MF, Blumenstein BA, Andrade WP, et al: Methotrexate in the treatment of corticosteroid dependent asthma. A double-blind crossover study. *N Engl J Med* 318:603–606, 1988.

330. Erzurum SC, Leff JA, Cochran JE, et al: Lack of benefit of methotrexate in severe steroid dependent asthma. *Ann Intern Med* 114:353–360, 1991.

331. Carmichael J, Paterson IC, Diaz P, et al: Corticosteroid resistance in chronic asthma. *Br Med J* 282:1419–1422, 1981.

332. Dykewicz MS, Greenberger PA, Patterson R, et al: Natural history of asthma in patients requiring long-term systemic corticosteroids. *Arch Intern Med* 146:2369–2372, 1986.

333. Corrigan CJ, Brown PH, Barnes NC, et al: Glucocorticoid resistance in chronic asthma. *Am Rev Respir Dis* 144:1016–1032, 1991.

334. NIH conference: Syndromes of glucocorticoid resistance. Moderator: Chrousos GP. *Ann Intern Med* 119:1113–1124, 1994.

335. Barnes PJ: New drugs for asthma. *Eur Respir J* 5:1126–1136, 1992.

336. Lane DJ, Lane TV: Alternative and complementary medicine for asthma. *Thorax* 46:787–797, 1991.

337. Schwartz YA, Kinity S, Ilfeld DN, et al: A clinical and immunologic study of colchicine in asthma. *J Allergy Clin Immunol* 85:578–582, 1990.

338. Mazer BD, Gelfand EW: An open-label study of high-dose intravenous immunoglobulin in severe childhood asthma. *J Allergy Clin Immunol* 87:976–983, 1991.

339. Mullarkey MF, Lammert JK, Blumenstein BA: Long-term methotrexate treatment in steroid dependent asthma. *Ann Intern Med* 112:577–581, 1990.

340. Dyer P, Vaughan T, Weber R: Methotrexate in the treatment of steroid-dependent asthma. *J Allergy Clin Immunol* 88:208–212, 1991.

341. Shiner RJ, Nunn AJ, Chung KF, et al: Randomized, double-blind, placebo controlled trial of methotrexate in steroid dependent asthma. *Lancet* 336:137–140, 1990.

342. Coffey MJ, Sanders G, Eschenbacher WL, et al: The role of methotrexate in the management of steroid-dependent asthma. *Chest* 105:117–121, 1994.

343. Bernstein DI, Bernstein IL, Bodenheimer SS, et al: An open study of auranofin in the treatment of steroid dependent asthma. *J Allergy Clin Immunol* 81:6–16, 1988.

344. Nierop G, Gijzel WP, Bel EH, et al: Auranofin in the treatment of steroid dependent asthma: a double blind study. *Thorax* 47:349–354, 1992.

345. Muranaka M, Miyamoto T, Shida T, et al: Gold salts in the treatment of bronchial asthma—a double-blind study. *Ann Allergy* 40:132–137, 1978.

346. Klaustermeyer WB, Noritake DT, Kwong FK: Chrysotherapy in the treatment of corticosteroid dependent asthma. *J Allergy Clin Immunol* 79:720–725, 1987.

347. Spector SL, Katz FH, Farr RS: Troleandomycin: Effectiveness in steroid dependent asthma. *J Allergy Clin Immunol* 54:367–379, 1974.

348. Szefler SJ, Rose JQ, Elliott EF, et al: The effect of troleandomycin on methylprednisolone elimination. *J Allergy Clin Immunol* 66:447–451, 1980.

349. Zeiger RS, Schatz M, Sperling W, et al: Efficacy of troleandomycin in outpatients with severe, corticosteroid-dependent asthma. *J Allergy Clin Immunol* 66:438–446, 1980.

350. Wald JA, Friedman BF, Farr RS: An improved protocol for the use of troleandomycin in the treatment of steroid requiring asthma. *J Allergy Clin Immunol* 78:36–43, 1986.

351. Kamada AK, Hill MR, Ikhe DN, et al: Efficacy and safety of low-dose troleandomycin therapy in children with severe, steroid-requiring asthma. *J Allergy Clin Immunol* 91:873–882, 1993.

352. Nelson HS, Hamilos DL, Corsello PR, et al: A double-blind study of troleandomycin and methylprednisolone in asthmatic subjects who require daily corticosteroids. *Am Rev Respir Dis* 147:398–404, 1993.

353. Calderon E, Lockey RF, Bukantz SC, et al: Is there a role for cyclosporine in asthma? *J Allergy Clin Immunol* 89:629–636, 1992.

354. Finnerty NA, Sullivan TJ: Effect of cyclosporine on corticosteroid-dependent asthma [abstract]. *J Allergy Clin Immunol* 87:297, 1991.

355. Alexander AG, Barnes NC, Kay AB: Trial of cyclosporin in corticosteroid dependent chronic severe asthma. *Lancet* 339:324–327, 1992.

356. Holtzman MJ: Arachidonic acid metabolism. *Am Rev Respir Dis* 143:188–203, 1991.

357. Samuelsson B, Dahlen SE, Lindgren JA, Rouzer CA, Serhan CN: Leukotrienes and lipoxins: structures, biosynthesis, and biological effects. *Science* 237:1171–1176, 1987.

358. Drazen JM, Austen KF: Leukotrienes and airway responses. *Am Rev Respir Dis* 136:985–998, 1987.

359. Drazen JM: Inhalation challenge with sulfidopeptide leukotrienes in human subjects. *Chest* 89:414–419, 1986.

360. Drazen JM, O'Brien JB, Sparrow D, Weiss ST, Martins MA, Israel JE, et al: Recovery of leukotriene $E_4$ from the urine of patients with airway obstruction. *Am Rev Respir Dis* 146:104–108, 1992.

361. Smith CM, Hawksworth FCK, Thien PE, et al: Urinary leukotriene $E_4$ in bronchial asthma. *Eur Respir J* 5:693–699, 1992.

362. Busse WW, Gaddy JN: The role of leukotriene antagonists and inhibitors in the treatment of airway disease. *Am Rev Respir Dis* 143:S103–S107, 1991.

363. Cloud ML, Enas GC, Kemp J, Platts-Mills T, Altman LC, Townley R, et al: A specific LTD4/LTE4-receptor antagonist improves pulmonary function in patients with mild, chronic asthma. *Am Rev Respir Dis* 140:1336–1339, 1989.

364. Taylor IK, O'Shaughnessy KM, Fuller RW, Dollery CT: Effect of cysteinyl-leukotriene receptor antagonist ICI 204.219 on allergen-induced bronchoconstriction and airway hyperreactivity in atopic subjects. *Lancet* 337:690–694, 1991.

365. Manning PJ, Watson RM, Margolskee DJ, Williams VC, Schwartz JI, O'Bryne PM: Inhibition of exercise-induced bronchoconstriction by MK-571, a potent leukotriene D4-receptor antagonist. *N Engl J Med* 323:1736–1739, 1990.

366. Israel E, Dermarkarian R, Rosenberg M, Sperling R, Taylor G, Rubin P, et al: The effects of 5-lipoxygenase inhibitor on asthma induced by cold, dry air. *N Engl J Med* 323:1740–1744, 1990.

367. Dahlen B, Kumlin M, Margolskee DJ, et al: The leukotriene-receptor antagonist MK-0679 blocks airway obstruction induced by inhaled lysine-aspirin in aspirin-sensitive asthmatics. *Eur Respir J* 6:1018–1026, 1993.

368. Israel E, Rubin P, Kemp JP, et al: The effect of inhibition of 5-lipoxygenase by zileuton in mild-to-moderate asthma. *Ann Intern Med* 119:1059–1066, 1993.

369. Asthma: the important questions, part 2. *Am Rev Respir Dis (Suppl)* 146:1249–1366, 1992.

Chapter **10**

# Chronic Obstructive Lung Diseases:
## Emphysema, Chronic Bronchitis, Bronchiectasis, and Cystic Fibrosis

## James K. Stoller
## Loutfi S. Aboussouan

THE TERM "chronic obstructive pulmonary disease" (COPD) describes a heterogeneous and overlapping group of disorders. Indeed, standards of the American Thoracic Society define COPD as "a disorder characterized by abnormal tests of expiratory flow (structural or functional) that do not change markedly over periods of several months' observation" (1). As such, this definition subsumes chronic bronchitis (a clinical diagnosis), emphysema (a pathological diagnosis), and peripheral airway disease, but excludes specific causes of air flow obstruction such as bronchiectasis or cystic fibrosis.

In addressing the issue of chronic obstructive lung diseases, this chapter considers a broader spectrum of COPD, and includes bronchiectasis and cystic fibrosis. As a background to this discussion and rationale for the broader focus of this chapter, it is noteworthy that "COPD and allied conditions" (subsuming emphysema, chronic bronchitis, asthma, bronchiectasis, and hypersensitivity pneumonitis) have recently been ranked the fourth leading cause of death among Americans, rising from their prior fifth ranking and surpassing accidental deaths for the first time (2).

This chapter first considers definitions of COPD, then turns to epidemiology, pathology, and current theories of pathogenesis. Attention then turns to diagnosis, prognosis, and treatment of COPD. Finally, bronchiectasis and cystic fibrosis are addressed.

## EMPHYSEMA AND CHRONIC BRONCHITIS

### DEFINITIONS

Various consensus panels have defined chronic bronchitis and emphysema (1, 3–6).

### Chronic Bronchitis

The clinical hallmarks of chronic bronchitis are chronic mucus hypersecretion and cough, and these features are reflected in all of the available definitions. Perhaps the most widely used of these is the American Thoracic Society (ATS) definition (1, 4), which further specifies the duration of symptoms as "persistence of cough and excessive mucus secretion for most days out of 3 months in at least 2 successive years." In contrast to the definition of emphysema, the definition of chronic bronchitis omits any specific pathologic feature, though mucous gland hypertrophy is sometimes suggested. Also, air flow obstruction is not a requisite part of the definition of chronic bronchitis, though air flow obstruction is frequently present in such patients. The last key feature of the definition of chronic bronchitis is that it excludes clinical conditions that could also give rise to chronic cough and phlegm production but that are not chronic bronchitis (6); for example, lung cancer, tuberculosis, and chronic congestive heart failure.

### Emphysema

Definitions of emphysema have evolved since the first symposium convened to formulate a definition in 1959 (1, 3–6), but all available definitions specify pathologic rather than clinical features as diagnostic criteria. Key pathologic features of emphysema include air space enlargement beyond the terminal bronchiole and destruction of the alveolar wall. Refinements of the earlier 1962 ATS definition (4) have included specifying that the air space enlargement is permanent and that fibrosis is not a feature of true emphysema (1, 3).

Respiratory air space enlargement subsumes both emphysema alone and other entities in which acini are generally enlarged but not on the basis of alveolar destruction (e.g., Down's syndrome, congenital lobar overinflation, and so-called "senile" emphysema). Air space enlargement may also occur when adjacent areas of fibrosis cause traction on alveolar walls, though frank destruction may not be present. Though previously called "paracicatricial emphysema," the stricter criteria of the 1985 ATS definition (3) exclude air space enlargement due to fibrosis from the spectrum of emphysema.

"Senile" and "paracicatricial" emphysema no longer satisfy diagnostic criteria for emphysema, but three anatomic categories of emphysema are recognized (7, 8), based on the pattern of destruction within the acinus. These three pathologic types of emphysema are centriacinar emphysema (also known as centrilobular or proximal acinar emphysema), panacinar emphysema, and paraseptal or distal acinar emphysema. Considerable overlap between these subtypes may exist, especially when emphysema is advanced (8), but to the extent that purer forms of these subtypes can be recognized clinically and may have specific diagnostic and therapeutic implications, the distinction seems justified.

Centriacinar (or proximal acinar) emphysema implies central emphysema, with enlargement of the proximal portion of the acinus, the respiratory bronchiole. Usually, centriacinar emphysema results from long-term cigarette smoking and begins in the upper lung zones on the chest radiograph. In contrast, panacinar emphysema involves the whole acinus and is classically associated with $\alpha_1$-antitrypsin deficiency. Unlike centriacinar emphysema, panacinar emphysema may be most apparent in the bases of the lung on the chest radiograph. Finally, as the name implies, distal acinar (or paraseptal) emphysema has a different distribution, with involvement of the alveolar ducts and sacs farther out in the acinus. To the extent that these more distal acinar elements abut the pleura, paraseptal emphysema may present as pneumothorax, as in the spontaneous pneumothorax that can occur in young patients. Also, because air-conducting elements of the airways are spared in the distal acinar form, emphysema can be extensive with little accompanying air flow obstruction.

Although these subclasses of emphysema do permit some clinically useful distinctions, diagnosing emphysema on clinical grounds poses the difficult task of recognizing *clinical* features deemed to reflect the *pathologic* features that define emphysema. As is discussed in subsequent sections, clinical methods (e.g., physical examination, pulmonary function tests, and chest radiographs) often fall short of this goal.

### Epidemiology of Chronic Bronchitis and Emphysema

With over 14.1 million Americans currently afflicted, chronic obstructive pulmonary disease (as considered in this chapter, i.e., excluding asthma) remains common in the United States and has substantial associated morbidity and mortality.

Data from the National Health Interview Survey

(NHIS) of 1991 suggest that chronic bronchitis is the most prevalent cause of COPD among these conditions (12.5 million Americans or 50.5/1000 persons), followed by emphysema (1.6 million Americans or 6.6/1000 persons) (9).

Trends over the past two decades suggest a 60.4% increase in the prevalence of COPD through 1987. Individually, the prevalence of chronic bronchitis increased by 52%, emphysema increased by 34.8%, and asthma by 19.9% (10). However, more recent data from the NHIS indicate a 20% decrease in the prevalence of emphysema between 1990 and 1991 (from 8.2 cases/1000 Americans in 1990 to 6.6/1000 in 1991), while the prevalence of chronic bronchitis has remained stable (51.5/1000 in 1990 and 50.5/1000 in 1991) (9, 11).

In 1991, chronic obstructive lung disease (including asthma, bronchiectasis, and hypersensitivity pneumonitis) became the fourth leading cause of death of Americans, surpassing accidents, which had been the fourth leading cause between 1979 and 1990 (2). Chronic obstructive pulmonary disease now accounts for 4.2% of all deaths in 1991 (90,650 individuals), and an age-adjusted mortality rate of 20.1/100,000 persons in 1991 (Fig. 10.1). Mortality trends suggest recent increases in age-adjusted mortality from COPD (which has risen by 37.7% from 1979 to 1991), in contrast to declining mortality trends from other leading causes of death, for example, heart and cerebrovascular disease (Fig. 10.2). Among specific causes of age-adjusted death rates, emphysema (3.8/100,000) surpasses chronic bronchitis (0.8/100,000) and asthma (1.5/100,000). Also, in contrast to asthma, which shows relatively flat age-specific mortality rates with advancing

**TABLE 10.1**

**COPD AND ASTHMA: AGE-SPECIFIC PREVALENCE RATES PER 1000 PERSONS, 1991**

| Age Group | Chronic Bronchitis | Emphysema | Asthma |
|-----------|--------------------|-----------|--------|
| Total rate | 50.5 | 6.6 | 47.2 |
| <18 | 53.1 | [a] | 62.5 |
| 18–44 | 46.7 | 0.6[b] | 43.4 |
| 45–64 | 53.9 | 12.8 | 40.7 |
| 65+ | 52.5 | 32.4 | 52.5 |

Adapted from Adams PF, Benson V. Current estimates from the National Health Interview Survey, 1991. *Vital Health Stat* 10(184), 1992.

[a] No cases in sample.

[b] Estimate for which the numerator has a relative standard error of more than 30%.

age, death rates from COPD rise sharply with advancing age to a peak rate of 26.6/100,000 for chronic bronchitis and 60.8/100,000 for emphysema among Americans older than 85 years (2).

In addition to the substantial mortality and morbidity impact of these diseases, the economic impact of COPD in the United States is striking. The total 1986 cost of all lung diseases collectively was $40.9 billion, with COPD (23.5%) second only to lung cancer (26.4%) as the largest component (10).

Finally, data from the National Health Interview Survey clarify the demographic and geographic patterns of COPD in the United States. As shown in Table 10.1, chronic bronchitis and asthma are diseases of all ages, with fairly even distribution across age strata. In contrast, emphysema is a disease of the elderly, with 59.6% of all cases occurring in patients over 65 years and 96.2% of all cases occurring in patients over 45 years. Emphysema and chronic bronchitis also differ in gender distribution, with greater frequency of chronic bronchitis among women than men and greater prevalence of emphysema among men than women (9).

Racial differences between chronic bronchitis and emphysema are less striking, with age-specific increases in both blacks and whites. Overall, both diseases are more common among white than black persons. Geographic patterns of occurrence also differ for chronic bronchitis and emphysema. Chronic bronchitis has the greatest prevalence in the Midwest (55.8 cases/1000 Americans), followed by the Northeast (52.8/1000), the South (48.2/1000), and finally the West (46.0/1000). Emphysema is least common in the West (4.8/1000) and most common in the southern United States (7.9/1000) (9).

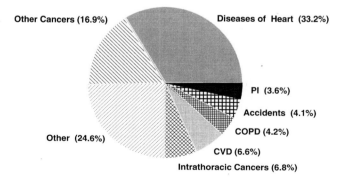

**FIGURE 10.1.** Leading causes of death, 1991. *CVD,* cerebrovascular disease; *PI,* pneumonia and influenza; *COPD,* COPD and allied conditions (includes asthma). (Data from National Center for Health Statistics: Advance report of final mortality statistics, 1991. *Monthly Vital Statistics Report* 42[2] [suppl], 1993.)

Other Cancers (16.9%)

Diseases of Heart (33.2%)

PI (3.6%)

Accidents (4.1%)

COPD (4.2%)

Other (24.6%)

CVD (6.6%)

Intrathoracic Cancers (6.8%)

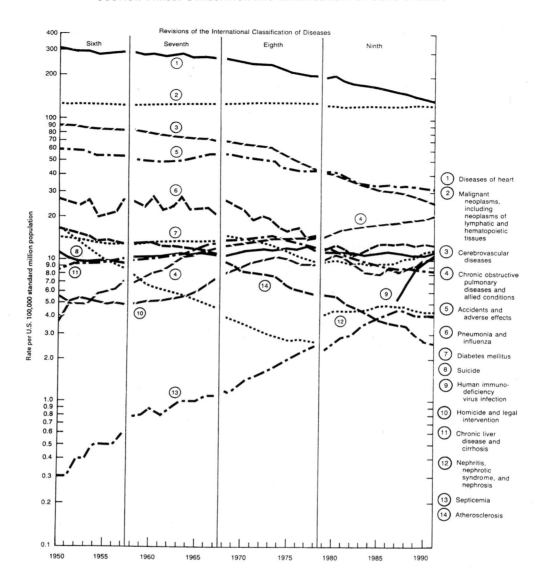

**FIGURE 10.2.** Leading causes of death, 1950–1991. COPD and allied conditions includes asthma. (Data from National Center for Health Statistics: Advance report of final mortality statistics, 1991. *Monthly Vital Statistics Report* 42[2] [Suppl], 1993.)

## PATHOLOGY OF CHRONIC BRONCHITIS AND EMPHYSEMA

### Chronic Bronchitis

Cardinal pathologic features of chronic bronchitis (8, 12–15) include

1. Enlargement of the mucus-secreting elements in the airways,
2. A disproportionate increase in the fraction of mucous versus serous glands
3. Accumulation of mucus in the small airways,
4. Narrowing and inflammation (i.e., bronchiolitis) of small (2-mm diameter or smaller) airways,

5. Development of bronchoscopically visible diverticula in the airways, and
6. Colonization of normally sterile airways with bacteria, often *Streptococcus pneumoniae, Haemophilus influenzae,* and *Moraxella catarrhalis.*

Enlargement of the mucus-secreting elements consists of an increase both in the number of glands and in their size (hypertrophy), characterized by dilation of the ducts and enlargement of the secretory cells (Fig. 10.3). The magnitude of glandular hypertrophy has been studied extensively (12–14) and was first quantified by the Reid index (Fig. 10.4), which compares the

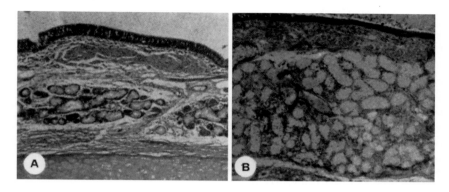

**FIGURE 10.3.** **A,** Normal bronchus. The epithelium (*top*) is delicately ciliated pseudostratified columnar. The basement membrane is thin. The gland layer occupies about one-third of the distance from cartilage to epithelium and is composed of about equal numbers of mucous (*clear*) and serous (*solid*) acini (hematoxylin and eosin stain; original magnification, ×50). **B,** Bronchial mucous gland hyperplasia. The epithelium is partly occupied by patches of metaplastic squamous epithelium, and the basement membrane is thickened. The bronchial wall is thickened and the lumen narrowed by an increased gland layer that occupies about three-fourths of the wall thickness and is composed mostly of mucous acini (hematoxylin and eosin stain; original magnification, ×50). (From Mitchell RS, Ryan SF, Petty TL, Filley GF: The significance of morphologic chronic hyperplastic bronchitis. Reprinted with permission of the *American Review of Respiratory Disease* 93:720–729, 1966.)

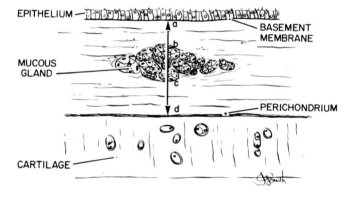

**FIGURE 10.4.** The Reid index is calculated by measuring the maximum thickness of a bronchial seromucous gland internal to the cartilage (*b–c*) and dividing this by the bronchial wall thickness. The latter is the distance from basement membrane to inner perichondrium (*a–d*). (From Thurlbeck WM: Chronic obstructive lung disease. In Sommers SC [ed]: *Pathology Annual.* East Norwalk, CT, Appleton-Century-Crofts, 3:367–398, 1968.)

ratio of gland thickness to bronchial wall thickness and, as originally described, permitted a distinction between normal non-bronchitic subjects (mean Reid index 0.26, range 0.14 to 0.36) and patients with chronic bronchitis (mean Reid index 0.59, range 0.41 to 0.79). Although initial reports suggested that the Reid index permitted clear-cut separation of non- bronchitics from bronchitic patients with no overlap, subsequent studies by Thurlbeck (8) have suggested that the Reid index displays a unimodal distribution and therefore fails to discretely separate bronchitic patients from non-bronchitics. Although overlap exists between the two populations in these more recent studies, these investigations do confirm that, in aggregate, chronic bronchitics have a higher Reid index than non-bronchitics (i.e., mean Reid index of 0.52 versus 0.44). Besides the Reid index, other systems for pathologic grading of chronic bronchitis include the proportional area of the bronchus occupied by mucous glands and the thickness and area of the mucous glands, but these have not been found to be as useful as the Reid index.

A second cardinal pathologic feature of chronic bronchitis is the disproportionate increase in the number of the mucous versus serous glands in the airways. For example, Thurlbeck observed that in non-bronchitics, mucous secreting cells accounted for 39% of the volume of the bronchial gland (range 16 to 55%), whereas in patients with chronic bronchitis, the proportion increased to 48% (range 26 to 62%) (8, 12). Another glandular element is the goblet cell, which is less common than either mucous or serous glands (i.e., 1% or less of the total glandular population) and is found more distally in the airways. Reports about goblet cell hyperplasia in chronic bronchitis are conflicting.

Airway obstruction by mucus is another pathologic feature of chronic bronchitis, and postmortem studies of patients with both chronic bronchitis and emphysema suggest an eightfold increase in airway mucus above normal (approximately 1.0 ml of mucus is found in the normal airways) (7, 8).

Narrowing and inflammation of small airways and a deficit of small airways with specific size ranges are also pathologic features in chronic bronchitis (14). For example, careful postmortem studies suggest that the average small airway diameter decreases in chronic bronchitis (0.66 mm versus 0.81 mm) and that this narrowing causes a loss of small airway cross-sectional lumen from 1.43% of the total lung volume to 1.09%, as well as a deficit of airways between 0.6 and 2.0 mm in diameter.

The development of bronchoscopically visible diverticula in the walls of the airways is another pathologic hallmark of chronic bronchitis. Dubbed "mucous pits," these diverticula are believed to represent dilated openings of mucous glands, and they range in size from 0.2 to 1.2 mm in diameter. They occur commonly in larger airways and at carinae and may be visible through the bronchoscope or on bronchograms.

### Emphysema

As noted above, emphysema is characterized by destructive loss of alveolar walls (3, 7) within the acinus. Three distinctive patterns of alveolar destruction are recognized and are further described below:

1. Centriacinar emphysema (also known as proximal acinar or centrilobular emphysema), in which the respiratory bronchioles are primarily affected (Fig. 10.5);
2. Panacinar emphysema (also known as panlobular

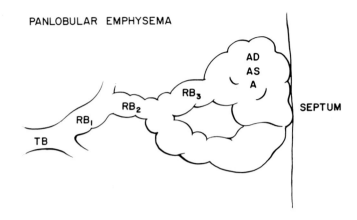

**FIGURE 10.6.** In panlobular (panacinar) emphysema, the enlargement and destruction of air spaces involve the acinus more or less uniformly. Abbreviations are as in Figure 10.5. (From Thurlbeck WM, Dunnill MS, Hartung W, et al: A comparison of three methods of measuring emphysema. *Hum Pathol* 1:215–226, 1970.)

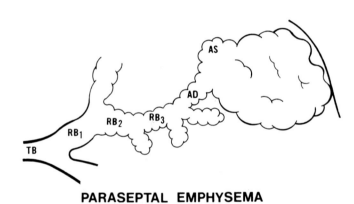

**FIGURE 10.7.** In paraseptal (distal acinar) emphysema, the peripheral part of the acinus (alveolar ducts and sacs) is dominantly or selectively involved. Abbreviations are as in Figure 10.5. (From Thurlbeck WB: *Chronic Airflow Obstruction in Lung Disease.* Philadelphia, WB Saunders, 1976.)

### CENTRILOBULAR EMPHYSEMA

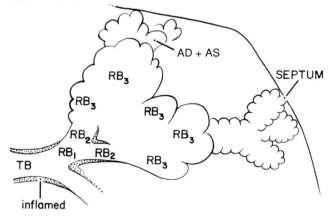

**FIGURE 10.5.** In centrilobular (proximal acinar) emphysema, respiratory bronchioles are selectively and dominantly involved. *TB,* terminal bronchiole; *RB₁, RB₂, RB₃,* respiratory bronchioles of the first, second, and third orders; *AD,* alveolar duct; *AS,* alveolar sac. (From Thurlbeck WM, Dunnill MS, Hartung W, et al: A comparison of three methods of measuring emphysema. *Hum Pathol* 1:215–226, 1970.)

emphysema), in which the whole acinus is affected (Fig. 10.6); and
3. Distal acinar (also known as paraseptal emphysema), in which the major site of involvement is the alveolar sacs and ducts (Fig. 10.7).

### Centriacinar Emphysema

Cardinal pathologic features of centriacinar emphysema include patchy involvement throughout the lung, with some lobules affected and adjacent ones spared, and predominantly upper lobe involvement, especially the posterior and apical segments of the upper lobes, and superior segments of the lower lobes. Black pigment frequently appears in the walls of the affected lung tissue, and centriacinar emphysema may be superficially confused with simple coal workers' pneumoconiosis, though distinctive pathologic features of coal workers' pneumoconiosis include more acinar dilation than destruction and a more regular pattern of acinar involvement. Strikingly, alveolar inflammation is not a prominent pathologic feature of centriacinar emphysema. Also, centriacinar emphysema is almost uniformly related to smoking (8).

*Panacinar Emphysema*

As suggested by its name, panacinar emphysema involves the entire acinus, progressing from early diffuse destruction, in which the distinction between alveolar ducts and alveoli is lost, to total effacement of the alveolus, with only strands of lung tissue remaining. Unlike centrilobular emphysema, panlobular emphysema most frequently affects the lower lobes of the lungs, and unlike other pathologic types of emphysema is distinctly associated with $\alpha_1$-antitrypsin deficiency (8, 16). This is a condition that predisposes to early emphysema and is characterized by lower lobe bullous changes on chest x-ray (see section on $\alpha_1$-Antitrypsin Deficiency, below). Panacinar emphysema may also accompany bronchial and bronchiolar obstruction and focal lung scarring, when the adjacent lung parenchyma is not only distended (as in so-called paracicatricial emphysema) but actually destroyed.

*Distal Acinar Emphysema*

The third anatomic type of emphysema is distal acinar emphysema, also called paraseptal or periacinar emphysema. These various terms for the same entity reflect the predominant involvement of alveolar sacs and ducts, in contrast to more proximal involvement of respiratory bronchioles in centriacinar emphysema. Paraseptal emphysema often abuts the pleural surface and, like centriacinar emphysema, usually involves the upper lobes. Because only the distal portions of the alveolus are effaced, paraseptal emphysema characteristically does not cause significant air flow obstruction but, by the same token, the subpleural location predisposes to spontaneous pneumothorax (8).

Other pathologic features of emphysema include bullae and blebs. By definition, bullae are emphysematous spaces exceeding 1 cm in diameter that may be seen in all types of emphysema (7). In both centriacinar and paraseptal emphysema, they most frequently appear in the upper lobes and may cause a subpleural scalloped appearance on the plain chest x-ray. In panacinar emphysema, the bullae more commonly occur in the lower lobes. In both centriacinar and panlobular emphysema, bullae may compound air flow obstruction by compressing adjacent normal lung, which can be suggested by several radiographic and physiologic features (17): displacement and compression of nearby vessels, mediastinal displacement to the contralateral side on expiration (as in patients with the Swyer-James syndrome or unilateral hyperlucent lung), decreased diffusing capacity for carbon monoxide, surprisingly rapid declines in $FEV_1$ on serial spirometry, and marked discrepancies between lung volumes measured by helium dilution and body plethysmography.

Blebs are collections of air within the layers of the pleura. These may occur as a consequence of paraseptal emphysema, when air dissects into the pleura after rupture of distal alveolar elements.

## Pathologic Overlap between Emphysema and Chronic Bronchitis

Though chronic bronchitis and emphysema demonstrate distinctive pathologic features and may be seen in "pure" form, pathologic features of both entities often coexist in the same individual. This frequent overlap between emphysema and chronic bronchitis has been suggested in several different ways. First, as the extent of emphysema increases in resected papermounted lungs, the Reid index rises (8, 15). Second, as the degree of emphysema increases among resected lungs, the frequency of chronic bronchitis in these patients increases. Observations by Thurlbeck suggest that among patients with postmortem evidence of severe emphysema, premortem chronic bronchitis is universally present (7). Finally, among patients satisfying the clinical definition of chronic bronchitis, emphysema of at least 25% of the examined lung was 6 times more prevalent (72% of chronic bronchitics) than in non-bronchitic patients (18).

### PATHOGENESIS OF CHRONIC OBSTRUCTIVE PULMONARY DISEASE

## Role of Cigarette Smoking

Several lines of evidence suggest that cigarette smoking is a major cause of chronic obstructive pulmonary disease in the United States. First, the risk of developing COPD in smokers has been estimated to be 9.7 to 30 times higher than in nonsmokers, in whom COPD is relatively uncommon (19, 20). By the same token, cigarette smoking was responsible for 80 to 90% of the more than 60,000 deaths ascribed to COPD in 1983 (19). Second, longitudinal studies confirm a dose-response relationship between cigarette smoking and the rate of pulmonary function decline (21). Third, cessation of smoking may result in some improvement in lung function (especially measures of small airways dysfunction, though improvement in $FEV_1$ may be observed in some young smokers after cessation) (22–26). Fourth, even though pulmonary function does not improve with smoking cessation, the accelerated decline of pulmonary function seen in smokers is restored to the usual age-related decline once smoking is stopped (27). Among the most instructive reports of pulmonary function decline in smokers is a longitudinal study of 792 British transport workers who were followed over 8 years (21, 27). The emergent model of the effect of smoking on pulmonary function decline is shown in Figure 10.8 and suggests that the rate of $FEV_1$ decline in susceptible smokers may be several times higher than in nonsmokers and that, with cessation of smoking, the rate of $FEV_1$ decline is restored to that in nonsmokers (27). This study also emphasizes that other features of the host and the environment affect whether or not pulmonary damage occurs with cigarette smoking, since the accelerated decline of $FEV_1$ has only been observed in a minority (10 to 15%) of smokers, the so-called "susceptible" group. While uncertainty persists about ancillary risk factors for COPD, strong possibilities include air pollution and environmental exposure,

passive smoking and exposure to sidestream smoke, genetic predisposition to COPD, and airway hyperreactivity. Emphysema has also been observed in association with other diseases, including hypocomplementemic urticarial vasculitis (28), cutis laxa (a genetically acquired disorder of elastin) (29), Salla disease (a recessively inherited disorder of sialic acid metabolism) (30), Down's syndrome, Marfan's syndrome, and intravenous methylphenidate abuse (31). Infection with the HIV virus has also been reported to cause an emphysema-like condition (32). Speculation that these conditions cause emphysema requires further study.

### PATHOGENESIS OF EMPHYSEMA: THE PROTEASE-ANTIPROTEASE HYPOTHESIS

Current understanding of the pathogenesis of emphysema is summarized by the protease-antiprotease hypothesis (33–37), depicted in Figure 10.9. According to this model, alveolar effacement in emphysema occurs when the balance between lung matrix breakdown and defenses against lung breakdown is tipped in favor of destruction. Lung breakdown is caused by proteases, the major threat being neutrophil-derived elastase, a normal component of neutrophil granules (34). Though several circulating antiproteases can be found in human serum and in the airways (e.g., secretory leukoprotease inhibitor, $\alpha_1$-antichymotrypsin, $\alpha_2$-macroglobulin), most of the defense against alveolar breakdown is provided by $\alpha_1$-antitrypsin, a 52-kilodalton glycoprotein that inactivates neutrophil elastase by tightly binding the protease, thereby inactivating both proteins. Under normal circumstances, the antiprotease screen exceeds the proteolytic threat to the lung, and little alveolar breakdown occurs, but this normal balance may be tipped unfavorably toward increased alveolar destruction, such as when the neutrophil elastase burden increases (e.g., by neutrophil recruitment to lung), or when endogenous $\alpha_1$-antitrypsin defenses are inactivated. As a major risk factor for emphysema, cigarette smoking promotes alveolar breakdown in several ways:

1. By recruiting elastase-rich neutrophils to alveoli (35);
2. By inactivating $\alpha_1$-antitrypsin, both directly by oxidant products of combustion and indirectly through oxidant products of neutrophils (e.g., HOCl, superoxide, etc.) (33); and
3. By opposing elastin resynthesis, a result of diminished activity of the enzyme (lysyl oxidase) responsible for cross-linking newly synthesized elastin fibrils (38).

Bronchoalveolar lavage fluid in cigarette smokers shows evidence of neutrophil recruitment to the lung

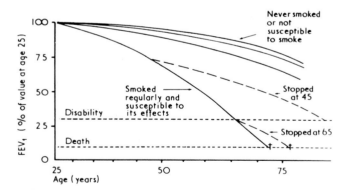

**FIGURE 10.8.** Risks for various men if they smoke; differences between these lines illustrate effects that smoking, and stopping smoking, can have on $FEV_1$ of a man who is liable to develop chronic obstructive lung disease if he smokes. †, Death, the underlying cause of which is irreversible chronic obstructive lung disease, whether the immediate cause of death is respiratory failure, pneumonia, cor pulmonale, or aggravation of other heart disease by respiratory insufficiency. Although this shows the rate of loss of $FEV_1$ for one particular susceptible smoker, other susceptible smokers will have different rates of loss, thus reaching "disability" at different ages. (From Fletcher C, Peto R: The natural history of chronic airflow obstruction. *Br Med J* 1: 1645–1648, 1977.)

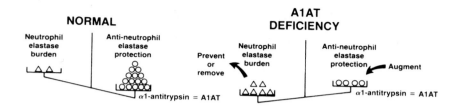

**FIGURE 10.9.** Pathogenesis of the lung destruction associated with $\alpha_1$-antitrypsin (A1AT) deficiency and strategies for its prevention. In normal persons (*left*), a mild but chronic burden of neutrophil elastase in the lower respiratory tract is balanced by an excess of A1AT that provides ample antineutrophil elastase protection. In A1AT deficiency (*right*), there is a mild increase in the neutrophil elastase burden and a marked reduction in the antineutrophil elastase screen secondary to the deficiency of A1AT, leaving the lung vulnerable to destruction by the elastase. Theoretically, two strategies could be used to prevent the lung destruction: prevent the accumulation of neutrophils and hence diminish the burden of elastase, or augment the antineutrophil elastase screen. (From Hubbard RC, Crystal RG: Alpha 1-antitrypsin augmentation therapy for alpha 1-antitrypsin deficiency. *Am J Med* 84[Suppl 6A]:52–62, 1988.)

as a 5- to 10-fold increase in the percentage of neutrophils retrieved (35). Along with the smoking-related increased elastase burden in the lung, oxidation of the crucial methionine residue at position 358 of the $\alpha_1$-antitrypsin molecule by cigarette smoke or by neutrophil oxidation products impairs the ability of $\alpha_1$-antitrypsin to inactivate neutrophil elastase. Specifically, once oxidized, the rate at which $\alpha_1$-antitrypsin can inactivate neutrophil elastase is slowed 2000-fold.

Overall, several lines of evidence support the protease-antiprotease hypothesis, as follows:

1. A threshold value for serum $\alpha_1$-antitrypsin levels has been identified (11 $\mu$M), above which the emphysema risk is not deemed to be increased and below which emphysema risk and severity increase as serum levels of $\alpha_1$-antitrypsin fall. For example, patients with serum $\alpha_1$-antitrypsin levels below normal but above this "protective" threshold of 11 $\mu$M (e.g., PiMZ heterozygotes) are not considered to be at increased risk of developing emphysema (16).

2. Numerous animal studies suggest that proteases applied to explanted lung tissue or instilled directly into the trachea in vivo can produce emphysema experimentally (36, 37). The first observations that intratracheal papain (a plant protease) could produce emphysema in hamsters spawned many other studies of different proteases (e.g., pancreatic elastase, neutrophil elastase from various species) in different animal models, including hamsters, dogs, and rats. Species-specific studies have shown that canine neutrophil elastase instilled intratracheally can produce emphysema in dogs. Finally, more recent studies have shown that intratracheal instillation of human neutrophil elastase can produce experimental emphysema in animals (37).

Thus, much circumstantial evidence supports the protease-antiprotease model of emphysema, though the development of emphysema in individuals with normal $\alpha_1$-antitrypsin levels and function suggests that other inadequately understood factors play a role as well.

## CLINICAL ASSESSMENT OF CHRONIC OBSTRUCTIVE PULMONARY DISEASE

### Clinical Presentation and Physical Examination

In the years since the original distinction between "pink puffers" and "blue bloaters" was made (Table 10.2) (39), it has become apparent that the patient with COPD can present with features of both syndromes as well as with asthmatic features. Initial symptoms of chronic obstructive pulmonary disease may include dyspnea, cough, and wheezing. Chronic bronchitis features also include mucoid phlegm production, which may become more copious and purulent during acute exacerbations. Hemoptysis may also accompany these bronchitic exacerbations but must also raise concern about lung cancer. Although it has been disputed by some, bronchoscopy plays an important role in confirming the absence of lung cancer in the chronic bronchitic with hemoptysis.

For patients with longstanding hypoxemia, symptoms of right heart failure may be prominent, such as pedal edema, liver enlargement and tenderness, and cyanosis. Notably, digital clubbing is not a feature of chronic bronchitis or emphysema and should prompt consideration of other comorbid conditions such as bronchiectasis, lung cancer, interstitial disease, congenital heart disease, or inflammatory bowel disease.

Weight loss can be a presenting complaint of patients with COPD and occurs in about a third of the

TABLE **10.2**
CLINICAL FEATURES OF CHRONIC OBSTRUCTIVE PULMONARY DISEASE: DISTINCTIONS BETWEEN CHRONIC BRONCHITIS AND EMPHYSEMA

| Features | Chronic Bronchitis (Alternate Names: Blue Bloater, Type B COPD) | Emphysema (Alternate Names: Pink Puffer, Type A COPD) |
|---|---|---|
| Symptoms, signs | | |
| Chronic cough, phlegm | Common | Less common |
| Cor pulmonale | Present (often with multiple exacerbations) | Present (but generally only in late disease stage) |
| Physiologic function | | |
| Air flow | | |
| $FEV_1$ | Decreased | Decreased |
| $FEV_1/FVC$ | Decreased | Decreased |
| Lung volumes | | |
| Residual volume | Normal | Increased, consistent with air trapping |
| Total lung capacity | Normal | Increase |
| Functional residual capacity | Mild increase | Increased |
| Gas exchange, diffusion | | |
| $Pa_{O_2}$ | Often decreased | Often preserved until end stage |
| $Pa_{CO_2}$ | Often decreased | Often preserved |
| Diffusing capacity | Normal | Decreased |
| Other | | |
| Static compliance | Normal | Often increased |

more severely impaired patients, but correlates only weakly with $FEV_1$. Notably, weight loss is an independent predictor of mortality in patients with COPD (40, 41). The mechanism of weight loss appears to be a 10 to 20% increase in resting energy expenditure without a matched increase in dietary intake, although the total caloric intake may actually exceed the estimated daily requirements (41, 42). This hypermetabolism can only partially be explained by increased work of breathing, and additional factors such as circulating catecholamines, cytokines, and drug therapy may contribute (41). Unlike malnourished patients without lung disease, patients with emphysema do not appear to be hypercatabolic (41, 43).

Visual examination of the patient may be unremarkable in patients with early, stable COPD or may reveal features characteristic of "pink puffers" (e.g., a thin, tachypneic patient, often barrel-chested, using accessory muscles of respiration and pursed-lip breathing) or "blue bloaters" (a more heavy-set, less distressed-appearing but cyanotic patient, possibly with visual evidence of right heart failure). In using accessory muscles of respiration, the patient may lean forward with the elbows out and the neck extended (so-called "tripod sign") to place the sternocleidomastoid and scalene muscles at maximum mechanical advantage for assisting inspiration. Inspection of the chest of hyperinflated patients may also show a paradoxic retraction or dimpling at the lower lateral chest wall during inspiration (44). Sometimes called "Hoover's sign," this finding reflects contraction of a flattened diaphragm, which pulls medially rather than moving caudally during contraction.

Auscultation of the chest may show diminished breath sounds when air flow obstruction is very severe or in areas with large bullae. With bronchitis and asthma, coarse inspiratory sounds corresponding to large-airway secretions and wheezing may be prominent. Signs of cor pulmonale may include jugular venous distention, a right ventricular heave with a loud pulmonic valve component of the second heart sound, ascites, and sacral or pedal edema.

Besides changes in pulmonary function tests and chest radiographs (see below), laboratory assessment may show polycythemia in chronically hypoxemic individuals and metabolic alkalosis, which may reflect chronic diuretic use or compensation for hypercapnia of at least a day's duration. The electrocardiogram is an insensitive tool in detecting cor pulmonale, because electrocardiographic changes develop late. However, characteristic electrocardiographic features include evidence of a P pulmonale pattern (prominent P waves in inferior leads), right axis deviation, evidence of right ventricular hypertrophy (ratio of R to S wave in $V_1$ greater than 1), and an incomplete or complete right bundle-branch block. Doppler flow echocardiography is a sensitive technique for detecting cor pulmonale, based on estimation of pulmonary artery pressures and the presence of right ventricular hypertrophy.

## Pulmonary Function Tests in Chronic Bronchitis

Table 10.2 presents the classic features of types A and B chronic obstructive pulmonary disease, which have been considered by some to be synonymous with emphysema and chronic bronchitis, respectively. However, as emphasized by Thurlbeck (8), types A and B COPD (or the "pink puffer" and "blue bloater" syndromes, respectively) prove more useful as descriptors of syndromes than as diagnoses to characterize individual patients, especially because many patients exhibit characteristics of both the type A and type B syndrome.

As suggested in Table 10.2, studies of patients with chronic phlegm production but little radiographic evidence of emphysema offer a physiologic picture of "pure" chronic bronchitis. Such patients show moderate air flow obstruction with mild degrees of hyperinflation (i.e., elevated residual volume and functional residual capacity), though less so than in patients with emphysema. In sharp contrast to patients with at least moderate emphysema, total lung capacity and diffusing capacity tend to be preserved in chronic bronchitis. Though Dornhorst's early description of "blue bloaters" (39) suggested a distinctive association between right ventricular hypertrophy or failure and chronic bronchitis, subsequent studies have suggested that right heart failure is not unique to chronic bronchitis and correlates poorly with mucus hypersecretion (8). Rather, cor pulmonale results from hypoxemia, which reflects the degree of ventilation-perfusion mismatching. Some studies even suggest a closer association between right ventricular hypertrophy and the degree of emphysema (8).

## Pulmonary Function Tests in Emphysema

Pulmonary function abnormalities in emphysema result from the loss of lung parenchyma and a reduction in the gas exchange surface. Specifically, loss of alveolar capillary units causes a reduction in the diffusing capacity, and loss of lung matrix decreases the radial traction on the airways, resulting in early airway closure. The loss of airway tethering affects both air flow and lung volume measurements in emphysema. As summarized in Table 10.2, early airway closure reduces the $FEV_1$, while decreased elastic recoil diminishes the lung's opposition to inspiratory muscle force, causing total lung capacity (TLC) to rise, although usually only slightly. Functional residual capacity (FRC), which is the amount of air in the lung after exhaling a normal tidal breath, is also increased as the elastic

recoil of the lung falls. Lung forces opposing the tendency of the chest wall to expand at end-expiration are decreased, and FRC therefore increases. Residual volume (RV), the amount of air left in the lung after a maximal exhalation, is increased in emphysema as well. Vital capacity (VC), the difference between TLC and RV, is often decreased in emphysema, as the rise in RV usually exceeds the rise in TLC. Loss of elastic recoil also causes an increase in the static compliance of the lung, and static pressure-volume curves can distinguish patients with emphysema from those with normal lungs (Fig. 10.10) and from those with "pure" chronic bronchitis. However, because elasticity changes correlate poorly with the pathologic degree of emphysema and because these measurements require placement of an esophageal balloon, static pressure-volume curves have had limited clinical popularity.

As therapy of COPD is directed at maximizing available lung function, assessing the presence of reversible air flow obstruction (conventionally defined as a post-bronchodilator increment of 12% and a rise in $FEV_1$ of 200 ml or more) has clinical appeal. While only a minority of patients with chronic obstructive pulmonary disease have reversible air flow obstruction as defined, the absence of reversibility during a single testing session does not discount its presence. For example, in a study of 985 patients with COPD, Anthonisen and coworkers (45) performed serial bronchodilator treatments and found that 68% of initially nonresponsive

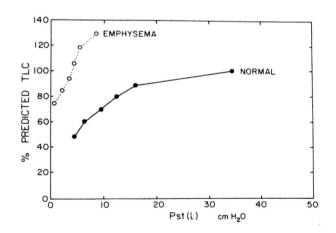

**FIGURE 10.10.** Static pressure-volume relationships in emphysema are contrasted with normal. Volume is expressed as percentage of predicted TLC, and Pst(L) is the static recoil pressure of the lung. At a given pressure, lung volumes are larger in emphysema (and at the same lung volume, recoil pressures are less). By contrast, in bronchitis, pressure-volume relationships should be normal. (From Thurlbeck WM: *Chronic Airflow Obstruction in Lung Disease.* Philadelphia, WB Saunders, 1976.)

patients eventually satisfied criteria for air flow reversibility when tested up to 7 times. In view of the insensitivity of a single bronchodilator trial for reversibility of air flow obstruction and the observation that bronchodilators may improve functional status in COPD patients without demonstrable reversibility (46, 47), the absence of a rise in $FEV_1$ should not interdict a bronchodilator trial in such patients.

As implied by the name "pink puffer," resting hypoxia tends to develop late in the course of emphysema, though clinically significant desaturation may occur when the diffusing capacity for carbon monoxide ($D_{LCO}$) falls markedly (e.g., less than 55% of predicted) (48). Preservation of gas exchange despite parenchymal loss in emphysema is best explained by the parallel loss of alveolocapillary units, so that ventilation-perfusion mismatch is not an early event.

### Correlations between Structure and Physiologic Function

The relationship between pathologic change and physiologic derangement in both emphysema and chronic bronchitis has been studied extensively and remains controversial. In emphysema, studies by Thurlbeck suggest that the pathologic degree of emphysema correlates intermediately ($r$ 0.7) with measures of air flow obstruction (e.g., $FEV_1$, $FEV_1/FVC$, mid-expiratory flow rate). Decline in mid-expiratory flow rates can occur in the presence of even little pathologic evidence of emphysema. Also, although loss of elastic recoil is one of the physiologic sequelae of parenchymal loss, derangement in elastic recoil correlates poorly with the pathologic degree of emphysema.

Of the physiologic function tests, derangement in the diffusing capacity for carbon monoxide, whether measured by single-breath or equilibrium techniques, has been proved to correlate strongly with the pathologic degree of emphysema in various studies. However, early emphysema may be unaccompanied by derangement in diffusing capacity. Overall, the difficulty of correlating structure and function simply in emphysema has been emphasized by Thurlbeck: "It is clear that no one test or combination will predict accurately the amount of emphysema in the lungs of living patients" (7). As will be discussed below, the advent of computed tomography with its sensitivity in detecting emphysema may challenge this earlier statement (49).

### Chest Imaging in Chronic Obstructive Pulmonary Disease: Plain Chest Radiography and Computed Tomography

#### The Plain Chest Radiograph

The plain chest radiograph plays an important role in evaluating patients with chronic obstructive pulmonary disease. Among the several clinical purposes served by a chest x-ray in the initial evaluation of the COPD patient are:

1. The chest x-ray can increase confidence in the diagnosis of COPD when several radiographic features characteristic of COPD are present and when other findings that may explain the patient's symptoms of dyspnea, cough, or phlegm production are absent (e.g., pneumonia, pleural effusions, interstitial infiltrates, etc.).
2. The distribution of radiographic abnormalities (e.g., lower-lobe bullous change versus upper-lobe change) can suggest the presence of panacinar emphysema and $\alpha_1$-antitrypsin deficiency (50).
3. Though the value of the chest x-ray as a screening maneuver is limited, the chest x-ray can help exclude other diseases for which smokers predisposed to emphysema are also at risk (e.g., lung cancer).

*Emphysema.* The plain chest radiographic features of emphysema are summarized in Table 10.3 and depicted in Figure 10.11. These features have been generally divided into features of hyperinflation (e.g., depression and flattening of the diaphragms, blunting

---

**TABLE 10.3**
**RADIOGRAPHIC SIGNS OF EMPHYSEMA**

Signs in the posteroanterior chest radiograph

1. Peripheral vessels: a reduction in the caliber and number of the peripheral branches of the pulmonary artery in the outer half of the lung field when compared with the radiographs of normal persons.
2. Flattened diaphragm: depression and flattening of the diaphragm with blunting of the costophrenic angles. The actual level of the diaphragm is not as significant as the contour. The body build of the patient should also be considered. For example, in a short, stocky person, emphysema might be diagnosable even if the diaphragm were at the level of the tenth rib posteriorly.
3. Irregular radiolucency of lung fields: this manifestation is the result of the irregularity in distribution of the emphysematous tissue destruction. It is sometimes more clearly recognizable in laminograms.

Signs in the lateral chest radiograph

4. Abnormal retrosternal space: this is defined as a space showing increased radiolucency and measuring 2.5 cm or more from the sternum to the most anterior margin of the ascending aorta.
5. Flattened diaphragm: flattening of even concavity of diaphragmatic contour. A useful index of the change is the presence of a 90 or larger sternodiaphragmatic angle. In most patients with emphysema, this junction is more readily seen than in subjects with a normal chest.

From Nicklaus DW, Stowell DW, Christiansen WR, Renzetti AD. The accuracy of the roentgenologic diagnosis of chronic pulmonary emphysema. *Am Rev Respir Dis* 1966;93:889–899.

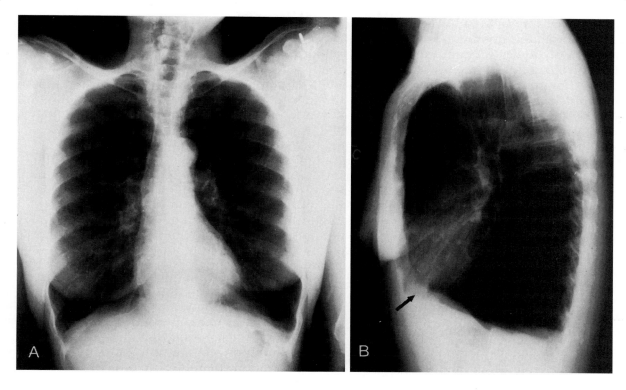

**FIGURE 10.11.** Chest radiograph (posteroanterior and lateral views) of a 62-year-old black female smoker with emphysema (FEV$_1$ = 0.70 liter) and a normal $\alpha_1$-antitrypsin level. Vascular attenuation, hyperlucency in the upper lung zones, and diaphragm flattening (flattened costophrenic angles and an oblique sternocostal angle [*arrow*]) are demonstrated.

of the costophrenic angles, increased length of the lung, and increased size of the retrosternal air space) and features of vascular attenuation and hyperlucency (e.g., loss of lung parenchyma, bullous change, and disappearance of vascular markings, especially in the lung periphery). Less commonly recognized features include alteration of the tracheal shadow with development of "saber sheath" trachea, characterized by marked coronal narrowing associated with sagittal widening of the trachea (51). Finally, other vascular changes may reflect the development of pulmonary hypertension as a result of COPD. In a study of 1085 normal chest x-rays, Chang reported that the upper limit of the inspiratory diameter of the descending right pulmonary artery in normal males is 16 mm (52). Enlargement of the descending right pulmonary artery (width greater than 16 mm) is associated with elevation of the mean pulmonary artery pressure above 20 mm Hg (53).

Because emphysema is a pathologic diagnosis, the most reliable studies of diagnostic criteria have assessed chest x-ray features in patients who subsequently come to necropsy (7, 54–58). Even with such studies, impediments to identifying a single ideal chest

x-ray marker of emphysema have included the trade-off between sensitivity (true positive rate) and specificity (1 − [false-positive rate]), interstudy variations in the pathologic criteria of emphysema, differences in study design and purpose, and intraobserver and interobserver variation in chest x-ray interpretation. Thus, controversy persists in the literature about the best radiographic marker of emphysema. On the one hand, proponents of using hyperinflation criteria (e.g., diaphragm flattening, increased retrosternal air space, etc.) suggest that hyperinflation is an early pathologic event in emphysema and that radiographic evidence of hyperinflation establishes emphysema, even in the absence of air flow obstruction or symptoms (57). On the other hand, more conservative observers use criteria for decreased vascularity and hyperlucency, because these are sensitive in moderate to severe emphysema without falsely identifying patients with trivial emphysema. Several studies have directly compared the diagnostic performance of the individual radiographic criteria mentioned above (Table 10.3). For example, Thurlbeck and Simon (54) examined chest x-rays from 696 patients with necropsy confirmation of emphysema and showed that objectively determined decreased vascularity or hyperlucency detected 40 to 65% of those with severe emphysema with almost no "false-positive" diagnoses (i.e., called emphysema by chest x-ray without pathologic evidence). More precise criteria, like the vertical length of the lungs, the width of the retrosternal air space, and the level of the diaphragm with respect to the ribs, did not enhance the radiographic diagnosis of emphysema, and "no combination of criteria resulted in better recognition of moderately severe and severe emphysema than did the subjective diagnosis of emphysema" in this series. A similar study by Nicklaus and coworkers (58) examined five radiographic criteria for emphysema—attenuation of pulmonary vessels in the periphery of the lung, diaphragmatic flattening on the posterior-anterior view and on the lateral view, irregular radiolucency of the lung fields, and depth of the retrosternal air space—and concluded that diaphragmatic flattening and increased retrosternal space were favored criteria, though no set of individual criteria performed as well as an experienced radiologist's overall impression. Proponents of hyperinflation criteria (57) also point out that these criteria show greater intraobserver and interobserver reproducibility (88 and 75%, respectively) than is seen with vascular attenuation criteria (80 and 53%, respectively).

In the face of persistent controversy about the most useful radiographic criterion of emphysema, it is important to recognize that all of the criteria can be misapplied to falsely diagnose emphysema, such as when hyperinflation occurs on the chest x-ray during acute asthma or when an increased retrosternal air space from a pectus excavatum deformity is ascribed incorrectly to emphysema. An overzealous radiographic diagnosis in the absence of clinical and physiologic signs has little therapeutic merit but can clearly impose undue worry. Weighing this potential for morbidity from overzealous diagnosis, more conservative plain radiographic criteria (e.g., signs of vascular attenuation) would seem more appropriate to use in evaluating individual patients.

*Chronic Bronchitis.* Radiographic criteria for chronic bronchitis have received less attention than emphysema, probably because chronic bronchitis is a clinical diagnosis and because the major role of the chest x-ray in chronic bronchitis is to exclude emphysema. Common chest x-ray features in chronic bronchitis (59) include hyperinflation; "tram lines," which are parallel line shadows corresponding to thickened bronchial walls seen in coronal section; and a diffuse increase in lung markings, especially at the bases, sometimes dubbed "dirty lungs." As with markers of emphysema, however, the reliability of these radiographic signs has been contested. For example, Fraser and Paré

(59) suggest that tram lines more often indicate bronchiectasis than chronic bronchitis. Furthermore, attempts by these authors to identify other radiographic markers of chronic bronchitis (e.g., thickening of bronchial walls when seen "end-on" or peribronchial cuffing) have not been successful to date.

*Computed Tomography*

Several studies have demonstrated the ability of computed tomography of the chest to diagnose emphysema, especially using high-resolution techniques. High-resolution computed tomography (CT) allows a display of fine anatomic details, and is therefore particularly well suited to describe and quantitate the structural abnormalities of emphysema in living subjects (Fig. 10.12) (59–62). The accuracy of high-resolution CT has been reported to rival direct pathologic examination, and may accurately diagnose emphysema in mild or even clinically silent emphysema (49, 63, 64). On the other hand, several investigators have shown that mild degrees of emphysema may be missed by computed tomography (60, 61, 64). For example, Gurney et al observed that 20% of their patients with functional emphysema (defined as a diffusion capacity less than 75% of predicted and an $FEV_1$ less than 80% of predicted) had no subjective findings of emphysema on high-resolution computed tomography (64). Despite these limitations, high-resolution computed tomography of the chest is being advocated for the early diagnosis of emphysema, particularly where intervention may have a clinical impact (e.g., smoking cessation in susceptible individuals, and augmentation therapy for patients with emphysema associated with $\alpha_1$-antitrypsin deficiency) (49, 65).

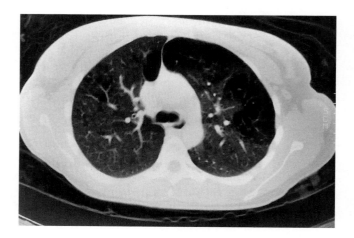

**FIGURE 10.12.** Computed tomographic section demonstrating extensive areas of lung destruction bilaterally consistent with the diagnosis of emphysema.

## TREATMENT OF CHRONIC OBSTRUCTIVE PULMONARY DISEASE

### General Goals of Therapy

The goals of treating chronic obstructive pulmonary disease are to prevent disease progression, to reverse acute complications, and, for patients with established but stable disease, to optimize pulmonary function and functional status. Therapy should also attempt to prolong life whenever possible.

Primary prevention consists of discouraging smoking, and secondary preventive maneuvers include smoking cessation (19–27, 66–70) as well as the administration of vaccines for prevention of influenza (71–74) and complications of pneumococcal pneumonia (75–81). Available therapies for managing acute exacerbations and stable disease include anticholinergic bronchodilators (82–99) and sympathomimetic drugs (45–47, 100–114), xanthines (e.g., theophylline-like drugs) (115–128), corticosteroids (129–165), antibiotics (166–169), oxygen (114, 170–188), and other agents (e.g., almitrine) (189, 190). Besides measures to optimize air flow, pulmonary rehabilitation (183, 191–199) and nutritional supplementation (200–203) can be important adjunctive treatments for improving patients' functional status. Some clinicians also advocate ventilatory muscle training (204–206) and intermittent ventilation (207–211) for patients with stable COPD. In a highly selected group with emphysema and local bullae, surgical treatment of emphysema (i.e., bullectomy) can be considered (17, 212, 213). Finally, lung transplantation is increasingly becoming an option for patients with very advanced COPD (214–216).

In the sections that follow, evidence regarding the role of each of these therapies will be discussed. Distinctions between treatment approaches for chronic bronchitis versus emphysema will be made where appropriate, and management of acute exacerbations will be distinguished from strategies for the stable but impaired patient.

### Preventive Strategies: Smoking Prevention and Cessation

Smoking prevention and cessation remain the foremost means of preventing chronic obstructive pulmonary disease and its attendant morbidity and mortality (19, 66), with up to 80% of the 60,000 estimated COPD-related deaths in 1983 ascribed to the effects of smoking. Careful surveys of current smoking trends among American adults suggest that as of 1990, 25.5% of adult Americans continue to smoke, but that the overall prevalence has shown a steady decline by 0.5% per year between 1965 and 1985, and by 1.1% annually

from 1987 to 1990 (67). The greatest declines in smoking prevalence have been in socioeconomically privileged groups with much slower declines in less educated and more economically disadvantaged populations (67). Also, although the yearly prevalence of smoking in young women (20 to 24 years) with fewer than 12 years of education remained unchanged (i.e. approximately 40%) prior to 1985, a sharp decrease to 24.3% was noted in 1990 in this group (67). The declining overall prevalence of smoking among adults aged 20 to 24 years is particularly encouraging, and the accelerated rate of decline of smoking may be due to several factors, including decreased social acceptability, increased cost of cigarettes, increased awareness of the risks of both active and passive smoking, as well as possible underreporting of smoking. Nevertheless, this rate will need to be maintained if the national health objective of reducing smoking prevalence in adults to 15% or less by the year 2000 is to be achieved (67). Projections of smoking rates to the year 2000 by educational strata suggest that prevalence rates will decline least among non–high school graduates (Fig. 10.13).

Smoking cessation counseling is another important

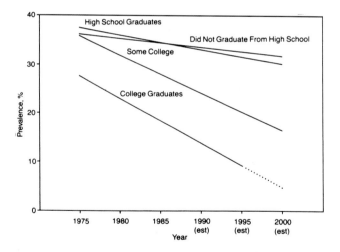

**FIGURE 10.13.** Smoking prevalence by educational status with projections to year 2000. Lines were computed via linear regression based on observed values from National Health Interview Surveys by National Center for Health Statistics in 1974, 1976, 1978 through 1980, 1983, and 1985. Slopes (percentage point change for year) are 0.19 ± 0.03 for persons who did not graduate from high school, −0.030 ± 0.07 for high school graduates, −0.78 ± 0.09 for persons with some college, and −0.91 ± 0.13 for college graduates. *est*, estimate. (From Pierce JP, Fiore MC, Morotny TE, et al: Trends in cigarette smoking in the United States: Projections to the year 2000. *JAMA* 261:61–65, 1989. Copyright 1989, American Medical Association.)

preventive maneuver for established smokers, especially because a large percentage (e.g., 71% of the 45.8 million current American smokers) are projected to see a physician during the course of a single year. This frequency of physician visits affords clinicians an opportunity to promote smoking cessation in the majority of current smokers (19, 66, 68, 69).

Unfortunately, despite evidence that even casual discussion of smoking cessation by a general practitioner can be associated with approximately 5% quit rates at 1 year (66), many physicians consider counseling about smoking cessation to be futile. It should be remembered that concerted efforts to promote smoking cessation can effect even higher quit rates (up to approximately 35%) and that, although this rate is still disappointing, the absolute number of patients that quit would be large (e.g., approximately 35% of 38 million patients per year) if smoking cessation counseling were employed routinely by all physicians seeing current smokers (69). A variety of smoking cessation strategies are available and have been recently reviewed (66, 68, 69): counseling, nicotine gum or patch, behavior modification techniques, acupuncture, and hypnosis. Though quit rates with these different maneuvers vary in different studies (presumably reflecting differences in patient motivation and clinical settings), a meta-analysis of 108 interventions in 39 published control trials suggests that smoking cessation efforts are most successful when multiple interventions are practiced by several health care providers over multiple reinforcing sessions (69).

As a general strategy to promote smoking cessation, the following steps have been proposed (66, 68):

1. Advise cessation;
2. Motivate the patient to make a quit attempt by informing the patient regarding the risks of smoking and relating these to the patient's current health status;
3. Assess prior attempts to stop smoking and problems encountered with those attempts;
4. Set agreement for a quitting date and record this date on the chart;
5. Discuss the patient's concerns about the effects of smoking cessation and advise possible strategies, emphasizing the health benefits of smoking cessation;
6. Emphasize the importance of follow-up by requesting a return visit specifically to assess smoking cessation or by arranging telephone follow-up;
7. Consider the role of additional steps, for example,
   a. A written contract with the patient regarding smoking cessation,
   b. Nicotine gum or patch,
   c. Formal smoking cessation programs, behavioral modification techniques, etc.

Specific literature to aid physicians in their encouragement of smoking cessation is available, as are a variety of patient materials, from the National Cancer Institute, the American Cancer Society, and the American Lung Association.

The nicotine transdermal delivery system or patch was introduced simultaneously in 1992 by several drug manufacturers and may be most beneficial for smokers with a high level of physical dependence defined as (a) smoking more than 20 cigarettes a day, (b) smoking within 30 minutes of rising, and (c) strong craving for cigarettes during previous quitting attempts (70). In addition, the smoker must be highly motivated to quit; i.e, he or she should be able to list reasons for quitting and express a strong desire to quit (70). The success rate of nicotine patches is high, with associated quit rates from 18 to 77%, twice those of placebo-treated subjects. Quit rates with nicotine patches can be further improved by counseling on smoking cessation (70).

### Prevention of Complications: Vaccination against Influenza and Pneumococcal Infections, Antiviral Agents

In addition to primary prevention of COPD by avoidance or cessation of smoking and treatment of sequelae (e.g., air flow obstruction, hypoxemia), secondary prevention of infection by vaccination is an important aspect of treating chronic obstructive pulmonary disease. Currently, two vaccines—the influenza vaccine (72–74) and the pneumococcal vaccine (75–81)—are widely used.

Because influenza infection poses an increased risk of hospitalization and death in patients with chronic obstructive pulmonary disease (71), current recommendations also call for administering the influenza vaccine yearly to patients with COPD (72, 74). The vaccine consists of an inactivated egg-grown virus, almost always a trivalent combination of two A virus strains and one B virus strain, and is administered each fall to avert the arrival of influenza by early December. Influenza B viruses were the predominant strains isolated worldwide during the 1992–1993 season (73). The influenza vaccine can be administered concurrently with the pneumococcal vaccine (though at a different site) and infrequently causes self-limited constitutional symptoms of fever, malaise, and myalgias. Patients allergic to egg protein should not receive the vaccine.

In the event of an influenza A outbreak in an unprotected group of COPD patients, amantadine hydrochloride (or its analogue rimantadine) can provide chemoprophylaxis with 70 to 90% efficacy (72). Amantadine may also reduce the duration of influenza

A–related constitutional symptoms if administered within 48 hours of the onset of viral disease. The usual adult dose of amantadine is 200 mg once daily, but the dose is reduced to 100 mg daily for patients aged 65 or above or for patients with impaired renal function. Amantadine is best used as an adjunct to late immunization in patients at high risk for influenza A infection, so treatment should persist only until an antibody response is expected (usually within 2 weeks of vaccination).

The available pneumococcal vaccine is a 23-valent preparation that contains capsular antigens from pneumococcal serotypes that are responsible for 87% of bacteremic pneumococcal infections (76, 77). Early controlled trials established the protective efficacy of pneumococcal vaccination in high-risk, healthy populations (efficacy rates of 60 to 82.3%) (77). Therefore, because of the increased risk for contracting pneumococcal infection and the increased mortality risk from infection in debilitated patients, pneumococcal vaccination has been recommended for adults with chronic illnesses (e.g., chronic pulmonary disease, cardiovascular disease, splenic dysfunction, Hodgkin's disease, myeloma, renal failure, and immunosuppression), as well as otherwise healthy adults aged 65 years and older (76). Individuals who received the earlier, 14-valent vaccine (available from 1977 to 1983) need not be revaccinated routinely with the 23-valent vaccine, but the Immunization Practices Advisory Committee recommends revaccination 6 years after the first dose for individuals considered to be at high risk for rapid decline in antibody levels (e.g., chronic renal failure, nephrotic syndrome, or transplanted organs) or for fatal pneumococcal infections (e.g., asplenic patients) (76).

Mild local reactions (e.g., erythema, pain at the injection site) occur in roughly one-half of vaccine recipients, severe reactions (fever, severe local reactions) occur rarely (less than 1%), and anaphylactoid reactions have been very rarely described (approximately 5 per million doses administered) (75).

Specific information about the efficacy of pneumococcal vaccination in patients with chronic obstructive pulmonary disease is sparse, and recommendations about routine vaccination for COPD patients are divided (77–80). Despite several suggestive reports (80, 81), clear-cut evidence of protective efficacy in COPD is lacking. Notably, COPD patients who are frequently colonized with streptococcal species frequently have prevaccination serum antibody titers to pneumococcal antigens that exceed protective thresholds (78), so the incremental value of vaccinating COPD patients may be small. However, based on the substantial information supporting the protective efficacy of the vaccine

in healthy populations as well as in other debilitated groups and the apparent lack of increased vaccine morbidity in patients with stable COPD (78), these authors favor routinely administering the pneumococcal vaccine to stable COPD patients.

## Anticholinergic Bronchodilators

Inhaled anticholinergic medications have been used for treating air flow obstruction for several centuries (82). The recent resurgence of interest in anticholinergic bronchodilators has been based on newer understanding of the role of cholinergic tone in the control of airways resistance (83–85) as well as the availability of quaternary anticholinergic drugs (e.g., ipratropium bromide), which cause less toxicity than the tertiary ammonium precursors, such as atropine sulfate (86). As a manifestation of the newer importance attached to anticholinergics in managing COPD, ipratropium bromide was the only bronchodilator studied in the Lung Health Study and has recently been proposed as the first-line bronchodilator in treating emphysema (Fig. 10.14) (87–89).

Though somewhat controversial, cholinergic innervation of the airways is thought to exert a tonic bronchoconstrictive effect that is mediated by postganglionic nerve endings (84). Large and central airways appear to be preferentially innervated by cholinergic fibers so that bronchodilation from anticholinergic drugs occurs centrally, in contrast to the effects of sympathomimetic agents, which are believed to act in more peripheral airways.

Currently available anticholinergic bronchodilators include both tertiary ammonium compounds (e.g., scopolamine and atropine sulfate) (85) as well as quaternary ammonium compounds such as atropine methonitrate, glycopyrrolate (90), and ipratropium bromide (86, 91). Unlike the more lipid-soluble, less polar tertiary ammonium compounds, the quaternary compounds are less well absorbed across the bronchial mucosa, so that inhalation is less likely to result in systemic absorption and attendant toxicity (e.g., mydriasis, constipation, urinary retention, and psychosis) (91).

In recent years, ipratropium bromide has become the most widely used inhaled anticholinergic bronchodilator based on its availability in metered dose inhalers and, in Europe, as a solution for nebulized administration. Using the metered dose inhaler, the recommended dose is 36 $\mu$g (2 puffs) 4 times a day. Although some authors suggest doubling or even tripling this dose for maximal bronchodilation (88), other studies have shown no incremental bronchodilation after doubling the dose from a metered dose inhaler

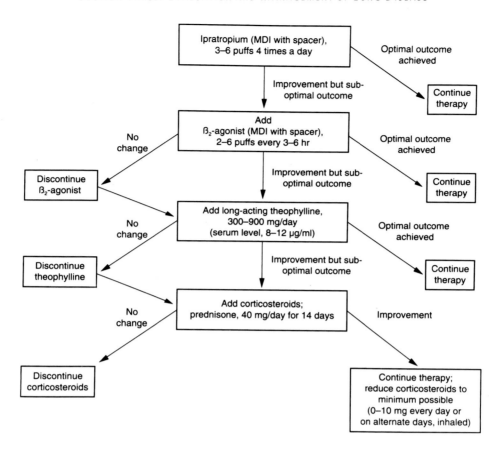

**FIGURE 10.14.** Proposed algorithm for the management of COPD. Outcome measure in terms of improvement in the $FEV_1$, $FEV_1/FVC$, and peak flow; improvement in the distance covered in a 6- or 12-minute walk; and objectively observed reduction in dyspnea, medication use, and nocturnal symptoms. *MDI*, me-

tered dose inhaler. (Reprinted, by permission of the New England Journal of Medicine, from Ferguson GT, Cherniack RM: Management of chronic obstructive pulmonary disease. *N Engl J Med* 328:1017–1022, 1993.)

(92). In contrast, dose-response studies using the nebulized solution suggest that an inhaled dose of 0.4 mg provides greater bronchodilation than inhalation of 36 $\mu$g using a metered dose inhaler. More extensive data on the nebulized solution must await greater experience with this preparation in the United States.

Recent evidence recommends anticholinergic bronchodilators over sympathomimetic agents in several clinical settings: bronchospasm precipitated by $\beta$-blockers, air flow obstruction in stable COPD (86, 103), and bronchospasm precipitated by psychogenic causes (93, 94). Some studies suggest the superiority of anticholinergic bronchodilators over sympathomimetic agents in acute exacerbations of COPD (95) and in severe COPD (96, 97).

Ipratropium bromide is the most extensively studied anticholinergic bronchodilator in stable chronic obstructive pulmonary disease, and most short-term

studies have found standard doses of ipratropium to be at least as effective as bronchodilators as the compared sympathomimetics, including albuterol (104, 105), metaproterenol (104), and fenoterol (106). For example, comparing the $FEV_1$ response to 200 $\mu$g of inhaled salbutamol versus 40 $\mu$g of inhaled ipratropium bromide in chronic bronchitics with reversible air flow obstruction, Lightbody and coworkers observed similar $FEV_1$ rises after administration of ipratropium and salbutamol (105). Other studies report that both atropine sulfate and ipratropium produced significant bronchodilation in patients with irreversible chronic obstructive pulmonary disease (that is, patients who fail to respond to an inhaled sympathomimetic), suggesting that as single agents, anticholinergics are superior bronchodilators in patients with stable COPD (97, 98, 106).

Though few long-term studies have been per-

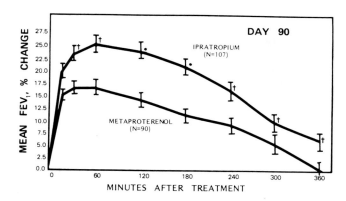

**FIGURE 10.15.** Mean percentage changes in $FEV_1$ at serial times after inhalation of ipratropium 40 $\mu$g or metaproterenol 1500 $\mu$g on day 90 of the 90-day trial period of daily drug administration. *, $p$ 0.01, comparison of adjusted group means from analysis of covariance. †, $p$ 0.05, comparison of adjusted group means from analysis of covariance. (From Tashkin DP, Ashutosh K, Blecker ER, et al: Comparison of the anticholinergic bronchodilator ipratropium bromide with metaproterenol in chronic obstructive pulmonary disease: a 90-day multi-center study. *Am J Med* 81[Suppl 5A]:81–90, 1986.)

formed, available evidence again favors ipratropium as a bronchodilator in patients with stable COPD (103). Specifically, in a multicenter trial comparing standard metered dose inhaler doses of metaproterenol and ipratropium over a 90-day period, Tashkin and coworkers (103) observed that ipratropium produced significantly greater and more longstanding bronchodilation than metaproterenol, an effect that persisted over 3 months of therapy (Fig. 10.15). Although fewer studies are available in acute exacerbations of chronic obstructive pulmonary disease, ipratropium and sympathomimetics appear comparably effective in some studies and additively effective in others (95, 104, 107). Based on the superiority of higher doses of ipratropium administered in a nebulized solution, these recommendations may evolve as ipratropium becomes more widely available for administration in solution.

Whether or not combining an anticholinergic with a sympathomimetic agent enhances bronchodilation in patients with stable COPD remains controversial (99, 107). Additive efficacy is predicted by observations that anticholinergic agents and sympathomimetic agents cause bronchodilation at different airway sites (i.e., large versus small airways, respectively) (84), and several studies report greater bronchodilation from coadministering these agents (99). On the other hand, at least one study in which maximal doses of inhaled ipratropium (120 $\mu$g) were added to maximal doses of inhaled albuterol (up to 800 $\mu$g) failed to show any

additive bronchodilation (107). Despite this finding, advocates of combination therapy suggest that the different pharmacologic properties of inhaled ipratropium and available sympathomimetic agents justify coadministering these drugs in stable COPD. Specifically, sympathomimetics tend to show an earlier onset of bronchodilation with a shorter duration, while ipratropium exerts a more delayed but prolonged effect (86, 103). In balance, coadministering an anticholinergic and a sympathomimetic agent can be recommended for patients with stable COPD for whom using multiple metered dose inhalers is acceptable.

**Sympathomimetic Agents**

$\beta$-Adrenergic bronchodilators are widely used in the treatment of COPD (101, 102). Agents like albuterol, metaproterenol, terbutaline, and newer drugs like fenoterol and bitolterol are the preferred sympathomimetic agents because they produce less acceleration of heart rate for a given degree of bronchodilation than nonselective adrenergic agonists. Many of these drugs can be administered in various forms (e.g., orally, by metered dose inhaler, or by nebulized solution), but inhalation appears to provide equivalent bronchodilation with less toxicity (e.g., tremor and tachycardia) and is therefore the preferred route of administration. Most patients can be instructed in the proper use of the metered dose inhaler, which offers more convenience than nebulizers and can provide equivalent bronchodilation, both in chronic stable COPD and during acute exacerbations (108).

Proper technique is very important with metered dose inhalers to ensure adequate drug administration (109–112). The recommended steps for use of metered dose inhalers are as follows (111, 112):

1. Remove inhaler cap.
2. Shake inhaler.
3. Hold inhaler upright.
4. Tilt head back or keep level.
5. Exhale (to either functional residual capacity or residual volume).
6. Close lips on inhaler, keeping tongue flat and teeth apart or keep mouthpiece 2 to 4 cm away from mouth.
7. Begin breathing then actuate device once.
8. Continue slow, deep inspiration.
9. Hold breath for 5 to 10 seconds at total lung capacity.
10. Breathe out (through either mouth or nose), and wait 20 to 30 seconds before next puff.
11. Shake inhaler again before next actuation.

Some authors further recommend holding the metered dose inhaler approximately two fingerbreadths outside the open mouth during inhalation, rather than in the mouth, to maximize drug delivery. Improper technique can compromise efficacy, since only 10 to 20% of the administered dose is delivered to the airways with optimal use. Because improper technique is common even in longstanding metered dose inhaler users, careful instruction on proper technique by health care providers is strongly encouraged (109–112).

Several lines of evidence support the use of sympathomimetic agents in chronic obstructive lung disease:

1. A component of reversible air flow obstruction is frequently present in patients with COPD, though reversible air flow obstruction may escape detection on any single bronchodilator test (45, 113). For example, Berger and Smith found evidence of a significant bronchodilator response (defined in this study as a greater than 15% rise in $FEV_1$) in 38% of tests in 517 patients with COPD (113). Furthermore, Anthonisen and coworkers performed serial isoproterenol inhalations in 985 COPD patients and found that 68% of patients whose $FEV_1$ failed to increase on the first bronchodilator trial showed a significant response on subsequent testing (up to seven serial tests) (45).

2. Even in the absence of reversible air flow obstruction, aggressive bronchodilator therapy can improve dyspnea and functional status in patients with COPD (46, 47). For example, Berger and Smith showed that walking distance could be significantly enhanced by metaproterenol inhalation, despite the absence of a rise in $FEV_1$ as experienced in a prior course of corticosteroids (47). Similarly, Guyatt and coworkers have reported that combined sympathomimetic and theophylline treatment improve air flow, walking capacity, and functional status in stable COPD patients who lack reversibility of air flow obstruction (46).

3. Aggressive bronchodilator treatment can improve gas exchange in stable COPD. As shown in the Nocturnal Oxygen Therapy Trial (173) and in subsequent studies (114), combined therapy with theophylline and sympathomimetics can improve oxygenation enough to eliminate the need for long-term oxygen therapy in at least 21% of COPD patients who are potential candidates for oxygen therapy.

## Theophylline

Despite continued uncertainty about its mechanism of action, theophylline is still used commonly in treating stable COPD and acute exacerbations (115).

Besides beneficial effects on air flow (116), right heart function in cor pulmonale (117, 118), and diaphragmatic function (119, 120), further support for using aminophylline in stable COPD comes from studies showing that theophylline can enhance patients' functional status and improve dyspnea even in the absence of bronchodilation (47, 121). For example, in a double-blind, crossover trial of theophylline versus placebo in patients with stable COPD, Mahler and coworkers observed improved Dyspnea Index scores in theophylline recipients, without any significant changes in $FEV_1$ or arterial oxygen tension (121). Though debate continues (122), more recent studies have confirmed these findings (46, 123) and have further suggested that the beneficial effects of theophylline on dyspnea and functional status in stable COPD correlate most closely with improvements in respiratory muscle function (123, 124).

Because theophylline may improve functional status in these stable COPD patients and because even small amounts of bronchodilation can produce large proportionate increases in air flow, theophylline remains a reasonable treatment in patients with stable COPD who have significant functional impairment.

The principles of using theophylline in stable COPD are the same as for managing asthma, and vigilance for toxicity (e.g., insomnia, tremulousness, irritability, nausea, seizures, and atrial and ventricular ectopy) is warranted, even when serum levels fall within the so-called "therapeutic range" of 10 to 20 $\mu g/ml$ (116, 125). Because of a log-linear relationship between bronchodilation and blood level, increasing the blood level above 10 $\mu g/ml$ may result in considerable toxicity without a significant increase in therapeutic benefit (126). A distinctive potential complication of theophylline in COPD is the development of multifocal atrial tachycardia, a rapid but irregular supraventricular tachycardia characterized by at least three separate P wave morphologies. Originally believed to reflect the sequelae of underlying lung disease, its occurrence as a manifestation of theophylline toxicity has more recently been suggested (127).

In contrast to the continued popularity of theophylline in treating stable COPD, its efficacy in acute exacerbations of COPD has been questioned recently (128). Comparative studies in acute asthma (116) suggest that aminophylline is less effective as an acute bronchodilator than either inhaled or parenteral sympathomimetic agents. In a randomized, double-blind, controlled trial in acute exacerbations of COPD (128), adding intravenous aminophylline to a regimen of oral antibiotics, inhaled metaproterenol, and intravenous methylprednisolone neither enhanced bronchodilation, improved arterial blood gases, nor ameliorated dyspnea. On the other hand, aminophylline recipients experienced more frequent side effects (especially gastrointestinal symptoms). Overall, recent data suggest that aminophylline confers at best only a marginal benefit in treating patients with acute exacerbations of COPD.

## Corticosteroids

In spite of longstanding clinical use and investigation, the efficacy of systemic corticosteroids for patients with stable chronic obstructive pulmonary disease remains controversial (129–132). Table 10.4 summarizes the results of one meta-analysis of 14 available randomized controlled trials of steroids in stable COPD (129, 133–148). Overall, eight of the 14 studies found corticosteroids more effective than placebo in improving at least one study outcome (e.g., air flow, walking distance). The $FEV_1$ was the most frequently considered outcome event, and six of the 13 trials evaluating $FEV_1$ showed that corticosteroids improved $FEV_1$ more than placebo. Following this meta-analysis, another study by Callahan et al reviewed 33 studies of corticosteroids for patients with stable COPD and concluded that corticosteroid recipients experienced more frequent $FEV_1$ increases (of 20% or more) than placebo recipients by 10% (132). Since these meta-analyses, several additional studies have examined whether inhaled corticosteroids offer long-term benefit to patients with stable COPD. In a 6-week randomized controlled trial of inhaled beclomethasone

(840 $\mu$g/day) versus placebo in patients with chronic bronchitis, Thompson et al showed that recipients of inhaled corticosteroids had improved spirometry values in association with decreased airway inflammation (as assessed by bronchoalveolar lavage and direct airway examination) (149). In a longer 2½-year controlled trial comparing beclomethasone (800 $\mu$g/day), ipratropium bromide (160 $\mu$g/day), and placebo in patients with a broad spectrum of obstructive airway disease, Kerstjens et al showed that beclomethasone but not ipratropium was associated with increased $FEV_1$ and decreased airway hyperresponsiveness (150). However, the largest improvements in $FEV_1$ were seen in the subset of patients with features of asthma (i.e., age less than 40, airway hyperresponsiveness with baseline $PC_{20}$ 0.6 mg/ml, nonsmokers), so the benefits of inhaled corticosteroids for patients with COPD were not conclusively demonstrated in this study (150). Similar findings have been reported by Weir et al (151). Corticosteroids (inhaled or oral) have also been suggested to slow the progression of chronic air flow obstruction (152–154). Finally, Sparrow et al recently showed that normal men with higher endogenous cortisol levels had a slower decline in FVC than subjects with lower cortisol levels, suggesting that cortisol may modulate the deterioration of lung function with aging (155). Though these lines of evidence suggest a benefit

## TABLE 10.4
### RESULTS OF 14 TRIALS: TYPES OF OUTCOMES EXAMINED, CONFIDENCE INTERVALS AROUND CHANGE IN $FEV_1$ ON STEROIDS, AND CATEGORICAL ANALYSIS OF $FEV_1$ RESPONSE

| | | | Shown to Improve More With Steroid Than Placebo? | | | | 95% Confidence Interval for ($FEV_1$ Rise after Steroids − $FEV_1$ Rise after Placebo) | | Categorical Analysis Proportion (%) of Patients with >15% $FEV_1$ Rise on | |
|---|---|---|---|---|---|---|---|---|---|---|
| Reference | Publication Date | No. Pts. Completing the Trial | $FEV_1$ | FVC | 12-Min Walk Distance | Any Measured Outcome? | Interval (ml) | "Width" of Interval | Placebo | Steroids |
| Trial 1  Ogilvie and Newell (146) | 1960 | 60 | — | — | — | 0 | ? | ? | ? | ? |
| Trial 2  Beerel et al (148) | 1963 | 10 | 0 | — | — | 0 | ? | ? | 4/10 (40) | 4/10 (40) |
| Trial 3  Hurford et al (147) | 1963 | 39 | + | — | — | + | 101.3 ± 45.3 | 90.6 | 2/20 (10) | 4/19 (21) |
| Trial 4  Morgan and Rusche (145) | 1964 | 12 | 0 | — | — | 0 | 64.4 ± 259.7 | 519.4 | 1/7 (14) | 1/7 (14) |
| Trial 5  Beerel and Vance (138) | 1964 | 17 | 0 | 0 | — | + | ? | ? | ? | ? |
| Trial 6  Evans et al (140) | 1974 | 10 | 0 | — | — | 0 | 36.0 ± 116.1 | 232.2 | 1/10 (10) | 1/10 (10) |
| Trial 7  Shim et al (137) | 1978 | 24 | + | — | — | + | 154.2 ± 45.6 | 91.1 | 4/24 (16) | 11/24 (46) |
| Trial 8  Mendella et al (133) | 1982 | 46 | + | — | — | + | ? | ? | 8/46 (17) | 13/46 (28) |
| Trial 9  O'Reilly et al (139) | 1982 | 10 | 0 | 0 | 0 | + | 74.0 ± 74.3 | 148.6 | 1/10 (10) | 3/10 (30) |
| Trial 10  Lam et al (141) | 1983 | 16 | + | + | + | + | 180.0 ± 71.5 | 143.0 | 2/26 (3) | 9/16 (56) |
| Trial 11  Mitchell et al (136) | 1984 | 43 | + | + | + | + | ? | ? | 8/43 (19)[b] | 15/43 (35)[b] |
| Trial 12  Blair and Light (142) | 1984 | 44 | + | + | — | + | ? | ? | 4/12 (33) | 16/20 (55) |
| Trial 13  Strain et al (143) | 1985 | 13 | 0 | 0 | — | 0 | ? | ? | ? | ? |
| Trial 14  Eliasson et al (144) | 1986 | 16 | 0 | 0 | — | 0 | ? | ? | ? | ? |

From Stoller JK, Gerbarg ZB, Feinstein AR. Corticosteroids in stable chronic obstructive pulmonary disease: reappraisal of efficacy. *J Gen Intern Med* 1987;2:29–35.

[a] +, yes; 0, no; —, does not apply, outcome not measured; ? cannot be determined from published report.

[b] 20% rise in $FEV_1$.

of corticosteroids in the long-term management of stable COPD, the issue remains controversial.

Overall, it appears that corticosteroids are beneficial in 10 to 56% of patients with stable chronic obstructive pulmonary disease, and that individual patients may sometimes respond much more substantially than the relatively small group mean responses seen in these trials. In the authors' view, corticosteroid trials should be considered when stable COPD patients remain functionally impaired despite optimal conventional therapy (e.g., inhaled $\beta_2$-adrenergic agonists and anticholinergics, theophylline, pulmonary rehabilitation). When used, corticosteroids should be given in moderate doses (e.g., 40 mg or more of prednisone daily or equivalent) for at least 1 week (156). In the absence of a clear-cut objective benefit of steroid therapy (e.g., a substantial $FEV_1$ increment, improved gas exchange), the clinician should consider a randomized crossover trial with the individual patient (*n*-of-1 trial) (157, 158), lest patients incur steroid-associated toxicity for benefits that do not exceed placebo effects. If a short course of corticosteroids does prove beneficial, the clinician should then determine the lowest dose of corticosteroids necessary to preserve this benefit. Tapering to an inhaled corticosteroid alone or to an every-other-day oral regimen are attractive options, which are sometimes successful and are associated with less morbidity than chronic high doses of systemic corticosteroids (159–162).

As with acute exacerbations of asthma, corticosteroids have been shown to be effective in accelerating recovery from acute exacerbations of chronic obstructive pulmonary disease (135). For example, studying 44 patients with severe chronic bronchitis during an acute exacerbation, Albert and colleagues (135) conducted a randomized placebo-controlled trial comparing intravenous corticosteroids (methylprednisolone, 0.5 mg/kg every 6 hours for 3 days) with placebo. All patients received standard therapy including intravenous aminophylline and an inhaled sympathomimetic, oral antibiotics (ampicillin or tetracycline), and oxygen. Recovery of $FEV_1$ was accelerated in the steroid recipients, supporting the use of intravenous corticosteroids for exacerbations of chronic obstructive pulmonary disease. However, this study has been criticized because of a lower initial $FEV_1$ in the steroid group despite randomization, and because of inadequate statistical methods (163). More recent studies (164) suggest that unlike a 3-day course of intravenous methylprednisolone, a single dose of 100 mg in the emergency room does not accelerate improvement during an acute exacerbation of chronic bronchitis. Though no clear information is available in COPD, conclusions regarding

corticosteroids and acute exacerbations of asthma suggest that oral corticosteroid tapers and repository forms of corticosteroids (i.e., methylprednisolone sodium acetate intramuscularly) may be useful alternatives to intravenous therapy. Information about the optimal dose of corticosteroids is scanty, but studies on asthma suggest that high doses of intravenous methylprednisolone (e.g., 125 mg every 6 hours) accelerate improvement in air flow more rapidly than lower doses (e.g., 15 mg every 6 hours) (165). Overall, because of the persisting uncertainty about the benefits of systemic corticosteroids in acute exacerbations of COPD, a multicenter randomized, placebo-controlled trial is currently being conducted.

### Antibiotic Therapy in Chronic Obstructive Pulmonary Disease

Acute exacerbations of COPD often present with worsened dyspnea and increased volume and purulence of phlegm. Sputum examination most frequently shows *Haemophilus influenzae*, *Streptococcus pneumoniae*, or *Moraxella catarrhalis*, although these are common organisms of the normal upper respiratory tract (166).

Despite a time-honored view that antibiotics are beneficial for acute exacerbations of COPD, evidence for their efficacy has only recently become available. Specifically, an earlier randomized, double-blind trial of tetracycline (500 mg orally 4 times daily for 1 week) versus placebo for acute exacerbations of chronic bronchitis failed to demonstrate significant benefit from adding tetracycline to a conventional regimen of bronchodilators, corticosteroids, chest physiotherapy, or diuretics (167). More recently, Anthonisen and coworkers (168) performed a double-blind, placebo-controlled trial in which 362 acute exacerbation episodes were treated with a 10-day course of an oral antibiotic (trimethoprim-sulfamethoxazole [one single-strength tablet daily], amoxicillin [250 mg 4 times daily] or doxycycline [200 mg once, then 100 mg daily]) or placebo. Successful resolution of the acute exacerbation was 1.24 times more likely in antibiotic recipients than in placebo recipients, and clinical deterioration beyond 72 hours after treatment was almost 2 times less likely in patients receiving antibiotics. The benefits of antibiotic therapy were greatest in patients who experienced the symptom triad of increased dyspnea, increased sputum volume, and increased purulence, and no differences between the three antibiotic regimens were observed. Based on this study, antibiotics are recommended in the short-term management of exacerbations of chronic obstructive pulmonary disease. Although Gram's stain and culture of the sputum have not been deemed helpful in the initial management of acute exacerbations of COPD (169), the emergence of

*Moraxella catarrhalis* may revise this view. Because 75% of *Moraxella catarrhalis* produce β-lactamase, identifying the characteristic Gram-negative diplococci suggesting this organism on a Gram's stain should alter the initial choice of antibiotic (166).

The role of prophylactic antibiotic therapy to prevent exacerbations has been extensively studied, with conflicting results. Overall, it appears that the value of antibiotic prophylaxis is limited, except possibly in patients with a large number of exacerbations (166).

## Supplemental Oxygen Administration

Supplemental oxygen administration is a key aspect of treating patients with hypoxic COPD, because oxygen has been shown to benefit patients with acute hypoxemic exacerbations of COPD, as well as patients with chronic, stable hypoxemic COPD (170–182).

In chronic hypoxemic COPD, the benefits of oxygen administration have been demonstrated by two important studies: the British Medical Research Council (MRC) study (174) and the American Nocturnal Oxygen Therapy Trial (NOTT) (173). Though these studies were designed differently, their aggregate results confirm that oxygen administration improves survival in patients with hypoxemic COPD. Specifically, the British study compared the benefits of 15 hours of oxygen daily (usually 2 liters/minute by nasal cannulae) versus no oxygen, and the NOTT trial compared nocturnal oxygen only (i.e., 12 hours/day) with "continuous" oxygen therapy, titrated to maintain the arterial oxygen tension (PaO$_2$) greater than 65 mm Hg. The mean daily duration of oxygen use in the "continuous" group was actually 19 hours/day.

As shown in Figure 10.16, both the British and American studies demonstrate that oxygen administration improves survival in patients with stable, hypoxemic COPD. In the British study, the crude 5-year mortality rate in oxygen recipients was 45.2% versus 66.7% in nonrecipients of oxygen, and in the NOTT trial, the 2-year crude mortality rate in the "continuous" oxygen group was 22.4% versus 40.8% in the nocturnal oxygen group (relative risk of death, 1.94). Other physiologic benefits of oxygen therapy in the American trial included significantly decreased pulmonary vascular resistance in the continuous oxygen recipients (mean reduction of 11.1% versus a mean rise of 6.5% in the nocturnal group), a greater amelioration of polycythemia in the "continuously" treated group (a mean hematocrit decline of 9.2% versus 2.0%), and improved neuropsychologic function in the continuously treated group, an effect that was observed only after approximately 1 month of continuous oxygen treatment. Based on the aggregate results of these

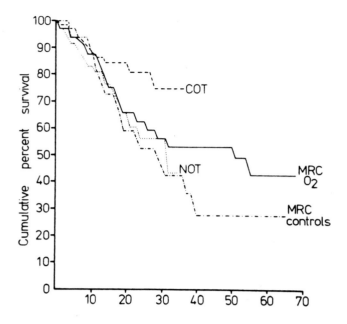

**FIGURE 10.16.** Cumulative percent survival of patients in the Nocturnal Oxygen Therapy Trial (NOTT) and Medical Research Council (MRC) controlled trials of long-term domiciliary oxygen therapy for men aged over 70. The MRC control subjects (– · –·–·) received no oxygen, NOTT subjects (···) received oxygen for 12 hours in the 24-hour day, including the sleeping hours; MRC O$_2$ subjects ( ) received oxygen for 15 hours in the 24-hour day, including the sleep hours, and continuous oxygen therapy (COT) subjects (– – –) received oxygen for 24 hours in the 24-hour day (on average, 19 hours). (From Flenley DC: Long-term oxygen therapy. *Chest* 87:99–103, 1985.)

two studies, it can be concluded that for stable, hypoxemic COPD patients, oxygen for part of the day is better than no oxygen, but continuous oxygen therapy affords the greatest advantage (178). Therefore, long-term oxygen therapy is recommended for stable COPD patients with the following indications:

1. Room air PaO$_2$  55 mm Hg,
2. Room air 55 mm Hg < PaO$_2$  59 mm Hg, with evidence of edema, polycythemia (hematocrit 55%), or cor pulmonale on the electrocardiogram.

Reimbursement guidelines accept an oxygen saturation level of 88% or less as qualifying for reimbursable supplemental oxygen, though oxygen saturation levels from oximetry may correlate inexactly with arterial blood gas values.

The importance of establishing stable hypoxemia before committing patients to long-term oxygen supplementation is emphasized by the fact that with aggressive bronchodilator treatment, oxygenation may improve in chronic obstructive pulmonary disease. For example, after 3 weeks of aggressive bronchodilator therapy (theophylline, sympathomimetic agents with antibiotics or diuretics as needed), 21% of patients initially eligible for the Nocturnal Oxygen Therapy Trial no longer met $PaO_2$ entry criteria (173). A more recent study suggests that this probationary period should be extended to 3 months for patients whose room air $PaO_2$ values fall between 50 and 60 mm Hg (114).

While the survival benefit of oxygen supplementation is evident from these studies, the mechanism by which this oxygen supplementation prolongs survival remains controversial, with some studies supporting a relationship between improved survival and decreased pulmonary artery pressures or pulmonary vascular resistance (173, 175), and others suggesting that oxygen promotes survival by improving oxygen delivery to tissues without concomitant pulmonary hemodynamic changes (180).

Oxygen therapy is also beneficial in the acute management of hypoxemic COPD exacerbations. Early studies (170, 171) suggested that by raising arterial oxygen content, oxygen administration increased tissue oxygen delivery in these patients. More recent and detailed hemodynamic studies of oxygen administration to hypoxemic acutely decompensated COPD patients suggests a heterogeneous response to oxygen administration (176, 177). In some patients, supplemental oxygen raises arterial oxygen content without altering cardiac output, and tissue oxygen delivery is concomitantly increased. In a second group of patients, the increase in arterial oxygen content is offset by a decrease in cardiac output in response to oxygen therapy, resulting in no net change in systemic oxygen delivery. Though markedly different in their response to oxygen therapy, these two groups of patients cannot be distinguished on usual clinical grounds. Baseline invasive measurements suggest that patients with a stable cardiac output on oxygen therapy tend to have a lower initial mixed venous oxygen tension (less than 35 mm Hg), suggesting increased tissue oxygen extraction to compensate for impaired delivery. Notably, acute oxygen administration may have little impact on observed pulmonary hypertension in these patients. Overall, supplemental oxygen is recommended for hypoxemic patients with acute exacerbations of chronic obstructive pulmonary disease, though the clinician must remain vigilant for hypercapnia resulting from the suppressive effect on hypoxic drive.

Whether supplemental oxygen should be prescribed for COPD patients with exercise desaturation alone with nocturnal desaturation but daytime $PaO_2$ exceeding 60 mm Hg remains controversial. Recent studies suggest that supplemental oxygen for patients with nocturnal desaturation but daytime $PaO_2$ of 60 mm Hg

or above can reduce pulmonary artery pressures and is associated with a trend toward increased survival (181–183). Though current Health Care Financing Administration (HCFA) guidelines allow reimbursement for nocturnal oxygen when saturations decrease by 5% or more during sleep, the paucity of evidence that nocturnal oxygen enhances survival has led many investigators to defer prescribing nocturnal oxygen for such patients in favor of organizing a large-scale randomized trial (like the NOTT or MRC studies) to settle the controversy.

Recent progress in oxygen therapy includes new apparatuses for delivering oxygen, which provide alternatives to traditional nasal cannulas (172, 184). Oxygen conservation devices (e.g., the Oxymizer Reservoir Cannula and the Oxymizer Pendant) permit equivalent oxygenation with a lower liter flow requirement by storing exhaled oxygen in a reservoir or by triggering oxygen flow with inspiratory demand. Another recent development is transtracheal oxygen therapy, in which a small catheter is inserted into the trachea through an anterior tracheal ring (185). Transtracheal oxygen therapy has been promoted on the basis of lower liter flow requirements, avoidance of the morbidity associated with the nasal cannula, and improved cosmesis. Other reported advantages include decreased dyspnea and increased exercise tolerance, possibly due to a decrease in inspired minute ventilation (186), and decreased hospitalization, possibly due to increased compliance with continuous therapy (187). Available experience with transtracheal oxygen therapy suggests that sequelae and complications are relatively infrequent and are only rarely clinically significant. Patients' acceptance of transtracheal oxygen therapy is generally high, though careful patient selection continues to seem prudent (188). In the authors' view, the major indication for transtracheal oxygen therapy is the inability to provide a sufficient level of arterial oxygen (e.g., $PaO_2$ greater than 55 mm Hg) despite a high liter flow (e.g., 6 liters/minute or more) by nasal cannula. Others have advocated transtracheal oxygen therapy for improved functional status (e.g., increased duration for a single oxygen tank or improved cosmesis) and to avoid the morbidity associated with nasal cannulas (irritation, etc.) (185).

### Almitrine Bismesylate

Excitement accompanied the introduction of almitrine bismesylate, a new drug that appears to improve oxygenation in COPD patients by improving ventilation-perfusion matching. For example, in a placebo-controlled trial, Bell and coworkers demonstrated a mean $PaO_2$ rise of 11.2 mm Hg in almitrine recipients (versus a 1.5 mm Hg rise in $Pa_{O_2}$ with placebo), accompanied by only a 3.8 mm Hg decrement in the $Pa_{CO_2}$ (190). Despite this initial appeal, however, subsequent evaluation has shown that almitrine can worsen dyspnea in a large minority of recipients and that almitrine use is associated with further elevation of pulmonary arterial pressure in patients with COPD (mean rise from $22 \pm 4$ mm Hg to $35 \pm 5$ mm Hg in one series) (189). Thus, improved ventilation-perfusion matching appears to be associated with adverse effects, which has dampened enthusiasm that almitrine will alter the current management of stable COPD.

## Pulmonary Rehabilitation

A pulmonary rehabilitation program can be a useful adjunct to medical therapy for patients with stable COPD (191, 192). Typical components of rehabilitation programs include exercise training (e.g., serial treadmill training, stationary bicycles, stair climbing, and upper-extremity exercises) (193); physical and occupational therapy (i.e., to review energy conservation techniques); didactic sessions with respiratory health care providers to review the pathophysiology of COPD, pharmacologic principles, inspiratory muscle training, and techniques for optimal medication use (e.g., metered dose inhaler techniques) (112); and support sessions with fellow patients and family members.

Demonstrated short-term benefits of rehabilitation include improved strength and/or endurance of the specific muscle groups trained (194), improved exercise capacity, and improved functional status (191, 192).

Because training benefits are specific for the muscle group trained (194), specific attention has been given to identifying important muscle groups that may affect respiratory status and for which training can enhance respiratory function. Many studies have examined the benefits of training the "traditional" ventilatory muscles of inspiration (e.g., diaphragm, external intercostal muscles, scalene muscles) and have shown that serial inspiratory training through threshold resistors can produce enhanced exercise tolerance and increased inspiratory muscle strength (205). More recently, a dual role of shoulder girdle and upper torso muscles to support both upper-extremity function and inspiration has been appreciated (195). For example, fatiguing arm exercise may cause dyspnea and disrupted thoracoabdominal muscle excursion. By the same token, upper-extremity training has been shown to enhance ventilatory muscle endurance and inspiratory muscle strength, while decreasing dyspnea and oxygen consumption for specific tasks (196). On this basis, upper-extremity training should be included as a routine part

of a comprehensive pulmonary rehabilitation program (183, 194, 196).

Reductions in air flow obstruction are generally meager, if they occur at all. A decrease in lactate and minute ventilation in response to exercise have recently been demonstrated in patients undergoing a rehabilitation program (197). Another study documented the benefit of upper-extremity training in reducing oxygen uptake, carbon dioxide production, and minute ventilation (196). These two studies thereby provide a physiologic rationale for improved exercise tolerance after rehabilitation.

Whether a rehabilitation program confers lasting benefit has been questioned, but recent studies suggest that when participants continue a regular training regimen at home following the program, enhanced exercise tolerance can be sustained over at least a year (191, 198). For patients who cannot participate in a formal rehabilitation program, a regimen of progressive stair climbing at home has also been shown to enhance exercise tolerance (199).

## Nutritional Supplementation

Malnutrition is common among patients with COPD and is estimated to affect between 27 and 71% of these patients. Furthermore, to the extent that malnutrition adversely affects prognosis in COPD (40, 41), attempts to improve outcome by improving nutrition are appealing. Initial studies in a spectrum of malnourished patients have shown that inspiratory muscle strength is impaired by malnutrition and that parenteral nutritional repletion can improve body mass and inspiratory muscle strength (203). In patients with chronic obstructive pulmonary disease, early reports were less promising, but more recent studies suggest that oral nutritional supplementation can also promote weight gain, which is accompanied by enhanced respiratory and nonrespiratory muscle function. Specifically, Wilson and coworkers showed that 2 weeks of nutritional repletion in patients with COPD (150% of caloric needs) resulted in a mean weight gain of 3.1 kg and concomitantly increased maximal inspiratory mouth pressure, transdiaphragmatic pressure, and handgrip strength (200). Extending these findings, Efthimiou and colleagues conducted a single-blind randomized trial of nutritional repletion versus usual diet for 3 months in COPD patients (201). After increasing caloric and protein intake by approximately 150% over baseline, mean weight rose by 4.2 kg, respiratory muscle strength and handgrip strength increased, and walking distance and functional status improved. No changes in air flow or gas exchange were observed. Unfortunately, follow-up after the 3-month trial showed that patients frequently reverted to their baseline inadequate diets, with a concomitant loss of improvements. In a recent review of five controlled studies of nutritional supplementation in patients with COPD, Muers et al concluded that only patients with caloric intake increases of over 30% seemed to benefit from supplementation (41).

Based on these data, it appears that high-protein, high-calorie diets can benefit patients with COPD, but that these benefits accrue only while the improved diet is followed. A recent study has shown that treating malnutrition in COPD with carbohydrate-rich meals (versus fat-rich diets or placebo) is associated with an increased minute ventilation, carbon dioxide production, oxygen consumption, and arterial $Pa_{CO_2}$, along with worsened dyspnea ratings on a Borg scale and a decrease in the 6-minute walk distance (202). This study provides a strong rationale for prescribing high-fat rather than high-carbohydrate supplementation to COPD patients. To ensure continued benefit from diet, follow-up reminders to patients and ongoing dietary monitoring should be a part of a dietary plan for these patients. Whether nutritional repletion also favorably affects prognosis remains unclear at the present time.

### Ventilatory Muscle Training

Because patients with COPD demonstrate impaired ventilatory mechanics and can develop inspiratory muscle fatigue, ventilatory muscle training is an appealing treatment for stable patients. As recently reviewed by Belman (204), the three available methods of ventilatory muscle training have been:

1. Resistive training, in which the patient breathes through progressively smaller apertures,
2. Hyperpneic training, in which high levels of ventilation are sustained for increasing durations, and
3. Threshold load training, in which the patient inspires against a resistance that permits inspiratory flow only after a threshold inspiratory pressure is reached.

Because of its technical ease, resistive training has been the most widely examined technique for ventilatory muscle training. Initial enthusiasm for this method was based on findings that patients could breathe through small orifices after a resistive training program, but more recently, Belman has pointed out that patients can breathe through small orifices by altering their breathing strategy (i.e., breathing more slowly), rather than as a result of improved ventilatory muscle strength (204). A recent meta-analysis of techniques for ventilatory muscle training has found little evidence for a clinical benefit of exercises involving resistive breathing or isocapnic hyperventilation (205). Secondary analyses of these same data suggest that

clinically significant improvements in strength and endurance may occur when the breathing pattern is controlled to ensure generating adequate mouth pressures (205). Studies with hyperpneic training and threshold load devices have shown modest improvements in patients' inspiratory muscle strength and walking capacity (206), but further study will be required before ventilatory muscle training can be endorsed routinely for patients with stable COPD. Specifically, basic questions are currently unanswered, for example:

1. Can ventilatory muscle training induce fatigue, and if so, in whom?
2. Is exercise capacity limited by inspiratory muscle strength or endurance in patients with stable COPD? and
3. Which method of ventilatory muscle training is preferable?

### Intermittent Mechanical Ventilation for Stable COPD

Intermittent mechanical ventilation to rest the inspiratory muscles has been proposed as an adjunct to managing patients with hypercapnic but stable COPD (207, 208). Despite the promising results of earlier short-term or uncontrolled studies (209), more recent randomized control trials have failed to show significant clinical benefit for noninvasive ventilation administered by either face mask ventilation (211) or negative-pressure ventilation (210). Thus, despite the demonstrable benefit of intermittent ventilation in patients with hypoventilatory respiratory failure from restrictive neuromuscular diseases or chest wall deformities, intermittent mechanical ventilation cannot currently be endorsed for patients with COPD (209).

### Surgical Therapy for Bullous Emphysema: Bullectomy and Reduction Pneumoplasty

A minority of patients with emphysema will have localized bullae on chest radiograph (1 to 22%) that may prompt consideration of bullectomy or surgical resection of bullae (17, 212). In view of the paucity of information on long-term efficacy of bullectomy, patient selection should be strict and confined to those who are markedly impaired (dyspnea, pneumothorax, and infected bullae have been common indications), who have large but localized bullae (i.e., more than one-third of the affected lung), and who have physiologic and radiographic features predictive of benefit from bullectomy. These features include (17):

1. A large (e.g., up to 4-liter) discrepancy between functional residual capacity determined by helium dilution and plethysmography, suggesting trapped air behind compressed airways,
2. Evidence of ipsilateral lung compression by a large

bulla (e.g., compression of lung markings, often with downward displacement of the hila by upper lung zone bullae), and

3. Evidence of vascular crowding adjacent to the bullae on pulmonary angiogram.

Predictors of poor surgical outcome include diffuse emphysema, chronic bronchitis (especially with hypercapnia), and $\alpha_1$-antitrypsin deficiency. However, the advent of augmentation therapy for $\alpha_1$-antitrypsin deficiency may eliminate this contraindication, especially if augmentation therapy proves effective in arresting the progression of emphysema in affected patients.

Operative mortality rates following bullectomy range from 1.5 to 9.0% (17, 212). Although data from long-term follow-up studies are scant, several series do suggest that bullectomy can improve air flow and functional status, though subsequent progression of lung disease does not appear to be altered by bullectomy. In a recent long-term study of 46 patients after bullectomy, Nickoladze concluded that although long-term (i.e., 5-year) improvement in respiratory function was apparent after removal of bullae affecting more than a third of the lung, no improvement was noted for smaller bullae, and deterioration of lung function was noted after resection of bullae associated with pneumonia (213).

More recently, reduction pneumoplasty (which involves removal of small portions of emphysematous lung) has been proposed to enhance pulmonary function and and patients' functional status. Although preliminary results in a small number of recipients have been promising (213a), more experience and critical evaluation will be needed before this procedure can be endorsed or selection criteria specified.

## Lung Transplantation

In recent years, lung transplantation has become a more widely available therapeutic option for patients with end-stage lung disease. Currently, although concerns about mediastinal shift with postoperative compression of the transplanted lung by the more compliant overinflated emphysematous lung led to the early recommendations that patients with emphysema undergo double lung transplantation (215), more recent experience with single lung transplantation for emphysema suggests that although mediastinal shift may occur, it rarely has significant clinical impact (216). In the International Lung Transplantation Registry, emphysema from COPD and $\alpha_1$-antitrypsin deficiency account for about 60% of all single lung transplantations performed (214). Actuarial survival curves after single lung transplantation for emphysema show a 2- and 3-year survival of 77% and 75%, respectively (214). Actuarial survival rates for single lung transplant patients with emphysema are significantly higher than the survival rates for transplant patients with interstitial pulmonary fibrosis or primary pulmonary hypertension (Fig. 10.17) (214). Survival after transplantation for emphysema is significantly higher after single lung transplantation than after double lung transplantation (214).

## PROGNOSIS IN CHRONIC OBSTRUCTIVE PULMONARY DISEASE

Establishing an accurate prognosis for the patient with chronic obstructive pulmonary disease remains a

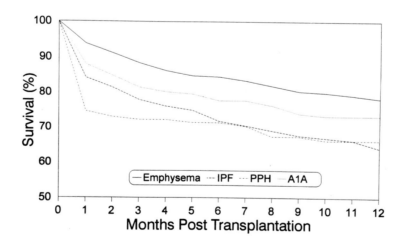

**FIGURE 10.17.** Actuarial survival from single lung transplantation by indication. The overall survival is significantly higher in patients with emphysema (including $\alpha_1$-antitrypsin deficiency) versus idiopathic pulmonary fibrosis or primary pulmonary hypertension. (Reproduced with permission from Hosenpud JD, Novick RJ, Breen TJ, Daily OP: The Registry of the International Society for Heart and Lung Transplantation: Eleventh Official Report—1994. *J Heart Lung Transplant* 13:561–570, 1994.)

formidable but important challenge for the clinician and has been the subject of both intense study and controversy. Of the many available series, studies employing a longitudinal design (i.e., in which the same patients are followed serially) have most clearly identified key prognostic determinants. Studies with the alternative cross-sectional design (i.e., different patient study groups are each examined once) are subject to bias that may underestimate the rate of disease progression (217).

Prognosis in both chronic bronchitis and emphysema is determined by several major factors, including the severity of air flow obstruction and its rate of decline (218, 219), the nature of the lung disease (e.g., chronic bronchitis, emphysema, or so-called chronic asthmatic bronchitis) (220), the activity and magnitude of smoking, the hemodynamic sequelae of lung disease (173, 180), and associated constitutional features (e.g., weight loss) (40, 41).

### Severity of Air Flow Obstruction and Its Rate of Decline

Many studies confirm that the degree of air flow obstruction is the strongest single predictor of outcome in chronic obstructive pulmonary disease. For example, in the long-term follow-up series by Diener and Burrows (219), 12-year survival rates declined from approximately 40% to nearly 5% in patients whose initial $FEV_1$ was greater than 1.25 and less than 0.75 liter, respectively. Whether or not the rate of change of $FEV_1$ further predicts outcome is controversial. Data from Diener and Burrows suggest that for comparable degrees of air flow obstruction, patients with lower yearly rates of $FEV_1$ decline fare better than those with more precipitously declining lung function. Other investigators have interpreted the low values of $FEV_1$ to simply reflect the antecedent effects of accelerated decline in pulmonary function, an effect dubbed the "horse racing effect" (21). Still other investigators have observed that the rate of $FEV_1$ decline is slower in patients with markedly impaired lung function than in those whose $FEV_1$ is higher, an observation in conflict with the "horse racing effect" (221). This slower rate of decline in patients with already markedly impaired lung function has been interpreted as the "survivor effect," suggesting that survival with a low $FEV_1$ reflects a low rate of $FEV_1$ decline before.

### Type of Lung Disease

Studies examining prognostic differences between emphysema and chronic bronchitis have focused on the impact of mucus hypersecretion, the clinical hallmark by which the diagnosis of chronic bronchitis is made. Overall, the weight of available evidence suggests that the type of lung disease is a less potent determinant of outcome than the magnitude of air flow obstruction, but that all other determinants being equal, chronic bronchitics may enjoy a more benign course than patients with emphysema. For example, Kanner and coworkers longitudinally studied 84 patients with a spectrum of obstructive lung diseases—emphysema, bronchiectasis, chronic bronchitis, asthma, and admixtures of these (222). Multivariate regression analysis showed that disease type was an independent predictor of outcome and that the mean yearly decline in $FEV_1$ was lower in chronic bronchitics ($-12.2$ ml/year) than in patients with emphysema ($-62.5$ ml/year) (222). Other studies confirm this observation (223). Furthermore, in the classic longitudinal study of 792 British postal and transit workers, Fletcher and coworkers (21) noted a strong correlation between mucus hypersecretion and the yearly decline in $FEV_1$, but because short-term increases in phlegm production were dissociated from changes in $FEV_1$, bronchitic symptoms were not believed to cause the $FEV_1$ decline. Patients with mucus hypersecretion but no air flow obstruction were found to have a quite favorable prognosis in this series (224).

Finally, some series suggest that patients with COPD and asthmatic features (i.e., so-called chronic asthmatic bronchitics) (220) have both a better survival rate (80% 10-year survival) and slower decline in $FEV_1$ than patients with emphysema or chronic bronchitis lacking asthmatic features. Because of competing theories about the pathogenesis of chronic air flow obstruction (i.e., the so-called Dutch versus British hypotheses) (225), the correlation between airway reactivity and the rate of $FEV_1$ decline has taken on special importance in the literature. Briefly stated, the British hypothesis suggests that mucus hypersecretion is an early event in the development of chronic bronchitis, resulting in a sequence of bronchial infection leading to bronchial obstruction and parenchymal loss (i.e., emphysema). In contrast, the Dutch hypothesis maintains that increased airway reactivity is the inciting event, resulting in mucosal edema and mucus hypersecretion. Irreversible air flow obstruction putatively follows.

Efforts to examine these alternative hypotheses have focused on the relationship between airway reactivity (i.e., bronchial hyperactivity to nonspecific bronchoconstrictors or reversibility of air flow obstruction by inhaled bronchodilators) and the rate of decline in lung function. Proponents of the Dutch hypothesis suggest the $FEV_1$ decline is accelerated in patients with increased bronchodilator responsiveness, even in patients without established baseline air flow obstruction.

Despite extensive study, the prognostic impact of bronchodilator responsiveness remains controversial. Some studies show accelerated loss of lung function in patients with bronchodilator responsiveness and others show slower than expected declines in these patients.

Like the most recent study by Burrows and coworkers (220), data from the Intermittent Positive Pressure Breathing (IPPB) Trial (226) suggest that bronchodilator responsiveness to inhaled isoproterenol correlated with slower declines in $FEV_1$. Although bronchodilator response also correlated with increased survival initially, using the postbronchodilator $FEV_1$ as a determinant of survival caused the correlation with bronchodilator responsiveness to disappear. These and other studies (227) have concluded that the degree of fixed air flow obstruction was the strongest determinant of survival in these patients.

In contrast, other studies have suggested that increased bronchodilator responsiveness is associated with more rapid declines in $FEV_1$ (222, 228) and lend support to the Dutch hypothesis. Most notable among these is the study by Vollmer and coworkers in which 795 patients with normal baseline values of $FEV_1$ were observed (228). Matched sample comparisons between patients with bronchodilator responsiveness (i.e., increase in postbronchodilator $FEV_1$ of 7.72% or greater) and those without this responsiveness showed more rapid declines in $FEV_1$ in the former group, especially among active and former smokers. Still other studies support this finding (229) but further confound the issue by suggesting that although bronchodilator responsiveness is associated with less rapid decline in $FEV_1$, increased airway activity to nonspecific bronchoconstrictors (e.g., inhaled histamine) is associated with an accelerated decline in $FEV_1$. Studies currently under way (e.g., the Lung Health Study) promise to clarify the prognostic impact of bronchodilator responsiveness and routine bronchodilator use in stable COPD.

## $\alpha_1$-ANTITRYPSIN DEFICIENCY

$\alpha_1$-Antitrypsin deficiency is an inherited disorder that predisposes to emphysema and accounts for 2 to 5% of all cases of emphysema (16, 230). Since the association between deficiency of a serum protein ($\alpha_1$-antitrypsin, also known as $\alpha_1$-antiprotease in recognition of its physiologic function) and emphysema was first proposed by Laurell and Eriksson in 1963 (231), study of $\alpha_1$-antitrypsin deficiency has clarified the biochemistry and molecular biology of this protein and has helped formulate the current protease-antiprotease hypothesis of emphysema.

## Molecular Biology of $\alpha_1$-Antitrypsin

$\alpha_1$-Antitrypsin is a 52,000-dalton (394–amino acid) glycoprotein that is synthesized in the liver and that serves as the major inactivator of neutrophil-derived elastase (232). The disorder is codominantly inherited, and as of this writing over 75 different alleles have been identified, which are categorized according to a Pi (protease inhibitor) nomenclature system. The most common allele is the M type, and the PiMM phenotype accounts for at least 85% of individuals in most populations and at least 95% of those of northern European ancestry. $\alpha_1$-Antitrypsin variants differ in protein structure or in gene expression, with some variants preserving antiprotease activity and others impairing either synthesis (e.g., Pi null null) or antiprotease activity (e.g., PiZZ) once circulating. Of the variants associated with decreased serum levels or protein activity, the S allele is most common, with a gene frequency of 3.4%, followed by the Z allele, which accounts for a gene frequency of 1.1%. Besides PiZZ, the most common allelic combinations are PiMZ and PiMS, neither of which has been clearly implicated as predisposing to emphysema. Based on epidemiologic studies, a serum level of 80 mg/dl (or 11 $\mu$M) of $\alpha_1$-antitrypsin is deemed a "protective" threshold against emphysema, and the most common phenotype with low levels and elevated risk is PiZZ. In contrast to normal serum levels of 180 to 240 mg/dl among PiMM patients, those with a PiZZ phenotype have serum levels that are consistently less than 50 mg/dl (or 12 to 15% of normal). Individuals with PiSZ phenotypes (serum levels of 30 to 35% of normal) are considered to be at moderate risk for developing emphysema, and those with Pi Null Null (in whom no $\alpha_1$-antitrypsin is synthesized in the liver) are considered to be an even higher risk than PiZZ individuals.

The biochemical defect in Z type $\alpha_1$-antitrypsin is a single amino acid substitution (lysine instead of glutamic acid) at residue 342 (232). The striking impact of this structural alteration is impaired hepatic synthesis and release of $\alpha_1$-antitrypsin, with resultant low serum levels, although some investigators have suggested impaired activity of circulating Z type $\alpha_1$-antitrypsin as well.

The antiprotease activity of $\alpha_1$-antitrypsin derives from its ability to bind and inactivate neutrophil-derived elastase, an action that depends on an intact "active" site on the glycoprotein. This active site surrounds a central methionine residue (at position 358), oxidation of which can severely compromise antielastase activity. As mentioned, the oxidant activity of cigarette smoke, therefore, presents a substantial threat to the antielastase defense of the lung parenchyma and may tip the protease-antiprotease balance in favor of lung destruction.

## Clinical Aspects of $\alpha_1$-Antitrypsin Deficiency

The most common clinical feature of affected individuals with $\alpha_1$-antitrypsin deficiency is emphysema of unusually early onset, commonly with chest x-ray evidence of basal bullae unlike the usual apical location of bullae in smoking-related centriacinar emphysema. Dyspnea is the most common pulmonary symptom present in virtually all affected individuals. Though symptoms may begin in even young nonsmoking PiZZ individuals, conventional wisdom suggests that those who have never smoked may develop symptoms somewhat later than smokers, with a mean delay in onset of 13 years (53 years versus 40 years of age) (233, 234). Chronic or episodic bronchitis has been reported in up to 37% of patients, and a minority (4 to 11%) may have asthma or other pulmonary symptoms (e.g., cough, pleurisy), though the relation of these other symptoms to $\alpha_1$-antitrypsin deficiency remains unclear (230, 233, 234).

Radiographically, evidence of emphysema on plain films of the chest has been observed in the majority of index cases (87%) in most series, but also in most (75%) patients identified by family studies (i.e., nonindex cases) (230). In the NIH series (234), 72% of PiZZ patients had basal bullous changes versus 26% with diffuse bullous changes and fewer than 1% with apical bullous changes. Diaphragmatic flattening and vascular attenuation are common features of the chest radiograph as well. Ventilation-perfusion lung scans characteristically show loss of basal perfusion and delayed washout of basal ventilation, consistent with greater involvement of dependent lung zones. Computerized tomographic studies confirm this distribution of abnormality.

Pulmonary function tests show the expected pattern of air flow obstruction with severe declines in $FEV_1$ (34 to 42% of predicted on average in several series) (230, 234) and relative preservation of forced vital capacity (FVC). Negative effort dependence is shown by lowering of the vital capacity during forced versus slow maneuvers (mean FVC 52% of predicted versus slow vital capacity 65% of predicted in the NIH series) (234), and lung volume measurements show evidence of air trapping, with plethysmographic thoracic gas volumes exceeding helium equilibration measures (116% versus 98% of predicted, respectively, in the NIH series) (234). Loss of alveolar-capillary units is reflected by a decline in diffusing capacity. Resting room air oxygen tension is variable but is often only mildly impaired, though the alveolar-arterial oxygen gradient is often widened.

In keeping with the presence of accelerated parenchymal loss with $\alpha_1$-antitrypsin deficiency, affected individuals show more rapid rates of $FEV_1$ decline than normal (mean decline of 51 ml/year $\pm$ 82 ml versus 20 to 30 ml/year loss seen in the normal nonsmoking population) along with accelerated decline in diffusing capacity (2.0 $\pm$ 2.0 ml/mm Hg/minute/year). Mean expected survival is shortened in affected individuals with $\alpha_1$-antitrypsin deficiency. In the NIH series, survival probability to age 50 was 52% and to age 60 was 16% (234). In other series in which the cause of death has been ascertained (233), most deaths (60%) have been attributed to respiratory insufficiency.

Besides emphysema, PiZZ $\alpha_1$-antitrypsin deficiency has been associated with a variety of other diseases. The strongest association is with liver disease, particularly neonatal hepatitis, cirrhosis, and hepatoma. In a screening study of 200,000 Swedish infants, Sveger reported liver function test abnormalities in approximately 15% of PiZZ homozygotes and a childhood risk of death from cirrhosis of 2 to 3% (235). In adult series of PiZZ homozygotes, liver function abnormalities occur in 8 to 12% of patients, with biopsy-proven cirrhosis in a large proportion (83%) of these adults (233, 234). Autopsy series have suggested that one-third of PiZZ individuals have cirrhosis, with hepatoma in half of these. While some patients with childhood liver disease appear to progress to adult cirrhosis, adult cirrhosis may develop in the absence of reported childhood disease. In the series by Larsson, only one of 29 PiZZ individuals with cirrhosis reported childhood hepatitis (233).

Positive associations between many other diseases and $\alpha_1$-antitrypsin deficiency have been reported, but the significance and strength of these associations remain less clear than with either liver disease or panniculitis, the latter seen as a rare complication in deficient individuals. One noteworthy exception is the development of a severe bleeding diathesis in a patient with an $\alpha_1$-antitrypsin variant called antitrypsin Pittsburgh. In this patient, substitution of the methionine residue (position 358) by alanine created an $\alpha_1$-antitrypsin variant with antithrombin III activity instead of activity to inactivate elastase, reflecting the considerable homology between various antiproteases (232).

## Treatment of $\alpha_1$-Antitrypsin Deficiency

Treatment options for $\alpha_1$-antitrypsin deficiency have included liver transplantation, use of various drugs to augment hepatic synthesis (e.g., danazol, tamoxifen) (236–238), and, most recently, augmentation therapy by infusion of purified $\alpha_1$-antitrypsin (239). While clearly effective, liver transplantation is a major intervention available to relatively few individuals, and drug therapy to promote protein synthesis has produced only modest increases in serum levels of $\alpha_1$-antitrypsin (236–238). As of 1988, a pooled human plasma purified $\alpha_1$-antitrypsin preparation has been commercially available and has been evaluated in several available series. Experience to date has shown that infusion of this purified $\alpha_1$-antitrypsin preparation is biochemically effective, in that $\alpha_1$-antitrypsin levels in serum and epithelial lining fluid (ELF) obtained by bronchoalveolar lavage fluid can be augmented above a protective threshold level (239). Also, antineutrophil elastase activity in serum and ELF can be successfully augmented. Both weekly and monthly infusion schedules have been examined, and both appear biochemically successful and safe. The biochemical efficacy of biweekly infusion is less certain at the present time. Currently available longitudinal follow-up of recipients of weekly or monthly infusion is inadequate to assess whether this therapy alters the progression of emphysema, and the clinical (versus biochemical) efficacy of augmentation therapy remains unproved. A National, Heart, Lung, and Blood Institute (NHLBI) sponsored Registry has been established to assess the natural history of lung disease in these patients, whether or not they are receiving augmentation therapy. While not a randomized clinical trial of the efficacy of augmentation therapy, this Registry (which is expected to complete 5-year follow-up in 1995–1996) is expected to provide data on the rate of $FEV_1$ decline in patients receiving versus not receiving augmentation therapy with pooled human antiprotease (240). Current treatment guidelines of the American Thoracic Society suggest augmentation therapy for patients satisfying the following criteria (241):

1. Serum $\alpha_1$-antitrypsin level less than 11 $\mu$M,
2. Age above 18 years except in the rare instance when obstructive lung disease is already present earlier,
3. Abnormal lung function consistent with emphysema, and
4. Expected patient compliance.

In view of the considerable expense and technical difficulties of infusion therapy, recent attention has turned to alternative routes of administration. Preliminary studies (242, 243) suggest that inhalation of a human recombinant DNA preparation of $\alpha_1$-antitrypsin can augment serum and alveolar levels and activity, and this is a promising treatment strategy for which further investigation is needed.

Recent exciting developments regarding "gene therapy" have involved the adenovirus-mediated transfer of a recombinant $\alpha_1$-antitrypsin gene to the lung epithelium of rats, with subsequent detection of $\alpha_1$-antitrypsin in epithelial lining fluid for at least 1 week

(244). Also, the human gene has been introduced into rabbit lung, liver, and endothelium by means of a plasmid-liposome complex (245). Because augmentation therapy is already available, safety issues pertaining to the use of a viral transfer factor will need to be answered before gene therapy can be implemented as a treatment option for $\alpha_1$-antitrypsin deficiency (246).

Finally, as with centriacinar emphysema, single lung transplantation has become an option for patients with end-stage panacinar emphysema due to $\alpha_1$-antitrypsin deficiency. Although earlier observations raised concern that actuarial survival among $\alpha_1$-antitrypsin deficient lung transplant recipients was lower than that of patients with centriacinar emphysema from smoking, more recent studies suggest similar survival rates following lung transplantation (Fig. 10.17) (214). The role of augmentation therapy to improve survival after lung transplantation has yet to be defined.

## Bronchiectasis

Defined anatomically, bronchiectasis is a condition characterized by chronic, irreversible dilation and distortion of the bronchi caused by inflammatory destruction of the muscular and elastic components of the bronchial walls. The postmortem appearance of bronchiectasis was described by Laennec in 1826 (247). Laennec's imagery anticipated by over a century the contemporary classification system of bronchiectasis, which was introduced by Reid in 1950 (248). This scheme divides bronchiectasis into cylindrical, varicose, and saccular (or cystic) varieties. Although this classification is helpful in roentgenographic and pathologic descriptions of the disorder, there appear to be very few, if any, epidemiologic, prognostic, or therapeutic distinctions among the various anatomic forms of bronchiectasis. The clinical utility of such classification systems is therefore minimal, at best.

Bronchiectasis is best classified according to the underlying cause or predisposing factor. Bronchiectasis is not a discrete disease entity, but rather represents the possible result of several different diseases or insults. Some conditions associated with the development of bronchiectasis are listed in Table 10.5. In large measure, the clinical features of a case of bronchiectasis such as the severity, distribution (localized versus diffuse), prognosis, and therapeutic potential are determined by the underlying cause. Another specific cause of bronchiectasis, cystic fibrosis, is discussed in this chapter, whereas allergic bronchopulmonary aspergillosis is discussed separately in Chapter 9.

**TABLE 10.5**

**CONDITIONS ASSOCIATED WITH THE DEVELOPMENT OF BRONCHIECTASIS**

Proximal airway obstruction
  Foreign body aspiration
  Middle lobe syndrome
  Benign airway tumors
Diffuse airway injury
  Inhalation of noxious gases (e.g., anhydrous ammonia, sulfur dioxide)
  Aspiration
Postinfection
  Bacterial pneumonia
  Tuberculosis
  Pertussis
  Measles
  Influenza
Genetic disorders
  Cystic fibrosis
  $\alpha_1$-Antitrypsin deficiency (?)
Abnormal host defense
  Ciliary dyskinesia (e.g., Kartagener's syndrome)
  Humoral immunodeficiency
Other conditions
  Allergic bronchopulmonary aspergillosis
  Yellow nail syndrome
  Congenital cartilage deficiency (Williams-Campbell syndrome)
  Tracheobronchomegaly (Mounier-Kuhn syndrome)
Idiopathic

## CLINICAL PRESENTATION

The hallmark of bronchiectasis is the production of large quantities of purulent and often foul-smelling sputum. The quantification of daily sputum production may serve as a helpful indicator of disease exacerbations or response to therapy. Ellis and colleagues (249) categorized less than 10 ml of sputum daily as indicating mild bronchiectasis, 10 to 150 ml as indicating moderate bronchiectasis, and greater than 150 ml as indicating severe bronchiectasis. Systemic manifestations of persistent infection—including fever, weight loss, and digital clubbing—may occur as well, but are now much less frequently observed in the antibiotic era.

Bronchiectasis is not always associated with sputum production, however. So-called "dry bronchiectasis" (to distinguish it from the more typical "wet" variety) may occur, especially when the involved area of the lung is limited to the upper lobes (such as with prior tuberculosis infection), presumably due to the beneficial effect of dependent drainage.

Hemoptysis is frequent in bronchiectasis and occurs more commonly in the dry variety than in the wet variety (250). Although hemoptysis is usually relatively mild, occurring most commonly as blood streaking of purulent sputum, the possibility of massive hemoptysis from dilated bronchial arteries or bronchial-pulmonary anastomoses under systemic pressure is ever present. In the pre-antibiotic era, hemoptysis accounted for about 7% of deaths (251) but was not the cause of a single fatality among 62 deaths analyzed in 1969 (252).

With modern treatment approaches, the average age at death is about 55 years (252). Most patients with bronchiectasis succumb to cor pulmonale, the underlying disease, or an incidental cause, rather than infectious complications.

## EVALUATION

### Roentgenographic Studies

The relative value and indications of plain chest radiography, bronchography, and computed tomography (CT) have recently been reviewed (253). Although patients with bronchiectasis rarely have an entirely normal chest radiograph, the typical findings (increase in size and number of bronchovascular markings) are quite nonspecific. In more severe forms of the disease, cystic spaces can be found and raise the suspicion that bronchiectasis is present. Overall, the chest film is unreliable in detecting and determining the anatomic distribution of bronchiectasis. Bronchography is the traditional "gold standard" technique for assessing bronchiectasis. This method can be easily and safely performed via fiberoptic bronchoscopy using oily contrast agents, such as Dionosil (Glaxo Products, Greenford, England). However, the advent of high-resolution CT techniques and discontinued production of some bronchography contrast agents has hampered the use of bronchography in the last decade. For example, in one large referral center, only one to five bronchograms are performed annually to evaluate or diagnose bronchiectasis (254). Bronchography has no role in the routine diagnosis or evaluation of bronchiectasis, because there is usually no impact on therapeutic approach. In particular, the performance of bronchography to distinguish mild bronchiectasis from chronic bronchitis should be discouraged.

Computed tomography using thin contiguous sections (2- to 4-mm sections at 5-mm intervals) has a very high sensitivity and specificity in the diagnosis of bronchiectasis (253). The recent availability of this imaging modality is one of the factors leading to a decline in bronchograms performed. However, use of CT scanning for this purpose should be reserved for instances in which the findings will affect clinical management.

## Bronchoscopy

Bronchoscopy is helpful in evaluating the proximal airways for lesions (obstructing tumors, foreign bodies, etc.) and for assessing the cause and localizing the source of hemoptysis.

## Ancillary Evaluation

With the decrease in pyogenic infections of the lungs, bronchiectasis is now more commonly due to abnormal host defenses such as is seen with cystic fibrosis, immunoglobulin deficiency states, and dyskinetic cilia syndromes (255). Cystic fibrosis is reviewed elsewhere in this chapter.

Congenital or acquired humoral immunodeficiency has long been recognized as a cause of recurrent sinopulmonary infections and bronchiectasis. The most common humoral immunodeficient state associated with bronchiectasis is panhypogammaglobulinemia, which can be detected easily by measurement of serum immunoglobulin levels. Identification of patients with such a deficiency is important, because replacement therapy may be effective in reducing the frequency and severity of infectious episodes and their sequelae. Recently, it has become apparent that patients with selective immunoglobulin deficiencies may be at risk for bronchiectasis. In particular, abnormalities in IgG subclasses may be significant. Absence of $IgG_4$, even with no abnormalities in other IgG subclasses or other immunoglobulins, is associated with bronchiectasis (256, 257). Reductions of $IgG_2$ and $IgG_3$, with or without IgA deficiency, are also associated with recurrent sinopulmonary infections (258, 259). It is not entirely clear whether a selective deficiency of IgA is an independent risk factor for bronchiectasis. One large series of IgA-deficient patients made no mention of bronchiectasis (260). Because IgA deficiency is relatively common (about 1 in 700 individuals), it is unlikely that this condition confers a major risk for bronchiectasis.

In the 1930s, Kartagener reported patients with a triad of situs inversus, recurrent sinusitis, and bronchiectasis. It is now apparent that such patients, as well as many others who do not have situs inversus, share a defect in ciliary structure that renders the cilia nonfunctional. This defect has been termed the immotile cilia syndrome (261). In addition to sinopulmonary infections, male infertility due to immotile sperm is an important clinical hallmark. It is likely that variations of this syndrome will be identified; the term dyskinetic cilia syndrome is gaining favor with the increasing recognition that in many patients the cilia are in fact motile, albeit with abnormal motions. Of interest, syndromes of male infertility (due to obstructive azoospermia) and recurrent respiratory infection have been identified that appear to be distinct from both cystic fibrosis and the dyskinetic cilia syndromes (262, 263). Diagnosis of the various syndromes associated with bronchiectasis, sinusitis, and male infertility may require evaluation of biopsies of the testis and the mucosa of the bronchi or nasopharynx. Electron microscopy may be needed to detect ultrastructural abnormalities. Generally, such a complete evaluation is not required in routine clinical practice.

### TREATMENT

## Medical Management

The general therapeutic approach to bronchiectasis includes antibiotics and chest physical therapy with postural drainage and chest clapping. Antibiotic therapy should be guided through the use of sputum Gram's stain and cultures. The more recent availability of recombinant DNAse, which may lyse the DNA that causes sputum to be viscous, offers new options, but requires further study before a recommendation can be made (264, 265).

## Surgical Therapy

Surgical therapy is indicated in bronchiectasis only when recurrent and refractory clinical symptoms are due to a focal area of disease involvement. Full lung imaging, either by fine-cut CT or, less commonly, bilateral full bronchograms, should usually be performed prior to consideration of surgical resection to ensure that significant diffuse bronchiectasis does not exist. Massive hemoptysis is a clear indication for surgery, but bronchial artery angiography and selective embolization may be considered instead, especially in patients whose suitability for surgery is poor (266).

### CYSTIC FIBROSIS

Cystic fibrosis (CF) is the most common fatal inherited disease in Caucasians. In the white population, about 5% of individuals carry the gene, and the disease occurs about once in every 2500 live births (267). Cystic fibrosis is inherited as a simple autosomal recessive trait. The main pathophysiologic abnormality in cystic fibrosis is a defect in electrolyte transport. Decreased secretion of chloride into the airway lumen and increased sodium reabsorption from the airway lumen lead to a decrease in water content and increased viscosity of airway secretions (268).

A milestone was reached in 1989 with the identification of the cystic fibrosis gene (269). The classic cystic fibrosis phenotype, characterized by diagnosis at childhood, pancreatic insufficiency, and meconium ileus, is due to a mutation resulting in the loss of a phenylalanine residue at codon 508, hence its designation as

ΔF508 (267). This mutation is responsible for 70% of all CF mutations, and results in an alteration in the secondary and tertiary structure of the "cystic fibrosis transmembrane conductance regulator" (CFTR) protein, which is thought to represent a chloride channel (267). About 170 other mutations of the CFTR gene account for the remaining 30%. The discovery of the cystic fibrosis gene and the ability to detect the common CFTR mutations now allow the routine screening of 33 mutations and the detection of 95% of carriers, and opens the avenue of genetic counseling for couples at risk (267). Another consequence of the discovery of the CF gene has been the development of the first animal model for cystic fibrosis (270).

Although cystic fibrosis is typically diagnosed in infancy or early childhood, a recent review of 142 patients found that 5% were diagnosed between 16 and 30 years of age (271). Less commonly, the diagnosis is made as late as 35 years of age (272, 273). While the correlation of genotype with phenotype is often imprecise, this variability may be ascribed to mutations outside the common ΔF508 locus. Milder mutations appear to be dominant in defining the phenotype of a compound heterozygote (267), but the genotype cannot be used to predict the severity of pulmonary disease (274).

Among the patients diagnosed after childhood, respiratory symptoms are frequently the major manifestation of the disease. Therefore, it is clearly important for pulmonary physicians, in particular, to have an awareness of cystic fibrosis and to be facile in its diagnosis.

## CLINICAL MANIFESTATIONS

The clinical manifestations are protean and are variably expressed from patient to patient. All organ systems that have exocrine gland function may be affected, including the exocrine pancreas, the small intestine, the biliary tract, the paranasal sinuses, the uterine cervix, the salivary glands, and the male reproductive tract. In young children, gastrointestinal problems often predominate. Meconium ileus occurs in 5 to 10% of newborns with cystic fibrosis. Clinical evidence of pancreatic insufficiency, including steatorrhea and failure to thrive, occurs in 85% of affected children but is a lesser problem for adults. Table 10.6 lists some clinical findings that should raise the suspicion that cystic fibrosis is present in the adult patient.

## PULMONARY MANIFESTATIONS

Pulmonary manifestations of cystic fibrosis include cough, sputum production, wheezing, and intermittent radiographic infiltrates. As the disease progresses,

**TABLE 10.6**
**CLUES TO CYSTIC FIBROSIS IN ADULTS**

Respiratory
  Atypical asthma or unexplained air flow obstruction
  Chronic bronchitis (cough and sputum)
  Mucoid *Pseudomonas aeruginosa* in sputum
  Pneumothorax
  Nasal polyps
  Sinusitis
  Bronchiectasis
Gastrointestinal
  Biliary cirrhosis
  Pancreatitis
  Cholelithiasis
  Fecal impaction or intussusception
Other
  Infertility (azoospermia in males)
  Clubbing

mucoid strains of *Pseudomonas aeruginosa* often appear in the sputum. Such a finding is an important clue to the underlying diagnosis, but it is not entirely specific because mucoid *Pseudomonas* is also found in patients with bronchiectasis not caused by cystic fibrosis (275). Upper respiratory tract manifestations include nasal polyps (45% of adults) and radiographic evidence of sinusitis (90% of adults) (273).

The chest roentgenogram is normal in only about 2% of adults with cystic fibrosis. Many patients show only hyperinflation or increased bronchovascular markings (276, 277). More advanced disease reveals evidence of bronchiectasis, including ring shadows and cysts, and mucoid impaction seen as branching, finger-like shadows. Bronchiectatic changes tend to occur first in the right upper lobe, followed by the left upper lobe and the right middle lobe (273, 278). The "end-stage" chest roentgenogram reveals bronchiectasis, large cystic lesions, fibrotic areas, and hyperinflation.

Pulmonary function tests almost always reveal an obstructive impairment (271). The tests of small-airway function are most sensitive to the early changes of cystic fibrosis, correlating with the pathologic findings showing that the initial lesion is in the peripheral airways. As the disease worsens, large-airway obstruction (including a decline in $FEV_1$), elevation of arterial $P_{CO_2}$, and cor pulmonale occur.

## DIAGNOSIS

### Sweat Chloride Test

In most instances, the diagnosis of cystic fibrosis is readily made by the presence of an elevated sweat chloride concentration (greater than 60 mEq/liter) in conjunction with a clinical picture of typical pulmonary and gastrointestinal manifestations (279). The sweat chloride test involves collection of sweat via pilocarpine iontophoresis. The use of a standardized methodology is important to avoid false-positive or false-negative results. Up to 40% of patients referred to cystic fibrosis centers may have had inaccurate previous testing (280). One cause of faulty values is failure to obtain an adequate sweat collection of at least 100 mg in 45 minutes.

### ATYPICAL OR DIFFICULT CASES

Clinicians need to be aware that an elevated sweat chloride level can occur in conditions other than cystic fibrosis, including hypothyroidism, hypoparathyroidism, adrenal insufficiency, nephrogenic diabetes insipidus, and glycogen storage diseases (280). Fortunately, these disorders are readily distinguished from cystic fibrosis on clinical grounds.

More problematic is the fact that a small number of patients with cystic fibrosis have sweat chloride concentrations less than 60 mEq/liter, and a small number of adults without cystic fibrosis have sweat chloride concentrations above 60 mEq/liter (Fig. 10.18). It is estimated that 1 to 2% of cystic fibrosis patients have values between 50 and 60 mEq/liter, and that one in 1000 of such patients will have values less than 50 mEq/liter (278, 279, 281). There has also been one recent report of siblings with a demonstrable mutation of the CFTR gene and mild disease with normal sweat electrolyte levels (282).

Boat has proposed criteria to help the clinician diagnose or exclude cystic fibrosis in the borderline or atypical situation (Table 10.7) (280). A DNA probe specific for the currently identified mutations of the CFTR gene can be used to clarify difficult diagnoses.

### TREATMENT

The prognosis of cystic fibrosis patients improved dramatically between 1940, when the median survival was about 2 years (280), and 1992, when the median survival reached about 29 years (267, 283). The projected survival by actuarial methods for a CF child born today is 40 years (267). Although enhanced diagnosis of mild or atypical cases probably accounts for a portion of this improvement, comprehensive and aggressive multidisciplinary management undoubtedly has contributed in a major way to the improved outlook. Nevertheless, most of the approaches currently used have not been tested in controlled trials. The major goals of treatment are to improve nutrition, control infection, promote clearing of mucus, and optimize

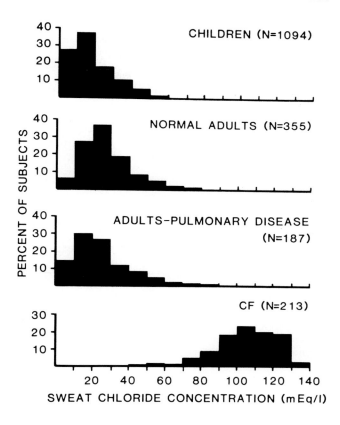

**FIGURE 10.18.** Distribution of sweat chloride concentrations in 1094 children without cystic fibrosis (*top panel*), 355 healthy normal adults (*second panel*), 187 adults with pulmonary disease (*third panel*), and 213 patients with cystic fibrosis (CF) (*bottom panel*). Even in the adult range, sweat chloride level is an excellent discriminant for cystic fibrosis. (From Davis PB, Sant'Agnese PA: Diagnosis and treatment of cystic fibrosis: an update. *Chest* 85:802–809, 1984.)

psychosocial factors. The recent discovery of the cystic fibrosis gene and the abnormal CFTR product open the prospects of gene therapy, studies of which are currently under way (267).

### Gene Therapy

In April 1993, the National Heart, Lung and Blood Institute (NHLBI) announced the start of the first gene therapy trials for treating cystic fibrosis. The gene therapy technique under study involves the instillation into the airway of an adenovirus containing the normal human gene for CFTR with the goal of transfecting the host CF patient's respiratory epithelial cells. Resultant expression of the normal gene is hoped to compensate for the abnormal gene. Periodic administration of the modified adenovirus may be necessary to maintain the benefit (246, 267).

**TABLE 10.7**
**CRITERIA FOR THE DIAGNOSIS OF CYSTIC FIBROSIS IN ATYPICAL CASES**[a]

Major criteria
    Sweat chloride >60 mEq/liter before age 20 (>80 mEq/liter in adults)
    Chronic obstructive lung disease with *Pseudomonas* infection of airways
    Unexplained obstructive azoospermia (confirmed by scrotal exploration and testicular biopsy)
Minor criteria
    Sweat chloride >40 mEq/liter (>60 mEq/liter in adults)
    Family history of classic cystic fibrosis
    Exocrine pancreas insufficiency before age 20
    Unexplained chronic obstructive lung disease before age 20
    Unexplained azoospermia (without scrotal exploration and testicular biopsy)

Reproduced with permission from Stern RC, Boat TF, Doershuk CF. Obstructive azoospermia as a diagnostic criterion for the cystic fibrosis syndrome. *Lancet* 1:1401–1404, 1982.

[a] The diagnosis is established by the presence of two major criteria or by one major and one minor finding. The two criteria used in diagnosis must involve different organ systems.

## Correction of Abnormal Salt Transport

Amiloride (a potassium-sparing diuretic) can block the uptake of sodium from the airway by respiratory epithelium, resulting in an increased mucus water content and improved clearance of secretions. Aerosolized amiloride has been shown to slow the deterioration in pulmonary function in moderately affected CF patients (284).

Similarly, triphosphate nucleotides (ATP or uridine triphosphate) applied to the apical surface of respiratory epithelium result in a chloride efflux, perhaps mediated through the $P_2$ nucleotide receptor. Clinical trials of aerosolized nucleotides are being designed (285).

## Decrease Viscosity of Airway Mucus

The presence of polymerized DNA from degenerating leukocytes significantly increases the viscosity of airway secretions. The use of aerosolized recombinant DNAse has been shown to be well tolerated and to result in significant improvement in lung function (264, 265).

## Modulation of Airway Inflammation

A recent study has shown that aerosolized leukoprotease inhibitor results in a significant decrease in interleukin-8, neutrophil elastase levels, and neutrophil numbers on the respiratory epithelial lining fluid of cystic fibrosis patients. This may result in decreased damage to epithelial cells (286).

Alternate-day corticosteroid administration decreased hospitalizations due to exacerbations of lung disease over a 4-year period in a double-blind controlled study (287). The routine use of corticosteroids cannot be advocated at the current time, however. The preliminary results of a multicenter trial currently under way suggest a significant risk of adverse side effects (glucose abnormalities, cataracts, and growth retardation), requiring discontinuation of the drug in 30% of patients receiving high-dose (2 mg/kg) alternate-day prednisone therapy (288).

## Control of Infections

Four bacterial species predominate as causes of lung infection in cystic fibrosis patients: *Staphylococcus aureus, Haemophilus influenzae, Pseudomonas aeruginosa,* and *Pseudomonas cepacia* (289, 290). Nontuberculous mycobacteria (291, 292), and viral infections (293–296) have also been implicated in exacerbations of cystic fibrosis.

Several aspects of antibiotic therapy in cystic fibrosis patients remain controversial. Specifically, a firm consensus is lacking with regard to indications for antibiotic therapy, the type of antibiotics to be used, or the route of administration. The interested reader is referred to a comprehensive review of this topic (297). The choice of antibiotics ideally should be based on results of sputum culture and sensitivity testing (289). In most instances, appropriate antibiotic therapy for *S. aureus* and *H. influenzae* will eliminate the organism from the sputum, at least temporarily. Suggested drugs for treating *H. influenzae* include trimethoprim-sulfamethoxazole, chloramphenicol, ampicillin (290), ampicillin-sulbactam, and ticarcillin-clavulanate. If *S. aureus* is present, the choice may include a cephalosporin, clindamycin, chloramphenicol, or a semisynthetic penicillin. *Pseudomonas* species are never completely eradicated from the sputum once chronic colonization and infection are initiated. Treatment is therefore aimed more at controlling clinical evidence of deterioration as might be manifested by fever (although patients are typically afebrile), cough, increased sputum, and changes in the chest roentgenogram or pulmonary function tests. Also, improvements in lung function have been found to correlate with the reduction of sputum *P. aeruginosa* bacterial density (298). Intravenous multidrug antibiotic therapy using an aminoglycoside and another antipseudomonal antibiotic (e.g., penicillin derivative, β-lactone drug, or third-generation cephalosporin) is commonly employed. To shorten hospitalization, home intravenous therapy should be considered. The duration of therapy for exacerbations should be over 14 days, as shorter courses of 5 to 7 days may result in rapid recurrence. Despite the earlier controversy surrounding the use of inhaled antibiotic therapy in cystic fibrosis (299, 300), a recent study has established the efficacy and safety of high-dose aerosolized tobramycin in the treatment of *P. aeruginosa* infections (301). The development of an oral antipseudomonal antibiotic effective for cystic fibrosis patients has been a major advance. In this regard, ciprofloxacin offers some promise (302) and is now commonly used. Although resistance to ciprofloxacin often rapidly emerges, the clinical virulence of the resistant organism may be less. Clearly, future research is required to resolve several issues concerning antibiotic use in cystic fibrosis.

## Chest Physiotherapy

Patients with a productive cough have traditionally received indoctrination in proper daily chest percussion and postural drainage techniques. Nevertheless, the short- and long-term efficacy of these procedures remains unclear (303, 304), although most physicians treating CF patients think they are clearly useful. Vigorous self-directed cough sessions are potentially as useful as more complex and time-consuming methods (305, 306), though newer methods of inducing secretion clearance (e.g., positive expiratory pressure [PEP] treatment, autogenic drainage, etc.) may provide patients more autonomy in managing secretions than traditional chest physiotherapy that requires assistance of a caregiver (307). Self-administration of high-frequency chest compression therapy has also been shown to be efficacious, and also offers the advantage of increased independence (308).

## Other Treatment

Patients should be immunized against influenza virus infection yearly.

Most CF centers routinely use $\beta$-agonist inhalers for non-bronchodilating effects on mucociliary clearance.

Mucomyst (acetylcysteine) is of questionable efficacy and is injurious to respiratory epithelium when used chronically. Inhalation of this substance should be used selectively and for short duration (280).

Promotion of adequate nutrition is extremely important. Many patients require the regular use of pancreatic enzyme preparations to aid digestion and nutrient absorption. Typically, supplementation of vitamins A, D, E, and K is also provided.

Double lung transplantation is an option for patients with cystic fibrosis. The overall survival is about the same as transplant recipients with idiopathic pulmonary fibrosis and primary pulmonary hypertension. Complications specific to this group of patients include

an increased rate of bacterial infections, and erratic absorption of cyclosporine with concomitant seizures (216).

## COMPLICATIONS

### Hemoptysis

Massive hemoptysis occurs in about 5 to 7% of cystic fibrosis patients and carries a mortality rate of about 11% (278, 309). Surgical therapy with lung resection is often contraindicated in many patients due to poor lung function. Even in those with adequate lung function, surgery should nevertheless be used only as a last resort. Sparing of lung tissue is important in the view of the chronic progressive nature of cystic fibrosis and the known high incidence of recurrent hemoptysis in these patients. Fortunately, acute control of massive hemoptysis can usually be achieved with endobronchial Fogarty balloon tamponade or bronchial artery embolization (309).

### Pneumothorax

Pneumothorax rarely occurs in cystic fibrosis patients who are less than 10 years of age but is reported in about 20% of patients over 14 years of age (273, 310). Treatment of pneumothorax in cystic fibrosis is similar to spontaneous pneumothorax due to other conditions, except that the high incidence of recurrence (50%) in cystic fibrosis argues for pleurodesis or other definitive therapy following the first large pneumothorax (273, 311). The occurrence of a pneumothorax in cystic fibrosis indicates severe underlying disease and heralds a poor prognosis. In one series, the mean survival after the initial pneumothorax was only 3.4 years (273). Pleurodesis in the management of a pneumothorax may complicate subsequent lung transplantation.

*Acknowledgments*

The authors thank Paul C. Stillwell, M.D., for his critical review and helpful suggestions on the Cystic Fibrosis section.

▼

## REFERENCES

1. American Thoracic Society: Standards for the diagnosis and care of patients with chronic obstructive pulmonary disease (COPD) and asthma. *Am Rev Respir Dis* 36: 225–228, 1987.
2. National Center for Health Statistics: Advance report of final mortality statistics, 1991. *Monthly Vital Statistics Report* 42(2) (Suppl), 1993.
3. Snider G, Kleinerman J, Thurlbeck WM, Bengali ZH: The definition of emphysema. *Am Rev Respir Dis* 132: 182–185, 1985.

4. American Thoracic Society: Chronic bronchitis, asthma and pulmonary emphysema. A statement by the committee on diagnostic standards for nontuberculous respiratory diseases. *Am Rev Respir Dis* 85:762–768, 1962.

5. CIBA Foundation Chest Symposium: Terminology, definitions, and classification of chronic pulmonary emphysema and related conditions. *Thorax* 14:286–299, 1959.

6. Fletcher CM, Pride NB: Definitions of emphysema, chronic bronchitis, asthma, and airflow obstruction: 25 years on from the CIBA Symposium [editorial]. *Thorax* 39:81–85, 1984.

7. Thurlbeck WM: *Chronic Airflow Obstruction in Lung Disease.* Philadelphia, WB Saunders, 1976, pp 31–95.

8. Thurlbeck WM, Henderson JA, Fraser R, Bates DV: Chronic obstructive lung disease: a comparison between clinical, roentgenologic, functional and morphologic criteria in chronic bronchitis, emphysema, asthma, and bronchiectasis. *Medicine* 49:81–145, 1970.

9. Adam PF, Benson V: Current estimates from the National Health Interview Survey, 1991. National Center for Health Statistics. *Vital Health Stat* 10(184), 1992.

10. *Statistical Compendium on Adult Lung Diseases.* New York, American Lung Association, 1987.

11. Adam PF, Benson V: Current estimates from the National Health Interview Survey, 1990. National Center for Health Statistics. *Vital Health Stat* 10(181), 1991.

12. Thurlbeck WM, Angus GE, et al: Mucous gland hypertrophy in chronic bronchitis and its occurrence in smokers. *Br J Dis Chest* 57:73–78, 1963.

13. Reid L: Measurement of the bronchial mucous gland layer: a diagnostic yardstick in chronic bronchitis. *Thorax* 15:132–141, 1960.

14. Matsuba KI, Thurlbeck WM: Disease of the small airways in chronic bronchitis. *Am Rev Respir Dis* 107:552–558, 1973.

15. Greenburg SD, Boushy SF, Jenkins DE: Chronic bronchitis and emphysema. Correlation of pathologic findings. *Am Rev Respir Dis* 96:918–928, 1987.

16. Gadek JE, Crystal RG: Alpha 1-antitrypsin deficiency. In Stanbury JB, Wyngaarden JB, Frederickson DS, et al, eds: *Metabolic Basis of Inherited Disease.* New York, McGraw-Hill, 1982, pp 1450–1467.

17. Gaensler EA, Cugell DW, Knudson RJ, FitzGerald MX: Surgical management of emphysema. *Clin Chest Med* 4:443–463, 1983.

18. Mitchell RS, Ryan SF, Petty TL, Filley GF: The significance of morphologic chronic hyperplastic bronchitis. *Am Rev Respir Dis* 93:720–729, 1966.

19. Fielding JE: Smoking: health effects and control. *N Engl J Med* 313:491–498, 1985.

20. Dresler C: Smoking cessation. *Pulmonary Perspectives* 10(2):1–3, 1993.

21. Fletcher C, Peto R, Tinker C, Speizer FE: *The Natural History of Chronic Bronchitis and Emphysema: An Eight-Year Study of Early Chronic Obstructive Lung Disease in Working Men in London.* New York, Oxford University Press, 1976.

22. Nemery B, Moavero NE, Brasseur L, Stanescu DC: Changes in lung function after smoking cessation: an assessment from a cross-sectional survey. *Am Rev Respir Dis* 125:122–124, 1982.

23. Bode FR, Dosman J, Martin RR, Macklem PT: Reversibility of pulmonary function abnormalities in smokers: a prospective study of early diagnostic tests of small airways disease. *Am J Med* 59:43–52, 1975.

24. Buist AS, Sexton GJ, Nagy JM, Ross BB: The effect of smoking cessation and modification on lung function. *Am Rev Respir Dis* 114:115–122, 1976.

25. Buist AS, Nagy JM, Sexton GJ: The effect of smoking cessation on pulmonary function: a 30-month follow-up of two smoking cessation clinics. *Am Rev Respir Dis* 120:953–957, 1979.

26. Camilli AE, Burrows B, Knudson RJ, et al: Longitudinal changes in forced respiratory volume in one second in adults: effects of smoking and smoking cessation. *Am Rev Respir Dis* 135:794–799, 1987.

27. Fletcher C, Peto R: The natural history of chronic airflow obstruction. *Br Med J* 1:1645–1648, 1977.

28. Schwartz HR, McDuffie FC, Black LF, Schroeter AL, Conn DL: Hypocomplementemic urticarial vasculitis: association with chronic obstructive pulmonary disease. *Mayo Clin Proc* 57:231–238, 1982.

29. Reed WB, Horowitz RE, Beighton P: Acquired cutis laxa: primary generalized elastolysis. *Arch Dermatol* 103:661–669, 1971.

30. Pääkkö P, Ryhänen L, Rantala H, Autio-Harmainen H: Pulmonary emphysema in a nonsmoking patient with Salla disease. *Am Rev Respir Dis* 135:979–982, 1987.

31. Sherman CB, Hudson LD, Pierson DJ: Severe precocious emphysema in intravenous methylphenidate (Ritalin) abusers. *Chest* 92:1085–1087, 1987.

32. Diaz PT, Clanton TL, Pacht ER: Emphysema-like pulmonary disease associated with human immunodeficiency virus infection. *Ann Intern Med* 116:124–128, 1992.

33. Janoff A: State of the art: elastases and emphysema: current assessment of the protease-antiprotease hypothesis. *Am Rev Respir Dis* 132:417–433, 1985.

34. Gadek JE, Fells GA, Zimmerman RL, et al: Antielastases of the human alveolar structures. Implications for the protease-antiprotease theory of emphysema. *J Clin Invest* 68:889–898, 1981.

35. Hunninghake GW, Crystal RG: Cigarette smoking and lung destruction: accumulation of neutrophils in the lungs of cigarette smokers. *Am Rev Respir Dis* 128:833–838, 1983.

36. Janoff A, Sloan B, Weinbaum G, et al: Experimental emphysema induced with purified human neutrophil elastase: tissue localization of the instilled protease. *Am Rev Respir Dis* 115:461–478, 1977.

37. Senior RM, Tegner H, Kuhn C, et al: The induction of pulmonary emphysema with leukocyte elastase. *Am Rev Respir Dis* 116:469–475, 1977.

38. Laurent P, Janoff A, Kagan HM: Cigarette smoke blocks cross-linking of elastin in vitro. *Am Rev Respir Dis* 127:189–192, 1983.

39. Dornhorst AC: Respiratory insufficiency. *Lancet* 1:1185–1187, 1955.

40. Wilson DO, Rogers RM, Wright EC, Anthonisen NR: Body weight in chronic obstructive pulmonary disease: the National Institutes of Health intermittent positive-pressure breathing trial. *Am Rev Respir Dis* 139:1435–1438, 1989.

41. Muers MF, Green JH: Weight loss in chronic obstructive pulmonary disease. *Eur Respir J* 6:729–734, 1993.

42. Schols AMW, Soeters PB, Mostert R, Saris WHM, Wouters EFM: Energy balance in chronic obstructive pulmonary disease. *Am Rev Respir Dis* 143:1248–1252, 1991.

43. Goldstein SA, Thomashow BM, Kvetan V, Askanazi J, Kinney JM, Elwyn DH: Nitrogen and energy relationships in malnourished patients with emphysema. *Am Rev Respir Dis* 138:636–644, 1988.

44. Hoover CF: Definitive percussion and inspection in estimating size and contour of heart. *JAMA* 75:1626–1630, 1920.

45. Anthonisen NR, Wright EC, the IPPB Trial Group: Response to inhaled bronchodilators in COPD. *Chest* 91:36S–39S, 1987.

46. Guyatt GH, Townsend M, Pugsley SO, et al: Bronchodilators in chronic air-flow limitation: effects on airway function, exercise capacity, and quality of life. *Am Rev Respir Dis* 135:1969–1074, 1987.

47. Berger R, Smith D: Effect of inhaled metaproterenol and exercise performance in patients with stable "fixed" airway obstruction. *Am Rev Respir Dis* 138:624–629, 1988.

48. Owens GR, Rogers RM, Pennock BE, Levin D: The diffusing capacity as a predictor of arterial oxygen desaturation during exercise in patients with chronic obstructive pulmonary disease. *N Engl J Med* 310:1218–1221, 1984.

49. Groskin SA: Emphysema: fact, fiction or just a lot of hot air? *Radiology* 183:319–320, 1992.

50. Gishen P, Sanders AJS, Tobin MJ, Hutchinson DCS: Alpha 1-antitrypsin deficiency: the radiological features of pulmonary emphysema in subjects of Pi Type Z and Pi Type SZ: a survey of the British Thoracic Association. *Clin Radiol* 33:371–377, 1982.

51. Greene R: "Saber-sheath" trachea: relation to chronic obstructive pulmonary disease. *AJR* 130:441–445, 1978.

52. Chang CH: The normal roentgenographic measurement of the right descending pulmonary artery in 1085 cases. *AJR* 87:929–935, 1962.

53. Matthay RA, Schwarz MI, Ellis JH, et al: Pulmonary artery hypertension in chronic obstructive pulmonary disease: determination by chest radiography. *Invest Radiol* 16:95–100, 1981.

54. Thurlbeck WM, Simon G: Radiographic appearance of the chest in emphysema. *AJR* 130:429–440, 1978.

55. Sutinen S, Christoforidis AJ, Klugh GA, et al: Roentgenologic criteria for the recognition of nonsymptomatic pulmonary emphysema. *Am Rev Respir Dis* 91:69–76, 1965.

56. Palmer WH, Gee JB, Mills JBL, et al: The accuracy of the roentgenologic diagnosis of chronic pulmonary emphysema. *Am Rev Respir Dis* 93:889–894, 1966.

57. Pratt PC: Role of conventional chest radiography in diagnosis and exclusion of emphysema. *Am J Med* 82:998–1006, 1987.

58. Nicklaus DW, Stowell DW, Christiansen WR, Renzetti AD: The accuracy of the roentgenologic diagnosis of chronic pulmonary emphysema. *Am Rev Respir Dis* 93:889–899, 1966.

59. Fraser RG, Paré JAP: Roentgenologic signs in the diagnosis of chest disease. In: *Diagnosis of Diseases of the Chest*, 2nd ed. Philadelphia, WB Saunders, 1977, pp 518–523.

60. Miller RR, Mueller NL, Morrison NJ, Staples CA: Limitations of computed tomography in the assessment of emphysema. *Am Rev Respir Dis* 139:980–983, 1989.

61. Kinsella M, Müller NL, Abboud RT, Morrison NJ, DyBuncio A: Quantitation of emphysema by computed tomography using a "density mask" program and correlation with pulmonary function tests. *Chest* 97:315–321, 1990.

62. Rienmüller RK, Behr J, Kalender WA, et al: Standardized quantitative high resolution CT in lung diseases. *J Comput Assist Tomogr* 15:742–749, 1991.

63. Kuwano K, Matsuba K, Ikeda T, et al: The diagnosis of mild emphysema. Correlation of computed tomography and pathology score. *Am Rev Respir Dis* 141:169–178, 1990.

64. Gurney JW, Jines KK, Robbins RA, et al: Regional distribution of emphysema: correlation of high-resolution CT with pulmonary function tests in unselected smokers. *Radiology* 183:457–463, 1992.

65. Snider GL: Emphysema: the first two centuries—and beyond. A historical overview, with suggestions for future research: part 1. *Am Rev Respir Dis* 146:1334–1344, 1992.

66. Stokes J, Rigotti NA: The health consequences of cigarette smoking and the internist's role in smoking cessation. *Adv Intern Med* 33:431–460, 1988.

67. Cigarette smoking among adults—United States, 1990. *MMWR* 41:354–362, 1992.

68. Nett LM, Dingus SM: Smoking cessation techniques. In: Kacmarek RM, Stoller JK, eds. *Current Respiratory Care.* Toronto, BC Decker, 1988, pp 107–116.

69. Kottke TE, Battista RN, De Friese GH, Brekke ML: Attributes of successful cessation interventions in medical practice: a meta-analysis of 39 controlled trials. *JAMA* 259:2882–2889, 1988.

70. Fiore MC, Jorenby DE, Baker TB, Kenford SL: Tobacco dependence and the nicotine patch. Clinical guidelines for effective use. *JAMA* 268:2687–2694, 1992.

71. Glezen WP, Decker M, Perrotta DM: Survey of underlying conditions of persons hospitalized with acute respiratory disease during influenza epidemics in Houston, 1979–1981. *Am Rev Respir Dis* 136:550–555, 1987.

72. Recommendations of the Immunization Practices Advisory Committee. Prevention and control of influenza. *Ann Intern Med* 107:521–525, 1987.

73. Influenza activity—United States and worldwide, and composition of the 1993–94 influenza vaccine. *JAMA* 269:1778–1779, 1993.

74. Prevention and control of influenza: part 1, vaccines. *MMWR* 38:297–311, 1989.

75. Update: pneumococcal polysaccharide vaccine usage—United States. *JAMA* 251:3071–3075, 1984.

76. Update on adult immunization. Recommendations of the Immunization Practices Advisory Committee (ACIP)—Pneumococcal disease. *MMWR* 40:42–43, 1991.

77. LaForce FM, Eickhoff TC: Pneumococcal vaccine: an emerging consensus. *Ann Intern Med* 108:757–759, 1988.

78. Davis AL, Aranda CP, Schiffman G, Christianson LC: Pneumococcal infection and immunologic response to pneumococcal vaccine in chronic obstructive pulmonary disease. *Chest* 92:204–212, 1987.

79. Williams JH, Moser KM: Pneumococcal vaccine and patients with chronic lung disease. *Ann Intern Med* 104:106–109, 1986.

80. Landesman SH, Smith PM, Schiffman G: Pneumococcal vaccine in elderly patients with COPD. *Chest* 84:433–435, 1983.

81. Riley ID, Tarr PI, Andrews M, et al: Immunization with a polyvalent pneumococcal vaccine: reduction of adult respiratory mortality in a New Guinea Highlands community. *Lancet* 1:1338–1341, 1977.

82. Gandevia B: Historical review of the use of parasympatholytic agents in the treatment of respiratory disorders. *Postgrad Med J* 51(suppl 7):13–20, 1975.

83. Douglas NJ, Davidson I, Sudlow MF, Flenley DC: Bronchodilatation and the site of airway resistance in severe chronic bronchitis. *Thorax* 34:51–56, 1979.

84. Bleeker ER: Cholinergic and neurogenic mechanisms in obstructive airways disease. *Am J Med* 81(suppl 5A): 93–102, 1986.

85. Ingram RH, McFadden ER Jr: Localization and mechanisms of airway responses. *N Engl J Med* 297:596–600, 1977.

86. Gross NJ: Ipratropium bromide. *N Engl J Med* 319: 486–494, 1988.

87. Connett JE, Kusek JW, Bailey WC, O'Hara P, Wu M: Design of the Lung Health Study: a randomized clinical trial of early intervention for chronic obstructive pulmonary disease. *Controlled Clinical Trials* 14(2 Suppl): 3S–19S, 1993.

88. Ferguson GT, Cherniack RM: Management of chronic obstructive pulmonary disease. *N Engl J Med* 328: 1017–1022, 1993.

89. Weinberger SE: Recent advances in pulmonary medicine. *N Engl J Med* 328:1389–1470, 1993.

90. Gal TJ, Suratt PM, Lu JY: Glycopyrrolate and atropine inhalation: comparative effects on normal airway function. *Am Rev Respir Dis* 129:871–873, 1984.

91. Pekes GE, Brogden RN, Heel RC, et al: Ipratropium bromide: a review of its pharmacological properties and therapeutic efficacy in asthma and chronic bronchitis. *Drugs* 20:237–266, 1980.

92. LeDoux EJ, Morris JF, Temple WP, Duncan C: Standard and double dose ipratropium bromide and combined ipratropium bromide and inhaled metaproterenol in COPD. *Chest* 95:1013–1016, 1989.

93. McFadden ER Jr, Luparello T, Lyons H, et al: The mechanism of action of suggestion in the induction of acute asthma attacks. *Psychosom Med* 31:134–143, 1969.

94. Neild JE, Cameron IR: Bronchoconstriction in response to suggestion: its prevention by an inhaled anticholinergic agent. *Br Med J* 290:674, 1985.

95. Karpel JP, Pesin J, Greenberg D, Gentry E: A comparison of the effects of ipratropium bromide and metaproterenol sulfate in acute exacerbations of COPD. *Chest* 98: 835–839, 1990.

96. Braun SR, McKenzie WN, Copeland C, Knight L, Ellersieck M: A comparison of the effect of ipratropium and albuterol in the treatment of chronic obstructive airway disease. *Arch Intern Med* 149:544–547, 1989.

97. Braun SR, Levy S: Comparison of ipratropium bromide and albuterol in chronic obstructive pulmonary disease: a three center study. *Am J Med* 91(suppl 4A):28S–32S, 1991.

98. Marini JJ, Lakshminarayan S: The effect of atropine inhalation in "irreversible" chronic bronchitis. *Chest* 77: 591–596, 1980.

99. Chervinsky P: Concomitant bronchodilator therapy and ipratropium bromide: a clinical review. *Am J Med* 81(suppl 5A):67–72, 1986.

100. Rebuck AS, Chapman KR, Abboud R, et al: Nebulized anticholinergic and sympathomimetic treatment of asthma and chronic obstructive airway disease in the emergency room. *Am J Med* 82:59–64, 1987.

101. Rossing TH, Fanta CH, Goldstein DH, et al: Emergency

therapy of asthma: comparison of the acute effects of parenteral and inhaled sympathomimetics and infused aminophylline. *Am Rev Respir Dis* 122:365–371, 1980.

102. Backman R, Hellstrom PE: Fenoterol and ipratropium bromide in respiratory treatment of patients with chronic bronchitis. *Curr Ther Res Clin Exp* 38:135–140, 1985.

103. Tashkin DP, Ashutosh K, Bleeker ER, et al: Comparison of the anticholinergic bronchodilator ipratropium bromide with metaproterenol in chronic obstructive pulmonary disease: a 90-day multi-center study. *Am J Med* 81(Suppl 5A):81–90, 1986.

104. Braun SR, McKenzie WN, Copeland C, et al: A comparison of the effect of ipratropium and albuterol in the treatment of chronic obstructive airway disease. *Arch Intern Med* 149:544–547, 1989.

105. Lightbody IM, Ingram CG, Legge JS, Johnston RN: Ipratropium bromide, salbutamol and prednisolone in bronchial asthma and chronic bronchitis. *Br J Dis Chest* 72:181–186, 1978.

106. Hughes JA, Tobin MJ, Bellamy D, Hutchinson DCS: Effects of ipratropium bromide and fenoterol aerosols in pulmonary emphysema. *Thorax* 37:667–670, 1982.

107. Easton PA, Jadve C, Dhingra S, Anthonisen NR: A comparison of the bronchodilating effects of a β-2 adrenergic agent (albuterol) and an anticholinergic agent (ipratropium bromide) given by aerosol alone or in sequence. *N Engl J Med* 315:735–739, 1986.

108. Turner JR, Corkery KJ, Eckman D, et al: Equivalence of continuous flow nebulizer and meters dose inhaler with reservoir bag for treatment of acute air flow obstruction. *Chest* 93:476–481, 1988.

109. Self TH, Brooks JB, Lieberman P, Ryan MR: The value of demonstration and role of the pharmacist in teaching the correct use of pressurized bronchodilators. *Can Med Assoc J* 128:129–131, 1983.

110. Allen SC, Prior A: What determines whether an elderly patient can use a metered dose inhaler correctly? *Br J Dis Chest* 80:45–49, 1986.

111. Kesten S, Zive K, Chapman KR: Pharmacist knowledge and ability to use inhaled medication delivery systems. *Chest* 104:1737–1742, 1993.

112. Hanania NA, Wittman R, Kesten S, Chapman KR: Medical personnel's knowledge of and ability to use inhaling devices. Metered-dose inhalers, spacing chambers, and breath-actuated dry powder inhalers. *Chest* 105: 111–116, 1994.

113. Berger R, Smith D: Acute postbronchodilator changes in pulmonary function parameters in patients with chronic airways obstruction. *Chest* 93:541–546, 1988.

114. Levi-Valensi P, Weitzenbaum E, Pedinelli JL, et al: Three month followup of arterial blood gas determinations in candidates for long-term oxygen therapy: a multicentric study. *Am Rev Respir Dis* 133:547–551, 1986.

115. Make B: Medical management of emphysema. *Clin Chest Med* 4:465–482, 1983.

116. Rossing TH: Methylxanthines in 1989. *Ann Intern Med* 110:502–504, 1989.

117. Matthay RA, Berger HJ, Loke J, et al: Effects of aminophylline upon right and left ventricular performance in chronic obstructive pulmonary disease: noninvasive assessment by radionuclide angiocardiography. *Am J Med* 65:903–910, 1978.

118. Matthay RA, Berger HJ, Davis R, et al: Improvement in

cardiac performance by oral long-acting theophylline in chronic obstructive pulmonary disease. *Am Heart J* 104: 1022–1026, 1982.

119. Aubier M, DeTroyer A, Sampson M, et al: Aminophylline improves diaphragm contractility. *N Engl J Med* 305: 242–252, 1981.

120. Murciano D, Aubier M, Lecocguic Y, et al: Effects of theophylline on diaphragmatic strength and fatigue in patients with chronic obstructive pulmonary disease. *N Engl J Med* 311:349–353, 1984.

121. Mahler D, Matthay RA, Snyder PE, et al: Sustained-release theophylline reduces dyspnea in nonreversible obstructive airway disease. *Am Rev Respir Dis* 131: 22–25, 1985.

122. Snider GL: Chronic bronchitis and emphysema. In Murray JF, Nadel JA, eds: *Textbook of Respiratory Medicine.* Philadelphia, WB Saunders, 1988, pp 1069–1106.

123. Murciano P, Audair MH, Pariente R, Aubier M: A randomized, controlled trial of theophylline in patients with severe chronic obstructive pulmonary disease. *N Engl J Med* 320:1521–1525, 1989.

124. Stoller JK, Ferranti R, Feinstein AR, et al: Further specification of a new clinical index for dyspnea. *Am Rev Respir Dis* 134:1129–1134, 1986.

125. Bukowskyj M, Nakatsu K, Munt PW: Theophylline reassessed. *Ann Intern Med* 101:63–73, 1984.

126. Snider GL: Theophylline in the ambulatory treatment of chronic obstructive pulmonary obstructive lung disease: resolving a controversy. *Cleve Clin J Med* 60: 197–201, 1993.

127. Levine JH, Michael JR, Guarnieri T: Multifocal atrial tachycardia: a toxic effect of theophylline. *Lancet* 1: 12–14, 1985.

128. Rice KL, Leatherman JW, Duane PG, et al: Aminophylline for acute exacerbations of chronic obstructive pulmonary disease: a controlled trial. *Ann Intern Med* 107: 305–309, 1987.

129. Stoller JK, Gerbarg ZB, Feinstein AR: Corticosteroids in stable chronic obstructive pulmonary disease: reappraisal of efficacy. *J Gen Intern Med* 2:29–35, 1987.

130. Stoller JK: Systemic corticosteroids in stable chronic obstructive pulmonary disease: do they work? *Chest* 91: 155–156, 1987.

131. Sahn S: Corticosteroids in chronic bronchitis and pulmonary emphysema. *Chest* 73:389–396, 1978.

132. Callahan CM, Dittus RS, Katz BP: Oral corticosteroid therapy for patients with stable chronic obstructive pulmonary disease. A meta-analysis. *Ann Intern Med* 114: 216–223, 1991.

133. Mendella L, Manfreda J, Warren CPW, Anthonisen NR: Steroid response in stable chronic obstructive pulmonary disease. *Ann Intern Med* 96:17–21, 1982.

134. Shim CS, William MH Jr: Aerosol beclomethasone in patients with steroid-responsive chronic obstructive pulmonary disease. *Am J Med* 78:655–658, 1985.

135. Albert RK, Martin TR, Lewis SW: Controlled clinical trial of methylprednisolone in patients with chronic bronchitis and acute respiratory insufficiency. *Ann Intern Med* 92:753–758, 1980.

136. Mitchell D, Rehahn M, Gildeh P, et al: Effects of prednisolone in chronic airflow limitation. *Lancet* 2:193–196, 1984.

137. Shim CS, Stover DE, Williams MH Jr: Response to corticosteroids in chronic bronchitis. *J Allergy Clin Immunol* 62:262–267, 1978.

138. Beerel R, Vance J: Prednisone treatment for stable pulmonary emphysema. *Am Rev Respir Dis* 104:264–266, 1971.

139. O'Reilly J, Shaylor JM, Fromings KM, Harrison BDW: The use of the 12 minute walking test in assessing the effect of oral steroid therapy in patients with chronic airway obstruction. *Br J Dis Chest* 76:374–382, 1982.

140. Evans JA, Morrison IM, Saunders KB: A controlled trial of prednisone in low dosage, in patients with chronic airway obstruction. *Thorax* 29:401–406, 1974.

141. Lam WK, Shun YS, Yu DYC: Response to oral corticosteroids in chronic airflow obstruction. *Br J Dis Chest* 77: 189–198, 1983.

142. Blair G, Light R: Treatment of chronic obstructive pulmonary disease with corticosteroids: comparison of daily vs. alternate-day therapy. *Chest* 86:524–528, 1984.

143. Strain DS, Kinasewitz GT, Franco DP, George RB: Effect of steroid therapy on exercise performance in patients with irreversible chronic obstructive pulmonary disease. *Chest* 88:718–721, 1985.

144. Eliasson O, Hoffman J, Trueb D, et al: Corticosteroids in COPD: a clinical trial and reassessment of the literature. *Chest* 89:484–490, 1986.

145. Morgan W, Rusche E: A controlled trial of the effect of steroids in obstructive airway disease. *Ann Intern Med* 61:248–254, 1964.

146. Ogilvie A, Newell D: A maintenance trial of combined steroid and antibiotic treatment in a series of asthmatics with chronic bronchitis. *Br J Dis Chest* 54:308–320, 1960.

147. Hurford J, Little GM, Loudon HWG: The use of prednisolone in chronic bronchitis. *Br J Dis Chest* 57:133–139, 1963.

148. Beerel F, Jick H, Tyler J: A controlled study of the effect of prednisone on airflow in severe pulmonary emphysema. *N Engl J Med* 268:226–230, 1963.

149. Thompson AB, Mueller MB, Heires AJ, et al: Aerosolized beclomethasone in chronic bronchitis. Improved pulmonary function and diminished airway inflammation. *Am Rev Respir Dis* 146:389–395, 1992.

150. Kerstjens HAM, Brand PLP, Hughes MD, et al: A comparison of bronchodilator therapy with or without inhaled corticosteroid therapy for obstructive airway disease. *N Engl J Med* 327:1413–1419, 1992.

151. Weir DC, Grove RI, Robertson AS, Burge PS: Corticosteroid trials in non-asthmatic chronic airflow obstruction: a comparison of oral prednisolone and inhaled beclomethasone dipropionate. *Thorax* 45:112–117, 1990.

152. Dompeling E, van Schayck CP, van Grunsven PM, et al: Slowing the deterioration of asthma and chronic obstructive pulmonary disease observed during bronchodilator therapy by adding inhaled corticosteroids. A 4-year prospective study. *Ann Intern Med* 118:770–778, 1993.

153. Postma DS, Steenhuis EJ, Van der Weele LT, Sluiter HJ: Severe chronic airflow obstruction: can corticosteroids slow down progression? *Eur J Respir Dis* 67:56–64, 1985.

154. Postma DS, Peters I, Steenhuis EJ, Sluiter HJ: Moderately severe chronic airflow obstruction. Can corticosteroids slow down obstruction? *Eur Respir J* 1:22–26, 1988.

155. Sparrow D, O'Connor GT, Rosner B, Demolles D, Weiss ST: A longitudinal study of plasma cortisol concentration and pulmonary function decline in men. The normative aging study. *Am Rev Respir Dis* 147:1345–1348, 1993.

156. Webb J, Clark TJH, Chilvers C: Time course of response to prednisolone in chronic airflow obstruction. *Thorax* 36:18–21, 1981.

157. Guyatt G, Sackett DL, Taylor DW, et al: Determining optimal therapy—randomized trials in individual patients. *N Engl J Med* 314:889–892, 1986.

158. Guyatt GH, Keller JL, Jaeschke R, Rosenbloom D, Adachi J, Newhouse MT: The *n*-of-1 randomized controlled trial: clinical usefulness. Our three-year experience. *Ann Intern Med* 112:293–299, 1990.

159. Dunlap NE, Fulmer JD: Corticosteroid therapy in emphysema. *Clin Chest Med* 5:669–683, 1984.

160. Toogood JH, Lefcoe NM, Haines DSM, et al: Dose requirement of steroid-dependent asthmatic patients for aerosol beclomethasone and oral prednisone. *J Allergy Clin Immunol* 61:355–364, 1978.

161. Williams MH: Beclomethasone dipropionate. *Ann Intern Med* 95:464–467, 1981.

162. Cooper EF, Grant IWB: Beclomethasone dipropionate aerosol in treatment of chronic emphysema. *Q J Med* 46:295–308, 1977.

163. Glenny RW: Steroids in COPD. The scripture according to Albert [Letter]. *Chest* 91:289–290, 1987.

164. Emerman CL, Connors AF, Lukens TW, et al: A randomized controlled trial of methylprednisolone in the emergency treatment of acute exacerbations of COPD. *Chest* 95:563–567, 1989.

165. Haskell RJ, Wong BM, Hansen JE: A double-blind, randomized clinical trial of methylprednisolone in status asthmaticus. *Arch Intern Med* 143:1324–1327, 1983.

166. Murphy TF, Sethi S: Bacterial infection in chronic obstructive pulmonary disease. *Am Rev Respir Dis* 146:1067–1083, 1992.

167. Nicotra MB, Rivera M, Awe RJ: Antibiotic therapy of acute exacerbations of chronic bronchitis: a controlled study using tetracycline. *Ann Intern Med* 97:18–21, 1982.

168. Anthonisen NR, Manfreda J, Warren CPW, et al: Antibiotic therapy in exacerbations of chronic obstructive pulmonary disease. *Ann Intern Med* 106:196–204, 1987.

169. Paterson IC, Petrie GR, Crompton CK, Robertson JR: Chronic bronchitis: is bacteriological examination of sputum necessary? *Br Med J* 2:537–538, 1978.

170. Flenley DC, Miller HC, King AJ, et al: Oxygen transport in acute pulmonary edema and in acute exacerbations of chronic bronchitis. *Br Med J* 1:78–81, 1973.

171. Warrel DA, Edwards RHT, Godfrey S, Jones NL: Effect of controlled oxygen therapy on arterial blood gases in acute respiratory failure. *Br Med J* 1:452–455, 1970.

172. Christopher KL: At-home administration of oxygen. In: Kacmarek RM, Stoller JK, eds: *Current Respiratory Care*. Toronto, BC Decker, 1988, pp 9–18.

173. Nocturnal Oxygen Therapy Trial Group: Continuous or nocturnal oxygen therapy in hypoxemic chronic obstructive lung disease: a clinical trial. *Ann Intern Med* 93:391–398, 1980.

174. British Medical Research Council Working Party: Long-term domiciliary oxygen therapy in chronic hypoxic cor pulmonale complicating chronic bronchitis and emphysema. *Lancet* 1:681–685, 1981.

175. Ashutosh K, Mead G, Dunsky M: Early effects of oxygen administration and prognosis in chronic obstructive pulmonary disease and cor pulmonale. *Am Rev Respir Dis* 127:399–404, 1983.

176. Degaute JP, Domenighetti G, Naeije R, et al: Oxygen delivery in acute exacerbation of chronic obstructive pulmonary disease: effects of controlled oxygen therapy. *Am Rev Respir Dis* 124:26–30, 1981.

177. Wiedemann HP, Matthay RA: Cor pulmonale in chronic obstructive pulmonary disease: circulatory pathophysiology and new concepts of therapy. *Curr Pulmonol* 8:127–162, 1987.

178. Petty TL: Home oxygen therapy. *Mayo Clin Proc* 62:841–847, 1987.

179. Conference Report. Further recommendations for prescribing and supplying long-term oxygen therapy. *Am Rev Respir Dis* 138:745–747, 1988.

180. Kawakami Y, Kishi F, Yamamoto H, et al: Relation of oxygen delivery, mixed venous oxygenation, and pulmonary hemodynamics to prognosis in chronic obstructive pulmonary disease. *N Engl J Med* 308:1045–1049, 1983.

181. Fletcher EC, Luckett RA, Goodnight-White S, Miller CC, Qian Wei, Costarangos-Galarza C: A double-blind trial of nocturnal supplemental oxygen for sleep desaturation in patients with chronic obstructive pulmonary disease and a daytime $PaO_2$ above 60 mmHg. *Am Rev Respir Dis* 145:1070–1076, 1992.

182. Fletcher EC, Donner CF, Midgren B: Survival in COPD patients with a daytime $PaO_2$ >60 mmHg with and without nocturnal oxyhemoglobin desaturation. *Chest* 101:649–655, 1992.

183. Fletcher EC: Controversial indications for long-term oxygen therapy. *Respir Care* 39:333–346, 1994.

184. Barker AF, Burgher LW, Plummer AL: Oxygen conserving methods for adults. *Chest* 105:248–252, 1994.

185. Christopher KL, Spofford BT, Petrun MD, et al: A program for transtracheal oxygen delivery: assessment of safety and efficacy. *Ann Intern Med* 107:802–808, 1987.

186. Couser JI, Make BJ: Transtracheal oxygen decreases inspired minute ventilation. *Am Rev Respir Dis* 139:627–631, 1989.

187. Hoffman LA, Wesmiller SW, Sciurba FC, et al: Nasal cannula and transtracheal oxygen delivery. A comparison of patient response after 6 months of each technique. *Am Rev Respir Dis* 145:827–831, 1992.

188. Adamo JP, Mehta AC, Stelmach K, Meeker D, Rice T, Stoller JK: The Cleveland Clinic's initial experience with transtracheal oxygen therapy. *Respir Care* 35:153–160, 1990.

189. MacNee W, Connaughton JJ, Rhind GB, et al: A comparison of the effects of almitrine or oxygen breathing on pulmonary arterial pressure and right ventricular ejection fraction in hypoxic chronic bronchitis and emphysema. *Am Rev Respir Dis* 134:559–565, 1986.

190. Bell RC, Mullins RC, West LG, et al: The effect of almitrine bismesylate on hypoxemia in chronic obstructive pulmonary disease. *Ann Intern Med* 105:342–346, 1986.

191. Holle RHO, Williams DV, Vandree JC, et al: Increased muscle efficiency and sustained benefits in an outpatient community hospital-based pulmonary rehabilitation program. *Chest* 94:1161–1168, 1988.

192. Stelmach K, Stoller JK, Meeker DP, Curtis PS: The impact of a pulmonary rehabilitation program on functional status of patients with lung disease [Abstract]. *Respir Care* 33:926, 1988.

193. Ries AL, Ellis B, Hawkins RW: Upper extremity exercise training in chronic obstructive pulmonary disease. *Chest* 93:688–692, 1988.

194. Lake FR, Henderson K, Briffa T, Openshaw J, Musk AW: Upper-limb and lower-limb exercise training in patients with chronic airflow obstruction. *Chest* 97:1077–1082, 1990.

195. Martinez FJ, Couser JI, Celli BR: Respiratory response to arm elevation in patients with chronic airflow obstruction. *Am Rev Respir Dis* 143:476–480, 1991.

196. Couser JI Martinez FJ, Celli BR: Pulmonary rehabilitation that includes arm exercise reduces metabolic and ventilatory requirements for simple arm elevation. *Chest* 103:37–41, 1993.

197. Casaburi R, Patessio A, Ioli F, Zanaboni S, Donner CF, Wasserman K: Reductions in exercise lactic acidosis as a result of exercise training in patients with obstructive lung disease. *Am Rev Respir Dis* 143:9–18, 1991.

198. Guyatt GH, Berman LB, Townsend M: Long-term outcome after pulmonary rehabilitation. *Can Med Assoc J* 137:1089–1095, 1987.

199. McGavin CR, Gupta SP, Lloyd EL, et al: Physical rehabilitation for the chronic bronchitic: results of a controlled trial of exercises in the home. *Thorax* 32:307–311, 1977.

200. Wilson DO, Rogers RM, Sanders MH, et al: Nutritional intervention in malnourished patients with emphysema. *Am Rev Respir Dis* 134:672–677, 1986.

201. Efthimiou J, Fleming J, Gomes C, et al: The effect of supplementary oral nutrition in poorly nourished patients with chronic obstructive pulmonary disease. *Am Rev Respir Dis* 137:1075–1082, 1988.

202. Efthimiou J, Mounsey PJ, Benson DN, Madgwick R, Coles SJ, Benson MK: Effect of carbohydrate rich versus fat rich loads on gas exchange and walking performance in patients with chronic obstructive lung disease. *Thorax* 47:451–456, 1992.

203. Kelly SM, Rosa A, Field S, et al: Inspiratory muscle strength and body composition in patients receiving total parenteral nutrition therapy. *Am Rev Respir Dis* 130:33–37, 1984.

204. Belman MJ: Ventilatory muscle training. In Kacmarek RM, Stoller JK, eds: *Current Respiratory Care.* Toronto, BC Decker, 1988 pp 223–226.

205. Smith K, Cook D, Guyatt GH, Madhavan J, Oxman AD: Respiratory muscle training in chronic airflow limitation: a meta-analysis. *Am Rev Respir Dis* 145:533–539, 1992.

206. Larson JL, Kim MJ, Sharp JT, et al: Inspiratory muscle training with a pressure threshold breathing device in patients with chronic obstructive pulmonary disease. *Am Rev Respir Dis* 138:689–696, 1988.

207. Cropp A, DiMarco AF: Effects of intermittent negative pressure ventilation on respiratory muscle function in patients with severe chronic obstructive pulmonary disease. *Am Rev Respir Dis* 135:1056–1061, 1987.

208. Gutierrez M, Beroiza T, Contreras G, et al: Weekly cuirass ventilation improves blood gases and inspiratory muscle strength in patient with chronic air-flow limitation and hypercarbia. *Am Rev Respir Dis* 138:617–623, 1988.

209. Hill NS: Noninvasive ventilation: Does it work, for whom, and how? *Am Rev Respir Dis* 147:1050–1055, 1993.

210. Shapiro SH, Ernst P, Gray-Donald K, et al: Effect of negative pressure ventilation in severe chronic obstructive pulmonary disease. *Lancet* 340:1425–1429, 1992.

211. Strumpf DA, Millman RP, Carlisle CC, et al: Nocturnal positive-pressure ventilation via nasal mask in patients with severe chronic obstructive pulmonary disease. *Am Rev Respir Dis* 144:1234–1239, 1991.

212. FitzGerald MX, Keelan PJ, Cugell DW, Gaensler EA: Long-term results of surgery for bullous emphysema. *J Thorac Cardiovasc Surg* 68:566–585, 1974.

213. Nickoladze GD: Functional results of surgery for bullous emphysema. *Chest* 101:119–122, 1992.

213a. Trulock EP, Cooper JD: Reduction pneumoplasty for COPD. *Chest* 106(Suppl 2):52S, 1994.

214. Hosenpud JD, Novick RJ, Breen TJ, Daily OP: The Registry of the International Society for Heart and Lung Transplantation: Eleventh Official Report—1994. *J Heart Lung Transplant* 13:561–570, 1994.

215. Patterson GA: Double lung transplantation. *Clin Chest Med* 11:227–233, 1990.

216. Patel SR, Kirby TJ, McCarthy PM, et al: Lung transplantation: The Cleveland Clinic experience. *Cleve Clin J Med* 60:303–319, 1993.

217. Glindmeyer HW, Diem JE, Jones RN, Weill H: Noncomparability of longitudinally and cross-sectionally determined annual change in spirometry. *Am Rev Respir Dis* 125:544–548, 1982.

218. Burrows B, Earle RH: Course and prognosis of chronic obstructive lung disease. *N Engl J Med* 280:397–404, 1969.

219. Diener CF, Burrows B: Further observations on the course and prognosis of chronic obstructive lung disease. *Am Rev Respir Dis* 111:719–723, 1975.

220. Burrows B, Bloom JW, Traver GA, Cline MG: The course and prognosis of different forms of chronic airways. Obstruction in a sample from the general population. *N Engl J Med* 317:1309–1314, 1987.

221. Burrows B, Knudson RJ, Camilli AE, et al: The "horse-racing effect" and predicting decline in forced expiratory volume in one second from screening spirometry. *Am Rev Respir Dis* 135:788–793, 1987.

222. Kanner RE, Renzetti AD, Klauber MR, et al: Variables associated with changes in spirometry in patients with obstructive lung diseases. *Am J Med* 67:44–50, 1979.

223. Mitchell RS, Webb NC, Filley GF: Chronic obstructive bronchopulmonary disease: factors influencing prognosis. *Am Rev Respir Dis* 89:878–896, 1964.

224. Peto R, Speizer FE, Cochrane AL, et al: The relevance in adults of air-flow obstruction, but not of mucous hypersecretion, to mortality from chronic lung disease. *Am Rev Respir Dis* 128:491–500, 1983.

225. Weiss ST: Atopy and airways responsiveness in chronic obstructive pulmonary disease. *N Engl J Med* 317:1345–1347, 1987.

226. Anthonisen NR, Wright EC, Hodgkin JE, and the IPPB Trial Group: Prognosis in chronic obstructive pulmonary disease. *Am Rev Respir Dis* 133:14–20, 1986.

227. Traver GA, Cline MG, Burrows B: Predictors of mortality in chronic obstructive pulmonary disease. *Am Rev Respir Dis* 119:895–902, 1979.

228. Vollmer WM, Johnson LR, Buist AS: Relationship of response to a bronchodilator and decline in forced expiratory volume in one second in population studies. *Am Rev Respir Dis* 132:1186–1193, 1985.

229. Postma DS, De Vries K, Koeter GH, Sluiter HJ: Independent influence of reversibility of air-flow obstruction and nonspecific hyperreactivity on the long-term course

of lung function in chronic air-flow obstruction. *Am Rev Respir Dis* 134:276–280, 1986.

230. Tobin MJ, Hutchinson DCS: An overview of the pulmonary features of alpha 1-antitrypsin deficiency. *Arch Intern Med* 142:1342–1348, 1982.

231. Laurell CB, Eriksson S: The electrophoretic alpha 1-globulin pattern of serum in alpha 1-antitrypsin deficiency. *Scand J Lab Clin Invest* 15:132–140, 1963.

232. Brantly M, Nukiwa T, Crystal RG: Molecular basis of alpha 1-antitrypsin deficiency. *Am J Med* 84(Suppl 6A):13–31, 1988.

233. Larsson C: Natural history and life expectancy in severe alpha 1-antitrypsin deficiency, PiZ. *Acta Med Scand* 204:345–351, 1978.

234. Brantly ML, Paul LR, Miller BH, et al: Clinical features and history of the destructive lung disease associated with alpha 1-antitrypsin deficiency of adults with pulmonary symptoms. *Am Rev Respir Dis* 138:327–336, 1988.

235. Sveger T: The natural history of liver diseases in alpha 1-antitrypsin deficient children. *Acta Paediatr Scand* 77:847–851, 1988.

236. Wewers MD, Gadek JE, Keogh BA, et al: Evaluation of danazol therapy for patients with PiZZ alpha 1-antitrypsin deficiency. *Am Rev Respir Dis* 134:476–480, 1986.

237. Wewers MD, Brantly ML, Casolaro MA, Crystal RG: Evaluation of tamoxifen as a therapy to augment alpha 1-antitrypsin concentrations in Z homozygous alpha 1-antitrypsin deficient subjects. *Am Rev Respir Dis* 135:401–402, 1987.

238. Eriksson S: The effect of tamoxifen in intermediate alpha 1-antitrypsin deficiency associated with the phenotype PiSZ. *Ann Clin Res* 15:95–98, 1983.

239. Hubbard RC, Crystal RG: Alpha 1-antitrypsin augmentation therapy for alpha 1-antitrypsin deficiency. *Am J Med* 84(Suppl 6A):52–62, 1988.

240. Stoller JK: α1-antitrypsin deficiency and augmentation therapy in emphysema. *Cleve Clin J Med* 56:683–689, 1989.

241. American Thoracic Society: Guidelines for the approach to the patient with severe hereditary alpha-1-antitrypsin deficiency. *Am Rev Respir Dis* 140:1494–1497, 1989.

242. Hubbard RC, Casolaro MA, Mitchell M, et al: Fate of aerosolized recombinant DNA-produced alpha 1-antitrypsin: use of the epithelial surface of the lower respiratory tract to administer proteins of therapeutic importance. *Proc Natl Acad Sci USA* 86:680–684, 1989.

243. Hubbard RC, McElvaney NG, Sellers SE, et al: Recombinant DNA-produced α1-antitrypsin administered by aerosol augments lower respiratory tract antineutrophil elastase defenses in individuals with α1-antitrypsin deficiency. *J Clin Invest* 84:1349–1354, 1989.

244. Rosenfeld MA, Siegfried W, Yoshimura K, et al: Adenovirus-mediated transfer of a recombinant α1-antitrypsin gene to the lung epithelium in vivo. *Science* 252:431–434, 1991.

245. Canonico AE, Conary JT, Meyrick BO, Brigham KL: Aerosol and intravenous transfection of human α1-antitrypsin gene to lungs of rabbits. *Am J Respir Cell Mol Biol* 10:24–29, 1994.

246. Crystal RG: Gene therapy strategies for pulmonary disease. *Am J Med* 92 (suppl 6A):44S–52S, 1992.

247. Laennec RTH: *Traité de l'Auscultation Mediate et des Maladies des Poumons et du Coeur*, 2nd ed. Paris, Brosson et Chaude, 1826; cited by Lindskog GE: Bronchiectasis revisited. *Yale J Biol Med* 59:41–53, 1986.

248. Reid LM: Reduction in bronchial subdivision in bronchiectasis. *Thorax* 5:233–247, 1950.

249. Ellis DA, Thornley PE, Wightman AF, et al: Present outlook in bronchiectasis: clinical and social study and review of factors influencing prognosis. *Thorax* 36:659–664, 1981.

250. Moll HH: A clinical and pathological study of bronchiectasis. *Q J Med* 25:457–469, 1932.

251. Bradshaw HH, Putrey FJ, Clerf CH, et al: The fate of patients with untreated bronchiectasis. *JAMA* 116:2561–2563, 1941.

252. Konietzko NFJ, Carton RW, Leroy EP: Causes of death in patients with bronchiectasis. *Am Rev Respir Dis* 100:852–858, 1969.

253. Stanford W, Galvin JR: The diagnosis of bronchiectasis. *Clin Chest Med* 9:691–699, 1988.

254. Swartz MN: Bronchiectasis. In Fishman AP, ed: *Pulmonary Diseases and Disorders*. New York, McGraw-Hill, 1988, pp 1553–1581.

255. Barker AF, Bardana EJ Jr: Bronchiectasis: update of an orphan disease. *Am Rev Respir Dis* 137:969–978, 1988.

256. Beck CS, Heiner DC: Selective immunoglobulin G$_4$ deficiency and recurrent infections of respiratory tract. *Am Rev Respir Dis* 124:94–96, 1981.

257. Heiner DC, Moyer AS, Beck AS: Deficiency of IgG$_4$: a disorder associated with frequent infections and bronchiectasis that may be familial. *Clin Rev Allergy* 1:259–266, 1983.

258. Umetsu DT, Ambrosino DM, Quinti I, et al: Infection and impaired antibody response to bacterial capsular polysaccharide antigen in children with selective IgG-subclass deficiency. *N Engl J Med* 313:1247–1251, 1985.

259. Bjorkander B, Bake B, Oxelius V, et al: Impaired lung function in patients with IgA deficiency and low levels of IgG$_2$ or IgG$_3$. *N Engl J Med* 313:720–724, 1985.

260. Ammann AJ, Hong RR: Selective IgA deficiency: presentation of 30 cases and a review of the literature. *Medicine* 50:223–236, 1971.

261. Eliasson R, Mossberg B, Camner P, et al: The immotile-cilia syndrome: a congenital ciliary abnormality as an etiologic factor in chronic airway infections and male sterility. *N Engl J Med* 297:1–6, 1977.

262. Handelsman D, Conway A, Boylan L, et al: Young's syndrome: obstructive azoospermia and chronic sino-pulmonary infections. *N Engl J Med* 310:3–9, 1984.

263. Schanker HMJ, Rajfer F, Saxon A: Recurrent respiratory disease, azoospermia, and nasal polyposis. *Arch Intern Med* 145:2210–2203, 1985.

264. Fuchs HJ, Borowitz DS, Christiansen DH, et al: Effects of aerosolized recombinant human DNase on exacerbations of respiratory symptoms and on pulmonary function in patients with cystic fibrosis. *N Engl J Med* 331:637–642, 1994.

265. Ramsey BW, Astley SJ, Aitken ML, et al: Efficacy and safety of short-term administration of aerosolized recombinant human deoxyribonuclease in patients with cystic fibrosis. *Am Rev Respir Dis* 148:145–151, 1993.

266. Uflacker R, Kaemmerer A, Neves C, et al: Management of massive hemoptysis by bronchial artery embolization. *Radiology* 146:627–634, 1983.

267. Collins FS: Cystic fibrosis: molecular biology and therapeutic implications. *Science* 256:774–779, 1992.

268. Davis PB: Cystic fibrosis from bench to bedside. *N Engl J Med* 325:575–577, 1991.

269. Rommens JM, Iannuzzi MC, Kerem B, et al: Identification of the cystic fibrosis gene: chromosome walking and jumping. *Science* 245:1059–1065, 1989.

270. Snouwaert JN, Brigman KK, Latour AM, Malouf NN, Boucher RC, Smithies O, Koller BH: An animal model for cystic fibrosis made by gene targeting. *Science* 257:1083–1088, 1992.

271. Huang NN, Schidlow DV, Szatrowski TH, et al: Clinical features, survival rate, and prognostic factors in young adults with cystic fibrosis. *Am J Med* 82:871–879, 1987.

272. Stern RC, Boat TF, Doershuk CF, et al: Cystic fibrosis after age 13: twenty-five teenage and adult patients including three asymptomatic men. *Ann Intern Med* 87:188–191, 1977.

273. Murphy S: Cystic fibrosis in adults: diagnosis and management. *Clin Chest Med* 8:695–710, 1987.

274. The Cystic Fibrosis Genotype-Phenotype Consortium: Correlation between genotype and phenotype in patients with cystic fibrosis. *N Engl J Med* 329:1308–1313, 1993.

275. Rivera M, Nicotra MB: Pseudomonas aeruginosa mucoid strain. Its significance in adult chest disease. *Am Rev Respir Dis* 126:833–836, 1982.

276. Brasfield S, Hicks G, Soong SJ, et al: The chest roentgenogram in cystic fibrosis: a new scoring system. *Pediatrics* 63:24–29, 1979.

277. Friedman PJ, Harwood IR, Ellenbogen PH: Pulmonary cystic fibrosis in the adult: early and late radiologic findings with pathologic correlation. *AJR* 136:1131–1144, 1981.

278. di Sant'Agnese PA, Davis PB: Cystic fibrosis in adults: 75 cases and a review of 232 cases in the literature. *Am J Med* 66:121–132, 1979.

279. Davis PB, di Sant'Agnese PA: Diagnosis and treatment of cystic fibrosis: an update. *Chest* 84:802–809, 1984.

280. Boat TF: Cystic fibrosis. In Murray JF, Nadel JA, eds: *Textbook of Respiratory Medicine.* Philadelphia, WB Saunders, 1988, pp 1126–1152.

281. Davis PB, Hubbard VS, di Sant'Agnese PA: Low sweat chloride electrolytes in a patient with cystic fibrosis. *Am J Med* 69:643–646, 1980.

282. Strong TV, Smit LS, Turpin SV, et al: Cystic fibrosis gene mutation in two sisters with mild disease and normal sweat electrolyte levels. *N Engl J Med* 325:1630–1634, 1991.

283. FitzSimmons SC: The changing epidemiology of cystic fibrosis. *J Pediatr* 122:1–9, 1993.

284. Knowles MR, Church NL, Waltner WE, et al: A pilot study of aerosolized amiloride for the treatment of lung disease in cystic fibrosis. *N Engl J Med* 322:1189–1194, 1990.

285. Knowles MR, Clarke LL, Boucher RC: Activation by extracellular nucleotides of chloride secretion in the airway epithelia of patients with cystic fibrosis. *N Engl J Med* 325:533–538, 1991.

286. McElvaney NG, Nakamura H, Birrer P, et al: Modulation of airway inflammation in cystic fibrosis. In vivo suppression of interleukin-8 levels on the respiratory epithelial surface by aerosolization of recombinant secretory leukoprotease inhibitor. *J Clin Invest* 90:1296–1301, 1992.

287. Auerbach HS, Williams M, Kirkpatrick JA, et al: Alternate day prednisone reduces morbidity and improves pulmonary function in cystic fibrosis. *Lancet* 2:686–688, 1985.

288. Rosenstein BJ, Eigen H: Risks of alternate-day prednisone in patients with cystic fibrosis. *Pediatrics* 87:245–246, 1991.

289. Michel BC: Antibiotic therapy in cystic fibrosis: a review of the literature published between 1980 and February 1987. *Chest* 94(Suppl):129S–140S, 1988.

290. Thomassen MJ, Demko CA, Doershuk CF: Cystic fibrosis: a review of pulmonary infections and interventions. *Pediatr Pulmonol* 3:334–351, 1987.

291. Hjelte L, Petrinin B, Kallenius G, Strandvik B: Perspective study of mycobacterial infections in patients with cystic fibrosis. *Thorax* 45:397–400, 1990.

292. Aitken ML et al: Non-tuberculous mycobacterial disease in adult CF patients. *Chest* 103:1096–1099, 1993.

293. Wang EEL, Prober CG, Manson B, et al: Association of respiratory viral infections with pulmonary deterioration in patients with cystic fibrosis. *N Engl J Med* 311:1653–1658, 1984.

294. Shale DJ: Viral infections: a role in the lung disease of cystic fibrosis? *Thorax* 47:89, 1992.

295. Conway SP, Simmonds EJ, Littlewood JM: Acute severe deterioration in cystic fibrosis associated with influenza A virus infection. *Thorax* 47:112–114, 1992.

296. Pribble CG, Black PG, Bosso JA, Turner RB: Clinical manifestations of exacerbations of cystic fibrosis associated with nonbacterial infections. *J Pediatr* 117:200–204, 1990.

297. Kerrebijn KF, ed: Pulmonary infection and antibiotic therapy in patients with cystic fibrosis. *Chest* 94(Suppl):97S–169S, 1988.

298. Regelmann WE, Elliott GR, Warwick WJ, Clawson CC: Reduction of sputum *Pseudomonas aeruginosa* density by antibiotics improves lung function in cystic fibrosis more than do bronchodilators and chest physiotherapy alone. *Am Rev Respir Dis* 141:914–921, 1990.

299. Hodson ME, Penketh ARL, Batten JC: Aerosol carbenicillin and gentamicin treatment of Pseudomonas aeruginosa infection in patients with cystic fibrosis. *Lancet* 2:1137–1139, 1981.

300. Wall MA, Terry AB, Eisenberg J, et al: Inhaled antibiotics in cystic fibrosis. *Lancet* 1:1325, 1983.

301. Ramsey BW, Dorkin HL, Eisenberg JD, et al: Efficacy of aerosolized tobramycin in patients with cystic fibrosis. *N Engl J Med* 328:1740–1746, 1993.

302. Hodson ME, Butland RJA, Roberts CM, et al: Oral ciprofloxacin compared with conventional intravenous treatment for Pseudomonas aeruginosa in adults with cystic fibrosis. *Lancet* 1:235–237, 1987.

303. Zapletal A, Stefanova J, Horak J, et al: *Chest* physiotherapy and airway obstruction in patients with cystic fibrosis—a negative report. *Eur J Respir Dis* 64:426–433, 1983.

304. Desmond KJ, Schwenk F, Thomas E, et al: Immediate

and long-term effects of chest physiotherapy in patients with cystic fibrosis. *J Pediatr* 103:538–542, 1983.

305. Rossman CM, Waldes R, Sampson D, et al: Effect of chest physiotherapy on the removal of mucus in patients with cystic fibrosis. *Am Rev Respir Dis* 126: 131–135, 1982.

306. Zinman R: Cough versus chest physiotherapy: a comparison of the acute effects on pulmonary function in patients with cystic fibrosis. *Am Rev Respir Dis* 129: 182–184, 1984.

307. Hardy K: A review of airway clearance: new techniques, indications, and recommendations. *Respir Care* 39: 440–455, 1994.

308. Warwick WJ, Hansen LG: The long-term effect of high-frequency chest compression therapy on pulmonary complications of cystic fibrosis. *Pediatr Pulmonol* 11: 265–271, 1991.

309. Porter DK, Van Every MJ, Anthracite RF, et al: Massive hemoptysis in cystic fibrosis. *Arch Intern Med* 143: 287–290, 1983.

310. Penketh A, Knight RK, Hodson ME, et al: Management of pneumothorax in adults with cystic fibrosis. *Thorax* 37:850–853, 1982.

311. Stern RC: Cystic fibrosis: recent developments in diagnosis and treatment. *Pediatr Rev* 7:276–286, 1986.

# Chapter 11

# Sleep-Related Breathing Disorders

## Richard B. Berry

SLEEP ARCHITECTURE
VENTILATION AND SLEEP
RESPIRATORY DEFINITIONS
SLEEP MONITORING
   Multiple Sleep Latency Test
SLEEP DISORDERS

Narcolepsy
Idiopathic Hypersomnia
Periodic Limb Movement Disorder
Sleep Apnea Syndromes
Sleep and Asthma
Sleep and COPD

I~N THE LAST~ few decades there has been an explosion of knowledge about sleep and sleep disorders. Consequently, the topic of sleep disorders is much too broad to be covered in any detail in a single chapter. Therefore, the goal of this chapter is to present the elements of sleep physiology and monitoring that are relevant to sleep-related breathing disorders and to discuss these disorders with an emphasis on the sleep apnea syndromes.

## SLEEP ARCHITECTURE

Sleep is not a homogeneous state and therefore has been divided into sleep stages. This is relevant for the study of breathing during sleep, because each stage has a characteristic impact on respiration. Furthermore, disease processes frequently alter not only the total sleep time but also the relative amount of time spent in the various sleep stages.

Sleep is composed of non–rapid eye movement (NREM) sleep and rapid eye movement (REM) sleep. Non–rapid eye movement sleep is further divided into stages 1 to 4. Stages 1 and 2 are referred to as light sleep and stages 3 and 4 as deep or slow-wave sleep. A given night of sleep is divided into periods of time called epochs (usually 30 seconds in duration). The predominant stage in a given epoch names that epoch.

Staging is based on electroencephalographic (EEG), electro-oculographic (EOG) (eye movement), and electromyographic (EMG) criteria (1, 2). Usually only one or two sets of EEG leads are required for staging sleep. The EOG leads are positioned near the eyes. Because a potential difference exists across each eyeball (positive anterior and negative posterior), eye movements result in voltage changes that are detected in the EOG leads. Surface EMG leads, usually in the chin area, detect electrical activity whose amplitude reflects the relative amount of muscle tone. The EMG tracing is useful in detecting stage REM, which is characterized by generalized skeletal muscle hypotonia and a low-amplitude EMG signal. The EEG, EOG, and EMG lead placement and terminology will be discussed in a later section.

The awake EEG (Fig. 11.1) is characterized by low-amplitude, high-frequency activity. With the onset of drowsiness, the EEG reveals alpha waves (8 to 13 Hz), which are associated with eye closure and are best detected by leads in the occipital area. The stage 1 EEG (Fig. 11.2) is characterized by low-voltage, mixed-frequency activity (3 to 7 Hz). Stage 1 is scored when less than 50% of an epoch contains alpha waves. Slow rolling eye movements in the EOG tracing may also be present, and the level of muscle tone (EMG) is equal or diminished compared to that in the awake state. Stage 2 is characterized by the presence of either sleep

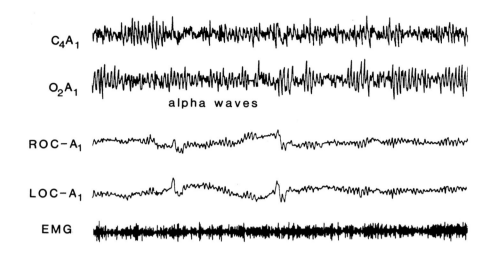

**Figure 11.1.** One epoch (30 seconds) of drowsy wakefulness (stage 0 or W). $C_4A_1$ and $O_2A_1$ are central and occipital EEG tracings, and ROC-$A_1$ and LOC-$A_1$ are right and left EOG tracings. The alpha waves are more prominent in the occipital EEG.

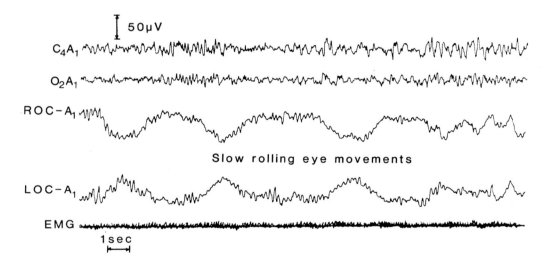

**Figure 11.2.** An epoch (30 seconds) of stage 1 sleep. Alpha wave activity is present in less than 50% of the EEG tracings. Slow, rolling eye movements are present in the right and left tracings (ROC-$A_1$, LOC-$A_1$). No sleep spindles or K complexes are present.

spindles (Fig. 11.3), which are bursts of 12- to 14-Hz activity, or K complexes, which are large-amplitude biphasic EEG deflections (Fig. 11.4). To qualify as stage 2, an epoch must contain less than 20% of slow (delta) wave EEG activity. Slow waves are large-amplitude (greater than 75-$\mu$V) deflections with a frequency of less than 2 Hz. An epoch is scored as stage 3 when it contains 20 to 50% slow-wave EEG activity and as stage 4 when it consists of more than 50% slow-wave activity (Fig. 11.5). The EMG usually falls progressively

on transition from wakefulness (stage W) to stage 4. Stage REM is defined by the presence of rapid eye movements (REMs) in the EOG tracings, low-voltage, mixed-frequency EEG activity, and low muscle tone (Fig. 11.6). A similar EEG pattern and eye movements can occur with relaxed, eyes-open (suppresses alpha activity) wakefulness, but the muscle tone is higher. More-detailed discussions of the rules of sleep staging are available (1–3).

There is a normal progression of sleep stages during

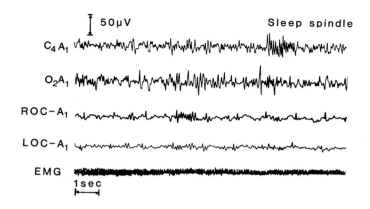

**FIGURE 11.3.** An epoch of stage 2 sleep. A sleep spindle is noted in the EEG tracing. Less than 20% of the EEG tracing is composed of slow-wave activity.

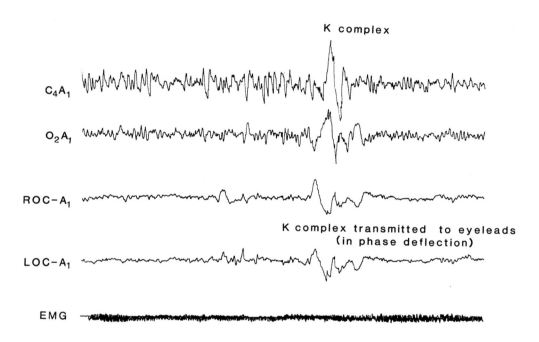

**FIGURE 11.4.** An epoch of stage 2 sleep. A K complex is noted in the EEG tracing. Note that this activity is transmitted to the EOG leads and results in deflections that are in phase (both up or down) in the EOG tracings.

the night (2–5). Usually two to four cycles of stages 1 → 2 → 3 → 4 → 3 → 2 → REM of 90 to 120 minutes' duration are present in the first portion of the night. Then the remainder of the night is spent in either stage 1, 2, or REM, with the REM episodes tending to increase in length. Periods of wakefulness (stage wake) may also occur during the remainder of the night.

Total sleep time (TST) is the total minutes of REM and NREM sleep. Sleep period time (SPT) equals TST plus any stage wake that occurs after sleep onset but before the final awakening. The sleep latency is the time from lights out (beginning of monitoring) to the onset of sleep. A sleep latency of more than 30 minutes is typical of patients complaining of difficulty falling asleep (insomnia). The REM latency is defined as the time from sleep onset until the first epoch of stage REM. A normal REM latency is around 90 minutes (70 to 120 minutes). The time in bed (TIB) is the time from lights out to lights on. Sleep efficiency is defined as TST/TIB. It is customary to express the time spent in

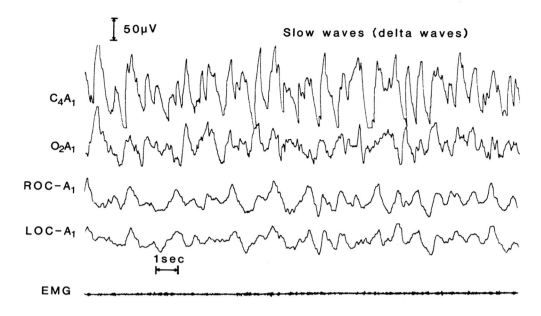

**FIGURE 11.5.**   An epoch of stage 4 sleep. More than 50% of the EEG tracings contain high-voltage, slow-wave activity. Note that the EMG activity has also decreased.

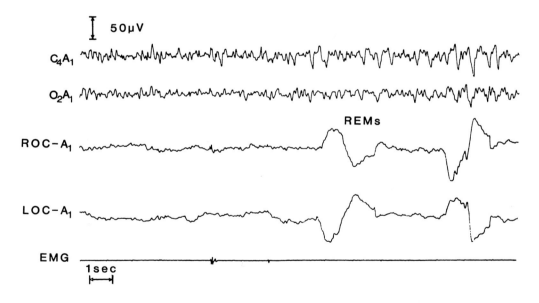

**FIGURE 11.6.**   An epoch of stage REM sleep. The EEG tracing shows low-voltage, mixed-frequency activity. The rapid eye movements (REMs) result in out-of-phase deflections in the right and left EOG leads (ROC-$A_1$ and LOC-$A_1$). The EMG level of activity is quite reduced.

each stage (including the stage wake present during the SPT) as a percentage of SPT. A young adult typically spends less than 5% of SPT in stage wake, 5 to 10% in stage 1, 50% in stage 2, 20 to 30% in stages 3 and 4, and 20 to 25% in stage REM. A normal 60-year-old has a greater percentage of stage wake and stage 1 sleep and reduced stage 3 and 4 sleep (less than 10%), but about the same percentage of stage REM (2).

An arousal is defined as an abrupt shift in EEG frequency that may include theta (4 to 8 Hz), alpha, and/or frequencies greater than 16 Hz (but not spindles). The EMG amplitude also commonly increases. Recently, a task force of the American Sleep Disorders Association (ASDA) has proposed a set of rules for scoring arousals (6). The EEG frequency shift must be at least 3 seconds in duration to be scored as an arousal. In NREM sleep an arousal can be scored without an increase in EMG amplitude. However, in REM sleep an increase in EMG amplitude is required as well as an EEG frequency shift. The rationale for this rule is that bursts of alpha waves are common in REM sleep. When sleep is filled with many brief arousals it is not restorative. Thus, daytime sleepiness can occur even if the TST (as scored by standard criteria) is not markedly shortened (7). Sleep interrupted by frequent arousals and stage shifts is said to be fragmented.

## VENTILATION AND SLEEP

Respiratory drive is reduced during NREM sleep due to loss of the stimulatory effect of wakefulness and decreases in chemosensitivity. There is a decrease in the ventilatory responses to hypoxia and hypercapnia (8–9). In most studies a further decrease in chemosensitivity has been present in stage REM. Stages 1 and 2 are often characterized by a periodic waxing and waning of tidal volume and respiratory rate (periodic breathing). This is thought to be due to transition between the awake set point for $P_{CO_2}$ and the sleep set point, which is somewhat higher (10). Stages 3 and 4 are characterized by a regular pattern of tidal volume and respiratory rate. Compared to awake values, ventilation is reduced by 1 to 2 liters/minute, $P_{CO_2}$ increased by 2 to 8 mm Hg, and $P_{O_2}$ decreased by 5 to 10 mm Hg. While animal studies have consistently shown a fall in tidal volume and an increase in respiratory rate during NREM sleep, studies in humans are less consistent. Most studies have shown a reduction in minute ventilation associated with a decrease in tidal volume and either a decrease in respiratory rate or an increase not large enough to compensate for the fall in tidal volume (11).

Stage REM is characterized by an irregular pattern of varying tidal volume and respiratory rate; short periods of central apnea may be seen. Frequently, periods of reduced ventilation may coincide with bursts of phasic eye movements (REMs). Intercostal and accessory muscle activity is reduced and functional residual capacity may also decrease (12, 13). Upper-airway resistance increases during NREM sleep, and this acts as a resistive load on the ventilatory system (14). During REM sleep it is believed that upper-airway resistance may increase further. In the study of Hudgel and co-workers (14), however, the upper-airway resistances in REM and NREM sleep were not significantly different. The loss of intercostal muscle activity during REM sleep makes the diaphragm less efficient (12). This is especially important in patients with diaphragmatic weakness or a mechanical disadvantage due to hyperinflation (chronic obstructive pulmonary disease). Indeed, stage REM is usually the stage of sleep associated with the most severe oxygen desaturation in patients with sleep-related respiratory disorders.

## RESPIRATORY DEFINITIONS

An apnea is defined as the cessation of air flow at the nose and mouth for 10 seconds or longer. Obstructive apnea (Fig. 11.7) is present when there is continued respiratory effort (evidence of central respiratory drive such as chest and abdominal movement) during the absence of air flow. Central apneas are characterized by absence of both air flow and respiratory effort. Mixed apneas are those in which the initial portion of the apnea is central (no respiratory effort) and the remaining portion obstructive (respiratory effort present). Desaturations are usually defined as a fall in arterial oxygen saturation of 4% or more from baseline. It is important to remember that the change in $P_{O_2}$ associated with a 4% change in saturation depends critically on the initial $P_{O_2}$ (position on the oxyhemoglobin saturation curve). The above definitions are arbitrary but widely used (3, 15).

Periods of reduced tidal volume or air flow may also be associated with desaturations or sleep disturbance. These events are called hypopneas. Definitions of hypopnea vary among clinicians (15, 16). Some require only a fall in air flow or tidal volume to between one-third and one-half of the baseline value, while others require that an associated desaturation be present. Although hypopneas could be due to a fall in central drive (central hypopneas) or partial airway obstruction (obstructive hypopneas), such a separation is not always possible from routine measurements. Obstructive hypopneas are often associated with paradoxical movements of the chest and abdomen, although in

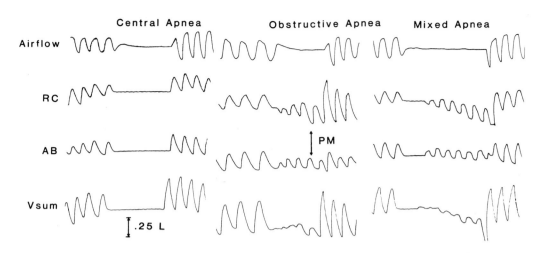

**FIGURE 11.7.** Illustrations of central, obstructive, and mixed apnea. Respiratory inductance plethysmography is used to monitor respiratory effort. The three lower channels are rib cage (chest) (*RC*), abdomen (*AB*), and the summed signal (*Vsum*). After calibration, changes in the Vsum approximate tidal volume. Note the paradoxical movement (*PM*) of the chest and abdomen during obstruction.

some patients only more subtle changes in phase between chest and abdominal movements can be detected (16). The apnea index (or apnea plus hypopnea index) is defined as the number of events per hour of sleep (number of events/TST in hours). An alternate term for the apnea plus hypopnea index (AHI) is the respiratory disturbance index (RDI).

## SLEEP MONITORING

The detailed monitoring of sleep is called polysomnography. The standard positions of the EEG, EOG, and EMG leads are illustrated in Figure 11.8. The central EEG leads are termed $C_3$ and $C_4$ in the international 10–20 system. The odd and even numbers in this system refer to the left and right sides of the body, respectively. The leads are usually referenced to electrodes in the mastoid area ($A_1$, $A_2$). The term *derivation* refers to the signal obtained from a pair of electrodes amplified with a differential amplifier. Although both $C_3$ and $C_4$ are usually placed, only one derivation is monitored at a time ($C_4$-$A_1$ or $C_3$-$A_2$), and the other is available in case of lead failure. In these derivations sleep spindles, slow waves, and alpha waves may be recorded (1–3). Although the central derivation alone is adequate to stage sleep, an additional set of leads in the occipital area ($O_1$ or $O_2$) is useful because alpha waves are best recorded there. These are also referenced to a mastoid electrode ($O_1$-$A_2$, $O_2$-$A_1$). While one set of eye leads can detect eye movements, the two-set scheme depicted in Figure 11.8 is recommended. The right and left EOG electrodes are placed near the outer corner (outer canthus) of the eyes and are abbreviated ROC and LOC (right and left outer canthus). One electrode is placed above and the other below the canthi so that vertical as well as horizontal eye movements can be detected. In this lead configuration, eye movements (which are conjugate) result in out-of-phase deflections (one up, one down), while deflections due to artifacts or high-voltage EEG activity are in phase. One set of surface EMG electrodes in the submental area is adequate for assessing muscle tone. A typical scheme is to reference EEG and EOG electrodes to a common mastoid electrode ($C_4$-$A_1$, ROC-$A_1$, LOC-$A_1$, $EMG_1$-$EMG_2$). Another method references the EOG leads to the contralateral mastoid (ROC-$A_1$, LOC-$A_2$). For more technical information the reader is referred to the references (1–3).

Air flow is detected qualitatively by using thermistors or thermocouples at the nose and mouth (3). Air flow across these devices changes their temperature and hence their resistance (thermistor) or voltage output (thermocouple). With appropriate circuitry, air flow results in a signal that can be recorded on a polygraph. Pneumotachographs inserted in a face mask can be used if quantitative measurements of air flow are required. Air flow can also be detected by using $CO_2$ measuring devices that detect the increased $CO_2$ content in exhaled gas. This method can be misleading because small exhalations rich in $CO_2$ may occur during obstructive apneas despite the absence of inspiratory air flow. The resulting substantial fluctuations in

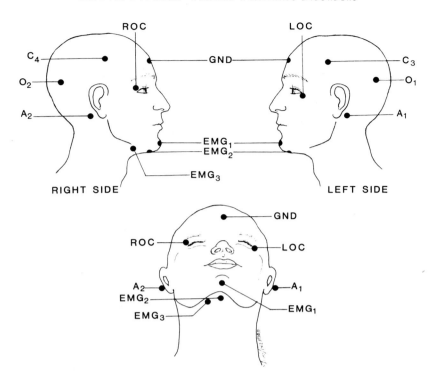

**FIGURE 11.8.** Electrode placement for EEG, EOG, and EMG leads.

$CO_2$ may give the appearance of significant air flow (3).

Respiratory effort is commonly monitored by devices that detect chest and abdominal movement. Such devices include impedance plethysmography, strain gauges, or respiratory inductance plethysmography (3, 17, 18). In some obese individuals, respiratory effort during obstructive apnea does not result in easily discernible motion of the chest wall or abdomen. A more sensitive method for detecting respiratory effort employs a catheter placed in the esophagus to detect changes in pleural pressure due to inspiratory muscle contraction (17). This method is not routinely used, although a small percentage of apneas will be misclassified as central on the basis of surface measurements of respiratory effort. Recently, many laboratories are using small, soft, fluid-filled catheters to detect pleural pressure changes rather than the more uncomfortable esophageal balloons. If the respiratory inductance plethysmography (RIP) technique is used, the signals from the chest (RC) and abdominal (AB) bands can be added to provide a signal (Vsum) whose changes can be calibrated to estimate tidal volume (18). Obstructive apnea results in paradoxical movements of the chest and abdomen. With proper calibration, apneas may be detected by absence of a deflection in the Vsum signal (RC = −AB), and hypopneas as a reduction in tidal volume. Obstructive hypopneas are associated either with frank chest-abdominal paradox or chest and abdominal movements that are out of phase (17, 18). However, tight calibration of RIP is usually difficult with very obese individuals.

Arterial oxygen saturation is continuously measured by pulse oximetry using ear or finger probes. One should note that the nadir of a desaturation associated with a respiratory event usually occurs after the event has ended. The delay is due to the circulation time to the sensing device as well as instrumental delay. An electrocardiographic lead is monitored to detect sleep-associated arrhythmias.

Leg movements are detected by monitoring leg electromyograms using surface electrodes placed over the anterior tibialis muscles. Periodic leg movements during sleep can cause sleep disturbance and result in symptoms that can mimic the sleep apnea syndromes (see later section). All of the parameters described above are recorded on a polygraph, which usually runs at a paper speed of 10 mm/second. This speed is not optimum for either respiratory or ECG recording but is commonly used to stage sleep.

## MULTIPLE SLEEP LATENCY TEST

In addition to nocturnal polysomnography, daytime tests are used to document the degree of daytime sleepiness (19). The multiple sleep latency test (MSLT) consists of four or five short naps, usually spaced across the day in 2-hour intervals (for example, 8:00 AM, 10:00 AM, noon, 2:00 PM, and 4:00 PM). Patients are given 20 minutes to fall asleep. If sleep occurs, patients are given another 15 minutes to reach REM sleep. Once REM sleep is reached or the period of time has run out, the test is terminated. The subject then gets out of bed until the next nap. The sleep latency (time from lights out to initial sleep) and the presence or absence of REM sleep are determined. Mean sleep latencies of less than 5 minutes, 5 to 10 minutes, and 10 to 15 minutes document severe, moderate, and mild degrees of sleepiness. A sleep latency of greater than 15 minutes is considered "normal," although normal healthy controls can exhibit a sleep latency of 10 to 15 minutes. Normally there are no (rarely one) periods of REM during the brief naps. For correct interpretation, the MSLT should always follow an all-night polysomnogram. Medications that affect sleep (especially REM sleep) such as stimulants, sedatives (ethanol), and tricyclic antidepressants should be withdrawn, if possible, for 2 weeks before testing. In a variation of the MSLT termed the maintenance of wakefulness test (MWT), subjects are requested to stay awake in a dark, quiet room during multiple 40-minute periods while semirecumbent and monitored for sleep (20). The correlation between the sleep latencies determined on the MSLT and the MWT is rather low but statistically significant (20). For example, certain patients will have a short sleep latency on the MSLT but are able to stay awake for 40 minutes during the MWT. These tests may well measure different aspects of the same process. While the MSLT is considered the standard test for assessing daytime sleepiness, the MWT may be more sensitive for demonstrating an effect of treatment or evaluating a given patient's ability to function in the tasks of daily living (21). If the sleep latency on the MWT is 15 minutes or less, the patient may have a difficult time performing tasks requiring attention.

## SLEEP DISORDERS

The International Classification of Sleep Disorders (22) provides a scheme for classifying an extensive number of disease processes. The reader is referred to this reference. This chapter discusses only processes

**TABLE 11.1**
**CONDITIONS PRESENTING WITH EXCESSIVE DAYTIME SLEEPINESS**

| |
|---|
| Sleep apnea syndromes |
| Narcolepsy |
| Idiopathic hypersomnia |
| Periodic limb movements (PLMs) in sleep |
| Psychiatric disorders (depression) |
| Drug and alcohol dependency |
| Insufficient sleep syndrome |
| Circadian disorders (jet lag, shift work) |

that are commonly associated with complaints of excessive daytime sleepiness (Table 11.1). In a large cooperative study of sleep-wake disorder centers, 42% of patients presented with complaints of excessive daytime sleepiness (EDS), and 43% of those with EDS had sleep apnea (23). Any physician providing care for patients with sleep apnea should be familiar with the other conditions presenting with EDS. One should not assume that every sleepy, snoring patient has sleep apnea. In addition, patients with sleep apnea can also have narcolepsy or periodic limb movements (PLMs) in sleep. Therefore the evaluation of any sleepy patient should include questions relevant to narcolepsy, PLMs, and depression as well as to sleep apnea. A careful history of medications and the use of ethanol, stimulants (including caffeine), and sedatives must be obtained. A recording of the patient's usual amount and pattern of sleep may also be instructive. Most sleep centers use a sleep log that the patient completes before coming for evaluation. A brief discussion of the first three nonrespiratory disorders listed in Table 11.1 will precede a discussion of sleep apnea.

### NARCOLEPSY

Narcolepsy (24, 25) is a syndrome associated with the tetrad of sleep attacks, cataplexy, hypnagogic hallucinations, and sleep paralysis. The first two are the most common. When cataplexy is unequivocal, the diagnosis can be made with confidence. Unfortunately, the sleep attacks may be present for several years before cataplexy. In addition, cataplexy is often subtle and difficult to document. All four components of the tetrad are present in only 11 to 14% of cases.

The attacks of sleepiness usually begin in adolescence or early adulthood and can occur at any time of the day. After a brief nap the patient may awaken completely refreshed. Patients with narcolepsy may also complain of chronic sleepiness as well as sleep attacks. Cataplexy refers to the sudden loss of muscle tone or strength following a period of high emotion such as surprise, laughter, or anger. The cataplectic attacks may vary from subtle weakness of an isolated muscle group (loss of facial muscle tone) to sudden paralysis of all skeletal muscles and postural collapse. Some prolonged episodes of cataplexy are also associated with hallucinations. Hypnagogic (sleep onset) and hypnopompic (at awakening) hallucinations are vivid, dreamlike experiences often associated with fear. Sleep paralysis also occurs at the transitions between wakefulness and sleep and involves an inability to move even though awake that lasts from a few seconds to 20 minutes. Fortunately, respiration is usually not affected, although some patients complain of dyspnea during the paralysis episodes. Sleep paralysis can also occur in non-narcoleptics.

The polysomnographic hallmark of narcolepsy is sleep-onset stage REM (SOREM). Whereas the normal REM latency is about 90 minutes, patients with narcolepsy often have a REM latency of less than 15 minutes. The MSLT is very useful for supporting the diagnosis of narcolepsy. The standard criteria are a mean sleep latency of less than 5 minutes and two or more REM onsets in five nap opportunities. Over 80% of patients with narcolepsy will meet this diagnostic criterion. An occasional patient will fail to have a sleep latency less than 5 minutes or two SOREM periods on an initial test but will demonstrate this on a second MSLT (19). A negative MSLT does not absolutely rule out narcolepsy. In such cases, a firm diagnosis of narcolepsy would require that a history of both daytime sleepiness and unequivocal cataplexy be present. The MSLT should follow a night of polysomnography to document that the SOREM is not due to preceding REM deprivation (and to rule out other sleep pathology). Sleep-onset REM may also be seen in some patients with sleep apnea (which can reduce the amount of REM sleep), depression, schizophrenia, and following withdrawal of REM-suppressing medications.

Narcolepsy occurs in about four of 10,000 people and has a definite familial basis. In a national cooperative study of sleep disorders centers, narcolepsy was present in about 25% of the patients complaining of increased daytime sleepiness (23). Studies have found that 80 to 95% of patients with classic narcolepsy were positive for the HLA-DR2 antigen, depending on their ethnic background (25, 26). Unfortunately, 25 to 36% of the general population is positive for this antigen. Therefore, the utility of the HLA-DR2 antigen in diagnosing narcolepsy remains to be determined. The etiology of narcolepsy is still unknown.

The treatment of narcolepsy depends on which symptoms are bothering the patient. Treatment of the sleep attacks usually includes the use of stimulants such as methylphenidate (Ritalin) or pemoline (Cylert). Methylphenidate is started at a dose of 15 to 20 mg/day divided into three or four doses and must be given on an empty stomach to be effective. The drug is most effective if given before sleep attacks characteristically occur. Once a sleep attack is in progress, the best treatment is a short nap. Most patients are controlled on 15 to 60 mg/day. Higher doses are associated with side effects and are rarely effective. A drug holiday of 2 weeks may restore the effectiveness of the drug, and many clinicians prescribe such a holiday every 6 months. The attacks of cataplexy may be decreased by tricyclic antidepressants in doses below those used for depression. Protriptyline (Vivactil) (15 to 30 mg/day in three divided doses) and imipramine (Tofranil) (75 mg/day) are the most commonly used agents (24). If stimulants and tricyclics are used together, careful monitoring is needed, because serious side effects such as hypertension can result.

### IDIOPATHIC HYPERSOMNIA

This syndrome was formerly called idiopathic central nervous system hypersomnolence. It is characterized by daytime somnolence but no other manifestations of narcolepsy (22). Unlike narcolepsy, the daytime naps are not refreshing and the night sleep period is usually long. It is sometimes associated with other symptoms such as headaches or syncope and has been reported after viral infection, mononucleosis, hepatitis, or the Guillain-Barré syndrome. Multiple sleep latency testing shows a short sleep latency but no SOREM. These patients made up about 10% of all patients complaining of EDS in a large cooperative study (23). Treatment with CNS stimulants is usually attempted but is less effective than with narcolepsy.

### PERIODIC LIMB MOVEMENT DISORDER

The syndrome of periodic limb movements (PLMs) (also known as nocturnal myoclonus or periodic leg movements) consists of stereotypic periodic leg (or arm) movements during sleep that may or may not be associated with arousals (27). If enough arousals occur, sleep may be so fragmented that daytime sleepiness results. While about 10 to 12% of patients seen in sleep centers for insomnia complaints have PLMs as the etiology, only 2 to 3% of the patients presenting with excessive daytime sleepiness are found to have PLMs as the major cause of their sleepiness. Probably a much higher percentage of elderly patients have PLMs but no symptoms (27). Because narcoleptics frequently have PLMs, any patient with excessive daytime sleepiness and PLMs on a polysomnogram should be questioned carefully concerning narcoleptic manifestations.

PLMs can also appear after withdrawal of anticonvulsants, benzodiazepines, barbiturates, or other hypnotics (22). Patients with sleep apnea on occasion exhibit a large increase in PLMs after treatment with nasal continuous positive airway pressure (29).

Patients with EDS due to PLMs may or may not remember the awakenings during the night but almost never remember the leg movements. The movements usually consist of dorsiflexion of the foot at the ankle, extension of the big toe and partial flexion of the knee and hip. A small portion of the patients have the restless leg syndrome (RLS), which involves a creeping sensation in the legs associated with a desire to move them. These sensations commonly occur at bedtime. It is important to question patients about these sensations, because if a patient has RLS symptoms he or she frequently also has PLMs.

The diagnosis of the PLM syndrome requires monitoring of leg EMGs. Leg movements may occur in one or both legs, and therefore monitoring of both legs is suggested. Not all events are associated with arousals. Only movements leading to arousals are considered detrimental. New guidelines (28) for scoring leg movements (LMs) differ somewhat from previous criteria (27) and suggest that all LMs—whether occurring individually or in groups (periodic)—be counted in both sleep and wakefulness. This recognizes that all LMs can potentially disturb sleep. An LM is identified when there is a 0.5- to 5-second burst of anterior tibialis activity with an amplitude greater than 25% of that recorded during polygraph calibration when the patient moves his or her legs on command. To be scored as part of a "PLM sequence," an LM must occur during sleep, must not follow an arousal due to other events, and must occur in a group of four or more LMs separated by more than 5 seconds and less than 90 seconds (event onset to onset). The number of these events per hour of sleep (PLM index) and the number per hour of sleep followed by an arousal (PLMAr index) are still used to diagnose the periodic leg movement syndrome. A PLM index greater than 5 is considered abnormal; 5 to 24, mild; 25 to 49, moderate; and 50 or more, severe (22). The true impact of this disorder is probably more accurately assessed by looking at the PLM-arousal index. Severe daytime sleepiness is usually associated with a PLM-arousal index greater than 25 (22).

Treatment of PLM syndrome is usually with benzodiazepines, which suppress the awakenings but not the PLMs. The most commonly used agent is clonazepam 0.5 mg taken a half hour before bedtime. The dose may be titrated upward to 1.5 mg. Recently the combination of levodopa and carbidopa has been used by some clinicians with success (30).

## SLEEP APNEA SYNDROMES

The sleep apnea syndromes may be divided into the obstructive sleep apnea syndromes (OSAS) and the central sleep apnea syndromes (CSAS). Patients with predominantly mixed apneas or repetitive hypopneas (16) due to partial airway obstruction behave like those with pure obstructive apneas and are considered to have the OSAS. While patients with obstructive sleep apnea may have some central apneas, the diagnosis of central sleep apnea requires that a majority of apneas be central in nature. The OSAS is much more common than the CSAS, with the latter accounting for less than 10 to 15% of patients treated for sleep apnea in most centers (23, 31).

### Obstructive Sleep Apnea

The true incidence of obstructive sleep apnea is unknown, but estimates of 1 to 4% have been quoted (31, 32). Over 40% of patients seen in sleep disorder centers complaining of daytime sleepiness are found to have sleep apnea (23). Patients with the OSAS usually present with a complaint of excessive daytime sleepiness (EDS). They typically have a long history of snoring, and bedmates frequently report pauses in breathing terminated by snorts. A history of chronic nasal obstruction or congestion, hypertension, or recent weight gain preceding an exacerbation of daytime sleepiness is common. Other manifestations or associations include impotence, enuresis, and morning headaches (31). Conditions known to predispose patients to sleep apnea include the male sex (15), increasing age (15), alcohol use (33), obesity (34), hypothyroidism (35), acromegaly (36), and hypnotic use (37). Recent studies have suggested that the OSAS may be more common in female subjects than was formerly suspected (32).

Symptoms and signs of right heart failure are present in a minority (10 to 15%) of cases (38). Physical examination frequently reveals nasal obstruction, a large tongue, retrognathia (posterior displacement of the mandible), a dependent soft palate, or a hypertrophied uvula. Many patients have a short, thick neck. In fact, neck circumference correlates better with the AHI than body weight. Up to 40% of patients in some sleep centers are not obese. The laboratory evaluation of patients suspected of having OSA should always include thyroid studies. The majority of patients do not have either polycythemia or evidence of $CO_2$ retention on arterial blood gas analysis. We reserve arterial blood gas analysis for patients who have low awake oxygen saturations or unexplained elevations in serum bicarbonate.

A small subset of patients with obstructive sleep

apnea are very obese and manifest daytime hypoventilation (increased $P_{CO_2}$). These patients, formerly called Pickwickian, are now said to have the obesity hypoventilation syndrome (OHS). Most (but not all) patients with this syndrome have severe obstructive sleep apnea. Occasionally a patient will not have discrete apneas or hypopneas during sleep but will simply manifest hypoventilation during the day, which worsens during sleep. Most patients with sleep apnea and a normal daytime $P_{CO_2}$ and $P_{O_2}$ have normal ventilatory responses to hypercapnia and hypoxemia (39), although their responses to resistive loads may be reduced (40). Those with the obesity hypoventilation syndrome have reduced ventilatory responses to hypoxemia and hypercapnia (41, 42) and have a lower compliance of the respiratory system compared to non-hypercapnic patients with equivalent obesity (43). With adequate treatment of the sleep apnea, the daytime $CO_2$ retention will improve in some but not all OHS patients (44, 45). This implies both acquired (reversible) and congenital dysfunction of ventilatory control.

*Polysomnography in the OSAS*

Polysomnography of patients with OSAS reveals repetitive obstructive apneas and hypopneas (Fig. 11.9). Apneas are followed by resumption of air flow, which usually coincides with evidence of arousal and often

movement. The nadir of oxygen saturation usually occurs after apnea termination. During the apnea the chest and abdomen move in a paradoxical manner. The heart rate usually slows during the apnea and then speeds up during the post-apnea arousal. The fall in heart rate appears to be secondary to a combination of increased vagal tone and hypoxia (46, 47). The bradycardia is blocked by atropine and improved with oxygen therapy when the latter prevents arterial oxygen desaturation. Heart block (all types) and atrial and ventricular arrhythmias may also be associated with sleep apnea (48). Apnea-associated sudden death during sleep can occur, although it is probably not common.

Because many totally asymptomatic elderly males may have a small amount of obstructive apnea, defining exact criteria for normality based on the apnea index (or apnea plus hypopnea index) is difficult (15, 32, 33). Although some have suggested that an apnea index greater than five per hour or 30 apneas per night should be considered abnormal, an apnea plus hypopnea index from 5 to 10 may be normal if symptoms are absent. A retrospective study (49) found an increase in mortality when the apnea index exceeded 20 per hour. An arbitrary but useful scheme is to consider a combined apnea plus hypopnea index less than 20 as mild, 20 to 40 as moderate, and greater than 40 as severe. Occasionally a sleepy, snoring patient will have

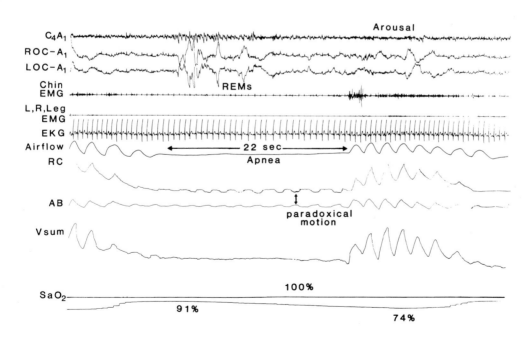

**FIGURE 11.9.** A complete polysomnographic tracing of an obstructive apnea during REM sleep. Note that the EEG and EMG change at apnea termination, signifying an arousal, and that the nadir of arterial oxygen saturation ($Sa_{O_2}$) occurs after the apnea has terminated.

relatively few apneas when studied. Patients with mild degrees of apnea may show more night-to-night variability in the apnea plus hypopnea index. The physician should rule out the confounding influences of ethanol and posture. If the patient abstains from his or her usual dose of ethanol or does not sleep supine during the sleep study, this may lead to a "falsely" low amount of apnea. One must also consider the impact of periodic leg movements and the possibility of unsuspected narcolepsy. If the physician feels that the amount of apnea or PLMs is inadequate to explain the degree of daytime sleepiness, an MSLT should be ordered both to document the degree of sleepiness and to rule out narcolepsy. In such a patient, a short sleep latency on the MSLT but no REM onsets would also be compatible with idiopathic hypersomnia or inadequate sleep. Recently, a group of patients with few discrete apneas and hypopneas but with recurrent brief arousals due to increased upper-airway resistance has been described (50). Not all of these patients with the "upper-airway resistance syndrome" snored. These patients all had symptoms of EDS and a reduced sleep latency, which improved when treated as if they had obstructive sleep apnea. Definitive diagnosis of this syndrome requires demonstration of an increase in supraglottic or esophageal pressure defections and/or fall in tidal volume preceding the brief arousals. However, if frequent unexplained brief arousals are consistently preceded by changes in respiratory effort or tidal volume, one should suspect that the upper-airway resistance syndrome is present.

The degree of arterial oxygen desaturation in patients with OSA is not necessarily correlated with the apnea index and must also be considered in assessing the severity of disease. A study of the factors determining the severity of desaturation found that (*a*) a lower baseline $P_{O_2}$, (*b*) a greater percentage of sleep time spent in apnea, and (*c*) a smaller expiratory reserve volume (functional residual capacity minus residual volume) all tended to produce more severe desaturation (51). This is consistent with the observation that patients with baseline hypoxemia due to obesity (with or without $CO_2$ retention) or superimposed chronic obstructive pulmonary disease tend to desaturate more rapidly during apnea.

Pulmonary arterial blood pressure rises during apneas and then falls when the oxygen saturation returns to normal after apnea (52). The main cause of these episodic increases in pulmonary arterial blood pressure is hypoxic vasoconstriction. Studies have suggested that *daytime* pulmonary hypertension (53) and right heart failure (38) are generally confined to obstructive sleep apnea patients with daytime hypoxemia. Patients with obstructive sleep apnea and daytime hypoxemia usually have either the obesity hypoventilation syndrome or a mixture of obstructive sleep apnea and chronic obstructive pulmonary disease (COPD).

Systemic arterial blood pressure falls during normal sleep. In contrast, an increase in systemic blood pressure is associated with each obstructive apnea. There is a slow rise in blood pressure during the apnea and a steeper increase at the time of arousal (52). Arterial blood pressure also increases during heavy snoring (54). Do these nocturnal increases in blood pressure result in daytime hypertension? In one study of 50 patients referred to a hypertension clinic, 30% had obstructive sleep apnea (55). Some studies have found that 60 to 80% of patients with severe sleep apnea have hypertension (31), and sometimes treatment of their sleep apnea results in improved blood pressure control. Does the association between hypertension and sleep apnea indicate causality or simply that both entities are due to other factors such as obesity? This question remains unanswered.

### Upper-Airway Obstruction—Pathophysiology

The pathophysiology of upper-airway obstruction is still under active investigation. During normal inspiration the brain sends impulses to the muscles maintaining upper-airway patency as well as to the muscles of respiration. Thus airway patency is maintained despite a negative intraluminal pressure. During sleep, muscle tone decreases and upper-airway resistance increases, even in normal subjects (14). The supine posture also predisposes to airway closure due to the effect of gravity. If the forces tending to close the airway (gravity, narrow airway opening, negative intraluminal pressure) exceed those maintaining airway patency, airway closure occurs. During sleep an obstruction to air flow occurs in patients with OSA at one or several locations in the upper airway (56).

The upper airway of OSA patients is abnormal even during wakefulness. The supraglottic resistance is increased (57), and a higher than normal percentage of the maximal upper-airway muscle tone is required to preserve airway patency (58). Thus at sleep onset a loss of upper-airway muscle tone is likely to have greater consequences in OSA patients. Studies of the upper airway in awake patients with OSA by cephalometric radiographs, computed tomography, acoustic reflection techniques, and magnetic resonance imaging have usually shown smaller than normal upper airways (59). However, there is considerable overlap between normals and patients with OSA, and the importance of anatomy in causing obstruction varies between patients. Some patients have bony abnormality, while in others a long soft palate, increased fat deposition, or tissue edema may all play a role in narrowing the airway. A major problem is that all of the above imaging techniques are done with the patient awake. The airway size that is present after airway tone decreases with sleep onset is what is relevant to airway closure or patency.

Other factors besides the loss of the wakeful stimulus contribute to a decrease in upper-airway muscle tone pre-apnea. In patients with OSA there is a periodic fluctuation in neural drive to both the upper airway and muscles of respiration (60). The amount of drive falls with the return to sleep and the onset of apnea, rises during the terminal phase of apnea, and is high at apnea termination and in the early post-apneic ventilatory period. This high ventilatory drive in the early post-apnea period may lead to an "overshoot" in ventilation and hypocapnia as the patient falls back asleep. Hypocapnia then contributes to the fall in ventilatory drive as the patient falls asleep. If the $P_{CO_2}$ falls below a point called the "apneic threshold" (usually 1 to 3 mm Hg below the awake $P_{CO_2}$ set point), then respiratory drive ceases, resulting in central apnea (61). This is thought to be the origin of the central portion of mixed apnea (62). While the fluctuations in ventilatory drive described above undoubtedly contribute to the perpetuation of cycles of obstructive apnea, they may not be the initiating cause. When the upper airway is stabilized using nasal continuous positive airway pressure (CPAP), fluctuations in drive vanish in most patients with OSA.

During obstructive apnea, the genioglossal and diaphragmatic EMGs progressively increase as the apneic period continues. However, the increasingly negative intraluminal pressure maintains airway collapse. Upper-airway opening appears to occur only after arousal and a preferential increase in upper-airway tone (56). The fact that arousal does not occur despite prolonged periods of apnea and arterial oxygen desaturation suggests that a defect in arousal mechanisms is present (63). The magnitude of the stimulus for arousal appears to depend on the level of inspiratory effort (ventilatory drive), rather than the individual levels of $P_{O_2}$ or $P_{CO_2}$ (64). In summary, anatomic factors and fluctuating and inadequate upper-airway muscle tone allow airway closure to occur, and impairment in arousal permits the apnea to persist.

### Daytime Sleepiness in the OSAS

The sleep architecture of patients with OSAS is impaired, with reduced amounts of REM and stage 3 and 4 sleep as well as frequent arousals and a reduced sleep efficiency. On daytime MSLT testing, a shortened sleep latency is usually noted. Two or more naps may contain REM sleep. This occurs much more commonly in patients with narcolepsy than in those with OSA. However, because two or more REM onsets in OSA is not

rare, a diagnosis of narcolepsy (in addition to sleep apnea) cannot be made with confidence unless unequivocal cataplexy is present. The MSLT should be repeated after the sleep apnea is treated (see below).

The exact causes of the excessive daytime somnolence in the obstructive sleep apnea syndrome are still under investigation. Sleep fragmentation is probably the most important factor, although hypoxemia may also play a role. In one study the apnea plus hypopnea index did not differ between a group of hypersomnolent and nonhypersomnolent patients with OSA (65). In another study, the respiratory arousal index (arousals related to respiratory events per hour of sleep) correlated best with the sleep latency on the MSLT (66). Measures of sleep fragmentation such as the arousal frequency or alterations in sleep architecture (increased stage 1 and decreased stages 3 and 4) appear to be more abnormal in sleepy OSA patients (67). In clinical practice one occasionally sees patients with very mild desaturation who have frequent arousals and significant daytime sleepiness. Oximetry monitoring alone may not reflect the severity of these patients' sleep disorder. At the other extreme, some patients with profound arterial oxygen desaturation have only mild to moderate symptoms of daytime sleepiness. Cognitive impairment does appear to be more severe in patients with sleep apnea who have hypoxemia (68).

Treatment with tracheostomy or nasal continuous positive airway pressure frequently results in long periods of stages 3, 4, and REM on the first night when airway obstruction is prevented and a rapid improvement in daytime alertness in many patients (69-71). The sleep latency on the MSLT after nasal CPAP treatment usually improves but not always to the normal range. In one study the MWT sleep latency improved from 18 to 32 minutes after treatment with nasal CPAP (71).

### Treatment of Obstructive Sleep Apnea

The treatment of obstructive sleep apnea begins with an identification and elimination of exacerbating factors such as hypothyroidism and ethanol ingestion as well as an examination of the patient's upper-airway anatomy. Surgical and medical therapies are discussed below followed by general guidelines for selecting an appropriate treatment.

The gold standard of therapy for obstructive sleep apnea has been tracheostomy (70). This bypasses the upper-airway obstruction and results in almost uniform abolition of obstructive apneas and symptoms. However, in addition to the psychological morbidity, the procedure has frequent complications, especially in patients with fat necks. Now that nasal continuous positive airway pressure is available, tracheostomy is rarely performed for sleep apnea. A less drastic surgical procedure is uvulopharyngopalatoplasty (UPPP).

The uvula, portions of the soft palate, and redundant pharyngeal tissue are removed. If nasal obstruction is present, this is often repaired. Unfortunately, the UPPP significantly reduces the severity of apnea and desaturation in only about 50% of the patients (72, 73). Often the AHI remains above 20 events/hour. It is a very effective procedure for snoring. Several methods of evaluation of the upper airway while patients are awake or asleep have suggested that patients who have significant airway narrowing mainly in the retropalatal area are more likely to improve after UPPP (74). However, no method can predict with absolute certainty which patients will benefit from this surgery. Because of dissatisfaction with UPPP, several new surgical procedures have been developed to treat obstruction behind the tongue or in the lower pharynx (75). With anterior mandibular osteotomy, a window of bone where the genioglossus inserts on the mandible is cut and pulled anteriorly, which results in the tongue moving forward. This procedure is usually combined with a hyoid suspension in which the hyoid bone is pulled up and suspended from the mandible. If this fails, the next step is maxillary mandibular osteotomy (MMO). In this procedure the maxilla and mandible are moved forward and the orthodontic occlusion is preserved. Either tracheotomy or nasal CPAP is needed in the immediate postoperative period. This extensive procedure appears to be effective, but it is expensive and is available only at specialized centers.

Medical therapy should always include weight loss if the patient is obese. Some patients will have a significant improvement after moderate weight loss (76). Position therapy (elevation of the head and avoidance of the supine position) may be effective in selected patients (77). Drug therapy with protriptyline (Vivactil), a nonsedating tricyclic antidepressant, is only mildly effective (78), and up to 50% of patients must discontinue using this medication due to side effects (urinary retention, etc.). Like all tricyclic antidepressants, protriptyline decreases the amount of stage REM sleep. Medroxyprogesterone (Provera) is a progestational agent with respiratory stimulant activity. Treatment with this drug appears to benefit patients with the obesity hypoventilation syndrome mainly by lowering the daytime $P_{CO_2}$ with a subsequent improvement in the $P_{O_2}$ (79, 80). Little if any effect on the frequency of apnea has been demonstrated (81), although the severity of desaturation and the associated right heart failure may improve in some patients. Side effects include impotence, hair loss, and hyperglycemia.

Nocturnal oxygen therapy has also been tried in patients with obstructive sleep apnea (82). An early report noted a profound increase in apnea length after oxygen was administered (83). Other acute and chronic studies using continuous low-flow oxygen have usually found small increases in event duration. With oxygen therapy, oxygenation usually improves, but the frequency of respiratory events usually decreases only slightly or remains unchanged. Therefore, it is not surprising that oxygen therapy does not improve the sleep latency on MSLT testing (84). No long-term studies have shown an improvement in morbidity or mortality with oxygen therapy. However, if the patient refuses or cannot tolerate more effective therapy, oxygen therapy may be tried to improve oxygenation and therefore reduce cardiac sequelae. It may improve cor pulmonale or arrhythmias associated with nocturnal desaturation in selected patients. Sleep monitoring during oxygen administration is warranted before this therapy is prescribed to patients with sleep apnea to document efficacy. Oxygen therapy can dramatically increase the amount of $CO_2$ retention during sleep in patients with both hypercapnic COPD and sleep apnea (85).

Medical therapy for obstructive sleep apnea was revolutionized by the introduction of nasal continuous positive airway pressure (nasal CPAP) by Sullivan and coworkers (86). With this method, a flow of pressurized room air via the nose maintains a positive pressure in the upper airway (Fig. 11.10). Therefore airway closure is prevented by a "pneumatic splint." Although a nasal mask is most commonly used, an alternative device (nasal pillows) fits into the external nares, providing a seal. The amount of pressure needed to maintain airway patency is determined by a sleep study (nasal CPAP trial) in which the level of CPAP is increased until apnea, hypopnea, desaturation, and snoring are prevented. Pressures in the range of 5 to 17 cm $H_2O$ are commonly used. Usually higher CPAP pressures are needed during REM sleep or when the patient is supine. In patients with awake hypoxemia

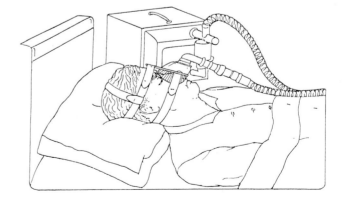

**Figure 11.10.**   A typical nasal CPAP apparatus in use. The mask covers only the nose.

or severe obesity, hypoxemia may persist during sleep despite the reversal of upper-airway obstruction with nasal CPAP. This can be especially severe during the prolonged REM episodes (REM rebound) that occur on the first night of CPAP. In such cases, oxygen can be added (and may be needed on a regular basis during sleep in a few patients in addition to nasal CPAP). Due to economic constraints, many sleep laboratories use partial night or "split" studies (87). In such studies, the initial part of the night is used to document the presence and severity of sleep apnea and the second part of the night is a nasal CPAP trial. Such a strategy may be satisfactory in patients with clear-cut severe OSA, provided that the patients receive adequate education about nasal CPAP before bedtime and are allowed to become familiar with the equipment.

The main difficulty with nasal CPAP therapy is the problem with patient acceptance. Long-term compliance is at best around 60%. Common complaints include dryness of the nose/mouth, difficulty with the mask seal (or mask discomfort), claustrophobia (difficulty tolerating the pressure), and noise. Improvements in mask and machine design have been made in an attempt to reduce these problems. Recent innovations include bilevel CPAP, in which different levels of pressure may be provided for inspiration and expiration (for example, 16 cm $H_2O$ during inspiration and 12 $H_2O$ during expiration). This allows a lower level of pressure during expiration and potentially less discomfort and better tolerance (88). Another useful innovation is the "ramp" system, in which the pressure slowly increases to the preset goal. This allows patients to fall asleep on lower pressures and increases the tolerance to higher pressures. Humidification systems have also been introduced. Devices that automatically titrate the amount of pressure needed to maintain airway patency ("smart CPAP") will soon be available.

Nasal CPAP can dramatically reduce symptoms of daytime sleepiness (69) and has also been shown to increase the sleep latency on MSLT testing and maintenance of wakefulness testing (71). He and coworkers (49) found a decrease in mortality when patients with obstructive sleep apnea were treated with tracheostomy or nasal CPAP but not UPPP. These findings need to be confirmed by other studies, but they are reasonable, since both tracheostomy and nasal CPAP essentially abolish obstructive apnea and desaturation.

Recently, there has been considerable interest in the use of dental/oral devices as a treatment for obstructive sleep apnea (89). Most of these devices work by moving the lower jaw (and hence the tongue) forward. One problem to date has been a lack of standardization. Long-term studies to document efficacy are also needed. Most devices require the involvement of a qualified dentist to ensure that occlusion or temporomandibular joint problems do not occur. Nevertheless, these devices do appear effective in selected patients. To date they appear most effective in patients with mild to moderate sleep apnea.

With the different treatment modalities in mind, one can select an appropriate therapy depending on the severity of the patient's symptoms and the results of the polysomnogram. In assessing the severity of disease one must consider the apnea plus hypopnea index, the severity of sleep fragmentation and arterial oxygen desaturation, the presence of significant arrhythmias during sleep, any evidence of right heart failure, and the severity of daytime sleepiness. The patient's own estimate of the degree of daytime sleepiness is very unreliable. There is no substitute for good physician judgment. The significance of a mild degree of sleepiness in an elderly sedentary individual is entirely different from that in a commercial truck driver. Mild disease can be treated with weight loss if the patient is obese, avoidance of ethanol, position therapy, dental devices, or possibly protriptyline. In some cases in which there appears to be little impact of disease, observation may be warranted. Conversely, even if the apnea plus hypopnea index is in the mild range, significant symptoms may warrant a trial of nasal CPAP. One should remember that such patients may fit the recently described "upper-airway resistance syndrome." Moderate disease can be treated with nasal CPAP or possibly UPPP if the patient's upper-airway anatomy is appropriate. If UPPP is used as treatment, a follow-up polysomnogram is essential to document a clinical response. Severe disease should be treated with tracheostomy or nasal CPAP. In OSA patients with daytime hypoxemia due to the obesity hypoventilation syndrome or COPD, desaturation may occur during sleep even if apnea is eliminated. This can be treated by the addition of oxygen to nasal CPAP (or tracheostomy).

Unfortunately, some patients with severe OSA find neither nasal CPAP nor tracheostomy acceptable. Although an occasional patient will respond to dental devices or UPPP, the only commonly effective alternative to nasal CPAP or tracheostomy in severe OSA is major upper-airway surgery. Such surgery is best performed in specialized centers. In patients with OSA and significant cor pulmonale who refuse or do not tolerate more effective therapy, nocturnal oxygen may be considered. The safety and efficacy of oxygen therapy in a given patient should be documented with a sleep study before this treatment is prescribed.

In patients with daytime $CO_2$ retention due to the

obesity hypoventilation syndrome, medroxyprogesterone may be useful in lowering the level of $CO_2$ retention and reducing the severity of nocturnal desaturation. However, medroxyprogesterone does not reduce the apnea plus hypopnea index or improve sleep quality. Treatment with nasal CPAP or tracheostomy is more effective and may normalize the daytime $P_{CO_2}$ in many patients.

*Persistent Daytime Sleepiness on Nasal CPAP*

Today, because a majority of patients with significant sleep apnea are treated with nasal CPAP, the physician is often presented with the problem of the patient continuing to complain of daytime sleepiness despite using nasal CPAP. One must consider several possibilities. These include lack of compliance (not using CPAP or using it for only part of the night), inadequate pressure, poor mask seal (therefore inadequate pressure), an inadequate sleep period, and other sleep pathology. Narcolepsy and periodic leg movements are not rare in patients with OSA. An all-night polysomnogram using CPAP and an MSLT (also using CPAP) should be performed (19). The polysomnogram would determine if the prescribed level of CPAP was adequate and if significant PLM-associated arousals were present. If the MSLT was normal, one would consider the possibility that the patient was not truly compliant or habitually had an inadequate sleep period at home. If the nocturnal polysomnogram documented adequate sleep but the MSLT showed a short sleep latency and no SOREM, one might consider poor compliance, inadequate sleep period at home, or the idiopathic hypersomnia syndrome. A diagnosis of narcolepsy could be made if the polysomnogram documented adequate sleep (including a normal amount of REM sleep) but the MSLT met the criteria for narcolepsy. In such cases, stimulant medications as well as nasal CPAP may be indicated.

*Prognosis and Mortality in OSA*

Little information has been available concerning the natural history of the disorder or the effect of therapy. One recent study found an increase in mortality in patients with moderate to severe obstructive sleep apnea (apnea index greater than 20/hour) and that both tracheostomy and nasal CPAP decreased both mortality and morbidity (49). Another study found no evidence of an increase in mortality, and no patients with sleep apnea died in their sleep (90). Both studies were retrospective. While the former study included a larger group of patients, many were lost to follow-up and the precise cause of death was not presented. Therefore, conclusive evidence of an increase in mortality in patients with obstructive sleep apnea is not available. This is an important question, because some patients

with substantial sleep apnea are relatively asymptomatic. It may be difficult to insist that they undergo treatment if they lack evidence of apnea-induced arrhythmias or heart failure when the natural history of their disorder is still unclear.

Another difficult issue is whether patients with OSA are fit to drive an automobile. Patients with OSA are at increased risk for automobile accidents (91). State laws vary on the physician's responsibility to report patients with "impaired consciousness." The physician must balance such responsibilities with the patient's right for confidentiality. It seems prudent to instruct patients with OSA and severe sleepiness not to drive until adequate treatment has begun. It has been our practice to report only those patients with severe daytime sleepiness who do not adequately comply with therapy. The physician treating patients with OSA should consult their local physician organizations for standard of practice guidelines.

## Central Sleep Apnea and Periodic Breathing

A diagnosis of central sleep apnea (CSA) requires that a majority of apneas be central in nature (92, 93). Usually only 10 to 15% of sleep apnea patients in large series are classified as having CSA. One complicating factor is that CSA is a heterogeneous group of disorders, each having different clinical presentations and pathophysiology and requiring different therapy. In fact, the only common characteristic is apnea due to a loss of central respiratory drive. In some patients, CSA may be a component of periodic breathing. In periodic breathing there is a regular (periodic) waxing and waning of the respiratory drive (and tidal volume). The term Cheyne-Stokes breathing (CSB) is used to describe a severe form of periodic breathing in which central hypopneas or apneas occur at the nadir in ventilatory drive. It is important to realize that CSA can exist in the absence of periodic breathing. In CSA not associated with periodic breathing there is an abrupt absence of ventilatory effort, and the resumption of ventilatory effort is usually associated with an arousal. In CSA associated with periodic breathing, there is a gradual increase then a decrease in tidal volume (crescendo-decrescendo pattern) preceding the central apnea (Fig. 11.11). Following the apnea, the tidal volume again gradually increases, and the pattern repeats. If arousal occurs after apnea, it is usually several breaths after the apnea has ended and during a period of maximal ventilatory effort.

*Pathogenesis of Central Sleep Apnea*

A detailed discussion of the pathogenesis of CSA is beyond the scope of this chapter and can be found in the literature (92). Briefly, the respiratory muscles are

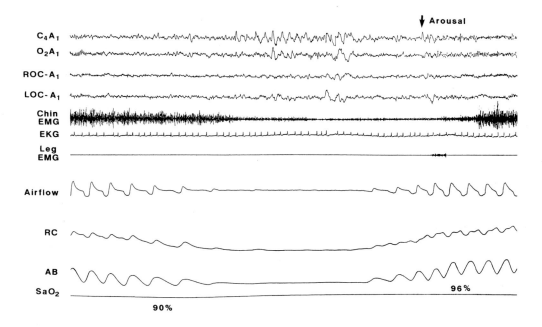

**FIGURE 11.11.** A polysomnographic tracing of a patient with cardiomyopathy and atrial fibrillation while on nasal CPAP of 10 cm $H_2O$. This level of CPAP eliminated upper-airway obstruction (on lower pressures a mixed apnea pattern was present), but central apnea with a Cheyne-Stokes breathing pattern persisted. Note that arousal occurred several breaths after termination of the central apnea. Higher levels of CPAP did not eliminate Cheyne-Stokes breathing in this patient.

controlled by three systems: the metabolic control system (responding to $CO_2$, pH, and $O_2$), the behavioral control system (phonation etc.), and the waking neural drive (a generalized stimulatory influence). With sleep onset, only the metabolic control system is active. The loss of the waking stimulus results in a higher $P_{CO_2}$ set point. During sleep onset, if the $P_{CO_2}$ is below this set point (apneic threshold), ventilatory drive will cease, causing central apnea. Some patients with CSA have defective metabolic control that results in hypoventilation during wakefulness and thus even more hypoventilation or central apnea during sleep. Another group of patients have neuromuscular weakness that is partially compensated by increased respiratory drive during wakefulness. With sleep onset this compensatory drive ceases and hypoventilation worsens. Other groups of patients with CSA have normal waking metabolic control and normal or low daytime $P_{CO_2}$. In some of these patients transient loss of ventilatory drive occurs at sleep onset because the $P_{CO_2}$ is below the sleeping apneic threshold. The apneas are terminated by arousals and transition to wakefulness. The arousals may also induce an increase in ventilation and reduce the $P_{CO_2}$, which tends to increase the likelihood of central apnea as the patient returns to sleep. In patients with CSA associated with periodic breathing, the normal fluctuations of breathing at sleep onset are exaggerated and persistent due to an instability in the

ventilatory control and feedback systems. Factors predisposing to such instability include a high ventilatory response to hypoxia and hypercapnia, awake hypoxia and hypocapnia, a long circulation time (delayed feedback), and low oxygen stores. For example, periodic breathing is common during sleep when normal subjects go to high altitude (hypoxia).

Normally, increases in ventilatory drive result in decreases in $P_{CO_2}$ and increases in $P_{O_2}$ that feed back and eventually decrease ventilatory drive. In the CSA associated with periodic breathing, the system "overshoots," and the $P_{CO_2}$ is decreased below the apneic threshold. In addition to the mechanisms described above, some have hypothesized that upper-airway obstruction may induce a reflex leading to central apnea. The fact that CSA is more likely to occur in some patients in the supine position (where gravity favors upper-airway collapse) suggests that the upper airway may be involved in the pathogenesis of central apnea in some patients.

### Hypercapnic Central Sleep Apnea

To discuss the different groups of patients with CSA it is convenient to divide them into groups with and without daytime $CO_2$ retention (94). Those with daytime hypoventilation usually have evidence of abnormalities in awake ventilatory control, neuromuscular weakness, or an abnormality in chest wall compliance (kyphoscoliosis). The defects in ventilatory control (central alveolar hypoventilation) may be primary or secondary to brain stem dysfunction (cerebrovascular infarction, neoplasm, or infection). Neuromuscular diseases include poliomyelitis (95), amyotrophic lateral sclerosis, diaphragmatic paralysis, and myopathies. These hypercapnic patients with CSA usually present with episodes of hypercapnic respiratory failure and cor pulmonale. Morning headaches and daytime sleepiness are common. Polysomnography reveals worsening hypoventilation and periods of central hypopnea and apnea. The degree of arterial oxygen desaturation tends to be rather severe, especially during REM sleep.

Treatment of this group of CSA patients depends on the underlying disease. In those with central alveolar hypoventilation, respiratory stimulants may be tried but are rarely effective. Supplemental oxygen may prevent nocturnal desaturation and improve symptoms (96). A sleep study is required to demonstrate efficacy and to rule out a worsening of hypoventilation with oxygen therapy. If the respiratory muscles are intact, diaphragmatic pacing has been effective in some patients. Negative-pressure ventilation can also be attempted. Unfortunately, these last two modes of therapy frequently tend to induce obstructive sleep apnea, because respiratory efforts are not coordinated with increases in upper-airway tone. Nocturnal positive-pressure ventilation, either via a nasal mask or tracheostomy, is probably the most effective therapy. If a nasal mask is used, some positive end-expiratory pressure may be needed to maintain airway patency. In milder cases, bilevel CPAP used in a mode similar to pressure support ventilation may also prove effective.

*Nonhypercapnic Central Sleep Apnea*

The second group of patients with central sleep apnea has no evidence of daytime hypoventilation. They usually present with complaints of disturbed sleep (awakenings, choking), insomnia, or excessive daytime sleepiness. A history of snoring is also common. Cor pulmonale and polycythemia are usually not present. This group can be further divided into those with idiopathic CSA and those with CSA associated with Cheyne-Stokes breathing.

The group with idiopathic CSA tends to be elderly males. Polysomnography shows CSA usually in stage 1 sleep or following arousals and awakenings. The desaturations are very modest. This group tends to have daytime hypocapnia and a prolonged transition from wakefulness to sleep. The apneas are terminated by arousals, and this causes sleep fragmentation. The arousals also tend to worsen the awake hypocapnia. Some have suggested that sedatives might be efficacious in this specific group of CSA patients. In fact, a

small study found the benzodiazepine hypnotic triazolam was of modest benefit (97). However, wider experience is necessary before this therapy can be recommended. Diamox (acetazolamide) also proved effective at least acutely in a small group of patients with nonhypercapnic CSA, presumably by inducing metabolic acidosis (98). Issa and Sullivan found that nasal CPAP was efficacious in idiopathic CSA (99). Two explanations for the efficacy of nasal CPAP are (*a*) CPAP prevents airway collapse and subsequent reflex central apnea, and (*b*) nasal CPAP is an expiratory load and induces mild increases in $P_{CO_2}$.

The causes of CSA associated with periodic breathing (CSB) include sleeping at altitude, renal failure, brain lesions, and congestive heart failure. CSB is more common during sleep stages 1 and 2. The therapy of CSA in this group is discussed below.

*Congestive Heart Failure and Sleep*

It is important for physicians to recognize that patients with congestive heart failure (CHF) may have significant arterial oxygen desaturations during sleep in the absence of daytime hypoxemia. Complaints of poor nocturnal sleep and daytime sleepiness may be erroneously assumed to be due to CHF. When a group of patients with dilated cardiomyopathy and obstructive sleep apnea were treated with nasal CPAP, not only were sleep quality and oxygen saturation improved, but the left ventricular ejection fraction during wakefulness increased significantly (100). The mechanisms by which nighttime nasal CPAP improve daytime cardiac function are not clear. Although only a small fraction of patients with CHF have obstructive apnea, it is important to recognize and treat OSA in such patients. Another group of patients with CHF have Cheyne-Stokes breathing. It has been estimated that up to 40% of patients with severe heart failure have CSB (101). Although CSB is more common in severe left ventricular (LV) dysfunction, there is no clear correlation between the severity of LV dysfunction and the presence of CSB. CSB results in periodic desaturations during sleep and sleep disturbance. Evidence is accumulating that the episodic hypoxia and arousals can cause a further decline in cardiac function. In most studies, CSB in these patients was primarily confined to sleep stages 1 and 2. Although the traditional explanation is that an increase in circulation time produces the instability in ventilatory control, this mechanism may not be the sole cause of CSB in these patients.

Improvement in cardiac function may reduce the amount of CSB. Therefore, the treatment of CSB in these patients begins with an effort to optimize the medical management of CHF. Studies have also shown that the amount of CSB can be reduced and oxygenation improved with theophylline (102), supplemental oxygen (103), and nasal CPAP (104). However, the potential for exacerbating arrhythmias has limited the use of theophylline. While oxygen can usually prevent desaturation, some patients will continue to have some CSB and sleep disturbance. Unfortunately, all patients with CSB and CHF may not benefit from nasal CPAP (105). To date, nasal CPAP seems most useful in patients with airway obstruction or high filling pressures (101). In the absence of long-term studies showing the superiority of any one treatment, the physician should treat each case on an individual basis with a sleep study to document efficacy. In addition, the first step is to maximize other medical therapy for CHF.

Patients with congestive heart failure and CSB can present with symptoms that mimic the traditional obstructive sleep apnea syndrome (102). A typical pattern of Cheyne-Stokes breathing may be present. However, sometimes the polysomnogram shows mixed obstructive apnea, often with a long central portion. This means that upper-airway closure is occurring during the waxing period of respiratory effort. Two subtle clues for the presence of CSB in the setting of mixed apnea are that the maximal breaths tend to occur several breaths after the apnea is broken (rather than immediately postapnea) and the nadir in oxygen saturation is markedly delayed (increased circulation time). Recognition that CSB (as well as obstructive apnea) is present may direct attention to better treatment of congestive heart failure. In addition, nasal CPAP treatment may be more difficult in patients with CSB. For example in some patients, a low level of CPAP may eliminate the obstructive component, but CSB and central apneas may persist (Fig. 11.11). Further increases in pressure may eliminate CSB in some but not all patients.

## SLEEP AND ASTHMA

Nocturnal asthma is a significant problem both for asthmatic patients and for their physicians. In a large survey of asthmatics, 74% responded that they awoke from sleep at least one night each week with symptoms of asthma (106). The study of the effect of sleep on asthma has been complicated by the time-related rhythms in bronchomotor tone. In normal persons the best pulmonary function occurs at 4:00 PM and the worst at 4:00 AM. This fluctuation in airway function is even more dramatic in asthmatics. Thus, studies must consider the effects of the 24-hour clock as well as those of recumbency and sleep. It appears that sleep induces an independent worsening of lung function, although no sleep stage–specific effects have been documented (107). Arterial oxygen desaturation is usually mild and most severe during REM sleep. Polysomnography is

not indicated unless sleep apnea is suspected. The simplest way to document a patient's predisposition for nocturnal asthma is to have the patient record a peak expiratory flow rate (PEFR) at bedtime, during nocturnal awakening, and in the morning. A detailed discussion of the pathophysiology of the nocturnal worsening of asthma is beyond the scope of this chapter and is available in the literature (108). Briefly, nocturnal falls in circulating epinephrine and corticosteroids and increases in histamine and vagal tone may be important. In patients with nocturnal asthma, the $\beta$-adrenergic receptor function decreases at night. In addition, a recent study suggests that patients with significant worsening of lung function at night have a circadian influx of effector cells into the lung. In those patients, a significant increase in neutrophils and eosinophils was noted in the bronchoalveolar lavage fluid at 4:00 AM (109). The ideal treatment for nocturnal asthma would require bronchodilators with a long duration of action that do not disturb sleep. Unfortunately, most oral long-acting bronchodilators also have stimulant effects, and most available inhaled bronchodilators do not retain full activity for 8 hours. Although theophylline could potentially disturb sleep quality due to its central stimulant effects, therapy with sustained-action theophylline was more effective than a long-acting (8 hours' duration) inhaled $\beta$ agonist (bitolterol) without impairing sleep quality (110). In patients with nocturnal asthma, theophylline dosing should be arranged so that maximum serum levels occur at night. Long-acting oral $\beta$ agonists are also of potential benefit but also have the potential for sleep disturbance (111). Corticosteroid therapy can also decrease the nocturnal worsening of lung function (112). The timing as well as the dose appears to be important. Preliminary results suggest that a 3:00 PM steroid dose may be more efficacious than one in the morning or at bedtime in preventing the nocturnal worsening of lung function (113) and the influx of inflammatory cells into the lung. As vagal tone is increased at night, anticholinergics such as ipratropium bromide are of potential benefit (114). A higher bedtime dose may be needed so that the duration of action is long enough to last for most of the night. If an asthmatic patient has obstructive sleep apnea, nasal CPAP may actually reduce asthmatic attacks (115). Snoring and recurrent upper-airway obstruction may be triggering mechanisms in these patients.

## SLEEP AND COPD

Some patients with chronic obstructive pulmonary disease (COPD) may have nocturnal desaturation without the cyclic apnea-desaturation-arousal pattern common in obstructive sleep apnea. Others have considerable obstructive sleep apnea as well as airway disease (the overlap syndrome). This latter group of patients may have particularly severe oxygen desaturation since their pre-apnea saturations may be quite low.

A typical pattern of nocturnal arterial oxygen saturation in a COPD patient (116–119) without substantial obstructive apnea includes (a) a fall in the baseline arterial oxygen saturation on transition from wakefulness to sleep, (b) small transient fluctuations in oxygen saturation (3 to 5%) during NREM sleep, and (c) larger drops in saturation during REM sleep (10 to 50%) that may last from several minutes to a half hour or more. One should recall that even normal persons have a small fall in $P_{O_2}$ during sleep but, due to their position on the flat portion of the oxyhemoglobin saturation curve, little desaturation occurs. Conversely, patients with an awake $P_{O_2}$ in the 55 to 60 mm Hg range (the steep portion of the curve) will have significant desaturation from small falls in $P_{O_2}$. It appears that in some COPD patients the fall in $P_{O_2}$ with sleep is within the normal range (119) but desaturation is worse because of a lower baseline $P_{O_2}$. Patients with $CO_2$ retention or low awake $P_{O_2}$ are more likely to exhibit severe desaturation (120).

The episodes of profound desaturation during stage REM are usually associated with periods of hypopnea in which tidal volume is reduced but respiratory rate is essentially unchanged (121). There is a reduction in pleural pressure swings in most cases, implying a reduction in central drive. However, one should note that during stage REM a loss of intercostal muscle tone makes the diaphragm less effective, especially in patients with hyperinflation which places this muscle at a mechanical disadvantage. Thus, even if the neural output to the diaphragm was constant, less inspiratory pressure might be generated. The reduction in minute ventilation during hypopneas is thought to lead to alveolar hypoventilation, with a resulting increase in $P_{CO_2}$ and fall in $P_{O_2}$. Some investigators have attempted to determine if increases in ventilation-perfusion mismatch also contribute to the dramatic falls in the oxygen saturation. During stage REM, a loss of intercostal muscle tone is believed to decrease the functional residual capacity, and this may increase ventilation-perfusion mismatch. The importance of increases in ventilation-perfusion mismatch is difficult to prove experimentally, because the ventilation in REM sleep varies widely and the standard analysis using the ideal gas equation applies to steady-state conditions. On the basis of limited studies, it appears that both hypoventilation and increases in ventilation-perfusion mismatch are important (122).

Hypoxemia leads to pulmonary vasoconstriction and pulmonary hypertension. Some have hypothesized that prolonged nocturnal hypoxemia and pulmonary hypertension may lead to cor pulmonale in the absence of daytime desaturation (123). This interesting hypothesis remains unproven. In the group of COPD patients with daytime $P_{O_2}$ above 60 mm Hg, desaturation occurs most commonly in REM sleep. The REM sleep desaturation may be severe, but the total duration of this type of desaturation typically lasts less than an hour per night. Is treatment of this type of desaturation beneficial? Nocturnal supplemental oxygen or room air was administered in a double-blind manner to a group of COPD patients with daytime $P_{O_2}$ above 60 mm Hg and documented REM sleep desaturation. At 3 years the oxygen group showed nearly a 4 mm Hg decrease in daytime mean pulmonary pressure, while the room air group showed about a 4 mm Hg rise (124). However, no study has documented that supplemental nocturnal oxygen will decrease mortality or morbidity in this group of patients with desaturations confined to REM sleep.

Nocturnal low-flow oxygen therapy prevents the episodes of nonapneic desaturation associated with COPD without markedly increasing the $P_{CO_2}$ (85). The exception is COPD patients with significant obstructive sleep apnea in whom large increases in $P_{CO_2}$ may occur. While oxygen therapy definitely improves the mortality and morbidity of patients with daytime desaturation, the benefits of treatment of isolated nocturnal desaturation remain unproved. Until the clinical importance of isolated nocturnal desaturation in patients with COPD is clarified, widespread sleep monitoring in these patients cannot be justified except to rule out obstructive sleep apnea (120). A possible exception is to document the need for nocturnal oxygen therapy when evidence of cor pulmonale unexplained by daytime arterial blood gas analysis is present. Even then, no firm guidelines exist concerning the amount of nocturnal desaturation required to justify nocturnal administration of oxygen. Patients whose baseline saturation remains below 85% for a majority of the night or who have evidence of cor pulmonale unexplained by other factors probably should be treated. As stated above, the importance of treating isolated and often short periods of desaturation associated with REM sleep is less clear.

The sleep quality in patients with significant COPD is frequently poor. A shortened TST, low sleep efficiency, and frequent arousals are common. Many patients complain of coughing or difficult breathing during the night. Like asthmatics, the diurnal variation in pulmonary function may be exaggerated in these patients, and many patients have the greatest difficulty breathing in the early morning hours. There are conflicting data on whether the sleep quality of patients with COPD is improved by oxygen therapy (125, 126). As with asthmatics, bronchodilators, while improving lung function, could potentially worsen sleep quality due to central stimulation. However, in one study, sustained-action theophylline improved early-morning spirometry and the oxygen saturation in NREM sleep without impairing sleep quality (127). Many patients request hypnotics to improve sleep quality. The benzodiazepine triazolam appears to increase sleep length without significantly worsening oxygenation (128). Caution is still advised. Sedatives of any type are probably contraindicated in hypercapnic or unstable patients.

The group of patients with both COPD and OSA (overlap syndrome) tend to have more severe cardiopulmonary sequelae than those with equivalent amounts of sleep apnea (129). Furthermore, these patients may continue to have impressive nocturnal desaturation during REM sleep even after treatment of obstructive apnea with a tracheostomy (130). Alternatively, oxygen alone rarely completely reverses the hypoxemia and may lead to considerable $CO_2$ retention and morning headache (85). One approach is to treat the OSA with nasal CPAP and then add oxygen as needed if nocturnal desaturation persists even though airway patency during sleep is restored. If daytime hypoxemia is present, oxygen will almost certainly be needed in addition to nasal CPAP.

▼

## REFERENCES

1. Rechtschaffen A, Kales A (eds): *A Manual of Standardized Terminology Techniques and Scoring System for Sleep Stages of Human Sleep*. Los Angeles, Brain Information Service/ Brain Research Institute, UCLA, 1968.
2. William RL, Karacan I, Hursch CJ: *Electroencephalography (EEG) of Human Sleep: Clinical Applications*. New York, John Wiley & Sons, 1974.
3. West P, Kryger MH: Sleep and respiration: terminology and methodology. In Kryger MH (ed): *Symposium on Sleep Disorders: Clinics in Chest Medicine*. Philadelphia, WB Saunders, 1985, pp 691–712.
4. Hauri P: *Current Concepts: The Sleep Disorders*. Kalamazoo, Michigan, Upjohn, 1982.
5. Baker TL: Introduction to sleep and sleep disorders. In Thawley SE (ed): *Symposium on Sleep Apnea Disorders: Medical Clinics of North America*. Philadelphia, WB Saunders, 1985, pp 1123–1152.
6. ASDA Task Force. EEG Arousals: Scoring rules and examples. *Sleep* 15:173–184, 1992.
7. Downey R, Bonnet MH: Performance during frequent sleep disruption. *Sleep* 10:354–363, 1987.
8. Phillipson EA: Control of breathing during sleep. *Am Rev Respir Dis* 118:909–937, 1978.
9. Douglas NJ: Control of ventilation during sleep. In Kryger MH (ed): *Symposium on Sleep Disorders: Clinics in Chest Medicine*. Philadelphia, WB Saunders, 1985, pp 563–575.
10. Phillipson EA: Sleep disorders. In Murray JF, Nadel JA (eds): *Textbook of Respiratory Medicine*. Philadelphia, WB Saunders, 1988, pp 1841–1860.
11. Krieger J: Breathing during sleep in normal subjects. In Kryger M (ed): *Symposium on Sleep Disorders: Clinics in Chest Medicine*. Philadelphia, WB Saunders, 1985, pp 577–594.
12. Tabachnik E, Muller NL, Bryan C, et al: Changes in ventilation and chest wall mechanics during sleep in normal adolescents. *J Appl Physiol* 51:557–564, 1981.
13. Hudgel DW, Devadatta P: Decrease in functional residual capacity during sleep in normal humans. *J Appl Physiol* 57:1319–1322, 1984.
14. Hudgel DW, Martin RJ, Johnson B, et al: Mechanics of the respiratory system and breathing pattern during sleep in normal humans. *J Appl Physiol* 56:1–137, 1984.
15. Block AJ, Boysen PG, Wynne JW, et al: Sleep apnea, hypopnea, and oxygen desaturation in normal subjects. A strong male predominance. *N Engl J Med* 300:513–517, 1979.
16. Gould GA, Whyte KF, Rhind GB, et al: The sleep hypopnea syndrome. *Am Rev Respir Dis* 137:895–898, 1988.
17. Staats BA, Bonekat HW, Harris CD, Offord KP: Chest wall motion in sleep apnea. *Am Rev Respir Dis* 130: 59–63, 1984.
18. Cohn M: Respiratory monitoring during sleep— respiratory inductance plethysmography. In Guilleminault C (ed): *Sleeping and Waking Disorders: Indications and Techniques*. Boston, Butterworths, 1982, pp 213–223.
19. Standards of Practice Committee of the American Sleep Disorders Association, Thorpy MJ, Chairman. The clinical use of the Multiple Sleep Latency Test. *Sleep* 15: 268–276, 1992.
20. Sangal RB, Thomas L, Mitler MM: Maintenance of Wakefulness Test and Multiple Sleep Latency Test. *Chest* 101:898–902, 1992.
21. Sangal RB, Thomas L, Mitler MM: Disorders of excessive sleepiness. Treatment improves ability to stay awake but does not reduce sleepiness. *Chest* 102: 699–703, 1992.
22. ICSD-Diagnostic Classification Committee, Thorpy MJ, Chairman: International Classification of sleep disorders: diagnostic and coding manual. Rochester, Minnesota, American Sleep Disorders Association, 1990.
23. Coleman RM, Roffwarg HP, Kennedy SJ, et al: Sleep-wake disorders based on a polysomnographic diagnosis—a national cooperative study. *JAMA* 247:997–1003, 1982.
24. Kales A, Vela-Bueno A, Kales JD: Sleep disorders: sleep apnea and narcolepsy. *Ann Intern Med* 106:434–443, 1987.
25. Mitler M, Nelson S, Hajudukovic R: Narcolepsy— diagnosis, treatment and management. In Erman MK (ed): *Sleep Disorders: The Psychiatric Clinics of North America*. Philadelphia, WB Saunders, 1987, pp 593–606.
26. Kramer RE, Dinner DS, Braun WE, et al: HLA-DR2 and narcolepsy. *Arch Neurol* 44:853–855, 1987.
27. Coleman RM: Periodic movements in sleep (nocturnal myoclonus) and restless legs syndrome. In Guilleminault C (ed): *Sleeping and Waking Disorders: Indications and Techniques*. Boston, Butterworths, 1982, pp 265–295.

28. ASDA Atlas Task Force: Recording and scoring leg movements. *Sleep* 16:749–759, 1993.

29. Fry JM, Diphillip MA, Pressman MR: Periodic leg Movements in sleep following treatment of obstructive sleep apnea with nasal CPAP. *Chest* 96:89–91, 1989.

30. Monteplaisir J, Lapierre O, Warnes H, Pelletier G: The treatment of the Restless Leg Syndrome with or without Periodic Leg Movements in Sleep. *Sleep* 15:391–395, 1992.

31. Sullivan CE, Issa FG: Obstructive sleep apnea. In Kryger MH (ed): *Symposium on Sleep Disorders—Clinics in Chest Medicine*. Philadelphia, WB Saunders, 1985, pp 633–650.

32. Young T, Palta M, Dempsey J, Skatrud J, Weber S, Badr S: The occurrence of sleep-disordered breathing among middle-aged adults. *N Engl J Med* 328:1230–1235, 1993.

33. Block AJ, Hellard DW, Slayton PC: Effect of alcohol ingestion on breathing and oxygenation during sleep. *Am J Med* 80:595–600, 1986.

34. Harman E, Wynne JW, Block AJ, et al: Sleep-disordered breathing and oxygen desaturation in obese patients. *Chest* 79:256–260, 1981.

35. Rajagopal KR, Abbrecht PH, Derderian SS, et al: Obstructive sleep apnea in hypothyroidism. *Ann Intern Med* 101:491–494, 1984.

36. Mezon BJ, Maclean JP, Kryger MH: Sleep apnea in acromegaly. *Am J Med* 69:615–618, 1980.

37. Dolly FR, Block AJ: Effect of flurazepam on sleep-disordered breathing and nocturnal oxygen desaturation in asymptomatic subjects. *Am J Med* 73:239–243, 1982.

38. Bradley TD, Rutherford R, Grossman R, et al: Role of daytime hypoxemia in the pathogenesis of right heart failure in obstructive sleep apnea syndrome. *Am Rev Respir Dis* 131:835–839, 1985.

39. Garay SM, Rapoport D, Sorkin B, et al: Regulation of ventilation in the obstructive sleep apnea syndrome. *Am Rev Respir Dis* 124:451–457, 1981.

40. Rajagopal KR, Abbrecht PH, Tellis CJ: Control of breathing in obstructive sleep apnea. *Chest* 85:174–180, 1984.

41. Zwillich CW, Sutton FD, Pierson DJ, et al: Decreased hypoxic ventilatory drive in the obesity-hypoventilation syndrome. *Am J Med* 59:343–348, 1975.

42. Rochester DF, Enson Y: Current concepts in the pathogenesis of the obesity hypoventilation syndrome. *Am J Med* 57:402–420, 1974.

43. Sharp JT: The chest wall and respiratory muscles in obesity, pregnancy, and ascites. In Roussos C, Macklem PT (eds): *The Thorax*. New York, Marcel Dekker, 1985, pp 999–1016.

44. Rapoport DM, Garay SM, Epstein H, et al: Hypercapnia in the obstructive sleep apnea syndrome. *Chest* 89: 627–635, 1986.

45. Sullivan CE, Berthon-Jones M, Issa FG: Remission of severe obesity-hypoventilation syndrome after short-term treatment during sleep with nasal continuous positive airway pressure. *Am Rev Respir Dis* 128:177–181, 1983.

46. Zwillich C, Devlin T, White D, et al: Bradycardia during sleep apnea. *J Clin Invest* 69:1286–1292, 1982.

47. Guilleminault C, Connolly S, Winkle R, et al: Cyclical variation of the heart rate in sleep apnoea syndrome. *Lancet* 1:126–131, 1984.

48. Tilkian AG, Guilleminault C, Schroeder JS, et al: Sleep-induced apnea syndrome. Prevalence of cardiac arrhythmias and their reversal after tracheostomy. *Am J Med* 63:348–358, 1977.

49. He J, Kryger MH, Zorick FJ, et al: Mortality and apnea index in obstructive sleep apnea. *Chest* 94:9–14, 1988.

50. Guilleminault C, Stoohs R, Clerk A, Cetel M, Saltros P: A Cause of excessive daytime sleepiness: the upper airway resistance syndrome. *Chest* 104:781–787, 1993.

51. Bradley TD, Martinez D, Rutherford R: Physiological determinants of nocturnal arterial oxygenation in patients with obstructive sleep apnea. *J Appl Physiol* 59: 1364–1368, 1985.

52. Shephard JW JR: Hemodynamics in obstructive sleep apnea. In Fletcher EC (ed): *Abnormalities in Respiration during Sleep*. Orlando, FL, Grune & Stratton, 1986, pp 39–61.

53. Weitzenblum E, Krieger J, Apprill M, et al: Daytime pulmonary hypertension in patients with obstructive sleep apnea syndrome. *Am Rev Respir Dis* 138:345–349, 1988.

54. Lugaresi E, Coccagna G, Cirignotta F: Snoring and its clinical implications. In Guilleminault C, Dement WC (eds): *Sleep Apnea Syndromes*. New York, Alan R Liss, 1978, pp 13–21.

55. Kales A, Bixler EO, Cadieux RJ, et al: Sleep apnea in a hypertensive population. *Lancet* 2:1005–1008, 1984.

56. Remmers JE, Degroot WJ, Sauerland EK, et al: Pathogenesis of upper airway occlusion during sleep. *J Appl Physiol* 44:931–938, 1978.

57. Anch AM, Remmers JE, Bunce H III: Supraglottic resistance in normal subjects and patients with occlusive sleep apnea. *J Appl Physiol* 53:1158–1163, 1982.

58. Mezzanotte WS, Tangel DJ, White DP: Waking Genioglossal electromyogram in sleep apnea patients versus normal controls. *J Clin Invest* 89:1571–1579, 1992.

59. Fleetham JA: Upper airway imaging in relation to obstructive sleep apnea. In Phillipson EA and Bradley TD (eds): *Breathing Disorders in Sleep: Chest Clinics of North America*. Philadelphia, WB Saunders, 1992, pp 399–416.

60. Onal E, Lopata M, O'Connor T: Pathogenesis of apneas in hypersomnia–sleep apnea syndrome. *Am Rev Respir Dis* 125:167–174, 1982.

61. Iber C, Davies SF, Chapman RC, Mahowald MM: A possible mechanism for mixed apnea in obstructive sleep apnea. *Chest* 89:800–805, 1986.

62. Dempsey JA, Skatrud JB: A sleep induced apneic threshold and it consequences. *Am Rev Respir Dis* 133: 1163–1170, 1986.

63. Phillipson EA, Sullivan CE: Arousal: the forgotten response to respiratory stimuli [Editorial]. *Am Rev Respir Dis* 118:807–809, 1978.

64. Gleeson K, Zwillich CW, White DP: The influence of increasing ventilatory effort on arousal from sleep. *Am Rev Respir Dis* 142:295–300, 1990.

65. Orr WC, Martin RJ, Imes NK, et al: Hypersomnolent and nonhypersomnolent patients with upper airway obstruction during sleep. *Chest* 75:418–422, 1979.

66. Roehrs T, Zorick F, Wittig R, Conway W, Roth T: Predictors of objective level of daytime sleepiness in patients with sleep-related breathing disorders. *Chest* 95: 1202–1206, 1989.

67. Guilleminault C, Partinen M, Quera-Salva MA, et al: Determinants of daytime sleepiness in obstructive sleep apnea. *Chest* 94:32–37, 1988.

68. Findley LJ, Barth JT, Powers DC, et al: Cognitive impairment in patients with obstructive sleep apnea and associated hypoxemia. *Chest* 90:686–690, 1986.

69. Rajagopal KR, Bennett LL, Dillard TA: Overnight nasal CPAP improves hypersomnolence in sleep apnea. *Chest* 90:172–176, 1986.

70. Guilleminault C, Simmons FB, Motta J, et al: Obstructive sleep apnea syndrome and tracheostomy—long term follow up and experience. *Arch Intern Med* 126:14–20, 1982.

71. Poceta JS, Timms RM, Jeong D, Ho S, Erman MK, Mitler MM: Maintenance of Wakefulness Test in Obstructive sleep apnea syndrome. *Chest* 101:893–897, 1992.

72. Fujita S, Conway W, Zorick F, Roth T: Surgical correction of anatomic abnormalities in obstructive sleep apnea syndrome: uvulopalatopharyngoplasty. *Otolaryngol Head Neck Surg* 89:923–934, 1981.

73. Fujita S, Conway WA, Zorick FJ, et al: Evaluation of the effectiveness of uvulopalatopharyngoplasty. *Laryngoscope* 95:70–74, 1985.

74. Launois SH, Feroah TR , Campbell WN, Issa FG, Morrison D, Whitelaw WA, Isono S, Remmers JE: Site of pharyngeal narrowing predicts outcome of surgery for obstructive sleep apnea. *Am Rev Respir Dis* 147:182–189, 1993.

75. Riley RW. Powell NB, Guilleminault C: Maxillary, Mandibular, and Hyoid Advancement for Treatment of Obstructive Sleep Apnea. *J Oral Maxillofac Sur* 48:20–26, 1990.

76. Smith PL, Gold AR, Moyers DA, Haponik EF, Bleecker ER: Weight loss in mildly to moderately obese patients with obstructive sleep apnea. *Ann Intern Med* 103:850–855, 1985.

77. McEvoy RD, Sharp DJ, Thornton AT: The effects of posture of obstructive sleep apnea. *Am Rev Respir Dis* 133:662–666, 1986.

78. Smith PL, Haponik EF, Allen RP, Bleecker ER: The effects of protriptyline in sleep disordered breathing. *Am Rev Respir Dis* 127:8–13, 1983.

79. Sutton FD, Zwillich CW, Creagh CE et al: Progesterone for outpatient treatment of the Pickwickian syndrome. *Ann Intern Med* 83:476–479, 1975.

80. Strohl KP, Hensley MJ, Saunders NA et al: Progesterone administration and progressive sleep apneas. *JAMA* 245:1230–1232, 1981.

81. Rajagopal KR, Abbrecht PH, Jabbari B: Effects of medroxyprogesterone acetate in obstructive sleep apnea. *Chest* 90:815–821, 1986.

82. Fletcher EC, Munafo D: Role of Nocturnal oxygen therapy in obstructive sleep apnea. *Chest* 98:1497–1504, 1990.

83. Motta J, Guilleminault C: Effects of oxygen administration in sleep-induced apneas. In Guilleminault C, Dement WC (eds): *Sleep Apnea Syndromes.* New York, Alan Liss, 1978, pp 137–144.

84. Smith PL, Haponik EF, Bleecker ER: The effects of oxygen in patients with sleep apnea. *Am Rev Respir Dis* 130:957–963, 1984.

85. Goldstein RS, Ramcharan V, Bowes G, et al: Effect of supplemental nocturnal oxygen on gas exchange in patients with severe obstructive lung disease. *N Engl J Med* 310:425–429, 1984.

86. Sullivan CE, Issa FG, Berthon-Jones M, Eves L: Reversal of obstructive sleep apnoea by continuous positive airway pressure applied through the nares. *Lancet* 1:862–865, 1981.

87. Sanders MH, Kern NB, Costantino JP, Stiller RA, Studnicki K, Coates J, Orris S, Schimerman S: Adequacy of prescribing positive airway pressure therapy by mask for sleep apnea on the basis of a partial-night trial. *Am Rev Respir Dis* 147:1169–1174, 1993.

88. Sanders MH , Kern N: Obstructive sleep apnea treated by independently adjusted inspiratory and expiratory positive airway pressures via nasal mask. *Chest* 98;317–324, 1990.

89. Schmidt-Nowara WW, Meade TE, Hays MB: Treatment of Snoring and Obstructive sleep apnea with a dental orthosis. *Chest* 99:1378–1385, 1991.

90. Gonzales-Rothi RJ, Foresman AJ, Block AJ: Do patients with sleep apnea die in their sleep? *Chest* 94:531–538, 1988.

91. Findley LJ, Unverzagt ME, Suratt PM: Automobile accidents involving patients with Obstructive Sleep Apnea. *Am Rev Respir Dis* 138:337–340, 1988.

92. Phillipson EA: Hypoventilation syndromes. In Murray JF, Nadel JA (eds): *Textbook of Respiratory Medicine.* Philadelphia, WB Saunders, 1988, pp 1831–1840.

93. Bradley TD and Phillipson EA: Central sleep apnea. In Bradley TD and Phillipson EA (eds): *Breathing Disorders in Sleep: Clinics in Chest Medicine.* Philadelphia, WB Saunders, 19992, pp493–505.

94. Bradley TD, McNicholas WT, Rutherford R, et al: Clinical and physiologic heterogeneity of the central sleep apnea syndrome. *Am Rev Respir Dis* 134:217–221, 1986.

95. Hill R, Robbins AW, Messing R, et al: Sleep apnea syndrome after poliomyelitis. *Am Rev Respir Dis* 127:129–131, 1983.

96. McNicholas WT, Carter JL, Rutherford R, et al: Beneficial effect of oxygen in primary alveolar hypoventilation with central sleep apnea. *Am Rev Respir Dis* 125:773–775, 1982.

97. Bonnet MH, Dexter JR, Arand DL: The effect of triazolam on arousal and respiration in central sleep apnea patients. *Sleep* 13:31–41, 1990.

98. White DP, Zwillich CW, Pickett CK, et al: Central sleep apnea: improvement with acetazolamide therapy. *Arch Intern Med* 142:1816–1819, 1982.

99. Issa FG, Sullivan CE: Reversal of central sleep apnea using nasal CPAP. *Chest* 90:165–171, 1986.

100. Malone S, Liu PP, Holloway R, Rutherford R, Xie A, Bradley TD: Obstructive sleep apnea in patients with dilated cardiomyopathy: effects of continuous positive airway pressure. *Lancet* 338:1480–1484, 1991.

101. Yamashiro Y, Kryer MH: Sleep in heart failure. *Sleep* 16:513–523, 1993.

102. Dowdell WT, S Javaheri, Mcginnis W: Cheyne-Stokes Respiration presenting as sleep apnea syndrome. *Am Rev Respir Dis* 871–879, 1990.

103. Hanly PJ, Millar TW, Steljes DG, Baer R, Frais M, Kryger MH: The effect of oxygen of respiration and sleep in patients with congestive heart failure. *Ann Intern Med* 1111:777–782, 1989.

104. Takasaki Y, Orr D, Popkin J, Rutherford R, Liu P, Bradley TD: Effect of nasal continuous positive airway pressure on sleep apnea in congestive heart failure. *Am Rev Respir Dis* 140:1578–1584.

105. Davies RJ, Harrington KJ, Ormedrod OJM, Stradling JR: Nasal continuous positive ariway pressure in chronic heart failure with sleep-disordered breathing. *Am Rev Respir Dis* 147:630–634, 1993.

106. Turner-Warwick M: Epidemiology of nocturnal asthma. *Am J Med* 85:6–8, 1988.

107. Ballard RD, Saathoff MC, Patel DK, Kelly PL, Martin RJ: Effect of sleep on nocturnal bronchoconstriction and ventilatory patterns in asthmatics. *J Appl Physiol* 67:243–249, 1989.

108. Martin RJ. Nocturnal asthma. In Phillipson EA, Bradley TD: *Breathing Disorders in Sleep; Clinics in Chest Medicine.* Philadelphia 1992, pp 533–550.

109. Martin RJ, Cicutto LC, HR Smith, RD Ballard, Szefler SJ: Airways inflammation in nocturnal asthma. *Am Rev Respir Dis* 143:351–357, 1991.

110. Zwillich CW, Nealgley SR, Cicutto L, White DP: Nocturnal asthma therapy: inhaled bitolerol versus sustained release theophylline. *Am Rev Respir Dis* 139:470–474, 1989.

111. Stewart IC, Rhind GB, Power JT, Flenley DC, Douglas NJ: Effect of sustained release terbutaline on symptoms and sleep quality in patients with nocturnal asthma. *Thorax* 42:797–800, 1987.

112. Beam WR, Ballard RD, Martin RJ: Spectrum of Corticosteroid sensitivity in Nocturnal asthma. *Am Rev Respir Dis* 145:1082–1086, 1992.

113. Beam WR, Weiner DE, Martin RJ: Timing of Prednisone and Alterations of Airways Inflammation in Nocturnal asthma. *Am Rev Respir Dis* 146:1524–1536, 1992.

114. Coe CI, Barnes PJ: Reduction of nocturnal asthma by an inhaled Anticholinergic drug. *Chest* 90:485–488, 1986.

115. Chan CS, Woolcock AJ, Sullivan CE: Nocturnal asthma: role of snoring and obstructive sleep apnea. *Am Rev Respir Dis* 137:1502–1504, 1988.

116. Phillipson EA, Goldstein RS: Breathing during sleep in chronic obstructive pulmonary disease. State of the art. *Chest* 85:24S–30S, 1984.

117. Flenley DC: Sleep in chronic obstructive lung disease. In Kryger MH (ed): *Symposium on Sleep Disorders: Clinics in Chest Medicine.* Philadelphia, WB Saunders, 1985, pp 651–661.

118. Fletcher EC: Sleep, breathing, and oxyhemoglobin saturation in chronic lung disease. In Fletcher EC (ed): *Abnormalities of Respiration during Sleep.* Orlando, FL, Grune & Stratton, 1986, pp 155–179.

119. Catterall JR, Calverley PMA, Mac Nee W, et al: Transient hypoxemia during sleep is not a sleep apnea syndrome. *Am Rev Respir Dis* 128:24–29, 1983.

120. Connaughton JJ, Catterall JR, Elton RA, Stradling JR, Douglas NJ: Do sleep studies contribute to the management of patients with severe chronic obstructive pulmonary disease. *Am Rev Respir Dis* 138:341–344, 1988.

121. Hudgel DW, Martin RD, Capehart M, Johnson B, et al: Contribution of hypoventilation to sleep oxygen desaturation in chronic obstructive pulmonary disease. *J Appl Physiol* 55:669–677, 1983.

122. Fletcher EC, Gray BA, Levin DC: Nonapneic mechanisms of arterial oxygen desaturation during rapid-eye-movements sleep. *J Appl Physiol* 54:632–639, 1983.

123. Block AJ, Boysen PG, Wynne JW: The origins of cor pulmonale: a hypothesis. *Chest* 300:513–517, 1979.

124. Flethcher EC, Luckett RA, Goodnight-White S, Miller CC, Quan W, Costarangos-Galarza C: A double blind trial of nocturnal supplemental oxygen for sleep desaturation in patients with chronic obstructive pulmonary disease and a daytime $PO_2$ above 60 mmHg. *Am Rev Respir Dis* 145:1070–1076, 1992.

125. Calverley PMA, Brezinova V, Douglas NJ, et al: The effect of oxygenation on sleep quality in chronic bronchitis and emphysema. *Am Rev Respir Dis* 126:206–210, 1982.

126. Fleetham J, West P, Mezon B, et al: Sleep, arousals, and oxygen desaturation in chronic obstructive pulmonary disease. The effect of oxygen therapy. *Am Rev Respir Dis* 125:429–433, 1982.

127. Berry RB, Desa MM, Branum JP, Light RW: Effect of theophylline on sleep and sleep-disordered breathing in patients with chronic obstructive pulmonary disease. *Am Rev Respir Dis* 143:245–250, 1991.

128. Timms RM, Dawson A, Hajdukovic R, Mitler MM: Effect of triazolam on sleep and arterial oxygen saturation in patients with chronic obstructive pulmonary disease. *Arch Intern Med* 148:2159–2163, 1988.

129. Fletcher EC, Schaaf JW, Miller J, et al: Long-term cardiopulmonary sequelae in patients with sleep apnea and chronic lung disease. *Am Rev Respir Dis* 135:525–533, 1987.

130. Fletcher EC, Brown DL: Nocturnal oxyhemoglobin desaturation following tracheostomy for obstructive sleep apnea. *Am J Med* 79:35–42, 1985.

# Chapter 12

# Pulmonary Thromboembolism and Other Pulmonary Vascular Diseases

**Alejandro C. Arroliga**
**Michael A. Matthay**
**Richard A. Matthay**

ABNORMALITIES OF THE pulmonary vascular bed may be caused by various diseases, ranging from chronic obstructive lung disease to interstitial fibrosis (1, 2). If the disease is extensive, pulmonary hypertension may ensue (1). Pulmonary hypertension is also a feature of many congenital and acquired heart diseases and such systemic disorders as scleroderma and systemic lupus erythematosus (1). This chapter reviews the disorders associated with pulmonary vascular disease, focusing on pulmonary thromboembolism and infarction, primary pulmonary hypertension, and pulmonary heart disease (cor pulmonale); congenital and acquired pulmonary arteriovenous malformations and neoplasia of the pulmonary vascular bed are also discussed briefly.

## Pulmonary Thromboembolism and Infarction

A crucial function of the pulmonary circulation is to act as a filter for particulate matter transported to the lung by venous blood (3). Particles that are too large to pass through the pulmonary capillary bed lodge in the lung as emboli, and smaller "sticky" materials (e.g., leukocytes or tumor cells) also may adhere to pulmonary vessels. Nonparticulate agents, such as irritant drugs that can induce vasculitis or vasospasm, may also reach the pulmonary circulation (3). However, the material most commonly filtered out by the lung is the bland thromboembolus transported from its origin by venous circulation (3).

### Incidence

Pulmonary embolism is the most common acute pulmonary disorder among hospitalized patients in the United States, occurring in approximately 650,000 patients per year (4–8). It ranks third as a cause of death in this country, accounting for at least 50,000 to 100,000 deaths annually (5–7).

Approximately one-third of the deaths from pulmonary embolism occur within 1 hour of the onset of symptoms, and the diagnosis is not even suspected in nearly 60% of the patients who die (6). Between one-quarter and one-half of fatal cases occur in patients with a good prognosis (9). Patients in whom the diagnosis is made and therapy is instituted account for only about 7% of the deaths due to thromboembolism; therefore, a simple, inexpensive screening test to detect asymptomatic deep venous thrombosis, the precursor of pulmonary embolism, would be invaluable (4, 6).

In a recent autopsy study, pulmonary embolism was the major cause of death in 10% of 239 patients (10). Eighty-three percent had lower-extremity deep venous thrombosis and only 19% of these patients were diagnosed with deep venous thrombosis before death. Furthermore, only 3% of these patients underwent diagnostic testing for deep venous thrombosis (10). These data emphasize the underdiagnosis of venous thromboembolic disease. Multiple injuries, immobilization, and bed rest put patients, especially the elderly, at high risk for deep venous thrombosis (10–13) (Tables 12.1 and 12.2).

### Pathogenesis

Most pulmonary emboli arise from detached portions of venous thrombi that form in the deep veins of

**Table 12.1**

**Frequency of Deep Venous Thrombosis in Various Hospitalized Patient Groups**

| Group | Frequency (%) |
|---|---|
| Orthopedic (fractured hip) | 54–67 |
| Urologic (prostatectomy) | 25 |
| Surgical patients over the age of 40 | 28 |
| Gynecologic | 18 |
| Cardiovascular (acute myocardial infarction) | 39 |
| Obstetric | 3 |

Data from references 5, 10, 11, and 12.

**Table 12.2**

**Conditions Predisposing to Venous Thrombosis and Pulmonary Thromboembolism**

Advanced age
Postoperative status
Previous venous thrombosis
Trauma
Congestive heart failure
Cerebrovascular accidents
Thrombocytosis
Erythrocytosis
Homocystinuria
Sickle-cell anemia
Oral contraceptive use
Pregnancy
Prolonged bed rest
Long periods of travel
Carcinoma
Obesity
Antiphospholipid syndrome

Data from references 5, 10, 11, and 12.

the lower extremities or the pelvis and in the right side of the heart (5, 13, 14). Thrombus formation is fostered by blood stasis, hypercoagulable states, and vessel wall abnormalities. Stasis may be caused by local pressure, venous obstruction, or immobilization after a fracture or surgery; stasis commonly occurs in patients with congestive heart failure, shock, hypovolemia, dehydration, and varicose veins. An enlarged fibrillating right atrium frequently contains blood clots.

Several conditions enhance the intravascular coagulability of blood (14–17). In polycythemia the blood viscosity increases, with resultant sluggish flow next to the vessel wall. In other hypercoagulable states, abnormalities of the platelets and dysfunction of the endothelium mediated by cytokine activation may be important (15). Activation of endothelium may lead to loss of its normal anticoagulant surface functions, resulting in a pro-inflammatory thrombogenic phenotype (15). Certain abnormalities of the coagulation or fibrinolytic system are associated with recurrent venous thromboembolism, including increased platelet adhesiveness, increased platelet survival time, and abnormalities of the coagulation cascade, such as unusually high levels of factor V or factor VII or deficiency of antithrombin III, protein C, or protein S (14–16). Deficiency in one of the latter three anticoagulants has been identified in as many as 50% of patients in families with recurrent thrombosis (15). Other groups at risk for venous hypercoagulability are patients with primary or secondary antiphospholipid syndrome (15, 17). Healthy men with high anticardiolipin antibody titer have a higher risk of developing deep venous thrombosis or pulmonary embolism than men without anticardiolipin antibodies (17). The magnitude of this risk is similar to that of other well-established risk factors such as obesity and use of oral contraceptives (17). The pathophysiologic mechanism in these patients is not fully understood, but inhibition of endothelial cell production of prostacyclin by autoantibodies and block in endothelial-cell thrombomodulin mediated protein C activation have been suggested (15). Other less common congenital causes of venous hypercoagulability include dysfibrinogenemias, disorders of plasmin generation, homocystinuria, and possibly heparin cofactor II deficiency (15). Of all these hematologic causes of recurrent thrombosis, antithrombin III deficiency, the antiphospholipid syndrome, polycythemia, and thrombocythemia are probably the most common (15).

Malignancy-associated phlebitis (Trousseau's syndrome) should be considered in patients 50 years of age or older without risk factors who develop deep venous thrombosis and/or pulmonary embolism or in whom thrombosis or embolism recurs during warfarin therapy (16, 18). The pathophysiology in Trousseau's syndrome is not understood, but tumor cells interacting with thrombin and plasmin-generating systems can influence thrombus formation (15). Patients who present with deep venous thromboses and no known risk factors should have a minimal workup for malignancy, including measurement of serum carcinoembryonic antigen as well as a test for fecal occult blood and measurement of prostate-specific antigen in men and mammography in women (15, 18).

Local trauma or inflammation may damage a vessel wall. In instances of marked local phlebitis with tenderness, redness, warmth, and swelling, the thrombus may be more securely attached to the wall. When the thrombus fragment is released, it is carried into one of the pulmonary arteries (5). Large thrombi may become lodged in a large artery or break up and block several smaller vessels. Distribution is probably related to the normal regional blood flow in the upright position; the lower lobes are predominantly involved because of their higher blood flow (6).

## PATHOLOGY

Autopsies reveal that fewer than 10% of pulmonary emboli cause a pulmonary infarction (6). Infection and left heart failure increase the likelihood of pulmonary infarction, as do poor premortem functional status, emboli in multiple lobes, and lung cancer (6, 19).

Upon microscopic examination, a pulmonary infarct shows coagulative necrosis of alveolar walls, alveoli filled with erythrocytes, and a mild inflammatory response (6). On chest radiograph, this type of true infarct appears as an infiltrate that lasts longer than 1 week and frequently leaves a linear scar. An incomplete infarct demonstrates extravasation of erythrocytes into alveoli without necrosis of the alveolar wall. This condition manifests itself as a transient infiltrate on the chest radiograph and usually clears within 2 to 4 days, leaving no residual scar (6).

## PATHOPHYSIOLOGY

Whatever the source of the embolic material, the acute pathophysiologic results of a sudden pulmonary arterial branch obstruction are similar and have been well defined (8, 14). A total cessation of blood flow to the distal lung zone is the initial effect of embolic obstruction, and this leads to respiratory and hemodynamic consequences (8).

### Respiratory Consequences

Embolic obstruction of a pulmonary artery is followed by three primary respiratory events: an increase in alveolar dead space, pneumoconstriction, and loss of alveolar surfactant (8, 20). Alveolar dead space is ventilated but receives no blood flow. Because gas exchange cannot occur in a nonperfused zone, any ventilation to it is wasted. Adequate alveolar ventilation requires an increase in total ventilation, and this contributes to the patient's dyspnea (8, 21). However, pneumoconstriction reduces the functional size of the ventilated, nonperfused lung zone. Because the terminal airways, including the alveolar zones, themselves are involved, the dead space is increased.

Among the factors contributing to the development of lung constriction is reduced carbon dioxide tension ($P_{CO_2}$) in the embolic zone. $P_{CO_2}$ decreases in a lung zone that is ventilated with essentially $CO_2$-free inspired air and receives no pulmonary blood flow. It has been demonstrated that severely hypocapnic areas constrict; inhalation of air containing carbon dioxide reverses this process (22), and inflation of the lungs overcomes the constriction temporarily. Additional studies have indicated that regional hypoxia is involved, since inhalation of oxygen can also reverse the constriction (23). It is also possible that humoral agents released from the lung or embolus itself (serotonin, histamine) promote pneumoconstriction (24).

The activity of alveolar surfactant begins to decline shortly after pulmonary artery occlusion, resulting within 24 hours in alveolar collapse and regional atelectasis (25, 26).

A secondary respiratory consequence of embolic obstruction is arterial hypoxemia (20). Not all patients with embolism have arterial hypoxemia, but a wide alveolar-arterial oxygen tension gradient and a reduced arterial oxygen tension are common, particularly in massive embolism. Ventilation-perfusion mismatch, or intrapulmonary shunting of mixed venous blood (perfusion of nonventilated lung units due to atelectasis), alveolar hypoventilation, and preexistent cardiopulmonary disease may contribute to hypoxemia (20). In massive embolic obstruction, hypoxemia may be aggravated by a reduction of cardiac output with a subsequent drop in mixed venous oxygen tension (20). Right ventricular failure accompanied by a patent foramen ovale in some patients may contribute to severe hypoxemia (20).

### Hemodynamic Consequences

The main hemodynamic consequence of pulmonary embolism is a decrease in the functional cross-sectional area of the pulmonary arterial bed, causing increased resistance to blood flow. To maintain the same flow at a higher pressure, the right ventricle must work harder. Therefore, in patients with substantial occlusion of the pulmonary vascular bed due to pulmonary embolism, there is an increase in pulmonary arterial resistance, pulmonary artery pressure, and right ventricular work (20).

The severity of these hemodynamic consequences depends on the extent of the embolic obstruction, operation of reflex humoral factors, and the patient's condition before the embolic event (8). Pulmonary vascular resistance and right ventricular work correlate directly with the extent of pulmonary vascular bed obstruction (20). The substantial reserve capacity of the pulmonary vascular bed provides some protection to the right ventricle; the vascular bed must be reduced by more than 50% before significant pulmonary hypertension develops at normal pulmonary blood flow levels. When more than 50% of the pulmonary vascular bed is occluded, pulmonary arterial pressure rises, requiring

additional right ventricular work to maintain cardiac output. In patients with acute pulmonary embolism, pulmonary arterial pressures rarely exceed a mean of 40 mm Hg (20, 27, 28). The thin-walled right ventricle is not designed to accept acute heavy pressure loads, which may result in right ventricular failure and cardiovascular collapse (20).

The role of reflex vasoconstriction in the pathogenesis of pulmonary hypertension associated with acute pulmonary embolism is uncertain (20). However, vasoactive amines such as the vasoconstrictors serotonin and thromboxane $A_2$ may play a role in the development of pulmonary hypertension after acute pulmonary embolism (20). Furthermore, experimental data suggest that administration of a serotonin antagonist (ketanserin) reduces mean pulmonary artery pressure (20, 29–31).

### Infarction

A rare consequence of embolism is ischemic death of the pulmonary parenchyma, i.e., pulmonary infarction (19, 20). Fewer than 10% of all pulmonary emboli result in the death of distal pulmonary parenchyma (8). The infrequency of infarction is not surprising, because the lung obtains oxygen from the bronchial arterial system and the airways in addition to the pulmonary arterial system. Studies indicate that at least two of the three oxygen sources must be compromised to promote infarction.

Infarction is most common in patients with pre-existing left ventricular failure or pulmonary disease, because bronchial arterial flow and ventilation are most likely to be compromised simultaneously in these patients (19, 20). Occasionally and for unknown reasons, infarction occurs in patients without overt cardiopulmonary disease (19). Clinical and laboratory data suggest that pulmonary infarction occurs more commonly in patients with occluded small pulmonary arteries (20).

### Resolution of Pulmonary Thromboembolism

Like venous thrombi, pulmonary emboli tend to resolve rapidly. Beyond the acute stage the most frequent course of thromboembolic obstruction is restoration of vascular patency (32–35). As with deep venous thrombosis, the removal of embolic material from the pulmonary vascular bed depends on fibrinolysis and organization of the thrombus.

Emboli are lysed by the action of circulating fibrinolytic factors in the blood and fibrinolytic factors released by the intima of pulmonary arteries. Several factors influence the speed of fibrinolytic dissolution, and a thrombus that has aged or become organized before being released is less sensitive (or even completely resistant) to fibrinolytic attack (36).

Vascular patency is also restored by organization of thrombus, a slower process than fibrinolysis, requiring days to weeks for completion. Factors governing the organization are not understood, but clinical and animal studies have revealed significant variations in its speed and degree. Residual embolic obstruction ranges from small areas of intimal thickening to permanent and complete obstruction, with retraction of vessel walls around the organizing thrombus (8).

The less thrombus that is removed through fibrinolysis, the more that remains for organization and the more likely residual pulmonary artery obstruction becomes. Regardless of the mechanisms involved in the removal of embolic material, vascular patency is generally restored to normal (8). Studies in dogs have demonstrated substantial resolution of emboli within hours and established that administration of heparin can accelerate this rate (35, 36). Perfusion lung scans and angiographic studies in humans have confirmed substantial resolution of emboli within a few days, with a progressive reduction in residual emboli within 4 to 6 weeks (32–34). Permanent residual emboli do occur, although the exact incidence is unknown (37–39). Fewer than 10% of patients appear to retain perfusion defects after 6 weeks (8). The rate and degree of resolution observed in humans are probably related to age, the composition and volume of the thrombus, and individual differences in fibrinolytic activity. Even massive emboli are likely to resolve within days or weeks, particularly in young persons without coexisting cardiopulmonary disease.

Two groups of patients may develop late pulmonary hypertension: those with major "central" obstruction of main or lobar arteries, and those with obstruction of several more distal vessels. Their embolic events are not always recognized clinically, and incorrect diagnoses ranging from chronic lung disease to primary pulmonary hypertension are often made (3, 38, 39).

## CLINICAL MANIFESTATIONS

It is important to maintain a high index of suspicion for deep venous thrombosis and pulmonary thromboembolism, particularly in patients at risk (Tables 12.1 and 12.2) (4, 12, 40). Clinical diagnosis of deep venous thrombosis can be difficult, but nearly all patients with deep venous thrombosis have pain or swelling in the affected leg. Physical findings include erythema and warmth in one-third of patients, and swelling and tenderness in three-fourths. The presence of Homan's sign or a palpable cord is variable. Moreover, proximal

**TABLE 12.3**

**SYMPTOMS IN 117 PATIENTS WITH PULMONARY EMBOLISM AND NO PRE-EXISTING CARDIAC OR PULMONARY DISEASE**

| Symptom | Frequency (%) |
|---|---|
| Dyspnea | 73 |
| Pleuritic pain | 66 |
| Cough | 37 |
| Leg swelling | 28 |
| Leg pain | 26 |
| Hemoptysis | 13 |
| Palpitations | 10 |
| Wheezing | 9 |
| Angina-like pain | 4 |

Data from reference 42.

deep venous thrombosis is observed on venograms in only 42% of patients with two or more of the following clinical findings: swelling above and below the knee, fever, and a history of immobility and cancer (41).

Dyspnea, the most common symptom of pulmonary embolism (Table 12.3) (8, 42), was present in 73% of patients with angiographically proven pulmonary embolism in a recent study of 117 patients (42). The severity of dyspnea is related to the extent of embolic obstruction of the pulmonary vasculature, resulting primarily from the sudden appearance of alveolar dead space in the lung and likely being a response to changes in lung mechanics caused by the emboli. In some patients, dyspnea lasts only a few minutes, and both patient and physician may consider this an episode of nonspecific hyperventilation. Massive embolism, however, tends to cause striking and persistent dyspnea.

Pleuritic chest pain and hemoptysis occur secondary to infarction or congestive atelectasis and develop after vascular occlusion. Massive embolism can cause severe chest pain, mimicking coronary insufficiency. Although these clinical findings are nonspecific and can occur in various cardiopulmonary disorders, the context in which they occur (e.g., in the postoperative period, after lower-extremity trauma, or in the postpartum period) may increase the likelihood that they are due to pulmonary embolism (3).

Characteristic physical findings associated with embolism are few (Table 12.4) (8, 40). Tachypnea and tachycardia may, like dyspnea, be transient. Sustained marked tachycardia and tachypnea occur in patients with extensive embolism (8, 42). Fine crackles on lung examination arise from pneumoconstriction and atelectasis (42), but the lungs are usually clear to auscultation and percussion (3).

**Table 12.4**
**Signs in 117 Patients with Pulmonary Embolism and No Pre-existing Cardiac or Pulmonary Disease**

| Sign | Frequency (%) |
|------|---------------|
| Tachypnea (respiration rate 20/min) | 70 |
| Rales (crackles) | 51 |
| Tachycardia (pulse >100/min) | 30 |
| Fourth heart sound | 24 |
| Increased pulmonary component of second sound | 23 |
| Deep venous thrombosis | 11 |
| Diaphoresis | 11 |
| Fever (temperature >38.5 C) | 7 |
| Wheezes | 5 |
| Homan's sign | 4 |
| Right ventricular lift | 4 |
| Pleural friction rub | 3 |
| Third heart sound | 3 |
| Cyanosis | 1 |

From Stein PD, Terrin MC, Hales CA, et al: Clinical, laboratory, roentgenographic and electrocardiographic findings in patients with acute pulmonary embolism and preexisting cardiac or pulmonary disease. *Chest* 100:598–608, 1991.

Additional physical findings may be present in up to 10% of embolic incidences in which congestive atelectasis or infarction occurs. These include pleural friction rub, evidence of a pleural effusion, and fever (3, 43). The friction rub generally is audible over the lung bases because embolism occurs most frequently in the lower lobes. Rarely is the effusion massive (42).

Patients with massive embolism may have cardiac findings suggestive of acute cor pulmonale (right heart disease), including large A waves in the jugular venous pulse, a "lift" palpable over the right ventricle, a right ventricular diastolic gallop ($S_3$), a scratchy systolic murmur in the pulmonary valve area, and an accentuated pulmonary valve closure sound (loud $P_2$). However, the intensity of the closure sound may not reflect the extent of embolism. In massive obstruction, the right ventricle may fail, pulmonary blood flow may decrease, pulmonary arterial pressure may fall to or below normal values, and the pulmonic closure sound may be barely audible (8).

Fixed splitting of the second heart sound is an ominous finding because it evolves only in patients with marked right ventricular compromise (44). Its development is controlled by two factors: premature closure of the aortic valve as the reduced volume of blood from the lungs rapidly flows out of the left ventricle, and delayed pulmonary valve closure as high resistance in

the pulmonary vasculature delays the right ventricular ejection time (44).

## Arterial Blood Gases

Most patients with acute pulmonary embolism have a respiratory alkalosis. Carbon dioxide retention is rare unless pulmonary embolism occurs in a comatose or paralyzed patient on assisted ventilation. Some investigators have reported arterial oxygen tension ($PaO_2$) in patients with pulmonary embolism to be uniformly 80 mm Hg or less, whereas others have found $PaO_2$ values higher than 80 mm Hg on room air in 10 to 15% of patients with angiographically proven pulmonary emboli (6).

## By-products of Thrombin and Plasmin

Until anticoagulation therapy is initiated for pulmonary embolism, clot formation associated with thrombin generation occurs simultaneously with clot lysis secondary to plasmin generation. Fibrin degradation products in serum are increased in more than 90% of patients with angiographically proven pulmonary emboli if sensitive detection techniques are used; however, this finding is nonspecific (6). Measurement of D-dimer, an epitope present after the stabilization of the fibrin network and subsequent lysis by plasmin, has been used to diagnose pulmonary embolism and deep venous thrombosis (45). Although the specificity of the test is only 39%, a value below 500 $\mu$g/liter has been shown to rule out deep venous thrombosis and pulmonary embolism in 98% of patients studied (45).

## Electrocardiogram

The electrocardiogram (ECG) can rule out other serious diagnoses, such as acute myocardial infarction or pericarditis, in patients with pulmonary embolism. Only 13% of ECG results are normal in such patients, but abnormalities are nonspecific in 70 to 75% of cases (6). The ECG is most likely to be abnormal in massive pulmonary embolism. In a study of 35 patients with massive pulmonary emboli, 20 had the classic SIQ3T3 pattern and nine had a right bundle-branch block pattern (6).

## Chest Radiograph

The plain chest radiograph cannot be used by itself to diagnose or exclude pulmonary embolism, but it may rule out other potentially life-threatening conditions such as tension pneumothorax (46). In a dyspneic patient, however, a normal chest radiograph may be a clue to the presence of pulmonary embolism (46). A parenchymal density and even evidence of pleural reaction or effusion are often present in patients with pulmonary embolism who have infarction or atelectasis (42). These densities vary in configuration, ranging from patchy infiltrates to round nodular lesions; abutment against a pleural surface is their only unique feature. This may not be noted until multiple views are obtained.

Subtle chest radiographic signs are more common than frank infiltration. Comparable vessels may be of unequal size (e.g., one main pulmonary artery may be enlarged while the other is smaller or normal). A major pulmonary artery with a "rat tail" appearance is indicative of an organizing thrombus within it. Oligemia of the lung zone also suggests embolic obstruction, particularly in association with increased flow to other lung areas. The presence of a prominent central pulmonary artery or cardiomegaly (in the absence of previous cardiopulmonary disease) is suggestive of pulmonary hypertension (46).

**Thoracentesis**

Pulmonary embolism exhibits no diagnostic pleural fluid findings (6, 47). Sixty-five percent of pleural effusions in patients with pulmonary embolism are sanguineous, and these are usually associated with infiltrates on the chest radiograph. Total leukocyte count varies from 22,000 to 57,000 per microliter. Approximately half of the effusions are exudates, even in the absence of an infiltrate. Thoracentesis is used primarily to exclude empyema and to look for a grossly bloody pleural effusion, which occurs in up to 27% of patients with pulmonary embolism (47). Trauma, malignant neoplasms, and pulmonary embolism are the main causes of a grossly bloody pleural effusion, the presence of which is not a contraindication to therapy for pulmonary embolism.

### LUNG SCANNING AND PULMONARY ANGIOGRAPHY (ALSO SEE CHAPTER 7)

The mortality of patients with untreated pulmonary embolism is as high as 30%; patients appropriately diagnosed and treated have a mortality of 2.5 to 8%, substantiating the need for prompt and accurate diagnosis (48). Standard laboratory tests are of little help in the diagnosis, but the combination of history, physical examination, and the specific laboratory tests mentioned excludes many other possibilities, allowing therapy to be initiated (3, 40, 42). However, only the ventilation-perfusion ($\dot{V}/\dot{Q}$) lung scan and pulmonary angiography are reasonable, sensitive, and reliable in the diagnosis of pulmonary embolism. Because of the current

emphasis on pulmonary embolism as merely the respiratory manifestation of venous thromboembolism, the diagnostic approach includes clinical evaluation, combination of diagnostic modalities for pulmonary embolism ($\dot{V}/\dot{Q}$ scan and pulmonary angiogram) as well as noninvasive modalities for detecting deep venous thrombosis (impedance plethysmography and B-mode imaging ultrasound) (48–54).

The perfusion lung scan is usually performed after intravenous injection of 10- to 50-$\mu$m particles radiolabeled with a $\gamma$-emitting isotope, usually technetium-99m macroaggregate of albumin (48). The particles are trapped in the pulmonary arteriolar capillary bed, their distribution representing pulmonary blood flow. A $\gamma$-detecting system records the radioactivity and provides an accurate visual display of pulmonary blood flow distribution. Embolic obstruction is manifested as zones of reduced or absent blood flow or perfusion defects (see Fig. 7.21**B**). However, any process that destroys or constricts pulmonary arterial vessels (e.g., old or recent necrotizing infection or regional hypoventilation) can also cause perfusion defects (3, 48). Therefore, although the scan is a sensitive detector of changes in regional blood flow, it lacks specificity; however, a normal scan essentially eliminates clinically significant thromboembolic obstruction (3, 48–54). The specificity of an abnormal perfusion scan is improved when it is combined with a ventilation scan. Most ventilation scans are done with xenon-133, but xenon-127, krypton-181m, and technetium-99m aerosols have been used (48). Embolism often causes regions of high or infinite $\dot{V}/\dot{Q}$ ratio—areas with reduced to absent blood flow but normal ventilation (see Fig. 7.21 **A** and **B**) (3, 48). In contrast, parenchymal disorders that cause perfusion defects are generally associated with decreased or absent ventilation in the same lung zones (3, 48). Thus, embolism tends to cause a ventilation-perfusion "mismatch," whereas parenchymal diseases result in "matched" ventilation-perfusion abnormalities (3, 48). Furthermore, if the $\dot{V}/\dot{Q}$ scan is abnormal, the result can be classified as high probability, intermediate or indeterminate probability, and low probability for pulmonary embolism based on the size of the defect and the degree of "mismatch" between the $\dot{V}/\dot{Q}$ scan and chest radiography abnormalities (Table 12.5) (48–54). Concomitant cardiopulmonary disease does not diminish the diagnostic utility of a $\dot{V}/\dot{Q}$ scan in acute pulmonary embolism (55).

In a recent major prospective multicenter study, the usefulness of the $\dot{V}/\dot{Q}$ lung scan in the diagnosis of acute pulmonary embolism was assessed (56). The study protocol consisted of a standardized history,

**Table 12.5**
**Revised PIOPED V̇/Q̇ Scan Interpretation Criteria**

| | |
|---|---|
| High probability | Two or more large (>75% of a segment) segmental perfusion defects without corresponding ventilation or abnormalities on chest radiograph. |
| | One large segmental perfusion defect and two or more moderate (25–75% of a segment) segmental perfusion defects without corresponding ventilation or abnormalities on chest radiograph. |
| | Four or more moderate segmental perfusion defects without corresponding ventilation or abnormalities on chest radiograph. |
| Intermediate probability | One moderate or up to two large segmental perfusion defects without corresponding ventilation defect or abnormalities on chest radiograph. |
| | Corresponding V̇/Q̇ defects and parenchymal opacity in lower lung zone on chest radiograph. |
| | Corresponding V̇/Q̇ defects and small pleural effusion. |
| | Single moderate matched V̇/Q̇ defects with normal findings on chest radiograph. |
| | Difficult to categorize as normal, low, or high probability. |
| Low probability | Multiple matched V̇/Q̇ defects, regardless of size, with normal findings on chest radiograph. |
| | Corresponding V̇/Q̇ defects and parenchymal opacity in upper or middle lung zone on chest radiograph. |
| | Corresponding V̇/Q̇ defects and large pleural effusion. |
| | Any perfusion defects with substantially larger abnormality on chest radiograph. |
| | Defects surrounded by normally perfused lung (stripe sign). |
| | Single or multiple small (<25% of a segment) segmental perfusion defects with a normal chest radiograph. |
| | Nonsegmental perfusion defects (cardiomegaly, aortic impression, enlarged hila) |
| Normal | No perfusion defects, and perfusion outlines the shape of the lung seen on chest radiograph. |

Data from reference 48.

physical examination, chest radiograph, electrocardiogram, lung scan, and pulmonary angiogram (56). Clinicians estimated the probability of pulmonary embolism before the lung scan was done, and the clinical estimate was combined with the finding of the V̇/Q̇ scan to determine the probability of pulmonary embolism on the pulmonary angiogram (56). The V̇/Q̇ in-

terpretive criteria are shown in Table 12.5. The likelihood of pulmonary embolism diagnosed by angiography as determined by the result of the scan and the clinical probability is shown in Table 12.6. Patients with a high-probability V̇/Q̇ scan and high clinical probability of pulmonary embolism had a 96% chance of having the embolism confirmed by pulmonary angiogram; on the other hand patients with a normal scan, independent of the clinical probability, had a very low likelihood of having a pulmonary embolism. Patients with an intermediate- or low-probability scan still have a substantial probability of having pulmonary embolic disease, independent of the clinical probability, and pulmonary angiography was critical in establishing the diagnosis.

The study did not systematically evaluate the lower extremities for deep venous thrombosis. Other investigators have shown that combining the lung scan with impedance plethysmography and B-mode imaging ultrasound is diagnostically useful in patients suspected of having pulmonary embolism (48, 53) (Figure 12.1 presents an algorithm for a combined diagnostic approach). Impedance plethysmography and B-mode ultrasound have been shown to correlate positively with the leg venogram in 83 to 94% of cases in the diagnosis of proximal deep venous thrombosis (femoral and popliteal) (50, 53, 57–59). The correlation for distal (calf) venous thrombosis is less reliable (50, 57). B-mode imaging has been used for the diagnosis of upper-extremity venous thrombosis, an increasing cause of pulmonary embolism; however, venography remains the most reliable technique (57).

**Table 12.6**
**Likelihood of Identifying Pulmonary Embolism on Pulmonary Angiogram Based Upon V̇/Q̇ Lung Scan Reading and Clinical Probability Assessment**

| | Probability of Pulmonary Embolism (%) | | |
|---|---|---|---|
| Scan Interpretation | High Clinical Probability | Intermediate Clinical Probability | Low Clinical Probability |
| High probability | 96 | 88 | 56 |
| Intermediate probability | 66 | 28 | 16 |
| Low probability | 40 | 16 | 4 |
| Near normal/ normal | 0 | 6 | 2 |

Modified from The PIOPED investigators: Value of the ventilation/perfusion scan in acute pulmonary embolism. Results of the prospective investigation of pulmonary embolism diagnosis (PIOPED). *JAMA* 263:2753–2759, 1990.

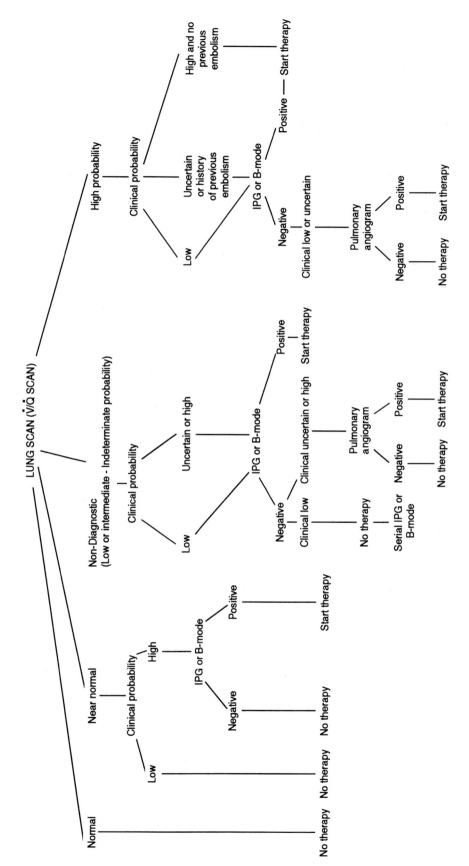

**FIGURE 12.1.** Strategy for diagnosis of pulmonary embolism in stable patients based on clinical suspicion, lung scan, pulmonary angiogram, and noninvasive tests for deep venous thrombosis. *IPG*, impedance plethysmography; *B-mode*, duplex, compression ultrasound. (Modified from Stein PD, Hull RS, Saltzman HA, Pineo G: Strategy for diagnosis of patients with suspected acute pulmonary embolism. *Chest* 103:1553–1559, 1993.)

The pulmonary angiogram is the definitive test for diagnosing pulmonary embolism (53, 60). When this procedure is performed and interpreted by experts, the false-negative rate is only 1 to 2% (53). The death rate from the procedure is 0.5%, and 1% of patients develop major complications (60).

On the angiogram pulmonary embolism is diagnosed by finding an abrupt cutoff of a major vessel due to full embolic obstruction. However, since most emboli are not totally obstructive, the most common angiographic abnormality is a filling defect resulting from the flow of contrast medium around a partial obstruction (see Fig. 7.22) (60). Additional angiographic signs include absent, decreased, or delayed filling of a lung zone, delayed venous emptying, "pruning" (absence of small branches), and abnormal vessel tapering, as well as dilation of the right ventricle and great vessels. None of these findings is as specific as cutoff and filling defects, particularly in the presence of other cardiopulmonary diseases (60).

When performed with a cardiac catheter inserted into the pulmonary artery, pulmonary angiography provides the opportunity to assess the hemodynamic status of the patient. Right atrial, right ventricular, pulmonary artery, and pulmonary artery wedge pressure measurements and the assessment of cardiac output may provide information vital to therapeutic decisions (60). In those whose condition is unstable, segmental injection can be made into the abnormal area seen on perfusion scan (6, 61). Patients who have had an allergic reaction to the contrast medium tolerate pulmonary angiography if they are pretreated with high-dose corticosteroids or diphenhydramine before the procedure (6).

The diagnostic approach to pregnant patients is generally similar; however, the perfusion scan is done with a low dose of radioisotope (1 to 2 mCi), and if impedance plethysmography of the lower extremities is positive, a venogram is obtained to rule out a false-positive result of the impedance study caused by the compression of the iliac vein by the gravid uterus, especially during the third trimester (62). During the performance of venography, the patient's abdomen is covered with a lead-lined apron.

## DIFFERENTIAL DIAGNOSIS

The sudden onset of atrial fibrillation in a patient with pre-existing cardiac disease is commonly caused by pulmonary embolism, although the mechanisms involved are not clear. Sudden or progressive worsening of congestive heart failure also suggests embolic disease. Similarly, embolism may occur in a patient with chronic obstructive pulmonary disease (COPD) whose condition suddenly deteriorates or in a patient with worsening hypoxemia and dyspnea in the absence of infection or other obvious cause (8).

Attacks of syncope and dizziness in an apparently healthy person may indicate embolic phenomena, particularly in association with dyspnea (8), and recurrent attacks of hyperventilation should arouse suspicion. Moser observed patients with hyperventilation and fleeting episodes of chest discomfort who had recurrent embolization rather than psychological problems (3).

Bacterial or viral pneumonitis may mimic embolism in a clinical context that predisposes to pulmonary embolism. For example, in the postoperative period, a low-grade fever, dyspnea, and tachycardia may develop, and the chest radiograph may show a nonspecific infiltrate, possibly representing atelectasis, pneumonia, or pulmonary embolism (8).

Infarction secondary to embolism may be confused with any disorder capable of producing acute pleuritis, including collagen vascular diseases as well as infectious diseases. An exudative sanguineous pleural effusion with no organisms on Gram stain is typical of embolism but is not definitive (8).

Finally, patients with other acute cardiopulmonary disorders (e.g., myocardial infarction, dissecting aortic aneurysm, and pneumothorax) can present with substernal discomfort, dyspnea, tachycardia, and electrocardiographic abnormalities (8). Pulmonary thromboembolism should be included among the differential diagnoses in these contexts, for once the possibility of this diagnosis is considered, it can be confirmed.

## PREVENTION AND TREATMENT

### Prophylaxis of Deep Venous Thrombosis

The frequency of deep venous thrombosis perioperatively ranges from 7% in general surgery patients to 80% in patients after hip and knee surgery (63, 64). Patients with acute spinal cord injury (38%), myocardial infarction (24%), ischemic stroke (47%), and such other medical conditions as heart failure and pneumonia (20%) have an intermediate frequency (63).

Despite the availability of agents that prevent deep venous thrombosis, a recent survey showed that only one-third of patients with multiple risk factors received prophylaxis (63, 64, 65). There are two basic kinds of prophylaxis of deep venous thrombosis: mechanical and pharmacologic (63, 64). The mechanical approaches, which reduce venous stasis, include early ambulation (desirable in all patients at risk for venous thrombosis), the use of elastic stockings, pneumatic calf compression, and electrical stimulation of calf muscles (64). The pharmacologic agents, which combat

**TABLE 12.7**
**PROPHYLAXIS OF DEEP VENOUS THROMBOSIS AND PULMONARY EMBOLISM**

| Type of Operation or Condition | Usual-Risk Patient[a] | High-Risk Patient (e.g., prior DVT or PE)[a] |
|---|---|---|
| General abdominothoracic surgery | <40 y/o, surgery <30 minutes: no risk factors. No prophylaxis, early ambulation<br>All other patients: LDH, SC q 12 hr starting 2 hr preoperatively plus ES<br>**OR**<br>IPC | Very high risk with multiple risk factors: LDH or LMW or dextran plus IPC |
| Orthopedic surgery<br>Hip replacement | Low-dose warfarin (2 mg qd) or Warfarin (INR 2–3)<br>**OR**<br>LMW or adjusted-dose heparin (aPTT 31–36 sec) | Combination of methods<br>**OR**<br>Selected patients: IVCF? |
| Hip fractures | Warfarin or LMW | Selected patients: IVCF? |
| Knee operations | IPC or LMW or warfarin | Selected patients: IVCF? |
| Eye surgery or neurosurgery | IPC ± ES | |
| Acute spinal cord injury with paralysis | Adjusted-dose heparin (aPTT 31–36 sec)<br>**OR**<br>LMW, warfarin? IPC? | Adjusted-dose heparin (aPTT 31–36 sec)<br>**OR**<br>LMW, warfarin? IPC? |
| Multiple trauma | IPC? or warfarin? or LMW? | IPC? or warfarin? or LMW? |
| General medical patient<br>Myocardial infarction | LDH or warfarin (INR 2–3)<br>LMW ? IPC ? ES ? | LDH or warfarin (INR 2–3)<br>LMW ? IPC ? ES ? |
| Ischemic stroke and lower-extremity paralysis | LMW or LDH<br>Warfarin? IPC? ES? | LMW or LDH<br>Warfarin? IPC? ES? |
| Other medical condition (heart failure, pneumonia, malignancy, etc.) | LDH? | LDH? |
| Long-term indwelling catheter and malignancy | Warfarin 1 mg qd | Warfarin 1 mg qd |

Data from Clagett GP, Anderson FA Jr, Levine MN. Prevention of venous thrombi embolism. *Chest* 102:391S-407S, 1992.
[a] Abbreviations: LDH, low-dose heparin 5000 units per dose; LMW, low–molecular weight heparin; ES, graduated compression elastic stockings; INR, international normalized ratio; IVCF, inferior vena cava filter; IPC, intermittent pneumatic compression; ?, probably indicated but insufficient data; DVT, deep venous thrombosis; PE, pulmonary embolism.

hypercoagulability of the blood, include warfarin, dextran, low–molecular weight heparin, heparinoids, and heparin (63, 64). Standard heparin is given in low doses or adjusted doses to maintain the activated partial thromboplastin time (aPTT) between 31 and 36 seconds 6 hours after therapy is administered. Low-molecular weight heparin, a derivative of standard heparin, has restricted molecular weight distribution around 5000 daltons (66); heparinoids are a mixture of glycosaminoglycans, including heparin sulfate and dermatan sulfate (67). Table 12.7 summarizes the current recommendations for prophylaxis of deep venous thrombosis, as set forth by the Third Conference of the American College of Chest Physicians (63).

**Treatment of Acute Deep Venous Thrombosis**

Heparin is the drug of choice for acute deep venous thrombosis because of its immediate action, relative safety, and specific inhibitory effects on the coagulation system (14, 68, 69). Heparin catalyzes the effect of antithrombin III, a coagulation inhibitor that inactivates thrombin and factors Xa and IXa. Moreover, heparin inhibits the activation of factors V and VIII by thrombin (68). Heparin does not lyse existing clots, but prevents formation and propagation of further clots. Although there is disagreement regarding the most effective method of administration, continuous intravenous therapy is generally preferred to intermittent intravenous bolus administration, and probably is associated with fewer bleeding complications (68). If intravenous therapy is not possible, a good alternative is adjusted-dose subcutaneous therapy, usually starting at 17,500 units every 12 hours and adjusting the dose to give an aPTT of 55 to 60 seconds within 1 hour of the next scheduled dose (68).

In patients with venous thromboembolic disease, heparin is frequently underdosed (68, 70). The goal of heparin therapy is to maintain the aPTT at 55 to 60 seconds (71). Recently, nomograms have been used to facilitate dosing (70, 71). In a recent study, patients treated according to a weight-based nomogram achieved therapeutic levels of heparin in a short period of time in three-fourths of patients with no major hemorrhagic complications (70).

In the first 24 to 36 hours of heparin therapy, when adequate anticoagulation is often difficult to achieve and sustain, the aPTT should be determined every 4 hours, and the heparin dose should be adjusted according to the aPTT (Table 12.8).

The incidence of major bleeding complications with this continuous intravenous heparin therapy is approximately 1% (68). Factors associated with an increased risk for bleeding complications are advanced age, uncontrolled hypertension, underlying coagulation abnormality, recent gastrointestinal hemorrhage, active vasculitis, chronic liver disease, uremia, and recent surgery or major arterial cannulation. It is prudent to maintain the aPTT at 45 to 50 seconds in patients with one or more of these risk factors. In patients without significant risk for bleeding complications, an aPTT of 55 to 60 seconds should be maintained.

The current recommendations for the duration of heparin therapy include the initiation of oral anticoagulation on the first or second day of heparin therapy to reduce in-hospital days. Once anticoagulation has been achieved with the oral agent, heparin is continued for at least two additional days. The minimal treatment with heparin is 5 to 7 days, and in patients with massive pulmonary embolism or extensive iliofemoral thrombosis a longer period of heparin therapy may be considered (68).

The coumarin derivatives are orally administered drugs that inhibit vitamin K–dependent clotting proteins in the liver (factors II, VII, IX, and X); the most commonly used coumarin derivative is racemic warfarin sodium (68, 72). These agents must be given for 6 to 7 consecutive days for a full antithrombotic effect (68). Coumarin derivatives are suitable for outpatient therapy and can provide long-term anticoagulation for patients with thrombotic problems. Early introduction of warfarin on day 1 or 2 in small loading doses of 10 mg can decrease the duration of heparin therapy to less than 7 days (68). The prothrombin time (PT) must be monitored during coumarin therapy to ensure anticoagulation is adequate. An effective level of anticoagulation is reflected by a PT prolongation by an International Normalized Ratio (INR) of 2 to 3 (68). If coumarin therapy is contraindicated (for example, in pregnant patients), adjusted-dose heparin to maintain the aPTT beyond 1.5 times normal is indicated (68).

Patients who need long-term anticoagulation are easily identified. For example, a patient with a fracture of the pelvis or lower extremities requires anticoagulation until he or she is fully ambulatory. In patients with congestive heart failure, the cardiac problem should be stabilized and the patient mobilized before therapy is discontinued. The patient with a history of recurrent thromboembolism requires continued anticoagulation, and although the appropriate duration has not been established, a 6- to 9-month period is generally employed. Treatment in these patients needs to be individualized, and further studies are needed to establish the appropriate duration of therapy (68).

Low–molecular weight heparin preparations have been developed for the treatment of patients with proximal deep venous thrombosis (68, 73, 74). These preparations can provide simple, safe, and effective treatment, in some uncomplicated cases, with the potential advantage of outpatient management (68). More studies are needed before a definitive recommendation on the use of low–molecular weight heparin is made.

**Table 12.8**
**Heparin Infusion Nomogram. Adjustment to Infusion after a Bolus of 5000 Units[a]**

| aPTT (sec) | Dose Change (U/hr) | Additional Action |
| --- | --- | --- |
| 45 | ↑240 | Repeat aPTT in 4 hr |
| 46–54 | ↑120 | Repeat aPTT in 4 hr |
| 55–85 | 0 | None |
| 86–110 | ↓120 | Stop heparin for 1 hr, repeat aPTT in 4 hr after restarting heparin. |
| >110 | ↓240 | Stop heparin for 1 hr, repeat aPTT in 4 hr, after restarting heparin. |

Adapted from Elliott CG, Hiltunen SJ, Suchyta M, et al. Physician-guided treatment compared with a heparin protocol for deep vein thrombosis. *Arch Intern Med* 154:999–1004, 1994.
[a] Concentration 20,000 U in 500 ml. Initial rate of 1240 U/hr (31 ml/hr) in patients with risk of bleeding and at 1680 U/hr in those without identified risk of bleeding.

## Thrombolytic Therapy in Deep Venous Thrombosis

The role of thrombolytic therapy in deep venous thrombosis is not defined, although streptokinase, urokinase, and tissue plasminogen activator have been used (68). Early use of streptokinase can decrease subsequent pain, the loss of venous valves, and the incidence of postphlebitic syndrome (68). Evidence of partial or complete lysis is found in 80 to 90% of patients treated with streptokinase compared with 0 to 28% for heparin (75). Best results are achieved within the first 5 days of onset of the clinical problem; after 10 days, results are poor (75). Proximal thrombi (iliofemoral veins) respond better than distal thrombi. Streptokinase is given in a dose of 250,000 units in 30 minutes, followed by 100,000 units/hour for 72 hours, through an intravenous line preferably in the affected limb distal to the thrombus (75). The thrombin time should be checked at 6 hours; if supratherapeutic, the infusion can be discontinued for a few hours and then reinitiated at a lower rate (75). In patients receiving streptokinase, the incidence of minor bleeding is increased; however, major bleeding episodes (requiring 2 or more units of blood) are apparently no more common than in patients receiving heparin only (75). Concomitant therapy with acetaminophen and intravenous corticosteroids are suggested to minimize allergic reaction (less than 5%) in patients receiving streptokinase therapy (75). After streptokinase therapy, heparin infusion (without a bolus) is needed (75). Although some authors suggest that all patients with deep venous thrombosis without contraindications should receive thrombolytic therapy (75), a recent report of the Third Conference of the American College of Chest Physicians suggests that such therapy needs to be highly individualized and that further clinical studies are needed before a definitive recommendation is made (68).

## Treatment of Pulmonary Thromboembolism

The treatment plan for pulmonary embolism depends on the extent and sites of the obstruction and the hemodynamic condition of the patient. The first step is to stop the thrombotic process by instituting heparin therapy in a regimen similar to that established for deep venous thrombosis (68).

Additional supportive measures may be necessary. If arterial hypoxemia is present, supplemental oxygen should be administered. Mild sedation or analgesia may be required to alleviate anxiety or pain. In patients with hypotension and shock, fluid therapy to increase right ventricular preload is the first line of treatment. Second, vasopressor support will usually be needed.

Isoproterenol has the advantage of lowering pulmonary vascular resistance but may be associated with tachyarrhythmias and may aggravate systemic hypotension. Dopamine and Neo-Synephrine, the vasopressors of choice, maintain systemic blood pressure and increased cardiac output. Mechanical ventilation is often needed to support the patient because of the high work of breathing, increased dead-space fraction, and the metabolic acidosis that may be associated with the decline in cardiac output (8).

Streptokinase, urokinase, and tissue plasminogen activator can rapidly lyse pulmonary thromboemboli, and these agents should be considered for patients with massive embolism who are hemodynamically unstable and have no contraindication (e.g., bleeding) (68). These thrombolytic agents must not be administered concurrently with heparin (68). Thrombolytic therapy has been shown by angiography to result in early clot lysis, but it has not been shown to reduce the mortality from pulmonary embolism (68). In patients with submassive and massive life-threatening pulmonary emboli, streptokinase is administered in the same dose utilized for deep venous thrombosis for 24 hours (75). Therapy with urokinase, 4400 units/kg over 30 minutes followed by 4400 units/kg/hour for 24 hours, is an alternative and is the preferred agent in massive emboli because it produces more rapid thrombolysis (75). After thrombolysis, heparin should be given without a bolus to maintain the aPTT at 55 to 60 seconds.

Emergency surgical embolectomy is rarely done; it has a high mortality rate (50 to 94%), and good medical management may result in a lower mortality, especially with the availability of thrombolytic therapy to supplement other supportive treatment. Factors associated with enhanced mortality from submassive and massive emboli include cardiac arrest and history of cardiopulmonary disease (68). Transvenous catheter extraction of emboli has a mortality rate of 27% (68, 76) and a success rate of 61% (77). Surgical embolectomy should be considered in otherwise healthy patients with large emboli who cannot receive thrombolytic therapy because of recent surgery or some other contraindication (68).

In patients with proximal leg deep venous thrombosis in whom anticoagulation is contraindicated, has failed, or has caused complications, inferior vena cava interruption is indicated (68, 78). It is also indicated for large free-floating caval thrombi, for chronic pulmonary embolism, and in patients undergoing pulmonary embolectomy or pulmonary endarterectomy (68). In patients with a vena cava filter, the reported rate of pulmonary embolism is less than 2%, and insertion of a filter causes fatal complications in approximately 0.1%

(78). Insertion of a vena cava filter has been suggested for prophylaxis of pulmonary embolism in patients at high risk of bleeding in extensive trauma, cancer, or hip or knee surgery and in paraplegic patients with spinal cord injury (78, 79). However, trials that compare filters with other prophylactic therapy are lacking (78). Although patients with an inferior vena cava filter do not require anticoagulation, continuous warfarin therapy (if it is not contraindicated) is recommended to prevent the development and propagation of thrombi below the filter (68, 78).

## Prognosis

Even with massive pulmonary embolism and hypotension, most patients will survive with only anticoagulation (80). The mortality from pulmonary embolism among patients with shock is 18% (80). In patients without shock in whom the diagnosis is made and treatment administered, the mortality from pulmonary embolism is only 2.5% (81). The overall in-hospital mortality rate from treated pulmonary embolism without associated shock is 24%, due mostly to underlying cardiopulmonary disease, cancer, and sepsis (81). The recurrence rate of pulmonary embolism is approximately 17% in studies that include follow-up lung scans (81). Recurrence is most common during the first week of follow-up and is associated with a case fatality rate of 45% (81).

## Chronic Thromboembolic Pulmonary Hypertension

Chronic thromboembolic pulmonary hypertension, a disease of the major pulmonary arteries, is the result of a single embolus or recurrent emboli that fail to resolve (82, 83). It is a rare disorder, the prevalence being estimated at 0.1% (83, 84). The majority of affected patients have a history consistent with venous thrombosis or pulmonary embolism. When the pulmonary vessels become occluded, with extensive loss of cross-sectional area of the vascular bed, pulmonary hypertension develops at rest or with minimal exertion (82). Dyspnea on exertion is common, and other symptoms are conspicuously absent (82–84). In some patients the physical examination reveals only a systolic or continuous murmur heard over the lung fields (82). The murmur, which is due to partial obstruction of major pulmonary arteries, is rare in other pulmonary vascular diseases and absent in primary pulmonary hypertension (82, 83). Other physical findings late in the disease are suggestive of elevated right heart pressure (e.g., hepatomegaly, leg edema, loud $P_2$, murmur of tricuspid insufficiency) (83).

Laboratory tests are in general unremarkable. Fewer than 1% of affected patients have deficiencies of antithrombin III and protein C and S, and lupus anticoagulant is present in 10% (82). The chest radiograph is often normal, although such subtle findings as unequal central pulmonary vascular shadows and zones of avascularity are occasionally found (82). Right ventricle enlargement is a late finding (82). The electrocardiogram is normal early in the disease; later, right axis deviation, right ventricular hypertrophy, and T-wave inversion in the precordium may be present (82, 83). Echocardiography shows elevated pulmonary arterial systolic pressure and increase in size of the right heart chambers (82). Pulmonary function tests are normal or show a restrictive ventilatory defect. The diffusing capacity for carbon monoxide ($D_{LCO}$) is normal or reduced (82). The arterial oxygen tension is normal at rest and declines during exercise (82). The most important noninvasive test in chronic thromboembolic pulmonary hypertension is the $\dot{V}/\dot{Q}$ lung scan (82). All affected patients have a segmental or larger perfusion-ventilation mismatch (82). In patients with primary pulmonary hypertension, the perfusion scan is normal or shows only patchy subsegmental defects (82, 83). The pulmonary angiogram confirms the diagnosis (82–85); confirmatory findings include intraluminal bands, webs, intimal irregularities, vascular narrowing and obstruction, and "pouching defects" (occlusive thrombi that organize in a concave configuration) (85). The pulmonary arterial pressures are elevated with a normal wedge pressure (82).

The prognosis of chronic thromboembolic disease is related to the degree of pulmonary hypertension (84). The only successful therapy is thromboendarterectomy of the pulmonary arteries; the presence of comorbid conditions, such as coronary disease, increases the risk of this surgical procedure (82). The overall perioperative mortality is 13% in leading centers (83).

## Septic Thromboembolism

Septic thromboembolism is encountered primarily after gynecologic-obstetric procedures and as a complication of intravenous drug use (3). The classic inciting event in gynecologic-obstetric procedures is a septic abortion, but septic thromboembolism may occur after a normal delivery and after in-hospital sterile gynecologic procedures such as dilation and curettage. Additional potential sources of infected emboli are related to medical technology; for example, infection may develop from catheters placed in peripheral and central veins, ventriculoatrial shunt catheters, transvenous pacemakers, and catheters for hemodialysis. Patients with the acquired immunodeficiency syndrome

(AIDS) and organ transplant recipients are at risk for pulmonary septic emboli (86).

In septic thromboembolism, a traumatized vein is invaded by microorganisms. In drug users, the vein is used for intravenous drug administration; in gynecologic-obstetric patients, the pelvic veins are involved; in patients with catheters, the cannulated vein is affected (3). The involved veins become occluded by mixtures of blood clot and bacteria, and small emboli are dislodged from such foci. The process may gradually resolve, with or without specific therapy, but if embolism develops, the already septic patient becomes more dyspneic; cough, sputum production, hemoptysis, and pleuritic chest pain often develop (3). The drug abuser often presents with severe sepsis and multiple pulmonary infiltrates (septic infiltrates) that tend to cavitate (86).

The chest radiograph characteristically shows multiple small, nodular densities, usually with fuzzy outlines (3). The number of these lesions may increase rapidly, and radiographs taken at 24-hour intervals often show striking changes that reflect the occurrence of repetitive, small infected emboli. There may be so many lesions that they become confluent. Cavitation usually appears within the nodules after hours or days and may lead to rapid development of thin-walled cavities. Computed tomographic scans may show multiple peripheral nodules of various sizes, predominantly basilar in distribution. These nodules may be cavitated and have air bronchograms (86). A blood vessel leading to a nodule (feeding vessel sign) is present in two-thirds of the patients (86). Wedge-shaped peripheral lesions abutting the pleura or extending into the pleural space are common.

Bacteremia is a common complication, sometimes resulting in endocarditis involving the tricuspid and, rarely, pulmonary valves (3). Echocardiography may be helpful in these cases. The friable valvular vegetations may subsequently embolize to the lungs and produce the clinical and radiographic features described above.

Both the infection and the thromboembolism must be treated with vigorous antibiotic therapy combined with heparinization. The value of adding heparin to the antibiotic regimen has been established (3). Because blood cultures may be negative, antibiotic selection must be made empirically; antibiotic coverage should include Gram-negative and Gram-positive organisms, including penicillinase-producing staphylococci (3). Any indwelling venous catheter should be removed immediately and cultured.

The use of heparin in patients with right-sided endocarditis is controversial because of the risk of hemorrhage. However, most evidence indicates that heparin plays a major role in the therapeutic regimen in these patients and that hemorrhagic risk is minor (3).

If antibiotic-heparin therapy fails to reverse the embolic process within 24 to 48 hours, surgical procedures to isolate drainage from the infected area should be considered (3). Ligation of the inferior vena cava and the left ovarian vein is necessary in septic pelvic thrombophlebitis. The source of the embolism determines the other sites of venous ligation. Combined antibiotic-heparin therapy usually precludes the necessity for ligation and other surgical procedures such as hysterectomy or extirpation of an infected valve (3).

## PULMONARY EMBOLI OTHER THAN THROMBOEMBOLI

Causes of pulmonary emboli other than venous thromboemboli are shown in Table 12.9. This chapter briefly discusses certain of these entities; for a more detailed discussion the interested reader is referred to other reviews of the subject (3, 87–89).

### Fat Emboli

Of the many types of tissue that obstruct the lungs, fat has received the most attention and is subject to some controversy (3, 90). Fat cells and neutral fat are often found in the lungs of patients who have died after long-bone fractures and other types of severe trauma, burns, and surgery. In addition, intravenous infusion of large quantities of neutral fat can induce dyspnea, pulmonary hypertension, and gas exchange abnormalities in animals (3). However, the link between these facts and the fat embolism syndrome is open to question.

**TABLE 12.9**
**PULMONARY EMBOLI OTHER THAN THROMBOEMBOLI**

Fat emboli
Bone marrow emboli
Amniotic fluid emboli
Foreign-body emboli
Air emboli
Tumor emboli
Trophoblast emboli
Brain emboli
Liver emboli
Bile thromboemboli
Plastic emboli (from intravenous tubing)
Cotton-fiber emboli
Lymphangiographic (Ethiodol) emboli
Parasitic emboli (schistosomal flukes—*Schistosoma haematobium, S. mansoni, S. japonicum*)

The typical case history involves a patient with long-bone fractures who, on admission, is alert, oriented, and in good condition with the exception of the traumatized areas. Within 12 to 36 hours, however, mental status changes occur and may progress to delirium and coma; high fever and marked dyspnea, tachypnea, and tachycardia may occur and a petechial rash may develop, particularly over the thorax and upper extremities. Fine rales may fill the lungs, and the chest radiograph shows a diffuse alveolar filling-type pattern throughout both lung fields. Arterial hypoxemia and hypocapnia develop; thrombocytopenia is common. Fat may be recovered from sputum and urine—a nonspecific finding that may occur in other conditions as well. Bronchoalveolar lavage specimens, when stained with oil red O, show fat droplets in 63% of the cells recovered from affected patients compared with less than 2% in patients who do not have fat embolism (91).

A mechanical theory of the pathogenesis of the syndrome proposes that bone marrow contents enter the venous system, lodge in the lungs, and may "cross" to the systemic circulation through the pulmonary capillaries or through a patent foramen ovale (92–94). A biochemical theory suggests that direct damage of pneumocytes by circulating free fatty acid causes the abnormalities of gas exchange (92). These two theories may not be mutually exclusive, but further studies are necessary (92). Treatment of suspected fat embolism is supportive, as with any form of adult respiratory distress syndrome. Infusion of heparin, ethanol, and low–molecular weight dextran seems to be ineffective, whereas corticosteroid therapy has been associated with ambiguous results (3, 92).

### Bone Marrow Emboli

Bone marrow is probably the most common tissue source of emboli. Marrow fragments sometimes lodge in the lungs after trauma to marrow-containing bones or after surgical procedures that involve bone transection or compression (thoracotomy, sternal splitting). The introduction of closed cardiac massage, which involves considerable sternal and rib trauma and often fractures, has led to a marked increase in the incidence of marrow embolism and invariably is associated with autopsy evidence of this entity (3, 94).

### Amniotic Fluid Embolism

Amniotic fluid embolism usually occurs during or shortly after delivery. The exact incidence is unknown, but the mortality is high (80 to 90%), accounting for 10 to 20% of peripartum maternal deaths (95). The clinical presentation consists of sudden onset of dyspnea, restlessness, chills, and vomiting. Most patients are cyanotic, hypoxic, tachycardic, and hypotensive (95). Noncardiogenic pulmonary edema develops quickly, and

mechanical ventilation is required. Grand mal seizures and disseminated intravascular coagulation occur in 10 to 15% of affected patients (95). All women in labor are at risk, but amniotic fluid embolism is more common in women with prolonged and tumultuous labor. Uterine stimulants have been used in 22% of cases (95). In patients with suspected amniotic fluid embolism, cytologic examination of a specimen obtained from a pulmonary artery catheter in the wedge position may help confirm the diagnosis. The specimen reveals large numbers of fetal squames coated with neutrophils, and less frequently mucin and hair (95). The management of these patients is supportive, and most require mechanical ventilation and diuresis. Corticosteroids, anticoagulants, and antibiotics have no role in the initial management (95).

### Foreign Body Emboli

Various irritant agents used to "cut" heroin may enter the circulation and pulmonary arteries of narcotic addicts. Talcum powder is one of these agents; it has a marked effect on the pulmonary vessels, causing a granulomatous reaction in the lumina of small pulmonary arteries or causing an interstitial granulomatous reaction with few granulomas in the pulmonary arteries (88). These insults may be extensive enough to cause pulmonary hypertension. Perfusion lung scans and pulmonary function tests are often abnormal, and thrombi-obliterative changes are frequently seen at autopsy (3).

### Air Emboli

Air can enter the pulmonary circuit after entering via the systemic veins. Small quantities of air are removed rapidly from blood and lungs without causing symptoms, although repeated small air injections have induced pulmonary vascular lesions (3) and even acute noncardiogenic pulmonary edema experimentally (96). Rapid entry of a large bolus of air into the heart can obstruct pulmonary blood flow. Head, neck, and thorax wounds are particularly hazardous owing to the strong suction exerted during inspiration on veins in these areas. Air embolism may complicate cardiopulmonary bypass procedures and is always a possibility when intravenous catheters or needles are in place if the infusions are allowed to run out or if leaks in the tubing occur (3). Patients treated with mechanical ventilation for the adult respiratory distress syndrome may be at high risk of developing air embolism as a form of barotrauma. In these patients, a high index of suspicion is necessary, particularly in the presence of livedo reticularis, angioedema of the face or neck, and cerebral and cardiac dysfunction (97). Air embolism must be treated promptly to prevent air entering into the heart. The patient must be placed immediately in the left lateral decubitus position to allow collection of air in the superiorly placed right atrium. If this is unsuccessful, compression in a hyperbaric chamber may be useful (3).

## PULMONARY HYPERTENSION

Pulmonary hypertension may be defined as an increase in mean pulmonary artery pressure at rest or during exercise, as measured during catheterization (98). Pulmonary hypertension is present when the systolic/diastolic pressure in the pulmonary artery exceeds 30/15 mm Hg at rest or when the mean pulmonary artery pressure exceeds 18 to 20 mm Hg (99). A minor rise in pulmonary artery pressure usually causes no clinical, radiographic, or electrocardiographic changes (100). At catheterization, additional pressure increases may be reflected as elevation not only of pulmonary artery and right ventricular systolic pressures but also of right ventricular end-diastolic pressure.

In theory, pulmonary hypertension could result from either increased pulmonary vascular resistance or increased pulmonary blood flow alone; however, even a large increase in pulmonary blood flow seldom leads to more than a mild elevation of the pressure as long as there are no vascular changes. Because of the elasticity of the pulmonary vasculature the pulmonary vessels dilate in response to a large flow, causing the resistance to fall. The other factor explaining the low resistance of the pulmonary vessels is the capacity for recruitment of additional vessels (101). If flow increases, additional vessels open (usually in the upper lobes), decreasing pulmonary vascular resistance (101). Generally, pulmonary hypertension derives from either an increased resistance in the precapillary vessels or impedance to the pulmonary venous inflow. The resistance in the pulmonary arteries and arterioles may increase because of either functional changes (e.g., hypoxic vasoconstriction) (102) or organic changes (e.g., thromboemboli) (103, 104).

### PATHOLOGIC CHARACTERISTICS

Pulmonary vessels undergo various pathologic changes in pulmonary hypertension; these changes depend on the cause of the hypertension and partially on the duration of exposure to high pressure (103–105). Both elastic and muscular pulmonary arteries are affected (106). In the elastic arteries, the muscular tunica media hypertrophies and the intimal connective tissue thickens. Medial hypertrophy may be followed by a form of mucoid degeneration, which, in conjunction with atrophy of the medial elastic tissue, may lead to

aneurysmal dilation or even rupture. These conditions have been described in patent ductus arteriosus, mitral stenosis, and chronic pulmonary hypertension developing after corrective surgery for relief of tetralogy of Fallot (106). In addition to the medial changes, marked intimal atheromas usually develop, particularly at bifurcations. The atheroma may promote local thrombus formation, from which distal embolism may develop. Focal media aplasia is an additional feature resulting either from organization of mural thrombi or from healing of mural necrosis secondary to hypertensive pulmonary polyarteritis (106).

Although morphologic characteristics of the vessels may vary depending on the cause of hypertension, some changes develop regardless of the cause. These changes are most striking in arterioles and in arteries less than 500 $\mu$m in diameter. In the arterioles, changes consist of muscular thickening and intimal proliferation. Whereas arterioles normally have no tunica media, in mild to moderate pulmonary hypertension a distinct muscular tunica media develops, constituting up to 25% of the external diameter of the vessel and separated by internal and external elastic laminae (107). Later, intimal proliferation occurs, which is initially cellular but subsequently becomes fibrous. Finally, elastic tissue may develop and intimal proliferation may completely block the lumen. The tunica intima of the pulmonary trunk and the large elastic vessels become atherosclerotic, and muscular hyperplasia may thicken the tunica media (98).

### PATHOGENESIS

The underlying process of pulmonary hypertension varies, and multiple factors are often responsible. The rise in pulmonary arterial pressure may be due to vasoconstriction and thus should be reversible. In other cases, obstruction of the pulmonary vascular tree is largely or totally organic and thus irreversible (98). In Table 12.10, the causes of pulmonary hypertension are divided into three general groups, each with somewhat different clinical, physiologic, and radiologic characteristics: (*a*) precapillary hypertension, (*b*) postcapillary hypertension, and (*c*) combined precapillary and postcapillary hypertension, a group in which the significant physiologic disturbance arises from vessels on both sides of the capillary bed. The capillaries may be involved to some extent in each case and may play a major role in the increase in vascular resistance. In emphysema or idiopathic pulmonary fibrosis, pressure rises as a result of obstruction of the capillary bed. In postcapillary venous hypertension, however, edema surrounding the capillaries may become organized, thus limiting elasticity of the capillary bed (98).

## TABLE 12.10
### Classification of Pulmonary Hypertension

**PRECAPILLARY PULMONARY HYPERTENSION**
Primary vascular disease
  Increased flow (large left-to-right shunts)
  Decreased flow (tetralogy of Fallot)
  Primary pulmonary hypertension
  Pulmonary thromboembolic disease
    Thrombotic
    Metastatic neoplastic
    Parasitic
    Trophoblastic
    Foreign bodies; fat embolism; talc granulomatosis
  Pulmonary arteritides
Primary pleuropulmonary disease
  Emphysema
  Diffuse interstitial or air-space disease of the lungs
    Granulomatous
    Fibrotic
    Neoplastic: metastatic, bronchioloalveolar
    Miscellaneous: alveolar microlithiasis, idiopathic hemosiderosis, alveolar proteinosis, mucoviscidosis, bronchiectasis
    Postresection changes
  Pleural disease (fibrothorax)
  Chest deformity
    Thoracoplasty
    Kyphoscoliosis
  Alveolar hypoventilation
    Neuromuscular
    Obesity
    Idiopathic
    Chronic upper-airway obstruction in children
  High-altitude pulmonary hypertension
**POSTCAPILLARY PULMONARY HYPERTENSION**
Cardiac
  Left ventricular failure
  Mitral valvular disease
  Myxoma (or thrombus) of the left atrium
  Cor triatriatum
Pulmonary venous
  Congenital stenosis of the origin of the pulmonary veins
  Mediastinal granulomas and neoplasms
  Idiopathic veno-occlusive disease
  Anomalous pulmonary venous return
**COMBINED PRECAPILLARY AND POSTCAPILLARY HYPERTENSION**

Reproduced with permission from Fraser RG, Paré JAP: Pulmonary hypertension and edema. In Fraser RG, Paré JAP (eds): *Diagnosis of Diseases of the Chest,* ed 2. Philadelphia, WB Saunders, 1978, vol 2, p 1201.

## Precapillary Pulmonary Hypertension

### Increased Flow

Disorders classified in this group include congenital heart defects with left-to-right shunt such as atrial septal defect, ventricular septal defect, patent ductus arteriosus, aortopulmonary window, and partial anomalous pulmonary venous return. A substantial increase in pulmonary artery flow may be undetected for an extended period before increased resistance results in pulmonary artery hypertension. The heightened peripheral resistance is believed to result from an increase in vasomotor tone, with subsequent development of morphologic changes of increased flow and pulmonary hypertension. The major chest radiographic sign is enlarged pulmonary arteries throughout the lungs; the corresponding hemodynamic change is increased flow, and the main and hilar pulmonary arteries usually are distended. Normally invisible vascular markings in the peripheral 2 cm of the lungs may be seen. Fluoroscopic observation of greater pulsation amplitude of the enlarged pulmonary arteries (which usually is greatest in atrial septal defect and least in patent ductus arteriosus) and distention of individual cardiac chambers suggests the diagnosis of left-to-right shunt. The cardiac murmur may be distinctive, and specific signs may strongly suggest a particular anomaly, but accurate assessment often requires cardiac catheterization, with or without angiocardiography (98).

### Primary Pulmonary Hypertension

Primary pulmonary hypertension is a disease or group of diseases clinically characterized by a mean pulmonary artery pressure greater than 25 mm Hg at rest and 30 mm Hg during exercise, with a normal pulmonary artery wedge pressure and absence of secondary causes (101, 108, 109). The pathogenesis of primary pulmonary hypertension is unknown, but the initial insult in a predisposed individual is probably at the pulmonary endothelium by shear forces, viruses, drugs, hypoxia, or autoimmune disorders (101, 109). Damage to the endothelium probably alters the balance between vasoconstrictive mediators such as thromboxane and vasodilators such as endothelial-derived relaxing factors, the end result being vasoconstriction (101, 109). Vasoconstriction may not be the primary event, but it is an important component in the pathophysiology of primary pulmonary hypertension (109).

Most of the structural changes are confined to the small pulmonary arterial branches and result in a progressive increase in pulmonary vascular resistance and thus pulmonary hypertension. Pharmacologic and pathologic evidence supports the view that functional and reversible vasoconstriction occurs in the early stages of primary pulmonary hypertension, with the development of irreversible vascular damage as the disease progresses (106).

### Primary Thromboses

Thromboses are occasionally generated in the pulmonary arterial circulation itself. Decreased flow and increased blood viscosity typical of polycythemia probably contribute to their development. Pulmonary vascular changes caused by increased vasomotor tone, inflammation of the vessel wall, and sickling due to hemoglobin SC and hemoglobin SS disease also are contributing factors. Pulmonary vasoconstriction due to low $PaO_2$ and pH renders the lung vessels particularly susceptible to the increased viscosity caused by sickling, and various nonthrombotic emboli may occlude the vessels of the lungs and lead to pulmonary hypertension (Table 12.10).

## Pulmonary Arteritides

Pulmonary arterial hypertension occurs in 6 to 60% of patients with scleroderma secondary to severe interstitial fibrosis (110). In a subgroup of patients with limited scleroderma, isolated pulmonary hypertension occurs independent of the degree of fibrosis (110). Occasionally, rheumatoid arthritis, systemic lupus erythematosus, and mixed connective tissue disease cause pulmonary hypertension (111). Pulmonary artery involvement in Takayasu's arteritis results in an uncommon and often unrecognized form of pulmonary hypertension (112). Compression of the main pulmonary artery or its branches, sometimes as a result of an acquired mediastinal disorder, causes diffuse pulmonary oligemia of "central" origin (98). For example, a mediastinal mass exerting pressure on a pulmonary artery may compromise pulmonary artery flow (113). Dissecting aneurysms of the pulmonary artery or of the aorta, primary chondrosarcoma of the sternum, and fibrosing mediastinitis may have the same effect (98).

## Primary Pleuropulmonary Disease

Numerous primary diseases of the lungs, pleura, chest wall, and respiratory control center may increase pulmonary arterial pressure and yet have no significant effect on pulmonary venous pressure (Table 12.10). Less arterial and arteriolar narrowing due to intimal thickening and medial hypertrophy occurs, and pulmonary artery pressures seldom reach the levels attained in cases of primary vascular disease. The hypertension may in fact be transient, reflecting pulmonary infection and associated hypoxia (98).

Hypoxemia, with or without respiratory acidosis, may be the main cause of pulmonary artery hypertension in this group of conditions. Ventilation-perfusion inequality or generalized alveolar hypoventilation may be the source of reduced oxygen saturation. When arterial oxygen saturation is increased through treatment of pulmonary infections or the administration of oxygen, the pulmonary artery pressure usually falls

significantly. Other contributory factors include hypervolemia and polycythemia, especially in cases of pulmonary emphysema and chronic bronchitis (98).

Pulmonary capillary destruction also may be associated with increased pulmonary artery pressure. The most common entities in this form of precapillary pulmonary hypertension include emphysema and chronic bronchitis and diffuse interstitial or airspace disease of the lungs (102). Severe degrees of kyphoscoliosis or thoracoplasty may lead to pulmonary artery hypertension and cor pulmonale due to a poorly ventilated but relatively well-perfused lung. Finally, there is a group of hypoventilation syndromes usually associated with sleep-disordered breathing that may be associated with severe arterial hypoxemia and hypercapnia. Patients with these disorders may present clinically in right-sided heart failure (114, 115).

Pulmonary hypertension has been described in humans and animals living at high altitude and is known as chronic mountain sickness or Monge's disease (102, 116, 117). Affected individuals have a decreased sensitivity to carbon dioxide, and their alveolar carbon dioxide tensions are higher than those of healthy highlanders (118). The symptoms and signs are similar to those of other causes of pulmonary hypertension due to alveolar hypoventilation, although secondary polycythemia is more constant and severe.

### POSTCAPILLARY HYPERTENSION

There are two major forms of postcapillary hypertension: cardiac and pulmonary venous (Table 12.10). The most common causes of cardiac-induced postcapillary hypertension are failure of the left ventricle, mitral valve disease, myxoma (or thrombus) of the left atrium, and, rarely, cor triatriatum. The pulmonary venous causes of postcapillary hypertension include congenital stenosis at the origin of the pulmonary veins, mediastinal granulomas and neoplasms, idiopathic veno-occlusive disease (119–121), and anomalous pulmonary venous return. Any condition that raises pulmonary venous pressure above a critical level can result in postcapillary hypertension. Mitral stenosis is the chief cause of this disorder (98, 122).

Symptoms related to postcapillary hypertension usually are easily distinguished from those of precapillary origin. In left ventricular failure, perhaps the most common cause of pulmonary venous hypertension, symptoms and signs predominantly arise from acute or subacute pulmonary edema. Postcapillary hypertension causes orthopnea, dyspnea, and occasionally paroxysmal nocturnal dyspnea, reflecting interstitial and air space edema. In mitral stenosis, the pink frothy expectoration characteristic of acute cardiogenic pulmonary edema may be accompanied by bright red blood from hemorrhaging varicosities of the bronchial veins. Pulmonary vascular pressure remains steady until the mitral valve orifice shrinks to less than half its normal size (123). The symptoms and signs of pulmonary edema—the characteristic long opening snap of the first heart sound and the rumbling diastolic murmur—permit differentiation between this form of hypertension and primary pulmonary hypertension (98).

Pulmonary venous hypertension may occur from blockage of the left atrium by a myxoma or a thrombus. Episodes of pulmonary edema or syncope that can be relieved by a change in position are frequent. Left atrial myxomas may be the source of systemic embolization or may be associated with fever, weight loss, increased sedimentation rate, anemia, or elevated γ-globulin levels.

## DIAGNOSIS OF PULMONARY HYPERTENSION

### Clinical Manifestations

Chronic, progressive pulmonary hypertension is generally characterized clinically by increasing exertional dyspnea, precordial discomfort, attacks of syncope, anginal pain, hoarseness, and occasional hemoptysis. Chest radiographs and electrocardiograms demonstrate enlargement of the right ventricle and subsequent evidence of right-sided heart failure (106).

Primary pulmonary hypertension is characterized by a slow, insidious onset of vague symptoms (101). On average the diagnosis is delayed for almost 2 years, and frequently patients have been misdiagnosed as having hyperventilation and depression (101). Primary pulmonary hypertension is rare and can occur at any age, although it is more common in the third and fourth decades. The female to male ratio is 1.2:1, and familial disease represents 6% of all cases. The disease may have a genetic basis, with dominant features and incomplete penetrance (101, 108, 109). The most common symptom is dyspnea, present in 60% of patients on initial presentation (101, 108). Angina, probably as a result of underperfusion of the right ventricle or due to stretching of the large pulmonary arteries, is present in 47% of patients (101, 109). Syncope is an early symptom in 8% of patients (109). Other symptoms include cough, hemoptysis, hoarseness resulting from compression of the recurrent laryngeal nerve by the pulmonary vessels, and Raynaud's phenomenon in 10% of patients (101, 109). Physical findings are similar in all patients with pulmonary hypertension. A loud second heart sound and right-sided fourth heart sounds are common (109). Other common signs are right ventricular heave, palpable systolic impulse of

the pulmonary artery, pulmonary ejection, and pulmonary tricuspid regurgitation murmur (101, 109). Signs of right ventricular failure such as distended jugular veins, enlarged and pulsatile liver, ascites, and peripheral edema may be present (101, 109). Cyanosis is present, due to low cardiac output and right-to-left shunting across a patent foramen ovale. Clubbing does not occur in primary pulmonary hypertension (101, 109).

Chest radiographic findings often include a small aorta, significant enlargement of the main and hilar pulmonary arteries, pruning of the peripheral arteries, and variable expansion of the right ventricle and atrium (98, 101, 109). Chest radiograph is normal in 6% of affected patients (101, 109). Pleural effusions do not occur with right-sided heart failure alone (124).

In pulmonary veno-occlusive disease, a form of postcapillary hypertension, the signs and symptoms are similar (119, 120). This form of primary pulmonary hypertension carries a poor prognosis (101, 109). Radiographically, the main pulmonary artery and primary pulmonary branches are prominent, and there is evidence of increased bronchovascular markings and Kerley B lines (101). This contrasts with the radiolucent peripheral lung fields seen in classic pulmonary hypertension. In addition, there is no radiographic evidence of increased regional blood flow to the upper zones of the lungs such as that observed in pulmonary hypertension resulting from left atrial hypertension (e.g., mitral stenosis) (106). Electrocardiographic findings in both forms are right axis deviation with right ventricular hypertrophy and strain.

The physician must be aware of secondary forms of pulmonary hypertension because mitral valve disease or other treatable lesions may be present. Patients with rheumatic mitral stenosis may present with severe pulmonary hypertension; subtle findings may indicate the presence of mitral valve obstruction. The symptoms, which suggest decreased cardiac output rather than mitral stenosis, reflect elevated pulmonary capillary pressure: severe exertional dyspnea, orthopnea, exertional cough, acute paroxysmal pulmonary edema, and hemoptysis. The murmur may not be evident at auscultation owing to low cardiac output and the rotation of the heart caused by right ventricular hypertrophy. The chest radiograph may show only a prominent main pulmonary artery and right-sided enlargement, with little evidence of left atrial enlargement. Cardiac catheterization may reveal only increased pulmonary artery pressure, low cardiac output, and limited increase in pulmonary artery wedge pressure, which on rare occasions may be within normal limits (125).

Radiographic studies, including fluoroscopy, may

help detect underlying lesions. Even minor enlargement of the left atrium may suggest mitral stenosis; Kerley B lines, if present, are helpful, and the mitral valve area should be assessed for calcification, which if present generally confirms the presence of mitral valve disease until proved to result from other causes. P waves compatible with left atrial enlargement are an electrocardiographic abnormality suggestive of mitral valve disease. Echocardiography has largely replaced catheterization of the left side of the heart as a final study for detecting mitral stenosis (125).

## Differential Diagnosis

Frequently, severe pulmonary hypertension secondary to increased vascular resistance is the obvious diagnosis. However, the specific cause may be difficult to define clinically. Symptoms developing after pregnancy, deep venous thrombosis, or a surgical operation likely represent thromboembolic obstructive hypertension. Systemic lupus erythematosus, scleroderma, and schistosomiasis should be considered, and appropriate laboratory tests should be performed.

Excluding diseases of the pulmonary parenchyma requires careful assessment of the clinical picture and radiographic findings. Pulmonary function tests, particularly in the case of obstructive airways disease, may be helpful. High-resolution computed tomography may be useful in the group of patients with chronic interstitial lung disease and normal chest radiograph (126). A rise in pulmonary artery pressure, like that seen in patients with primary pulmonary hypertension, is rare in pulmonary parenchymal disease. Even moderate elevation in pulmonary artery pressure appears late in the course of the disease, well after the clinical picture has suggested primary pulmonary parenchymal disease (125). Primary pulmonary hypertension provides no clinical leads to diagnosis, and most laboratory tests are negative (106).

## Hemodynamic Studies in Patients with Pulmonary Hypertension

Figure 12.2 illustrates pressure relationships in pulmonary hypertension, either primary or secondary to emphysema and chronic bronchitis (127). The left ventricular end-diastolic pressure (5 mm Hg), left atrial pressure (3 to 6 mm Hg), and pulmonary venous pressure (6 to 10 mm Hg) are all normal. Pulmonary arterial pressure is increased; the right ventricular end-diastolic pressure remains normal until right heart failure develops. Because the pulmonary venous pressure is normal, the pulmonary artery wedge pressure is normal, in contrast to the elevation found in left heart failure and mitral stenosis.

These pressure relationships differ from those seen in postcapillary pulmonary hypertension caused by mitral stenosis (Fig. 12.3) (128). Left ventricular end-diastolic pressure is normal (5 mm Hg). However, left atrial pressure increases to 20 mm Hg or more owing to obstruction at the mitral valve, which results in elevation of pulmonary venous pressure. Secondary increased resistance in the pulmonary vascular bed, shown here in the pulmonary artery, results in additional increase in pulmonary arterial systolic and diastolic pressure. The right ventricular systolic pressure reaches 65 mm Hg; the diastolic pressure remains at a normal level near zero as long as there is no right heart failure.

Figure 12.4 illustrates pressure relationships during left ventricular failure (128). The left ventricular end-diastolic pressure (20 mm Hg) is increased, and left atrial pressure (20 mm Hg) and pulmonary venous pressure (25 mm Hg) are elevated. Secondary increased pulmonary vascular resistance in the pulmonary arteries produces even greater elevation in pulmonary arterial pressure. Right ventricular systolic pressure rises, but unless right ventricular failure develops, right ventricular end-diastolic pressure remains normal. The pressure relationships are similar

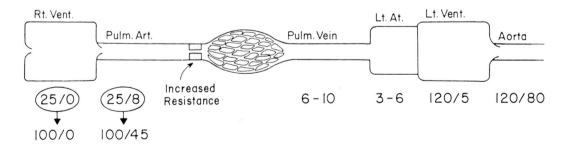

**FIGURE 12.2.** Pulmonary hypertension. Pressure relationships in cor pulmonale caused by primary pulmonary hypertension or COPD. (Adapted with permission from Fowler ND: Chronic cor pulmonale caused by lung dise... . In Baum GL [ed]: *Textbook of Pulmonary Diseases*, ed 2. Boston, Little, Brown, 1974, p 745.)

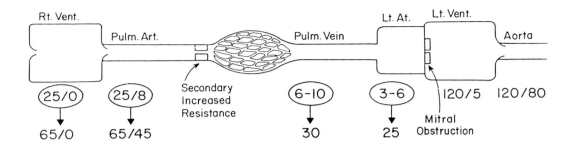

**FIGURE 12.3.** Pulmonary hypertension pressure relationships in mitral stenosis. (Adapted with permission from Fowler NO: Pulmonary hypertension. In Baum GL [ed.]: *Textbook of Pulmonary Diseases,* ed 2. Boston, Little, Brown, 1974, p 701.)

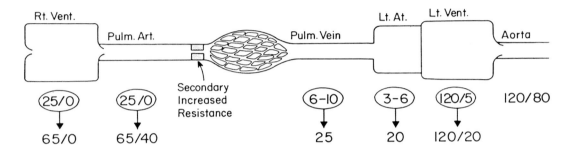

**FIGURE 12.4.** Pulmonary hypertension pressure relationships during left ventricular failure. (Adapted with permission from Fowler NO: Pulmonary hypertension. In Baum GL [ed]: *Textbook of Pulmonary Diseases,* ed 2. Boston, Little, Brown, 1974, p 701.)

to those in mitral stenosis, except that in mitral stenosis the left ventricular diastolic pressure is normal.

### TREATMENT OF PULMONARY HYPERTENSION

Primary pulmonary hypertension is progressive and often fatal (129). During the last decade, significant improvements have been made in the treatment of affected patients. The mainstay of treatment consists of supplemental oxygen, anticoagulation, and vasodilators. Supplemental oxygen must be given to patients who are hypoxemic at rest or during exercise. The arterial oxygen saturation needs to be maintained above 90% to attenuate hypoxic pulmonary vasoconstriction (109). Chronic warfarin therapy has been shown to improve survival in patients with primary pulmonary hypertension (130, 131). The prothrombin time must be monitored to maintain the INR between 2 and 3 when warfarin is being used (109). Adjusted-dose heparin may be an alternative to warfarin therapy (109).

Vasodilators have been advocated as a treatment of primary pulmonary hypertension for four decades; several of them have been tested, with mixed results

(101). The basis for vasodilator therapy in pulmonary hypertension is the assumption that reversible pulmonary vasoconstriction is present. The goal with vasodilator therapy is to reduce mean pulmonary artery pressure and pulmonary vascular resistance by at least 20%, with a concomitant rise in cardiac output, while not inducing systemic hypotension (101, 109). Unfortunately, only 26% of patients have a therapeutic response to oral vasodilators (109). Calcium channel blockers are the oral vasodilators most frequently used (131), and nifedipine and diltiazem are preferred because they have fewer negative inotropic actions (101). Titration of nifedipine or diltiazem is done with hourly doses under close hemodynamic monitoring (pulmonary arterial catheter) until maximal effects or adverse effects are present. Patients who respond to vasodilator therapy have a 5-year survival rate of 94% compared with 55% for nonresponders (109, 131). The average daily dose of sustained-release nifedipine is 120 to 240 mg/day; diltiazem in doses up to 900 mg/day is an alternative in tachycardiac patients (131). Intravenous prostacyclin, initially used as a screening agent for vasoreactivity, has recently been used in a continuous infusion with some benefits in patients who failed to respond to conventional vasodilator therapy (132). Patients receiving continuous prostacyclin need close monitoring, because tachyphylaxis occurs with chronic use (132). Other therapeutic agents used in pulmonary hypertension include digoxin and diuretics. The role of digoxin is unclear, but it may be used to counteract the negative inotropism of calcium channel blockers (109). Diuretics may be used in low doses to control hepatic congestion and leg edema (109).

Single-lung, double-lung, and combined heart-lung transplantation offer new hope for patients with primary pulmonary hypertension (109, 133–135). Although there is no consensus on whether single-lung is preferred to double-lung transplantation and the timing is controversial, consideration should be given to transplantation for patients in functional class III or IV (New York Heart Association) refractory to medical management (109). (Lung transplantation is discussed in Chapter 19).

## COR PULMONALE (PULMONARY HEART DISEASE)

The terms ''cor pulmonale'' and ''pulmonary heart disease'' refer to enlargement of the right ventricle (hypertrophy or dilation) secondary to disorders affecting lung structure or function (136). In general, the manifestations of cor pulmonale vary from initial adaptations of the right ventricle in response to the demands of increased pulmonary artery pressures to frank right ventricular failure. In cor pulmonale, the cause of the heart disease may be either intrinsic pulmonary disease (e.g., interstitial lung disease or COPD), inadequate function of the chest bellows (e.g., kyphoscoliosis), or insufficient ventilatory drive from the respiratory centers. Anatomic adaptation (dilation or hypertrophy) is confined predominantly to the right ventricle. The degree and duration of pulmonary arterial hypertension determine the relative effects of dilation or hypertrophy on right ventricular enlargement (137, 138).

### INCIDENCE

Cor pulmonale is common, being closely associated with chronic bronchitis and emphysema, which are major causes of disability and death (137). In the United States, approximately 86,000 persons die of chronic bronchitis and emphysema each year. However, the incidence of cor pulmonale is difficult to determine because of unreliable reporting. In addition, anatomic hallmarks, particularly right ventricular hypertrophy, are often overlooked at autopsy. Of patients with COPD, approximately 50% of those older than 50

years develop pulmonary hypertension (137). In these patients, when pulmonary vascular resistance is more than 550 dynes-second-cm$^{-5}$, survival approximates that of patients with inoperable lung cancer (137). (Chronic bronchitis and pulmonary emphysema are discussed in detail in Chapter 10.)

### SYMPTOMS AND SIGNS

Symptoms of cor pulmonale are nonspecific, although increases in pulmonary artery pressures frequently result in increasing dyspnea and easy fatigability. As the right ventricle loses its ability to meet mechanical work demands, symptoms related to fluid retention and weight gain may emerge. Upon physical examination, the patient is commonly cyanotic and dyspneic, often with audible wheezing and tachypnea (137). If considerable carbon dioxide is retained, the patient may be confused, somnolent, or even comatose. Hand flapping and tremors (asterixis) similar to those observed in hepatic decompensation (139) are common. Examination of the ocular fundi occasionally reveals papilledema (140), a finding that is more likely if carbon dioxide retention has produced increased cerebral blood flow and increased intracranial pressure. Except in patients with overt right ventricular failure—who have cyanosis, peripheral edema, and hepatomegaly—important physical findings may be limited to the cardiovascular system. The cardiac examination is frequently inhibited by hyperinflated lungs or adventitious breath sounds. There may be a prominent left parasternal lift due to an enlarged right ventricle. The pulmonary second sound (P$_2$) may be palpable. Low-frequency diastolic gallops arising from the right heart may be heard to the left of the sternum; a presystolic or right atrial gallop sound (S$_4$) indicates increased right ventricular filling pressures and may coincide with prominent A waves in the jugular venous pulse. A protodiastolic gallop (S$_3$) is evidence of right ventricular failure and is usually accompanied by other signs of right heart failure. Less frequently, a diastolic decrescendo murmur of pulmonary insufficiency indicates dilation of the pulmonary valve ring due to excessive pulmonary artery pressure (137).

In patients with severe right ventricular failure, the functional insufficiency of the valve due to ventricular dilation gives rise to the holosystolic murmur of tricuspid regurgitation, a murmur that may increase with inspiration. Palpable pulsations in an enlarged, tender liver and prominent V waves in the jugular venous pulse are often seen as well (137).

### ELECTROCARDIOGRAPHIC ABNORMALITIES

The diagnostic value of the electrocardiogram in cor pulmonale depends on the underlying pulmonary ventilatory disorder. Electrocardiographic findings are reliable if pulmonary artery hypertension is due to primary pulmonary vascular or interstitial disease. However, characteristic electrocardiographic patterns of right ventricular enlargement are uncommon when cor pulmonale complicates chronic bronchitis and emphysema, due to pulmonary hyperinflation with rotation and displacement of the heart, expanded distances between electrodes, or intrinsic cardiac disease and cardiac enlargement. A distinctive pattern of right ventricular enlargement indicates severe heart involvement (141, 142).

## THE CHEST RADIOGRAPH

In patients with pulmonary heart disease, manifestations of the underlying disease may dominate the chest film. Investigators have attempted to establish criteria for the radiographic diagnosis of pulmonary hypertension in severe COPD and have concluded that the chest radiograph can identify the presence, but not the degree, of pulmonary artery hypertension. The most convincing evidence of the disorder is the combination of a large main pulmonary artery, a large right descending pulmonary artery (greater than 16 mm) on the posteroanterior chest radiograph (Fig. 12.5), and a

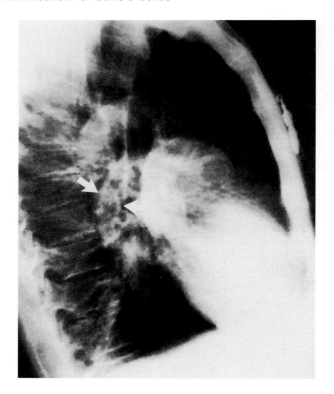

**FIGURE 12.6.** Enlarged left descending pulmonary artery (*arrows*) on left lateral chest radiograph in a patient with COPD and pulmonary artery hypertension. (Reproduced with permission from Matthay RA, Schwarz MI, Ellis JH Jr, et al: Pulmonary hypertension in chronic obstructive pulmonary disease: determination by chest radiography. *Invest Radiol* 16:95–100, 1981.)

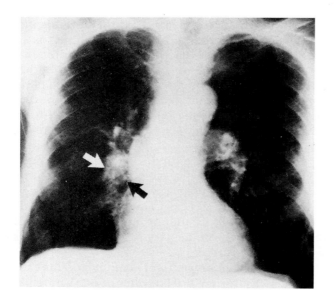

**FIGURE 12.5.** Enlarged right descending pulmonary artery (*arrows*) on posteroanterior chest radiograph in a patient with COPD. Note also the large left main pulmonary artery. The mean pulmonary artery pressure is 57 mm Hg (normal is 18 to 20 mm Hg). (Reproduced with permission from Matthay RA, Schwarz MI, Ellis JH Jr, et al: Pulmonary hypertension in obstructive pulmonary disease: determination by chest radiography. *Invest Radiol* 16:95–100, 1981.)

large left descending pulmonary artery (greater than 19 mm) on the lateral chest radiograph (Fig. 12.6) (143). An additional clue is an enlarged right ventricular silhouette. Generally, cardiomegaly is more readily detected through serial chest films than on a single examination. This is particularly true in chronic bronchitis and emphysema, since dramatic changes in heart size may occur with the onset of acute respiratory failure (2).

Pleural effusions do not occur in the setting of cor pulmonale alone. The presence of pleural effusions should suggest left heart failure or a primary pleural process such as infection, malignancy, or pulmonary embolism (124).

## OTHER TESTS FOR EVALUATING PATIENTS WITH COR PULMONALE

Patients with cor pulmonale have arterial hypoxemia with a resting $P_{O_2}$ usually ranging from 40 to 60 mm Hg. In some patients the $P_{O_2}$ falls further at night, so the patient has periods of marked oxygen desaturation. The hypoxemia further aggravates the pulmonary hypertension, which then worsens the cor pulmonale. The arterial $P_{CO_2}$ is usually in the range of 40 to 70 mm Hg. The degree of alveolar hypoventilation does not correlate well with the severity of airway obstruction. However, if the $P_{CO_2}$ rises at night, then the acidemia (associated with the increase in $P_{CO_2}$) can further potentiate the pulmonary hypertension and cor pulmonale (2).

First-pass radionuclide angiocardiography has been used to study the right and left ventricles in COPD (144, 145). This method has provided reproducible values for right ventricular ejection fraction, which correlates well with clinical and electrocardiographic evidence of cor pulmonale. The technique appears to be sensitive enough to provide a noninvasive method for early detection of right ventricular performance abnormalities secondary to occult pulmonary hypertension before they are manifested clinically in chronic bronchitis and cystic fibrosis (144, 146).

## THERAPY FOR ACUTELY DECOMPENSATED COR PULMONALE

The goal of therapy in cor pulmonale is to decrease the workload of the right ventricle by lowering pulmonary artery pressure. However, cor pulmonale caused by anatomic lesions such as primary pulmonary hypertension is not usually amenable to treatment. The disorders in which hypoxic pulmonary vasoconstriction is of primary importance are more responsive and include chronic bronchitis and emphysema.

### Oxygen

The initial treatment for acutely decompensated cor pulmonale is supplemental oxygen therapy to restore arterial oxygen to acceptable levels (2, 136). An end point of 90% arterial oxygen saturation (or an arterial $P_{O_2}$ of 60 mm Hg or greater) is adequate in most settings. The coexistence of hypercapnia imposes constraint on administering oxygen; a practical approach consists of a cautious trial of a modestly enriched oxygen mixture (e.g., 25 to 30% oxygen), monitored by observance of the ventilation and sampling of arterial blood to detect an unacceptable rise in arterial $P_{CO_2}$. In the event of decreased ventilation with a rising arterial $P_{CO_2}$, mechanical ventilation may be necessary to improve oxygenation and to avoid progressive respiratory acidosis (2).

### Diuretics

Oxygen is the best diuretic. As arterial $P_{O_2}$ rises, pulmonary hypertension decreases and cardiac output rises, owing to a reduced right ventricular afterload.

In some instances, diuretics are important in the management of cor pulmonale and heart failure (136). The lungs may share in accumulation of excess water in the body; this excess fluid may compromise pulmonary gas exchange and heighten pulmonary vascular resistance. In this setting, an initial diuresis can lower pulmonary artery pressure by decreasing total blood volume. Diuretics must be administered cautiously to avoid volume depletion and possible reduction in cardiac output (2). Another potential complication of diuretic therapy is a hypochloremic metabolic alkalosis, which can diminish the effect of the $CO_2$ stimulus on the respiratory centers and depress ventilatory drive. Therefore, serum electrolytes must be measured after diuretic administration or during periods of intensive salt and water retention. In some clinical circumstances, bed rest, modest salt restriction, and improved oxygenation alone may relieve significant water accumulation (2).

### Digitalis

There is little proof that digitalis therapy is useful in patients with cor pulmonale. Digitalis therapy is considered appropriate only in the presence of coincident left heart failure or supraventricular arrhythmia (2, 136, 138).

### Bronchodilators

Oral or intravenous theophylline enhances biventricular performance in patients with COPD, particularly patients with cor pulmonale (136, 147, 148). Bronchodilators also alleviate reversible airway obstruction, and theophylline may improve diaphragmatic contractility and help prevent inspiratory muscle fatigue in acute respiratory failure in patients with COPD (149). Moreover, selective $\beta$-adrenergic bronchodilating agents, such as terbutaline, may reduce afterload on the right and left ventricles and thereby improve cardiac output (150). Therefore, these drugs should be given along with the theophylline preparation.

### Antibiotics

Antibiotic therapy must be considered early in patients with acutely decompensated cor pulmonale and chronic bronchitis who have severe underlying disease or experience severe exacerbations (151). Sputum should be stained and cultured to identify the infecting organism and determine appropriate drug therapy. Therapy directed at *Moraxella catarrhalis, Haemophilus influenzae,* and *Streptococcus pneumoniae* should be considered in the previously nonhospitalized patient with purulent sputum, with or without pulmonary infiltrates, until culture results or clinical course indicate another pathogen or process (151).

## Corticosteroids

The need for corticosteroid therapy is determined by its likely effect on pulmonary function; for example, pulmonary function improves more rapidly in patients with acutely decompensated COPD if corticosteroids are given in addition to routinely used agents (152). In theory, improvement in underlying lung disease and gas transport problems will lead to reduced load on the right ventricle and subsequent improvement in performance.

## Phlebotomy

The benefit of phlebotomy may be due to a reduction in total blood volume rather than to a change in viscosity. In practice, the former is best achieved by diuresis. In patients with severe erythrocytosis and stable cor pulmonale, reduction in hematocrit is accompanied by reduction in mean pulmonary artery pressure and pulmonary vascular resistance (136, 137). However, in the setting of acute decompensation, the effect of phlebotomy is unknown. Accordingly, the procedure is best limited to cases with marked or refractory erythrocytosis (hematocrit greater than 65%) in which supplemental oxygen has failed to reduce the hematocrit or to cases in which there is concern regarding thrombotic or central nervous system manifestations (137).

### Long-Term Management of Cor Pulmonale

For many patients, reversing the acute precipitating factors of cor pulmonale restores satisfactory, or even normal, limits of pulmonary artery pressures and right ventricular function until additional causes of decompensation supervene or the underlying lung disease becomes more severe. However, in some patients qualitative disturbances of pulmonary vascular and myocardial function continue, although to a less marked degree. Persistent alveolar hypoxia sometimes contributes significantly to chronic elevation of pulmonary artery pressure; in these cases, continuous low-flow oxygen therapy has emerged as a useful tool. Long-term continuous administration of supplemental oxygen to carefully selected patients to relieve hypoxia can significantly decrease hematocrit and resting pulmonary artery pressure and improve right ventricular performance without risking significant oxygen toxicity or carbon dioxide retention. Such therapy has been shown to improve quality of life, reduce hospital admissions, and improve survival (153, 154). Candidates for long-term oxygen therapy are patients with a $Po_2$ below 55 mm Hg or 88% oxygen saturation. Patients with a $Po_2$ above 55 mm Hg but below 59 mm Hg or

oxygen saturation below 89% in the presence of cor pulmonale, heart failure, or erythrocytosis (hematocrit above 55%) are candidates for supplemental oxygen therapy as well. The $Pao_2$ must be re-evaluated at 1, 3, and 6 months to document the need for supplemental oxygen (137, 138).

## Congenital Pulmonary Vascular Disorders and Acquired Aneurysms

A variety of congenital abnormalities are manifested in the pulmonary arteries and pulmonary veins (Table 12.11) (155). Further details on these congenital disorders are in Perloff's textbook on congenital heart disease (156).

### Pulmonary Arteriovenous Malformations

Because arteries and veins develop from a common embryonic capillary plexus, persistent connections may develop even after birth (155, 156). Shunts between large blood vessels and between chambers of

**Table 12.11**
**Congenital Abnormalities of the Pulmonary Arteries and Pulmonary Veins**

Pulmonary Artery Abnormalities
  Complete absence of the main trunk of the pulmonary artery
  Absence of one main pulmonary artery
  Hypoplasia of one or more pulmonary arteries or lobar divisions
  Postvalvular pulmonary stenosis of the pulmonary artery
  Aberrant pulmonary artery
Pulmonary Vein Abnormalities
  Failure of the stem of the common pulmonary vein to become incorporated into the atrium, resulting in cor triatriatum
  Failure of the pulmonary veins to join normally with the lung venous plexus or, in case of established union, subsequent atresia
  Drainage of the pulmonary veins or of a common pulmonary vein into the atrium of the heart
  Drainage of the right pulmonary vein into the superior vena cava, azygos vein, or right innominate vein
  Drainage of left pulmonary veins into a persistent left superior vena cava, coronary sinus, or anomalous pulmonary vein
  Persistent connections between the pulmonary veins and the adult portal vein (fetal vitelline-umbilical venous system, including the ductus venosus)
  Drainage of the pulmonary veins of the right lung into the inferior vena cava (scimitar syndrome)

Reproduced with permission from Spencer H: Congenital abnormalities of the lung, pulmonary vessels and lymphatici. In: *Pathology of the Lung*, ed 3. Oxford, Pergamon Press, 1977, vol 1, p 71.

the heart normally exist during fetal life. Trauma, chest surgery, infection, and metastatic carcinomas are the chief causes of abnormal vascular shunts after birth (157). Multiple arteriovenous and other intervascular connections may also develop in the lungs as a result of chronic infection, such as bronchiectasis.

Small arteriovenous communications occur among the vascular systems of most tissues; in the lung these connections protect against increases in the pulmonary vascular flow and pressures (157). From 5 to 7% of the total pulmonary blood flow does not become arterialized to the maximum extent, and thus functions as venous admixture. In certain pathologic disorders, a large volume of blood may be shunted from the pulmonary artery to the pulmonary vein, resulting in considerable hypoxemia. Pulmonary arteriovenous malformation, a rare congenital lesion, is typical of true venous admixture. The shunt occurs from a pulmonary artery to a pulmonary vein. Such malformations may be single or multiple, and most of them are localized in the lower lobes and near the visceral pleura (157).

Pulmonary arteriovenous malformation may be isolated or, as in 36 to 57% of cases, associated with hereditary hemorrhagic telangiectasia (Osler-Weber-Rendu disease) (157). Localized dilations of small vessels forming telangiectasias or angiomata that tend to bleed are characteristic of the condition. These tiny lesions generally occur on the face, the nasopharyngeal and buccal mucous membranes, the lips, the skin, and the nail beds. The respiratory, gastrointestinal, or genitourinary tract and even the brain and spinal cord may be involved as well.

The cause of this inherited disorder is unknown. Women are more frequently affected than men, and the mean age at presentation is 40 years (157). Although the disease may be static for years, it is frequently progressive. Two distinct types have been identified; one is unrelated to any clinical signs, and the other is associated with dyspnea on exertion, palpitations, hemoptysis, and chest pain. Cyanosis, clubbing of the fingers and toes, pulmonary vascular bruits, and systolic murmur are frequently present (157). If the shunt is large, the primary symptoms are due to the chronic hypoxemia caused by shunting of unoxygenated blood through the aneurysm.

Neurologic effects of pulmonary arteriovenous shunts are headaches, confusion, dizziness, convulsions, syncope, paresthesia, diplopia, thick speech, and paresis, as well as cerebrovascular accidents. Such complications have been attributed to cerebral hypoxia and polycythemia as well as to telangiectasia in the brain with or without associated cerebral thrombosis. Brain abscess due to paradoxical emboli always needs to be considered as well (157).

In patients with hereditary hemorrhagic telangiectasias, an important complication is bleeding, most commonly epistaxis from telangiectatic lesions in the nasal mucous membranes. Hemoptysis, hematuria, melena, and cerebral hemorrhage may also occur owing to telangiectasis in the tracheobronchial tree, genitourinary and gastrointestinal tracts, and central nervous system (157).

The lesions may be so small as to be barely discernible on chest radiograph, but a large pulmonary arteriovenous malformation can be seen on a routine posteroanterior chest film. Typically, it is a lobulated or spherical opacity with smooth, discrete margins. It may be connected to the hilus by band-like linear or sinuous opacities, although the afferent and efferent vessels may not be visible. The aneurysm may involve any segment of either lung, although there appears to be a predilection for the lower and middle lobes. Fluoroscopic examination may demonstrate pulsations in the lobulated density as well as in the hilus (157). Chest computed tomography, contrast echocardiography, and pulmonary angiography are important in the evaluation of patients with pulmonary arteriovenous malformations (157).

Physiologically, the presence of a true right-to-left shunt can be confirmed by the failure of the arterial $P_{O_2}$ to rise above 500 mm Hg when a patient inhales 100% oxygen. Cardiac output is usually normal, although it may rise if the oxygen tension is very low. Pulmonary hypertension is present in 1% of affected patients (157). Therapy can range from conservative management to surgical resection (157). Recently, embolization of the malformation has been achieved with low morbidity and no mortality (157, 158). Embolization reduces the shunting, alleviates dyspnea, and improves exercise capacity and gas exchange (158). Therapeutic embolization is now the modality of choice in patients with single or multiple pulmonary arteriovenous malformations (158).

## PULMONARY ARTERY ANEURYSMS

Pulmonary artery aneurysms are rare saccular dilatations of the walls of the pulmonary artery that are usually detectable on a chest radiograph (159). Risk factors for acquired aneurysms are infection (bacterial, fungal, tuberculosis, and syphilis); congenital and acquired cardiac abnormalities; abnormalities of the vessel walls like cystic medionecrosis and atherosclerosis; vasculitis; trauma; and other conditions such as Hughes-Stovin syndrome, Behçet's syndrome, and primary pulmonary hypertension (159). The clinical presentation is nonspecific, but dyspnea, chest pain, cough, and hemoptysis may be present (159). Surgical resection of the aneurysm is the treatment of choice in most cases (159).

## NEOPLASIA OF THE PULMONARY VASCULAR BED

True neoplasms of the pulmonary arteries, veins, and lymphatic vessels are rare. Sarcoma of the pulmonary arteries carries a poor prognosis, and surgical resection is the treatment of choice (160).

Metastatic lymphangitic carcinoma involves not only the lymphatic vessels of the lung but also the pulmonary arteries (161, 162). Lymphangitic cancer is usually a complication of adenocarcinoma; primary sites are the stomach, pancreas, breasts, prostate, ovaries, colon, and endometrium. In early reports, the most common primary tumor was carcinoma of the stomach, but now nearly 50% of metastatic lymphangitic carcinomas in North America arise from breast cancer (161). Lymphangitic carcinoma has been described as a complication of breast cancer in 24% of such patients (161).

Embolization of the tumor to the branches of the pulmonary artery with subsequent invasion of the arterial wall is regarded as the cause of lymphangitic cancer. Subsequent extension into the adjacent lymphatic vessels is followed by centripetal spread of the tumor. This theory is supported by the frequency with which tumor emboli are found in pulmonary arteries, 20 of 23 cases of one series (161). Further evidence of systemic hematogenous spread of tumor to other organs is often found in patients with lymphangitic carcinoma. The former belief that hilar lymph nodes were involved with retrograde spread of tumor has been disproved, and it is now apparent that hilar lymph nodes are free of tumor in as many as half of the patients (161).

▼

## REFERENCES

1. Gregoratos G, Karliner JS, Moser KM: Mechanisms of disease and methods of assessment. In Moser KM (ed): *Pulmonary Vascular Diseases.* New York, Marcel Dekker, 1979, pp 279–339.
2. Fishman AP: Chronic cor pulmonale. *Am Rev Respir Dis* 224:775–794, 1976.
3. Moser KM: Pulmonary vascular obstruction due to embolism and thrombosis. In Moser KM (ed): *Pulmonary Vascular Disease.* New York, Marcel Dekker, 1979, pp 341–386.
4. Mohr DN, Ryu JH, Litin SC, et al: Recent advances in the management of venous thromboembolism. *Mayo Clin Proc* 63:281–290, 1988.
5. Raskob GE, Hull RD: Diagnosis and management of pulmonary thromboembolism. *Q J Med* 76:787–797, 1990.
6. Wilson JE III: Pulmonary embolism: diagnosis and treatment. *Clin Notes Respir Dis* 19:3–7, 1981.
7. Bell WR, Simon TL: Current status of pulmonary thromboembolic disease: pathophysiology, diagnosis, prevention and treatment. *Am Heart J* 103:239–262, 1982.
8. Moser K: State of the art: venous thromboembolism. *Am Rev Respir Dis* 141:235-249, 1990.
9. Wolfe WB, Sabiston DC Jr: Pulmonary embolism. *Major Probl Clin Surg* 25:1–180, 1980.
10. Sandler DA, Martin JF: Autopsy proven pulmonary embolism in hospital patients: are we detecting enough deep vein thrombosis? *J R Soc Med* 82:203–205, 1989.
11. Kudsk KA, Fabian TC, Baum S, et al: Silent deep vein thrombosis in immobilized multiple trauma patients. *Am J Surg* 158:515–519, 1989.
12. Belenkie I: Pulmonary vascular disease. In Guenter CA, Welch MH (eds): *Pulmonary Medicine.* Philadelphia, JB Lippincott, 1982.
13. Kinasewitz GT: Thrombophlebitis and pulmonary embolism in the elderly patient. *Clin Chest Med* 14:523–536, 1993.
14. Carter BL, Jones ME, Waickman LA: Pathophysiology and treatment of deep-vein thrombosis and pulmonary embolism. *Clin Pharm* 4:279–296, 1985.
15. Nachman RL, Silverstein R: Hypercoagulable states. *Ann Intern Med* 119:819–827, 1993.
16. Prandoni P, Lensing AWA, Buller HR, et al: Deep-vein thrombosis and the incidence of subsequent symptomatic cancer. *N Engl J Med* 327:1128–1133, 1992.
17. Ginsburg KS, Liang MH, Newcomer L, et al: Anticardiolipin antibodies and the risk for ischemic stroke and venous thrombosis. *Ann Intern Med* 117:997–1002, 1992.
18. Prandoni P: Deep vein thrombosis and occult cancer. *Ann Med* 25:447–450, 1993.
19. Schraufnagel DE, Tsao MS, Yao YT, et al: Factors associated with pulmonary infarction. A discriminant analysis. *Am J Clin Pathol* 84:15–18, 1985.
20. Elliott CG: Pulmonary physiology during pulmonary embolism. *Chest* 101:163S–171S, 1992.
21. Kakkar VV, Corrigan TP: Detection of deep venous thrombosis: survey and current status. *Prog Cardiovasc Dis* 17:207–217, 1974.
22. Severinghaus JW, Swenson EW, Finley TN, et al: Unilateral hypoventilation produced in dogs by occluding one pulmonary artery. *J Appl Physiol* 15:53–60, 1961.
23. Tisi GM, Wolfe WG, Fallat RJ, et al: Effects of $O_2$ on airway smooth muscle following pulmonary vascular occlusion. *J Appl Physiol* 28:570–573, 1970.
24. Thomas D, Stein M, Tanabe G, et al: Mechanisms of bronchoconstriction produced by thromboemboli in dogs. *Am J Physiol* 206:1207–1212, 1964.
25. Finley TN, Swenson EW, Clements JA, et al: Changes in mechanical properties, appearance and surface activity of extracts of one lung following occlusion of its pulmonary artery in the dog. *Physiologist* 3:56, 1960.
26. Finley TN, Tooley WH, Swenson EW, et al: Pulmonary surface tension in experimental atelectasis. *Am Rev Respir Dis* 89:372–378, 1964.
27. Dexter L, Smith GT: Quantitative studies of pulmonary embolism. *Am J Med Sci* 247:641–648, 1964.
28. Parmley LF Jr, North RL, Ott BS: Hemodynamic alterations of acute pulmonary thromboembolism. *Circ Res* 11:450–465, 1962.

29. Nelson JR, Smith JR: The pathologic physiology of pulmonary embolism. *Am Heart J* 58:916–932, 1959.

30. Huval WV, Mathieson MA, Stemp LJ, et al: Therapeutic benefits of 5-hydroxytryptamine inhibition following pulmonary embolism. *Ann Surg* 197:3220–3225, 1983.

31. Huet Y, Brun-Buisson C, Lemaire F, et al: Cardiopulmonary effects of ketanserin infusion in human pulmonary embolism. *Am Rev Respir Dis* 135:114–117, 1987.

32. Mathur VS, Dalen JE, Evans H, et al: Pulmonary angiography one to seven days after experimental pulmonary embolism. *Invest Radiol* 2:304–312, 1967.

33. Wessler S, Freeman DG, Ballon JS, et al: Experimental pulmonary embolism with serum induced thrombi. *Am J Pathol* 38:89–101, 1961.

34. Fred HL, Axelrod MA, Lewis JM, et al: Rapid resolution of pulmonary thromboemboli in man. *JAMA* 196:1137–1139, 1966.

35. Moser KM, Guisan M, Bartimmo EE, et al: In vivo and postmortem dissolution rates of pulmonary emboli and venous thrombi in the dog. *Circulation* 48:170–178, 1973.

36. Freiman DG, Wessler S, Lertzman M: Experimental pulmonary embolism with serum-induced thrombi aged in vivo. *Am J Pathol* 39:95–102, 1961.

37. Moser KM, Daily PO, Peterson K, et al: Thromboendarterectomy for chronic, major-vessel thromboembolic pulmonary hypertension. Immediate and long term results in 42 patients. *Ann Intern Med* 107:560–565, 1987.

38. Rich S, Levitsky S, Brundage BH: Pulmonary hypertension from chronic pulmonary thromboembolism. *Ann Intern Med* 108:425–434, 1988.

39. Weir EK, Archer SL, Edwards JE: Chronic primary and secondary thromboembolic pulmonary hypertension. *Chest* 93:(Suppl 3)149S–154S, 1988.

40. Fulkerson WJ, Coleman RE, Ravin CE, et al: Diagnosis of pulmonary embolism. *Arch Intern Med* 146:961–967, 1986.

41. Landefeld CS, McGuire E, Cohen AM: Clinical findings associated with acute proximal deep vein thrombosis: a basis of quantifying clinical judgement. *Am J Med* 88:382–388, 1990.

42. Stein PD, Terrin MC, Hales CA, et al: Clinical, laboratory, roentgenographic and electrocardiographic findings in patients with acute pulmonary embolism and preexisting cardiac or pulmonary disease. *Chest* 100:598–608, 1991.

43. Hull RD, Raskob GE, Carter CJ, et al: Pulmonary embolism in outpatients with pleuritic chest pain. *Arch Intern Med* 148:838–844, 1988.

44. Cobbs BW Jr, Logue RB, Dorney EG: The second heart sound in pulmonary embolism and pulmonary hypertension. *Am Heart J* 71:843–844, 1966.

45. Goldhaber SZ, Simons GR, Elliott CG, et al: Quantitative plasma D-dimer levels among patients undergoing pulmonary angiography for suspected pulmonary embolism. *JAMA* 270:2819–2822, 1993.

46. Stein PD, Athanasoulis C, Greenspan RH, Henry JW: Relation of plain chest radiographic findings to pulmonary arterial pressure and arterial blood oxygen levels in patients with acute pulmonary embolism. *Am J Cardiol* 69:394–396, 1992.

47. Bynum LJ, Wilson JE III: Characteristics of pleural effusions associated with pulmonary embolism. *Arch Intern Med* 136:159–162, 1976.

48. Worsley DF, Alavi A, Palevsky JH: Role of radionuclide imaging in patients with suspected pulmonary embolism. *Radiol Clin North Am* 31:849–858, 1993.

49. Huisman MV, Buller HR, Ten-cate JW, et al: Unexpected high prevalence of silent pulmonary embolism in patients with deep venous thrombosis. *Chest* 95:498–502, 1989.

50. Hull RD, Raskob GE, Ginsberg JS, et al: A noninvasive strategy for the treatment of patients with suspected pulmonary embolism. *Arch Intern Med* 154:289–297, 1994.

51. Oudkerk M, van Beek EJR, van Putten WLJ, Bullen HR: Cost-effectiveness analysis of various strategies in the diagnostic management of pulmonary embolism. *Arch Intern Med* 153:947–954, 1993.

52. Kelley MA, Carson JL, Palevsky HI, Schwartz JS: Diagnosing pulmonary embolism: New facts and strategies. *Ann Intern Med* 114:300–306, 1991.

53. Stein PD, Hull RS, Saltzman HA, Pineo G: Strategy for diagnosis of patients with suspected acute pulmonary embolism. *Chest* 103:1553–1559, 1993.

54. Hull RD, Raskob GE: Low-probability lung scan findings: a need for change. *Ann Intern Med* 114:142–143, 1991.

55. Stein PD, Coleman RE, Gottschalk A, et al: Diagnostic utility of ventilation/perfusion lung scans in acute pulmonary embolism is not diminished by preexisting cardiac or pulmonary disease. *Chest* 100:604–606, 1991.

56. The PIOPED investigators. Value of the ventilation/perfusion scan in acute pulmonary embolism. Results of the prospective investigation of pulmonary embolism diagnosis (PIOPED). *JAMA* 263:2753–2759, 1990.

57. Cronan JJ: Venous thromboembolic disease: the role of U.S. *Radiology* 186:619–630, 1993.

58. Heijboer H, Buller HR, Lensing AWA, et al: A comparison of real-time compression ultrasonography with impedance plethysmography for the diagnosis of deep-vein thrombosis in symptomatic outpatients. *N Engl J Med* 329:1365–1369, 1993.

59. Rosner NH, Doris PE: Diagnosis of femoropopliteal venous thrombosis: comparison of Duplex sonography and plethysmography. *AJR* 150:623–627, 1988.

60. Stein PD, Athanasoulis C, Alavi A, et al: Complication and validity of pulmonary angiography in acute pulmonary embolism. *Circulation* 85:462–468, 1992.

61. Quinn MF, Lundell CJ, Klotz TA, et al: Reliability of selective pulmonary arteriography in the diagnosis of pulmonary embolism. *AJR* 149:469–471, 1987.

62. Demers C, Ginsberg JS: Deep venous thrombosis and pulmonary embolism in pregnancy. *Clin Chest Med* 13:645–656, 1992.

63. Clagett GP, Anderson FA Jr, Levin MN, et al: Prevention of venous thromboembolism. *Chest* 102:391S–407S, 1992.

64. Kumar R, McKinney WP, Raj G: Perioperative prophylaxis of venous thromboembolism. *Am J Med Sci* 306:336–344, 1993.

65. Anderson FA, Wheeler HB, Goldberg RJ, et al: Physician practices in the prevention of venous thromboembolism. *Ann Intern Med* 115:591–595, 1991.

66. Triplett DA: Low-molecular-weight heparins. Is smaller better? [Editorial] *Arch Intern Med* 153:1525–1526, 1993.

67. Salzman EW: Low-molecular-weight heparin and other new antithrombotic drugs [Editorial]. *N Engl J Med* 326:1017–1019, 1992.

68. Hyers TM, Hull RD, Weg JG: Antithrombotic therapy for venous thromboembolic disease. *Chest* 102: 408S–425S, 1992.

69. Hirsh J: Heparin. *N Engl J Med* 324:1565–1574, 1991.

70. Raschke RA, Reilly BM, Guidry JR, et al: The weight-based heparin dosing nomogram compared with a "standard care" nomogram. A randomized controlled trial. *Ann Intern Med* 119:874–881, 1993.

71. Elliott CG, Hiltunen SJ, Suchyta M, et al: Physician-guided treatment compared with a heparin protocol for deep vein thrombosis. *Arch Intern Med* 154:999–1004, 1994.

72. Hirsh J: Oral anticoagulant drugs. *N Engl J Med* 324:1865–1875, 1991.

73. Hull RD, Raskob GE, Pineo GF, et al: Subcutaneous low-molecular-weight heparin compared with continuous intravenous heparin in the treatment of proximal-vein thrombosis. *N Engl J Med* 326:975–982, 1992.

74. Simonneau G, Charbonier B, Decousus H, et al: Subcutaneous low-molecular-weight heparin compared with continuous intravenous unfractionated heparin in the treatment of proximal deep vein thrombosis. *Arch Intern Med* 153:1541–1546, 1993.

75. Bell WR, Streiff MB: Thrombolytic therapy: a comprehensive review of its use in clinical medicine, Part II. *J Intensive Care Med* 8:115–129, 1993.

76. Greenfield LJ: Catheter pulmonary embolectomy. *Chest* 100:593–594, 1991.

77. Timsit JF, Reynaud P, Meyer G, Sors H: Pulmonary embolectomy by catheter device in massive pulmonary embolism. *Chest* 100:655–658, 1991.

78. Becker DM, Philbrick JT, Selby JB: Inferior vena cava filters. Indications, safety, effectiveness. *Arch Intern Med* 152:1985–1994, 1992.

79. Golueke PJ, Garrett WV, Thompson JE, et al: Interruption of the vena cava by means of the Greenfield filter: expanding the indications. *Surgery* 193:111–117, 1988.

80. Hall RJC, Sutton GC, Kerr IH: Long-term prognosis of treated acute massive embolism. *Br Heart J* 39: 1128–1134, 1979.

81. Carson JL, Kelley MA, Duff A, et al: The clinical course of pulmonary embolism. *N Engl J Med* 326:1240–1245, 1992.

82. Moser KM, Auger WR, Fedullo PF, Jamieson SW: Chronic thromboembolic pulmonary hypertension: Clinical picture and surgical treatment. *Eur Respir J* 5: 334–342, 1992.

83. Moser KM, Auger WR, Fedullo PF: Chronic major-vessel thromboembolic pulmonary hypertension. *Circulation* 81:1735–1743, 1990.

84. Widimsky J: Acute pulmonary embolism and chronic thromboembolic pulmonary hypertension: is there a relationship? [Editorial]. *Eur Respir J* 4:137–140, 1991.

85. Auger WR, Fedullo PF, Moser KM, et al: Chronic major-vessel thromboembolic pulmonary artery obstruction: appearance at angiography. *Radiology* 182:393–398, 1992.

86. Kuhlman E, Fishman EK, Teigen C: Pulmonary septic emboli: diagnosis with CT. *Radiology* 174:211–213, 1990.

87. Bloor CM: Acute pulmonary thromboembolism and other forms of pulmonary embolization. In Saldana MJ (ed): *Pathology of Pulmonary Disease*. Philadelphia, JB Lippincott, 1994, p 171.

88. Virmani R, Farb A, Burke AP, Popek EJ: Thromboembolic pulmonary hypertension, intravenous drug addiction, and rare forms of pulmonary embolization. In Saldana MJ (ed): *Pathology of Pulmonary Disease*. Philadelphia, JB Lippincott, 1994, p 225.

89. Chan CK, Hutcheon MA, Hyland RH, et al: Pulmonary tumor embolism: a critical review of clinical, imaging and hemodynamic features. *J Thorac Imaging* 2:4–14, 1987.

90. Guenter CA, Braun TE: Fat embolism: changing prognosis. *Chest* 79:143–145, 1981.

91. Chastre J, Fagon JY, Soler P, et al: Bronchoalveolar lavage for rapid diagnosis of the fat embolism syndrome in trauma patients. *Ann Intern Med* 113:583–588, 1990.

92. Fabian TC: Unraveling the fat embolism syndrome [Editorial]. *N Engl J Med* 329:961–963, 1993.

93. Pell ACH, Hughes D, Keating J, et al: Brief report: Fulminating fat embolism syndrome caused by paradoxical embolism through a patent foramen ovale. *N Engl J Med* 329:926–929, 1993.

94. Ereth MH, Weber JG, Abel MD, et al: Cemented versus noncemented total hip arthroplasty—embolism, hemodynamics and intrapulmonary shunting. *Mayo Clin Proc* 67:1066–1974, 1992.

95. Masson RG: Amniotic fluid embolism. *Clin Chest Med* 13:657–665, 1992.

96. Ohkuda K, Nakahara K, Binder A, et al: Venous air emboli in sheep: reversible increase in lung microvascular permeability. *J Appl Physiol* 51:887–894, 1981.

97. Marini JJ, Culver BH: Systemic gas embolism complicating mechanical ventilation in the adult respiratory distress syndrome. *Ann Intern Med* 110:699–703, 1989.

98. Fraser RG, Paré JAP: Pulmonary hypertension and edema. In Fraser RG, Paré JAP (eds): *Diagnosis of Diseases of the Chest*, ed 3. Philadelphia, WB Saunders, 1988, vol 2.

99. Fowler NO, Westcott RN, Scott RC: Normal pressure in the right heart and pulmonary artery. *Am Heart J* 46: 264–267, 1953.

100. Sasamoto H, Hosono K, Viatayam K, et al: Electrocardiographic findings in patients with chronic cor pulmonale. *Respir Circ* 9:55, 1961.

101. Olivari MT: Primary pulmonary hypertension. *Am J Med Sci* 302:185–198, 1991.

102. Watanabe S: Pathophysiology of hypoxemic pulmonary vascular diseases. *Bull Eur Physiopathol Respir* 23 (Suppl 11):207S–209S, 1987.

103. Wagenvoort CA, Wagenvoort N: *Pathology of Pulmonary Hypertension*. New York, John Wiley & Sons, 1977, p 9.

104. Fishman AP, Renkin EM: *Pulmonary Edema*. Bethesda, Maryland, American Physiological Society, 1979.

105. Edwards WD: Pathology of pulmonary hypertension. *Cardiovasc Clin* 18:321–359, 1988.

106. Crofton J, Douglas A: Pulmonary hypertension. In Crofton J, Douglas A: *Respiratory Diseases*, ed 2. London, Blackwell Scientific Publications, 1975, p 360.

107. Harris P, Heath D: *The Human Pulmonary Circulation: Its Form and Function in Health and Disease*. Baltimore, Williams & Wilkins, 1962.

108. Rich S, Dantzker DR, Ayres SM, et al: Primary pulmonary hypertension. A national prospective study. *Ann Intern Med* 107:216–223, 1987.

109. Rubin LJ: Primary pulmonary hypertension. *Chest* 104: 236–250, 1993.

110. Arroliga AC, Podell DN, Matthay RA: Pulmonary manifestations of scleroderma. *J Thorac Imaging* 7:30–45, 1992.

111. Wiedemann HP, Matthay RA: Pulmonary manifestations of the collagen vascular diseases. *Clin Chest Med* 10:677–722, 1989.

112. Lupi HE, Sanchez TG, Horwitz S, et al: Pulmonary artery involvement in Takayasu's arteritis. *Chest* 67:69–74, 1975.

113. Del Castillo JJ, Gianfrancesco H, Mannix EP Jr: Pulmonary stenosis due to compression by sternal chondrosarcoma. *J Thorac Cardiovasc Surg* 52:255–260, 1966.

114. Krieger J, Sforza E, Apprill M, et al: Pulmonary hypertension, hypoxemia, and hypercapnia in obstructive sleep apnea patients. *Chest* 96:729–737, 1989.

115. Kaplan J, Staats BA: Obstructive sleep apnea syndrome. *Mayo Clin Proc* 65:1087–1094, 1990.

116. Saldana MJ, Arias-Stella J: Pulmonary hypertension and pathology at high altitudes. In Saldana MJ (ed): *Pathology of Pulmonary Disease.* Philadelphia, JB Lippincott, 1994, p 247.

117. Singh I, Khanna PK, Lal M, et al: High-altitude pulmonary hypertension. *Lancet* 2:146–150, 1965.

118. Hurtado A: Some clinical aspects of life at high altitudes. *Ann Intern Med* 53:247–358, 1960.

119. Haselton PS, Ironside JW, Whittaker JS, et al: Pulmonary veno-occlusive disease. A report of four cases. *Histopathology* 10:933–944, 1986.

120. Wagenvoort CA, Wagenvoort N, Takahashi T: Pulmonary veno-occlusive disease: involvement of pulmonary arteries and review of the literature. *Hum Pathol* 16:1033–1041, 1985.

121. Burke AP, Virmani R, Far B: Primary pulmonary hypertension and veno-occlusive disease. In Saldana MJ (ed): *Pathology of Pulmonary Disease.* Philadelphia, JB Lippincott, 1994, p 235.

122. Farb A, Burke AP, Virmani R: Pulmonary hypertension caused by chronic left heart failure, obstruction of pulmonary venous return and parenchymal lung disease. In Saldana MJ (ed): *Pathology of Pulmonary Disease.* Philadelphia, JB Lippincott, 1994, p 203.

123. Gorlin R, Gorlin SG: Hydraulic formula for circulation of the area of the stenotic mitral valve, other cardiac valves, and central circulatory shunts. *Am Heart J* 41:1–29, 1951.

124. Wiener-Kronish JP, Goldstein R, Matthay RA, et al: Lack of association of pleural effusion with chronic pulmonary arterial and right atrial hypertension. *Chest* 92:967–970, 1987.

125. Blount SG, Grover RF: Pulmonary hypertension. In Hurst JW (ed): *The Heart.* New York, McGraw-Hill, 1978, p 1456.

126. Mueller NL, Ostrow DN: High-resolution computed tomography of chronic interstitial lung disease. *Clin Chest Med* 12:97–114, 1991.

127. Fowler NO: Chronic cor pulmonale caused by lung disease. In Baum GL (ed): *Textbook of Pulmonary Disease,* ed 2. Boston, Little, Brown, 1974, p 737.

128. Fowler NO: Pulmonary hypertension. In Baum GL (ed): *Textbook of Pulmonary Diseases,* ed 2. Boston, Little, Brown, 1974, p 701.

129. D'Alonzo GE, Barst RJ, Ayres SM, et al: Survival in patients with primary pulmonary hypertension. Results from a national prospective registry. *Ann Intern Med* 115:343–349, 1991.

130. Fuster V, Steele PM, Edwards WD, et al: Primary pulmonary hypertension: natural history and the importance of thrombosis. *Circulation* 70:580–587, 1984.

131. Rich S, Kaufmann E, Levy PS: The effect of high dose of calcium-channel blockers on survival in primary pulmonary hypertension. *N Engl J Med* 327:76–81, 1992.

132. Rubin LJ, Mendoza J, Hood M, et al: Treatment of primary pulmonary hypertension with continuous intravenous prostacyclin (epoprostenol): results of a randomized trial. *Ann Intern Med* 112:485–491, 1990.

133. Reitz BA, Wallwork JL, Hunt SA, et al: Heart-lung transplantation: successful therapy for patients with pulmonary vascular disease. *N Engl J Med* 306:557–564, 1982.

134. Pasque MK, Kaiser LR, Dresler CM, et al: Single-lung transplantation for pulmonary hypertension: technical aspects and immediate hemodynamic results. *J Thorac Cardiovasc Surg* 103:475–482, 1992.

135. Levine SM, Gibbons WJ, Bryan CL, et al: Single-lung transplantation for primary pulmonary hypertension. *Chest* 98:1107–1115, 1990.

136. Wiedemann HP, Matthay RA: Cor pulmonale in chronic obstructive pulmonary disease: circulatory pathophysiology and new concepts of therapy. *Curr Pulmonol* 8:127–162, 1987.

137. Salvaterra CG, Rubin LJ: Investigation and management of pulmonary hypertension in chronic obstructive pulmonary disease. *Am Rev Respir Dis* 148:1414–1417, 1993.

138. Matthay RA, Arroliga AC, Wiedemann HP, et al: Right ventricular function at rest and during exercise in chronic obstructive pulmonary disease. *Chest* 101:255S–262S, 1992.

139. Conn HO: Asterixis: its occurrence in chronic pulmonary disease, with a commentary on its general mechanism. *N Engl J Med* 259:564, 1958.

140. Westlake EK, Simpson T, Kaye M: Carbon dioxide narcosis in emphysema. *Q J Med* 24:155–173, 1955.

141. Butler PM, Leggett SI, Howe CM, et al: Identification of electrocardiographic criteria for diagnosis of right ventricular hypertrophy due to mitral stenosis. *Am J Cardiol* 57:639–643, 1986.

142. Behar JV, Howe CM, Wagner NB, et al: Performance of new criteria for right ventricular hypertrophy and myocardial infarction in patients with pulmonary hypertension due to cor pulmonale and mitral stenosis. *J Electrocardiol* 24:231–237, 1991.

143. Matthay RA, Schwarz MI, Ellis JH Jr, et al: Pulmonary hypertension in chronic obstructive pulmonary disease: determination by chest radiography. *Invest Radiol* 16:95–100, 1981.

144. Berger HJ, Matthay RA, Loke J, et al: Assessment of cardiac performance with quantitative radionuclide angiography. Right ventricular ejection fraction with reference to findings in chronic obstructive pulmonary disease. *Am J Cardiol* 41:897–905, 1978.

145. Matthay RA, Berger HJ: Imaging techniques for assessing cardiovascular performance in chronic obstructive pulmonary disease. *J Thorac Imag* 1:61–74, 1986.

146. Matthay RA, Berger HJ, Loke J, et al: Right and left ventricular performance in cystic fibrosis: assessment by noninvasive radionuclide angiocardiography. *Br Heart J* 43:478–480, 1980.

147. Matthay RA, Berger HJ, Loke J, et al: Effects of aminophylline upon right and left ventricular performance in chronic obstructive pulmonary disease. Non-invasive assessment by radionuclide angiocardiography. *Am J Med* 65:903–910, 1978.

148. Matthay RA, Berger HJ, Loke J, et al: Augmentation of right ventricular performance by oral sustained-release theophylline in chronic obstructive pulmonary disease: non-invasive assessment by radionuclide angiocardiography. *Am Heart J* 104:1022–1026, 1982.

149. Aubier M, Detroyer A, Sampson M, et al: Aminophylline improves diaphragmatic contractility. *N Engl J Med* 305:249–252, 1981.

150. Brent BC, Mahler D, Berger HJ, et al: Augmentation of right ventricular performance in chronic obstructive pulmonary disease by terbutaline: a combined radionuclide and hemodynamic study. *Am J Cardiol* 50:313–319, 1982.

151. Murphy TF, Sethi S: Bacterial infections in chronic obstructive pulmonary disease. *Am Rev Respir Dis* 146:1067–1083, 1992.

152. Albert RK, Martin TR, Lewis SW: Controlled clinical trial of methyl-prednisolone in patients with chronic bronchitis and acute respiratory insufficiency. *Ann Intern Med* 92:753–758, 1980.

153. Nocturnal Oxygen Therapy Trial Group: Continuous or nocturnal oxygen therapy in hypoxemic chronic obstructive lung disease. *Ann Intern Med* 93:391, 1980.

154. The Medical Research Council Working Party: Long-term domiciliary oxygen therapy in chronic hypoxic cor pulmonale complicating chronic bronchitis and emphysema. *Lancet* 1:682, 1981.

155. Spencer H: Congenital abnormalities of the lung, pulmonary vessels and lymphatics. In Spencer H: *Pathology of the Lung,* ed 3. Philadelphia, WB Saunders, 1978, vol 1, p 71.

156. Perloff JK: *The Clinical Recognition of Congenital Heart Disease,* ed 2. Philadelphia, WB Saunders, 1987.

157. Burke CM Safai C, Nelson DP, Raffin TA: Pulmonary arteriovenous malformations: a critical update. *Am Rev Respir Dis* 134:334–339, 1986.

158. Pennington DW, Gold WM, Gordon RL, et al: Treatment of pulmonary arteriovenous malformations by therapeutic embolizations. Rest and exercise physiology in six patients. *Am Rev Respir Dis* 145:1047–1051, 1992.

159. Bartter T, Irwin RS, Nash G: Aneurysms of the pulmonary arteries. *Chest* 94:1065–1075, 1988.

160. Baker PB, Goodwin RA: Pulmonary artery sarcoma: a review and report of a case. *Arch Pathol Lab Med* 1098:35–39, 1985.

161. Janower ML, Blennerhasset JB: Lymphangitic spread of metastatic cancer to the lungs. A radiologic-pathologic classification. *Radiology* 101:267–273, 1971.

162. Filderman AE, Coppage L, Shaw C, et al: Pulmonary and pleural manifestations of extrathoracic malignancies. *Clin Chest Med* 10:747–807, 1989.

# Chapter 13

# Diffuse Interstitial and Alveolar Inflammatory Diseases

**Herbert Y. Reynolds**
**Richard A. Matthay**

THE INTERSTITIAL LUNG diseases are a diverse group of disorders that affect the supporting or architectural tissue of the lung, especially structural portions of the alveolar walls. They have many common features, including similarity of patient symptoms, comparable appearance of chest radiographs, consistent derangements in pulmonary physiology, and typical histologic features (1, 2). Although lung inflammation is an early phase of the disease, no known infectious agent is associated with the cause or onset of most of the various diseases. Exceptions include certain fungal and mycobacterial lung infections. For many of the diseases, the etiology is unknown.

The alveolar spaces (Fig. 13.1), which are lined by type I epithelial cells, bring inspired air into close proximity with circulating blood contained in capillaries lined with endothelial cells, thus creating the air-exchange units of the lung. Surrounding these units is the supporting tissue called the interstitium. This area is a potential space that can accumulate fluid and can contain such cells as fibroblasts, lymphocytes, dendritic cells, and monocytes that are undergoing maturation into macrophages; but few inflammatory cells are present in the normal interstitial space. In early phases of disease, inflammation is localized predominantly in the alveoli, and type II pneumocytes and alveolar macrophages may slough and accumulate in the air spaces (alveolitis). Other inflammatory cells, polymorphonuclear granulocytes (PMNs) and eosinophils, also collect in the alveoli. In later stages of disease, interstitial abnormalities occur of which derangement in the noncellular supporting structures, especially collagen, is most serious and causes fibrosis and distortion of lung architecture (3).

Although all the diffuse interstitial lung diseases share the common morphologic characteristic of an ab-

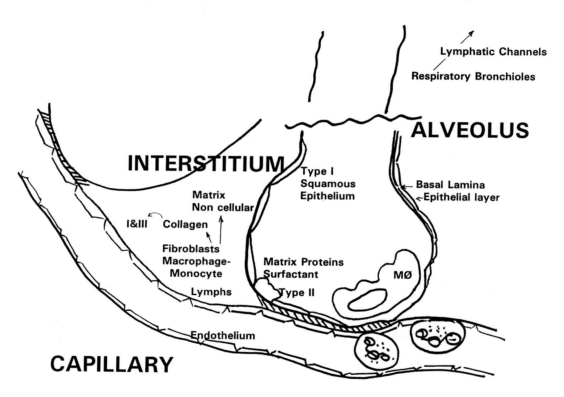

**FIGURE 13.1.** The diffuse interstitial lung diseases (DILDs) primarily involve the air exchange portion of the respiratory tract—the alveolar structures. Although there can be an element of bronchiolitis, this is not the site of inflammation or injury for most diseases. Bronchiolitis obliterans with organizing pneumonia is an exception. For DILD the initial process may involve the lining cells of the alveoli, after which inflammation spreads to the alveolar walls and their supporting structure, the interstitium, normally composed of fibroblasts capable of producing several forms of collagen and noncellular matrix glycoproteins and a few mononuclear cells, perhaps undergoing maturation before emerging as macrophages destined for the alveoli. Because of the proximity of the capillaries, the vascular component can be involved with inflammation as well. With chronicity the fibrotic reaction develops in which the discrete architecture of the alveolar unit becomes deranged and scarred or cytic changes result. In addition to inflammation, a granulomatous reaction may also occur concomitantly for many important diseases in the DILD group.

TABLE **13.1**
MAJOR CATEGORIES OF DIFFUSE INTERSTITIAL AND ALVEOLAR INFLAMMATORY LUNG DISEASE

| Lung Response | Unknown Cause | Known Cause |
|---|---|---|
| Interstitial inflammation and fibrosis without granuloma formation | Idiopathic pulmonary fibrosis[a]<br>Bronchiolitis obliterans pneumonia (BOOP)[a]<br>Collagen vascular diseases[a]<br>Pulmonary hemosiderosis[a]<br>Goodpasture's syndrome[a]<br>Pulmonary alveolar proteinosis[a]<br>Ankylosing spondylitis<br>Lymphocytic infiltration diseases<br>Eosinophilic lung syndromes[a] | Asbestos[b]<br>Fumes, gases[b]<br>Drugs (antibiotics, chemotherapy drugs)[a]<br>Radiation<br>Neoplasia (lymphangitic)<br>Cardiac failure<br>Aspiration (pneumonia) |
| With granuloma also | Sarcoidosis[a]<br>Langerhans cell granulomatosis[a]<br>  (histiocytosis X or eosinophilic<br>  granuloma)<br>Granulomatous vasculitides[a]<br>• Wegener's granulomatosis<br>• Lymphomatoid granulomatosis<br>• Allergic granulomatosis of Churg-Strauss | Hypersensitivity pneumonitis (organic<br>  dusts)[a]<br>Beryllium[b]<br>Silica[b]<br>Mycobacteria/fungi[c] |

[a] Discussed in this chapter.
[b] Discussed in Chapter 14.
[c] Discussed in Chapter 16.

normal lung interstitium, a satisfactory classification of them has been difficult to construct. This is because approximately 150 individual diseases have a component of interstitial lung involvement, either as a primary disease or as a significant part of a multiorgan process, such as a collagen-vascular disease. This diversity precludes a tight and orderly classification. One reasonable approach broadly separates the interstitial lung diseases into two groups, those with known causes and those with unknown causes; each of these groups can be subclassified further according to the presence or absence of granuloma in interstitial or vascular areas as viewed in histologic specimens (Table 13.1) (2).

Interstitial lung diseases of known cause include several major subcategories. By far the largest group comprises occupational and environmental inhalant diseases; these include diseases due to inhalation of inorganic dusts, organic dusts (hypersensitivity pneumonitis), gases, fumes, vapors, and aerosols (see Chapter 14). Other categories include lung diseases caused by drugs, irradiation, poisons, neoplasia, and chronic cardiac failure. The number of diseases with an unknown cause is likewise very large. The major subgroups within this category are idiopathic pulmonary fibrosis (IPF) and connective tissue (collagen vascular) disorders with interstitial lung disease, including rheumatoid arthritis, systemic lupus erythematosus, progressive systemic sclerosis, polymyositis-dermatomyositis, and Sjögren's syndrome. Systemic

vasculitides often have granulomas in tissue and include a variant of polyarteritis nodosa called allergic granulomatosis, lymphomatoid granulomatosis, and hypersensitivity vasculitis (leukocytoclastic). A number of inherited disorders such as tuberous sclerosis and neurofibromatosis can have a component of interstitial lung disease. Forms of familial pulmonary fibrosis have been described (4), and amyloidosis can occasionally involve the lung (1).

Six major entities that are most frequently associated with diffuse interstitial lung disease are reviewed in this chapter: idiopathic pulmonary fibrosis, connective tissue (collagen vascular) diseases, systemic granulomatous vasculitis, sarcoidosis, hypersensitivity pneumonitis, and drug-related hypersensitivity disease or fibrosis. In addition, bronchiolitis obliterans organizing pneumonia (BOOP), Goodpasture's syndrome, idiopathic pulmonary hemosiderosis, pulmonary alveolar proteinosis, and eosinophilic syndromes, representing diseases associated with both alveolar and interstitial abnormalities, will be discussed briefly.

## IDIOPATHIC PULMONARY FIBROSIS (CRYPTOGENIC FIBROSING ALVEOLITIS)

Because idiopathic or cryptogenic implies an unknown cause, idiopathic pulmonary fibrosis (IPF) sounds like a nebulous, poorly identified disease. On the contrary, however, whereas the descriptive name may be poor, IPF is a well-recognized clinical entity.

Initially the disease was described about 40 years ago by Hamman and Rich (5) as a fulminant, fatal form of so-called capillary alveolar block syndrome in which proliferating fibrotic tissue virtually occluded the peripheral airways. Thereafter, the disease was recognized more frequently, but considerable variation was noted in the clinical progression and morbidity it produced. Clinicians recognized that a spectrum of disease severity could occur. The disease has become known as diffuse interstitial pulmonary fibrosis in the United States, but in Europe it may be referred to as cryptogenic fibrosing alveolitis.

IPF is a syndrome of uncertain cause that is largely limited to the lungs. Clinical features include symptoms of nonproductive cough, and breathlessness (dyspnea) increasing with exertion; finding arterial hypoxemia is expected. Lung function tests reflect a pattern of restrictive and occasionally obstructive ventilatory dysfunction. Radiographically, a pattern of alveolar filling may evolve into one of reticular or reticulonodular densities that produces a distinctive but nondiagnostic sequence of chest radiographs. With high-resolution computed chest tomography (HRCT), areas of ground-glass appearance, denoting inflammation and cellularity on lung histology, and of a reticular pattern correlating with fibrosis and cystic changes of traction bronchiectasis can be observed in portions of the lung (6). Histologically, an early phase of lung pathology may show predominantly alveolitis; later this progresses to interstitial inflammation and to fibrosis with collagen derangement. Considerable distortion of lung architecture occurs, with thickening of alveolar septa and formation of cystic spaces in the parenchyma. Recent attempts have been made to study the kinetics of the fibrosis process (7) and to quantitate cellularity and fibrosis better in the biopsy specimen (8).

Among the interstitial diseases listed in Table 13.1, IPF should be considered as a diagnosis of exclusion, after common diseases such as collagen-vascular ones and diseases with a more distinctive radiographic presentation (stage I sarcoidosis with symmetrical hilar adenopathy) or with a characteristic clinical pattern (hypersensitivity pneumonitis) have been eliminated. However, this subtraction method for arriving at the diagnosis of IPF should not be construed to mean that the disease is uncommon. In fact, when the differential diagnoses suggested by the list of interstitial diseases in Table 13.1 are worked through, about 25% of patients presenting with a chest radiographic pattern of lower lung zone reticular markings will eventually end up in the IPF category. To repeat, IPF is a distinct clinical entity and not a wastebasket diagnosis to conveniently categorize patients with unusual or obscure lung disease.

## CLINICAL PRESENTATION AND EVALUATION

At the inception of disease, the patient feels short of breath or notes a change in his or her tolerance to some prescribed or accustomed amount of exercise. A dry cough frequently occurs. Unless there are systemic symptoms or other organ involvement suggesting a generalized illness, the patient may do nothing more than try to adjust to the episodic dyspnea. The symptoms and physical signs can be very nebulous in the early phase of disease, and the physician may not immediately put the diagnosis together. This breathlessness will have no other obvious cause such as asthma, obstructive airway disease, bronchitis, or heart failure. Other respiratory signs such as pleuritis, chest pain, wheezing, or hemoptysis, do not usually occur. Although sputum production is not present in many patients, about half may have mucus hypersecretion and expectoration. This occurrence has been correlated with glandular hypertrophy in the airway mucosa and accumulated mucus in the airways (9). Cigarette smokers are not apt to reduce their habit. Many patients have an occupational history that includes exposure to one or a variety of toxic inhalation products, and this may add uncertainty to the precise onset of symptoms and may suggest the contribution of several etiologic factors. A detailed work history, including each job dating back even to summer employment during school, is essential. Casual exposure to asbestos decades ago may provide a crucial link. Worker compensation and not respiratory symptoms per se may be a motivating factor for some people who seek evaluation.

A surprising percentage of patients, perhaps 30%, can pinpoint their awareness of breathlessness as an aftermath of a respiratory infection that is usually described as a viral illness. Even minor upper respiratory tract infections (influenza A) cause acute small-airway changes, and these changes can take several months to clear completely, which emphasizes the widespread impact of even mild viral disease in the lungs (10). An association between IPF and serum antibodies to hepatitis C has been noted (11) but needs further confirmation. Whether viruses can actually initiate the cellular inflammatory response that sets off the interstitial disease process is unknown. To date, adequate experimental models that simulate IPF have been difficult to create, so the viral hypothesis remains untested. Months to several years (mean about 1 to 3 years) may elapse between the onset of dyspnea and its progression to the point of symptomatic breathlessness that is sufficient to bring the patient to the physician's attention. When dyspnea is noticeable and imposes physical limitation, other constitutional symptoms may be present, such as fatigue, poor appetite, weight loss, and arthralgias. Fever is infrequent. Patients are usually in middle age (average age about 50 years), although the range includes young adults and some people in the sixth or seventh decade. The disease has been described in infants (12). Because several family clusters have been noted, it is likely that genetic factors can determine susceptibility to the disease.

Initially, the physical examination may not be revealing. Auscultation of the chest may be normal; but with disease progression, adventitial rales or crackles are usually heard. Vivid adjectives have been used to describe these lung sounds—"Velcro," crackling or cellophane paper, or "close to the ear." Other findings may include tachypnea at rest (50% of patients), ability to speak only in phrases of a few words because of breathlessness, and finger clubbing (70%) without hypertrophic osteoarthropathy (2). Occasionally, cyanosis can be detected. In later stages, cardiac involvement is frequent, and signs pointing to pulmonary artery hypertension and right heart failure are noted in many (60 to 70%). An augmented pulmonic second heart sound, right-sided lift, and S(sub 3) gallop, in addition to peripheral signs of heart failure, signal the presence of pulmonary hypertension and cor pulmonale. Right ventricular ejection fraction by radionuclide scan is often depressed in the face of normal left ventricular performance. Except for clubbing and evidence of heart failure, physical signs are limited to the chest, and other organ systems are not prominently involved.

The chest radiograph is still important in establishing an initial diagnosis, for it usually reveals a pattern of diffuse reticular markings, prominent in the lower lung zones (Fig. 13.2). A most important consideration at this point is to retrieve any existing chest radiographs and compare them for prior changes. Again, for emphasis, it is important to investigate the patient's occupational and recreational history for evidence of a toxic environmental exposure. Not all patients with a chronic diffuse interstitial lung disease will have an abnormal chest radiograph. In one series of 458 patients with biopsy-established forms of diffuse interstitial lung disease, about 10% had normal chest radiographs prior to a diagnostic lung biopsy (13). Patients with desquamative interstitial pneumonitis (an early pathologic form of alveolitis in IPF), sarcoidosis, and allergic alveolitis accounted for most of the patients with a clear chest radiograph. This retrospective study still leaves the clinician with two problems: (*a*) What physical signs and symptoms make one suspicious enough of the diagnosis to pursue it with a bronchoscopy and transbronchial biopsy or with an open lung biopsy in spite of the normal chest radiograph? (*b*)

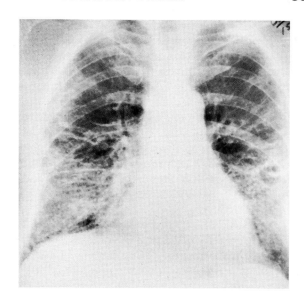

**FIGURE 13.2.** Idiopathic pulmonary fibrosis. Posterior-anterior (PA) chest radiograph of a 71-year-old man with end-stage pulmonary fibrosis. There are diffuse, bilateral interstitial infiltrates that form a honeycombing pattern.

What ancillary tests can establish that the lung parenchyma is in fact abnormal? In 22 of the 44 patients reviewed by Epler and coworkers (13), unexplained dyspnea and impaired lung function prompted the biopsy, and appropriately so. In the remainder, the biopsy was performed for other valid indications—pleural plaques, recurrent effusions, pneumothoraces, or possible hemoptyses—and in three cases autopsy tissue was obtained. Unsuspected interstitial lung pathology was a chance finding in these cases. The message is clear, however, that the standard chest radiograph can be normal in appearance, so we recommend continued evaluation in patients who have significant exercise intolerance, abnormal pulmonary function tests (including the diffusing capacity), and abnormal physical findings on examination of the chest (crackles).

In addition to the standard chest radiographs, interpretation of the HRCT may improve diagnostic accuracy from about one-third to about 46% for a form of diffuse interstitial lung disease when a group of pulmonary clinicians and radiologists compared both kinds of imaging studies (14).

Serologic and routine blood tests are indicated but may reveal few abnormalities of specific help. The erythrocyte sedimentation rate is elevated in most (90%), circulating immune complex titers may be high (15), serum immunoglobulin levels are increased by 30% or so, and cryoimmunoglobulins may be found in a surprisingly high number (41%) (2). Serologic tests to screen for collagen-vascular diseases are necessary to exclude these diagnoses with confidence. In IPF, however, serum rheumatoid factor, lupus erythematosus cell preparations, low levels of complement activity, antinuclear antibodies, and autoimmune parameters can be detected (10% frequency or less), but the titers are low and usually do not cause confusion with the collagen-vascular diseases, for which such serologic tests are much more important in establishing a diagnosis. Despite hypoxemia, at times profound, red cell mass is not usually increased and polycythemia is unusual (15% or less) (2).

Use of $^{67}$Ga gallium citrate isotope to scan the lungs has been touted to be helpful in assessing the overall inflammation in the lung parenchyma of many patients. In this disease, gallium uptake in lung was found to correlate with the presence of polymorphonuclear granulocytes in the airways and lung tissue (16). Initially, it was thought that lung scans might be a useful way to monitor treatment aimed at suppressing inflammation, but this has not developed (17). Recently, the proportional grading of the ground-glass and reticular patterns found in lung parenchyma by HRCT images has seemed to predict the long-term outcome of patients with IPF (6), which is notable but needs more substantiation in other series.

Lung function tests in virtually all patients with advanced disease reveal a reduction in total lung capacity and residual volume, indicating small, contracted lungs (18–20). Usually evidence of airway obstruction is minimal and the FEV(sub 1)/FVC ratio is within normal limits. The restrictive respiratory function pattern is characteristic of stiff, noncompliant lungs. The diffusing capacity, assessed by a single-breath carbon monoxide method (DLCO), is often reduced by 50 to 75% and is relied on heavily to support the diagnosis. The effect of cigarette smoking has to be factored into the lung function results, and this can produce obstructive changes. Thus, smoking introduces variability into these tests for lung volumes, pressure-volume characteristics and respiratory rate (21, 22). There is usually resting arterial hypoxemia, but the carbon dioxide tension is not elevated.

Exercise performance to measure the alveolar-arterial oxygen gradient is helpful in monitoring the course of disease and in assessing the effectiveness of various forms of treatment. Direct investigation of the airways by fiberoptic bronchoscopy is usually part of the evaluation, and transbronchial biopsy is an established means of obtaining samples of lung tissue for diagnosis. Bronchoalveolar lavage can be part of this procedure (23–31). Biopsies obtained through the bronchoscope can be taken from several places in a particular

lung but suffer from the fact that they are only several millimeters in size. Whereas an adequate number of alveoli may be visualized in a biopsy specimen, vessels and larger airways are not usually obtained; moreover, such specimens are inadequate for metal or inorganic fiber analysis of the tissue. Transbronchial biopsy usually does not give a sufficient amount of tissue for a definitive diagnosis. However, since it is a low-risk procedure in terms of significant bleeding and development of pneumothorax, transbronchial biopsy offers a reasonably safe attempt for a moderate yield of diagnostic tissue. In some diffuse, granulomatous interstitial diseases, such as sarcoidosis, the transbronchial biopsy will provide a tissue diagnosis in about 70% of cases. Moreover, bronchoscopy allows one to do a lung lavage, which gives helpful information about cells and proteins in the airways that seem to correlate with histologic changes present in the interstitial and alveolar areas (25–32).

If a transbronchial biopsy does not yield sufficient tissue for a confident diagnosis, the decision to proceed with an open biopsy must be weighed (32). Because an open lung biopsy is a once-only tissue procedure for most patients, this specimen is best obtained as part of the initial evaluation that establishes the diagnosis. Moreover, such a tissue specimen can give valuable information about inorganic contaminants in the lungs that might be causing concomitant disease. As occupational injury and worker's compensation are often factors that complicate many of these cases of diffuse interstitial lung disease, analysis of metals, silicates, and such substances is relevant. The importance of an adequate sample of lung tissue to permit a full histologic evaluation, good microbial cultures, tissue immunologic or immunofluorescence identification of lymphocytes and other inflammatory cells and electron microscopy study, sufficient analysis of inorganic substances, and a specimen for storage for future reference or study cannot be emphasized enough.

Less invasive ways of obtaining lung tissue are being evaluated, including video-guided thoracoscopic lung biopsy. Comparing this method with a modified open thoracotomy approach (33), it was found that comparable numbers of biopsies and amount of tissue were obtained and that length of the patient's hospital stay, duration of chest tube placement, and complications were less with the thoracoscopic technique. Whether the surgical fees and cost are less is hard to determine; certainly hospital stay is shortened. Some have said that losing the ability to palpate the areas of lung selected for biopsy is a drawback for any procedure short of the wider exposure with a formal thoracotomy. Patient morbidity must be weighed also.

## Lung Histology and Staging Disease Activity

Although general characteristics of lung pathologic changes are presented for each of the interstitial diseases discussed, a detailed description such as may be found in a pathology textbook is not given. For an excellent review of histologic changes in ILD, the article by Fulmer and Katzenstein is recommended (34). Presented here are a few concepts that correlate the patient's clinical status with findings present in lung tissue in an attempt to integrate pathophysiology and histology. The concepts include staging and activity of lung disease, characterizing inflammatory and immune effector cells in airways and lung parenchyma, and monitoring these immunologic parameters in a dynamic way that will allow the natural progression of the disease to be assessed or the effects of immunosuppressive or cytotoxic therapy to be evaluated in an objective way (35).

Usually patients with very early forms of IPF are not extensively evaluated because of the mild or possibly confusing complex of signs and symptoms. Tissue histology is rarely available. Most undergo definitive workup in the midperiod of disease. Thus, staging or assessing the activity of the cellular inflammatory reaction in the lungs becomes paramount because cellular forms of the disease usually respond best to therapy or have a higher rate of spontaneous regression (35–37). More advanced, acellular forms of disease in which excessive collagen deposition and fibrotic distortion of alveolar and interstitial architecture are pronounced are minimally responsive to therapy, as might be anticipated. Thus, the patient's clinical prognosis is determined largely by the histologic characteristics of lung tissue. Other factors that give the patient a better chance of response include younger age, recent onset of disease, female sex, finding of inflammatory cells in lung lavage analysis, and, especially, a relative increase in lymphocytes (17).

Three histologic features seem important. First is the degree of cellularity. Does the lung sample contain an abundance of inflammatory or reactive cells that suggest initial phases of disease, or is fibrosis already extensive? Second, what is the pattern or distribution of the cellular reaction? Collections of cells primarily in the alveolar spaces consisting of macrophages, type II pneumocytes, and inflammatory cells (polymorphonuclear granulocytes [PMNs] and eosinophils) suggest an alveolitis phase (3, 30, 38–40). Such histologic findings, when predominant, have been used to diagnose a desquamative form of interstitial pneumonitis (DIP), as described by Liebow and colleagues (36). Since the histology is usually not uniform throughout an entire lung, this rather rigid and formal method of histologic classification is not as accurate as it once seemed. Moreover, the appearance on the HRCT may give a better clue (6). However, the distinction between DIP and usual interstitial pneumonitis (UIP) has proved to be helpful in predicting the clinical course of patients so subdivided (37). The survival and corticosteroid responsiveness of patients with DIP are strikingly different than those of patients with UIP.

Third, the type of inflammatory or immune effector cells that are prevalent in the lung tissue is important and once again will give insight into the proposed efficacy of therapy. Biopsies that contain many PMNs, eosinophils, and especially lymphocytes (27, 31) often correlate with a response to corticosteroid therapy. This third feature is usually synonymous with that found in the previously described cellular lung specimen.

For staging the immune reactivity of lung tissue, sampling the peripheral airways and alveoli by bronchoalveolar lavage (BAL) is a helpful method for assessing airway inflammation and the accumulation of immune effector cells and proteins in the alveoli. Such BAL results correlate surprisingly well with cellular reactivity occurring in the interstitial tissue (2, 29–32). BAL analysis seems useful in gauging the degree of alveolitis present. Bronchoalveolar lavage is done in conjunction with diagnostic fiberoptic bronchoscopy and transbronchial biopsy, which are indicated for evaluation of patients with interstitial lung disease (40). Sterile saline is infused through the wedged bronchoscope in 20- to 50-ml aliquots, which are immediately aspirated by syringe; for adult patients a total of about 150 to 300 ml is instilled. Methods for handling the lavage fluid; separating respiratory cells from the lavage supernatant; preparing the fluid for measurement of protein, immunoglobulins, lipids (surfactant), and enzymes; and enumerating the respiratory cells have all been described in detail (27, 29, 30, 40–42). How many of these BAL constituents can be analyzed depends on the availability of the assays in the clinical laboratory. However, total cells and a differential count can be readily obtained on the respiratory cells in BAL and offer the most useful parameter at present. Quantitation of lymphocyte subclasses and macrophage secretory proteins, enzymes, or phospholipids (43) requires special laboratory facilities.

The recovery of increased percentages of inflammatory cells in lavage (i.e., 20% or more polymorphonuclear granulocytes in nonsmokers and 3 to 4% or more eosinophils) is characteristic of IPF and correlates well with interstitial inflammation in lung biopsy tissue (23–30). High-intensity alveolitis is defined by 10% or more PMNs in the BAL cell differential counts; patients with low-intensity alveolitis have 10% PMNs or less.

TABLE 13.2
IDIOPATHIC PULMONARY FIBROSIS—CELLULAR AND IMMUNOLOGIC CHANGES IN BLOOD, BRONCHOALVEOLAR LAVAGE FLUID, AND LUNG TISSUE

| Blood | Bronchoalveolar Fluid | Lung Tissue |
|---|---|---|
| Ig (IgG$_{1,3}$)<br>Immune complexes<br>Cryoglobulins<br>Serologic titers (low)<br>T-lymphs (sensitized to type I collagen) | Alveolitis (characterized by more macrophages and increased percentage of PMNs [20%] and eosinophils [2–4%], but lymphs can be increased also [20%])<br>Alveolar macrophages (active with numerous secretory components)<br>    Chemotaxins to attract PMN (Il-8 and LTB4) and smooth muscle cells<br>    Plasminogen activator<br>    Fibroblast growth factor<br>    Fibronectin<br>    Platelet-derived growth factor<br>    Steroid receptors increased<br>    Mitosis index increased<br>Collagenase (PMN origin)<br>IgG G$_3$, G$_1$ subclasses<br>Immune complexes<br>IgG-releasing cells<br>Histamine elevated<br>Abnormal content of surfactant Protein A<br>N-Terminal type III procollagen peptides | Interstitial inflammation<br>    Plasma cells<br>    Fibroblasts<br>        Collagen synthesis (type 11 > 1)<br>Fibrosis but no granulomas<br>Bronchiolitis obliterans can develop |

Evidence also indicates that the number of IgG-containing plasma cells (28) isolated from BAL fluid of IPF patients is quite high; after treatment with corticosteroids, the number decreases, giving some "cellular" substance to the prior observation that IgG levels may decrease as the disease responds or stabilizes with immunosuppressive therapy. Weinberger and coworkers (24) examined the PMN and IgG-albumin indices in eight patients who had repeated bronchoscopy with BAL analysis. Seven of these patients showed reduction in one or both of these measurements in response to therapy.

In airway secretions, ever-increasing numbers of enzymes and soluble proteins are being measured and identified as specific secretion products of alveolar macrophages or characteristic of certain lung disease (26, 44–53 ) (Table 13.2). Not only is the list of new substances found in BAL fluid lengthening (48–51), but the source of their secretion, often the alveolar macrophage, is being examined at the gene and molecular levels (52, 53).

## IMMUNOPATHOGENIC CONCEPTS OF IPF

Idiopathic pulmonary fibrosis seems to be an immunologically mediated disease set in motion after an initial acute injury or infection and driven or perpetuated in a chronic phase by activated or poorly regulated macrophages. The inciting antigen still remains unknown, but it might be a viral protein or some residual of a viral respiratory infection or hepatitis, since the association between a viral infection and the onset of symptoms that culminate in the IPF syndrome is quite clear in some patients. IgG in airway secretions and in blood, often in the form of immune complexes (15, 44), is increased in most patients; specific antibody reactivity in the IgG fraction has not been identified. IgG-secreting plasma cells can be recovered in increased numbers in bronchoalveolar lavage. The intervening steps between immune complex formation and their localization in lung tissue and the influx of such cells as PMNs and eosinophils into alveoli and interstitial spaces are still incompletely known (44).

Referring to Table 13.2, the combination of airway cells retrieved by BAL reflects an alveolitis characterized by an abundance of macrophages and a mixture of PMNs and eosinophils; increased lymphocytes are unusual unless the IPF is associated with a collagen vascular disorder. The macrophages are activated cells and are capable of producing a number of mediators that help to explain the inflammatory and fibrotic process. What activates the macrophages is not certain; but, should it be an IgG-containing immune complex on their cellular membranes, this would be a potent stimulus for the secretion of chemotaxins (44, 50–52, 54) and perhaps of the other fibrogenic factors (44, 45). Chemotaxins could attract PMNs into the alveoli, and subsequent elastolytic injury to the epithelial lining might develop. Likewise, substances like platelet-derived growth factor could attract smooth muscle cells and mesenchymal cells such as fibroblasts (46, 53). Fibroblast proliferation, occurring either in the interstitial areas of the alveolar units or in the intraluminal alveolar spaces as buds that form from rents in the type I cell epithelial lining (55), is the essence of the fibrotic process. What is intriguing now is the possibility that other alveolar-located cells may be participating in attracting and stimulating fibroblasts, so a new role for epithelial cells and for type II pneumocytes is evolving in addition to the one of the macrophage (56). The alveolar macrophage still seems to be a pivotal cell in the process, and new things continue to be uncovered about its activity (57, 58).

## TREATMENT AND PROGNOSIS

Plans and expectations that the physician and the patient develop and share about the response of IPF to therapy are predicated on how well some of the foregoing information has been collected and analyzed. An accurate diagnosis based on good histologic conclusions, attempted staging of the disease, assembly of good baseline physiologic and immunologic parameters to compare with later values for objectively assessing "improvement," and a perspective of the natural history of the disease are all essential before therapy is undertaken. A decision not to pursue an adequate lung tissue biopsy because it entails the unpleasantness of chest surgery or thoracoscopic biopsy and instead just to give the patient an empiric trial of corticosteroid therapy may not be advantageous to the patient in the long run. If definitive tissue must then be obtained after failure of treatment, or if proper staging and baseline data have not been established, the clinician may have no basis for discontinuing treatment should significant side effects from corticosteroids or cytotoxic drugs develop. In general, cellular stages of IPF respond best, but such histologic findings suggest an early phase of disease and are often noted in the young patient, both being circumstances that improve prospects for suppressing or arresting the disease. Desquamative alveolar stages of the disease also have about a 20% rate of spontaneous remission (37), and this must temper one's enthusiasm for strongly advocating that a particular regimen of therapy is efficacious. Finally, therapy for a disease of still-undiscovered etiology is nonspecific by definition, so the current strategy is directed at interrupting some step in the host's tissue response to the inciting agent and attacking the perceived injurious sequence. The drugs currently in use are far from specific in this respect.

Corticosteroids are the mainstay of therapy for IPF at present, and a trial with them is reasonable, even for patients who seem to be in an advanced stage of disease with relatively acellular and fibrotic changes in lung tissue. The concept of a trial must be emphasized. Immunosuppressive therapy will be given for a prescribed period and discontinued unless objective parameters show that it is effective; then maintenance therapy seems advisable. Such parameters include blood counts, erythrocyte sedimentation rate (ESR), pulmonary function testing, especially exercise tests with measurement of arterial oxygen desaturation and diffusing capacity for carbon monoxide ($D_{LCO}$), perhaps changes in the HRCT scan images and the patient's symptoms. A satisfactory regimen to use follows: Prednisone, 1 mg/kg/day, is given as a single oral dose for 6 to 8 weeks; then the dose is tapered slowly by reducing the daily dose by 0.05 mg/kg per week until a maintenance dose of 0.25 mg/kg/day is reached (1). This maintenance dose, which ranges from 15 to 30 mg/day of prednisone for the majority of patients, may be continued for another 6 months or so. After a total of 1 year of corticosteroid therapy, a careful decision should be made about weaning or continuing therapy. Some flexibility can be exercised in tailoring the maintenance therapy, and an alternate-day dose may be used if corticosteroid side effects are a significant management problem.

For patients who do not seem to be controlled with or responsive to corticosteroids (59), additional immunosuppressive therapy needs consideration. Cyclophosphamide, an alkylating drug, is a potent immunosuppressant and seems to be effective in some patients who are not controlled with corticosteroids (17, 60). Some information substantiates the use of cyclophosphamide as the preferred treatment for IPF, and hence it has been tried as the initial treatment instead of corticosteroids. The drug is taken orally in graduated amounts (50 mg/day initially, with 50-mg dose increments at approximately weekly intervals until a dose of 150 to 200 mg/day is reached for most patients) until a controlled and stable degree of peripheral blood lymphopenia is achieved. Ideally, a dose that suppresses the total lymphocyte count by half its baseline amount, yet preserves a circulating polymorphonuclear granulocyte count of 500/mm$^3$ or more to prevent bacterial infection, should be the goal. With frequent patient follow-up for side effects and blood counts, reasonably tight control can be maintained with cyclophosphamide. If improvement in the lung disease is documented after 3 months of this therapy, it should be continued for a 12-month interval. Alternatively, an intermittent schedule every 2 weeks using intravenous administration beginning with a 500-mg dosage seems to be a very successful protocol as well (60).

Azathioprine has been used as an alternative to cyclophosphamide. Penicillamine has been used in some patients in preliminary trials, with the rationale that it might prevent the cross-linking of abnormal collagen being synthesized in the interstitium and prevent or retard fibrosis (61). Patients who seem to show improvement with penicillamine tend to be those with earlier stages of disease, which suggests that this therapy is valuable in arresting disease rather than in improving established fibrosis. Patients with connective tissue diseases and interstitial fibrosis seem to show more improvement with penicillamine than those with IPF. Recently, the use of colchicine has been found effective for some patients with IPF (62) and needs evaluation in a larger group of patients in a prospective trial. This medication suppresses the release of a fibroblast factor from alveolar macrophages in vitro (63).

In addition to suppressing the patient's alveolitis and stabilizing the inflammatory process, several other measures may help respiratory function. It is imperative that these patients stop cigarette smoking. Although patients can have relatively normal oxygen saturation at rest, with exercise there is frequently a marked drop in arterial oxygen tension (Pao(sub 2)). Therefore, exercise tolerance may be significantly improved with supplemental oxygen therapy. When oxygen requirements are high (more than 4 liters/minute flow), direct administration of oxygen in the trachea may be preferred. Several modes of transtracheal catheter oxygen delivery are available (64). In addition to attaining a high local concentration of oxygen in the lungs, the cosmetic effect of not wearing obvious nasal prongs can be important. As the pulmonary vascular bed is impaired by progressive fibrosis, pulmonary hypertension and cor pulmonale can develop; right-sided congestive heart failure can be difficult to control. Judicious use of diuretics is advised, for a significant decrease in intravascular volume may be deleterious for lung perfusion. Digitalis or antiarrhythmic drugs might be required, although adequate oxygenation is probably the best treatment for heart failure. Some patients may also develop obstruction to air flow and be troubled with wheezing and coughing that may respond to bronchodilators. As infection may occur during immunosuppressive therapy, it is important to maintain a high index of suspicion and to treat infection aggressively. Prophylactic use of pneumococcal and influenza vaccines is encouraged. Finally, with refractory disease limited to the chest, the question of

lung transplantation arises. Recent success with single-lung transplantation for IPF (65–68) will make this therapy a reality for some patients, and already more medical institutions are offering the service.

In summary, the long-term prognosis of IPF is variable, and some patients may live 5 to 10 years with the disease. The stage at which the diagnosis is established and the degree of fibrosis are important features. Having a certain diagnosis based on an adequate specimen of lung tissue is important and may prevent some of the pitfalls of management and complications from inappropriate immunosuppression.

The identification of cellular mediators in the affected lung tissue and improved concepts of how these may injure tissue and promote fibrosis will lead to different forms of specific antimediator therapy in the future. For a selected few, lung transplantation may be a hope for improved health. The smoldering fibrotic disease continues to create health problems chronically. Terminal problems experienced by patients include increasing dyspnea, severe hypoxemia requiring supplemental home oxygen therapy, right heart failure, and complications from prolonged immunosuppressive therapy. Approximately 10% of patients will develop lung cancer, which means that patients with IPF have approximately a 6-fold (females) or 14-fold (males) increased risk of cancer (69).

## BRONCHIOLITIS OBLITERANS ORGANIZING PNEUMONIA (BOOP)

In 1985, Epler and coworkers (70) reported 94 patients with bronchiolitis obliterans, of whom 50 had patchy organizing pneumonia and no apparent cause or associated disease. Histologic characteristics of this bronchiolitis pneumonia (BOOP) included polypoid masses of granulation tissue in lumens of small airways, alveolar ducts, and some alveoli. Clinically, patients had a cough or flu-like illness for 4 to 10 weeks, and crackles were heard in the lungs of 68% of the patients. Chest radiographs showed an unusual pattern of patchy densities with a "ground-glass" appearance in 81%. There was a restrictive ventilatory defect in 72% and an abnormal diffusing capacity in 86%. Only cigarette smokers had evidence of airway obstruction on pulmonary function tests. Corticosteroid treatment was efficacious, and over a mean follow-up period of 4 years, complete clinical and physiologic recovery occurred in 65% of patients; only two died of progressive disease. BOOP is most often confused with idiopathic pulmonary fibrosis (70–74), which generally has a poorer prognosis and does not respond in most cases to corticosteroids. Moreover, IPF has a more insidious onset and the chest radiograph shows bilateral interstitial opacities, while localized air space densities are a feature in BOOP (73).

## CONNECTIVE TISSUE (COLLAGEN VASCULAR) DISEASES

Connective tissue is an extracellular material composed of a physiologically active ground substance containing fibrils of elastin, collagen, and reticulin. Alteration in the chemical composition and physical constitution of the ground substance leads to edema, fibrinoid degeneration, and vascular lesions characteristic of the connective tissue diseases (75, 76). The lungs may be the first organ involved in these diseases. In this section, the pulmonary manifestations of four connective tissue diseases are reviewed: systemic lupus erythematosus, rheumatoid arthritis, diffuse progressive systemic sclerosis (scleroderma), and polymyositis-dermatomyositis). Sjögren's syndrome (77–79) and mixed connective tissue disease (79–85) also have pleuropulmonary manifestations.

### SYSTEMIC LUPUS ERYTHEMATOSUS

Systemic lupus erythematosus (SLE) is a disease of unknown etiology that most often affects young women (86, 87). Connective tissues of any organ in the body can be involved, but the vascular system, the epidermis, and the serous and synovial membranes are most common. Pulmonary illness, however, may be the presenting manifestation of SLE (75, 88–99). Pleuropulmonary manifestations of SLE are summarized in Table 13.3 (79). The lungs and pleura are frequently affected in SLE, with involvement occurring in 50 to 70% of SLE patients (79, 88). Respiratory muscle dysfunction (100), including diaphragmatic muscle weakness (101), has been described in patients with SLE. This may in part explain the well-described basilar atelectasis and so-called vanishing lung syndrome noted in patients with this disease. Chest radiographic

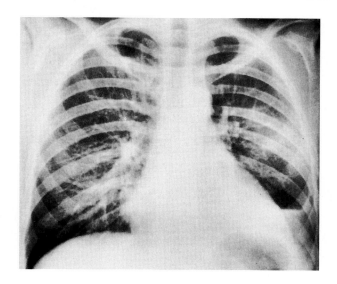

**FIGURE 13.3.** Systemic lupus erythematosus. PA chest radiograph of a 19-year-old man with an established diagnosis of systemic lupus erythematosus (SLE) who developed fever and shortness of breath acutely. Note the left pleural effusion and enlarged cardiac silhouette. An echocardiogram revealed pericardial fluid. Corticosteroid therapy was instituted, and within 5 days the chest radiograph returned to normal.

changes in patients with SLE include cardiac enlargement, pericardial effusion, pleuritis with or without effusion, and pulmonary infiltrates (Figs. 13.3 and 13.4) (75, 79, 88, 93, 102–104). The lung bases are most frequently involved with patchy areas of increased density, focal atelectasis with diaphragmatic elevation, and acute acinar or chronic interstitial infiltrates. The pulmonary infiltration tends to be recurrent and migratory in nature.

Pleural effusions, usually small but sometimes massive, are frequently bilateral (75, 79, 97, 103, 105–107). Winslow and coworkers (103) emphasized the importance of pleuritis as an early manifestation of SLE. Pleural effusion occurred in 42 (81%) of their 57 patients; in three it was an isolated first sign, and in 16 others it was associated with only minor antecedent symptoms. Such pleural effusions are inflammatory exudates, containing both mononuclear and polymorphonuclear cells. The glucose concentration and pH of the pleural fluid are within normal range. The finding of LE cells in the fluid is diagnostic. Moreover, a high pleural fluid antinuclear antibody (ANA) titer (1:160 or greater) and a pleural fluid to serum ANA titer ratio of greater than 1 strongly support the diagnosis (106). Low total and individual complement components are also characteristic of pleural effusion in SLE (85). Due

### TABLE 13.3
### PLEUROPULMONARY MANIFESTATIONS OF SYSTEMIC LUPUS ERYTHEMATOSUS

Pleurisy with or without effusion
Diaphragmatic dysfunction with reduced lung volume
Acute lupus pneumonitis
Diffuse alveolar hemorrhage
Diffuse interstitial disease
Pulmonary hypertension
Pulmonary thromboembolism

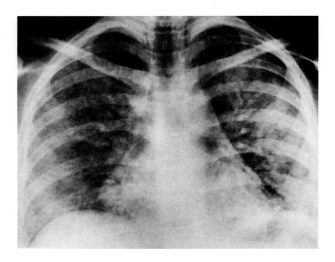

**FIGURE 13.4.** Systemic lupus erythematosus. PA chest radiograph of an 18-year-old woman with acute lupus pneumonitis. Note the bilateral alveolar filling process. Two weeks after corticosteroid and azathioprine therapy was instituted the chest radiograph had cleared markedly.

to the excellent response to corticosteroids, pleural fibrosis and resultant pleural entrapment and restrictive lung disease are uncommon sequelae (85).

Although many patients develop pulmonary infiltrates unrelated to infection (88, 102, 104), infection still appears to be the most frequent cause of pulmonary infiltrates in SLE (75, 102). Some cases with pulmonary infiltrates not caused by infection have an acute onset; others are chronic. Acute lupus pneumonitis (ALP) is characterized by severe dyspnea, a cough productive of scant sputum, fever (100 to 104 F), negative sputum and blood cultures, hypoxemia, and a bilateral alveolar filling process on the chest radiograph (Fig. 13.4) (88). Associated findings include cardiomegaly and pleuritis, with or without effusion. Clearing of the pulmonary infiltrates in response to corticosteroids is frequently rapid. Azathioprine has been administered with success to a small group of patients who did not respond to corticosteroids alone (88). ALP can develop during the course of the illness or can be the initial manifestation of SLE in 50% of cases with this complication (85, 88). In half of the patients surviving the acute illness, the chest radiograph clears completely. In the other half, the disease progresses to chronic interstitial pneumonitis, with hypocapnia, restrictive pulmonary function, and decreased DLCO (88).

Diffuse alveolar hemorrhage, which can be confused with ALP, is characterized by the acute onset of fever, cough, dyspnea, and hemoptysis (85, 105, 108). The concomitant occurrence of a fall in hematocrit and a diffuse alveolar filling pattern on the chest radiograph support the diagnosis (105). Unlike ALP, diffuse alveolar hemorrhage is not associated with pleural or pericardial disease and is not a presenting manifestation of SLE (105). The incidence of this complication is low, but may be rising (105). In spite of treatment with corticosteroids, immunosuppressives, and plasmapheresis, the mortality rate is high (85, 105).

In 1973, Eisenberg and coworkers (104) reported 18 patients and in 1990 Weinrib, Sharma, and Quismorio (109) reported 14 patients with SLE and chronic diffuse interstitial lung disease. Pulmonary symptoms in these patients included dyspnea, a nonproductive cough, and pleuritic chest pain. Physical findings were poor diaphragmatic movement and basilar crackles, but clubbing was not a feature in these patients. Hypoxemia, a restrictive ventilatory defect, and reduced diffusing capacity were evident on pulmonary function tests. Huang and coworkers (110) and Andonopoulos and coworkers (111) noted that patients with SLE may demonstrate these abnormalities in the absence of clinical symptoms or abnormal chest radiographs. In fact, Andonopoulos and coworkers (111) found normal function in only one-third of 70 nonsmoking patients with SLE, and an isolated reduction in DLCO was the most commonly detected functional abnormality (31% of patients).

Pulmonary hypertension in SLE can be secondary to progressive interstitial pneumonitis with resultant lung destruction and hypoxia, or it can be due to a primary fibroproliferative pulmonary vasculopathy (105). Fewer than 50 cases of the latter, primary form have been reported (105). This entity must be differentiated from recurrent pulmonary embolism. Raynaud's phenomenon is present in 75% of the cases, and women are affected in more than 90% of the cases (105). There is an associated glomerulonephritis in 63% of patients and cutaneous vasculitis in 33% (112).

Although most patients who die of SLE have severe pathologic changes in their lungs, there are no features that are considered unique (113–119). Gross and coworkers (119) found a high frequency of interstitial pneumonitis (98%), interstitial fibrosis (70%), and chronic pleuritis (95%) in 44 autopsy specimens. Acute inflammation of small pulmonary arteries and arterioles was found in 19%. Other common but nonspecific changes in those who die of SLE include alveolar hyaline membranes, hemorrhage (114–117), and capillary thrombi (88, 113). The pleural lesions often seen in this disease are usually manifested pathologically by a fibrinous pleuritis (119).

Treatment of SLE is usually directed at control of the systemic disease and preservation of renal function if the kidneys are seriously involved. Corticosteroids and cyclophosphamide are the main immunosuppressive drugs used, and in severe cases plasmapheresis is indicated (75, 79, 88). A general statement about therapy of lung disease can be made for SLE and other collagen-vascular diseases. When therapy is required because of pulmonary involvement, corticosteroids are usually tried first in doses similar to those used in IPF (i.e., 1 mg/kg). Scleroderma lung involvement is an exception, since it does not respond to corticosteroids, and therefore such therapy is not indicated.

An additional important complication in patients with SLE and a circulating lupus anticoagulant (antiphospholipid antibody) is venous thrombosis and pulmonary thromboembolism (85, 112, 120). A 25% incidence of pulmonary emboli has been reported in patients with SLE in whom a circulating anticoagulant is present (120).

## RHEUMATOID ARTHRITIS

Rheumatoid arthritis is a disease that primarily affects the joints, but it also involves other organs and tissues, including the lungs and pleura (79, 121–132). Pleuropulmonary disease is more common in patients with rheumatoid arthritis who have severe chronic articular disease, high titers of rheumatoid factor, subcutaneous nodules, and other systemic manifestations such as Felty's syndrome, cutaneous vasculitis, myopericarditis, and ocular inflammation (85, 129). There are several pleuropulmonary abnormalities associated with the rheumatoid process (Table 13.4) (75, 97, 121, 122, 133–140). Pleural involvement by the rheumatoid process is the most common thoracic complication of rheumatoid arthritis and accounts for attacks of pleurisy with or without effusion. Such pleurisy has a remarkable predilection for males, despite the fact that rheumatoid arthritis occurs predominantly in females in a ratio of 2:1. Pleural disease secondary to rheumatoid arthritis is discussed in more detail in Chapter 18. It appears that pleural disease is one of the systemic manifestations of rheumatoid arthritis. Such pleural

**TABLE 13.4**
**PLEUROPULMONARY MANIFESTATIONS OF RHEUMATOID ARTHRITIS**

| |
| --- |
| Pleurisy with or without effusion |
| Interstitial lung disease |
| Pulmonary nodules |
| Bronchiolitis obliterans organizing pneumonia |
| Bronchiolitis obliterans |
| Pulmonary hypertension |

disease rarely causes complications except for the occasional case of fibrothorax and restrictive lung disease that necessitates decortication. However, all patients with rheumatoid arthritis who present with pleurisy and effusion should have appropriate studies to exclude empyema, tuberculosis, and malignancy.

The prevalence of interstitial lung disease as detected by chest radiographic screening of rheumatoid patients is small. In one series of 516 cases, only eight patients (2%) had radiographic evidence of interstitial lung disease (126). A much higher prevalence is detected by pulmonary function tests (126, 135). Restrictive ventilatory impairment and a reduction of the diffusing capacity have been found in as many as 41% of a group of patients with rheumatoid arthritis (126). High-resolution CT (HRCT) may also identify clinically silent interstitial lung disease (85). A higher prevalence of interstitial lung disease occurs in men with rheumatoid arthritis than in women.

No specific pattern of arthritis is associated with interstitial lung disease, although 50% of such patients have subcutaneous nodules. Interstitial pneumonitis and pleural disease may precede articular manifestations (85). Cough and dyspnea are often present, and clubbing is found in up to 75% of cases (136). The chest radiograph shows diffuse interstitial infiltrates, most marked in the lung bases, and in far-advanced disease, small cysts (honeycomb lung) appear accompanied by loss of lung volumes (85). Histopathologic examination of tissue may be helpful, especially when rheumatoid nodules are present in the lung interstitium in addition to the interstitial pneumonitis (75). Large amounts of rheumatoid factor in alveolar walls and pulmonary capillaries have been demonstrated by direct immunofluorescent staining of rheumatoid lung tissue. This suggests a possible immune mechanism for the development of pulmonary disease associated with rheumatoid arthritis (89). Moreover, recent studies suggest a pathogenic role of neutrophils (94) and collagenase (95) in rheumatoid interstitial lung disease. In patients with rheumatoid arthritis and interstitial pneumonitis in whom a cellular lung biopsy is obtained, there is a positive objective response to corticosteroids or other immunosuppressive medications (85, 121). The mean survival for all patients with rheumatoid arthritis and interstitial pneumonitis is 5 years (121).

The intrapulmonary rheumatoid or necrobiotic nodule, which is pathologically identical to the subcutaneous nodule in rheumatoid arthritis, is more common in men than in women (75, 121, 122). On the chest radiograph, necrobiotic nodules appear as single lesions or as bilateral, multiple, varying-sized coin lesions, with a predilection for the upper lung zones (85). Since the nodular form of rheumatoid lung disease may precede the arthritic manifestations, it must be differentiated from other granulomatous diseases. In the case of a single nodule, it may correlate with the activity and treatment status of the disease, and it must be differentiated from malignancy. Nodules may coexist with rheumatoid pleural effusions; spontaneous pneumothorax may also occur.

Caplan (128) has described a syndrome in coal miners with rheumatoid arthritis. This rheumatoid pneumoconiosis (Caplan's syndrome) is characterized by the appearance on chest radiograph of rounded densities that evolve rapidly and can undergo cavitation—in contrast to the massive fibrosis of coal workers' pneumoconiosis. A similar syndrome has been reported in rheumatoid arthritis patients who are sandblasters, asbestos workers, potters, boiler scalers, and brass and iron workers (75, 121, 122). The pneumoconiotic nodule consists of layers of partially necrotic collagen and dust. Occasionally there are foci of tuberculosis. The pulmonary disease may precede or coincide with the onset of the arthritis.

Bronchiolitis obliterans organizing pneumonia (BOOP) has been reported in a few patients with rheumatoid arthritis, and its frequency in this disease remains unknown (85, 130). Treatment with corticosteroids has been effective (85).

Bronchiolitis obliterans, a disease of the terminal airways characterized by progressive air flow limitation with preservation or increase of lung volumes, has been described in patients with rheumatoid arthritis (85, 131, 132). Patients complain of cough and dyspnea, and in most cases the chest radiograph is clear or shows hyperinflation (85). Chest examination reveals rhonchi with an inspiratory squeak or diminished breath sounds (85). An autoimmunopathogenesis has been suggested (85). Unfortunately, no effective therapy is available for this disorder, and survival is usually less than 2 years following diagnosis (131).

In rare cases, pulmonary vasculitis may cause pulmonary hypertension in rheumatoid arthritis; more commonly, pulmonary hypertension is the result of advancing fibrosing alveolitis. Raynaud's phenomenon has been present in a few reported cases of rheumatoid arthritis and pulmonary vasculitis (75, 121, 122).

## Progressive Systemic Sclerosis (Scleroderma)

Scleroderma is an inflammatory-fibrotic disorder of connective tissue that results in fibrosis and vascular abnormalities (85, 141). The skin, gastrointestinal tract, musculoskeletal system, kidneys, heart, and lungs are frequently involved (141–143). The majority of patients are affected in their fourth through sixth decades; the disease is three times more common in females than in males. Prognosis is unfavorable, and the cause of death is usually either renal, cardiovascular, or pulmonary.

Among the visceral organs involved in scleroderma, the lungs are second only to the esophagus (79, 141, 142, 144–151). Clinical or autopsy evidence of pulmonary involvement is found in at least 70% of cases (146, 151). Chest radiographic abnormalities have been reported in up to 25% of cases. Pulmonary symptoms have been found at some time during the course of the illness in 50% of patients. One series using pulmonary function tests reported abnormalities in 21 of 22 patients (145). Postmortem studies on 196 cases revealed that only 18% were free of pleuropulmonary involvement (146). Pulmonary fibrosis was found in 77%, pulmonary vascular disease in 30%, and pleural disease in 32%. Two recent studies (152, 153) suggest an increased risk of malignancy, particularly lung cancer, in patients with scleroderma.

The most prominent respiratory symptoms are dyspnea and, less commonly, a cough, which may be slightly productive (146). The most frequent signs are fine basilar crackles and limited expansion of the chest. Signs of cor pulmonale may appear as a result of pulmonary vascular and interstitial disease (149, 150).

The most common abnormality on chest radiograph is an interstitial reticular pattern, particularly affecting the lung bases. As the disease progresses, the pulmonary infiltration becomes denser, with subsequent honeycombing and cyst formation (141). The cysts are most often subpleural in the basal and paravertebral areas and are usually bilateral. Although they tend to be small (5 mm or less in diameter), large cysts may form and rupture, resulting in a pneumothorax. Other findings include micronodulation, increased vascular markings, and pulmonary edema. Disseminated pulmonary calcification or calcification of the soft tissue of the thorax may be seen on the chest radiograph (75, 142, 144). The latter may also demonstrate the presence of pleural thickening, pleural effusion, and signs of pulmonary hypertension secondary to scleroderma lung disease. Disturbance of esophageal motility may result in retention of food and recurrent aspiration pneumonia. HRCT of the chest has been utilized to detect early interstitial lung disease (154) and to distinguish patients with predominantly fibrotic lung disease from those with significant inflammation (6, 155). Moreover, HRCT has been successful in detecting mediastinal adenopathy (156, 157) and asymptomatic esophageal involvement in patients with scleroderma (156).

Pulmonary function abnormalities include a restrictive pattern with reduction of vital capacity and normal flow rates (141, 142, 144, 151, 153–161). The compliance of the lung is reduced. A reduced $D_{LCO}$ is frequently the earliest abnormality noted and may be present prior to recognized chest radiographic abnormalities (146, 162). Owens and coworkers (163) and Silver and coworkers (164) found a significant correlation between bronchoalveolar lavage cellular recovery and the single-breath $D_{LCO}$. Sackner and coworkers (145) showed that scleroderma involvement of the chest wall does not interfere with pulmonary function.

Pathological changes in the lung occur frequently, with or without clinical or chest radiographic abnormalities (146, 162). In an autopsy study, Weaver and coworkers (146) found pulmonary abnormalities in all their 28 cases of scleroderma. A progressive, nonspecific, bilateral lower-lobe interstitial fibrosis with bronchiectasis and cyst formation was the most prominent finding. Marked intimal thickening by loose myxomatous connective tissue occurred in small pulmonary arteries and arterioles.

In reviews of vascular disease in scleroderma, Norton and Nardo (149) and Shuck and coworkers (165) point out that involvement of the arterioles and capillary bed in many tissues, particularly the lungs, is the basis of scleroderma. They conclude that scleroderma must be regarded as a vascular disease. It is clear that the pulmonary vascular lesions are not merely an extension of interstitial fibrosis, since many scleroderma lungs have areas of severe interstitial fibrosis without arterial lesions, as well as areas of vascular changes without interstitial disease (150). Thus, there are two predominant lung lesions in scleroderma: interstitial and pulmonary vascular (141). Other pathological findings in patients with scleroderma include pleural thickening or effusion, cardiomegaly, vascular congestion, pulmonary edema, and pneumonitis.

In general, corticosteroids are not beneficial in treating pulmonary disease in scleroderma (141). However, two studies (166, 167) demonstrated improvement in $D_{LCO}$ following penicillamine therapy, and one study (168) suggested this drug may arrest worsening of pulmonary dysfunction. Moreover, in a 12-month trial of recombinant gamma-interferon therapy in 14 patients, nine of whom completed the trial, significant improvement was observed in skin involvement and in arterial oxygen tension (169). Nifedipine may be useful for treating patients with early pulmonary vascular disease (141). The 5-year survival rate for patients with scleroderma following the detection of lung disease is less than 50% (158, 170).

## POLYMYOSITIS-DERMATOMYOSITIS

Polymyositis and dermatomyositis (PM-DM) include a group of diffuse inflammatory and degenerative disorders of striated muscle that cause symmetrical weakness and atrophy of proximal muscle groups (171–177). The disease is twice as common in females as in males. It shows two peak age incidences: the first decade and the fifth and sixth decades (76). Patients commonly present with erythematous skin lesions accompanied by weakness and pain of proximal muscle groups.

The pulmonary complications of PM-DM may precede, follow, or occur simultaneously with the muscle and skin parenchymal disease (85). There are three mechanisms for the development of pulmonary parenchymal disease in polymyositis: (*a*) primary interstitial pneumonitis; (*b*) aspiration pneumonia due to a hypotonic esophagus; and (*c*) hypostatic pneumonia secondary to chest wall involvement, with resultant hypoventilation (178).

Respiratory muscle dysfunction due to the inflammatory myopathy of PM-DM can lead to respiratory failure (alveolar hypoventilation) in up to 10% of patients (85). Subclinical respiratory muscle dysfunction is more frequent (85). These latter patients have tachypnea and dyspnea with exercise, and may develop the aforementioned hypostatic pneumonia due to failure to generate an adequate cough (85).

In contrast to the other connective tissue diseases, pleural disease is not common in polymyositis (85, 179). In one review of polymyositis lung, a total of 31 well-documented cases of interstitial pneumonitis was found in the world's literature (179). The exact prevalence of interstitial pneumonitis in polymyositis lung is difficult to determine; however, in a series from the Mayo Clinic, primary interstitial pneumonitis was present in 5% (180), likely an underestimate, since HRCT was not utilized to detect disease not seen on the plain chest radiograph.

The clinical presentation of this form of lung disease is quite variable. It may present as an acute pneumonitis with a mixed alveolar-interstitial pneumonitis in association with skin and muscle manifestations or as an asymptomatic finding on the chest radiograph. The most common presentation is one of gradual onset of dyspnea and cough with development of diffuse pulmonary infiltrates most prominent at the lung bases. Diffuse soft tissue calcification may be present, a finding more often seen in children with PM-DM than in adults. Histopathology is similar to that described for idiopathic pulmonary fibrosis (179). BOOP, usual interstitial pneumonia (UIP), diffuse alveolar damage, and pulmonary arteriolitis may be present (179).

In approximately 40% of patients, the pulmonary disease precedes the skin and muscle manifestations by 1 to 24 months (179). Clubbing is not often present. In most cases, the lung disease is progressive, causing severe restrictive lung disease and cor pulmonale. Corticosteroids have caused remission, with either stabilization or improvement in the symptoms, chest films, and physiologic abnormalities in 50% of patients (179).

## SYSTEMIC GRANULOMATOUS VASCULITIDES

### WEGENER'S GRANULOMATOSIS

Wegener's granulomatosis (WG) has a distinctive clinicopathologic triad of (a) necrotizing granulomatous vasculitis of the upper and lower respiratory tracts, (b) glomerulonephritis, and (c) variable degrees of disseminated small vessel vasculitis affecting arteries and veins (181–209). A localized form of WG limited primarily to the respiratory tract has been reported (195) but probably represents an early stage that, if not treated, eventually would involve the kidney and become a generalized Wegener's granulomatosis. However, some patients may have a forme fruste of the disease that never disseminates.

### Clinicopathologic Features

Fauci and his colleagues (194) have described the clinical features of Wegener's granulomatosis. The mean age at diagnosis was 41, range 14 to 75 years. The disease occurs in males almost twice as frequently as in females (187, 194, 195). Initially, clinical presentations vary widely among patients but generally are related to the upper respiratory tract. Typical findings include sinusitis (67%), otitis media (29%), rhinitis or nasal symptoms (22%), epistaxis (11%), and ulcers (6%) and hearing impairment (6%) (194). Although chest radiographic abnormalities are present in 71%, fewer than one-half of Fauci's patients had noticed respiratory symptoms (cough in 33%, hemoptysis in 18%, chest pain in 8%, dyspnea in 7%, and pleurisy in 5%) (194, 209). In one series (210), 8% of 77 patients with Wegener's granulomatosis presented with diffuse hemorrhage. Pulmonary function studies show loss of lung volume with a restrictive ventilatory defect in association with significant parenchymal lesions (76). More than 50% of patients with WG also have an obstructive ventilatory abnormality that cannot be related to cigarette smoking (79). In patients with obstructive changes, granulomatous lesions that have blocked a major airway may be found during fiberoptic bronchoscopy, and the severity of airflow obstruction has been shown to correlate with the extent of endobronchial disease (209, 211).

Renal disease is the sine qua non of generalized Wegener's granulomatosis. Prior to the use of cytotoxic agents as therapy in this disorder, most patients succumbed to renal disease, with a mean survival of 5 months from the onset of clinically evident renal involvement (184, 189). The urinary findings in generalized WG are of acute glomerulonephritis with hematuria, red blood cell casts, and proteinuria. Any of the other organ systems involved in WG may also be the focus of initial complaints (Table 13.5) (183, 184, 194). Among systemic signs and symptoms at presentation are fever (34%), weight loss (16%), and anorexia or malaise (8%) (194). Extrathoracic organ involvement at presentation includes arthritis (44%), skin rash (13%), ocular inflammation (6%), and proptosis (7%) (194, 209).

Wegener's granulomatosis presents a characteristic complex of laboratory findings (184, 187, 194). The mild anemia of subacute or chronic diseases is seen frequently, as is mild leukocytosis. Thrombocytosis (up to 1 million platelets per cubic millimeter) can be present and probably represents an acute reaction (184). The results of antinuclear antibody and lupus erythematosus (LE) cell preparation tests are uniformly negative. The total complement level is normal or mildly elevated. Mild hyperglobulinemia, particularly involving the serum IgA fraction, occurs commonly (196). Almost all patients have strikingly elevated erythrocyte sedimentation rates, usually 100 mm/hour or more (Westergren method) (184). In 1982, a serum IgG against cytoplasmic components of polymorphonuclear leukocytes was described in eight patients with necrotizing granulonephritis (212). Subsequent studies have established the specificity of this antineutrophilic cytoplasmic antibody (c-ANCA) for WG (213, 214). Among 277 patients with WG and 1,657 control patients the specificity of ANCA was 99% (214). However, sensitivity is dependent on disease activity; thus, when only limited disease is present the sensitivity drops to 67%, and in patients in remission the sensitivity is between 32 and 40% (214). There is a good correlation between disease activity and c-ANCA titer (215). The antigen for the Wegener's granulomatosis–specific c-ANCA is a 29-kd molecule found in the azurophilic granules of human neutrophils (216). A second antibody, reacting to the myeloperoxidase, forms a perinuclear pattern (p-ANCA) by immunofluorescence. p-ANCA occurs in a wide range of necrotizing vasculitides such as Churg-Strauss syndrome, polyarteritis nodosa with visceral involvement, and crescentic glomerulonephritis (215).

The etiology of WG remains unknown, although antineutrophilic cytoplasmic antibodies (ANCAs) are

**TABLE 13.5**

**CHARACTERISTIC FEATURES OF ORGAN SYSTEM INVOLVEMENT IN WEGENER'S GRANULOMATOSIS**

| Organ System | Approximate % Frequency | Typical Features |
|---|---|---|
| Nasopharynx | 75 | Necrotizing granulomas with ulceration, saddle nose deformity |
| Paranasal | 90 | Parasinusitis, necrotizing granulomas, secondary bacterial infection |
| Eyes | 60 | Keratoconjunctivitis, granulomatous sclerouveitis |
| Ears | 35 | Serous otitis media, secondary bacterial infection |
| Lungs | 95 | Multiple nodular cavitary infiltrates, necrotizing granulomatous vasculitis |
| Kidney | 85 | Focal and segmental glomerulitis, necrotizing glomerulonephritis (later in course) |
| Heart | 15 | Coronary vasculitis, pericarditis |
| Nervous system | 20 | Mononeuritis multiplex, cranial neuritis |
| Skin | 40 | Dermal vasculitis with secondary ulcerations |
| Joints | 50 | Polyarthralgias |

Adapted from Wolff SM, Fauci AS, Horn RG, et al: Wegener's granulomatosis. *Ann Intern Med* 81:513–525, 1974, and Fauci AS, Wolff SM: Wegener's granulomatosis and related diseases. *Dis Mon* 23:1–36, 1977.

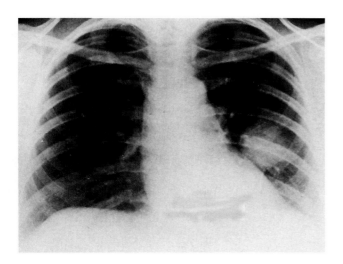

**FIGURE 13.5.** Wegener's granulomatosis. PA chest radiograph shows bibasilar lung nodules.

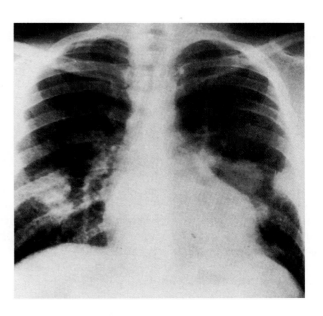

**FIGURE 13.6.** Wegener's granulomatosis. PA chest radiograph shows multiple large bilateral lung nodules. No cavitation, adenopathy, or pleural effusion is present.

thought to play a role in the pathogenesis of this disease (217). Many research groups are attempting to create an animal model of ANCA-induced disease that might resemble human autoimmune diseases such as WG (218).

### Chest Radiographic Manifestations

The pulmonary infiltrates of Wegener's granulomatosis are heterogeneous and may be of any size, shape, or lobar location (79, 181–186, 194, 195, 198–206). The most characteristic patterns (although not the most common) are solitary or multiple nodular densities or infiltrates, either poorly defined or sharply circumscribed (Figs. 13.5 and 13.6) (181). These opacities vary in size from less than 1 cm to greater than 9 cm (181, 199, 200), and occasionally air-fluid levels are found (148). The infiltrates may be quite transient, with one disappearing in one lung field and another appearing in a different location (200).

Atypical radiographic manifestations of WG include focal areas of collapsed lung adjacent to infiltrates (200) and mediastinal lymph node enlargement (201). The combination of hilar and mediastinal adenopathy on the chest radiograph should suggest an alternative diagnosis. Other occasional signs include bronchopleural fistula; narrow areas in the larger airways, which may lead to lobar collapse (202); and pleural thickening and pleural effusions (79, 199).

### Diagnosis and Pathologic Findings

An important aspect of Wegener's granulomatosis is its pathologic and clinical similarity to a variety of other disorders characterized by granulomatous inflammation, vasculitis, or both (181, 184, 194). These include disorders such as polyarteritis nodosa; hypersensitivity vasculitis; the spectrum of connective tissue diseases; granulomatous diseases, such as sarcoidosis and midline granuloma; mixed granulomatous and vasculitis diseases, such as allergic granulomatosis; infectious granulomatous diseases, such as tuberculosis, leprosy, and fungal disease; Goodpasture's syndrome; and a variety of neoplasms accompanied by a granulomatous or vasculitic inflammatory response (184). The diagnosis of Wegener's granulomatosis is established when typical pathologic features accompany a characteristic clinical syndrome (209). The American College of Rheumatology criteria for WG include the presence of vasculitis (tissue or angiographically demonstrated) and any two of the following four findings: (*a*) painful or painless oral ulcers, or purulent or bloody nasal discharge; (*b*) chest radiograph showing the presence of nodules, fixed infiltrates, or cavities; (*c*) microhematuria (more than five red blood cells per high power field) or red cell casts in urine sediment; (*d*) histologic changes showing granulomatous inflammation within the wall of an artery or in the perivascular or extravascular area (218). These criteria have an 88% sensitivity and 92% specificity in recognizing WG (218). Although c-ANCA was not used in developing these criteria, the presence of this highly specific, moderately sensitive marker of Wegener's granulomatosis may obviate the need for histologic confirmation (209).

Open lung biopsy is the procedure of choice for histologic confirmation of WG. This method has the added advantage of making specimens available to rule out infectious diseases. The outstanding pathologic feature in all cases is the presence of inflammatory masses (0.5 to 5 cm) within the parenchyma of one or both lungs (207). Generally, the masses are few and sharply circumscribed on gross examination. Microscopically, they consist of necrotic areas surrounded by zones of granulation tissue. The earliest lesion in the kidney is a focal and segmental glomerulitis (184, 208). If not treated properly, the lesions progress to a fulminant, necrotizing, and proliferative glomerulonephritis and eventually can lead to renal failure. At very early stages, glomerulitis may go undetected because the urinary sediment and renal function

may be normal. Therefore, percutaneous renal biopsies are recommended when there is a high index of suspicion of WG, even when the urinary sediment is normal (184). Renal biopsies not only aid in establishing a diagnosis but also serve to monitor response to therapy as measured by subsequent biopsies.

### Treatment and Prognosis

Untreated, Wegener's granulomatosis pursues a rapidly fatal course, with a mean survival time of 5 months in most cases (194, 219, 220). Eighty-two percent of patients die within 1 year and more than 90% within 2 years. Although corticosteroids increase mean survival to 12 months, the long-term prognosis is not significantly altered by this therapy, especially in patients with clinically apparent renal disease.

The current drug of choice in treating Wegener's granulomatosis is cyclophosphamide (79, 181, 182, 184, 186, 192, 194, 196, 209). Fauci reported a complete remission in 79 of 85 patients (93%) using cyclophosphamide (194). The drug is administered orally or, in cases of rapidly progressive disease, intravenously. A clinical response is usually seen after 1 to 3 weeks of therapy. The dose of cyclophosphamide must be monitored continually and adjusted to keep the white blood cell count above 3000 cells/mm$^3$ (79, 182, 192, 194). In patients who cannot tolerate cyclophosphamide because of severe leukopenia or hemorrhagic cystitis, or in young women who are not willing to accept the ovarian damage associated with cyclophosphamide, azathioprine and methotrexate are alternative agents (79, 182).

In 1985, De Remee et al (221) described improvement in 11 of 12 patients with WG treated with trimethoprim-sulfamethoxazole. Since then the use of this agent in WG has been reported in additional patients, including 31 patients unresponsive to standard therapy (222). Twenty-six patients responded and five remained unresponsive to therapy. The role of this therapy for early limited disease, as an adjunct in generalized disease, or as maintenance therapy during remission for prevention of relapses has yet to be elucidated (209).

### Lymphomatoid Granulomatosis

Lymphomatoid granulomatosis (LYG) is a systemic disease characterized by an angiocentric, angiodestructive, and lymphoreticular granulomatous vasculitis, primarily of the lungs but also frequently involving the kidneys (45%), skin (45%), and central nervous system (20%) (79, 188, 192, 204, 205, 223, 224). Although any organ system can be involved, the spleen, lymph nodes, and bone marrow usually are spared. This disorder resembles an indolent lymphoma, and in many instances it progresses to an atypical disseminated lymphoproliferative disease (79, 204, 223, 224). LYG has been described as a late complication of Epstein-Barr viral infection (225, 226). The cellular infiltrates are mixed, demonstrating normal as well as atypical lymphocytes, plasmacytoid cells, and cells apparently of reticuloendothelial origin (79, 224).

## Clinicopathologic Features

The male to female ratio is about 2:1, and most patients are in early middle age (204, 224). Lung involvement is a sine qua non of LYG and is usually manifested as multiple pulmonary infiltrates of various sizes that tend to cavitate (79, 186, 204, 223, 224). Most patients present with chest symptoms (cough and shortness of breath) or systemic complaints (fever, weight loss, malaise) or both. Upper airway disease is uncommon in LYG (209). The skin and central nervous system are the two most common extrathoracic sites of involvement (209, 223). Skin lesions occur in 30 to 50% of patients. A papular erythematous rash is typical, but painful and sometimes ulcerative nodules may develop (209). Central nervous system involvement occurs in 30% of patients and is usually manifested by signs and symptoms of a mass lesion (209–223).

There is no striking pattern of laboratory abnormalities. Most patients have a normal or only slightly reduced hematocrit. In the series of Katzenstein and coworkers (157), the presenting leukocyte count was normal in 50%, elevated in 30% (range, 9,000 to 38,000), and reduced in 20% (range, 1,200 to 3,900). A relative lymphocytopenia was noted in 33% and lymphocytosis in 6%. Serum immunoglobulins were normal in 53% of cases, and nonspecific increases, usually in IgG or IgM, were seen in the remainder (223).

## Chest Radiographic Manifestations

The chest radiographic manifestations of lymphomatoid granulomatosis depend in part on the duration of the disease. Lesions may appear and disappear without relation to therapy, as also occurs in Wegener's granulomatosis (79, 182, 186, 204). The pulmonary lesions predominate in the lower lung fields peripherally and are usually bilateral (Fig. 13.7) (204). Typically, the early lesions present as multiple, bilateral, ill-defined densities (203). Later, they become better defined and resemble nodular metastases of various malignancies (79, 204).

## Diagnosis and Pathologic Findings

The definitive diagnosis of lymphomatoid granulomatosis is made histologically. Plasma cells, lymphocytic cells, and large "atypical" mononuclear cells in various stages of maturity infiltrating perivascular tissue are characteristic (227). Occlusion by infiltration of the vessels and subsequent tissue necrosis are frequent findings. With peripheral nerve involvement, the infiltrate is seen surrounding the nerve, and spotty demyelination is present. When the skin is involved, small-vessel destruction with a lymphoreticular infiltrate is most often seen surrounding the dermal appendages (227).

This disorder is often confused clinically with Wegener's granulomatosis. However, granulomata are less copious and less distinct, and the vasculitis is remarkable in that it is not the characteristic leukocytoclastic or fibrinoid necrotic type seen in WG and other systemic vasculitides (79, 182, 188, 204). In contrast, there is an angiotrophic invasion of blood vessels of various sizes with a bizarre cellular infiltrate. Blood supply through the involved vessels is compromised, and infarction and necrosis occur as in other vasculitides.

In addition to its characteristic histopathologic features, lymphomatoid granulomatosis differs from Wegener's granulomatosis in several other ways (79, 188, 192, 193). As stated previously, sinus and upper airway involvement is unusual in lymphomatoid granulomatosis (184, 204, 208, 224). In addition, renal involvement in lymphomatoid granulomatosis takes the form of a diffuse nodular infiltrate of the renal parenchyma with a characteristic cellular infiltrate, in contrast to the necrotizing glomerulonephritis seen in Wegener's granulomatosis (184, 204, 208, 224). Leukopenia and anergy before therapy are rare in patients with WG but are seen frequently in lymphomatoid granulomatosis (181, 182, 196); the erythrocyte sedimentation rate may be normal or only mildly elevated in patients with active disease (209).

## Etiology and Pathogenesis

The etiology of lymphomatoid granulomatosis is unknown (188). It may be an acquired abnormality of the lymphocyte in a susceptible host, as is Sjögren's syndrome. Evidence for this includes absent delayed hypersensitivity, as demonstrated by nonreactivity to skin test antigens and the response of the lung lesions to corticosteroids (227). Like Sjögren's syndrome, lymphomatoid granulomatosis can terminate in a neoplastic disease (Fig. 13.7) (224, 227). In fact, Colby and Carrington (228) classified lymphomatoid granulomatosis as a malignant lymphoma.

Other diseases, such as lymphoma and mycosis fungoides, can have years of symptoms, with a biopsy showing nonspecific lymphoid and plasma cell infiltrates, before they assume the unusual features of neoplastic disease. Renal homotransplantation can be

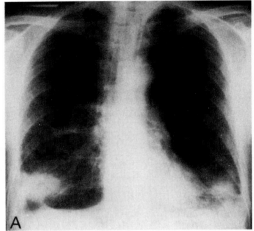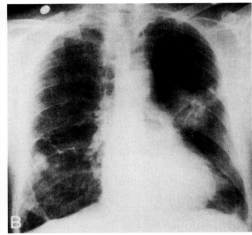

**FIGURE 13.7.** Lymphomatoid granulomatosis. **A,** PA chest radiograph shows bibasilar lung nodules. **B,** PA chest radiograph 2½ years later, after therapy with corticosteroids and chlorambucil, shows clearing of the bibasilar densities and appearance of at least two new lesions, one in the left midlung zone, the other in the lower third of the right lung. The left-sided lesion contains an air bronchogram. Open lung biopsy of the new, large left lung mass revealed lymphoma.

followed by lymphoreticular proliferation with involvement of the central nervous system (229–231). Antigenic exposure in an immunosuppressed host may alter the cell membrane and produce an autoimmune disease (224). With continued immunosuppression, neoplastic disease may result (232).

### Therapy and Prognosis

Untreated, lymphomatoid granulomatosis is usually rapidly progressive and fatal (182, 188, 192, 193). Death is often related to pulmonary or central nervous system complications (224). Preliminary reports (182, 192, 193, 233) indicate that a relatively high rate of long-term remissions (54%) can be achieved if patients are treated early with cyclophosphamide and corticosteroids in the same regimen used for Wegener's granulomatosis.

### ALLERGIC ANGIITIS AND GRANULOMATOSIS (CHURG-STRAUSS SYNDROME)

Churg and Strauss (234) in 1951 and Rose and Spencer (235) in 1957 described an uncommon granulomatous inflammation and vascular necrosis primarily involving the heart, lungs, skin, nervous system, and kidneys (188, 192, 193, 236). This entity, commonly referred to as allergic angiitis and granulomatosis, occurs primarily in patients with an allergic background, often with asthma. Characteristically, high degrees of blood eosinophilia are found (236).

### Clinicopathologic Features

In the 30 cases of the Churg-Strauss syndrome reported by Chumbley et al (237), 21 were men and nine were women. Ages ranged from 16 to 69 years; the average was 47 years. The mean duration of asthma was 8 years. It began at the same time as the manifestations of systemic vasculitis in six cases but preceded it in all others. Allergic rhinitis occurred in 21 of the 30 cases (70%). Most patients with Churg-Strauss syndrome have a fever at some point in their clinical course. Anemia and weight loss are common, as is leukocytosis. The elevation of the erythrocyte sedimentation rate and the degree of peripheral blood eosinophilia are good indicators of disease activity.

### Chest Radiographic Manifestations

Chest radiographic abnormalities range from transient patchy densities to massive bilateral nodular infiltrates throughout the lung fields (238, 239). New lesions may appear while older ones are disappearing; some remain stable after an initial period of improvement. Complete regression of a widespread active pulmonary process is sometimes seen with corticosteroids. Frequently, asthmatic symptoms recede as evidence of necrotizing vasculitis becomes prominent. The radiographic patterns are so varied that radiographic differential in this entity is not useful.

### Diagnosis and Pathologic Findings

Histologically, the lung typically shows fibrinoid, necrotizing, and eosinophilic granulomatous lesions, which frequently involve the pulmonary arteries (239). In about half of their cases Churg and Strauss (234) found parenchymal lesions in the form of an extensive pneumonic process involving septa and alveoli. In the acute stage, the exudate in the lungs had a predominance of eosinophilic leukocytes mixed with giant cells. Frequently, healing terminated in focal fibrosis. Histologic evidence of bronchial asthma (hyalinization of basement membrane, increased mucus secretion, and eosinophilic infiltration of the bronchial walls) was present in most cases but generally was not very marked (234).

Allergic granulomatosis (Churg-Strauss syndrome) strongly resembles classic polyarteritis nodosa, with some obviously distinguishing features. Churg-Strauss syndrome almost invariably is associated with an allergic diathesis, particularly severe asthma (182). Reports of the incidence of asthma with polyarteritis nodosa have ranged from 4% to as high as 54% (239). In general, unlike classic polyarteritis nodosa, in which pulmonary abnormalities are rare, lung involvement is invariable in Churg-Strauss syndrome. Also, this syndrome is characterized by high levels of peripheral eosinophilia (usually higher than 1500/mm$^3$), eosinophilic tissue infiltration and granulomatous reactivity (235, 237, 238). In contrast, the predominant cellular infiltrate in polyarteritis nodosa is the polymorphonuclear leukocyte. In addition to the fibrinoid necrosis of small and medium-sized muscular arteries that is the hallmark of classic polyarteritis nodosa, a substantial degree of involvement of small vessels such as capillaries and venules is present in Churg-Strauss syndrome. Apart from these differences, the presentation, clinicopathologic manifestations, organ system involvement, and clinical course of these two syndromes are similar (182).

The "overlap" syndrome of the systemic vasculitides combines many features that are characteristic of classic polyarteritis nodosa, other systemic vasculitides of the small- and medium-sized vessels, such as allergic angiitis and granulomatosis (Churg-Strauss syndrome), and the small-vessel hypersensitivity vasculitides (79, 182, 192, 193). Large and small arteries, as well as capillaries and venules, may be involved in the vasculitic process. One patient may have features that would be considered characteristic or even pathognomonic of either classic polyarteritis nodosa or allergic granulomatosis. The overlap syndrome is a multisystem disease, with protean clinical manifestations. The same patient may have small-vessel involvement (arterioles, capillaries, and venules), as well as the classic small- and medium-sized muscular artery involvement with characteristic angiographic findings of small

aneurysms. A history of allergy, peripheral eosinophilia, eosinophilic tissue infiltration, granulomatous reactions, and lung involvement described for Churg-Strauss syndrome may all be seen in the same patient, or one or more of these may be seen to the exclusion of the others (79, 182). This syndrome is the most difficult to classify.

### Therapy and Prognosis

Well-controlled experience with therapy for the Churg-Strauss syndrome is lacking. Chumbley and co-workers (237) treated 27 of their 30 patients with prednisone; most received 40 to 60 mg daily, others 100 to 120 mg daily. Fifteen of these 30 patients died, three within a year after symptoms of vasculitis appeared. The interval from onset of signs and symptoms of vasculitis to death ranged from 6 months to 15 years; the average was 4.6 years. A recent prospective, randomized study failed to establish that plasma exchange adds to corticosteroids in preventing disease relapses (240). Cyclophosphamide and azathioprine therapy have theoretical rationale, since they are effective in treating another necrotizing vasculitis, Wegener's granulomatosis. Although experience with these agents is minimal, one prospective, randomized study showed that cyclophosphamide added to prednisone–plasma exchange therapy enhanced the relapse-free interval during long-term follow-up (241).

## GOODPASTURE'S SYNDROME

Goodpasture's syndrome is characterized by pulmonary hemorrhage with hemoptysis, diffuse alveolar filling on the chest radiograph, anemia, and glomerulonephritis (often rapidly progressive) (79, 98, 189, 190, 242–250). Wilson and Dixon (244) extended this definition to include the presence of anti–glomerular basement membrane (anti-GBM) antibodies, which are found in most patients with Goodpasture's syndrome (245). While the catalyst is unknown, production of these antibodies is usually self-limited, and the syndrome apparently is inactive when the antibody is not detected (245, 248). Although the term Goodpasture's syndrome has gained wide popularity, to avoid confusion with a variety of other disorders (e.g., Wegener's granulomatosis and systemic lupus erythematosus) with similar clinical findings, Young (251) has recommended using the term anti-GBM antibody disease. This latter term describes pulmonary hemorrhage, with or without associated glomerulonephritis, due to circulating antibodies directed against basement membrane epitopes (251).

## CLINICOPATHOLOGIC FEATURES

Early reports on Goodpasture's syndrome indicated a marked male predominance of 9:1, but more recent studies describe lower male to female ratios of 3.5:1 and 2:1 (243). Seventy-five percent of patients are between the ages of 17 and 27 years at the onset of the illness, while the remainder range in age up to 75 years (243).

In most cases, the initial symptom is hemoptysis, which occurs at some point during the course of the disease in 99% of cases (189, 190, 242, 243). Bouts of hemoptysis range in severity from slightly blood-streaked sputum to massive hemorrhage (242). In about one-fifth of the patients, upper respiratory tract infections of a nonspecific (viral) nature precede the appearance of the syndrome (242). Chills and fever occur acutely with pulmonary hemorrhage but are not otherwise prominent. Substernal chest pain occurs without relation to activity, although it can be aggravated by coughing.

Renal abnormalities may occur before pulmonary symptoms. Urinary findings, present on admission in over 80% of patients (242), include proteinuria, microscopic hematuria, and, less commonly, pyuria (242, 243, 245). In 26 (81%) of Wilson and Dixon's patients, renal failure requiring dialysis occurred within 1 to 14 months of onset (mean 3.5 months) (244).

Anemia is universally present early in the disease. The anemia is apparently not hemolytic, although a decreased erythrocyte life span has been demonstrated (242). Neither hemolysis nor jaundice is present.

## CHEST RADIOGRAPHIC FINDINGS

The radiographic appearance of Goodpasture's syndrome is closely related to the distribution, volume, and temporal sequence of pulmonary hemorrhage. Both interstitial and alveolar involvement occur. Confluent densities are seen shortly after hemorrhage and may be indistinguishable from hypervolemia associated with azotemia or from noncardiogenic pulmonary edema of another origin (Fig. 13.8). All these conditions produce rapid alterations in the chest radiograph. Localized air space changes may progress to diffuse opacification within hours, while complete clearing may occur during remission. However, accentuated interstitial markings tend to persist in Goodpasture's syndrome after repeated episodes of bleeding due to the presence of siderophages in the interstitium. If the bleeding is of sufficient duration, permanent reticulonodular infiltrates develop, resembling those seen in idiopathic pulmonary hemosiderosis. Generally these changes are diffuse, but they may be localized. The

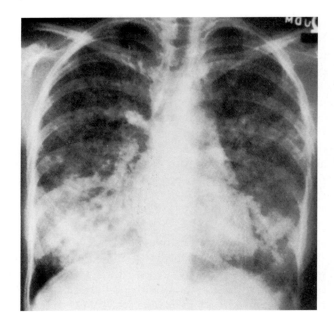

**FIGURE 13.8.** Goodpasture's syndrome. PA chest radiograph shows a characteristic alveolar filling pattern in a patient with hemoptysis and renal failure. The heart, pulmonary vascularity, and pleura are normal.

superimposition of fluffy alveolar densities on a reticulonodular background suggests recurrent pulmonary hemorrhage.

Goodpasture's syndrome demonstrates a predilection for perihilar involvement, while, in contrast to the pulmonary venous congestion and edema of left ventricular failure, Kerley B lines and pleural effusions are not characteristic.

## PULMONARY FUNCTION ABNORMALITIES

The diffusing capacity for carbon monoxide ($D_{LCO}$) may be useful in following the course of this disease (251, 252). Because intra-alveolar blood will bind carbon monoxide, the $D_{LCO}$ may be raised above baseline levels during lung hemorrhage (252). Thus, serial measurements of $D_{LCO}$ may help distinguish fresh pulmonary hemorrhage from other causes of radiographic opacities (e.g. infection) (251, 252).

## DIAGNOSIS AND PATHOLOGIC FINDINGS

Diagnosis of Goodpasture's syndrome depends on the demonstration of circulating anti-GBM antibodies and/or the finding of linear deposits of immunoglobulin along glomerular or alveolar basement membranes (245, 248, 251, 253). These findings are coupled with evidence of lung hemorrhage in a patient who typically presents with recurrent hemoptysis, dyspnea, and anemia (245, 248). The erythrocyte sedimentation rate, though often slightly elevated, is usually not strikingly elevated as in most cases of systemic vasculitis (e.g., Wegener's granulomatosis) (251). The degree of renal injury is mirrored by elevations in serum creatinine and blood urea nitrogen, and active glomerulonephritis is almost always accompanied by proteinuria, hematuria (gross or microscopic), and red blood cell casts (251). Histologically, the renal abnormality in patients with Goodpasture's syndrome is an actively proliferating, often necrotizing, crescent-forming type of glomerulonephritis (245). This is accompanied by variable, probably secondary tubular alterations and interstitial infiltrative processes.

### ETIOLOGY AND PATHOGENESIS

The presence of antibodies is clearly involved in the glomerulonephritis and probably the pulmonary hemorrhage of Goodpasture's syndrome (189, 190, 245). The mechanism responsible for these antibodies, however, is not known, although environmental factors are thought to be instrumental in triggering their production (245, 251). For example, antigens such as the influenza A2 virus might cause the production of antibodies that cross-react with the basement membrane structures (250). Many patients have a history of preceding viral syndromes, either of the upper respiratory tract or gastrointestinal tract. Infectious agents or chemical substances such as hydrocarbon solvents might uncover or alter some self-antigens so that they become immunogenic (244, 254).

### THERAPY AND PROGNOSIS

The prognosis for Goodpasture's syndrome is generally poor (98, 189, 190, 241, 242, 248, 249). Patients die of either renal failure or lung hemorrhage. In Wilson and Dixon's study (244), in which the diagnosis was based on the presence of circulating anti-GBM antibodies, 28 of 32 patients developed renal failure and over half died within 1 year of diagnosis.

The most successful therapy includes (*a*) plasmapheresis and treatment of the inflammatory response in tissues and (*b*) suppression of further antibody production through the use of corticosteroids and cyclophosphamide or azathioprine (191, 247, 251, 255–259). Because of the lack of controlled studies, the exact effects of this combined therapy are not clear. Since production of anti-GBM antibodies may be short-lived, plasma exchange should reduce damage to the glomerulus by lowering the levels of circulating anti-GBM antibody. Lockwood and coworkers (247) reported on

seven patients treated with plasma exchange, cytotoxic drugs, and corticosteroids. Renal function improved in three who were not already receiving dialysis at the initiation of therapy. Five patients had pulmonary hemorrhage that appeared to respond to therapy. These investigators reported that, although the fall in anti-GBM antibody titer was variable, there was also depletion of fibrinogen and complement. They believed that the reduction of the latter two substances could have been important therapeutically. Swainson and coworkers (258) noted a rebound increase in anti-GBM antibody levels following periods of plasma exchange. They concluded that plasma exchange was only effective in substantially reducing the circulating amounts of complement or fibrinogen when performed on consecutive days. The rapid rise in concentrations after exchange reflects rapid turnover and distribution from extravascular pools.

In general, plasma exchange may be useful in the early treatment of severe forms of Goodpasture's syndrome by controlling pulmonary hemorrhage and preventing irreversible renal damage from the high anti-GBM antibody levels. However, the removal of anti-GBM antibodies does not lead to recovery of renal function. Furthermore, there is considerable variation in the amount of reduction of anti-GBM levels in the serum produced by serial plasma exchange and immunosuppression.

### IDIOPATHIC PULMONARY HEMOSIDEROSIS

Although it is likely that idiopathic pulmonary hemosiderosis (IPH) is a separate entity, its chest manifestations are identical to those of Goodpasture's syndrome. Both diseases are of unknown etiology and are characterized by repeated episodes of pulmonary hemorrhage, iron-deficiency anemia, and, in longstanding cases, pulmonary insufficiency. In contrast to IPH, Goodpasture's syndrome includes renal disease with circulating anti-GBM antibodies, in addition to the pulmonary manifestations (190, 260–262).

IPH occurs most commonly in children, frequently below the age of 10 years; in this age group there is no sex predominance (262). When it develops in adults (and the incidence in adults appears to be increasing, especially in patients aged 40 years and more) (263–266), it occurs twice as often in men as in women (261).

### CLINICOPATHOLOGIC FEATURES

The onset of IPH may be acute or insidious, with anemia, pallor, weakness, lethargy, and sometimes a dry cough; typical changes of air-space hemorrhage may be apparent radiographically without a clear-cut episode of hemoptysis (261). Rarely, patients present with unexplained iron-deficient hypochromic anemia without a history of hemoptysis. Fever may be present, possibly due to elaboration of pyrogenic cytokines by pulmonary parenchymal cells (251).

Physical examination during an acute stage of pulmonary hemorrhage may reveal fine rales and dullness to percussion over the affected areas of lung. Liver, spleen, and lymph nodes are enlarged to palpation in 20 to 25% of cases.

Iron-deficiency anemia usually develops but may not be present when intrapulmonary hemorrhage is small, and it does not generally deplete the bone marrow iron stores. Serum iron and iron-binding capacity results are characteristic of iron-deficiency anemia, and it is generally agreed that hemolysis does not occur in this disease (261).

As in pulmonary hemorrhage of any cause, the D$_{LCO}$ may be increased (251). Other tests of pulmonary function may be normal initially, but may reveal a progressive restrictive ventilatory defect in chronic cases (251).

At the time of an acute episode of IPH, histologic material from the lungs reveals intraalveolar hemorrhage that may be extensive (267). Hemorrhage is typically confined to the peripheral air spaces; in fact, massive blood loss can occur into the lungs without hemoptysis, and the trachea and major bronchi may contain little or no blood. Sputum or lavage material may contain hemosiderin-laden macrophages. With repeated episodes of hemoptysis, interstitial fibrosis is present in most cases (262). The structural alteration of elastic fibers appears to be the consequence of intraalveolar bleeding rather than its cause; in fact, specimens of lung obtained by biopsy early in the course of the disease reveal morphologically normal elastic tissue (268). Alveolitis and alveolar necrosis are absent unless secondary pneumonia has been superimposed. In contrast to other syndromes considered to be immunologic, such as Wegener's granulomatosis, vasculitis is not an invariable pathologic feature of IPH and when present is usually minor (269, 270).

IPH can be differentiated from Goodpasture's syndrome by the absence of renal disease, the absence of circulating anti-GBM antibodies, and the absence of an antigen-antibody reaction (i.e., the lack of anti–glomerular basement membrane antibody on immunofluorescent staining of lung tissue) (271, 272).

## CHEST RADIOGRAPHIC FINDINGS

As mentioned, the changes apparent on the chest radiograph are identical in IPH and Goodpasture's syndrome. In the early stages, the pattern is one of diffuse mottled opacities characteristic of patchy air space consolidation throughout the lungs (261). An air bronchogram should be visualized in areas of major air space consolidation, and at this stage the radiographic pattern may simulate that of pulmonary edema.

During an acute episode, the fluffy deposits characteristic of acinar consolidation disappear within 2 to 3 days and are replaced by a reticular pattern whose distribution is identical to that of the air space disease (262, 263). The appearance of the chest radiograph usually returns to normal about 10 to 12 days after the original acute episode (261).

With repeated similar episodes, increasing amounts of hemosiderin are deposited within interstitial tissue and there is progressive interstitial fibrosis. Thus, after subsequent fresh hemorrhage there is only partial clearing of the chest radiograph, which reveals a fine reticular pattern (261).

## DIAGNOSIS, TREATMENT, AND OUTCOME

Although the diagnosis of IPH may be strongly suspected in young patients who manifest recurrent episodes of hemoptysis, iron-deficiency anemia, and the typical chest radiographic changes, definitive diagnosis may require lung biopsy. Examination of the sputum for hemosiderin-laden macrophages can provide supportive evidence. Lung biopsy specimens are obtained by transbronchial techniques or by limited thoracotomy.

The prognosis of IPH varies, with an interval from onset of symptoms until death of 2½ to 20 years (190, 262, 264). Remission can be permanent, with or without corticosteroid therapy and immunosuppressives such as azathioprine (251). To date, no therapy has been shown in a prospective, controlled trial to alter outcome.

## PULMONARY ALVEOLAR PROTEINOSIS

Pulmonary alveolar proteinosis is a disease of unknown etiology characterized by accumulation of periodic acid–Schiff (PAS)-positive, lipid-rich, proteinaceous material in the distal air spaces of the lungs (273–283). Rosen, Castleman, and Liebow (283) first described this entity in 1958 on the basis of human lung biopsies. Subsequent demonstrations that similar abnormalities could be produced in experimental animals by exposing them to a variety of dusts and fumes suggest that the disorder is a distinct but nonspecific response of pulmonary tissue to diverse inhaled injurious agents (275, 284).

## Clinicopathologic Features

Grossly, the lungs contain multiple, firm, yellow nodules ranging in size from several millimeters to 2 or 3 cm in diameter (276). Microscopically, large groups of alveoli and small distal bronchioles are filled with a granular, floccular PAS-positive material (Figs. 13.9 and 13.10) (276, 281). Generally, the alveolar walls are normal, but cellular infiltration and areas of fibrosis occur in the interstitial spaces of the lungs, particularly with longstanding disease (275–278). Electron microscopic examination of the proteinaceous material reveals alveolar macrophages that contain numerous lamellar osmiophilic inclusions within the cytoplasm. This lamellar material, rich in phospholipid, is found not only with macrophages but also lying free in amorphous debris in the alveolar spaces (275, 276). The marked PAS positivity of this material is probably due to the presence of large amounts of surfactant protein A, a heavily glycosylated surfactant constituent (285).

The age of onset is generally between 20 and 50 years, but the disorder also occurs in infants and the elderly (274, 277, 280–282, 285). There is a male preponderance of greater than 3:1. Many, but not all, patients have been exposed to a variety of dusts and fumes, such as wood dust and silica (275). The onset is usually gradual and insidious, but occasionally the disorder follows an acute febrile illness. Dyspnea during exertion is characteristically the first manifestation, gradually evolving into a dyspnea at rest. Cough is common and is often associated with the production of a thick, white to yellow sputum. In those with extensive lung

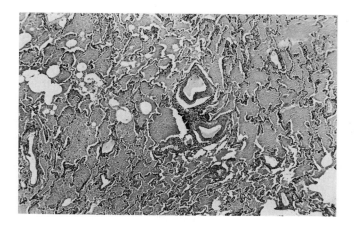

**Figure 13.10.** Pulmonary alveolar proteinosis. Open lung biopsy reveals diffuse alveolar flooding with a granular-like material that stained PAS positive. Note that the alveolar walls are relatively normal.

involvement, fatigability and weight loss are common. Chest pain and hemoptysis are unusual.

Abnormal physical findings are few. The resonance of the percussion note over the thorax is diminished, and breath sounds have a coarse bronchovesicular quality; coarse crackles are audible over affected areas. Fingers and toes become clubbed in some patients (277).

There are no distinctive hematologic abnormalities associated with pulmonary alveolar proteinosis. Anemia does not occur; in fact, erythrocythemia may result if hypoxemia is severe. Leukocyte counts vary from normal to a brisk leukocytosis (i.e., to as high as 15,000 to 20,000 cells/mm$^3$); this usually signifies the coexistence of an acute pulmonary infection. Hyperlipidemia, hyperglobulinemia, and elevated serum lactic dehydrogenase levels occur in some patients with pulmonary alveolar proteinosis (274, 277, 280–282).

Pulmonary function tests characteristically show a restrictive ventilatory pattern (207, 209). The accumulation of the proteinaceous material in the air spaces reduces the number of functioning lung units, thereby altering the overall pressure-volume relationships of the lung and causing pulmonary compliance to decrease (275). The vital capacity, residual volume, and functional residual capacity are all proportionally reduced. Flow rates are usually normal during a forced expiratory maneuver (274).

Marked ventilation-perfusion ratio abnormalities occur in pulmonary alveolar proteinosis. Many areas of lung are perfused with mixed venous blood but receive little or no ventilation. As a result, the alveolar-arterial difference for oxygen widens, and arterial hypoxemia is prominent. Moreover, because abnormal

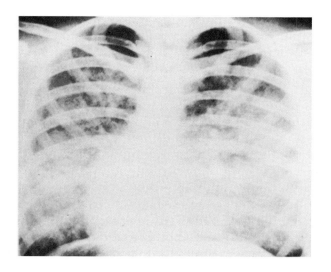

**Figure 13.9.** Pulmonary alveolar proteinosis. PA chest radiograph of a 21-year-old woman with a diffuse, bilateral alveolar filling process and a normal cardiac silhouette.

material in the alveolar spaces effectively amputates some gas-exchange surface and interferes with gas transfer across the alveolar axillary membrane, the DLCO is reduced and a fall in arterial oxygen saturation can be demonstrated regularly during exercise (285). Moreover, in most cases a shunt fraction greater than 17% is demonstrated while the patient is breathing 100% oxygen (285).

Serum laboratory values are usually within normal limits except for an elevation in the serum lactic dehydrogenase (LDH) level (285, 286). In fact, the combination of an elevated shunt fraction and an elevated serum LDH level suggests the diagnosis of pulmonary alveolar proteinosis (285). Of note, elevated serum LDH levels are also found in *Pneumocystis carinii* pneumonia.

### CHEST RADIOGRAPHIC FINDINGS

The chest radiograph shows a diffuse alveolar filling process characterized by scattered patchy, confluent, nodular infiltrates (Fig. 13.9) (280–282). The pattern and distribution are similar to those of cardiogenic pulmonary edema, except that the cardiac silhouette is usually normal in alveolar proteinosis and the alveolar filling pattern resembles a bat wing (285). The involvement is usually bilateral and symmetrical, but asymmetrical or unilateral patterns are seen occasionally. Hilar adenopathy, Kerley's B lines and pleural effusions do not occur (274, 285).

### DIAGNOSIS

Based on clinical, functional, and chest radiographic findings (i.e., dyspnea, diffuse alveolar filling on chest radiograph, elevated serum LDH level, and arterial hypoxemia with an increased shunt fraction), a presumptive diagnosis can often be made (285). However, definitive diagnosis is generally established by histologic examination of a lung biopsy obtained at bronchoscopy or thoracotomy (279, 280). The diagnosis has also been made by the demonstration of PAS-positive material on light microscopic examination of sputum or lung washings. Electron microscopy of sputum or lung washings is also useful diagnostically by revealing granular material and lamellar bodies (287–290). Findings on light microscopy and the clinical presentation can be confused with those of *P. carinii* infection; a methenamine-silver stain is needed to exclude this possibility.

### COURSE AND TREATMENT

Spontaneous recovery with complete resolution of clinical findings and chest radiographic changes occurs in about 25% of patients with pulmonary alveolar proteinosis (274, 277, 280–282, 285). In others, the disorder is progressive, although the rate of progression is variable. In about 15 to 20% of patients, this disease runs a rapid, fulminant course with marked arterial hypoxemia, cor pulmonale, and respiratory failure. In others, progression is over months to years, and in some patients with longstanding disease, interstitial fibrosis develops.

Pulmonary infections with mycotic organisms are common in alveolar proteinosis, which suggests impaired lung defenses. In fact, the alveolar macrophage, the principal cellular defense against intracellular organisms, has been found to be defective in this disease (275, 291, 292). The most frequently encountered infections are nocardiosis, cryptococcosis, aspergillosis, and mucormycosis (280–282).

The management of pulmonary alveolar proteinosis is made difficult by the fact that many patients improve spontaneously, which renders therapeutic intervention difficult to assess (280–282, 293). Moreover, there have been no properly controlled studies of therapy in this disease. Corticosteroids are of no proven benefit. A few patients appear to improve following administration of agents that presumably thin or liquefy bronchial secretions (e.g., potassium iodide, aerosolized streptokinase-streptodornase, trypsin, and a combination of saline, heparin, and acetylcysteine delivered by intermittent positive-pressure breathing) (274, 277, 280–282).

In patients with advanced disease and severe ventilatory compromise, lavage of an entire lung with large volumes of a saline solution has been proposed (280, 281, 285, 294). The procedure is performed under general anesthesia. The airway is intubated with a double-lumen bronchospirometric tube, and mechanical ventilation is instituted with a high inspired oxygen concentration. The details of the procedure have been described at length (285, 294, 295). Usually amelioration of symptoms, with improvement in pulmonary function, begins within hours after lavage, and by 24 to 48 hours pulmonary function and arterial $P_{O_2}$ exceed prelavage levels.

## DRUG-INDUCED PULMONARY DISEASE

The development of antibiotics, cytotoxic antineoplastic agents, and various immunosuppressive drugs has had a remarkable impact on medical therapeutics and has made control of infection, cancer, collagen-vascular diseases, and organ transplant rejection everyday realities in medicine. One undesirable by-product of drug therapy, albeit a rather minor one in the overall scheme, is related to iatrogenic and adverse complications of their use. Development of an allergy to drugs is common, and specific drug-induced pulmonary reactions occur frequently. In fact, almost every therapeutic agent used has (or may have) been noted to cause pulmonary disease; the lists compiled are impressive (296–309). A list of some of these drugs is provided in Table 13.6; the antineoplastic chemotherapy drugs and immunosuppressants are the most prominent offenders (300, 301, 310–319). Occasionally, lung toxicity results from a very commonly used drug such as hydrochlorothiazide (310) or from an antibiotic such as nitrofurantoin, penicillin, or a sulfonamide drug (301).

The host reaction often seems to be a hypersensitivity one, for contact with the drug may eventually cause sensitization to occur (300, 301, 305, 319). Subsequently an immune response develops in the form of antibody or an exaggerated lymphocytic mitogenic response when the host is challenged with the offending drug antigen. However, the precise mechanisms are poorly understood, and for this reason experimental models have been difficult to develop, except for bleomycin, discussed below.

Most drugs are organic compounds of low molecular weight (less than 1000). To become "antigenic" they must couple to larger carrier substances, which are usually serum proteins; in the process of drug-protein binding, the structure of the protein is denatured in that its tertiary molecular configuration is altered. The immune response that is elicited, however, is usually directed to the drug determinant, although a metabolite of the drug might be the actual antigen. Since the antigenic form is usually not known, this complicates selection of the correct metabolite to use in assaying the reaction in vitro or to use in an experimental model. Most of the drug reactions that affect the lung do not elicit IgE-antibody or cause a type 1 immediate hypersensitivity reaction as they do in other reactions, for example to penicillin, in which immediate or accelerated allergic reactions occur. Although asthmatic symptoms can be severe, it is the insidious onset of cough and dyspnea that characterizes most of the reactions caused by the drugs listed in Table 13.6.

Principal emphasis will be given to pulmonary disease caused by cytotoxic, immunosuppressive drugs, since the clinical setting of patients receiving them is complicated and the specific effect of drug toxicity is often difficult to factor out (297, 300, 311, 312). Pulmonary infection (often with nosocomial or opportunistic microorganisms), radiation therapy to the thorax and lung, or progression of the disease under treatment can confuse and compound the issue of drug toxicity. For example, gold (313, 314) or penicillamine, both of which can cause interstitial lung injury, may be used

to treat patients with rheumatoid arthritis, a disease with a 0 to 15% incidence of associated interstitial pulmonary fibrosis; whether disease progression or concomitant pulmonary drug toxicity is responsible may be difficult to decide. Moreover, a latent period may occur between the cessation of drug therapy and the onset of pulmonary symptoms that are in retrospect attributed to a toxic drug effect. A period of months to perhaps years, as noted with busulfan use, may elapse before the untoward drug reaction is evident (299, 300, 312).

Gradual development of shortness of breath and a nagging, dry, nonproductive cough are characteristic complaints of most patients with drug-related pulmonary disease (299, 300). Tachypnea and lung crackles may be found on physical examination. The connection between the drug and the symptoms may be overlooked if the patient has progressive signs of the primary lung disease process or a systemic disease. Subtle development of congestive heart failure may occur from use of potentially myotoxic drugs such as adriamycin, now used frequently in multiple-agent chemotherapy protocols. Chest radiographic abnormalities are not usually noted until the patient experiences respiratory symptoms; then, diffuse linear densities and streaks occur, predominantly in the lower lung zones. The chest radiograph may have an appearance similar to those characteristic of the group of interstitial diseases (Table 13.1). However, certain drug-induced pulmonary reactions have individual features that can heighten one's suspicion that they are causative or contributing to lung symptoms.

### CYTOTOXIC AGENTS

Bleomycin, a mixture of glycopeptides isolated from *Streptomyces verticillus*, is a versatile and effective drug used against squamous cell carcinoma, malignant lymphomas, and testicular tumors and is a popular drug to include in multiple-agent regimens (299, 300). It is a rather predictable cause of interstitial pulmonary fibrosis, and for this reason it has provided one of the best experimental models of this disease. Toxicity correlates with the total dose of bleomycin given, for significant drug-related pulmonary illness is infrequent (less than 10%) if the cumulative dose is less than 150 to 200 mg; for doses of more than 300 to 500 mg, toxicity may approach 50% with approximately 10% mortality (315). Several factors seem to enhance pulmonary toxicity from bleomycin, and these should alert the physician to expect complications. Older people will have more toxicity. Simultaneous administration of bleomycin and thoracic radiation increases the likelihood of toxicity, which will also occur at a lower cumulative dose of the drug. Prior use of radiation also increases the risk. Administration of high oxygen

Table 13.6
Drugs or Drug Groups that Cause Pulmonary Reactions

| Drug | Syndrome(s)[a] | Frequency |
|---|---|---|
| **CYTOTOXIC DRUGS** | | |
| Azathioprine | HP | <1% |
| Bleomycin | PF, NPE, HP, AP | 3% to 25% (PF) |
| Busulfan | PF | <1% |
| Carmustine | PF, AP | 10% to 30% |
| Cyclophosphamide | PF, NPE, HP | <1% |
| Cytosine arabinoside | NPE | <1% |
| Methotrexate | HP, NPE, PF, pleuritis | 7% (HP) |
| Mitomycin | PF, AP | 3% to 12% |
| Procarbazine | HP | <1% |
| Vinca alkaloids[b] | AP | 20% to 40% |
| **NONCYTOTOXIC DRUGS** | | |
| Amiodarone | PF, NPE, AP | 6% to 15% |
| Aspirin | NPE,[c] bronchospasm | 22%[c] (NPE) |
| β-Adrenergic blockers | Bronchospasm | Variable |
| Bromocriptine | PF, pleuritis | <1% |
| Captopril | Cough | 10% |
| Carbachol | Bronchospasm | <1% |
| Carbamazepine | HP | <1% |
| Chlorambucil | PF | <1% |
| Chlordiazepoxide | NPE[c] | <1% |
| Dantrolene | Pleuritis | <1% |
| Diphenylhydantoin | HP | <1% |
| Enalapril | Cough | 10% to 20% |
| Ethchlorvynol | NPE[c] | <1% |
| Gold salts | HP, PF, BO | <1% |
| Hydrochlorothiazide | NPE | <1% |
| Lidocaine | NPE | <1% |
| Methysergide | Pleuritis | <1% |
| Naloxone | NPE | <1% |
| Neuromuscular blocking agents | Bronchospasm | <1% |
| Nitrofurantoin | HP, PF | <1% |
| Nonsteroidal anti-inflammatory agents | Bronchospasm, HP | 4% to 20% |
| Opiates | NPE | <1% |
| Penicillamine | BO, PRS, PF, HP | <1% |
| Protamine | NPE | <1% |
| Pyrimethamine-chloroquine | HP | <1% |
| Pyrimethamine-dapsone | HP | <1% |
| Sulfasalazine | PF, HP, BO | <1% |
| Tocolytic agents | NPE | <1% |
| Tocainide | PF, NPE | <1% |

Adapted from Cooper JA Jr: Drug-related pulmonary diseases. In Bone RC, Dantzker DR, George RB, Matthay RA, Reynolds HY (eds): *Pulmonary and Critical Care Medicine,* vol 2. Chicago: Mosby-Year Book, 1993, pp M8:1–9.
[a] PF, pulmonary fibrosis; HP, hypersensitivity pneumonitis; BO, bronchiolitis obliterans; NPE, noncardiogenic pulmonary edema; PRS, pulmonary renal syndrome; AP, acute pneumonitis.
[b] Not as single agent, in conjunction with mitomycin only.
[c] Overdose only.

concentrations produces synergistic toxicity with bleomycin, and a fulminant form of interstitial pneumonitis and fibrosis can develop. Oxygen given during surgical procedures seems sufficient to trigger the response. Patients with esophageal carcinoma who have received radiation and bleomycin therapy and undergo subsequent surgery are at high risk to develop lung toxicity (316).

Whereas interstitial fibrosis is the usual manifestation of pulmonary toxicity, an apparent hypersensitivity form of toxicity can develop (317) that is more amenable to improvement with corticosteroid therapy than the fibrotic form. Finally, the route of bleomycin administration accounts for a striking difference in lung susceptibility to injury. In experimental animals, a single intratracheal dose may cause a progressive form of pulmonary fibrosis to develop (318). In contrast, if the drug is given parenterally, much larger and repetitive doses can be tolerated; in fact, continuous intravenous administration of the drug in low doses may lower the incidence of toxicity somewhat. Pulmonary functional abnormalities generally include arterial hypoxemia and a restrictive ventilatory pattern with decreased lung volumes and a diminished diffusing capacity for carbon monoxide (299, 300, 315).

The lung response to the three cytotoxic agents busulfan, cyclophosphamide, and methotrexate shows similarities and is different from other forms of pulmonary toxicity. A considerable latent period may occur before pulmonary symptoms suggesting toxicity develop; often the patient is under treatment for a hematologic malignancy, and several years of rather stable drug usage may have elapsed before toxicity appears for inapparent reasons. Cough, dyspnea, and fever set in and the chest radiograph may show a combined alveolar filling and interstitial pattern and occasionally a pleural effusion. The troublesome differential is that of a drug reaction versus a leukemic infiltration of the lung, and an opportunistic infection may be present as well. The onset of illness in patients taking methotrexate can be quite variable, occurring within a few days of beginning therapy or after a latent period; the dosage of drug per week may be an important determinant of this illness (299). In all these drug reactions fever is an important part of the toxic syndrome. Sputum or bronchial washings may yield unusual-appearing type II pneumocytes that can be identified by cytology and are characteristic of these particular drug-induced toxic pulmonary reactions.

### NONCYTOTOXIC AGENTS

Amiodarone, a powerful antiarrhythmic agent, causes lung disease in between 4 and 27% of patients (305). Pulmonary fibrosis and hypersensitivity or acute pneumonitis can be induced by this drug (305). A major risk factor is a maintenance dose(s) of more than 400 mg/day (305). Diffuse reticular infiltrates are most commonly seen on the chest radiograph, although diffuse acinar infiltrates have also been described (305). A restrictive ventilatory defect with a diffusion impairment is the most common physiologic abnormality (320). The $D_{LCO}$ is highly sensitive for amiodarone toxicity (320). Moreover, a $D_{LCO}$ greater than 80% of pretreatment level virtually excludes amiodarone toxicity (320). Discontinuation of the drug or reduction in drug dosage in conjunction with corticosteroid therapy can reduce the pulmonary disease (305, 320).

The antibiotic nitrofurantoin is one of the most widely recognized drugs causing pulmonary toxicity (296, 299, 301, 319). The acute onset of fever, chills, cough, and dyspnea can occur after a few days of therapy or within a few hours of the first dose in patients who have received the drug on previous occasions. Blood eosinophilia is likely and the symptom complex points to an allergic or hypersensitivity-type lung reaction, although the response has not been well characterized histologically. The pulmonary response seems to be one of pulmonary edema, with diffuse crackles heard in the lungs. A chest radiograph supports the impression of noncardiogenic pulmonary edema. Pleural effusion may be noted. The reaction will clear within 48 hours after discontinuing the drug; the disease is self-limited without mortality. Episodes of recurrent pneumonia can occur if the patient resumes use of the drug. To conclusively prove the drug-disease relationship, a challenge dose will elicit the reaction. A chronic form of nitrofurantoin disease can occur that does not include fever, pleural effusion, and eosinophilia but rather an insidious onset of cough and dyspnea months after the drug has been taken on a regular basis, usually for suppression of chronic bacteriuria. In this form, the lung disease is virtually indistinguishable from interstitial pneumonitis and fibrosis. Discontinuance of the drug plus corticosteroid therapy will arrest the process.

A variety of drugs are known to induce systemic lupus erythematosus; among the more than 20 drugs incriminated (99, 296, 299, 301), procainamide, hydralazine, diphenylhydantoin, and sulfonamides are among the ones most frequently encountered. Drug-induced SLE differs from the spontaneous disease in that there is less kidney and skin involvement and more pleuropulmonary reaction. The lung reaction and the entire syndrome remit if the causative drug is discontinued.

## SARCOIDOSIS

Sarcoidosis remains one of the most enigmatic diseases in the field of internal medicine. It occurs frequently, is variable in its severity, can affect multiple organs but has a propensity to involve the respiratory tract initially, and remains of unknown cause (321, 322). Pulmonary sarcoidosis is often a clinical diagnosis made from the clinical presentation and compatible chest radiographic pattern; laboratory studies and tissue histology are obtained to confirm and support the diagnosis. It is also a diagnosis of exclusion after such diseases as lymphoma, bronchogenic carcinoma, beryllium exposure, tuberculosis, histoplasmosis, and coccidioidomycosis have been eliminated, for each may mimic the clinical picture and the tissue histology of sarcoidosis.

Sarcoidosis was once stereotyped as a disease that was considered to usually affect young black people, often women, who lived in rural parts of the southern United States. This is now recognized as a faulty categorization, for Caucasians frequently have the disease and geography is not specific. The hallmark of the host's immune response to the disease is a delayed type of hypersensitivity and formation of tissue granuloma in affected organs. The peculiar noncaseating inflammation in the sarcoid granuloma, in contrast to those of tuberculosis, is not a specific histologic finding, contrary to the usual interpretation. However, sarcoidosis does feature many abnormalities in lymphocyte function, and these will be described in detail.

### CLINICAL AND RADIOGRAPHIC PRESENTATIONS

Sarcoidosis is protean in its clinical expression and at times can affect a variety of organs or begin with recurrent fever (323) and vague constitutional symptoms. However, respiratory tract findings are by far the most common (Table 13.7).

Sarcoidosis probably begins in the respiratory tract in response to some still-unknown inhaled substance or agent; certainly the lungs have a predilection to be involved with disease, although many other organs can be affected. The chest radiograph may provide the first clue, often in an asymptomatic person. Certain features of the disease vary between black and Caucasian patients, especially skin and ocular manifestations (324). After respiratory signs or symptoms, other findings are decidedly less frequent. Critical organ involvement may be striking and can confuse the diagnosis; when one is involved, this usually dictates prompt immunosuppressive therapy. Uveitis, cardiac arrhythmias (325, 326), neurologic signs (327, 328)—occasionally manifested as palsy of a single cranial nerve (the

**TABLE 13.7**
**MODE OF PRESENTATIONS OF SARCOIDOSIS**

| Presentation | Caucasian Patients (N = 105) | Black Patients (N = 103) |
|---|---|---|
| Respiratory symptoms | 36 | 43 |
| Routine chest film | 25 | 6 |
| Skin sarcoidosis | 5 | 15 |
| Arthralgia | | |
| With erythema nodosum | 5 | 2 |
| Without erythema nodosum | 8 | 5 |
| Ocular symptoms | 3 | 13 |
| Fatigue, weight loss | 8 | 5 |
| Peripheral adenopathy | 6 | 3 |
| Fever | 4 | 4 |
| Cardiac symptoms | 2 | 2 |
| Neurologic symptoms | 3 | 2 |
| Hepatic symptoms | 0 | 1 |
| Nasal symptoms | 1 | 0 |

Adapted from Israel H: Sarcoidosis. In Simmons DH (ed): *Current Pulmonology.* New York, John Wiley & Sons, 1979, vol 1, p 153.

seventh with Bell's palsy)—and hypercalcemia are the major concerns. Although liver dysfunction is not a usual presentation, this organ is often involved and is the source of diagnostic tissue in many patients (329, 330). Respiratory symptoms are not distinctive for sarcoidosis and are similar to those noted with other interstitial pulmonary diseases—breathlessness, often with minimal exertion, and nonproductive cough. Signs of pleural involvement or wheezing are unusual.

Sarcoidosis in the chest is suggested by a pattern of symmetrically enlarged bilateral hilar lymph nodes with ostensibly clear lung parenchyma on the chest radiograph (Fig. 13.11) (331). In such cases about half of the chest radiographs will also reveal enlarged paratracheal nodes (usually right-sided and unilateral). In fact, sarcoidosis is one of the few chest diseases that commonly involves nodes in the lung (hilar) and mediastinum simultaneously. In some instances bilateral hilar adenopathy found on a routine chest radiograph may be the only manifestation of sarcoidosis (322, 332). Approximately 5 to 9% of patients may present with only unilateral hilar adenopathy (333). In later stages of pulmonary sarcoidosis the lymph node response diminishes and progressive involvement of the lung parenchyma ensues; end stages of lung sarcoidosis may leave upper-zone cystic spaces and extensive linear streaking and infiltrates throughout but reveal little residual adenopathy. Such disease progression has led to a still-applicable radiographic classification of sarcoidosis (334). Stage I disease features symmetrical, bilateral hilar adenopathy (Fig. 13.11); stage II has hilar

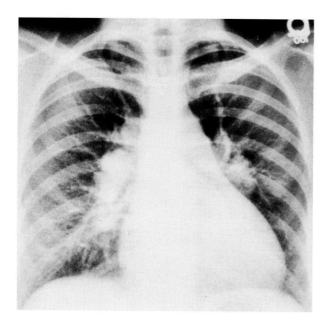

**FIGURE 13.11.** Sarcoidosis. PA chest radiograph of a 36-year-old woman with bilateral hilar and mediastinal adenopathy manifested by obliteration of the aortopulmonary window (ductus space). There is also right paratracheal adenopathy. The lung zones are normal; however, the cardiac silhouette is enlarged. The patient developed corticosteroid-responsive pulmonary infiltrates and cardiac arrhythmias, consistent with sarcoid cardiopulmonary involvement.

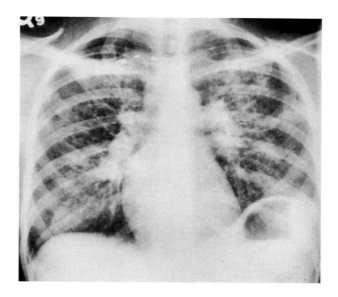

**FIGURE 13.12.** Sarcoidosis. PA chest radiograph of a 24-year-old woman with stage II sarcoidosis. Note the bilateral hilar adenopathy and interstitial infiltrates. (Clips from a previous surgical procedure are present in the right upper thorax.)

adenopathy and diffuse parenchymal changes (Fig. 13.12); and stage III has diffuse pulmonary infiltrates without adenopathy. This latter stage is often a burned-out, relatively stable period of disease in which extensive residual lung changes persist.

The classic chest radiographic sequence described above is not observed in every patient. When the hilar adenopathy stage is missed, clinicians often seem suspicious of the diagnosis of sarcoidosis and tend to think that the case is atypical. Dyspnea is roughly equated with higher radiographic stages of the disease (334) that feature greater involvement of conducting airways and air-exchange tissue; however, some patients may not have respiratory symptoms despite obvious changes in the radiograph. The nonuniform, patchy distribution of sarcoid lesions in lung tissue can leave areas of parenchyma virtually normal, and this probably accounts for the preservation of good lung function and lack of symptoms in some patients. Unusual radiographic patterns can be present, and one must be very alert to this possibility. Conglomerate infiltrates that give the appearance of pulmonary nodules or an alveolar filling pattern can occur, and evidence of pleural

effusion may exist. In one series of 89 patients with an established tissue diagnosis of sarcoidosis, 15% had an atypical-appearing chest radiograph with one of the features listed above noted (333).

## LABORATORY FINDINGS IN BLOOD AND LUNG

For patients with overt lung tissue involvement and radiographic changes of the parenchyma, tests of pulmonary function usually reveal a restrictive pattern, small lung volumes, and diminished DLCO as found with other forms of diffuse interstitial pulmonary fibrosis. Patients with adenopathy and ostensibly clear lung fields may have normal lung function. As a rule, a decrement of at least 20% below a patient's predicted values for lung volumes and spirometric parameters must be present before any immunosuppressive therapy would be considered to control or arrest a decline in lung function. Other organs that require laboratory screening include the heart for possible arrhythmias, liver with a liver enzyme profile, and kidneys. Serum calcium should be monitored. Kveim antigen skin testing and subsequent biopsy of the skin papule for typical sarcoid histology has long been useful for confirming the diagnosis. Because of the general scarcity of a well-characterized and reliable antigen, the Kveim test may be virtually impossible to perform nowadays.

Other changes in blood can be linked with the immunopathology occurring in affected organs such as

**TABLE 13.8**
**CELLULAR AND IMMUNOLOGIC CHANGES IN SARCOIDOSIS**

| Blood | Bronchoalveolar Fluid | Lung Tissue |
|---|---|---|
| Skin test anergy | Lymphocytes increased (T cells, cells with T helper cell activity high) | Granulomas (giant epithelioid cells, few eosinophils) |
| Lymphopenia with low number of T cells but increased T suppressor cells | Lymphocytes with gamma or delta receptor increased | |
| Immune complexes | Peripolesis noted (lymphocytes clustering around a macrophage) | |
| IgG elevated | Secretion of interleukin-2 and spontaneous secretion of lymphokines (monocyte chemotactic factor, interferon gamma) | |
| Interferon gamma may be increased | B lymphocytes and IgG secreting cells elevated | |
| Angiotensin-converting enzyme and lysozyme elevated | IgG increased | |
| | Activated alveolar macrophages (can secrete interleukin-1 and angiotensin-converting enzyme) | |
| | Prostaglandin $E_2$ | |
| | Tumor necrosis factor | |
| | PMNs in late stages of disease | |

the lung; Table 13.8 contrasts findings in blood and lung tissue (335).

Skin test anergy to common fungal and tuberculin antigens is a usual feature of active sarcoidosis; the cause of this faulty delayed hypersensitivity probably reflects the paucity of circulating T lymphocytes among the blood mononuclear cells. Leukopenia (total white cell count less than 4000/mm$^3$) occurs in about 30% of patients (322). Patients with both active and chronic forms of disease can have fewer blood lymphocytes than normals, and the proportions of T and B cells are abnormal (336). The fraction of T cells is likely to be decreased and the mitogenic response to phytohemagglutinin is reduced in sarcoid patients. B cells, in contrast, especially those with immunoglobulin identified on their surface, are often increased in acute, active disease; this increase can be correlated with elevated serum $\gamma$-globulins in about half of the patients. In addition to the lymphocyte alterations, blood monocytes are activated and may show depressed chemotactic responses (337). Excessive activity of the subpopulation of T lymphocytes has been documented in sarcoid patients (338, 339), and such activity may explain in part the skin anergy.

In serum, several enzyme and immunoglobulin changes can be documented. Serum globulin levels are increased in about half of patients with active disease (322) and immune complexes can be identified (339, 340). Two enzymes, lysozyme (341) and angiotensin-converting enzyme (ACE) (342) have been found to be elevated in patients with sarcoidosis and are used as diagnostic aids (343, 344). ACE, which acts to convert serum angiotensin I to angiotensin II and helps metabolize bradykinin, is produced primarily by capillary endothelial cells; however, other cells such as fibroblasts and alveolar macrophages can also produce it at times (345, 346). Whereas serum ACE is more helpful in the diagnosis of sarcoidosis because it is likely to be elevated in 60% or more of patients with active disease (an elevated value is greater than 2 standard deviations above the normal mean), it is not specific for sarcoidosis. Other diseases that may have elevated levels are Gaucher's disease; leprosy; coccidioidomycosis; some cases of silicosis, asbestosis, berylliosis, and *Mycobacterium intracellulare* infection; osteoarthritis; diabetes mellitus with retinopathy; and miliary tuberculosis, primary biliary cirrhosis, or inflammatory bowel disease. Unfortunately, the list of diseases associated with elevated ACE levels is large, yet sarcoidosis continues to be the most common disease with high serum values. Several reports have indicated the usefulness of serial ACE values in monitoring sarcoid disease activity (347–351).

Bronchoscopy is indicated to inspect the airways for possible endobronchial sarcoid, often recognized by a cobblestone appearance of whitish plaques on the airway mucosa, and to obtain transbronchial biopsies that have a high yield of granulomatous tissue in this disease—up to 70 to 80% (352, 353). Even though the chest radiograph may not show parenchymal evidence of

**TABLE 13.9**

**PROFILE OF RESPIRATORY CELLS RECOVERED IN BAL FLUID (FOR NONSMOKER NORMALS FOLLOWING 100- TO 300-ML LAVAGE)[a]**

| Cell Number Total | Viability | Macrophages | PMNs[b] | EOS/BASO[c] | Lymphocytes | Ciliated Cells | Erythrocytes |
|---|---|---|---|---|---|---|---|
| 15 × 10⁶ | <90 | 85 | 1–2 | <1 | 7–12 | 1–5 | <5% |
| Lymphocytes T cells (% of total) | Subsets (%) T helper/inducer[d] | T suppressor/ cytotoxic | | T killer lymphs | B lymphs[e] (Plasma cells) | Untypable lymphs | |
| 70 | 50[f] | 30 | | 7[g] | 5–10 | 5 | |

Adapted from Reynolds HY: Lung immunology and its contribution to the immunopathogenesis of certain diseases. *J Allergy Clin Immunol* 78:833–847, 1986.

[a] See references 41 and 42 for normal values.
[b] PMNs, polymorphonuclear granulocytes.
[c] EOS/BASO, Eosinophils/basophils.
[d] As percent of T cells. The $T_H/T_S$ ratio is about 1.5 : 1.8.
[e] Amount plasma cells are immunoglobulin releasing cells with the following frequency: IgG = IgA > IgE (see reference 28).
[f] The T helper subset contains about 7% of cells with HLA DR + antigen, and these can preferentially produce interleukin-2 (see reference 371).
[g] Killer lymphocytes seem inactive when retrieved from a normal lung (see reference 374).

disease, it is usually present, and parenchymal biopsies contain distinctive tissue changes.

The recovery of large numbers of lymphocytes in BAL fluid is a striking finding in many patients with active pulmonary sarcoidosis (24, 354), and this is the important cellular feature that separates the diverse group of interstitial lung diseases into two general categories, granulomatous and nongranulomatous (Table 13.1). As it is important to know the proportions of T lymphocyte subpopulations, a reference for normal cells is given in Table 13.9. For contrast with alveolar cells, in normal blood about 70% of the lymphocytes are T cells, and about the same ratio for T helper and T suppressor cells exists. Patients with active stages of pulmonary sarcoidosis usually have an increased percentage of lymphocytes in the mixture of respiratory cells retrieved by BAL (24, 355–358). This percentage can be quite high and has been noted to be about 40 to 60% (normal is less than 10%). Moreover, the vast majority of lymphocytes can be identified as T cells, and these may constitute 90% of the total lymphocyte population (359). Concomitant blood T lymphocyte numbers are reduced. Smoking status can influence the number of T cells and the CD4/CD8 ratio by decreasing them (360). In addition, the airway T cells are "activated" because they are capable of forming rosettes with sheep red blood cells at 37 C, instead of at 4 C as is the usual case, and they bear a surface receptor for IgG. Functionally, activated T cells spontaneously secrete a variety of lymphokines that affect other lymphocytes and monokines that interact with macrophages. Likewise, the macrophages are also activated and produce cytokines that modulate lymphocyte function. The sticking or clustering of lymphocytes around a macrophage (peripolesis) is complex and may reflect activity of the macrophage's membrane (361). These intraalveolar events probably mirror some of those ongoing in the tissue where the granuloma are formed. These cellular interactions are illustrated in Figure 13.13.

## IMMUNOLOGIC CONCEPTS

The inciting antigen or causative agent for sarcoidosis is still elusive, but evidence suggests that the T lymphocytes that accumulate in the lung have had surface antigen receptors stimulated (362). Whatever it is, it elicits a mononuclear cell lung response primarily of lymphocytes, especially of the T cell variety. Functionally these cells are activated, often adhere spontaneously to alveolar macrophages (361), forming rosettes, and secrete lymphokine substances. In examining Figure 13.13 and conceptually arranging the cell data for sarcoid immunopathogenesis, one might conclude that the alveolar macrophage may initiate the lung response.

Alveolar macrophages develop from circulating blood monocytes, which undergo further maturation or differentiation in the interstitial spaces before emerging on the alveolar surface. Vitamin D metabolites seem important in this process; lymphocytes are also affected (363). Although the first responsibility of the alveolar macrophage is to be a roving scavenger and phagocyte to clean debris from the alveolar surface, it is apparent that the macrophage, especially when activated as in sarcoidosis, can secrete a large

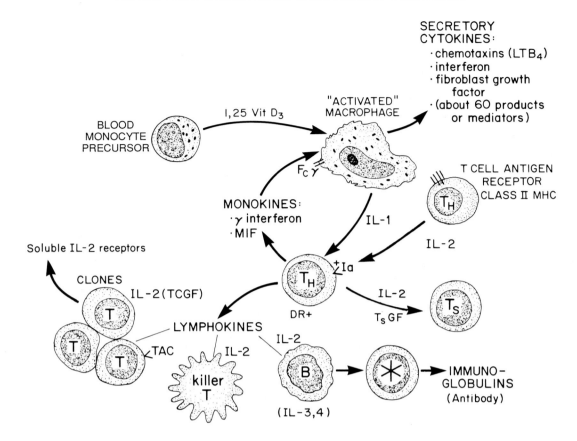

**Figure 13.13.**   An interaction between the "activated" alveolar macrophage and subpopulations of T lymphocytes, especially T helper cells, occurs in sarcoid lung disease, and this creates the alveolitis. Details about macrophage effects on lymphocyte activity (secretion of cytokines and antigen presentation) and T lymphocyte action that feeds back to the macrophage or directs the function of other immune cells through lymphokine and monokine mediators are given in the text. (Adapted from Reynolds HY: Lung immunology and its contribution to the immunopathogenesis of certain diseases. *J Allergy Clin Immunol* 78:833-847, 1986.)

array of cellular substances and mediators that affect the function of other cells (cytokines) (363a). As an example, macrophage chemotactic factors can attract other inflammatory cells to the alveoli, or fibroblast growth factors, such as platelet-derived growth factor and fibronectin, can influence fibroblast replication. Activated macrophages in sarcoidosis can secrete interleukin-1 (IL-1), which may attract lymphocytes into the alveoli (364). Such molecules as tumor necrosis factor and prostaglandin $E_2$ can have local effects that promote alveolitis (365), or they may diffuse into the systemic circulation as well. The list of enzymes, regulatory proteins, and inhibitors produced by macrophages continues to lengthen, as over 150 substances have been attributed to this heterogeneous cell population (366–368).

The macrophage also serves as an antigen presenting cell that can process an antigen, display it on its cell membrane where it is taken up by an appropriate T helper ($T_H$) lymphocyte and matched with respect to class II histocompatibility antigens. Antigen is received on the lymphocyte's membrane by a T cell antigen receptor that has an intricate structure composed of two $\beta$ and $\alpha$ chains. Whether or not the spontaneous lymphocyte-macrophage rosettes (361) seen in sarcoidosis lung fluid represent an initial phase of antigen presentation to T cells is uncertain. Antigen presentation by macrophages is enhanced in sarcoidosis (369, 370).

As noted, within the lumen of normal alveolar spaces, the majority of lymphocytes are T cells, and the T helper cells outnumber the suppressor cells by a ratio of about 1.5 to 1. Of the T helper cells, a small percentage (about 7% in normals) have an HLA-DR antigen; this subpopulation may increase when a lymphocytic alveolitis develops as in active sarcoidosis (371) and is responsible for most of the interleukin-2 produced (372, 373). Approximately 7% of the airway T cells are killer cells, but these seem dormant in normal subjects (374). In addition, about 5% of the lymphocytes are B cells or plasma cells. These cells can release various class-specific immunoglobulins from their surface as already mentioned. In sarcoidosis, the expanded number of DR-positive T helper cells is responsible for producing the large amount of IL-2 that may cause expansion of clones of lymphocytes, activate the killer cells, and stimulate immunoglobulin production (IL-4 is needed as well). No defects in the function of lung sarcoid suppressor cells have been noted, so lack of suppressor cell regulation is not the cause of the rather autonomous T helper cell function (375). In the activated T helper cell producing IL-2, increased expression of the IL-2 gene can be found (376). Thus, alveolar macrophages and lung T cells are selectively activated in the sarcoid lung (377).

In the other direction, the activated $T_H$ cells can secrete a variety of monokines, such as gamma interferon (378) and migration inhibition factor (MIF), that modulate macrophage activity in turn. Gamma interferon in particular can energize or activate the macrophage. Having considered intraalveolar events in active sarcoidosis, a crucial intermediate step between the alveoli and development of granulomas in interstitial areas might involve hilar and mediastinal lymph nodes, which characteristically enlarge in early radiographic stages of disease and then subside as parenchymal tissue becomes more involved. The precise stimulus for the development of the complex tissue granulomas with epithelioid cell differentiation and concentric layers of surrounding T and B lymphocytes and fibroblasts remains unclear. However, soluble mediators, T helper cell activity, and macrophage-derived substances such as ACE (379) may influence the kinetics of granuloma formation in the nodes and parenchymal tissue.

In advanced phases of sarcoid lung disease, an increased number of PMNs can be recovered in BAL fluid, and these inflammatory cells may contribute to the fibrotic stage of disease (380). Possibly, chemotactic factors produced by macrophages could have a role (381).

Thus, sarcoidosis involves complex cellular immune pathways; its pathogenesis is not simple. Peripheral blood findings do not reflect all the same changes noted in the airways; a compartmentalized immune response involving both macrophages and lymphocytes seems to occur. A relative excess of blood T suppressor cells probably contributes to the impaired cellular immunity often observed, whereas T helper cells are increased in the lungs of many patients with an active alveolar stage of disease. Finding evidence of numerous suppressor cells in the lung creating a CD8 alveolitis is unusual and may only be found in about 4% of patients when the diagnosis of sarcoidosis is made (382). In an early granulomatous stage some cases of sarcoidosis spontaneously resolve and granulomas regress, possibly under the impetus of serum chemotactic inactivating factor. In others the disease may progress, causing considerable tissue destruction and lung fibrosis.

## DISEASE COURSE AND THERAPY

Of 44 untreated, asymptomatic patients with symmetrical hilar adenopathy and no parenchymal infiltrates, spontaneous resolution of the radiographic disease occurred in most; 73% remitted and most did so in 6 to 17 months after diagnosis (331). Thus, advocacy of a particular form of therapy for patients in the earliest stages of disease must be tempered by the fact that spontaneous regression of the pulmonary process is frequent; this does not remove the lingering question about persistence of an inciting agent in a dormant stage. Since the cause of the disease is unknown, prevention or environmental control is not possible.

For extrapulmonary sarcoidosis involving such critical organs as eyes, heart, or nervous system, corticosteroid therapy is indicated. For the lungs, the decision to treat is more difficult. To assess the effect of corticosteroid therapy on pulmonary dysfunction in sarcoidosis, a prospective study (383) compared 6 months of moderate-dose prednisone therapy (60 mg/day for 1 month, then 20 mg/day for 5 months) with no treatment by monitoring pulmonary function for 1 to 2 years. Pulmonary dysfunction initially was rather modest in that mean $D_{LCO}$ was decreased 30% of predicted and mean arterial oxygen at rest was 80 mm Hg. Histologically, lung tissue had inflammatory changes and granulomas but was not severely distorted in most patients. In essence, treatment did nothing dramatic for these patients, for they neither improved nor worsened in pulmonary function when compared with the untreated control group.

If patients with pulmonary sarcoidosis, however, have troublesome respiratory symptoms and a 20 to 30% reduction in pulmonary function parameters (lung volumes, $D_{LCO}$, etc.), most clinicians will institute a trial of corticosteroid therapy for approximately 6 months (384). Such therapy will generally improve symptoms, variably improve pulmonary function tests, and often improve the appearance of the chest radiograph. Long-term use of small doses of corticosteroid does seem beneficial for many patients, and relapse and exacerbation of symptoms occur in some if the drug is tapered or withdrawn. However, the effectiveness of therapy for sarcoidosis remains controversial (383, 385, 386). Other cytotoxic and immunosuppressive drugs have been used to treat sarcoidosis but rarely in a controlled trial, and so none can be recommended as proven therapy for the disease. In the future, specific immunocytotoxic therapy that may obliterate certain hyperactive subsets of T cells, for example, may be developed and prove useful, or drug inhibitors or antibodies that neutralize enzymes such as ACE or that downregulate certain cell receptors (387) may suppress the formation of granulomas. It is noteworthy that corticosteroids will inhibit the secretion of IL-2 by T helper lymphocytes in active pulmonary sarcoidosis (388), so the effect of this drug in suppressing cellular activity in this disease is now better understood. For the present, only corticosteroids are recommended for therapy. Corticosteroids can be envisioned to act on the alveolitis and interstitial inflammatory component of the disease by suppressing T lymphocytes that accumulate in affected tissue and perpetuate the disease.

As discussed for idiopathic pulmonary fibrosis, objective assessment that therapy is actually suppressing disease activity can be difficult given the subjective nature of symptoms and the insensitivity of chest radiographs in showing improvement. Pulmonary physiology may not suffice either. At present, the serial application of such tests as ACE measurement, gallium lung scans (389), and various cellular or immunologic components in bronchoalveolar lavage have an uncertain role, since they do not always correlate with disease activity nor predict response to therapy (390–394). Other more sensitive parameters need to be identified and are being sought (371, 373, 376, 395). It remains important to find some mediator or cellular change that would identify the patient with sarcoidosis who may not have benign lung disease but will develop progressive fibrocystic debilitating lung changes. In addition, subgrouping of patients based on immunologic parameters in BAL fluid needs more investigation (396, 397).

For patients with established disease, the process eventually stabilizes and sarcoidosis seems to burn out. In this advanced stage, there is usually widespread cystic and fibrotic destruction of lung tissue, so the chest radiograph shows extensive honeycomb changes and diffuse interstitial markings. Pulmonary function is invariably impaired.

Sarcoidosis continues to be an enigmatic illness. Its cause remains elusive; it has a propensity to involve the respiratory tract, yet extrapulmonary disease can be severe and at times difficult to recognize; its course is unpredictable; and it is uncertain just how effective

anti-inflammatory therapy is. However, we are at an important juncture in understanding this disease. Continued investigation into ways of sampling the affected lung tissue (398) will undoubtedly uncover more details of deranged immunology at the molecular and genetic levels in a related disease caused by beryllium (399), which in turn will produce more specific therapy. It may be that the association between sarcoidosis and another immunologic infectious disease, AIDS, will give further insight into the mechanisms of lymphocytic alveolitis (400) that initiates the pulmonary phase.

## HYPERSENSITIVITY PNEUMONITIS (ALSO TERMED ALLERGIC ALVEOLITIS)

Inhalation of a variety of organic dusts can cause hypersensitivity pneumonitis (401–404). Although many people are exposed to these environmental substances and many become sensitized and develop precipitating serum antibodies to the causative antigens, only a few develop overt lung disease. These dusts can be derived from animal dander and proteins; from saprophytic fungi that contaminate vegetables, wood bark, or water-reservoir vaporizers; and from dairy and grain products (Table 13.10) (402). Colorful, descriptive names for the diseases underscore the frequent occupational nature of exposure. Either the inhaled dust itself causes respiratory disease or a microbial contaminant passively carried with it may be incriminated. Usually a species of thermophilic actinomycetes is found; these ubiquitous bacteria thrive at high ambient temperatures (45 to 60 C range) that are reached during the decomposition of vegetable matter. Perhaps about $10^9$ mold spores per cubic millimeter of air must be inhaled on a daily basis for allergic alveolitis to develop, as was found for a group of Swedish farmers (405).

Some forms of occupational disease are easily recognized. When the clinical symptoms are temporally related to workplace exposure, the index of suspicion is high that an environmental or inhalation source is causing illness. However, subtle forms of exposure may occur among office personnel or individuals in the home (called tight building syndrome), and putting clinical symptoms together with unsuspected and episodic exposure or with a lower dose but constant exposure can be most difficult. A considerable amount of medical detective work may be required to find that a water-cooled air conditioning unit or an infant's cold-mist vaporizer is the culprit or that an orchid grower is inhaling fungal spores from the bark chips he uses to mulch his flowers. The source may be obscure. In

**TABLE 13.10**
**SOME ETIOLOGIC AGENTS IN HYPERSENSITIVITY PNEUMONITIS**

| Disease | Source of Exposure | Major Antigens or Microbe |
|---|---|---|
| Farmer's lung | Moldy hay | *Micropolyspora faeni* (also *Faenia rectivirgula*) |
| Grain handler's lung | Moldy grain | *Micropolyspora faeni, Thermoactinomyces vulgaris* |
| Bagassosis | Moldy sugar cane fiber | *Thermoactinomyces sacchari* |
| Summer type hypersensitivity | House dust or bird droppings | *Trichosporon cutaneum* |
| Humidifier or air-conditioner lung | Contaminated forced-air system, heated water reservoirs | *M. faeni, T. vulgaris,* occasionally amoebae are implicated |
| Maple bark stripper's lung | Moldy bark | *Cryptostroma corticale* |
| Malt workers' lung | Moldy malt | *Aspergillus clavatus* |
| Sequoiosis | Moldy redwood dust | *Aureobasidium pullulans* and *Graphium* spp. |
| Wheat weevil disease | Wheat weevil disease | *Sitophilus granarius* |
| Cheese worker's lung | Cheese mold | *Penicillium caseii* |
| Suberosis | Moldy cork dust | *Penicillium frequentans* |
| Bird breeder's lung | Pigeons, parakeets, fowl, rodents | Avian or animal proteins (in excreta) |
| Chemical workers lung | Manufacture of plastics, polyurethane foam, or rubber | Trimellitic anhydride, diisocyanate, methylene diisocyanate |

our experience, a mold growing on a kitchen wall provided a chronic exposure for a symptomatic homemaker (23). The list of potential antigens that can be inhaled and cause airway sensitization is increasing, and recognition of these diseases is becoming more prevalent.

## CLINICAL PRESENTATION

Sensitization to an organic dust is usually insidious, and the potential patient is unaware of the detrimental effects it can cause. In certain avocations such as bird handling, almost all people intimately involved in care of the birds develop serum-precipitating antibodies to some avian antigens, but this immune response is not associated with disease in most (406). Likewise, farm workers may have serum antibodies to certain thermophilic bacteria (407). The onset of respiratory symptoms may not occur at first but may appear only later after an exposure pattern is well established. In the acute form of disease, respiratory and systemic symptoms develop explosively within 4 to 6 hours after dust is inhaled and consist of dyspnea, cough, chills, fever, and malaise. The symptoms may persist for 12 hours or so and abate spontaneously; with each reexposure the acute episode occurs again. When observed, the patient is acutely ill and dyspneic; inspiratory crackles can be heard prominently in the lower lung zones. Temperature may be alarmingly elevated and the peripheral blood leukocyte count can be in excess of

$25,000/mm^3$, with a left shift. The chest radiograph may appear normal but usually shows a fine, diffuse alveolar filling pattern and variable interstitial streaks.

Pulmonary function abnormalities, best measured in patients challenged with antigens in a pulmonary laboratory and followed with serial observations, appear in 4 to 6 hours when the clinical symptoms develop. A decrease in FVC and $FEV_{1.0}$ occurs; air trapping and hyperinflation may be documented; and the diffusing capacity for carbon monoxide is reduced. Also, pulmonary compliance decreases. These changes gradually return to normal as the clinical picture improves. Another pattern of pulmonary dysfunction may occur, involving a two-phase reaction. Initially, an immediate asthmatic-type reaction develops just after aerosol exposure to antigen that is characterized by air trapping and obstruction. This abates, to be followed in 4 to 6 hours by more restrictive and noncompliant lung function, as described.

Acute phases of the disease are seen infrequently, because a knowledgeable person will deduce the cause or make the connection between an airway exposure and subsequent respiratory symptoms. If the correlation is recognized, voluntary avoidance may solve the problem. On the other hand, if the exposure is continuous and protracted, a chronic form of disease may develop that does not include the acute exacerbations of respiratory symptoms (23, 408). Instead, patients will develop persistent symptoms of breathlessness, dyspnea with exertion, and cough that are indistinguishable from symptoms noted in other interstitial pulmonary diseases; fatigue, poor appetite, and weight loss can be significant in this disease. Symptoms and evidence of constitutional effects of disease may be evident for months and occasionally for years before the patient presents for evaluation. Many patients with hypersensitivity pneumonitis are not diagnosed until this more advanced stage of disease is present. Chest radiographs are abnormal and appear like other IPF films. Pulmonary function is characterized by a restrictive ventilatory pattern and a deficit in diffusing capacity for carbon monoxide. Such patients with this chronic form of inhalational hypersensitivity disease are difficult to separate from those with IPF and a host of similar diseases (Table 13.1) unless the exposure history happens to be obvious. A serum screen for hypersensitivity antigen precipitins will not establish a diagnosis but, if positive, might orient the clinician toward a possible environmental exposure. Physical examination does not provide any signs not found in other interstitial lung disease. Digital clubbing, initially considered an unusual occurrence (402, 403), has been noted to develop in about half the patients in one series (409).

## LABORATORY AND IMMUNOLOGIC FINDINGS

Except for the consequences of weight loss and poor appetite, the disease is limited to the respiratory tract, and most laboratory abnormalities relate to that organ system. Blood parameters reflect the effects of chronic disease in patients with advanced illness but do not necessarily mirror immunologic events occurring in the airways. With the exception of acute episodes of pneumonitis, the white cell count is not elevated and eosinophilia is not usual. The erythrocyte sedimentation rate may be elevated, and serum immunoglobulins are often increased. The presence of precipitating antibodies (in IgM, IgA, and IgG classes) in serum to antigens causing hypersensitivity disease can give a helpful clue; since many people develop such antibodies, this finding is not diagnostic but only indicates that prior exposure and sensitization have occurred. Skin testing with hypersensitivity antigens is not well standardized and can provide confusing conclusions. *Aspergillus* antigens may be useful in patients with bronchopulmonary aspergillosis, but other fungal preparations are not. Peripheral blood lymphocytes can be stimulated with appropriate antigens to give mitogenic responses, but generally the lymphocytes, especially ones recovered from the alveoli by lavage, have not been studied in the same detail as those from patients with sarcoidosis.

Most of the details about immune responses in the lungs have come from patients with farmer's lung with chronic hypersensitivity pneumonitis and from patients with pigeon breeder's (bird fancier's) lung (403, 410). These patients are evaluated with bronchoscopy like others with diffuse interstitial lung disease, and BAL and transbronchial biopsy help considerably to substantiate the diagnosis. Histologically, lung biopsy shows an infiltration with lymphocytes and inflammatory cells; granuloma formation and fibrosis are often evident as well. In patients with a chronic form of farmer's lung (23), the total recovery of cells from lung lavage was increased and reflected an increased number of lymphocytes. Of the respiratory cell population, 70% were lymphocytes, versus 8% customarily found in normal controls; most of the lymphocytes were T cells. Upon further analysis of subpopulations of T cells, a slight excess of T suppressor lymphocytes can be found (411–413). This is an interesting contrast to the striking increase in T helper cells that is characteristic of active sarcoidosis. There is a possibility that an elevated CD4-positive T-cell response is found with a more insidious onset of hypersensitivity pneumonitis (414), but this needs further study. Thus, there was an increase in the absolute number of lymphocytes found in bronchoalveolar lavage from patients with this form of chronic hypersensitivity pneumonitis. Moreover, lavage fluid from these patients contained high concentrations of immunoglobulin, especially IgG and IgM (23, 415). The presence of IgM is unusual because this immunoglobulin class is rarely found in measurable amounts in normal lung fluid and is infrequently present in lavage fluid obtained in other lung diseases. Specific precipitating antibody to inciting antigens was found in most sera and in the BAL fluid from a number of these patients. Patients with acute forms of hypersensitivity disease have not been studied extensively by lung lavage and biopsy, because the illness is usually transient. One would expect that alveolitis and inflammation are present in the early phase. The reaction seems to be one of mononuclear cells and an acute but transient increase in polymorphonuclear granulocytes and virtually no eosinophils (416). In more chronic stages of organic dust inhalation, the lung response is rather similar to that in sarcoidosis, which is the prototype of a granulomatous cellular response. Finally, an intermediate stage of the disease, or more accurately a stage of exposure, is an asymptomatic form in which the subject has no special symptoms of respiratory illness but has a subclinical form as alveolitis (417–419). An increased percentage of lung lymphocytes can be found as well as specific precipitating antibody. In such subjects this form of benign alveolitis or lung inflammation is well tolerated for periods of at least 2 years without overt disease developing (418). It appears that a lymphocytic alveolitis as sampled in BAL fluid from an asymptomatic farmer does not have any long-term clinical significance (420, 421).

### CONCEPTS OF IMMUNOPATHOGENESIS

Immunologic data from lung lavage studies in patients in a chronic phase of hypersensitivity pneumonitis (HP) are summarized in Table 13.11 (422–424). It is satisfying to know the etiology of the hypersensitivity diseases so that a specific antigen can be inserted to initiate the reaction. The prominent lymphocyte accumulation in the alveoli is impressive, and T cells predominate, especially T suppressor cells. Less is known about lymphocyte function and subsets of T cells in HP than in sarcoidosis, and the mediators have not been as well described (as shown in Fig. 13.13). Tissue granulomas develop in chronic forms of the disease. A striking contrast between hypersensitivity pneumonitis and sarcoidosis, however, is the apparent lack of hilar and mediastinal lymph node enlargement and absence of splenomegaly. The striking increase in airway IgG and IgM in chronic hypersensitivity pneumonitis is notable. As the inciting antigen is known, specific antibodies can be identified and the ingredients for immune complex formation are present.

### THERAPY

If the environmental source of inhaled antigen is identified, simple avoidance is sufficient treatment. The acute form of disease abates without specific therapy. Preventing disease by avoiding the causative antigen is not always easy, however, especially if an occupational exposure is identified. A change of job or relocation within a factory to decrease exposure may not be a simple matter. With chronic forms of disease accompanied by respiratory symptoms and abnormal pulmonary function, a trial of corticosteroids can be given with modest expectations that this form of immunosuppression will be effective.

## PULMONARY EOSINOPHILIC GRANULOMA AND EOSINOPHILIC SYNDROMES

The presence of eosinophils in lung tissue is a common occurrence and indicates that these inflammatory cells are part of the host's cellular response to a variety of inciting agents and systemic immunologic diseases (425, 426). Chemotactic factors released from degranulating mast cells attract eosinophils and localize them in sites of IgE-mediated reactions, whereupon eosinophils inactivate mediators and actually seem to control the extent of the reaction. Eosinophils are found in the

**TABLE 13.11**

**IMMUNOLOGIC FEATURES OF THE BLOOD, BRONCHOALVEOLAR LAVAGE FLUID, AND LUNG TISSUE IN CHRONIC STAGES OF HYPERSENSITIVITY PNEUMONITIS**

| Blood | Bronchoalveolar Fluid | Lung Tissue |
|---|---|---|
| Normal blood cell counts | Lung cell recovery increase | Alveolitis |
| Normal immunoglobulin levels, usually positive serum precipitins (IgG) | High lymphocyte percentages (50–70% of BAL cells) <br> • T lymphocytes predominate <br> • Possible to have an increased number of suppressor cells (slight reversal of $T_H/T_S$ cell ratio) | • Lymphocytes, plasma cells, granulomas (intraalveolar septal distribution) and foamy histiocytes <br> Bronchiolitis <br> Fibrosis possible |
| | Large and foamy macrophages, a minimal number of eosinophils, and an increased number (up to 1% of all lavage cells) of basophils | |
| | T-cell division high (RNA) | |
| | Total protein increased <br> • Elevated IgG and IgM levels <br> • IgG and IgA antibodies present | |
| | Abnormal surfactant composition | |
| | Fibrogenic factors increased (hyaluronic acid, type III procollagen, fibronectin and fibroblast growth factors) | |
| | Vitronectin | |
| | Laminin $P_1$ | |

airways and lung tissue of patients with idiopathic pulmonary fibrosis. In other interstitial diseases that seem to have an allergic component (such as hypersensitivity pneumonitis, drug-induced lung syndromes, and sarcoidosis), eosinophils are a minor component of the tissue reaction but can usually be identified in tissue sections. In contrast, eosinophils can be the most conspicuous inflammatory cell in certain primary lung or systemic diseases that have frequent lung involvement, and these are grouped together as eosinophilic syndromes. There is considerable overlapping among these syndromes, and precise separation is impossible because the etiology and pathogenesis are poorly understood. The classification developed by Crofton and colleagues (427) still seems to be useful. It includes the categories described below.

## TYPES OF EOSINOPHILIC SYNDROMES

### Simple Pulmonary Eosinophilia

This is a self-limited disease that features migratory, fleeting areas of infiltration in a peripheral pattern on the chest radiograph and is accompanied by minimal respiratory symptoms and blood eosinophilia (427, 428). The disease seems to be an allergic response that can result from parasitic infection; the human parasites *Ascaris lumbricoides* and *Strongyloides stercoralis*, and nonhuman ones such as dog and cat ascarids that produce visceral larva migrans, are known to be causative. Certain drugs such as sulfonamides have been implicated also. This pulmonary disease is known as Loeffler's pneumonia and the PIE syndrome (peripheral infiltrates with blood eosinophilia).

### Prolonged Pulmonary Eosinophilia

As suggested by its name, this disease differs from the simple form in that it is often chronic, and accompanying pulmonary and systemic symptoms can be severe. If this disease persists, it can lead to a form of interstitial pulmonary fibrosis that radiographically shows honeycombed lung changes and lung function abnormalities characteristic of other diseases in this group (Table 13.1).

Chronic eosinophilic pneumonia (429, 430) most commonly affects women and can present as a severe respiratory illness in which fever, night sweats, weight loss, and dyspnea are prominent symptoms. Blood eosinophilia is variable and often is not present. The disease is sometimes initially misdiagnosed as tuberculosis. A distinguishing feature in the first cases of eosinophilic pneumonia described (429) was deterioration in the patient's condition despite a trial of antituberculosis therapy. A lung biopsy is usually required

to establish the diagnosis. However, one helpful clue is often evident in the chest radiograph. Dense infiltrates develop that have a peculiar location in the peripheral portions of the lung. These peripheral infiltrates are not limited to a defined lobar or anatomical distribution but can extend across the usual anatomical barriers. Wheezing can be present or develop de novo in some patients. If the diagnosis is established, treatment with corticosteroids causes a striking regression in the radiographic findings and in clinical symptoms; a chest film taken a few weeks later may appear normal. Although the response to corticosteroid therapy is usually impressive, the disease may exacerbate after therapy is discontinued, and relapse can occur in about half of the patients during a 10-year follow-up period (431). The infiltrates tend to recur in the same locations on the chest radiograph. Two other pulmonary diseases that need careful consideration in the differential diagnosis are eosinophilic granuloma and the desquamative form of idiopathic interstitial pneumonitis.

### Tropical Pulmonary Eosinophilia (TPE)

Respiratory symptoms of cough, dyspnea, and in some patients attacks of asthma may be present in those with filarial infection. Systemic symptoms of malaise, fatigue, weight loss, and fever also occur; peripheral blood eosinophilia and high levels of antibody to filarial antigens are characteristic of laboratory abnormalities. The chest radiograph may reveal areas of patchy consolidation or bilateral streaking and increased parenchymal linearities in the hilar and lower lung zones. Histologically, microfilaria can be identified in areas of tissue nodules showing necrotic debris and eosinophils (429, 432, 433). Recently, the inflammatory process in the lung has been characterized (434). A striking recovery of eosinophils in bronchoalveolar lavage fluid was found; after therapy with diethylcarbamazine, these cells decreased and lung function tests improved (434).

In the BAL fluid obtained from patients with TPE is an increase of filaria-specific antibody to *Brugia malayi*, especially in the IgE class, but also in IgG, IgM, and, to a lesser degree, IgA (435). After therapy for 1 to 2 weeks with diethylcarbamazine, the parasite-specific antibodies in lung fluids were found to decrease. However, lung inflammation can persist (436).

### Pulmonary Eosinophilia with Asthma

Asthma is a frequent complaint in many forms of lung disease, including the eosinophilic syndromes; thus it is difficult to separate a single disease entity on this basis alone (437). Two diseases, allergic bronchopulmonary aspergillosis (438) and allergic angiitis with granulomatosis, as described by Churg and Strauss

(234), can fit this description. Since the eosinophilic component to the diseases seems incidental, it can be argued that these diseases are best discussed with respective asthma syndromes and systemic vasculitides affecting the lung, such as Churg-Strauss syndrome (see prior discussion in this chapter).

## Pulmonary Eosinophilia with Periarteritis Nodosa

In this form of systemic disease, the lung component is not a primary feature but represents one of many organ systems that are involved, usually with vasculitis (182, 192). Eosinophils are part of the inflammatory cell response and can be noted in granulomatous lesions and in tissue infiltrates.

## HISTIOCYTIC DISORDERS, INCLUDING EOSINOPHILIC GRANULOMA (LANGERHANS CELL GRANULOMATOSIS)

The histiocytoses are a group of diseases that feature proliferation and activation of mononuclear phagocytic cells, especially macrophages (439). The term *histiocyte* is synonymous with *macrophage* and emphasizes the fact that tissue macrophages can exist in many forms as alveolar or peritoneal cells, dermal Langerhans cells, hepatic Kupffer cells, osteoclasts, and microglial brain cells. Thus, the range of diseases and the principal organs affected are very broad. Often a form of cell-mediated immunity is evident and a granulomatous tissue reaction is found. Both findings suggest an intimate macrophage-lymphocyte interaction, as discussed already for sarcoidosis. Eosinophils may be contained in the granulomatous reaction, having been attracted to the inflammatory site by eosinophilic chemotactic factor (ECF-A), secreted by lymphocytes, but such a mechanism has not been proved. Immune complexes in blood can contribute to the lung reaction and perhaps stimulate macrophages or histiocytes, but this too remains uncertain. The proliferation and accumulation of histiocytes in affected tissue, often producing a granulomatous lesion, are part of the disease process in the histiocytic disorders.

A comprehensive classification of the histiocytic diseases based on macrophage involvement presents obvious overlapping with other syndromes readily explained by etiology or easily recognized clinically (439). The spectrum includes (a) reactive histiocytic proliferation with a known microorganism (tuberculosis, fungal, or parasitic agents) or with inert particles; (b) reactive proliferation in which the inciting agent is unknown, which includes such diverse entities as eosinophilic granuloma, Wegener's and lymphomatoid granulomatosis of lung, and sarcoidosis; (c) lipid storage diseases, which include Gaucher's disease, Niemann-Pick disease, sea blue histiocytosis, and

Fabry's disease; and (d) neoplastic disorders such as acute monocytic leukemia, chronic myelomonocytic leukemia, and histiocytic lymphoma. Eosinophilic granuloma is the only one that frequently affects the lungs, except for other granulomatous vasculitides and sarcoidosis.

Eosinophilic granuloma (EG) (or preferably called Langerhans cell granulomatosis [LCG]) can be a multifocal disease involving bones of the skull, extremities, ribs, pelvis, vertebrae, and mandible with lytic lesions. The triad of lytic skull lesions, exophthalmos, and pituitary involvement producing diabetes insipidus is known as Hand-Schüller-Christian disease and is a variant of multifocal LCG. A diffuse form of histiocytosis of the Letterer-Siwe type is a fulminant disease generally unresponsive to therapy. A unifocal or local extraosseous form of LCG involves the lungs and is a true cause of interstitial pulmonary fibrosis (439). Only the entity of LCG is discussed here in detail (440, 441).

LCG can affect all ages, but young adults, especially males, develop the disease most frequently. Symptoms may have an insidious onset, with cough and breathlessness with exertion as initial complaints. A spontaneous pneumothorax can be the presenting manifestation, although this is more likely to occur in advanced fibrotic stages of the disease when localized areas of airway obstruction lead to cyst formation and overdistention. Few constitutional symptoms may be present. Blood eosinophilia is unusual, but circulating immune complexes can be measured in serum in many patients with active disease, and the titer reflects the degree of cellular reactivity in a lung biopsy (442). The chest radiograph usually reveals a diffuse micronodular and interstitial-appearing infiltrate initially involving the middle and lower lung zones; later small cystic air spaces develop in the infiltrate, producing a honeycomb pattern (Fig. 13.14) (443). Adenopathy or pleural disease is unusual. The radiographic appearance differs from the one described for eosinophilic pneumonia, in which migratory infiltrates in the periphery of the lung are characteristic.

The course of LCG is quite variable in adults, and the prognosis is generally better for focal disease limited to the lungs than for multifocal disease and bone involvement. A bone scan is advisable as part of the initial evaluation of a patient with focal LCG and should certainly be made if bone symptoms occur later, because approximately 20% of patients eventually will develop a lytic bone lesion. Rarely, diabetes insipidus will occur. The lung disease does have a significant rate of spontaneous remission. Regression of pulmonary symptoms and chest radiographic infiltrates may occur in 10 to 25% of patients within several months of diagnosis, although the disease does not disappear

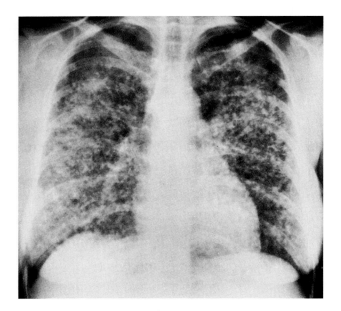

**FIGURE 13.14.** Eosinophilic granuloma of lung (Langerhans cell granulomatosis). A 31-year-old woman had a viral upper respiratory infection 3 months previously (a chest radiograph was not obtained), and a dry, nonproductive cough persisted. Dyspnea developed in the interim and shortness of breath limited her daily activities. Her chest radiograph shows extensive alveolar filling and interstitial infiltrates in all lung zones; also, small cystic spaces are evident. Tissue from an open lung biopsy revealed eosinophilic granuloma and evidence of cystic changes, suggesting that the disease process was chronic. Corticosteroid therapy improved the appearance of the chest radiograph and her symptoms. She also discontinued cigarette smoking which is an essential part of the therapy.

entirely without some residual symptoms. As most patients are cigarette smokers, cessation of smoking greatly helps. Corticosteroid treatment is not especially effective overall in suppressing the disease, except for the initial boost in subjective well-being associated with the "steroid effect." In many cases, the lung disease stabilizes and in effect burns out, leaving the patient with moderate pulmonary symptoms (dyspnea on exertion), residual lung fibrosis, cystic spaces in the parenchyma, and a restrictive pattern of lung function. Therapy at this stage of disease is symptomatic. Some patients are troubled with persisting bronchitis, which is superimposed on the quiescent interstitial fibrosis. If wheezing or obstructive airway changes on pulmonary testing are noted, judicious use of antibiotics and bronchodilators can be effective.

As indicated, the precise kind of immune mechanisms involved in developing the histiocytic-eosinophilic granulomatous response in the LCG lung is uncertain; failure to have an experimental animal model of the disease hampers investigative efforts. Because Hand-Schüller-Christian disease affects the head and airways, this form of disease is thought to be caused by some agent inhaled or concentrated in the nasooropharynx (439); multifocal osseous forms of the disease may reflect a different entry site. The disease does not seem to be a form of allergy, which seems important in the pathogenesis of certain eosinophilic lung syndromes, but instead features a granulomatous response (Fig. 13.14) and possibly an element of immune complex injury (442). Lung lavage analysis from patients has focused on the macrophages, which are usually increased in number; contained within this group are cells that can be identified as Langerhans cells. Using a monoclonal antibody, these cells can be found in increased numbers in LCG (444–446). This form of macrophage is considered to be a dendritic cell that has an added capability as an efficient antigen presenting cell (447, 448). Much more information has become available about the Langerhans cells that are involved in the granulomatous process. These macrophage-like cells seem to initiate or drive the immune response (449). Various growth factors such as granulocyte-macrophage colony-stimulating factor have a role in stimulating the cells (450).

## REFERENCES

1. Keogh BA, Crystal RG: Chronic interstitial lung disease. In Simmons DH (ed): *Current Pulmonology*. New York, John Wiley & Sons, 1981, vol 3, pp 237–340.
2. Crystal RG, Fulmer JD, Moss ML, et al: Idiopathic pulmonary fibrosis: clinical, histologic, radiographic, physiologic, scintigraphic, cytologic and biochemical aspects. *Ann Intern Med* 85:769–788, 1976.
3. Crystal RG, Bitterman PR, Rennard SI, et al: Interstitial lung diseases of unknown cause: disorders characterized by chronic inflammation of the lower respiratory tract. *N Engl J Med* 310:154–166, 235–244, 1984.
4. Bitterman PB, Rennard SI, Keogh BA, et al: Familial idiopathic pulmonary fibrosis—evidence of lung inflammation in unaffected family members. *N Engl J Med* 314:1343–1347, 1986.
5. Hamman L, Rich AR: Fulminating diffuse interstitial fibrosis of the lungs. *Trans Am Clin Climatol Assoc* 51:154–163, 1935.
6. Wells AU, Hansell DM, Rubens MB, et al: The predictive value of appearance of thin section computed tomography in fibrosing alveolitis. *Am Rev Respir Dis* 148:1076–1082, 1993.
7. Kuhn C III, Boldt J, King TE Jr, et al: An immunohistochemical study of architectural remodeling and connective tissue synthesis in pulmonary fibrosis. *Am Rev Respir Dis* 140:1693–1703, 1989.
8. Hyde DM, King TE Jr, McDermott T, et al: Idiopathic pulmonary fibrosis. Quantitative assessment of lung pathology. *Am Rev Respir Dis* 146:1042–1047, 1992.

9. Andoh Y, Aikawa T, Shimura S, et al: Morphometric analysis of airways in idiopathic pulmonary fibrosis patients with mucous hypersecretion. *Am Rev Respir Dis* 145:175–179, 1992.

10. Little JW, Hall WJ, Douglas RG Jr, et al: Airway hyperreactivity and peripheral airway dysfunction in influenza A infection. *Am Rev Respir Dis* 118:295–303, 1978.

11. Ueda T, Ohta K, Suzuki N, et al: Idiopathic pulmonary fibrosis and high prevalence of serum antibodies to hepatitis C. *Am Rev Respir Dis* 146:266–268, 1992.

12. Colin AA, Mark EJ: Lifelong progressive interstitial lung disease. Case records, Massachusetts General Hospital. *N Engl J Med* 329:1797–1805, 1993.

13. Epler GR, McLoud TC, Gaensler EA, et al: Normal chest roentgenograms in chronic diffuse infiltrative lung disease. *N Engl J Med* 298:934–939, 1978.

14. Nishimura K, Izumi T, Kitaichi M, et al: The diagnostic accuracy of high resolution computed tomography in diffuse interstitial lung diseases. *Chest* 104:1149–1155, 1993.

15. Dreisin RB, Schwarz MI, Theofilopoulos AN, et al: Circulating immune complexes in the idiopathic interstitial pneumonias. *N Engl J Med* 298:353–357, 1978.

16. Line BR, Fulmer JD, Reynolds HY, et al: Gallium-67 citrate scanning in the staging of idiopathic pulmonary fibrosis: correlation with physiologic and morphologic features and bronchoalveolar lavage. *Am Rev Respir Dis* 118:355–365, 1978.

17. Turner-Warwick M, Haslam PL: The value of serial bronchoalveolar lavages in assessing the clinical progress of patients with cryptogenic fibrosing alveolitis. *Am Rev Respir Dis* 135:26–34, 1987.

18. Fulmer JD, Roberts WC, von Gal ER, et al: Small airways and idiopathic pulmonary fibrosis. Comparison of morphologic and physiologic observations. *J Clin Invest* 60:595–610, 1977.

19. Epler GR, Saber FA, Gaensler ET: Determination of severe impairment (disability) in interstitial lung disease. *Am Rev Respir Dis* 121:647–659, 1980.

20. Keogh BA, Crystal RG: Pulmonary function testing in interstitial pulmonary disease. *Chest* 78:856–865, 1980.

21. Schwartz DA, Merchant RK, Helmers RA, et al: The influence of cigarette smoking on lung function in patients with idiopathic pulmonary fibrosis. *Am Rev Respir Dis* 144:504–506, 1991.

22. Hanley ME, King TE Jr, Schwarz MI, et al: The impact of smoking on mechanical properties of the lungs in idiopathic pulmonary fibrosis and sarcoidosis. *Am Rev Respir Dis* 144:1102–1106, 1991.

23. Reynolds HY, Fulmer JD, Kazmierowski JA, et al: Analysis of cellular and protein components of bronchoalveolar lavage fluid from patients with idiopathic pulmonary fibrosis and chronic hypersensitivity pneumonitis. *J Clin Invest* 58:165–175, 1977.

24. Weinberger SE, Kelman JA, Elson NA, et al: Bronchoalveolar lavage in interstitial lung disease. *Ann Intern Med* 89:459–466, 1978.

25. David GS, Brody AR, Craighead JE: Analysis of airspace and interstitial mononuclear cell populations in human diffuse interstitial lung disease. *Am Rev Respir Dis* 118:7–15, 1978.

26. Gadek JE, Kelman JA, Fells G, et al: Collagenase in the lower respiratory tract of patients with idiopathic pulmonary fibrosis. *N Engl J Med* 301:737–742, 1979.

27. Rudd RM, Halslam PL, Turner-Warwick M: Cryptogenic fibrosing alveolitis: relationship of pulmonary physiology and bronchoalveolar lavage to response to treatment and prognosis. *Am Rev Respir Dis* 124:1–8, 1981.

28. Lawrence EC, Martin RR, Blaese RM, et al: Increased bronchoalveolar IgG-secreting cells in interstitial lung diseases. *N Engl J Med* 302:1186–1188, 1980.

29. Hunninghake GW, Kawanami O, Ferrans VJ, et al: Characterization of inflammatory and immune effector cells in the lung parenchyma of patients with interstitial lung disease. *Am Rev Respir Dis* 123:407–412, 1981.

30. Reynolds HY: Idiopathic interstitial pulmonary fibrosis: contribution of bronchoalveolar lavage analysis. *Chest* 89:139–144, 1986.

31. Walters LC, Schwarz MI, Cherniack RM, et al: Idiopathic pulmonary fibrosis: pretreatment bronchoalveolar lavage cellular constituents and their relationships with lung histopathology and clinical response to therapy. *Am Rev Respir Dis* 135:696–704, 1987.

32. Reynolds HY: Idiopathic Pulmonary Fibrosis. In Lichtenstein LM, Fauci AS (eds): *Current Therapy in Allergy, Immunology and Rheumatology.* Toronto, BC Decker, 1988, vol 3, pp 214–220.

33. Bensard DD, McIntyre RC, Waring BJ, et al: Comparison of video thoracoscopic lung biopsy to open lung biopsy in the diagnosis of interstitial lung disease. *Chest* 103:765–770, 1993.

34. Fulmer JD, Katzenstein AA: The interstitial lung diseases. In Bone R, Dantzker D, George R, Matthay R, Reynolds H (eds): *Pulmonary and Critical Care Medicine.* St. Louis, Mosby Year Book, pp M1:1–15, 1993.

35. Reynolds HY: Classification, definition and correlation between clinical and histologic staging of interstitial lung diseases. *Semin Respir Med* 6:1–19, 1984.

36. Liebow AA, Steer A, Billingsley JG: Desquamative interstitial pneumonia. *Am J Med* 39:369–404, 1965.

37. Carrington CB, Gaensler EA, Coutu RD, et al: Natural history and treated course of usual and desquamative interstitial pneumonia. *N Engl J Med* 298:801–809, 1978.

38. Haslam PL, Cromwell O, Dewar A, Turner-Warwick M: Evidence of increased histamine levels in lung lavage fluids from patients with cryptogenic fibrosing alveolitis. *Clin Exp Immunol* 44:587–593, 1981.

39. Rankin JA, Kaliner M, Reynolds HY: Histamine levels in bronchoalveolar lavage fluids from patients with asthma, sarcoidosis and interstitial lung diseases. *J Allergy Clin Immunol* 79:371–377, 1987.

40. Reynolds HY: Bronchoalveolar lavage. *Am Rev Respir Dis* 135:250–263, 1987.

41. Cherniack RM (Coordinator) and other investigators, Bronchoalveolar lavage constituents in healthy individuals, idiopathic pulmonary fibrosis and selective comparison groups. *Am Rev Respir Dis* 141(Suppl)169–202, 1990.

42. Klech H, Hutter C (Editors): Clinical guidelines and indications for bronchoalveolar lavage—report of the European Society of Pneumology Task Group on BAL. *Eur Respir J* 3:937–974, 1990.

43. Robinson PC, Walters LC, King TE, Mason RJ: Idiopathic pulmonary fibrosis. Abnormalities in bronchoalveolar lavage fluid phospholipids. *Am Rev Respir Dis* 137:585–591, 1988.

44. Hunninghake GW, Gadek JE, Lawley TJ, et al: Mechanisms of neutrophil accumulation in the lungs of patients with idiopathic pulmonary fibrosis. *J Clin Invest* 68:259–269, 1981.

45. Bitterman PB, Rennard SI, Hunninghake GW, Crystal RG: Human alveolar macrophage growth factor for fibroblasts: regulation and partial characterization. *J Clin Invest* 70:806–822, 1982.

46. Martinet Y, Rom WN, Grotendorst GR, Martin GR, Crystal RG: Exaggerated spontaneous release of platelet derived growth factor by alveolar macrophages from patients with idiopathic pulmonary fibrosis. *Am Rev Respir Dis* 137:572–578, 1988.

47. Cantin AM, Boileau R, Begin R: Increased procollagen III aminoterminal peptide-related antigens and fibroblast growth signals in the lungs of patients with idiopathic pulmonary fibrosis. *Am Rev Respir Dis* 137: 572–578, 1988.

48. McCormack FX, King TE Jr, Voelker DR, et al: Idiopathic pulmonary fibrosis. Abnormalities in the bronchoalveolar lavage content of surfactant protein A. *Am Rev Respir Dis* 144:160–166, 1991.

49. Low RB, Giancola MS, King TE Jr, et al: Serum and bronchoalveolar lavage of N-terminal type III procollagen peptides in idiopathic pulmonary fibrosis. *Am Rev Respir Dis* 146:701–706, 1992.

50. Lynch JP III, Standiford TJ, Rolfe MW, et al: Neutrophilic alveolitis in idiopathic pulmonary fibrosis. The role of interleukin-8. *Am Rev Respir Dis* 145:1433–1439, 1992.

51. Ozaki T, Hayashi H, Tani K, et al: Neutrophil chemotactic factors in the respiratory tract of patients with chronic airway diseases or idiopathic pulmonary fibrosis. *Am Rev Respir Dis* 145:85–91, 1992.

52. Carr PC, Mortenson RL, King TE Jr, et al: Increased expression of the interleukin-8 gene by alveolar macrophages in idiopathic pulmonary fibrosis. *J Clin Invest* 88:1802–1810, 1991.

53. Shaw RJ, Benedict SH, Clark RAF, et al: Pathogenesis of pulmonary fibrosis in interstitial lung disease. Alveolar macrophage PDGF (B) gene activation and up-regulation by interferon gamma. *Am Rev Respir Dis* 143: 167–173, 1991.

54. Merrill WW, Naegel GP, Matthay RA, Reynolds HY: Alveolar macrophage-derived chemotactic factor—kinetics of in vitro production and partial characterization. *J Clin Invest* 65:268–276, 1980.

55. Basset F, Ferrans VJ, Soler P, et al: Intraluminal fibrosis in interstitial lung disorders. *Am J Pathol* 122:443–461, 1986.

56. Cherniack RM, Crystal RG, Kalica AR: Current concepts in idiopathic pulmonary fibrosis: a road map for the future. NHLBI Workshop Summary. *Am Rev Respir Dis* 143:680–683, 1991.

57. Janson RW, King TE, Hance KR, Arend WP: Enhanced production of Il-1 receptor antagonist by alveolar macrophages from patients with interstitial lung disease. *Am Rev Respir Dis* 148:495–503, 1993.

58. Meyer KC, Powers C, Rosenthal N, et al: Alveolar macrophage surface carbohydrate expression is altered in interstitial lung disease as determined by lectin-binding profiles. *Am Rev Respir Dis* 148:1325–1334, 1993.

59. Dayton CA, Schwartz DA, Helmers RA, et al: Outcome of subjects with idiopathic pulmonary fibrosis who fail corticosteroid therapy. *Chest* 103:69–73, 1993.

60. Baughman RP, Lower EE: Use of intermittent, intravenous cyclophosphamide for idiopathic pulmonary fibrosis. *Chest* 102:1090–1094, 1992.

61. Turner-Warwick M: Evaluation and treatment of cryptogenic fibrosing alveolitis. *IM-Internal Medicine for the Specialist* 2:34, 1981.

62. Peters SG, McDougall JC, Douglas WW, et al: Colchicine in the treatment of pulmonary fibrosis. *Chest* 103: 101–104, 1993.

63. Rennard SI, Bitterman RB, Ozaki T, et al: Colchicine suppresses the release of fibroblast growth factors from alveolar macrophages in vitro. *Am Rev Respir Dis* 137: 181–185, 1988.

64. Hoffman LA, Wesmiller SW, Sciurba FC, et al: Nasal cannula and transtracheal oxygen delivery. *Am Rev Respir Dis* 145:827–831, 1992.

65. Toronto Lung Transplant Group: Experience with single-lung transplantation for pulmonary fibrosis. *JAMA* 259:2258–2262, 1988.

66. Grossman RF, Frost A, Zamel N, et al: Results of single-lung transplantation for bilateral pulmonary fibrosis. *N Engl J Med* 322:727–733, 1990.

67. Trulock EP, Cooper JD, Kaiser LR, et al: The Washington University-Barnes Hospital experience with lung transplantation. *JAMA* 266:1943–1946, 1991.

68. ATS Statement, lung transplantation. *Am Rev Respir Dis* 147:772–776, 1993.

69. Turner-Warwick M, Lebowitz M, Burrows B, et al: Cryptogenic fibrosing alveolitis: clinical features and their influence on survival. *Thorax* 35:171–180, 1980.

70. Epler GR, Colby TV, McLoud TC, et al: Bronchiolitis obliterans organizing pneumonia. *N Engl J Med* 312: 152–158, 1985.

71. Guerry-Force ML, Muller NL, Wright JL, et al: A comparison of bronchiolitis pneumonia, and small airway diseases. *Am Rev Respir Dis* 135:705–712, 1987.

72. Muller NL, Guerry-Force ML, Staples CA, et al: Differential bronchiolitis diagnosis of bronchiolitis obliterans with organizing pneumonia and usual interstitial pneumonia; clinical, functional, and radiologic findings. *Radiology* 162:151–156, 1987.

73. Katzenstein AL, Myers JL, Prophet WD, et al: Bronchiolitis obliterans and usual interstitial pneumonia. A comparative clinicopathologic study. *Am J Surg Pathol* 10: 373–381, 1986.

74. Myers JL, Katzenstein AL: Ultrastructural evidence of alveolar epithelial injury in idiopathic bronchiolitis obliterans-organizing pneumonia. *Am J Pathol* 132: 102–109, 1988.

75. Matthay RA, Schwartz MI, Petty TL: Pleuro-pulmonary manifestations of connective tissue diseases. *Clin Notes Respir Dis* 16:3–9, 1977.

76. Boulware DW, Weissman DN, Doll NJ: Pulmonary manifestations of the rheumatic diseases. *Clin Rev Allergy* 3:249–267, 1985.

77. Constantopoulos SH, Drosos AA, Maddison PJ, et al: Xerotrachea and interstitial lung disease in primary Sjögren's syndrome. *Respiration* 46:310–314, 1984.

78. Fairfax AJ, Haslam PL, Vavia D, et al: Pulmonary manifestations of Sjögren's syndrome. *Chest* 70:354–361, 1976.

79. Hunninghake GW, Fauci AS: Pulmonary involvement

in collagen vascular diseases. *Am Rev Respir Dis* 119: 471–503, 1979.

80. Sullivan WD, Hurst DJ, Harmon CE, et al: A prospective evaluation emphasizing pulmonary involvement in patients with mixed connective tissue disease. *Medicine* 63: 92–107, 1984.

81. Prakash UB, Luthra HS, Divertie MB: Intrathoracic manifestations in mixed connective tissue disease. *Mayo Clin Proc* 60:813–821, 1985.

82. Derderian SS, Tellis CJ, Abbrecht PH, et al: Pulmonary involvement in mixed connective tissue disease. *Chest* 88:45–48, 1985.

83. Wiener-Kronish JP, Solinger AM, Warnock ML, et al: Severe pulmonary involvement in mixed connective tissue disease. *Am Rev Respir Dis* 124:499–503, 1981.

84. Martyn JB, Wong MJ, Huang SH: Pulmonary and neuromuscular complications of mixed connective tissue disease: a report and review of the literature. *J Rheumatol* 15:703–705, 1988.

85. Schwarz MI: Pulmonary manifestations of the collagen-vascular diseases. In Bone RA, Dantzker DR, George RB, Matthay RA, Reynolds HY (eds): *Pulmonary and Critical Care Medicine.* St. Louis, CV Mosby, 1993, vol 2, pp M4:1–16.

86. Steinberg AD, Gourley MF, Klinman DM, et al: NIH conference. Systemic lupus erythematosus. *Ann Intern Med* 115:548–559, 1991.

87. Tomer Y, Buskila D, Shoenfeld Y: Pathogenic significance and diagnostic value of lupus autoantibodies. *Int Arch Allergy Appl Immunol* 100:293–306, 1993.

88. Matthay RA, Schwarz MI, Petty TL, et al: Pulmonary manifestations of systemic lupus erythematosus: review of 12 cases of acute lupus pneumonitis. *Medicine* 54:397–409, 1975.

89. Brasington RD, Furst DE: Pulmonary disease in systemic lupus erythematosus. *Clin Exp Rheumatol* 3: 269–276, 1985.

90. Segal AM, Calabrese LH, Ahmad M, et al: The pulmonary manifestations of systemic lupus erythematosus. *Semin Arthritis Rheum* 14:202–204, 1985.

91. Turner-Stokes L, Turner-Warwick M: Intrathoracic manifestations of SLE. *Clin Rheum Dis* 8:229–242, 1982.

92. Schwartzberg M, Lieberman DH, Getzoff B, et al: Systemic lupus erythematosus and pulmonary vascular hypertension. *Arch Intern Med* 144:605–607, 1984.

93. Ansari A, Larson PH, Bates HD: Cardiovascular manifestations of systemic lupus erythematosus: current perspective. *Prog Cardiovasc Dis* 27:421–434, 1985.

94. Pines A, Kaplinsky N, Olchvsky D, et al: Pleuro-pulmonary manifestations of systemic lupus erythematosus: clinical features of its subgroups. Prognostic and therapeutic implications. *Chest* 88:129–135, 1985.

95. Wohlegelertner D, Loke J, Matthay RA, et al: Systemic and discoid lupus erythematosus: analysis of pulmonary function. *Yale J Biol Med* 51:57–164, 1978.

96. Perwz HD, Kramer N: Pulmonary hypertension in systemic lupus erythematosus: report of four cases and review of the literature. *Semin Arthritis Rheum* 11:177–181, 1981.

97. Sahn SA: Immunologic disease of the pleura. *Clin Chest Med* 6:83–102, 1985.

98. Leatherman SW, Davie SF, Hoidal JR: Alveolar hemorrhage syndromes: diffuse microvascular lung hemorrhage in immune and idiopathic disorders. *Medicine* 63: 343–361, 1984.

99. Cush JJ, Goldinas EA: Drug-induced lupus: clinical spectrum and pathogenesis. *Am J Med Sci* 290:36–45, 1985.

100. Martens J, Demedts M, Vanmeenen MT, et al: Respiratory muscle dysfunction in systemic lupus erythematosus. *Chest* 84:170–175, 1983.

101. Wilcox PG, Stein HB, Clarke SD, et al: Phrenic nerve function in patients with diaphragmatic weakness and systemic lupus erythematosus. *Chest* 93:352–358, 1988.

102. Harvey AM, Shulman LE, Tumulty PA, et al: Systemic lupus erythematosus: review of the literature and clinical analysis of 138 cases. *Medicine* 33:291–437, 1954.

103. Winslow WA, Ploss LN, Loitman B: Pleuritis in systemic lupus erythematosus: its importance as an early manifestation in diagnosis. *Ann Intern Med* 49:70–88, 1958.

104. Eisenberg H, Dubois EL, Sherwin RP, et al: Diffuse interstitial lung disease in systemic lupus erythematosus. *Ann Intern Med* 79:37–45, 1973.

105. Segal AM, Reardon EV: Systemic lupus erythematosus. In Cannon GW, Zimmerman G (eds): *The Lung in Rheumatic Diseases.* New York, Marcel Dekker, 1990, pp 261–278.

106. Good JT Jr, King TE, Antony VB, Sahn SA: Lupus pleuritis. Clinical features and pleural fluid antinuclear antibodies. *Chest* 84:714–718, 1983.

107. Bell R, Lawrence DS: Chronic pleurisy in systemic lupus erythematosus treated with pleurectomy. *Br J Dis Chest* 73:314–316, 1979.

108. Onomura K, Nakata H, Tanaka Y et al: Pulmonary hemorrhage in patients with systemic lupus erythematosus. *J Thorac Imag* 6:57–61, 1991.

109. Weinrib L, Sharma OP, Quismorio FP Jr: A long-term study of interstitial lung disease in systemic lupus erythematosus. *Semin Arthritis Rheum* 20:48–56, 1990.

110. Huang CT, Hennigar GR, Lyons HA: Pulmonary dysfunction in systemic lupus erythematosus. *N Engl J Med* 272:288–293, 1965.

111. Andonopoulos AP, Constantopoulos SH, Galanopoulos V, et al: Pulmonary function of nonsmoking patient with systemic lupus erythematosus. *Chest* 94:312–315, 1988.

112. Montes de Oca MA, Babron MC, Bletry O, et al: Thrombosis in systemic lupus erythematosus: a French collaborative study. *Arch Dis Child* 66:713–717, 1991.

113. Haupt HM, Moore GW, Hutchins GM: The lung in systemic lupus erythematosus. Analysis of the pathologic changes in 120 patients. *Am J Med* 71:791–798, 1981.

114. Abud-Mendoza C, Diaz-Jouanen E, Alarcon-Segovia D: Fatal pulmonary hemorrhage in systemic lupus erythematosus. Occurrence without hemoptysis. *J Rheumatol* 12:558–561, 1985.

115. Desnoyers M, Bernstein S, Cooper AG, Kopelman RI: Pulmonary hemorrhage in lupus erythematosus without evidence of an immunologic cause. *Arch Intern Med* 144:1398–1400, 1984.

116. Myers JL, Katzenstein AA: Microangiitis in lupus-induced pulmonary hemorrhage. *Am J Clin Pathol* 85: 552–556, 1986.

117. Carette S, Macher AM, Nussbaum A, Plotz PH: Severe, acute pulmonary disease in patients with systemic lupus erythematosus: ten years of experience at the National Institutes of Health. *Semin Arthritis Rheum* 14: 52–59, 1984.

118. Miller LR, Greenberg SD, McLarty JW: Lupus lung. *Chest* 88:265–269, 1985.

119. Gross M, Esterly JR, Earle RH: Pulmonary alterations in systemic lupus erythematosus. *Am Rev Respir Dis* 105:572–577, 1972.

120. Petri M, Rheinschmidt M, Whiting-O'Keefe Q, et al: The frequency of lupus anticoagulant in systemic lupus erythematosus: a study of sixty consecutive patients by activated portal thromboplastin time, Russell viper venom time, and anticardiolipin antibody. *Ann Intern Med* 106:524–531, 1987.

121. Walker WC, Wright V: Pulmonary lesions and rheumatoid arthritis. *Medicine* 47:501–520, 1968.

122. Scadding JG: The lungs in rheumatoid arthritis. *Proc R Soc Lond [Med]* 62:227–238, 1969.

123. Jones FL Jr, Blodgett RC Jr: Empyema in rheumatoid pleuropulmonary disease. *Ann Intern Med* 74:655–671, 1971.

124. Hunder GG, McDuffie FC, Hepper NG: Pleural fluid complement in systemic lupus erythematosus and rheumatoid arthritis. *Ann Intern Med* 76:357–363, 1972.

125. Turner-Warwick M, Haslam P: Antibodies in some chronic fibrosing lung disease. I. Non organ specific autoantibodies. *Clin Allergy* 1:83–95, 1971.

126. Frank ST, Weg JG, Harkleroad LE, et al: Pulmonary dysfunction in rheumatoid disease. *Chest* 63:27–34, 1973.

127. DeHoratius RJ, Abruzzo JL, Williams RC Jr: Immunofluorescent and immunologic studies of rheumatoid lung. *Arch Intern Med* 129:441–446, 1972.

128. Caplan A: Certain unusual radiological appearances in chest of coal miners suffering from rheumatoid arthritis. *Thorax* 8:29–37, 1953.

129. King TE, Dunn TL: Connective tissue disease. In Schwarz MI, King TE (eds): *Interstitial Lung Disease.* Philadelphia, BC Decker, 1988, pp 171–210.

130. Yousem SA, Colby TA, Carrington CB: Lung biopsy in rheumatoid arthritis. *Am Rev Respir Dis* 131:770–777, 1985.

131. Geddes DM, Corrin B, Brewerton DA, et al: Progressive airway obliteration in adults and its association with rheumatoid disease. *Q J Med* 46:427–444, 1977.

132. Herzog CA, Miller RA, Hoidal JR: Bronchiolitis and rheumatoid arthritis. *Am Rev Respir Dis* 124:636–639, 1981.

133. Shiel WC Jr, Prete PE: Pleuropulmonary manifestations of rheumatoid arthritis. *Semin Arthritis Rheum* 13:235–243, 1984.

134. Yousem SA, Colby TV, Carrington CB: Lung biopsy in rheumatoid arthritis. *Am Rev Respir Dis* 131:770–777, 1985.

135. Hakala M: Poor prognosis in patients with rheumatoid arthritis hospitalized for interstitial lung fibrosis. *Chest* 93:114–118, 1988.

136. Lee FI, Brain AT: Chronic diffuse interstitial fibrosis and rheumatoid arthritis. *Lancet* 2:693–695, 1962.

137. Weiland JE, Garcia JG, Davis WB, et al: Neutrophil collagenase in rheumatoid interstitial lung disease. *J Appl Physiol* 62:628–633, 1987.

138. Roschmann RA, Rothenberg RJ: Pulmonary fibrosis in rheumatoid arthritis: a review of clinical features and therapy. *Semin Arthritis Rheum* 16:174–185, 1987.

139. Sassoon CS, McAlpine SW, Tashkin DP, et al: Small airways function in nonsmokers with rheumatoid arthritis. *Arthritis Rheum* 27:1218–1226, 1984.

140. Garcia JG, James HL, Zinkgraf S, et al: Lower respiratory tract abnormalities in rheumatoid interstitial lung disease. *Am Rev Respir Dis* 136:811–817, 1987.

141. Arroliga AC, Podell DN, Matthay RA: Pulmonary manifestations of scleroderma. *J Thorac Imag* 7:30–45, 1992.

142. Barnett AJ: *Scleroderma.* Springfield, IL, Charles C Thomas, 1974.

143. Wilson RJ, Rodnan GP, Robin ED: An early pulmonary physiologic abnormality in progressive systemic sclerosis (diffuse scleroderma). *Am J Med* 26:361–369, 1964.

144. Sackner MA: *Scleroderma.* New York, Grune & Stratton, 1966.

145. Sackner M, Akgun N, Kimbel P, et al: The pathophysiology of scleroderma involving the heart and respiratory system. *Ann Intern Med* 60:611–630, 1964.

146. Weaver AL, Divertie MB, Titus JL: Pulmonary scleroderma. *Dis Chest* 54:490–498, 1968.

147. Konig G, Luderschmidt C, Hammer C, et al: Lung involvement in scleroderma. *Chest* 85:318–324, 1984.

148. Owens GR, Follansbee WP: Cardiopulmonary manifestations of systemic sclerosis. *Chest* 91:118–127, 1987.

149. Norton WL, Nardo JM: Vascular disease in progressive systemic sclerosis (scleroderma). *Ann Intern Med* 75:317–324, 1970.

150. Naeye RL: Pulmonary vascular lesions in systemic scleroderma. *Dis Chest* 44:374–380, 1963.

151. Steen VO: Systemic sclerosis. In Cannon GW, Zimmerman G (eds): *The Lung in Rheumatic Diseases.* New York, Marcel Dekker, 1990, pp 279–302.

152. Rosenthal AK, McLaughlin JK, Linet MS, et al: Scleroderma and malignancy: an epidemiological study. *Ann Rheum Dis* 52:531–533, 1993.

153. Abu-Shakra M, Guillemin F, Lee P: Cancer in systemic sclerosis. *Arthritis Rheum* 36:460–464, 1993.

154. Pianone A, Matucii-Cerinic M, Lombardi A, et al: High resolution computed tomography in systemic sclerosis. Real diagnostic utilities in the assessment of pulmonary involvement and comparison with other modalities of lung investigation. *Clin Rheumatol* 11:465–572, 1992.

155. Wells AU, Hansell DM, Corrin B, et al: High resolution computed tomography as a predictor of lung histology in systemic sclerosis. *Thorax* 47:738–742, 1992.

156. Bhalla M, Silver RM, Shepard JA, et al: Chest CT in patients with scleroderma: prevalence of asymptomatic esophageal dilatation and mediastinal lymphadenopathy. *AJR* 161:269-272, 1993.

157. Garber SJ, Wells AU, duBois RM, et al: Enlarged mediastinal lymph nodes in the fibrosing alveolitis of systemic sclerosis. *Br J Radiol* 65:983–986, 1992.

158. Peters-Golden M, Wise RA, Hochberg MC, et al: Carbon monoxide diffusing capacity as predictor of outcome in systemic sclerosis. *Am J Med* 77:1027–1034, 1984.

159. Greenwald GI, Tashkin DP, Gong H, et al: Longitudinal changes in lung function and respiratory symptoms in progressive systemic sclerosis. Prospective study. *Am J Med* 83:305–312, 1987.

160. Owens GR, Fino GJ, Herbert DL, et al: Pulmonary function in progressive systemic sclerosis. Comparison of CREST syndrome variant with diffuse scleroderma. *Chest* 84:546–550, 1983.

161. Peters-Golden M, Wise RA, Schneider P, et al: Clinical and demographic predictors of loss of pulmonary function in systemic sclerosis. *Medicine* 63:221–231, 1984.

162. Harrison NK, Myers AR, Corrin B, et al: Structural features of interstitial lung disease in systemic sclerosis. *Am Rev Respir Dis* 144:706–713, 1991.

163. Owens GR, Paradis IL, Gryzan S, et al: Role of inflammation in the lung disease of systemic sclerosis: comparison with idiopathic pulmonary fibrosis. *J Lab Clin Med* 107:253–260, 1986.

164. Silver RM, Metcalf JF, Stanley JH, et al: Interstitial lung disease in scleroderma. Analysis by bronchoalveolar lavage. *Arthritis Rheum* 27:1254–1262, 1984.

165. Shuck JW, Oetgen WJ, Tesar JT: Pulmonary vascular response during Raynaud's phenomenon in progressive systemic sclerosis. *Am J Med* 78:221–227, 1985.

166. Steen VD, Owens GR, Redmond C, et al: The effect of D-penicillamine on pulmonary findings in systemic sclerosis. *Arthritis Rheum* 28:882–888, 1985.

167. DeClerck LS, Dequeker J, Francx L, et al: D-penicillamine therapy and interstitial lung disease in scleroderma. A long-term follow-up study. *Arthritis Rheum* 30:643–650, 1987.

168. Akesson A, Blom-Bulow B, Scheja A, et al: Long-term evaluation of penicillamine or cyclofenil in systemic sclerosis. Results from a two-year randomized study. *Scand J Rheumatol* 21:238–244, 1992.

169. Hein R, Behr J, Hundgen M, et al: Treatment of systemic sclerosis with gamma-interferon. *Br J Dermatol* 126: 496–501, 1992.

170. Eason RJ, Tan PL, Gow PJ: Progressive systemic sclerosis in Aukland: a ten year review with emphasis on prognostic features. *N Engl J Med* 11:657–662, 1981.

171. Tuffanelli DL, Lavoie PE: Prognosis and therapy of polymyositis/dermatomyositis. *Clin Dermatol* 6:93–104, 1988.

172. Kasner CS, White CL, Freeman RG: Pathology and immunopathology of polymyositis/dermatomyositis. *Clin Dermatol* 6:64–75, 1988.

173. Sontheimer RD, Ziff M: Questions pertaining to the etiology and pathophysiology of polymyositis/dermatomyositis. *Clin Dermatol* 6:105–119, 1988.

174. Benedek JG: Neoplastic associations of rheumatic diseases and rheumatic manifestations of cancer. *Clin Geriatr Med* 4:333–355, 1988.

175. Callen JP: Dermatomyositis. *Dis Mon* 33:237–305, 1987.

176. Hochberg MC, Feldman D, Stevens MD: Adult onset polymyositis/dermatomyositis: an analysis of clinical and laboratory features and survival in 76 patients with a review of the literature. *Semin Arthritis Rheum* 15: 168–178, 1986.

177. Dickey BF, Myers AR: Pulmonary disease in polymyositis/dermatomyositis. *Semin Arthritis Rheum* 14:60–76, 1984.

178. Hepper NG, Ferguson RH, Howard FM Jr: Three types of pulmonary involvement in polymyositis. *Med Clin North Am* 48:1031–1042, 1964.

179. Schwarz MI, Matthay RA, Sahn SA, et al: Interstitial lung disease in polymyositis and dermatomyositis. Analysis of six cases and review of the literature. *Medicine* 55:89–104, 1976.

180. Frazier AR, Miller RD: Interstitial pneumonitis in association with polymyositis and dermatomyositis. *Chest* 65:403–407, 1974.

181. Fauci AS, Wolff SM: Wegener's granulomatosis: studies in 18 patients and a review of the literature. *Medicine* 52:535–561, 1973.

182. Fauci AS, Haynes BF, Katz P: The spectrum of vasculitis: clinical, pathologic, immunologic, and therapeutic considerations. *Ann Intern Med* 89:660–676, 1978.

183. Wolff SM, Fauci AS, Hom RG, et al: Wegener's granulomatosis. *Ann Intern Med* 81:513–525, 1974.

184. Fauci AS, Wolff SM: Wegener's granulomatosis and related diseases. *Dis Mon* 23:1–36, 1977.

185. Haworth SJ, Savage CO, Carr D: Pulmonary hemorrhage complicating Wegener's granulomatosis and microscopic polyarteritis. *Br Med J* 290:1775–1778, 1985.

186. Wechsler RJ, Steiner RM, Israel HL, et al: Chest radiograph in lymphomatoid granulomatosis: comparison with Wegener granulomatosis. *AJR* 142:79–83, 1984.

187. Littlejohn GO, Ryan PJ, Holdsworth SR: Wegener's granulomatosis: clinical features and outcome in seventeen patients. *Aust NZ J Med* 15:241–245, 1985.

188. Churg A: Pulmonary angiitis and granulomatosis revisited. *Hum Pathol* 14:868–883, 1983.

189. Salant DJ: Immunopathogenesis of crescentic glomerulonephritis and lung purpura. *Kidney Int* 32:408–425, 1987.

190. Leatherman JW: Immune alveolar hemorrhage. *Chest* 91:891–897, 1987.

191. Walker RG, Becker GJ, d'Apice AJ: Plasma exchange in the treatment of glomerulonephritis and other renal diseases. *Aust NZ J Med* 16:828–838, 1986.

192. Leavitt RY, Fauci AJ: Pulmonary vasculitis. *Am Rev Respir Dis* 134:149–166, 1986.

193. Chandler DB, Fulmer JD: Pulmonary vasculitis. *Lung* 163:257–273, 1985.

194. Fauci AJ, Haynes BF, Katz P, et al: Wegener's granulomatosis: prospective clinical and therapeutic experience with 85 patients for 21 years. *Ann Intern Med* 98:76–85, 1983.

195. Carrington CB, Liebow AA: Limited forms of angiitis and granulomatosis of Wegener's type. *Am J Med* 41: 497–527, 1966.

196. Fauci AS, Wolff SM, Johnson JS: Effect of cyclophosphamide upon the immune response in Wegener's granulomatosis. *N Engl J Med* 285:1493–1496, 1971.

197. Howell SB, Epstein WV: Circulating immunoglobulin complexes in Wegener's granulomatosis. *Am J Med* 60: 259–268, 1976.

198. Flye MW, Mundinger GH, Fauci AS: Diagnostic and therapeutic aspects of the surgical approach to Wegener's granulomatosis. *J Thorac Cardiovasc Surg* 77: 331–337, 1979.

199. Felson B: Less familiar roentgen patterns of pulmonary granulomas. *AJR* 81:211–223, 1959.

200. McGrego MB, Sandler G: Wegener's granulomatosis. A clinical and radiological survey. *Br J Radiol* 37:430–439, 1964.

201. Kornblum D, Feinberg R: Roentgen manifestations of necrotizing granulomatosis and angiitis of lungs. *AJR* 74:587–592, 1955.

202. Maguire R, Fauci AS, Doppman JL, et al: Unusual radiographic features of Wegener's granulomatosis. *AJR* 130: 233–238, 1979.

203. Landman S, Burgener F: Pulmonary manifestations of Wegener's granulomatosis. *AJR* 122:750–757, 1974.

204. Liebow AA: The J Burns Amberson Lecture: pulmonary angiitis and granulomatosis. *Am Rev Respir Dis* 108: 1–18, 1973.

205. Gonzales L, Van Ordstrand HS: Wegener's granulomatosis: review of 11 cases. *Radiology* 107:295–300, 1973.

206. Israel HL, Patchefsky AS: Wegener's granulomatosis of lung: diagnosis and treatment. Experience with 12 cases. *Ann Intern Med* 74:881–891, 1971.

207. Godman GC, Churg J: Wegener's granulomatosis: pathology and review of the literature. *Arch Pathol* 58:533–558, 1954.

208. Israel HL, Patchefsky AS, Saldama MJ: Wegener's granulomatosis, lymphoid granulomatosis, and benign lymphocytic angiitis and granulomatosis of lung. *Ann Intern Med* 87:691–699, 1977.

209. Winterbauer RH: Wegener's granulomatosis and other pulmonary granulomatous vasculitides. In Bone RA, Dantzker DR, George RB, Matthay RA, Reynolds HY (eds): *Pulmonary and Critical Care Medicine.* St Louis, CV Mosby, 1993, vol 2, pp M6:1–13.

210. Cordier JF, Valeyre D, Guillevin L, et al: Pulmonary Wegener's granulomatosis: a clinical and imaging study of 77 cases. *Chest* 97:906–912, 1990.

211. Rosenberg DM, Weinberger SE, Fulmer JD, et al: Functional correlates of lung involvement of Wegener's granulomatosis. Use of pulmonary function tests in staging and follow-up. *Am J Med* 69:387–394, 1980.

212. Davies DJ, Moran JE, Niall JF, et al: Segmental necrotizing glomerulonephritis with antineutrophil antibody. Possible arbor virus aetiology? *Br Med J* 285:606, 1982.

213. Vander Woude FJ, Rasmussen N, Lobatto S, et al: Autoantibodies against neutrophils and monocytes: tool for diagnosis and marker of disease activity in Wegener's granulomatosis. *Lancet* 1:425–429, 1985.

214. Nolle B, Specks U, Ludemann J, et al: Anticytoplasmic autoantibodies: their immunodiagnostic value in Wegener's granulomatosis. *Ann Intern Med* 111:28–40, 1989.

215. Kallenberg CG, Mulder AH, Tervaert JW: Antineutrophil cytoplasmic antibodies: a still-growing class of autoantibodies in inflammatory disorders. *Am J Med* 93:678–689, 1992.

216. Goldschmeding R, van der Schoot CE, ten Bokkel Huinink D, et al: Wegener's granulomatosis autoantibodies identify a novel diisopropylfluorophosphate-binding protein in the lysosomes of normal human neutrophils. *J Clin Invest* 84:1577–1587, 1989.

217. Jeanette JC, Ewert BH, Falk RJ: Do antineutrophil cytoplasmic autoantibodies cause Wegener's granulomatosis and other forms of necrotizing vasculitis? *Rheum Dis Clin North Am* 19:1–14, 1993.

218. Leavitt RY, Fauci AS, Bioch DA: The American College of Rheumatology 1990 criteria for the classification of Wegener's granulomatosis. *Arthritis Rheum* 33:1101–1107, 1990.

219. Walton EW: Giant-cell granuloma of the respiratory tract (Wegener's granulomatosis). *Br Med J* 2:265–270, 1958.

220. Hollander D, Manning RT: The use of alkylating agents in the treatment of Wegener's granulomatosis. *Ann Intern Med* 67:393–398, 1967.

221. DeRemee RA, McDonald TJ, Weiland LH: Wegener's granulomatosis: observations on treatment with antimicrobial agents. *Mayo Clin Proc* 60:27–32, 1985.

222. Specks U, De Remee RA: Granulomatous vasculitis. Wegener's granulomatosis and Churg-Strauss syndrome. *Rheum Dis Clin North Am* 16:377–397, 1990.

223. Katzenstein AA, Carrington CB, Liebow AA: Lymphomatoid granulomatosis: a clinicopathologic study of 152 cases. *Cancer* 43:360–473, 1979.

224. Liebow AA, Carrington CR, Friedman PJ: Lymphomatoid granulomatosis. *Hum Pathol* 3:457–558, 1972.

225. Meyers JL: Lymphomatoid granulomatosis. Past, present, future? *Mayo Clin Proc* 65:274–278, 1990.

226. Katzenstein AA, Peiper SC: Detection of Epstein-Barr virus genomes in lymphomatoid granulomatosis: analysis of 29 cases by the polymerase chain reaction technique. *Mod Pathol* 3:435–441, 1990.

227. Bone RC, Vernon M, Sobonya RE, et al: Lymphomatoid granulomatosis: report of a case and review of the literature. *Am J Med* 65:709–716, 1978.

228. Colby TV, Carrington CB: Pulmonary lymphomas: current concepts. *Hum Pathol* 14:884–887, 1983.

229. Schnek SA, Penn I: Cerebral neoplasms associated with renal transplantation. *Arch Neurol* 22:226–233, 1970.

230. Doak PB, Montgomerie JZ, North JDK, et al: Reticulum cell sarcoma after renal homotransplantation and azathioprine and prednisone therapy. *Br Med J* 4:746–748, 1968.

231. Pierce JC, Madge GE, Lee HM, et al: Lymphoma: a complication of renal allotransplantation in man. *JAMA* 219:1593–1597, 1972.

232. Fauci AS: Granulomatous vasculitides: distinct but related (editorial). *Ann Intern Med* 87:782–783, 1977.

233. Fauci AS, Haynes BC, Costa J, et al: Lymphomatoid granulomatosis: prospective clinical and therapeutic experience with 85 patients for 21 years. *N Engl J Med* 306:68–74, 1982.

234. Churg J, Strauss L: Allergic granulomatosis, allergic angiitis and periarteritis nodosa. *Am J Pathol* 27:277–301, 1951.

235. Rose GA, Spencer H: Polyarteritis nodosa. *Q J Med* 26:43–81, 1957.

236. Lanham JG, Elkon KB, Pusey CD, et al: Systemic vasculitis with asthma and eosinophilia: a clinical approach to the Churg-Strauss syndrome. *Medicine* 63:65–81, 1984.

237. Chumbley LC, Harrison EG Jr, Remee RA: Allergic granulomatosis and angiitis (Churg-Strauss syndrome): report and analysis of 30 cases. *Mayo Clin Proc* 52:477–484, 1977.

238. Levin DC: Pulmonary abnormalities in the necrotizing vasculitides and their rapid response to steroids. *Radiology* 97:521–526, 1970.

239. Churg J: Allergic granulomatosis and granulomatous-vascular syndromes. *Ann Allergy* 21:619–628, 1963.

240. Guillevin L, Fain O, Lhote F, et al: Lack of superiority of steroids plus plasma exchange to steroids alone in the treatment of polyarteritis nodosa and Churg-Strauss syndrome. A prospective, randomized trial in 78 patients. *Arthritis Rheum* 35:208–215, 1992.

241. Guillevin L, Jarrousse B, Lok C, et al: Long term follow-up after treatment of polyarteritis nodosa and Churg-Strauss angiitis with comparison of steroids, plasma exchange and cyclophosphamide to steroids and plasma exchange. A prospective randomized trial of 71 patients. *J Rheumatol* 18:567–574, 1991.

242. Teague CA, Doak PB, Simpson IJ, et al: Goodpasture's syndrome: an analysis of 29 cases. *Kidney Int* 13:492–504, 1978.

243. Schwartz EF, Teplick JG, Onesti G, et al: Pulmonary

hemorrhage in renal diseases: Goodpasture's syndrome and other causes. *Radiology* 122:39–46, 1977.

244. Wilson CB, Dixon FJ: Anti-glomerular basement membrane antibody induced glomerulonephritis. *Kidney Int* 3:74–89, 1973.

245. McPhaul JJ Jr, Dixon FJ: The presence of antiglomerular basement membrane antibodies in peripheral blood. *J Immunol* 103:1168–1175, 1969.

246. Matthew TH, Hobbs JB, Kalowski S, et al: Goodpasture's syndrome: normal renal diagnostic findings. *Ann Intern Med* 82:215–218, 1975.

247. Lockwood CM, Boulton-Jones JM, Lowenthal RM, et al: Recovery from Goodpasture's syndrome after immunosuppressive treatment and plasmapheresis. *Br Med J* 2: 252–254, 1975.

248. Whitworth JA, Lawrence JR, Meadows R: Goodpasture's syndrome: a review of nine cases and an evaluation of therapy. *Aust NZ J Med* 4:167–177, 1974.

249. Klasa RJ, Abboud RT, Ballon HS, et al: Goodpasture's syndrome: recurrence after a five-year remission. Case report and review of the literature. *Am J Med* 84: 751–755, 1988.

250. Wilson CB, Smith RC: Goodpasture's syndrome associated with influenza A2 virus infection. *Ann Intern Med* 76:91–94, 1972.

251. Young KR: Pulmonary hemorrhage syndromes. In Bone RA, Dantzker DR, George RB, Matthay RA, Reynolds HY (eds): *Pulmonary and Critical Care Medicine*. St. Louis, CV Mosby, 1993, vol 2, pp M10:1–13.

252. Ewan PLO, Jones HA, Rhodes CG, et al: Detections of intrapulmonary hemorrhage with carbon monoxide uptake. Application in Goodpasture's syndrome. *N Engl J Med* 295:1391–1396, 1976.

253. Hudson BG, Kalluri R, Gunwar S, et al: Molecular characteristics of the Goodpasture autoantigen. *Kidney Int* 43:135–139, 1993.

254. Bombassei GJ, Kaplan AA: The association between hydrocarbon exposure and anti-glomerular basement membrane antibody-mediated disease (Goodpasture's syndrome). *Am J Ind Med* 21:141–153, 1992.

255. Lang CH, Brown DC, Staley N, et al: Goodpasture's syndrome treated with immunosuppression and plasma exchange. *Arch Intern Med* 137:1076–1078, 1977.

256. McLeish KR, Maxwell DR, Luft FC: Failure of plasma exchange and immunosuppression to improve renal function in Goodpasture's syndrome. *Clin Nephrol* 10: 71–73, 1978.

257. Cove-Smith JR, McLeod AA, Blamey RW, et al: Transplantation, immunosuppression and plasmapheresis in Goodpasture's syndrome. *Clin Nephrol* 9:126–128, 1978.

258. Swainson CP, Robson JS, Urbaniak SJ, et al: Treatment of Goodpasture's disease by plasma exchange and immunosuppression. *Clin Exp Immunol* 32:233–242, 1978.

259. Johnson JP, Whitman W, Briggs A, et al: Plasmapheresis and immunosuppressive agents in antibasement membrane antibody-induced Goodpasture's syndrome. *Am J Med* 64:354–359, 1978.

260. Fraser RG, Paré JAP: Diseases of altered immunologic activity. In *Diagnosis of Diseases of the Chest*, ed 3. Philadelphia, WB Saunders, 1988, vol 2.

261. Soergel KH, Sommers SC: Idiopathic pulmonary hemosiderosis and related syndromes. *Am J Med* 32:499–511, 1962.

262. Boyd DHA: Idiopathic pulmonary hemosiderosis in adults and adolescents. *Br J Dis Chest* 53:41–51, 1959.

263. Bronson SM: Idiopathic pulmonary hemosiderosis in adults. Report of a case and review of the literature. *AJR* 83:260–273, 1960.

264. Ognibene AJ, Johnson DE: Idiopathic pulmonary hemosiderosis in adults. Report of a case and review of literature. *Arch Intern Med* 111:503–510, 1963.

265. Cooper AS: Idiopathic pulmonary hemosiderosis. Report of a case in an adult treated with triamcinolone. *N Engl J Med* 263:1100–1103, 1960.

266. Smith WE, Fienberg R: Early nonrecurrent idiopathic hemosiderosis in an adult. Report of a case. *N Engl J Med* 259:808–811, 1958.

267. Hyatt RW, Adelstein ER, Halazum JF, et al: Ultrastructure of the lung in idiopathic pulmonary hemosiderosis. *Am J Med* 52:822–829, 1972.

268. Soergel KH, Sommers SC: The alveolar epithelial lesion of idiopathic pulmonary hemosiderosis. *Am Rev Respir Dis* 85:540–552, 1962.

269. Overholt EL: Acute pulmonary-renal syndromes. *Dis Chest* 48:68–77, 1965.

270. Irwin RS, Cottrell TS, Hsu KC, et al: Idiopathic pulmonary hemosiderosis. An electron microscopic and immunofluorescent study. *Chest* 65:41–45, 1974.

271. Donlam CJ Jr, Srodes CH, Duffy FD: Idiopathic pulmonary hemosiderosis—electron microscopic, immunofluorescent, and iron kinetic studies. *Chest* 68:577–581, 1975.

272. Theros EG, Reeder MM, Eckert JF: An exercise in radiologic-pathologic correlation. *Radiology* 90:784–791, 1968.

273. Rosen SH, Castleman B, Liebow AA: Pulmonary alveolar proteinosis. *N Engl J Med* 258:1123–1146, 1975.

274. Claypool WD: Pulmonary alveolar proteinosis. In Fishman AP (ed): *Pulmonary Diseases and Disorders*. New York, McGraw-Hill, 1988, pp 893–900.

275. Gehle DW, Territo M, Finley TN, et al: Defective lung macrophages in pulmonary alveolar proteinosis. *Ann Intern Med* 85:304–309, 1976.

276. Costello JF, Moriarty DC, Branthwaite MA, et al: Diagnosis and management of alveolar proteinosis: the role of electron microscopy. *Thorax* 30:121–132, 1975.

277. Davidson JM, MacLeod WM: Pulmonary alveolar proteinosis. *Br J Dis Chest* 63:13–28, 1969.

278. Hudson AR, Halprin GM, Miller JA, et al: Pulmonary interstitial fibrosis following alveolar proteinosis. *Chest* 65:700–702, 1974.

279. Rubinstein I, Muller JB, Hoffstein V: Morphologic diagnosis of idiopathic pulmonary alveolar lipoproteinosis—revisited. *Arch Intern Med* 148:813–816, 1988.

280. DuBois RM, McAllister WA, Branthwaite MA: Alveolar proteinosis: diagnosis and treatment over a 10 year period. *Thorax* 38:360–363, 1983.

281. Claypool WD, Rogers RM, Matuschak GM: Update on the clinical diagnosis, management and pathogenesis of pulmonary alveolar proteinosis (phospholipidosis). *Chest* 85:550–558, 1984.

282. Kariman K, Kylstra JA, Spock A: Pulmonary alveolar proteinosis: prospective clinical experience in 23 patients for 15 years. *Lung* 162:223–231, 1984.

283. Rosen SH, Castleman B, Liebow AA: Pulmonary alveolar proteinosis. *N Engl J Med* 258:1123–1142, 1958.

284. Abraham JL, McEuen DD: Inorganic particulates associated with pulmonary alveolar proteinosis: SEM and x-ray microanalysis results. *Appl Pathol* 4:138–146, 1986.

285. Hoffman RM, Rogers RM: Pulmonary alveolar proteinosis. In Bone RC, Dantzker DD, George RB, Matthay RA, Reynolds HY (eds): *Pulmonary and Critical Care Medicine*. St. Louis, Mosby Year Book, 1993, vol 2, pp M12: 1–7.

286. Hoffman RM, Rogers RM: Serum and lavage lactate dehydrogenase isoenzymes in pulmonary alveolar proteinosis. *Am Rev Respir Dis* 143:42–46, 1991.

287. Haslam PL, Hughes DA, Dewar A, et al: Lipoprotein macroaggregates in bronchoalveolar lavage fluid from patients with diffuse interstitial lung disease: comparison with idiopathic alveolar lipoproteinosis. *Thorax* 43: 140–146, 1988.

288. Takemura T, Fukuda Y, Harrison M, et al: Ultrastructural, histochemical, and freeze-fracture evaluation of multilamellated structures in human pulmonary alveolar proteinosis. *Am J Anat* 179:258–268, 1987.

289. Hook GE, Gilmore LB, Talley FA: Dissolution and reassembly of tubular myelin-like multilamellated structures from the lungs of patients with pulmonary alveolar proteinosis. *Lab Invest* 55:194–208, 1986.

290. Hook GE, Gilmore LB, Talley FA: Multilamellated structure from the lungs of patients with pulmonary alveolar proteinosis. *Lab Invest* 50:711–725, 1984.

291. Nugent KM, Pesanti EL: Macrophage function in pulmonary alveolar proteinosis. *Am Rev Respir Dis* 127: 780–781, 1983.

292. Gonzalez-Rothi RJ, Harris JO: Pulmonary alveolar proteinosis. Further evaluation of abnormal alveolar macrophages. *Chest* 90:656–661, 1986.

293. Wilson DO, Rogers RM: Prolonged spontaneous remission in a patient with untreated pulmonary alveolar proteinosis. *Am J Med* 82:1014–1016, 1987.

294. Ramirez RJ: Bronchopulmonary lavage: new techniques and observations. *Dis Chest* 50:581–588, 1966.

295. Rogers RM, Szidon JP, Shelburne J, et al: Hemodynamic response of the pulmonary circulation to bronchopulmonary lavage in man. *N Engl J Med* 286:1230–1233, 1972.

296. Rosenow EC: The spectrum of drug-induced pulmonary disease. *Ann Intern Med* 77:977–234, 1972.

297. Cooper JA Jr, Zitnik RJ, Matthay RA: Mechanisms of drug-induced pulmonary disease. *Annu Rev Med* 39: 395–404, 1988.

298. Rosenow EC III: Drug-induced bronchopulmonary pleural disease. *J Allergy Clin Immunol* 80:780–787, 1987.

299. Cooper JA Jr, Matthay RA: Drug-induced pulmonary disease. *Dis Mon* 33:61–120, 1987.

300. Cooper JA Jr, White DA, Matthay RA: Drug-induced pulmonary disease. Part 1: cytotoxic drugs. *Am Rev Respir Dis* 133:321–340, 1986.

301. Cooper JA Jr, White DA, Matthay RA: Drug-induced pulmonary disease. Part 2: noncytotoxic drugs. *Am Rev Respir Dis* 133:488–505, 1986.

302. Rosenow EC III, Wilson WR, Cockerill FR III: Pulmonary disease in the immunocompromised host. *Mayo Clin Proc* 60:473–487, 1985.

303. Adamson IY: Drug-induced pulmonary fibrosis. *Environ Health Perspect* 55:25–36, 1984.

304. Gockerman JP: Drug-induced interstitial lung diseases. *Clin Chest Med* 3:521–536, 1982.

305. Cooper JA Jr: Drug-related pulmonary diseases. In Bone RC, Dantzker DR, George RB, Matthay RA, Reynolds HY (eds): *Pulmonary and Critical Care Medicine*. St. Louis, Mosby-Year Book, 1993, vol 2, pp M8:1–9.

306. Rosenow EC 3d, Myers JL, Swensen SJ, et al: Drug-induced pulmonary disease. An update. *Chest* 102: 239–250, 1992.

307. Israel-Biet D, Labrune S, Huchon GJ: Drug-induced lung disease: 1990 review. *Eur Respir J* 4:465–478, 1991.

308. Gregory SA, Grippi MA: The clinical diagnosis of drug-induced pulmonary disorders. *J Thorac Imaging* 6:8–18, 1991.

309. Zitnik RJ, Cooper JA Jr: Pulmonary disease due to antirheumatic agents. *Clin Chest Med* 11:139- 150, 1990.

310. Beaudry C, Laplante L: Severe allergic pneumonitis from hydrochlorothiazide. *Ann Intern Med* 78:251–253, 1973.

311. Sostman HD, Matthay RA, Putnam CE: Cytotoxic drug-induced lung disease. *Am J Med* 62:608–615, 1977.

312. Weiss RB, Muggia FM: Cytotoxic drug-induced pulmonary disease—update 1980. *Am J Med* 68:259–266, 1980.

313. Winterbauer RH, Wilske KR, Wheeis RF: Diffuse pulmonary injury associated with gold treatment. *N Engl J Med* 294:919–921, 1976.

314. McCormick J, Cole S, Lahirir B, et al: Pneumonitis caused by gold salt therapy: evidence for the role of cell-mediated immunity in its pathogenesis. *Am Rev Respir Dis* 122:145–152, 1980.

315. Pascual RS, Mosher MB, Sikand RS, et al: Effects of bleomycin on pulmonary function in man. *Am Rev Respir Dis* 108:211–217, 1973.

316. Goldiner PL, Carlon GC, Cvitkovic E, et al: Factors influencing postoperative morbidity and mortality in patients treated with bleomycin. *Br Med J* 1:1664–1667, 1978.

317. Holoye PY, Luna MA, Mackay B, et al: Bleomycin hypersensitivity pneumonitis. *Ann Intern Med* 88:47–49, 1978.

318. McCullough B, Collins JF, Johanson WG Jr, et al: Bleomycin-induced diffuse interstitial pulmonary fibrosis in baboons. *J Clin Invest* 61:79–88, 1978.

319. Hailey FJ, Glascock HW, Hewitt WF: Pleuropneumonic reactions to nitrofurantoin. *N Engl J Med* 281:1087–1090, 1969.

320. Kennedy JI Jr: Clinical aspects of amiodarone pulmonary toxicity. *Clin Chest Med* 11:119–130, 1990.

321. Mitchell DN, Scadding JG: Sarcoidosis (state of the art). *Am Rev Respir Dis* 110:774–802, 1974.

322. Mayock RL, Bertrand P, Morrison CE, et al: Manifestations of sarcoidosis (analysis of 145 patients with review of nine series selected from the literature). *Am J Med* 35: 67–89, 1963.

323. Nolan JP, Klatskin G: The fever of sarcoidosis. *Ann Intern Med* 61:455–461, 1964.

324. Israel H: Sarcoidosis. In Simmons DH (ed): *Current Pulmonology*. Boston, Houghton Mifflin, 1979, vol 1, pp 163–182.

325. Roberts WC, McAllister HA, Ferrans VJ: Sarcoidosis of the heart (114 necropsy patients). *Am J Med* 63:86–108, 1977.

326. Fleming HA: Sarcoid heart disease. *Br Heart J* 36:54–68, 1974.

327. Delaney P: Neurologic manifestations in sarcoidosis. *Ann Intern Med* 87:336–345, 1977.

328. Sharma OP, Sharma AM: Sarcoidosis of the nervous

system—a clinical approach. *Arch Intern Med* 151: 1317–1321, 1991.

329. Klatskin G, Yesner R: Hepatic manifestations of sarcoidosis and other granulomatous diseases—a study based on histological examination of tissue obtained by needle biopsy of the liver. *Yale J Biol Med* 23:207–248, 1950.

330. Israel HL, Goldstein RA: Hepatic granulomatosis and sarcoidosis. *Ann Intern Med* 79:669–678, 1973.

331. Winterbauer PH, Belic N, Moores KD: A clinical interpretation of bilateral hilar adenopathy. *Ann Intern Med* 78:65–71, 1973.

332. DeRemee RA, Andersen HA: Sarcoidosis—a correlation of dyspnea with roentgenographic stage and pulmonary function changes. *Mayo Clin Proc* 49:742–745, 1974.

333. Littner MR, Schachter EN, Putnam CE, et al: The clinical assessment of roentgenographically atypical pulmonary sarcoidosis. *Am J Med* 62:361–368, 1977.

334. Siltzbach LE, James DG, Neville E, et al: Course and prognosis of sarcoidosis around the world. *Am J Med* 57:847–852, 1974.

335. Prior C, Haslam PL: Increased levels of serum interferon-gamma in pulmonary sarcoidosis and relationship with response to corticosteroid therapy. *Am Rev Respir Dis* 143:53–60, 1991.

336. Daniele RP, Rowlands DT: Lymphocyte subpopulations in sarcoidosis. Correlation with disease activity and duration. *Ann Intern Med* 85:593–600, 1976.

337. Manderazo EG, Ward PA, Woronick CL, et al: Leukotactic dysfunction in sarcoidosis. *Ann Intern Med* 84:414–419, 1976.

338. Goodwin JS, DeHoratius R, Israel H, et al: Suppressor cell function in sarcoidosis. *Ann Intern Med* 90:169–173, 1979.

339. Daniele RP, Dauber JH, Rossman MD: Immunologic abnormalities in sarcoidosis. *Ann Intern Med* 92:406–416, 1980.

340. Daniele RP, McMillan LJ, Dauber JH, et al: Immune complexes in sarcoidosis—a correlation with activity and duration of disease. *Chest* 74:261–264, 1978.

341. Pascual RA, Gee JBL, Finch SC: Usefulness of serum lysozyme measurement in diagnosis and evaluation of sarcoidosis. *N Engl J Med* 289:1074–1076, 1973.

342. Lieberman J: Elevation of serum angiotensin converting enzyme level in sarcoidosis. *Am J Med* 59:365–372, 1975.

343. Zorn SK, Stevens CA, Schachter EN, et al: The angiotensin converting enzyme in pulmonary sarcoidosis and the relative diagnostic value of serum lysozyme. *Lung* 157:87–94, 1980.

344. Allen RK: A review of angiotensin converting enzyme in health and disease. *Sarcoidosis* 8:95–100, 1991.

345. Gee JBL, Bodel PT, Zorn SK, et al: Sarcoidosis and mononuclear phagocytes. *Lung* 155:243–253, 1978.

346. Hinman LM, Stevens C, Matthay RA, et al: Angiotensin convertase activities in human alveolar macrophages: effects of cigarette smoking and sarcoidosis. *Science* 205: 202–203, 1979.

347. Fanburg BL, Schoenberger MD, Bachus B, et al: Elevated serum angiotensin I converting enzyme in sarcoidosis. *Am Rev Respir Dis* 114:525–528, 1976.

348. Silverstein E, Friedland J, Ackerman T: Elevation of granulomatous lymph-node and serum lysozyme in sarcoidosis and correlation and angiotensin-converting enzyme. *Am J Clin Pathol* 68:219–224, 1977.

349. Lieberman J, Nosal A, Schlessner LA, et al: Serum angiotensin-converting enzyme for diagnosis and therapeutic evaluation of sarcoidosis. *Am Rev Respir Dis* 120: 329–335, 1979.

350. Nosal A, Schlessiner LA, Mishkin FS, et al: Angiotensin-I-converting enzyme and gallium scan in non-invasive evaluation of sarcoidosis. *Ann Intern Med* 90:328–331, 1979.

351. DeRemee RA, Rohrbach MS: Serum angiotensin-converting enzyme activity in evaluating the clinical course of sarcoidosis. *Ann Intern Med* 92:361–365, 1980.

352. Koontz CH, Joyner LR, Nelson RA: Transbronchial lung biopsy via the fiberoptic bronchoscope in sarcoidosis. *Ann Intern Med* 85:64–66, 1976.

353. Wall CP, Gaensler EA, Carrington CB, et al: Comparison of transbronchial and open biopsies in chronic infiltrative lung diseases. *Am Rev Respir Dis* 123:280–285, 1981.

354. Reynolds HY: The importance of lymphocytes in pulmonary health and disease. *Lung* 155:225–242, 1978.

355. Hunninghake GW, Fulmer JD, Young RC Jr, et al: Localization of the immune response in sarcoidosis. *Am Rev Respir Dis* 120:49–57, 1979.

356. Daniele RP, Dauber JH, Rossman MD: Lymphocyte populations in the bronchoalveolar air spaces: recent observations in asymptomatic smokers and nonsmokers. In Biserte G, Chretien J, Voisin C (eds): *International Symposium on Bronchoalveolar Lavage in Man*. Paris, L'Institut National de la Sante et de la Recherche Medicale, 1979, pp 193–209.

357. Hunninghake GW, Gadek JE, Young RC Jr, et al: Maintenance of granuloma formation in pulmonary sarcoidosis by T-lymphocytes within the lung. *N Engl J Med* 302:594–598, 1980.

358. Hunninghake GW, Crystal RG: Mechanisms of hypergammaglobulinemia in pulmonary sarcoidosis. Site of increased antibody production and role of T-lymphocytes. *J Clin Invest* 67:86–92, 1981.

359. Hunninghake GW, Crystal RG: T-suppressor cells in sarcoidosis. *N Engl J Med* 305:429–434, 1981.

360. Drent M, van Velzen-Blad H, Diamant M, et al: Relationship between presentation of sarcoidosis and T lymphocyte profile. A study in bronchoalveolar lavage fluid. *Chest* 104:795–800, 1993.

361. Van Maarsseveen TC, deGroot J, Stam J, et al: Peripolesis in alveolar sarcoidosis. *Am Rev Respir Dis* 147: 1259–1263, 1993.

362. DuBois RM, Kirby M, Balbi B, et al: T-lymphocytes that accumulate in the lung in sarcoidosis have evidence of recent stimulation of the T-cell antigen receptor. *Am Rev Respir Dis* 145:1205–1211, 1992.

363. Biyoudi-Vouenze R, Cadranel J, Valeyre D, et al: Expression of $1,25(OH)_2D_3$ receptors on alveolar lymphocytes from patients with pulmonary granulomatous diseases. *Am Rev Respir Dis* 143:1376–1380, 1991.

363a. Reynolds HY: Cytokines: role in respiratory illnesses and potential control with immunomodulatory therapy. *Focus & Opinion: Internal Medicine* 1(6):1–10, 1994.

364. Hunninghake GW: Release of interleukin-I by alveolar macrophages of patients with active pulmonary sarcoidosis. *Am Rev Respir Dis* 129:569–572, 1984.

365. Pueringer RJ, Schwartz DA, Dayton CS, et al: The relationship between alveolar macrophage TNF, I1-1, and $PGE_2$ release, alveolitis, and disease severity in sarcoidosis. *Chest* 103:832–838, 1993.

366. Fels AOS, Cohn ZA: The alveolar macrophage. *J Appl Physiol* 60:353–369, 1986.

367. Nathan CF: Secretory products of macrophages. *J Clin Invest* 79:319–326, 1987.

368. Sibille Y, Reynolds HY: Macrophages and polymorphonuclear neutrophils in lung defense and injury. *Am Rev Respir Dis* 141:471–501, 1990.

369. Venet A, Hance AJ, Saltini C, et al: Enhanced alveolar macrophage-mediated antigen-induced T-lymphocyte proliferation in sarcoidosis. *J Clin Invest* 75:295–301, 1985.

370. Lem VW, Lipscomb MF, Weissler JC, et al: Bronchoalveolar cells from sarcoid patients demonstrate enhanced antigen presentation. *J Immunol* 135:1766–1771, 1985.

371. Saltini C, Spurzem JR, Lee JJ, et al: Spontaneous release of interleukin 2 by lung T lymphocytes in active pulmonary sarcoidosis is primarily from the Leu + DR + T cell subset. *J Clin Invest* 77:1962–1970, 1986.

372. Pinkston P, Bitterman PB, Crystal RG: Spontaneous release of interleukin-2 by lung T-lymphocytes in active pulmonary sarcoidosis. *N Engl J Med* 308:783–800, 1983.

373. Hunninghake GW, Bedell BN, Zavala DC, et al: Role of interleukin 2 release by lung T-cells in active pulmonary sarcoidosis. *Am Rev Respir Dis* 128:634–638, 1983.

374. Robinson BWS, Pinkston P, Crystal RG: Natural killer cells are present in the normal human lung but are functionally impotent. *J Clin Invest* 74:942–950, 1984.

375. Saltini C, Spurzem JR, Kirby MR, et al: Sarcoidosis is not associated with a generalized defect in T cell suppressor function. *J Immunol* 140:1854–1860, 1988.

376. Muller-Quernheim J, Saltini C, Sondermeyer P, et al: Compartmentalized activation of the interleukin-2 gene by lung T lymphocytes in active pulmonary sarcoidosis. *J Immunol* 137:3475–3483, 1986.

377. Muller-Quernheim J, Pfeifer S, Männel D, et al: Lung-restricted activation of the alveolar macrophage/monocyte system in pulmonary sarcoidosis. *Am Rev Respir Dis* 145:187–192, 1992.

378. Robinson BWS, McLemore T, Crystal RG: Gamma interferon is spontaneously released by alveolar macrophages and lung T-lymphocytes in patients with pulmonary sarcoidosis. *J Clin Invest* 75:1488–1495, 1985.

379. Gilbert S, Steinbrech DS, Landas SK, et al: Amounts of angiotensin-converting enzyme mRNA reflect the burden of granulomas in granulomatous lung disease. *Am Rev Respir Dis* 148:483–486, 1993.

380. Roth C, Huchon GJ, Arnoux A, et al: Bronchoalveolar cells in advanced pulmonary sarcoidosis. *Am Rev Respir Dis* 124:9–12, 1981.

381. Sibille Y, Naegel GP, Merrill WW, et al: Neutrophil chemotactic activity produced by normal and activated human bronchoalveolar lavage cells. *J Lab Clin Med* 110:624–633, 1987.

382. Agostini C, Trentin L, Zambello R, et al: CD8 alveolitis in sarcoidosis: incidence, phenotypic characteristics, and clinical features. *Am J Med* 95:466–472, 1993.

383. Young RL, Harkleroad LE, Lordon RE, et al: Pulmonary sarcoidosis: a prospective evaluation of glucocorticoid therapy. *Ann Intern Med* 73:207–212, 1970.

384. Sharma OP: Pulmonary sarcoidosis and corticosteroids. *Am Rev Respir Dis* 147:1598–1600, 1993.

385. Johns CJ, MacGregor MI, Zachary JB, et al: Extended experience in the long-term corticosteroid treatment of pulmonary sarcoidosis. *Ann NY Acad Sci* 278:722–731, 1976.

386. DeRemee RA: The present status of treatment of pulmonary sarcoidosis: a house divided. *Chest* 71:388–393, 1977.

387. Rolfe MW, Standiford TJ, Kunkel SL, et al: Interleukin-1 receptor antagonist expression in sarcoidosis. *Am Rev Respir Dis* 148:1378–1384, 1993.

388. Pinkston P, Saltini C, Muller-Quernheim J, et al: Corticosteroid therapy suppresses spontaneous interleukin-2 release and spontaneous proliferation of lung T-lymphocytes of patient with active pulmonary sarcoidosis. *J Immunol* 139:755–760, 1987.

389. Israel HL, Albertine KH, Park CH, et al: Whole body gallium 67 scans–role in diagnosis of sarcoidosis. *Am Rev Respir Dis* 144:1182–1186, 1991.

390. Lawrence EC, Teague RB, Gottlieb MD, et al: Serial changes in markers of disease activity with corticosteroid treatment in sarcoidosis. *Am J Med* 74:747–756, 1983.

391. Ceuppens JL, Lacquet LM, Marien G, et al: Alveolar T-cells subsets in pulmonary sarcoidosis. Correlation with disease activity and effect of steroid treatment. *Am Rev Respir Dis* 129:563–568, 1984.

392. Baughman RP, Fernandez M, Boxken CH, et al: Comparison of gallium 67 scanning, bronchoalveolar lavage and serum angiotensin converting enzyme levels in pulmonary sarcoidosis. *Am Rev Respir Dis* 132:65–69, 1984.

393. Hollinger WM, Statton GW, Fajman WA, et al: Prediction of therapeutic response in steroid-treated pulmonary sarcoidosis. *Am Rev Respir Dis* 132:65–69, 1985.

394. Turner-Warwick M, McAllister W, Lawrence R, et al: Corticosteroid treatment in pulmonary sarcoidosis: do serial lavage lymphocyte counts, serum angiotensin converting enzyme measurements, and gallium-67 scans help management? *Thorax* 41:903–913, 1986.

395. Lawrence EG, Berger MB, Broussau KP, et al: Elevated serum levels of soluble interleukin-2 receptors in active pulmonary sarcoidosis: relative specificity and association with hypercalcemia. *Sarcoidosis* 4:87–93, 1987.

396. Reynolds HY: Pulmonary sarcoidosis. Do cellular and immunochemical lung parameters exist that would separate subgroups of patients for prognosis? *Sarcoidosis* 6:1–4, 1989.

397. Rankin JA, Huang SS, Sostman HD, et al: An analysis of the inter-relationships among multiple bronchoalveolar lavage and serum determinations, physiologic tests, and clinical disease activity in patients with sarcoidosis. *Sarcoidosis* 8:19–28, 1991.

398. Winterbauer RH, Wu R, Springmeyer SC: Fractional analysis of the 120-ml bronchoalveolar lavage. Determination of the best specimen for diagnosis of sarcoidosis. *Chest* 104:344–351, 1993.

399. Saltini C, Kirby M, Trapnell BC, et al: Biased accumulation of T lymphocytes with "Memory"-type CD45 leukocyte common antigen gene expression on the epithelial surface of the human lung. *J Exp Med* 171:1123–1140, 1990.

400. Lowery WS, Whitlock WL, Dietrich RA, et al: Sarcoidosis complicated by HIV infection: three case reports and a review of the literature. *Am Rev Respir Dis* 142:887–889, 1990.

401. Schatz M, Patterson R, Fink G: Immunopathogenesis of

hypersensitivity pneumonitis. *J Allergy Clin Immunol* 60: 27–37, 1977.

402. Reynolds HY: Hypersensitivity pneumonitis. *Clinics in Chest Medicine*. Philadelphia, WB Saunders, 1982, vol 3, pp 503–519.

403. Reynolds HY: Hypersensitivity pneumonitis: correlation of cellular and immunologic changes with clinical phases of disease. *Lung* 169:S109-S128, 1991.

404. Kaltreider HB: Hypersensitivity pneumonitis. Review. *West J Med* 159:570–578, 1993.

405. Malmberg P, Rask-Andersen A, Rosenhall L: Exposure to microorganisms associated with allergic alveolitis and febrile reactions to mold dust in farmers. *Chest* 103: 1202–1209, 1993.

406. Patterson R, Wang JLF, Fink JN, et al: IgA and IgG antibody activities of serum and bronchoalveolar fluid from symptomatic and asymptomatic pigeon breeders. *Am Rev Respir Dis* 120:1113–1118, 1979.

407. Treuhaft MW, Robert RC, Hackbarth C, et al: Characterization of precipitin response to *Micropolyspora faeni* in farmer's lung disease by quantitative immunoelectrophoresis. *Am Rev Respir Dis* 119:571–578, 1979.

408. Braun SR, doPico GA, Tsiatis A, et al: Farmer's lung disease: long-term clinical and physiologic outcome. *Am Rev Respir Dis* 119:185–191, 1979.

409. Sansoores R, Salas J, Chapela R, et al: Clubbing in hypersensitivity pneumonitis. *Arch Intern Med* 150:1849–1851, 1990.

410. Reynolds HY: Concepts of pathogenesis and lung reactivity in hypersensitivity pneumonitis (Louis E. Siltzbach Lecture). 10th International Conference on Sarcoidosis and Other Granulomatous Disorders. *Ann NY Acad Sci* 465:287–303, 1986.

411. Leatherman JW, Michael AF, Schwartz BA, et al: Lung T-cells in hypersensitivity pneumonitis. *Ann Intern Med* 100:390–392, 1984.

412. Costabel U, Bross KJ, Ruhle KH, et al: Ia-like antigens on T-cells and their subpopulations in pulmonary sarcoidosis and in hypersensitivity pneumonitis—analysis of bronchoalveolar and blood lymphocytes. *Am Rev Respir Dis* 131:337–342, 1985.

413. Semanzato G, Chilosi M, Ossi E, et al: Bronchoalveolar lavage and lung histology: comparative analysis of inflammatory and immunocompetent cells in patients with sarcoidosis and hypersensitivity pneumonitis. *Am Rev Respir Dis* 132:400–404, 1985.

414. Murayama J, Yoshizawa Y, Ohtsuka M, et al: Lung fibrosis in hypersensitivity pneumonitis. Association with CD4 + but not CD8 + cell dominant alveolitis and insidious onset. *Chest* 104:38–43, 1993.

415. Calvanico NJ, Ambegaonkar SP, Schlueter DP, et al: Immunoglobulin levels in bronchoalveolar lavage fluid from pigeon breeders. *J Lab Clin Med* 98:129–140, 1980.

416. Fournier E, Tonnel AB, Gesset P, et al: Early neutrophil alveolitis after inhalation challenge in hypersensitivity pneumonitis. *Chest* 88:563–566, 1985.

417. Solal-Celigny P, Laviolette M, Hebert J, et al: Immune reactions in the lungs of asymptomatic dairy farmers. *Am Rev Respir Dis* 126:964–967, 1982.

418. Cormier Y, Belanger J, Beaudoin J, et al: Abnormal bronchoalveolar lavage in asymptomatic dairy farmers—study of lymphocytes. *Am Rev Respir Dis* 130:1046–1049, 1984.

419. Cormier Y, Belanger J, Laviolette M: Persistent bronchoalveolar lymphocytosis in asymptomatic farmers. *Am Rev Respir Dis* 133:843–847, 1986.

420. Gariépy L, Cormier Y, Laviolette M, et al: Predictive value of bronchoalveolar lavage cells and serum precipitins in asymptomatic dairy farmers. *Am Rev Respir Dis* 140:1386–1389, 1989.

421. Lalancette M, Carrier G, Laviolette M, et al: Farmer's lung. Long-term outcome and lack of predictive value of bronchoalveolar lavage fibrosing factors. *Am Rev Respir Dis* 148:216–221, 1993.

422. Cormier Y, Laviolette M, Cantin A, et al: Fibrogenic activities in bronchoalveolar lavage fluid of farmer's lung. *Chest* 104:1038–1042, 1993.

423. Tescher H, Pohl WR, Thompson AB et al: Elevated levels of bronchoalveolar lavage vitronectin in hypersensitivity pneumonitis. *Am Rev Respir Dis* 147:332–337, 1993.

424. Pérez-Arellano JL, Pedraz MJ, Fuertes A, et al: Laminin fragment P1 is increased in the lower respiratory tract of patients with diffuse interstitial lung diseases. *Chest* 104:1163–1169, 1993.

425. Ottesen EA: Eosinophilia and the lung. In Kirkpatrick CH, Reynolds HY (eds): *Immunologic and Infectious Reactions in the Lung*. New York, Marcel Dekker, 1976, p 289.

426. Butterworth AE, David JR: Eosinophil function. *N Engl J Med* 304:154–156, 1981.

427. Crofton JW, Livingstone JL, Oswalk NC, et al: Pulmonary eosinophilia. *Thorax* 7:1–35, 1952.

428. Rossing TH: Pulmonary infiltrates with eosinophilia (PIE) syndrome and asthma. *Medical Grand Rounds* 4: 84–93, 1986.

429. Carrington CB, Addington WW, Goff AM, et al: Chronic eosinophilic pneumonia. *N Engl J Med* 280:787–798, 1969.

430. Sederlinic PJ, Sicilian L, Gaensler EA: Chronic eosinophilic pneumonia: a report of 19 and a review of the literature. *Medicine* 67:154–162, 1988.

431. Naughton M, Fahy J, Fitzgerald MX: Chronic eosinophilic pneumonia—a long term follow-up of 12 patients. *Chest* 103:162–165, 1993.

432. Webb JKG, Job CK, Gault EW: Tropical eosinophilia: demonstration of microfilaria in lung, liver and lymph nodes. *Lancet* 1:835, 1960.

433. Danaraj TJ, Pacheco G, Shanmugaratnum K, et al: The etiology and pathology of eosinophilic lung (tropical eosinophilia). *Am J Trop Med Hyg* 15:183–189, 1966.

434. Pinkston P, Vijayan VK, Nutman TB, et al: Acute tropical pulmonary eosinophilia—characterization of the lower respiratory tract inflammation and its response to therapy. *J Clin Invest* 80:216–225, 1987.

435. Nutman TB, Vijayan VK, Pinkston P, et al: Tropical pulmonary eosinophilia: analysis of antifilarial antibody localized to the lung. *J Infect Dis* 160:1042–1050, 1989.

436. Rom WN, Vijayan VK, Cornelius MJ, et al: Persistent lower respiratory inflammation associated with interstitial lung disease in patients with tropical pulmonary eosinophilia following conventional treatment with diethylcarbamazine. *Am Rev Respir Dis* 142:1088–1092, 1990.

437. Snider GL: In case records, Massachusetts General Hospital. *N Engl J Med* 303:1218–1225, 1980.

438. McCarthy DS, Pepys J: Allergic broncho-pulmonary aspergillosis. Clinical immunology: (1) clinical features. *Clin Allergy* 1:261–286, 1971.

439. Groopman JE, Golde DW: The histiocytic disorders: a pathophysiologic analysis. *Ann Intern Med* 94:95–107, 1981.

440. Marcy TW, Reynolds HY: Pulmonary histiocytosis. *Lung* 163:129–150, 1985.

441. Strieder DJ, Mark EJ: Pulmonary eosinophilic granuloma. In case records, Massachusetts General Hospital. *N Engl J Med* 298:327–332, 1978.

442. King TE, Schwarz MI, Dreisin RE, et al: Circulating immune complexes in pulmonary eosinophilic granuloma. *Ann Intern Med* 98:397–399, 1979.

443. Lacronique J, Roth C, Battesti JP, et al: Chest radiologic feature of pulmonary histiocytosis X: a report based on 50 adult cases. *Thorax* 37:104–109, 1982.

444. Chollet S, Dournovo P, Richard MS, et al: Reactivity of histiocytosis X cells with monoclonal anti T6 antibody. *N Engl J Med* 307:685–686, 1982.

445. Chollet S, Soler P, Dournovo P, et al: Diagnosis of pulmonary histiocytosis X by immunodetection of Langerhans' cells in bronchoalveolar lavage fluid. *Am J Pathol* 115:225–232, 1984.

446. Hance AJ, Basset F, Saumon G, et al: Smoking and interstitial lung disease. The effect of cigarette smoking on the incidence of pulmonary histiocytosis X and sarcoidosis. In Johns C (ed): Tenth International Conference on Sarcoidosis and Other Granulomatous Disorders. *Ann NY Acad Sci* 465:643–656, 1986.

447. Hance AJ, Cadranel J, Soler P, Basset F: Pulmonary and extrapulmonary manifestations of Langerhans' cell granulomatosis (histiocytosis X). *Semin Respir Med* 9:349–368, 1988.

448. Casolaro MA, Bernaudin JF, Saltini C, et al: Accumulation of Langerhans' cells on the epithelial surface of the lower respiratory tract in normal subjects in association with cigarette smoking. *Am Rev Respir Dis* 137:406–411, 1988.

449. Tazi A, Bonay M, Grandsaigne M, et al: Surface phenotype of Langerhans cells and lymphocytes in granulomatous lesions from patients with pulmonary histiocytosis X. *Am Rev Respir Dis* 147:1531–1536, 1993.

450. Tazi A, Bouchonnet F, Grandsaigne M, et al: Evidence that granulocyte macrophage colony stimulating factor regulates the distribution and differentiated state of dendritic cells/Langerhans cells in human lung and lung cancers. *J Clin Invest* 91:566–576, 1993.

# Chapter 14

# Occupational and Environmental Lung Disease

**Carrie A. Redlich**
**John Balmes**

THE PAST DECADE has seen a marked increase in concern about the adverse health effects of hazardous exposures in both the workplace and elsewhere in the environment. The lung with its extensive surface area, high blood flow, and thin alveolar epithelium is an important site of contact with substances in the environment. Such agents can cause direct toxicity or can be absorbed by or deposited in the respiratory tract. Because of the seemingly endless array of substances and/or lack of toxicologic, epidemiologic, and/or industrial hygiene expertise, many clinicians feel ill-prepared to recognize, diagnose, and treat occupational lung diseases.

This chapter discusses the major occupational respiratory tract disorders, with an emphasis on certain basic principles and the recognition and diagnosis of such disorders. The adverse health effects of environmental exposures such as passive smoking and domestic radon are also reviewed. Almost all respiratory diseases may be caused or exacerbated by factors in the workplace or environment. Thus, it is important to maintain a high level of suspicion when evaluating patients with any respiratory disorder. Several excellent recent occupational and environmental medicine textbooks provide a more extensive review of the topic (1–4).

## Principles of Occupational and Environmental Lung Disease

Certain principles apply broadly to the full range of respiratory disorders caused by inhalational exposure to agents in the workplace or environment:

1. Environmental and occupational lung diseases are difficult to distinguish from those of nonenvironmental origin. Almost any defined lung disease may have an environmental cause. Conversely, few environmental lung diseases will present with obvious or pathognomonic features.
2. A given substance in the workplace or environment can cause more than one clinical or pathologic entity. For example, cobalt can cause interstitial lung disease and airways disease.
3. The etiology of many lung diseases may be multifactorial, and occupational factors may interact with other factors. For example, asbestos-exposed workers who smoke have a much greater risk of developing lung cancer than those exposed to either asbestos or cigarettes alone.
4. The respiratory effects of occupational and environmental lung exposures occur following the exposure with a predictable latent interval that depends on the given exposure. For acute diseases, there is a short and usually predictable time period between exposure and resultant clinical manifestations, which should suggest an association. For chronic diseases such as cancer or most pneumoconioses, long latency between first exposure and subsequent clinical manifestations is common. Consequently, the patient's exposure to the offending agent(s) may have ceased long before the onset of the disease, making the diagnosis of such diseases much more of a challenge.
5. The dose of exposure is an important determinant of the proportion of individuals affected and/or the

severity of disease. Higher doses usually result in more affected individuals and/or greater disease severity. Dose will generally affect incidence in diseases with immunologic mechanisms and severity in those with nonimmunologic properties.
6. Individual differences in susceptibility to exposures exist. Adverse effects may occur in some individuals while others are spared. Host factors that determine susceptibility to environmental agents are poorly understood but likely include both inherited genetic factors and acquired factors, such as diet, the presence of other lung disease, and other exposures.

There are several compelling reasons to pursue the search for an occupational or environmental cause in all cases of pulmonary disease. Knowledge of cause may affect patient management and prognosis, and may prevent further disease progression. New associations between exposure and disease may be identified, such as new agents that can cause occupational asthma. A larger population at risk that may benefit from preventive measures may be identified. Finally, establishment of cause may have significant legal and financial implications for the patient.

### Clinical Approach to the Patient

There are two distinct phases of the workup of any patient with a potential occupational or environmental lung disease. First, as with any patient presenting with a potential disorder of the respiratory tract, its nature and extent must be defined and characterized, regardless of the suspected etiology. Second, whether the disease or symptom complex is caused or exacerbated by any exposures at work or in the environment must be determined.

The initial approach to all such patients includes a detailed history, physical examination, appropriate laboratory testing, chest radiograph, and pulmonary function testing. Initial exposure information can be used to direct the sequence of the workup and to obviate unnecessary procedures when the diagnosis is fairly straightforward. If the initial evaluation does not fully explain the patient's symptomatology, other tests are available to better characterize the nature and extent of the respiratory disorder, including computed chest tomography, laryngoscopy, flow-volume loops, cardiopulmonary exercise studies, nonspecific inhalation challenge, bronchoscopy, open lung biopsy, and various immunologic studies. However, few are specific for any given occupational or environmental diagnosis.

Prior medical records can be extremely helpful in the evaluation of a patient with a potential occupational or environmental lung disease. Such records can establish the patient's earlier complaints, may provide objective data such as prior pulmonary function tests or chest radiographs for comparison, and may clarify temporal relationships between exposure and effect, an important component of biologic plausibility.

## DIAGNOSTIC CRITERIA

After the disease process is characterized, then whether or not any occupational or environmental exposures are causative or contributory must be determined. The following criteria are used to determine whether a disease is caused or exacerbated by agents in the workplace or environment:

1. The clinical presentation and workup are consistent with the diagnosis.
2. A causal relationship (biologic plausibility) between the exposure and the diagnosed condition has been previously established or strongly suggested in the medical or toxicologic literature. Several different types of data can be used to establish a causal relationship. Epidemiologic studies (such as cohort or case control studies) can demonstrate associations between certain exposures or jobs and adverse effects. Clinical studies or case reports of similarly exposed patients can be used to determine the adverse effects of an exposure. Such studies may also provide useful information about the magnitude of the risk, the amount of exposure necessary for disease, and the latency between exposure and disease. Data from animal toxicologic studies can also be helpful, especially when human data are not available.
3. There is sufficient exposure to cause the disease, as assessed below.
4. The details of the particular case, such as the temporal relationship between exposure and disease, are consistent with known information about the exposure-disease association.
5. There is no other more likely diagnosis.

### Exposure Assessment

The occupational and environmental history is the single most helpful tool to determine whether exposure to one or more environmental agents has occurred and the magnitude and extent of the exposure. A detailed occupational history consists of a chronologic list of all jobs, including job title, a description of the

job activities, potential toxins at each job, and an assessment of the extent and duration of exposure. The length of time exposed to the agent, the use of personal protective equipment such as respirators, and a description of the ventilation and overall hygiene are helpful in attempting to quantify exposure from the patient's history.

Patients should be asked whether they think their problem is related to anything in the environment. Temporal associations between the patient's symptoms and exposures and the presence of similar symptoms among coworkers should be carefully determined. Information about potential exposures outside the workplace, such as in the home or encountered with hobbies, should also be obtained.

There are a number of sources available for obtaining additional exposure information. These include Material Safety Data Sheets (MSDSs) (employers are required by federal law to provide employees with information about the potential toxicity of the materials used in the workplace); exposure records from the employer or insurance companies; information from inspections by health and regulatory agencies such as the Occupational Safety and Health Administration (OSHA), unions and community groups, and direct site visits. For recent or current exposures, a site visit is usually most helpful in providing information about the nature and extent of potential exposures and other exposed workers. Epidemiologic data on coworkers or previous workers with similar types of jobs can be used to assess the nature and extent of exposures for a given patient. Finally, further information about the patient's exposure can be obtained from certain diagnostic tests, such as a positive radioallergosorbent test (RAST) or skin test to a specific antigen or tissue mineralogic analysis. For acute diseases such as occupational asthma, reproducing the disease manifestations by reexposure to the suspected environmental agent is additional evidence that supports the diagnosis.

Once this additional information is obtained, the clinician has to finally make a determination about whether any occupational or environmental exposures are causing or contributing to the patient's disease process. Although some diagnoses such as asbestosis are frequently very straightforward, others may be diagnostically more challenging and easily overlooked. There is always some degree of uncertainty in medical decision making. In most workers' compensation cases the standard of certainty is usually whether the patient's problem is more probably than not (a greater than 50% likelihood) related to an occupational or environmental exposure. This is a much lower standard of certainty than physicians generally use in making diagnostic decisions. Occupational or environmental diseases can be diagnosed even in the presence of a significant degree of uncertainty. Once such a diagnosis is made, the physician should consider the public health issues involved, i.e., that other individuals in that same environment may also be similarly affected, and consider appropriate action.

## CLASSIFICATION OF OCCUPATIONAL AND ENVIRONMENTAL LUNG DISEASE

Environmentally induced lung diseases can be classified by several schemes. Because these diseases so closely resemble other lung diseases, it may be helpful to classify them by the clinical presentation, as shown in Table 14.1. An overview of these acute and chronic disorders, and the adverse health effects of indoor and outdoor air pollutants, can be found in this chapter, with the exception of hypersensitivity pneumonitis and infectious diseases, which are discussed in Chapters 12 and 17, respectively.

## MAJOR ACUTE/SUBACUTE DISEASES

### UPPER RESPIRATORY TRACT IRRITATION

Symptoms of eye, nose, and throat irritation are frequently associated with environmental exposures (5). Numerous substances can cause upper respiratory tract irritation and inflammation, including dusts such as coal or manmade vitreous fibers (MMVF); irritant gases such as ammonia, chlorine, and ozone; metal fumes; and numerous solvents. Presenting symptoms can mimic common disorders such as upper respiratory infection, rhinitis, acute bronchitis, sinusitis, or hay fever. Many of these exposures can also cause lower respiratory tract disease, including occupational asthma, toxic pneumonitis, chronic bronchitis, or interstitial lung disease, depending on the particular agent and the dose and duration of exposure.

The diagnosis usually is made on the basis of a temporal association between exposure to the irritant substance(s) and symptoms. Improvement in symptoms away from work and similar symptoms in coworkers

**TABLE 14.1**
**CLASSIFICATION OF OCCUPATIONAL LUNG DISORDERS**

| Disease/Problem | Example of Causative Agent |
| --- | --- |
| Major acute or subacute diseases | |
|   Upper respiratory tract irritation | Irritant gases, solvents |
|   Airway disorders | |
|     Occupational asthma | |
|       Sensitization | Diisocyanates, animal dander |
|       Irritant-induced, RADS | Irritant gases |
|     Byssinosis | Cotton dust |
|     Grain dust effects | Grain |
|   Inhalation injury | |
|     Toxic pneumonitis | Irritant gases, metals |
|     Metal fume fever | Metal oxides—zinc, copper |
|     Polymer fume fever | Plastics |
|     Smoke inhalation | |
|   Hypersensitivity pneumonitis | Microbial agents |
|   Infectious disorders | Tuberculosis |
|   Acute pleural disease | Asbestos |
| Major chronic diseases | |
|   Interstitial fibrotic diseases (pneumoconioses) | Asbestos, silica, coal |
|   Beryllium/hard metal–related disease | Beryllium, cobalt |
|   Chronic bronchitis/COPD | Mineral dusts, coal |
| Malignancies of the respiratory tract and pleura | |
|   Sinonasal cancer | Wood dust |
|   Laryngeal cancer | Asbestos? |
|   Lung cancer | Asbestos, radon |
|   Mesothelioma | Asbestos |
| Air pollution | |
|   Ambient air pollution | Sulfur oxides, particulates |
|   Indoor air pollution | Environmental tobacco smoke |

are helpful clues. Atopic individuals appear to be at increased risk for upper respiratory tract irritation. It is important to determine whether there is any lower respiratory tract involvement, which usually can be determined by a patient's history and spirometry. RAST testing may be helpful if the history suggests IgE-mediated allergies. Successful treatment involves reducing or eliminating the offending exposures. Long-term sequelae generally do not develop.

## AIRWAY DISORDERS

### Occupational Asthma—Sensitization

*Definition and Causes*

Occupational asthma has been defined as variable air flow obstruction and/or airway hyperresponsiveness caused by a specific agent or process encountered in the workplace (6). This definition presumes nothing about pathogenic mechanism and is intended to include bronchospasm due to nonspecific stimuli, in addition to that caused by agents to which specific "sensitization" has developed. A broader definition would include aggravation of preexisting asthma by exposures in the workplace.

Many cases of occupationally caused asthma are due to sensitizing agents, which include both high–molecular weight (>1000 daltons) and low–molecular weight compounds (Table 14.2). High–molecular weight compounds include animal, plant, and fungal proteins. Low–molecular weight compounds are usually chemicals; most common are the diisocyanates, anhydrides, and plicatic acid (the putative cause of western red cedar–induced asthma). This distinction by size is justified by the differing clinical characteristics and pathogenic features of asthma induced by agents in the respective categories. The number of agents or processes that have been shown to cause occupational asthma is long and constantly growing (7). Environmental allergens generated by mites, cats, and cockroaches are also increasingly being recognized as important etiologic agents in asthma (8). The role of such environmental factors in asthma is discussed more fully in Chapter 9.

*Prevalence*

The prevalence of occupational asthma in the United States is unknown, but has been estimated to be 2 to 15% of all asthma cases (9, 10). An occupational etiology is more likely in those asthmatics with adult onset disease and with no history of atopy. The incidence of occupational asthma in different industrial settings varies. For example, 5 to 10% of isocyanate-exposed persons, 5 to 10% of those exposed to western red cedar, and up to 30% of animal handlers have been reported to develop occupational asthma (9, 10).

The single most important factor determining the prevalence of occupational asthma is exposure to a sensitizing or irritant agent. Only a portion of workers exposed to a sensitizing agent ever develop asthma. However, host susceptibility factors for occupational asthma are not well understood. Atopy is often a predisposing factor for the development of asthma due to high–molecular weight compounds such as animal- or plant-derived material (6, 11). However, atopy does not appear to be an important risk factor when low–molecular weight compounds such as diisocyanates or plicatic acid are the causative agents (6, 12). The role of cigarette smoking in the development of occupational asthma is unclear. Studies have suggested that both nonsmokers and smokers may be more susceptible (12, 13). It remains unclear whether preexisting nonspecific airway hyperresponsiveness predisposes to occupational asthma. Most patients with occupational asthma have nonspecific airway hyperresponsiveness that probably developed after exposure to the occupational agent (6).

*Clinical Features*

The most easily recognized presentation of occupational asthma consists of wheezing and dyspnea, which occur within minutes after contact with the offending agent at the workplace and typically disappear after work, the so-called immediate reaction. Productive cough or chest tightness rather than wheezing is also common. A delayed reaction may begin up to 12 hours after exposure, so that wheeze, cough, or chest tightness at night may be the only presenting symptoms. A delayed reaction is common with low–molecular weight compounds. Patients can have both immediate and delayed symptoms, i.e., a dual reaction. Symptoms frequently worsen over the course of the work week and improve on weekends and vacation. Sensitizer-induced occupational asthma develops after a latent period that can vary from months to years.

The relationship between symptoms and exposure may be unclear. Continued exposure to the causative agent may result in persistent airway obstruction and/or hyperresponsiveness, such that symptoms may persist after cessation of exposure. Failure of symptoms to improve during periods of time off work does not exclude the diagnosis of occupational asthma. However, lack of any improvement during a vacation of several weeks is unusual. Nonspecific triggers such as upper respiratory tract infections, exercise, cold, and emotional stimuli may precipitate asthmatic attacks in patients with occupational asthma, just as in those with asthma not related to the workplace.

TABLE **14.2**
OCCUPATIONAL ASTHMA[a]

| Asthma-Inducing Agents | Common Occupations |
|---|---|
| High-molecular-weight compounds | |
|   Animal-derived material (dander, excreta, secretions) | |
|     Laboratory animals | Laboratory workers |
|     Birds, bats | Breeders |
|     Shellfish | Food processors |
|     Insects | Laboratory workers |
|   Plants and vegetable products | |
|     Castor beans | Food processors |
|     Coffee beans | Food processors |
|     Grain dust | Grain handlers |
|     Cotton dust | Textile workers |
|     Flour | Bakers |
|     Psyllium | Laxative manufacturers |
|     Vegetable gums | Printers |
|   Enzymes | |
|     Alcalase | Detergent manufacturers |
|     Papain | Food processors |
|     Pancreatic extracts | Pharmaceutical workers |
| Low-molecular-weight compounds | |
|   Wood dusts | Woodworkers, carpenters |
|     Western red cedar | |
|     California redwood | |
|     Mahogany | |
|     Oak | |
|   Diisocyanates | Painters, printers, foam manufacturers |
|     Toluene (TDI) | |
|     Diphenylmethane (MDI) | |
|     Hexamethylene (HDI) | |
|   Acid anhydrides | Epoxy resin, paint, chemical workers |
|     Trimellitic (TMA) | |
|     Phthalic (PA) | |
|     Maleic (MA) | |
|   Amines | |
|     Ethylenediamine | Plastic workers |
|   Drugs | Pharmaceutical workers |
|     Cimetidine | |
|     Cephalosporins | |
|     Psyllium | |
|     Penicillins | |
|     Sulfonamides | |
|   Other chemicals | |
|     Azo dyes | Dye workers |
|     Formaldehyde | Nurses, laboratory workers |
|     Glutaraldehyde | Nurses, hospital workers |
|     Insecticides (organophosphates) | Manufacturers, farmers |
|     Persulfates | Hairdressers |
|     Polyvinyl chloride (decomposition) | Food wrappers |
|   Metal fumes and salts | Metal workers, metal platers, welders |
|     Chromium | |
|     Cobalt | |
|     Nickel | |
|     Platinum salts | |

[a] For a more comprehensive list see reference 6.

*Diagnosis*

The diagnosis of occupational asthma involves first establishing the diagnosis of asthma, and then determining whether or not it is associated with exposure to some substance or process in the workplace. There is no single simple diagnostic test for occupational asthma, and the diagnosis may be difficult to make. A high index of suspicion is key to the correct diagnosis.

A careful occupational history is the most effective, useful, and practical means of identifying workers with possible occupational asthma. The following should raise the suspicion for occupational asthma: new-onset asthma in an adult, worsening symptoms at or after work with deterioration over the course of the week, improvement away from work, and the presence of an agent in the workplace known to cause occupational asthma. Additional helpful information is the use of any new agents or processes at the worksite, similar symptoms in other workers, and the presence of preexisting asthma and/or atopy.

The diagnosis of asthma is confirmed, as with any asthmatic patient, by demonstrating reversible air flow obstruction on spirometry. Tests for nonspecific airway hyperresponsiveness, such as methacholine challenge, can be used to document hyperreactive airways if spirometry is normal.

Several methods are available to document the association between air flow obstruction and exposure to the suspected agent:

1. *Preshift and postshift measurement in $FEV_1$*
   Demonstration of a decrement of more than 10% in the forced expiratory volume in 1 second ($FEV_1$) across the workshift is a relatively specific test, but it is insufficiently sensitive because of the relatively frequent occurrence of delayed responses, and it can be logistically difficult to perform.
2. *Serial measurements of peak expiratory flow rates (PEFR)*
   Serial measurements of peak expiratory flow can be made by a worker throughout the workshift and later at home by means of a hand-held instrument, a Mini-Wright peak flowmeter (Fig. 14.1) (14). A reduction in peak flows associated with exposure to the suspected offending agent supports a diagnosis of occupational asthma. Visual interpretation is as useful as quantitative analysis. An example of a PEFR record supporting a diagnosis of occupational asthma is shown in Figure 14.2. Good-quality PEFR recordings with adequate off-work and work days may be difficult to obtain.
3. *Specific inhalation challenge*
   Workplace challenges can be performed under actual exposure conditions, but because multiple ex-

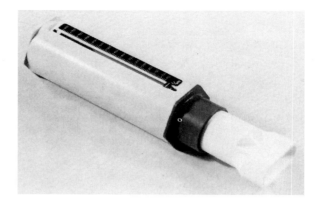

**FIGURE 14.1.** Peak flowmeter.

posures are common, they may not identify the specific agent. Specific challenge testing with the suspected agent(s) is considered the "gold standard" for diagnosing occupational asthma (15). A 20% fall in $FEV_1$ following exposure to the offending agent is diagnostic of occupational asthma. However, such testing requires a specialized chamber, carries certain risks, is time consuming, and is not widely available, and false negatives can occur. Specific inhalation challenge is helpful in documenting a previously unrecognized cause of occupational asthma and in establishing a specific etiologic diagnosis when the workup has been equivocal or multiple sensitizing exposures are present. However, specific challenge is unnecessary for the diagnosis of most cases of occupational asthma.

In practice, objective evidence of variable air flow obstruction in relation to workplace exposure can be difficult to obtain for multiple reasons, especially if the patient has changed jobs. A temporal association between asthmatic symptoms and a workplace exposure may provide sufficient evidence of work- relatedness if the suspect exposure is a documented cause of asthma (Table 14.2). One does not need to identify the specific causative agent to make a diagnosis of occupational asthma (16).

*Immunologic Tests*

Skin tests and detection of specific IgE antibodies in the serum by immunoassays such as the RAST to the suspected agent have varying degrees of usefulness. In the case of high–molecular weight allergens, such as flours or rodent proteins, the demonstration of a positive skin test and/or specific IgE antibodies is highly confirmatory of exposure. However, for low–molecular weight compounds, such as diisocyanates or plicatic acid, negative tests are common, and

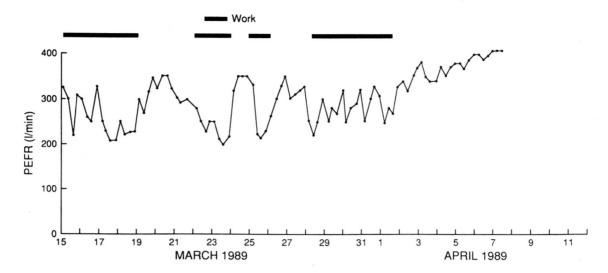

**FIGURE 14.2.** PEFR record of a hairdresser who developed symptoms of asthma from exposure to a bleaching reagent she used at work. PEFR showed improvement when she was away from work. (From Rosenstock K, Cullen MR: *Textbook of Clinical Occupational and Environmental Medicine.* Philadelphia, WB Saunders, 1994.)

the application of these techniques has limited clinical utility (12, 17).

*Outcome/Management*

Studies of workers with occupationally induced asthma, primarily due to diisocyanates and western red cedar, have shown that many of these workers (up to 80%) have persistent symptoms and airway hyperresponsiveness, even after removal from further exposure (6, 17, 18, 19). The factors that determine prognosis are not well defined, but persistent asthma following removal has been associated with longer duration of symptoms before diagnosis, abnormal spirometry, and more marked airway hyperresponsivenss. These patients clinically can be indistinguishable from intrinsic, non–occupationally induced asthmatics with acute exacerbations following viral infections and nonspecific irritants. Recovery is more likely with early diagnosis and removal from further exposure.

Since many exposures that cause occupational asthma are sensitizing agents, once symptomatic, exposure to minute quantities, even below regulatory permissible limits, can induce bronchospasm. Thus once occupational asthma has been diagnosed, attempts should be made to remove the patient from further exposure. Respiratory protective devices are rarely effective but can be tried with close monitoring. Medications used to treat occupational asthma are the same as those used with nonoccupational asthma.

*Reactive Airways Dysfunction Syndrome (RADS)*

The persistence of symptoms consistent with asthma and nonspecific airway hyperresponsiveness

in some individuals following a single high exposure to an irritating vapor, fume, gas, or smoke has been termed reactive airways dysfunction syndrome (RADS) (20). A number of examples of irritant-induced nonallergic asthma have been reported (7). The following criteria are used to diagnose RADS:

1. Absence of preceding asthma-like respiratory disease or complaints;
2. Onset of symptoms after a single or multiple high-level exposure(s) to a known irritant gas, vapor, fume, aerosol, or dust;
3. Onset of symptoms shortly (within 24 hours) of the exposure and lasting for at least 3 months, usually longer;
4. Symptoms and spirometric findings that simulate asthma;
5. Positive methacholine challenge if spirometry is normal;
6. Other asthma-like illnesses are ruled out.

The incidence of RADS is not well defined, but it is probably not uncommon. One study found that 10 of 59 workers diagnosed with occupational asthma had a history consistent with RADS (21). The evaluation of workers with RADS is similar to that for patients with sensitizer-induced occupational asthma. Exposure to respiratory irritants should be minimized. The worker may be able to return to the workplace if irritant exposures are limited. Close follow-up is necessary to monitor for persistent or progressive symptoms and air flow obstruction.

*Pathogenesis of Occupational Asthma*

Similar to non–work-related asthma, airway inflammation likely plays a crucial role in the pathogenesis of occupational asthma. Components of airway inflammation include alterations in airway epithelial and smooth muscle cells; airway infiltration by inflammatory cells including T lymphocytes, mast cells, eosinophils, and neutrophils; and thickening of the airway wall (22). How different exposures cause airway inflammation is not well understood but likely involves both immunologic and nonimmunologic mechanisms (6, 23). Airways may be injured directly by intense exposure to irritant chemicals such as chlorine or sulfur dioxide, resulting in epithelial damage, airway inflammation, and hyperresponsiveness. Such a mechanism is likely involved in the pathogenesis of RADS.

In most cases of occupational asthma caused by both low–molecular weight and high–molecular weight compounds, airway inflammation likely develops through immune-mediated processes (7). The following clinical characteristics all support an immune hypersensitivity-type reaction: asthma occurs in only a proportion of those exposed to the agent; asthma develops only after weeks to years of exposure; patients can have a dual, early or late response; and once "sensitized," very low levels of exposure to the agent can precipitate an asthmatic response. High–molecular weight animal- and plant-derived compounds can induce specific IgE responses in a high proportion of exposed individuals. Low–molecular weight chemicals such as diisocyanates may act as haptens, which have to be conjugated to a carrier protein to form a complete antigen. However, specific IgE or IgG antibodies are detected in only a small fraction of such patients. The immununologic mechanisms involved with exposure to low–molecular weight compounds are not well defined but may involve both IgE and T lymphocyte processes.

## Byssinosis—Textile Dust–Related Disease

*Definition*

Byssinosis, an occupational lung disease of textile workers, is caused by excessive inhalation of certain vegetable fiber dusts. First described by Ramazzini almost three centuries ago, it was essentially rediscovered by Richard Schilling in England in the 1950s (24, 25). The disease originally was recognized in cotton workers but also has been reported among other textile workers. In its early stages, byssinosis is characterized by symptoms of chest tightness, cough, wheezing, and dyspnea that are especially prominent on the first day back to work after a break in exposure. These symptoms initially tend to diminish over the first few days of the work week, but as the disease progresses, chronic chest tightness can develop. Acute and chronic obstructive changes in pulmonary function can occur. The term byssinosis refers to both the early and late manifestations of cotton dust–induced lung disease. In addition to byssinosis, textile workers can also develop hypersensitivity pneumonitis, chronic bronchitis, and febrile syndromes such as mill fever and mattress makers' fever.

*Risk Factors*

The risk of developing byssinosis is related to the intensity of dust exposure, duration of exposure, job, and particular mill and type of fiber. The highest incidence of disease traditionally has been found among workers involved in the dusty preparatory phases of the cotton textile manufacturing process. Workers engaged in the later phases of the process may also develop byssinosis, but the incidence is much lower. Exposure to the end product (e.g., cotton cloth) does not cause byssinosis.

There is some evidence that an atopic predisposition may increase the risk of developing byssinosis, but most textile workers who develop the typical symptom complex do not have a history of allergic reactions (26). Whether preexisting nonspecific airway hyperresponsiveness plays a role has not been well studied. Several studies have found that smokers have a greater incidence of byssinosis than nonsmokers (27).

*Clinical Features and Natural History*

During the early stages of byssinosis, symptoms of chest tightness and dyspnea tend to build gradually, with the onset usually noted about 1 hour after the beginning of work. When exposure ceases, these symptoms tend to disappear. The acute symptoms of byssinosis are correlated with a decline in $FEV_1$ over the work shift. This decrease in ventilatory function in the early stages of the disease is reversible (28). With further exposure, the periodic acute Monday exacerbations can progress to symptoms on every workday. After many years of textile work, respiratory symptoms can persist even in the absence of exposure, and disability may ensue (29). Several longitudinal studies have shown increased symptoms and accelerated loss of lung function in textile workers, independent of smoking history (29–31). Although byssinosis and occupational asthma share some features in common such as work-related reduction in $FEV_1$, byssinosis is felt by most to be a distinct entity on the basis of several features, including improvement in symptoms over the work week.

*Pathogenesis*

A number of studies have investigated the possible mechanisms by which cotton and other dusts cause acute and chronic byssinosis. These studies have been complicated by the large number of potentially toxic components of cotton dust, including bacteria, fungi, inorganic material, and organic chemicals. Several mechanisms have been suggested, including the release of pharmacologic mediators such as histamine, an immunologic IgE-mediated reaction, and bacterial endotoxins (29). It has been demonstrated that endotoxin is present in many cotton dusts and can cause bronchoconstriction, and that the acute symptoms and reduced lung function correlate with airborne endotoxin concentrations (32). However, there remains some uncertainty about the role of endotoxin, since inhalation of endotoxin-free cotton dust has also induced symptoms and bronchoconstriction (33).

### Diagnosis

There is no single test to diagnose byssinosis. The diagnosis depends primarily on the occupational history of the characteristic symptom pattern in association with exposure to cotton or other natural textile dusts (29). Spirometry documenting a cross-shift decline in $FEV_1$ supports the diagnosis but frequently can be difficult to obtain. Patients with more advanced chronic disease may have evidence of irreversible air flow obstruction.

### Treatment and Prevention

Antihistamines and standard asthma therapy have been used to treat the symptoms and airway obstruction. Attempts should be made to reduce exposures though improved hygiene. Removal should be considered in workers with evidence of progressive symptoms and loss of lung function (29). In the United States, the implementation of the OSHA cotton dust standard and the closure of older mills have reduced dust levels. However, in less developed countries, very dusty conditions still exist.

## Respiratory Effects of Grain Dust

Grain dust is a complex mixture consisting of various grains contaminated with fungi, mites, bacteria, insects, animal matter, endotoxins, various agricultural chemicals such as fungicides and pesticides, and inorganic matter, mainly soil. Acute and chronic respiratory disease in grain workers was first recognized by Ramazzini almost three centuries ago (24). Grain dust exposure can cause acute and chronic respiratory effects including asthma, acute febrile syndromes, hypersensitivity pneumonitis, chronic air flow obstruction, and chronic bronchitis (34). Although it is recognized that grain workers suffer from an excess incidence of acute and chronic respiratory disease, it is not clear what percentage of this excess disease is due to immunologically mediated "grain asthma,"

chronic irritant grain dust bronchitis, hypersensitivity pneumonitis, or chronic obstructive airway changes. Also unclear is which constituent(s) of grain dust are responsible for these acute and chronic effects.

### Risk Factors

Most grain workers who complain of respiratory symptoms do not have a history of atopy, possibly because of the healthy worker effect (35). Grain workers who are atopic are at increased risk of developing grain dust asthma (34). The combined effects of cigarette smoking and grain on lung function are probably additive (34).

### Clinical Effects of Grain Dust Exposure

There are several acute effects of grain dust exposure. *Grain fever* presents similarly to hypersensitivity pneumonitis, but without the chest radiographic changes that are typical of that disease. Acute upper airway symptoms including conjunctivitis, rhinitis, and pharyngitis have been noted to be excessively prevalent among grain workers.

True occupational asthma can develop in grain workers, likely caused by sensitization to any of a number of different allergens present in grain dust (34). Inhalation challenge tests with grain dusts or their extracts have documented classic immediate and/or delayed reactions. Precipitating antibodies and positive skin tests to grain dust extracts and various fungal antigens, as well as cross-shift decrements in lung function, have been found among grain workers. However, these immunologic tests have not been found to regularly correlate with the presence or absence of acute respiratory symptoms.

A number of studies have shown that chronic grain dust exposure is associated with both chronic bronchitic symptoms and reduced lung function (34, 36). Early, the initial decrements in lung function appear to be reversible, but with continued exposure, chronic irreversible changes in lung function can occur. Workers who experience acute respiratory symptoms and airway obstruction in response to grain dust may be at increased risk of developing chronic air flow obstruction (34). Evidence also exists to support a dose-response relationship for exposure to grain dust and annual decline of ventilatory function (36). Limited postmortem pathologic examination of grain dust workers has shown both diffuse emphysematous and fibrotic changes in the lungs.

Patients with grain dust asthma should be evaluated and treated like other patients with occupational asthma. Diagnosis and management of chronic grain dust disease are similar to those for byssinosis.

INHALATION INJURY

## Toxic Lung Injury/Toxic Pneumonitis

Excessive inhalational exposure to a large number of different irritant gases, mists, and fumes may produce inflammation of any portion of the respiratory tract, depending on the dose and duration of exposure and the anatomic level at which the toxin is deposited or absorbed (37). The latter is determined largely by the size of the particles and the solubility of gases in water. Highly soluble gases (such as ammonia) and large particles will affect the conjunctivae, pharynx, larynx, trachea, and major bronchi; small particles and insoluble gases (such as phosgene or nitrogen dioxide) will affect smaller distal airways and alveoli predominantly. Common irritant gases and metals are listed in Tables 14.3 and 14.4.

## Clinical Presentation and Long-Term Effects

Clinical signs appear after variable delays from the time of exposure; latency is shortest for the mucous membranes of the face and becomes progressively longer as one moves distally. Thus the eyes, nose, and throat are likely to become inflamed shortly after exposure, while evidence of pneumonitis may appear hours to days later. Because of variable latency, early results of blood gas analyses, chest radiographs, and lung function tests must be interpreted with caution.

Most patients who survive will recover completely. A chronic bronchitis with fixed or reversible airway obstruction may persist after the injury, usually with gradual improvement over the course of many months. RADS can develop and persist following acute irritant exposures, as discussed above. Progressive interstitial fibrosis and bronchiolitis obliterans are rare sequelae (38, 39).

## Treatment

There is no specific treatment for acute inhalational injury. Support and expectant management are the keys to treatment. Unless cardiorespiratory failure is imminent, emergency attention should proceed from the upper tract downward. Inflamed mucosal surfaces, especially the eyes, should be rinsed first. If hoarseness, stridor, or other signs are present, the vocal cords should be visualized and endotracheal intubation considered. Bronchospasm should be treated with bronchodilators. Pneumonitis, with onset as late as 72 hours after exposure, must be anticipated, especially if bronchospasm is present. Noncardiogenic pulmonary edema due to chemical pneumonitis should be managed in the same manner as other causes of severe pneumonitis and respiratory failure (see Chapter 22).

**TABLE 14.3**
**COMMON IRRITANT GASES AND VAPORS**

| Gas | Water Solubility | Lethality |
|---|---|---|
| Ammonia | High | Low |
| Acetaldehyde | High | Low |
| Chlorine | Medium | Medium |
| Hydrogen fluoride | High | Low |
| Hydrogen sulfide | High | Low |
| Methylisocyanate | (Highly reactive) | High |
| Oxides of nitrogen (NO, $NO_2$, $N_2O_4$) | Low | High |
| Ozone | Low | Low |
| Phosgene | Very low | Very high |
| Sulfur dioxide | High | Low |

## Specific Agents

### Irritant Gases

Common irritant gases are listed in Table 14.3. *Ammonia* is highly water soluble and thus extremely irritating to mucous membranes. Most cases of severe lower respiratory tract injury due to ammonia involve entrapment in confined spaces. *Sulfur dioxide* is generated during a wide range of industrial operations, including refining of petroleum products and paper manufacturing. It is relatively water soluble and causes sufficient upper respiratory tract irritation to warn anyone exposed to a high concentration. *Chlorine*, also widely used, is somewhat less soluble and is associated with a correspondingly increased risk of bronchiolitis or alveolitis. *Nitrogen dioxide*, reddish in color, is liberated whenever nitrogen-containing material is burned; it is also a byproduct of welding, store silage, and mining, as well as numerous chemical operations. It is relatively insoluble, so the risk of parenchymal lung injury is high. Recurrent episodes after exposure have been reported (40).

*Ozone* is is a highly toxic gas normally found in the atmosphere at very low concentrations. It can be generated by welding, and increased amounts are found at high altitude (airplanes) and in urban smog. It can cause substernal burning and transient changes in lung function (decreased $FEV_1$ and increased nonspecific airway responsiveness) but rarely pneumonitis or pulmonary edema. *Phosgene* is a poorly soluble gas originally developed for chemical warfare. It penetrates to the distal lung where it causes parenchymal injury.

### Toxic Metal and Polymer Fumes

Table 14.4 lists irritant metals encountered in industrial environments. *Cadmium* fumes from primary

**TABLE 14.4**
**IRRITANT METALS**

| Metal | Common Source of Exposure | Health Effects |
|---|---|---|
| Beryllium | Alloy production, metal refining | Pneumonitis, CBD |
| Cadmium | Smelting, brazing | Pneumonitis, COPD |
| Chromium | Alloy production | Pneumonitis |
| Mercury | Testing equipment | Pneumonitis |
| Manganese | Mining, welding | Metal fume fever |
| Nickel | Ore extraction, smelting | Asthma, pneumonitis |
| Osmium | Organic chemical manufacturing | Upper airway irritation |
| Vanadium | Chemical industry | Asthma, bronchitis |
| Zinc | Chemical industry | Metal fume fever |

smelting, electroplating, or welding can cause severe lower respiratory tract inflammation (41). Bronchitis and emphysema have been associated with chronic cadmium exposure (42). *Mercury* vapor and beryllium compounds can cause acute pneumonitis, and persistent symptoms can occur. Fumes and dusts of *manganese,* inhaled by welders, have been associated with acute airway and parenchymal lung inflammation.

*Metal Fume Fever*

Fumes of *zinc* and *copper,* generated from smelting, welding, or foundry work, contain fine particles of zinc and copper oxides. Several hours after an intense exposure, a flu-like illness with fever, myalgia, headache, and leukocytosis, called *metal fume fever,* can occur (43). Thirst and a metallic taste may also occur. In contrast to the toxic effects observed with the metals discussed above, chest infiltrates are not seen, and the illness generally runs a benign 24-hour course. "Tolerance" occurs with daily or continuous exposure; workers usually get the "fever" on Mondays after a few days away from exposure. Significant chronic changes in lung function have not been detected.

*Polymer Fume Fever*

Closely related to metal fume fever is *polymer fume fever* from inhalation of pyrolysis products of Teflon (polytetrafluorethylene) (44). Infiltrates do occur but clear spontaneously, along with the fever and constitutional symptoms. Symptoms may persist for weeks but typically resolve completely, although long-term studies have not been performed.

*Smoke Inhalation*

Smoke inhalation injury is common among burn patients, including firefighters. The pulmonary effects of smoke inhalation depend on the magnitude of the exposure and the specific chemical fumes released during combustion. The major components of fire smoke are toxic irritants such as acrolein and hydrogen chloride and chemical asphyxiants such as hydrogen cyanide (Table 14.5). Less commonly, thermal injury from high temperature can also occur, especially with aerosolized liquids (i.e., steam) or particles (i.e., metallic oxides), which have a greater heat capacity than dry air and can cause thermal injury to the lower airways. Fire victims are typically exposed to a number of different toxic inhalants because of the many potentially combustible products present at the site of a fire, such as furniture, plastics, carpets, and polyurethane materials.

*Evaluation and Management of Acute Smoke Inhalation*

Emergency evaluation of excessive smoke inhalation should include standard emergency principles and a careful assessment of risk factors for significant exposure. Initially, all smoke-exposed individuals should receive oxygen and have samples drawn for arterial blood gas and carboxyhemoglobin determinations. Physical examination should include a careful assessment for facial or oropharyngeal burns, wheezing on chest examination, or any neurologic abnormalities. A chest radiograph, ECG, and spirometry or peak flow determination are recommended. Patients with clinically significant smoke exposures need close observation for delayed pulmonary effects, even if initially asymptomatic.

Unless anoxic damage from hypoxemia or carbon monoxide poisoning supervenes, patients who survive smoke inhalation usually recover fully (45). However, as with other acute irritant gas exposures, respiratory symptoms and lung function abnormalities may persist. Permanent sequelae are not common but include interstitial pulmonary fibrosis, nonspecific airway

**TABLE 14.5**
**TOXIC INHALANTS COMMONLY ENCOUNTERED IN FIRES**

Chemical irritants
    Aldehydes (acrolein, formaldehyde)
    Ammonia
    Aromatic hydrocarbons (benzene)
    Hydrogen chloride
    Isocyanates
    Metals (lead, chromium, arsenic)
    Nitrogen dioxide
    Sulfur dioxide
Chemical asphxiants
    Hydrogen cyanide
    Carbon monoxide
    Hydrogen sulfide

hyperresponsiveness, bronchiolitis obliterans, and chronic bronchitis. Whether firefighters are at increased risk of developing chronic air flow obstruction or other nonmalignant respiratory disease is not resolved (46, 47). Individual firefighters can show accelerated loss of lung function, and removal from further exposure may be indicated.

### ACUTE PLEURAL DISEASE

Asbestos exposure can result in transient pleural effusions and, less commonly, recurrent attacks of pleurisy. Asbestos-induced pleural effusions typically are exudative and may be hemorrhagic and/or eosinophilic (48). The diagnosis depends on the history of asbestos exposure, the presence of an effusion, no other cause for the effusion, and no development of malignancy within 3 years of diagnosis. Benign asbestos effusions are frequently asymptomatic and occur with a latency of 10 years or more. They may result in the development of diffuse pleural thickening (see below).

## MAJOR CHRONIC DISEASES

### INTERSTITIAL FIBROSING DISEASES: Overview

Occupational and environmental interstitial lung diseases are a group of heterogeneous lung diseases that diffusely involve the lung parenchyma with varying degrees of chronic alveolitis and fibrosis. The term pneumoconioses has traditionally been defined as the accumulation of dust in the lung and the resulting tissue reaction. Originally used to describe inorganic dust-induced diseases such as asbestosis or silicosis, the term is also used more loosely to describe diseases resulting from the inhalation of other substances that may not accumulate in the lung, such as cobalt. There are a large number of occupational and environmental causes of pulmonary interstitial fibrosis, which are summarized in Tables 14.6 and 14.7.

**TABLE 14.6**
**MORE-COMMON CAUSES OF OCCUPATIONAL INTERSTITIAL LUNG DISEASES**

| |
|---|
| Free silica |
| Silicates |
|    Fibrous—asbestos |
|    Mixed dust |
| Coal |
| Metals |
|    Beryllium |
|    Hard metal (cobalt) |

**TABLE 14.7**
**LESS COMMON CAUSES OF OCCUPATIONAL INTERSTITIAL LUNG DISEASES**

| |
|---|
| Silicates |
|    Talc |
|    Kaolin |
|    Diatomaceous earth |
|    MMVF (?) |
|    Mica |
| Hydrocarbon-containing sedimentary rocks |
|    Graphite |
|    Oil shale |
| Metals |
|    Tin |
|    Aluminum |
|    Antimony |
|    Barium |
|    Iron |
|    Titanium |
| Irritant gases/fumes |
|    Sequela of toxic pneumonitis |
| Plastics |
|    Polyvinyl chloride |
|    Diisocyanates |
| Organic dusts |
|    Bacteria |
|    Fungi |
|    Animal proteins |
| Paraquat |

The fibrogenic potential of inorganic dusts varies considerably, with silica and asbestos having greater fibrogenic potential than coal dust or more benign agents such as iron. Most inorganic dusts, such as coal, asbestos, or silica, require prolonged exposure for at least 6 months, usually many years, at relatively high levels, for significant pulmonary disease to develop. However, disease can occur following shorter, more intense exposures (49). The response to agents such as beryllium or cobalt is much more idiosyncratic, and disease has been reported to occur after much lower exposures (50). The fibrogenic potential of a given exposure depends on various factors including the agent's ability to reach the lower respiratory tract; the dose, durability, and various physical and chemical properties of the agent; and individual host susceptibility factors.

Airway involvement in most pneumoconioses has traditionally been felt to be nonexistent and/or related to smoking. However, certain exposures such as asbestos can result in peribronchial fibrosis and some mild air flow obstruction, and many can cause chronic bronchitis, which may be associated with chronic airways disease (see below).

The overall prevalence of pneumoconioses in the

United States is unknown but varies significantly among different exposed populations. Historically, the most common interstitial lung diseases were due to inhalation of mineral dusts such as silica, asbestos, and coal dust. Worldwide, silicosis remains the most common pneumonoconiosis, and the incidence of pneumoconioses may still be rising in developing countries (51). With improved industrial hygiene and reduced use in the United States, heavy exposure to these dusts has declined. However, several recent reports demonstrate that high levels of exposure still exist, frequently in small uncontrolled workplaces, and can result in miniepidemics of disease (52). Even with overall improved control measures, the prevalence of these diseases remains high in many exposed populations because of the latency between exposure and disease.

Fibrotic lung diseases due to agents that appear to involve immune-mediated mechanisms and which have less clear dose-response relationships, such as beryllium or hard metal, are more difficult to both diagnose and control, as disease may occur at lower exposure levels and in a more sporadic fashion.

### Chest Radiography

The chest radiograph is the most important diagnostic test for occupational fibrotic disorders. It is critical that radiographs of high technical quality be obtained. The chest radiograph can be highly suggestive of a pneumoconiosis and is frequently sufficient, along with an appropriate exposure history, to establish a diagnosis. Chest radiography can be normal in approximately 10 to 20% or more of patients with interstitial lung disease (53).

An international uniform classification system, under the auspices of the International Labour Office (ILO) in Geneva, Switzerland, has evolved to evaluate chest radiographs for epidemiologic studies, clinical evaluation, and screening (54). The system classifies radiographic opacities according to shape, size, extent, and concentration. Pleural changes are also graded according to site, pleural thickening, and pleural calcification.

### Computed Tomography

Much has been written about the role of computed tomography (CT) scanning in the evaluation of patients with occupational interstitial lung disease, primarily asbestosis (55). Conventional CT scanning (8- to 10-mm-thick slices) and high-resolution computed tomographic scanning (HRCT) (1- to 3-mm-thick slices) can be used to better evaluate pleural and parenchymal abnormalities. Conventional CT scanning is more sensitive than chest radiography for the diagnosis of pleural disease. It is most useful for evaluating focal pulmonary masses. In patients with suspected interstitial lung disease but a normal chest radiograph, HRCT may be helpful in identifying parenchymal abnormalities. In most cases in which the diagnosis of an occupational interstitial lung disease is clear on the basis of the chest radiograph and history, CT and HRCT scanning is not indicated.

### Pulmonary Function and Cardiopulmonary Exercise Testing

Resting lung function testing is the most important tool to assess functional respiratory status. As with any interstitial fibrotic disease, physiologic testing in diffuse fibrotic occupational diseases typically shows a restrictive pattern with reduced lung volumes and decreased diffusing capacity (DLCO). Air flow rates and $FEV_1/FVC$ ratio are preserved unless there is coexisting airways disease. The findings on physiologic testing are not specific for a particular etiology, but they are important for evaluating dyspnea and assessing the degree of pulmonary impairment. In a given patient, chest radiographic findings, lung volumes, and DLCO may or may not be correlated in assessing the extent of disease and functional impairment. Patients with more severe disease should be evaluated for hypoxemia at rest and with exertion.

Cardiopulmonary exercise testing is helpful in evaluating a select group of patients with dyspnea and normal pulmonary function tests or dyspnea that appears out of proportion to the changes in lung function, and can help distinguish between cardiac, pulmonary, and deconditioning causes of dyspnea. However, in most patients with occupational interstitial lung disease, exercise testing is not indicated for diagnosis or management.

### Bronchoscopy

Under certain circumstances when the diagnosis is not straightforward, bronchoscopy with transbronchial biopsy and bronchoalveolar lavage (BAL) may be helpful. Transbronchial biopsies yield small tissue samples that may be adequate to diagnose the presence of interstitial fibrosis but usually can not determine specific etiology. They are most helpful in diagnosing granulomatous processes such as beryllium disease or hypersensitivity pneumonitis. Although not routinely performed in many institutions, under certain circumstances BAL can be helpful, such as in the diagnosis of beryllium disease, for which a positive lymphocyte transformation test is diagnostic. Cells obtained from BAL contain dust particles such as asbestos, which may reflect current and possibly past exposures. However, such assays primarily confirm the exposure history and have little clinical utility.

## Lung Biopsy

Although usually not needed diagnostically, open lung biopsy can be helpful when there is no clear cause of interstitial lung disease. To establish a diagnosis, histopathologic changes should be consistent with the known disease, and the suspected causative dusts or particles can, in most cases, be detectable in the lung. A number of methods to analyze dust content of tissue are available including light microscopic evaluation with polarization, bulk analytic techniques such as x-ray fluorescence, and microanalytic techniques such as scanning electron microscopy (56). If a patient with an interstitial lung disease of unclear etiology in whom an occupational or environmental cause is being considered undergoes open lung biopsy, more extensive particle analysis should be considered if light microscopic histologic examination is nondiagnostic. There are some serious limitations that should be remembered. Only particulates that are insoluble, retained in tissue, and at sufficient concentration will be detected. In addition, a positive finding indicates only some degree of exposure, not disease.

## SILICOSIS

Silicosis is a chronic fibrosing disease of the lungs, produced by excessive inhalation of free crystalline silica dust. The ores of most minerals, from coal to gold, are generally found embedded in silica-containing rock in the earth's crust. Mining and quarrying have long been associated with a high incidence of silicosis. Hazardous exposure to silica dust also may occur in a wide variety of other industries such as foundry work, tunneling, sandblasting, pottery making, and the manufacture of glass, tiles, and bricks. Finely ground silica, used in abrasive soaps, polishes, and filters, is especially dangerous.

Silica, or silicon dioxide, can exist unbound to other minerals (free silica) and in either crystalline or amorphous states. *Silicates* are minerals containing silicon dioxide combined with other elements, such as talc, asbestos, mica, or kaolin. Inhalational exposure to most silica-containing minerals has been associated with some risk of pneumoconiosis. However, free crystalline silica dust is more likely to cause pulmonary fibrosis than either amorphous silica or nonasbestiform silicates.

### Pathogenesis and Histologic Features

Respirable-sized silica particles deposited in the distal airways are readily ingested by scavenging alveolar macrophages or penetrate the interstitium. The alveolar macrophages become activated, can release a number of inflammatory mediators that initiate and perpetuate the processes of inflammation and fibrosis, and then may undergo cell death. Neutrophils, T lymphocytes, and other inflammatory cells probably contribute to the inflammatory and fibrotic processes, eventually resulting in the silicotic nodule (57).

Three types of silicosis have been described: (*a*) ordinary or simple chronic silicosis, in which exposure to relatively low concentrations of free silica dust has continued for 20 years or more; (*b*) accelerated silicosis, in which exposure to moderately high dust concentrations occurs, usually over a shorter period of time (4 to 8 years); and (*c*) acute silicosis, in which there is massive exposure to high concentrations of dust (58). These distinctions are important as far as clinical outcome is concerned.

Simple silicosis is characterized by the formation of silicotic nodules in the pulmonary parenchyma and the hilar lymph nodes. Particles of free silica may be demonstrated in the nodules by their birefringence under polarized light. Simple silicosis may be complicated by the development of progressive massive fibrosis (PMF). The lesions of PMF tend to be found in the upper lung zones and are composed of confluent nodules, often with obliterated blood vessels and bronchioles as well. With accelerated silicosis, the rate of progression is more rapid, and PMF occurs more frequently.

Acute silicosis is a relatively rare condition occurring only in workers exposed to very high concentrations of fine, particulate free silica dust without adequate ventilation or personal protective equipment. Unlike the situation in chronic silicosis, the lungs show consolidation without silicotic nodules, and the alveolar spaces are filled with fluid similar to that found in pulmonary alveolar proteinosis (59).

### Clinical Presentation

Silicosis is most commonly a chronic disease with a long latency. The most common form of silicosis is uncomplicated simple silicosis, which is usually asymptomatic and is diagnosed on the basis of chest radiographic findings. Pulmonary function testing in patients with simple silicosis can be normal or demonstrate abnormalities consistent with mild ventilatory restriction (60). A mild obstructive impairment is frequently found in patients with simple silicosis, presumably due to chronic bronchitis caused by silica or other dust and/or smoking (61).

Significant dyspnea on exertion generally is seen only with patients who have complicated disease characterized by PMF. Complicated silicosis is associated with reduced lung volumes and diffusing capacity, and arterial oxygen desaturation with exercise. Nodular lesions greater than 1 cm in diameter are seen on chest radiography and can become confluent and retract the hila upward. Constitutional symptoms such as malaise, anorexia, and weight loss can occur with complicated disease, as can respiratory failure.

The major features of accelerated silicosis are similar to those of complicated chronic silicosis, but the course of the disease is abbreviated, and there is a greater likelihood that significant disability will develop. Patients with acute silicosis present with marked dyspnea, fever, cough, and weight loss. There usually is rapid progression to respiratory failure.

### Diagnosis

The diagnosis of silicosis is based on (*a*) a history of sufficient silica exposure, (*b*) chest radiographic abnormalities consistent with silicosis, and (*c*) absence of other illnesses that mimic silicosis. Silica exposure occurs in a number of occupational settings, and the history of exposure may not always be obvious. The presence of diffuse nodular opacities on the chest radiograph of an individual known to have sustained prolonged exposure to silica is usually sufficient (Fig. 14.3). Calcification of hilar lymph nodes and a classic

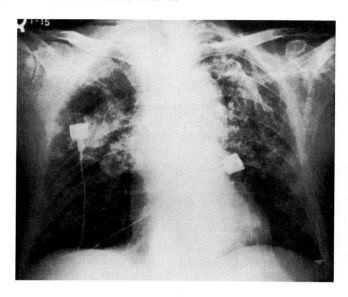

**FIGURE 14.4.**   Eggshell calcification of hilar lymph nodes.

"eggshell" pattern is not a consistent finding in silicosis, but when it is seen in patients with diffuse nodular lung disease, it generally excludes other diagnoses (Fig. 14.4). Histologic evaluation is usually not necessary.

### Associated Illnesses

Patients with silicosis have an increased risk of mycobacterial infection (involving atypical mycobacterial organisms as well as *Mycobacterium tuberculosis*) (62, 63). The decreased resistance of the silicotic lung to mycobacterial infection appears to be due in large measure to impaired macrophage function. Tuberculosis should be suspected in any patient with silicosis whose symptoms or chest radiograph change more acutely.

Various connective tissue disorders, particularly scleroderma, have been noted to occur with greater frequency in patients with silicosis (64). Caplan's syndrome (rheumatoid arthritis and large lung nodules) occurs with silicosis as well as with coal workers' pneumoconiosis. There is an increased prevalence of circulating autoantibodies, such as antinuclear antibody and rheumatoid factor, among silicotic patients. Patients with silicosis may be at increased risk of developing lung cancer (discussed below).

### Treatment

There is no specific treatment for silicosis except removal from further exposure, which may not affect progression of the disease. Supportive therapy with the aim of preventing debilitating complications such as tuberculosis can be offered. Patients with silicosis

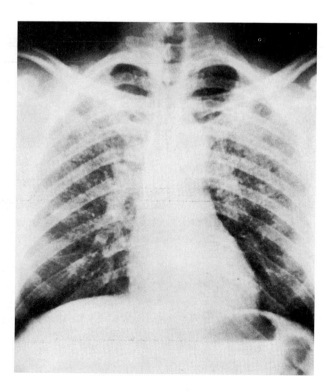

**FIGURE 14.3.**   Typical simple silicosis with diffuse, bilateral nodular densities.

should have annual screening for mycobacterial infection, i.e., PPD skin testing. At least 1 year of isoniazid therapy is recommended for patients with positive PPD tests without clinical evidence of active tuberculosis. Because of the decreased responsiveness of silicotuberculosis to chemotherapy, multidrug regimens are recommended (58). Different durations of therapy have been recommended, but generally longer durations than with tuberculosis alone (62). Establishing the diagnosis of tuberculosis in a patient with silicosis can be challenging; a high index of suspicion remains important. Tuberculosis should be suspected if any rapid changes occur on the chest radiograph. When tuberculosis is superimposed on complicated silicosis, there may be no obvious radiographic change at all. The use of induced sputum and fiberoptic bronchoscopy to obtain specimens for acid-fast staining and mycobacterial culture may increase the diagnostic yield.

The treatment of associated bronchitis is similar to that offered to any patient with chronic bronchitis (see Chapter 10). Bronchodilator therapy can be effective for patients in whom a reversible obstructive component is present. The cessation of cigarette smoking is of obvious importance. Whole-lung lavage has been reported to be helpful in patients with acute silicosis presenting with a clinicopathologic picture consistent with pulmonary alveolar proteinosis (65).

## NONMALIGNANT ASBESTOS-RELATED PULMONARY DISEASE

Asbestos is the generic name for a group of naturally occurring fibrous silicates. There are three main commercial types of asbestos. Chrysotile (serpentine) accounts for over 70% of the asbestos fiber consumed in the United States; much of the chrysotile used here is mined in Canada, but the former Soviet Union is the world leader in chrysotile production. Crocidolite (amphibole) and amosite (amphibole) are mined primarily in South Africa. Asbestos may cause several different types of disease involving the lungs and pleura and may also increase the risk of extrapulmonary neoplasms such as colon cancer. *Asbestosis* is a term that should be reserved for the diffuse interstitial pulmonary fibrosis caused by asbestos exposure.

### Epidemiology

Although asbestos has been valued since antiquity because of its resistance to fire, only during the last century has its mining and commercial use been extensive. Not until the 1930s did the magnitude of the asbestos hazard begin to be recognized. One reason for the delayed appreciation of the fibrogenic potential of asbestos is that there is a considerable latency period

between the initial exposure and the onset of clinical manifestations, often 20 to 30 years. It is estimated that up to 19 million U.S. workers have been significantly exposed to asbestos dust since 1940 and are at increased risk for asbestos-related disease (66). Use of asbestos in the United States has declined since the mid-1970s, but worldwide use continues to rise.

Workers with potentially significant asbestos exposure include asbestos miners and millers; many persons employed in the building trades and shipyards, such as insulation workers, pipefitters, sheet metal workers, welders, asbestos removal workers; and workers involved in the manufacture or repair of automotive friction products. While exposure to small amounts of asbestos fiber may contribute to the risk of malignancy, it is not generally associated with clinically significant, nonmalignant, asbestos-related pulmonary disease.

### Asbestos-Related Pleural Disease

Asbestos exposure can cause discrete pleural thickening (pleural plaques), diffuse pleural thickening, rounded atelectasis, and benign exudative effusions (discussed above). All types of asbestos have the potential to induce asbestos-related pleural disease.

#### Pleural Thickening

Circumscribed areas of pleural thickening, called pleural plaques, are the most common radiographic findings due to chronic asbestos exposure and most commonly occur without asbestosis. Individuals with isolated pleural plaques are usually asymptomatic. Pathologically, plaques usually involve the parietal pleural surface, are composed mostly of collagen, and are accompanied by an inflammatory reaction. Pleural plaques may become calcified. They have a latency of about 15 to 20 years following first exposure. Pleural plaques most often are visible on the PA chest radiograph along the lower lateral borders of the thoracic cavity and the central portions of the hemidiaphragms. Although there are other causes of unilateral pleural thickening and calcification (empyema, hemothorax, and thoracic trauma), the presence of bilateral pleural thickening is almost always due to asbestos exposure. Traditionally, it has been taught that circumscribed plaques, in the absence of parenchymal asbestosis, are not associated with respiratory impairment. However, there is evidence that workers with radiographic evidence of plaques but no asbestosis can have mildly reduced lung volumes (67).

Diffuse pleural thickening, involving visceral as well as parietal pleura, is less common than circumscribed plaques but is more likely to be associated with mildly reduced lung volumes and interstitial changes on HRCT (68, 69). Diffuse pleural thickening is believed to be a sequela of benign asbestos pleural effusions. Chest CT scanning provides the most sensitive and specific technique for identifying pleural plaques and diffuse pleural thickening. However, CT scanning is not required for routine clinical evaluation.

Whether asbestos-related pleural disease independent of exposure dose is a risk factor for lung cancer is an area of debate (70, 71). Progression to advanced asbestosis is not common. There is no evidence that pleural plaques undergo malignant transformation to mesothelioma.

### Rounded Atelectasis

Localized fibrosis of the pleura involving the visceral as well as the parietal surfaces can entrap the adjacent lung parenchyma and mimic the radiographic appearance of a solitary pulmonary nodule. This phenomenon, known as rounded atelectasis, occurs with asbestos-related pleural disease (72). Rounded atelectasis may be recognized radiographically by an irregular shadow that tapers toward the hilum, the so-called comet tail sign, and can usually be differentiated from a more serious mass lesion by use of CT scanning.

## Asbestosis

### Histologic Features and Pathogenesis

The light microscopic appearance of the pulmonary parenchyma in the early stages of asbestosis is similar to that seen with idiopathic interstitial pneumonitis. A mixed leukocyte infiltration of the interstitial spaces, accompanied by varying degrees of organizing fibrosis, is typically present. The initial areas of inflammation in asbestosis appear to center around the respiratory bronchioles. Peribronchial fibrosis may explain the observation of mild airways obstruction in nonsmoking workers exposed to asbestos dust.

Similar to silica, inhaled asbestos is phagocytosed by alveolar macrophages that become activated. Both asbestos and silica can generate reactive oxygen species such as superoxide anion, which can result in cell injury and altered function. Unlike silica, asbestos fibers generally are not cytotoxic to the macrophage. Activated macrophages release various cytokines and other inflammatory mediators that can directly injure the lung parenchyma or recruit additional inflammatory and mesenchymal cells, resulting in an alveolitis and fibrosis rather than normal healing. All major types of asbestos are fibrogenic, although some studies have provided support for the concept that it is the long, thin asbestos fibers that have the greatest fibrogenic potential.

## Clinical Presentation, Evaluation, and Diagnosis

The clinical presentation is indistinguishable from that of other forms of interstitial pulmonary fibrosis. The most common symptom in those with asbestosis is progressive dyspnea, usually over a period of years. Cough, either nonproductive or productive, is common. The physical examination findings are nonspecific; for example, bibasilar crackles and clubbing of the fingers can occur. Signs of pulmonary hypertension and cor pulmonale may be seen in advanced cases.

The diagnosis of asbestosis is based on a history of sufficient asbestos exposure with appropriate latency, and certain clinical, radiographic, and pulmonary function findings, not all of which may be present in a particular situation. The American Thoracic Society (ATS) has attempted to develop criteria for the diagnosis of asbestosis (73). A panel of ATS experts concluded that for the diagnosis of asbestosis to be made in the absence of pathologic examination of lung tissue (i.e., the usual situation), it is necessary that there be (*a*) a reliable history of exposure and (*b*) an appropriate time interval between exposure and detection (typically >15 years). The panel also regarded the following clinical criteria to be of recognized value: (*a*) chest radiographic evidence of small, irregular opacities; (*b*) a restrictive pattern of lung impairment with the forced vital capacity below the lower limit of normal; (*c*) a diffusing capacity below the lower limit of normal; and (*d*) bilateral late or pan-inspiratory crackles at the posterior lung bases not cleared with cough. Of these clinical criteria, the chest radiographic evidence is the most important. There is some controversy about what degree of profusion of small, irregular opacities is required. The certainty of the diagnosis of asbestosis increases as more of the criteria are met.

The occupational history of asbestos exposure is critical to the diagnosis of asbestosis. The onset, duration, and intensity of exposure are important to determine. There is a characteristic latency of 15 or more years between first exposure and disease manifestation. Exposure durations of less than 6 months rarely, but can result in asbestosis. The intensity of asbestos exposure can be determined by information on the job, industry, and use of personal protective equipment. Overall, exposures since the mid-1970s have been much reduced, although there are exceptions.

### Radiography

Chest radiograph and determination of lung volumes and diffusing capacity are usually sufficient to make a diagnosis of asbestosis once a history of occupational exposure is obtained. The characteristic chest

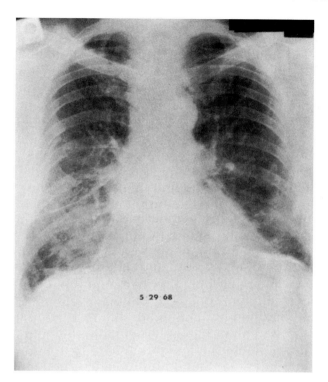

**FIGURE 14.5.** Typical asbestosis with "shaggy heart" and pleural plaques with diaphragm calcification.

radiograph shows irregular or linear opacities distributed throughout the lung fields but more prominent in the lower zones (Fig. 14.5). There can be loss of definition, or "shagginess," of the heart border. The most useful finding in the differential diagnosis of asbestosis is the presence of pleural thickening (Fig. 14.5). Diaphragmatic or pericardial calcification is almost a pathognomonic sign of asbestos exposure. However, asbestosis can occur without any visible pleural changes on chest radiography.

Histologic fibrosis can occur with a normal appearing chest radiograph. HRCT is more sensitive than either plain chest radiographs or conventional CT for the detection of parenchymal abnormalities (55). However, in most cases when the diagnosis is clear on the basis of the chest radiograph and history, HRCT is not necessary for either the diagnosis or the management of such patients.

*Pulmonary Function*

Pulmonary function abnormalities usually indicate the presence of a restrictive ventilatory defect with decreased lung volumes, decreased lung compliance, and decreased exercise tolerance. More-recent studies suggest that asbestos, in the absence of cigarette smoking, can result in a mild degree of air flow obstruction (74).

Although in population studies there is a correlation between pulmonary function and radiographic severity of asbestosis, in individual cases such correlation may not be present. The presence of a marked obstructive ventilatory defect usually indicates the influence of other factors, notably cigarette smoking. Because asbestosis and chronic air flow obstruction exert opposite effects on total lung capacity, the total lung capacity is an insensitive measure of impairment in patients with both asbestosis and obstructive airways disease (75).

*Other Tests*

Patients with asbestosis may have abnormal gallium uptake. However, such findings are not particularly sensitive or specific, and gallium scanning is not recommended in the evaluation of patients with asbestosis. Bronchoscopy and open lung biopsy are rarely indicated. Increased amounts of fibronectin and increased numbers of inflammatory cells (lymphoyctes, neutrophils) on BAL have been associated with reduced lung function (76, 77). However, the clinical utility of such findings is unclear. The presence of numerous asbestos bodies in a biopsy specimen confirms the exposure history and suggests that the pulmonary fibrosis seen is related to asbestos exposure (Fig. 14.6). However, asbestos bodies may also be found in lung tissue from individuals without significant histories of exposure (56). Fiber types other than asbestos may become coated with similar iron-containing material, hence the generic term *ferruginous body* has been coined. Analytic techniques can identify and quantify the specific type of fiber for research purposes but have little clinical utility.

*Prognosis and Treatment*

The natural history of patients with asbestosis is variable. Marked accelerated loss of pulmonary function can occur, but more stable disease with minimal or mild progression is more common (78). The risks that parenchymal scarring will develop and progress appear to increase with cumulative asbestos exposure (79). Progression of disease can occur following removal from exposure. A major concern is the increased risk of lung cancer, which is discussed below. In addition to its synergistic effects on lung cancer, it is possible cigarette smoking may also act to increase the fibrotic response to inhaled asbestos. Smoking cessation for active smokers is crucial.

Further asbestos exposure should be minimized. Steroids probably have little beneficial effect on the course of the disease, although no controlled trials have been reported in the literature. Appropriate therapy of superimposed respiratory tract infections is important, although it is not clear that patients with asbestosis are more susceptible to such infection.

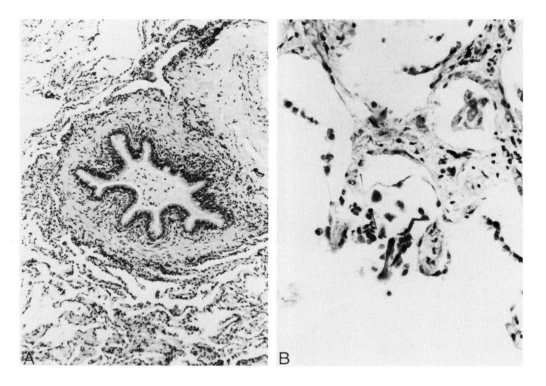

**FIGURE 14.6.** **A,** Lung biopsy from a patient with asbestos showing peribronchiolar fibrosis.
**B,** Intraalveolar asbestos bodies.

Bronchodilator therapy is indicated if there is evidence of a reversible obstructive component. Although there is no evidence that ongoing medical surveillance with annual chest radiography and spirometry is beneficial, such surveillance is commonly recommended.

## COAL WORKERS' PNEUMOCONIOSIS

Two different respiratory diseases can develop from the chronic excessive inhalation of coal dust: coal workers' pneumoconiosis (CWP) and chronic bronchitis. Chronic bronchitis secondary to mineral dust is treated in a separate section of this chapter, but it should be mentioned that this problem is more common among coal workers than CWP (80).

CWP occurs in either simple or complicated forms. Only a small percentage of miners with simple CWP ever develop complicated disease (81). The chest radiographic pattern of simple CWP is typically one of small nodular opacities. The opacities visible on chest radiographs of simple CWP are due to the presence of coal macules in the lungs. The diagnosis of complicated CWP is made when larger opacities (1 cm or larger in diameter) are seen on chest radiograph (Fig. 14.7). These large opacities represent masses of confluent fi-

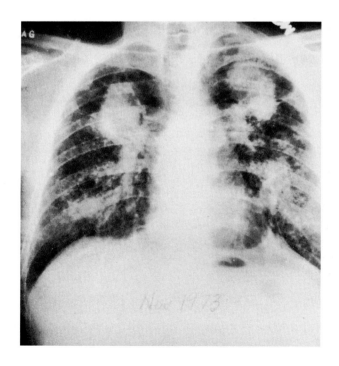

**FIGURE 14.7.** Coal workers' pneumoconiosis with progressive massive fibrosis.

brous tissue and may undergo cavitation secondary to either ischemic necrosis or superimposed tuberculous infection.

## History and Epidemiology

Pneumoconiosis was associated with coal mining in Great Britain early in the nineteenth century. The problem of respiratory disease in coal miners was given scant attention in the United States until the 1960s (80). Since 1969, there have been extensive efforts by the National Institute for Occupational Safety and Health (NIOSH) at surveillance of respiratory disease among coal miners. The popularization of the term *black lung disease* stems from the long-lasting struggle of coal miners in this country for public awareness of the serious respiratory health hazards involved in their work.

The prevalence of CWP varies from region to region within the United States, depending on the type of coal mined (anthracite being more hazardous than bituminous) and the method of mining (underground being more hazardous than open-strip). Since a heavy dust load usually is required to cause disease, CWP is seen more frequently among miners involved with work at the coal face. It is unusual to see significant pneumoconiosis in miners who have spent less than 20 years underground. Bronchitic symptoms from inhalation of coal dust are common among miners.

## Pathology and Pathogenesis

The initial response to the inhalation of coal dust into the terminal respiratory units involves phagocytosis of the deposited dust by alveolar macrophages. Coal appears to be less fibrogenic than asbestos or silica, but similar to these exposures, coal dust can result in increased oxidant production and macrophage activation. Dust-laden macrophages are generally able to reach the terminal bronchiole and be removed from the lung by the mucociliary clearance mechanism. When exposure is particularly heavy, this first-line defense is overwhelmed and significant retention of coal dust in the terminal respiratory units occurs. Lung fibroblasts can secrete a limiting layer of reticulin around the dust collection. Centrilobular emphysema may occur as the respiratory bronchioles in and immediately around the area of dust collection become destroyed or distorted (82). The coal macule, the basic pathologic lesion of CWP, appears to form in this manner. In contrast to the silicotic nodule described previously, the coal macule consists more of dust than of inflammatory reaction. The factors that determine whether simple CWP progresses to complicated CWP are not well understood. The presence of silica in the retained dust and superimposed tuberculous infection can stimulate fibrosis. However, cases of complicated CWP can occur in the absence of either of these factors.

## Clinical Evaluation and Diagnosis

Simple CWP is usually a relatively benign process unless superimposed pulmonary infections or other concomitant disease is present. Respiratory symptoms of cough and dyspnea are common among coal miners in general and may be present in a given individual miner regardless of whether the chest radiograph shows pneumoconiosis. Complicated disease is uncommon. Once the process of complicated disease begins, however, it generally results in PMF, even if there is no further exposure to coal dust. Miners with PMF are usually dyspneic to the point of being disabled. Pulmonary hypertension and cor pulmonale may be late sequelae.

The results of pulmonary function testing vary with the stage of CWP. With simple CWP, there are usually no gross abnormalities. However, small but statistically significant reductions in lung function in coal miners (compared with control populations) have been documented in several large epidemiologic studies (80, 83). Decline in $FEV_1$ and the presence of irregular opacities have been correlated with cumulative dust exposure (84). Miners with complicated CWP can have obstructive, restrictive, or mixed ventilatory defects. There is an increased prevalence of autoantibodies in the serum of miners with CWP, usually without clinical manifestation of collagen-vascular disease (85). Caplan's syndrome was first described in conjunction with CWP.

A diagnosis of CWP can usually be made on the basis of the exposure history and characteristic chest radiograph findings. A lung biopsy is rarely needed. Miners with CWP or bronchitis should try to minimize further mining exposures but do not necessarily have to leave mining, depending on the extent of their disease. Bronchospasm should be treated with standard bronchodilator therapy. For miners who smoke, smoking cessation should be strongly recommended.

### BERYLLIUM- AND HARD METAL–RELATED DISEASE

Beryllium and cobalt are both metals that may cause interstitial lung disease, probably through immunologically mediated mechanisms. Although more is known about the pathogenesis of chronic beryllium disease than about hard metal (cobalt)–related lung disease, these diseases share several features in common: only a fraction of exposed workers appear to be susceptible; disease can occur at relatively low exposure levels, compared with those necessary to cause traditional pneumoconioses such as asbestosis; and the exposure history is frequently less obvious than with exposures such as asbestos or coal dust. Thus, both the diagnosis and prevention of beryllium- and hard metal–related disease can be more challenging than with the traditional pneumoconioses.

## Chronic Beryllium Disease

Chronic beryllium disease (CBD) is a chronic pulmonary and systemic granulomatous disease that is similar to sarcoid but is caused by chronic beryllium exposure. Acute high beryllium exposures can cause an acute pneumonitis, which is not commonly seen.

### Epidemiology

Chronic granulomatous lung disease and systemic illness was first recognized in the United States among employees frosting fluorescent light bulbs with beryllium oxide (BeO) during World War II (86). As beryllium use has increased in aerospace, electronics, and other high technology industries, cases have become more widely dispersed. The reported prevalence of CBD in exposed workers is low, around 5% in most settings, but can be higher (87–89). As exposure is decreased, the incidence, but not necessarily the severity, appears to decrease. Cases of CBD from a metal refinery where exposures may have been below OSHA standards have been reported (50). Beryllium is usually present as an alloy with other metals such as copper, aluminum, and nickel, and workers may not be aware of beryllium exposure.

### Pathogenesis and Pathology

Noncaseating granulomas identical to those seen in sarcoidosis are the pathologic hallmark of CBD (Fig. 14.8). Although predominantly seen in the lung, these granulomas can be found in numerous peripheral sites such as the liver and skin. CBD is believed to be a disorder of cell-mediated immunity, a beryllium-specific delayed-type hypersensitivity reaction. This is supported by a number of findings, including lung and lymph node histology similar to that of other cell-mediated disorders, the presence of delayed hypersensitivity to beryllium salts, and animal models characterized by antigen-specific T-lymphocyte sensitization to beryllium (90, 91). Beryllium can be phagocytosed by macrophages that present beryllium antigen to lymphocytes, resulting in sensitization and proliferation of beryllium-specific CD4+ T cells. Beryllium-activated T cells may release various cytokines and other inflammatory mediators, resulting in granuloma formation.

Why only a small percentage of an exposed population becomes sensitized to beryllium is not well understood. A recent study has found a genetic marker that is an inherited risk factor for CBD (92). Ninety-seven percent of CBD cases expressed a certain MHC allele, HLA-DP$\beta$1, whereas only 30% of controls expressed this allele (92, 93). However, although almost every patient with CBD has this genetic marker, many beryllium-exposed people with this marker do not get the disease.

### Clinical Evaluation/Diagnosis

The most common symptom with CBD is progressive exertional dyspnea. The latency between exposure and manifestations of disease is more variable than with traditional pneumoconioses and can range from months to over 20 years. Nonproductive cough and systemic complaints such as fatigue or weight loss are common.

Chest radiographs typically show diffuse interstitial infiltrates, and bilateral hilar adenopathy in less than half the cases. Obstructive, restrictive, or mixed restrictive-obstructive patterns are seen on pulmonary function testing.

The Beryllium Case Registry established the following diagnostic criteria for CBD: (*a*) evidence of significant beryllium exposure; (*b*) presence of beryllium in lung or urine; (*c*) clinical picture consistent with CBD; (*d*) radiographic evidence of a pulmonary interstitial process; (*e*) abnormal pulmonary function testing; and (*f*) noncaseating granulomas in lung or lymph node (94). Four of these six criteria, including one of the first two, must be met for the Beryllium Case Registry (94). Newman and coworkers have proposed the following diagnostic criteria: (*a*) history of beryllium exposure; (*b*) beryllium-specific hypersensitivity (positive lymphocyte transformation test using peripheral blood or BAL lymphocytes); (*c*) consistent lung histopathology;

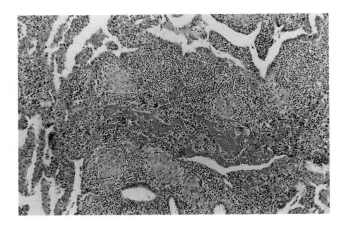

**FIGURE 14.8.** Lung biopsy from a patient with chronic beryllium disease showing lymphocytic alveolitis and noncaseating granulomas (hematoxylin and eosin).

and (*d*) clinical presentation including either respiratory symptoms, interstitial changes on chest radiograph, or restrictive and/or obstructive defects on pulmonary function testing (91).

The history of beryllium exposure can be difficult to obtain, as beryllium is frequently present as an alloy with other metals. Furthermore, because of the latency between exposure and clinical presentation, the relevant exposure history may be a job years in the past. A history of CBD in coworkers is very helpful in documenting exposure. Beryllium exposure can also be documented by measuring beryllium in tissues (especially in lung and lymph nodes) or in urine. Elevated tissue levels reflect body burden rather than recent exposure, and they document exposure, not disease. Adequate amounts of lung tissue for beryllium analysis can usually only be obtained from open lung biopsy, not from transbronchial biopsy. Urinary excretion of beryllium can be determined but usually indicates ongoing, rather than past, exposure.

Beryllium hypersensitivity can be documented by demonstrating the proliferation of either peripheral blood lymphocytes or lymphocytes obtained from BAL in response to beryllium salts in vitro (i.e., a positive lymphocyte transformation test). The test is more sensitive when performed on BAL lymphocytes (close to 100% sensitivity) than on peripheral blood lymphocytes (60–95%) (95, 96). The peripheral blood lymphocyte transformation test has been used to detect preclinical disease and to screen exposed workers for beryllium sensitization and early disease (91). The beryllium patch test is not recommended because it can cause hypersensitivity and exacerbate existing disease.

Clinically CBD can be difficult to distinguish from sarcoidosis. The presence of uveitis, erythema nodosum, a positive Kveim test, and asymptomatic hilar adenopathy favor a diagnosis of sarcoidosis; a history of beryllium exposure and evidence of beryllium hypersensitivity strongly support the diagnosis of CBD.

Although beryllium is the primary environmental cause of granulomatous lung disease, aluminum and titanium have been reported to induce pulmonary granulomatous reactions associated with specific T-lymphocyte sensitization (97, 98).

### Prognosis and Treatment

The natural history and prognosis with CBD can be quite variable and difficult to predict. CBD can progress to advanced, irreversible disease, even in the absence of ongoing exposure (90). Spontaneous improvement after removal from further exposure can also occur, and patients may respond to corticosteroids (90, 91). Earlier milder disease may be more reversible.

Patients with symptomatic CBD should be removed from further exposure, which may lead to improvement. Therapy follows the principles for sarcoidosis, including a trial of systemic steroids for symptomatic disease.

### Hard Metal Disease

Exposure to hard metal, a cemented alloy of tungsten carbide with cobalt, can result in interstitial pulmonary fibrosis and/or asthma (99). Cobalt is probably the etiologic agent for both processes. Cobalt dust has been shown experimentally to cause acute alveolitis, fibrosis, and bronchitis, while tungsten carbide without cobalt appears to be nontoxic (99). Positive responses to inhalational challenge with cobalt but not with tungsten also have been demonstrated among workers with occupational asthma (100). Furthermore, diamond workers exposed to cobalt without any tungsten carbide have developed an interstitial disease histologically identical to hard metal disease, as well as specific airway sensitization to cobalt (101, 102).

### Epidemiology and Pathogenesis

Exposure to cobalt is not uncommon and can occur during production or use of hard metal tools, and in industries such as diamond polishing. However, the reported prevalence of interstitial disease in exposed workers is relatively low, ranging from less than 1% (most studies) to 12.8% (99, 103). Cobalt-induced asthma is probably more common, around 5 to 10%. Although usually occurring separately, cobalt-induced interstitial lung disease and and asthma can occur in the same patient.

The histologic finding is a fibrosing alveolitis, with characteristic multinucleated giant cells consisting of macrophages and alveolar epithelial cells. Multinucleated macrophages can be seen on BAL but can be a nonspecific finding.

### Clinical Presentation, Diagnosis, and Management

Cobalt-exposed workers can present with symptoms of occupational asthma, slowly progressive interstitial lung disease, or rapidly progressive interstitial pneumonitis. Severe respiratory insufficiency can occur. The latency from exposure to onset of hard metal disease is variable, from a few to over 20 years. Chest radiographs in patients with hard metal disease typically demonstrate a diffuse reticulonodular pattern that tends to be more prominent in the mid and lower lung fields. Most commonly restrictive, but also obstructive or mixed, defects can be seen on pulmonary function testing.

A high level of suspicion and a careful occupational

history are key to the diagnosis of hard metal disease. An open lung biopsy is not uncommon. The characteristic lung pathology showing multinucleated giant cells is helpful. The detection of tungsten on lung biopsy confirms exposure. Cobalt, because it is more soluble than tungsten, is usually not detected. Cobalt in the blood and urine indicates current or recent exposure.

Hard metal disease can progress after removal from exposure. Removal from further exposure, steroids, and bronchodilator therapy if air flow obstruction is present are the mainstay of therapy.

## Other Pneumoconioses

A number of other silicates, dusts, and metals that are less common causes of pneumoconioses are listed in Table 14.7. Several of these are discussed below.

### Talcosis

Talc is a hydrated magnesium silicate that is chemically related to asbestos. Since asbestos and silica are found in conjunction with talc, there is some uncertainty about the magnitude of the fibrogenic potential of pure talc.

Pulmonary fibrosis can occur after many years of exposure to high concentrations of talc dust, usually in the course of mining soapstone. Significant talc exposure also can occur during the manufacture of ceramics, roofing materials, and rubber goods. Cases of talcosis have been reported to result from heavy exposure to commercial talcum powder (104). Pulmonary

**TABLE 14.8**
**Partial List of Agents That Cause Chronic Bronchitis**

Minerals
  Coal
  Oil mist
  Silica
  Silicates
  MMVF
Metals
  Welding fumes
Organic substances
  Cotton
  Grain
  Wood
Irritant gases
  Sulfur dioxide
  Chlorine
  Nitrogen dioxide
Smoke (firefighters)

fibrosis also may result from a microembolization process secondary to the intravenous injection of talc-containing pills by drug abusers (105). Pathologically, lesions similar to those of silicosis and asbestosis as well as foreign-body granulomas containing talc particles may be seen.

The clinical presentation is one of progressive dyspnea and productive cough. The initial chest radiographic appearance of talcosis is similar to that of asbestosis: the upper lung zones tend to be relatively spared, and mild pleural thickening and calcification may occur. However, talcosis may progress in a manner similar to that of silicosis with regard to the coalescence of lesions and the ultimate development of PMF. Studies of pulmonary function in patients with talcosis have demonstrated decreases in both lung volumes and diffusing capacity (106).

### Kaolin Pneumoconiosis

Kaolin, also called China clay, is a hydrated aluminum silicate used in the manufacture of ceramics, paint, paper, and cement. Epidemiologic studies are somewhat conflicting, but it appears that radiographic changes due to excessive kaolin dust exposure (diffuse nodular opacities) are more prominent than clinical manifestations of disease. However, cases of kaolin-associated PMF have been reported (107).

### Other Silicates

*Fuller's earth* (attapulgite) is an absorbent aluminum silicate clay now used primarily in oil refining and in the building of foundry molds. While massive fibrosis can occur, the pneumoconiosis associated with Fuller's earth generally runs a relatively benign course (108).

*Micas* are a group of complex aluminum silicates that have been associated with the development of interstitial pulmonary fibrosis in heavily exposed workers (109). Mica also has been associated with pleural thickening. It is unclear whether these findings may be due to contamination with silica or asbestos (110).

*Mixed-dust pneumoconiosis* refers to lung disease seen in workers exposed to crystalline silica and other dusts such as coal or iron oxides. The disease is similar to silicosis, the amount of fibrosis depending on the amount of free silica exposure.

### Manmade Vitreous Fibers

A variety of synthetic silicate mineral fibers (manmade vitreous fibers, MMVFs) have increasingly been used in substitution for asbestos. There are several types of MMVFs: mineral (slag or rock) wools, glass fibers, and ceramic fibers. Most common are mineral wools and glass fiber, which can cause skin and respiratory tract irritation and bronchitis but have not been shown to cause a pneumoconiosis. There is concern that the less common ceramic fibers may be more fibrogenic and carcinogenic, based on animal data and fiber shape (111). A possible relationship between pleural plaques and ceramic fiber exposure has been noted in a small number of workers (112). In view of the massive substitution of fiberglass for asbestos in insulation materials, it is understandable that there is concern about the long-term health risks of exposure to MMVF. Thus far, epidemiologic studies in populations exposed to MMVF have not revealed any evidence that symptomatic pneumoconiosis is a consequence of such exposure, although there may not yet be adequate followup time to entirely exclude the possibility (111, 113). The carcinogenic potential will be discussed below.

## Graphite Pneumoconiosis

Graphite is pure crystallized carbon, but most natural deposits are contaminated with some free silica. Graphite is used in the manufacture of steel, pencils, electrical equipment, and in the printing industry. Excessive carbon dust exposure may lead to chest radiographic changes identical to those of simple CWP, and concomitant silica exposure has been implicated as the cause for the more severe pulmonary fibrosis occasionally seen in graphite-exposed workers (114). However, PMF has been reported in carbon electrode workers who were not exposed to silica dust (115).

## Aluminum Pneumoconiosis

Aluminum is produced from bauxite, a naturally occurring hydrous aluminum oxide ore. Pulmonary fibrosis has been reported in workers exposed to aluminum oxide dust and fumes. This condition, known as Shaver's disease, typically presents as progressive dyspnea (116), and has been attributed to free silica contamination. However, exposure to aluminum powder that does not contain silica can result in pulmonary fibrosis and is associated with an increased incidence of spontaneous pneumothorax (117). The pathologic features of this uncommon pneumoconiosis are interstitial fibrosis, initially in the upper lobes, and emphysematous bleb formation on pleural surfaces. The aluminum content in the lung is greatly increased. Pulmonary function testing reveals a restrictive disorder.

Work in aluminum potrooms has been associated with obstructive lung disease, termed potroom asthma, although the exact causative agent is not clear (118).

## Miscellaneous Dusts

Exposure to the dusts of such metals as *iron, barium, tin, antimony*, and *titanium* may lead to radiographically visible deposits in the lungs without corresponding parenchymal fibrosis and pulmonary function impairment. Pneumoconiosis can also occur as a result of chronic exposure to dusts of synthetic materials such as *Bakelite* and polyvinyl chloride, but there is some controversy about the degree of functional impairment that may result (119, 120).

### CHRONIC BRONCHITIS AND CHRONIC AIRWAYS DISEASE

Occupational or industrial bronchitis is defined as bronchitis that is caused or aggravated by exposures at work. The pathophysiology and interrelationships between chronic bronchitis, emphysema, and asthma, all of which are associated with air flow obstruction, are discussed in Chapters 9 and 10. There is no question that a wide range of different occupational exposures can cause bronchitic symptoms, including gases, mineral dusts, metals, fumes, and organic substances (Table 14.8). Irritant exposures can cause airway inflammation and mucus hypersecretion, both of which can be associated with air flow obstruction.

Whether occupational exposure to chronic irritant exposures can cause air flow obstruction and/or accelerated loss of ventilatory function and not just bronchitic symptoms is an important question that has been a source of debate (121, 122). This has been difficult to determine because of the high prevalence of smoking, the limited size of some cohort studies, and the potential bias of the healthy worker effect in cross-sectional studies. A number of both community- and workforce-based epidemiologic studies have shown an association between chronic irritant exposures and air flow obstruction or accelerated loss of lung function in populations occupationally exposed to dusts and fumes (122, 123), such as miners or cotton workers. However, this occupational effect is usually of much lesser magnitude than the detrimental effect of cigarette smoke on lung function. Cigarette smoke is the major cause of bronchitic symptoms and chronic obstructive airways disease. Epidemiologic studies suggest that the interaction between smoking and occupational exposures in causing bronchitic symptoms and reduced lung function may be additive or multiplicative (122, 123). Certain host susceptibility factors such as preexisting nonspecific airway hyperresponsiveness may predispose certain workers to chronic airways obstruction. The presence of airway hyperresponsiveness is associated with a more rapid than expected annual rate of decline in lung function in certain exposed populations (124). However, it has been more difficult to determine whether the presence of industrial bronchitis itself causes air flow obstruction or is a marker for some other risk factor.

Pathologic data support the notion that occupational exposure to certain dusts is capable of causing chronic air flow obstruction. Coal miners, for example, had more centrilobular emphysema than controls in an autopsy study, and severity of emphysema was related to lung burden of coal dust (125).

Common exposures that can cause chronic bronchitis and are also associated with an accelerated loss of lung function include *asbestos, silica, coal dust, grain and wood dusts, and cotton dusts.* Chronic exposures that may cause chronic bronchitic symptoms but have not clearly shown any excess respiratory impairment include *MMVFs, welding fumes, firefighting exposures,* and *irritant gases.*

## Clinical Evaluation

The clinical evaluation of a patient with suspected occupational bronchitis is similar to that of any patient with chronic bronchitic symptoms. It is important to assess whether bronchitic symptoms alone are present or whether asthma, emphysema, or some other pulmonary process is involved. Any environmental or occupational exposures that may be causing or exacerbating the pulmonary condition should be identified. No specific diagnostic tests are available for occupational bronchitis, and a causal role for occupational exposures can be difficult to establish, especially in a smoker. The presence of eye and upper respiratory tract irritation/inflammation, a temporal association between symptoms and workplace exposures (especially early in the course), and coworkers with similar symptoms suggest work-relatedness. Chronic bronchitic symptoms can persist after removal from exposure.

Pulmonary function testing including D$_{LCO}$ is useful both diagnostically and to assess level of impairment. Methylcholine challenge testing may be indicated if the history suggests asthma and spirometry is normal. Chest radiography should also be performed.

When a patient's bronchitis is suspected to be work related, interventions to reduce or eliminate exposure to the putative agent(s) or process are justified. Engineering controls are preferable to the use of respirators. If the patient improves with such intervention, then the diagnosis of work-relatedness is supported. However, symptoms may persist after cessation of exposure. Commonly, bronchitis is of multifactorial etiology with smoking playing a role. Smoking cessation is key. Medical surveillance to detect accelerated loss of ventilatory function or airway hyperresponsiveness is recommended. The medical management of work-related chronic bronchitis is similar to that caused by smoking alone.

Data available concerning prognosis in patients with irritant-induced chronic bronchitis are limited. However, as discussed above, exposure to inhaled irritants may be associated with both symptoms of chronic bronchitis and small decrements in lung function.

## MALIGNANCIES OF THE RESPIRATORY TRACT AND PLEURA

This section addresses the occupational and environmental causes of lung carcinoma and other cancers of the respiratory tract and pleura. (See Chapter 15 for a more extensive discussion of the pathogenesis, evaluation and treatment of lung cancer.) An excellent extensive review of the causes of lung cancer can be found in a recently published monograph (126).

### Sinonasal Cancers

Squamous carcinoma and adenocarcinoma of the sinuses are rare in the general population but have been associated with several different exposures. Occupational exposures to nickel and wood dust are considered to be established risk factors for sinonasal cancers (127, 128). Increased risk of sinonasal cancers is also associated with exposure to chromium, cutting oils, formaldehyde, and wood smoke (129–132). The manufacture of leather goods and textiles, and furnace work also have been associated with increased risk of sinonasal cancers, although the specific causal agents have not been identified (133). Cigarette smoking and alcohol use are not major causes of sinonasal cancers.

### Laryngeal Cancer

Squamous carcinoma of the larynx usually is attributed to tobacco smoke and alcohol exposure. Data from several large cohorts, including insulators and friction product manufacturing workers, have provided evidence supporting a contributory role for asbestos fibers, possibly a twofold relative risk (134). Since synergism between asbestos exposure and cigarette smoking has been documented for lung cancer, it is possible that such synergism might apply to this related epithelial cancer. Additional possible occupational risk factors for laryngeal cancer include cutting oils, strong acids, nickel, and mustard gas (135, 136).

### LUNG CANCER (ALSO SEE CHAPTER 15)

Lung cancer, once a rare tumor, is now the leading cause of cancer death in both men and women in the United States. The dramatic increase in the incidence of lung cancers in the past 50 years has encouraged study of the modern environment for possible causal factors. Starting with the demonstration by Doll in the 1950s of a causal role for cigarette smoke, epidemiologic techniques have identified a number of respiratory tract carcinogens (137, 138). Although cigarette smoking is the single greatest risk factor for lung cancer, occupational and environmental exposures are important preventable causes. Estimates of the percentage of lung cancers attributable to occupational and environmental factors have varied widely, ranging from 5% to over 30% of all cases (138, 139). A number of agents are considered to be either known or suspected human lung carcinogens (Tables 14.9 and 14.10). Additionally, studies have shown an excess risk of lung cancer among members of several trades and industries, although identification of specific carcinogenic agents has not been possible.

There is considerable evidence that diet is also an important factor in the etiology and prevention of lung cancer. Most consistently, a diet high in fruit and vegetables has been shown to be associated with a reduced risk of lung cancer (140). What component(s) of such a diet, beta-carotene, retinoids, or other nutrient produce(s) the protective effect in unclear. Clinical trials of the efficacy of vitamin A and beta-carotene in preventing lung cancer among high-risk smokers and asbestos-exposed workers are in progress (141).

Potential causes of respiratory tract cancers have been demonstrated either by *case-control* or *cohort* studies. By either methodology, the idea of cause is expressed as *excessive relative risk* (ratio of the risk of a particular cancer in an exposed group to that in a comparable unexposed group).

From a public health standpoint, recognition of causal connections provides the first step in cancer control, reducing ongoing exposure to human carcinogens. For those already exposed, recognition of the degree of risk allows the intelligent application of smoking cessation and other interventions to reduce risk of lung cancer or screening strategies to identify early curable tumors.

### TABLE 14.9
#### KNOWN OCCUPATIONAL LUNG CARCINOGENS

| Substance | Examples of Exposure Settings |
|---|---|
| Asbestos | Insulation workers, shipyard workers |
| Arsenic | Smelting of copper, zinc, lead; pesticide production |
| Chloromethyl ether | Production workers |
| Chromium | Chromate production, pigment manufacture, electroplating |
| Mustard gas | Production workers, soldiers |
| Nickel | Nickel refining, plating |
| Polycylic aromatic hydrocarbons | Coke oven workers, rubber workers, aluminum reduction workers, roofers |
| Radon | Uranium mining, hard rock mining |

### TABLE 14.10
#### SUSPECTED OCCUPATIONAL LUNG CARCINOGENS

| Substance | Examples of Exposure Settings |
|---|---|
| Acrylonitrile | Plastics, petrochemicals |
| Beryllium | Beryllium production, processing |
| Cadmium | Smelting, battery production |
| Formaldehyde | Production formaldehyde resins |
| Silica | Mining, foundries |
| Synthetic fibers (MMVF) | Production, insulating |
| Vinyl chloride monomer | Polyvinyl chloride, plastic production |

### Clinical Evaluation and Management

The evaluation of any patient with lung cancer should include a careful occupational and environmental exposure history. To determine whether a given exposure caused the patient's cancer, the following guidelines are recommended. The clinician must determine what potential lung carcinogens the patient was exposed to and assess dose of exposure and latency as best as possible. A thorough smoking history is essential. When more than one carcinogen is present, it can be difficult to specify etiology, and one usually concludes that both exposures contributed to the patient's cancer. The management of a patient with occupationally induced lung cancer is similar to that of any patient with lung cancer.

### Known Lung Carcinogens

#### Asbestos

Asbestos was established as a cause of lung cancer in the 1950s (142). Lung cancer is a far more important cause of death than mesothelioma in asbestos-exposed workers, killing up to 40% of those with asbestosis

(143). Although numerous studies have confirmed a causal relationship between asbestos and lung cancer, a number of questions and areas of controversy remain, including the carcinogenic potential of different types of asbestos fibers, the magnitude of the synergistic effect between asbestos and cigarette smoke, whether asbestosis or asbestos exposure is the risk factor, whether a safe threshold exists, and the risks of low-level exposures.

There are no distinctive features of asbestos-related lung cancer to distinguish it from lung cancer due to smoking alone or other causes. Latency between exposure and disease peaks at 20 to 30 years. Although at one time it appeared that adenocarcinoma was the predominant histologic type, current data indicate a distribution of cell types comparable to that among the general population (144). While the location of tumors is more frequently in the lower lobes (two-thirds of asbestos-related tumors versus one-third of all lung cancers), this feature is insufficiently specific to determine etiology in an individual patient. Individuals with established asbestosis are clearly at highest risk, and most lung cancers related to asbestos occur in workers with asbestosis (145). Some studies have shown that individuals with asbestos exposure and only pleural plaques on chest radiographs without any parenchymal changes have an increased risk of lung cancer, although a number of epidemiologic and pathologic studies suggest that only those with fibrosis are at increased risk (146, 147).

Although the exact quantitative interaction may be debatable, cigarette smoke clearly potentiates the carcinogenic effects of asbestos. It is generally stated that asbestos and cigarette smoke act synergistically to increase risk for lung cancer. Some studies have shown more of an additive rather than a synergistic effect of asbestos and cigarettes. Among nonsmoking workers exposed to asbestos, the relative risk is increased by a factor of approximately five; among smokers who have not been exposed to asbestos, the risk is increased by a factor of approximately ten. However, among smoking asbestos workers, the relative risk is increased by a factor of at least 15 (additive) to greater than 50 (synergistic) (148). Cessation of smoking, therefore, is the most important step in cancer prevention for previously exposed individuals, although control of asbestos exposure is also imperative.

The data from epidemiologic studies of heavily exposed cohorts demonstrate a nearly linear relationship between estimates of exposure and mortality from lung cancer at high levels of asbestos exposure (147). However, the dose-response relationship at low levels of exposure is less clear. In some cohort studies the dose-response relationship does not include zero risk,

suggesting that there may be no threshold or "safe" level of exposure. There are also arguments that favor the existence of a safe threshold, including a number of cohort mortality studies showing no increased risk at low exposure, low-dose animal studies, negative studies among residents with low-level asbestos exposure, and data suggesting that asbestos-related lung cancers only occur in those with asbestosis. If there is an increased risk of lung cancer at low doses, the risk is small.

The mechanism of asbestos-related carcinogenesis is not clear but is probably linked to the processes of lung inflammation and fibrosis. Asbestos is a lung carcinogen that probably acts primarily as a promoting, rather than an initiating, agent. There is mounting evidence that both the physical dimensions and surface chemical characteristics of the fibers are important. Long, thin fibers appear to be the most carcinogenic. The length of time that fibers remain intact in the lungs (which probably is related to chemical characteristics) also is an important factor. All major forms of asbestos appear to be associated with an increased risk of lung cancer, although chrysotile appears to be less hazardous than the amphiboles (amosite, crocidolite, tremolite).

### Arsenic

Arsenic has been shown to increase lung cancer risk in workers engaged in smelting, pesticide manufacturing, and other industries with arsenic exposure (149). A clear dose-response relationship has been shown. The latency from onset of exposure to lung cancer is about 25 years on average. Arsenic is believed to be a late-stage promoter of lung cancer rather than an initiator.

### Chloromethyl Ethers and Mustard Gas

Alkylating agents used in the chemical and pharmaceutical industries, including bischloromethyl ether (BCME) and mustard gas (bis[2-chloroethyl] sulfide), are highly carcinogenic (150). A number of studies have documented that BCME exposure is strongly associated with an increased risk of lung cancer, especially small-cell carcinomas at a young age. Smoking does not appear to further increase the risk of cancer among BCME-exposed workers. BCME has also been shown to cause bronchogenic carcinoma in an animal model.

Large excesses of lung cancer cases have been found in mustard gas production workers, with smoking probably having an additive effect (151).

### Chromium

Hexavalent chromium, used in chromate production, electroplating, pigment manufacture, and the ferrochromium industry, has been associated with an increased relative risk of lung cancer (152).

### Nickel

Nickel exposure (among nickel mining and refinery workers) has been associated with excess lung cancer rates, with a mean latency of about 20 years (126). Metallic nickel has not been associated with an increased risk of lung cancer.

### Polyaromatic Hydrocarbons

Polyaromatic hydrocarbons (PAHs) are a complex mix of a number of widespread substances generated during the incomplete combustion of carbonaceous products such as coal, oil, pitch, and tar. PAHs are also present in cigarette smoke. Workers exposed to PAHs—including coke oven workers, printers, roofers, aluminum production workers, and drivers—have been found to have significant excess lung cancer rates (153).

### Radon

Radon is an inert gas that is a decay product of uranium-238. Radon decays with alpha particle emission to various short-lived radon daughters. Underground uranium miners exposed to radon and its decay products have a dramatically increased risk of developing lung cancer, with a preponderance of small cell carcinoma, although other cell types are also increased (154). Cigarette smoke and radon most likely interact more than additively in increasing the risk for lung cancer (154). Excess lung cancer rates have been found in other types of miners including tin, iron, and lead miners (155). The potential risk of domestic radon is discussed below.

## Suspected Lung Carcinogens

*Vinyl chloride monomer, beryllium,* and *acrylonitrile,* all animal carcinogens, are suspected respiratory tract carcinogens. *Vinyl chloride monomer* has been established as a cause of human angiosarcomas of the liver, and increased numbers of cancers of other organs, including the lungs, have been found in the vinyl plastics industry (156). Excess mortality due to lung cancer in human populations exposed to beryllium and acrylonitrile has been shown, but the magnitude of the effects for all three is relatively small (i.e., less than twofold increase in relative risk) (157, 158). There is some evidence that *cadmium* exposure is associated with increased risk of lung cancer (159).

Traditionally, *silica* has not been viewed as a carcinogen. However, there is increasing evidence of an excess of lung cancer associated with silica exposure. Several recent studies have reported an increased risk of lung cancer among miners, foundry workers, and other silica-exposed workers (160). The risk of lung cancer is probably greater in those with chronic silicosis than in those with only silica exposure.

*MMVFs* include rock and slag wool, glass fibers, and ceramic fibers. Some excess lung cancer risk has been reported in rock and slag workers but without a strong dose-response relationship (147, 161). Ceramic fibers, when instilled in the pleural space, can cause malignant mesothelioma in rodents.

A recent study of a large cohort of industrial workers exposed to *formaldehyde* showed a mildly increased risk of lung cancer (131). No increased lung cancer risk has been found among professional groups (pathologists, anatomists) exposed to formaldehyde.

Workers in several industries including foundries, rubber industry, welding and printing have been shown to be at increased risk of lung cancer in some studies (162). However, the etiologic agents are unclear, and confounding by smoking and other exposures can limit the findings.

## Risk Factors for Lung Cancer in the Environment

There has been increasing interest in the role of environmental exposures such as environmental tobacco smoke, air pollution, and domestic radon in the causation of lung cancer. The nonmalignant respiratory effects of these and other exposures present in indoor and ambient air are discussed in the final section of this chapter.

### Domestic Radon

The potential risk of lung cancer from exposure to radon in homes, derived primarily from rock, soil, and drinking water, is receiving increasing attention. Average domestic radon exposures in the United States range from 0.8 to 1.5 picocuries per liter (pCi/liter), well below the levels experienced by miners. However, cumulative lifetime exposures comparable to those of miners are likely to exist in a small percentage of American homes. It is believed that radon may act more than additively as a risk factor for lung cancer in smokers, possibly because radon decay particles can attach to respirable particles such as cigarette smoke (154).

Although there are a number of ongoing studies, most estimates of the risk of domestic radon are based on extrapolations from studies of miners to lower indoor levels (154). These risk assessments estimate that about 5,000 to 20,000 deaths annually in the United

States (approximately 3 to 15% of all lung cancer deaths) are attributable to radon (163). A recent case-control study in Sweden found an increased relative risk of lung cancer associated with increased domestic radon levels. A dose-response effect and an almost multiplicative interaction between radon and cigarette smoke was noted (164). However, other case-control studies have found no increased relative risk of lung cancer in relation to domestic radon exposure (165). In smokers, the best way to reduce the risk of lung cancer is to stop smoking, regardless of domestic radon levels. If very high domestic radon measurements are found (e.g., above 5–10 pCi/liter in a living area), it would be reasonable to consider home mitigation techniques such as improved ventilation.

### Environmental Tobacco Smoke

Environmental tobacco smoke (ETS) contains side-stream smoke (SS) released from the burning cigarette and mainstream smoke (MS) exhaled by the smoker. Passive smokers are exposed to the same carcinogenic constituents of tobacco smoke as smokers, although generally at lower doses and in different relative concentrations. A number of epidemiologic studies have shown a statistically significant increase in lung cancer risk in nonsmokers married to smokers of about 20 to 30% (166). A recent population-based case-control study of 191 nonsmokers with lung cancer found a twofold increased risk of lung cancer with exposure to 25 or more smoker-years during childhood and adolescence (167). Because of the large number of people exposed to ETS and the relatively high incidence of lung cancer, a small increase in lung cancer risk due to ETS risk is of great public health importance.

### Air Pollution

Outdoor air pollution is a complex and variable mixture of natural and manmade pollutants including sulfur oxides, particulates, carbon monoxide, and photochemical pollution (see below). Specific compounds found in air pollution are potentially carcinogenic, and there may be a small increased risk of lung cancer associated with air pollution (168). However, this has been difficult to confirm using epidemiologic data. There are numerous methodologic difficulties in attempting to determine whether air pollution is associated with an increased risk of lung cancer, including quantifying exposures and controlling for confounders such as cigarette smoking and occupational exposures.

Another concern is whether *indoor air pollution* such as household coal smoke or other heating or cooking smoke increases the risk of lung cancer. Studies from China suggest that household coal smoke may increase this risk (169).

### Asbestos in Buildings

Low-level asbestos exposure is ubiquitous. Exposures in buildings, especially schools and public buildings, which frequently contain friable and decaying asbestos, have created great anxiety. The primary concern about low-level exposure is the risk of mesothelioma and lung cancer. As discussed above, the magnitude of this risk, if any, is an area of controversy. Although the risk of cancer from such exposures is undoubtedly quite low, it is unlikely to be zero. In considering public policy and personal decisions, the risks of low-level asbestos exposure should be considered in the context of other risks in life, and the costs of remediation likewise need to be weighed against other costs and financial decisions.

## MALIGNANT MESOTHELIOMA

Malignant mesotheliomas are rare tumors of the pleura or peritoneum that in at least 80% of cases are associated with a history of asbestos exposure. Although there is some dose-response relationship between asbestos exposure and risk of mesothelioma, mesotheliomas may occur with relatively short-term and low-level exposures. Mesotheliomas have been reported to occur in family members of asbestos workers and persons living near shipyards. Many patients will be free of obvious radiographic evidence of asbestos exposure, unlike the situation with asbestos-related lung cancer (170). The latency period is in the range of 30 to 40 years. Pleural cases are more common than peritoneal.

The relative carcinogenicity of the different asbestos fiber types is an area of debate. Although all types probably can cause mesothelioma, chrysotile, the most common fiber type in the United States, is the least likely to cause mesothelioma, while the amphiboles crocidolite and amosite appear to have the highest potential for inducing mesotheliomas (170). Long, thin fibers appear to have the highest associated risk. In contrast to what has been observed with bronchogenic carcinoma, cigarette smoking does not increase the risk of mesothelioma.

The most common presenting symptom in patients with pleural mesothelioma is chest pain. Dyspnea, weight loss, and cough may also be present. A pleural effusion is frequently seen on the chest radiograph. CT scanning is frequently performed to confirm the presence of a pleural-based mass(es). The pleural fluid is exudative, and cytologic examination frequently is insufficiently sensitive or specific to confirm the diagnosis. Histologic differentiation from poorly differentiated adenocarcinoma metastatic to the pleura or reactive mesothelial cells is frequently difficult. Open pleural biopsy with adequate tissue specimens and an experienced pathologist capable of performing electron microscopic and histochemical studies are often required to make the diagnosis. Mesotheliomas extend locally and can also metastasize. There is no effective therapy for mesothelioma and most patients die within a year of diagnosis.

## AIR POLLUTION—NONMALIGNANT RESPIRATORY EFFECTS

There has been increasing concern about the adverse health effects of both outdoor ambient and indoor air pollution. Patients and the public frequently turn to physicians with questions concerning the risks of radon, environmental tobacco smoke, ozone, and other air pollutants, and for advice on what to do about such exposures. This section reviews the known nonmalignant pulmonary health effects of ambient (outdoor) and indoor air pollution and which populations may be more susceptible to these effects. The role of these exposures in contributing to lung cancer is addressed above.

### AMBIENT AIR POLLUTION

Numerous natural and manmade sources contribute to outdoor air pollution. There are four broad groups of exposures that may have adverse health effects: (a) combustion of sulfur-containing fossil fuels (sulfur oxides, particulates, acidic aerosols); (b) photochemical pollution (ozone); (c) carbon monoxide; and (d) toxic air pollutants (fossil fuel combustion and industrial products). The EPA has categorized pollutants as "criteria" pollutants (Table 14.11) and "hazardous" pollutants (primarily carcinogens such as asbestos), the levels of which are regulated by the Clean Air Act. Investigators have tried to determine the adverse effects of air pollution with both large-scale epidemiologic studies and experimental exposure chambers. It should be remembered that these exposures almost always occur as part of a complex mix of pollutants, not individually, and that interactions between different exposures probably exist but are difficult to determine.

Epidemiologic studies have shown that air pollution can be associated with increased respiratory symptoms and exacerbations of asthma and bronchitis (172, 173), although which particular component, such as fine particulates or ozone, is responsible can be difficult to determine from epidemiologic studies. Several recent studies have also shown an association between air pollution (primarily small particulates and sulfates) and daily mortality, largely from chronic respiratory

**TABLE 14.11**
**UNITED STATES AMBIENT AIR QUALITY CRITERIA POLLUTANTS AND PRINCIPAL HEALTH EFFECTS AT AMBIENT LEVELS**

| Pollutant | Health Effects |
|---|---|
| Ozone | Acute respiratory symptoms, decrements in lung function, and respiratory tract inflammation |
| Particulate matter (PM$_{10}$) | Asthma, COPD exacerbation, increased respiratory mortality |
| Sulfur oxides | Asthma exacerbation |
| Nitrogen dioxide | ? Asthma/COPD exacerbation; ? Increased susceptibility to respiratory tract infections |
| Carbon monoxide | Ischemic heart disease exacerbation |
| Lead | ? Decreased cognitive function in children |

diseases (COPD, pneumonia, and possibly lung cancer) (174, 175).

The effects of specific pollutants at ambient levels of exposure are summarized below (176, 177).

*Sulfur oxides* and *particulate matter* are produced by sulfur-containing fuels such as coal and petroleum and can probably exacerbate the status of patients with asthma and COPD and increase respiratory symptoms in children. Children and asthmatics also appear susceptible to *acid aerosols* (such as sulfuric acid, nitric acid) from various industrial operations.

Acute exposure to ambient levels of *ozone* has been shown to result in lung inflammation and transient reductions in lung function. However, the chronic effects of such exposures remain unclear. Asthmatics do not appear to have increased susceptibility to ozone.

Carbon monoxide (CO) can bind to hemoglobin and carboxyhemoglobin, reducing oxygen delivery to tissues. In patients with coronary artery disease, CO may exacerbate myocardial ischemia and arrhythmias.

In summary, current data suggest that ambient levels of certain pollutants may increase respiratory symptoms and exacerbate underlying lung disease, primarily in children, asthmatics, and persons with COPD. Cigarette smoking may have additive or synergistic effects with air pollutants, and exercise may also increase the likelihood of adverse effects.

### INDOOR AIR POLLUTION

Increasing concern is being raised about the adverse health effects of indoor air, and various symptoms have been attributed to exposures in the indoor environment. Illnesses that have been related to building exposures include allergic respiratory diseases such as sinusitis, rhinitis, asthma, and hypersensitivity pneumonitis due to exposures to molds, spores, chemicals or other substances (178, 179). Building-related infectious diseases such as Legionnaires' disease are well recognized. (These entities are discussed in Chapters 12 and 16.) It is important to obtain a careful occupational and environmental exposure history in any patient presenting with such an illness. Nonindustrial environments should not be assumed to be clean and free of significant exposures.

### Sick Building Syndrome (SBS)

Since the 1970s, nonspecific symptoms among employees in indoor, nonindustrial environments have increasingly come to medical attention. Because many SBS complaints are related to the respiratory tract, pulmonary physicians should be aware of this syndrome. The term SBS refers to nonspecific complaints that usually involve mucous membrane and upper respiratory irritative symptoms, headaches, fatigue, difficulty concentrating, and odor complaints, and which are associated with a particular building(s) (178). Symptoms generally improve away from that indoor environment. Similar symptoms in coworkers are common. Other causes for the patient's complaints should be evaluated and ruled out. The cause of SBS is likely multifactorial. Inadequate ventilation systems are clearly an important contributing factor in many cases. However, other factors such as ETS, job satisfaction, work stress, and lower pay scale may be involved. Physician recommendations concerning the workplace environment may facilitate ventilation improvements or other beneficial interventions in the work environment.

### Environmental Tobacco Smoke

As mentioned earlier, ETS contains most of the ingredients inhaled by the active smoker, but at lower concentrations. A number of studies have demonstrated that children of parents who smoke are at increased risk of respiratory infections, respiratory symptoms, asthma exacerbations, and reduced lung function, compared with children with nonsmoking parents (179, 180). The effects on respiratory symptoms, lung function, and underlying lung disease in adults is less clear.

### Biomass and Fossil Fuels

Indoor use of wood, coal, or kerosene for heating and cooking release various combustion products. Epidemiologic studies have shown an association between these exposures and childhood respiratory symptoms and also possibly an increased risk of childhood infections, asthma, and reduced lung function (178).

### Carbon Dioxide

Carbon dioxide, which is produced primarily by human respiration, is frequently measured as an indicator of adequate indoor ventilation and the results not uncommonly presented to physicians caring for patients with complaints of SBS. Normal $CO_2$ levels are frequently measured despite inadequate ventilation, and such measurements are usually not helpful in managing complaints of inadequate indoor air quality or SBS (178).

▼

## REFERENCES

1. Rosenstock L, Cullen MR: *Textbook of Clinical Occupational and Environmental Medicine.* Philadelphia, WB Saunders, 1994.
2. Rom WN: *Environmental and Occupational Medicine.* Boston, Little, Brown & Co, 1992.
3. Parkes WR: *Occupational Lung Disorders.* Oxford, Butterworth-Heinemann, 1994.
4. Harper P, Schenker M, Balmes J, (eds): *Occupational and Environmental Respiratory Disease.* St. Louis, Mosby-Year Book, 1995 (in press).
5. Cullen MR, Cherniack MG, Rosenstock L: Medical progress: occupational medicine. *N Engl J Med* 322: 594–601, (part 1), (part 2) 675–683, 1990.
6. Chan-Yeung M: Occupational asthma. *Chest* 98: 148S–161S, 1990.
7. Chan-Yeung M, Malo JL: Aetiological agents in occupational asthma. *Eur Respir J* 7:346–371, 1994.
8. Middleton E: Asthma, inhaled allergens, and washing the cat. *Am Rev Respir Dis* 143:1209–1210, 1991.
9. Chan-Yeung M, Lam S: Occupational asthma. *Am Rev Respir Dis* 133:686–703, 1986.
10. Becklake MR: Epidemiology and surveillance. *Chest* 165–172s, 1990.
11. Newman-Taylor AJ: Laboratory animal allergy. *Eur J Respir Dis* 63:123:60–64, 1982.
12. Chan-Yeung M: Immunologic and nonimmunologic mechanisms in asthma due to western red cedar (*Thuja plicata*). *J Allergy Clin Immunol* 70:32–37, 1982.
13. Venables KM, Dally MD, Nunn AJ, et al: Smoking and occupational allergy in workers in a platinum refinery. *Br Med J* 299:939–942, 1989.
14. Burge PS: Single and serial measurements of lung function in the diagnosis of occupational asthma. *Eur J Respir Dis* 63:(Suppl 123)47–59, 1982.
15. Cartier A: Definition and diagnosis of occupational asthma. *Eur Respir J* 7:153–160, 1994.
16. Cullen MR: Clinical surveillance and management of occupational asthma. *Chest* 98:196S–201S, 1990.
17. Vandenplas O, Malo J, Saetta M, et al: Occupational

asthma and extrinsic alveolitis due to isocyanates: current status and perspectives. *Br J Ind Med* 50:213–228, 1993.

18. Pisati G, Baruffini A, Zedda S: Toluene diisocyanate induced asthma: outcome according to persistence or cessation of exposure. *Br J Ind Med* 50:60–64, 1993.

19. Chan-Yeung M, Koerner S, Lam S: Clinical features and natural history of occupational asthma due to western red cedar (*Thuja plicata*). *Am J Med* 72:411–415, 1982.

20. Brooks SM, Weiss MA, Bernstein IL: Reactive airways dysfunction syndrome (RADS). *Chest* 88:376–384, 1985.

21. Tarlo SM, Broder I: Irritant-induced occupational asthma. *Chest* 96:297–300, 1989.

22. Pueringer RJ, Hunninghake GW: Inflammation and airway reactivity in asthma. *Am J Med* 92(6A):325–385, 1992.

23. Chan-Yeung M: Mechanism of occupational asthma due to western red cedar (*Thuja plicata*). *Am J Ind Med* 25:13–18, 1994.

24. Ramazzini B: De Morbis Artificum Diatriba (1713). Wright WC (trans). New York, Hafner, 1964.

25. Jones RN, Diem JE, Glindmeyer H, et al: Mill effect and dose-response relationships in byssinosis. *Br J Ind Med* 36:305–313, 1979.

26. Sepulveda, MJ, Castellan RM, Hankison JL, et al: Acute lung function response to cotton dust in atopic non-atopic individuals. *Br J Ind Med* 41:487–491, 1984.

27. Beck GJ, Maunder LR, Schachter EN, et al: Cotton dust and smoking effects on lung function in cotton textile workers. *Am J Epidemiol* 119:33–34, 1984.

28. Bouhuys A, Van de Woestyne KP: Respiratory mechanics and dust exposure in byssinosis. *J Clin Invest* 49: 106–118, 1970.

29. Schachter EN: Byssinosis and other textile dust-related lung diseases. In Rosenstock L, Cullen MR (eds): *Textbook of Clinical Occupational and Environmental Medicine*. Philadelphia, WB Saunders, 1994.

30. Merchant JA, Lumsden JC, Kilburn KH, et al: An industrial study of the biological effects of cotton dust and cigarette smoke exposure. *J Occup Med* 15:212–221, 1973.

31. Beck GJ, Schacter EN, Maunder LR: The relationship of respiratory symptoms and lung function loss in cotton textile workers. *Am Rev Respir Dis* 130:6–11, 1984.

32. Rylander R, Haglind P, Lundholm M: Endotoxin in cotton dust and respiratory function decrement among cotton workers in an experimental cardroom. *Am Rev Respir Dis* 131:209–213, 1985.

33. Buck MG, Wall JH, Schacter EN: Airway constrictor response to cotton bract extracts in the absence of endotoxin. *Br J Ind Med* 43:220–226, 1986.

34. Chan-Yeung M, Enarson DA, Kennedy SM: State of the art: the impact of grain dust on respiratory health. *Am Rev Respir Dis* 145:476–487, 1992.

35. Grzybowski S, Chan-Yeung M, Ashley JA: Atopy and grain dust exposure. In Dosman JA, Cotton DA (eds): *Occupational Pulmonary Disease: Focus on Grain Dust and Health*. New York, Academic Press, 1980.

36. Huy T, Schipper KD, Chan-Yeung M, et al: Grain dust and lung function: dose-response relationships. *Am Rev Respir Dis* 144:1314–1321, 1991.

37. Schwartz DA: Acute inhalational injury. *Occupational Medicine: State of the Art Review* 2(2):297–318, 1987.

38. Harkonen H, Nordman H, Korhonen O, et al: Long-term effects of exposure to sulfur dioxide. *Am Rev Respir Dis* 128:890–893, 1983.

39. Epler GR, Colby TV, McLoud TC, et al: Bronchiolitis obliterans organizing pneumonia. *N Engl J Med* 312: 152–158, 1985.

40. Jones GR, Proudfoot AT, Hall JI: Pulmonary effects of acute exposure to nitrous fumes. *Thorax* 28:61–65, 1973.

41. Barnhart S, Rosenstock L: Cadmium chemical pneumonitis. *Chest* 86:789–791, 1985.

42. Davison AG, Newman Taylor AJ, Darbyshire J, et al: Cadmium fume inhalation and emphysema. *Lancet* 1: 663–667, 1988.

43. Sperkazza SJ, Beckett WS: The respiratory health of welders: state of the art. *Am Rev Respir Dis* 143: 1134–1148, 1991.

44. Williams N, Smith, FK: Polymer fume fever: an elusive diagnosis. *JAMA* 219:1587–1589, 1972.

45. Whitener DR, Whitener LM, Robertson KJ, et al: Pulmonary function measurements in patients with thermal injury and smoke inhalation. *Am Rev Respir Dis* 122: 731–739, 1980.

46. Douglas DB, Douglas RB, Oakes D, et al: Pulmonary function of London firemen. *Br J Ind Med* 42:55–58, 1985.

47. Rosenstock L, Demers P, Heyer NJ, et al: Respiratory mortality among firefighters. *Br J Ind Med* 47(7):462–465, 1990.

48. Epler GR, McCloud TG, Gaensler EA: Prevalence and incidence of benign asbestos pleural effusion in a working population. *JAMA* 247:617–622, 1982.

49. Talcott JA, Thurber WA, Kantor AF, et al: Asbestos-associated diseases in a cohort of cigarette-filter workers. *N Engl J Med* 321:1220–1223, 1989.

50. Cullen MR, Kominsky JR, Rossman MD, et al: Chronic beryllium disease in a precious metal refinery: clinical epidemiologic evidence for continuing risk from exposure to low level beryllium fume. *Am Rev Respir Dis* 135: 201–208, 1987.

51. van Sprundel MP: Pneumoconioses: the situation in developing countries (review). *Exp Lung Res* 16:5–13, 1990.

52. Nugent K, Perrotta D, Dodson RF, et al: A cluster of silicosis in sandblasters [Letter]. *Am Rev Respir Disease* 142:1466, 1990.

53. Epler GR. Normal chest roentgenograms in chronic diffuse infiltrative lung disease. *N Engl J Med* 27:934–939, 1978.

54. International Labour Office: *Guidelines for the use of ILO International Classification of Radiographs of Pneumoconioses*. Occup Safety and Health Series No 22 (revised) Geneva, 1980.

55. Begin R: Computed tomography in the early detection asbestosis. *Br J Ind Med* 50:689–698, 1993.

56. Churg A, Green FHY (eds): *Pathology of Occupational Lung Disease*. New York, Igaku-Shoin, 1988.

57. Lapp NL, Castranova V: How silicosis and coal workers' pneumoconiosis develop—a cellular assessment. *Occup Med—State of the Art Rev* 8(1):35–55, 1993.

58. Weber SL, Banks DE: Silicosis. In Rosenstock L, Cullen MR (eds): *Clinical Occupational and Environmental Medicine*. Philadelphia, WB Saunders, 1994, pp 264–274.

59. Xipel JM, Ham KN, Price CG, et al: Acute silicolipoproteinosis. *Thorax* 104–111, 1977.

60. Teculescu DB, Stanescu DC, Pilot L: Pulmonary mechanics in silicosis. *Arch Environ Health* 14:461–468, 1967.

61. Irwig L, Rocks P: Lung function and respiratory symptoms in silicotic and non-silicotic gold miners. *Am Rev Respir Dis* 117:429–435, 1978.

62. Balmes J, Cullen MR, Gee JBL: What infections occur with occupational lung disease? *Clin Chest Med* 2: 111–120, 1981.

63. Snider DE: The relationship between tuberculosis and silicosis. *Am Rev Respir Dis* 455–460, 1978.

64. Ziskind M, Jones RN, Weill H: Silicosis: state of the art. *Am Rev Respir Dis* 113:643–665, 1976.

65. Costello JF, Moriarty DC, Branthwaite MA, et al: Diagnosis and management of alveolar proteinosis: the role of electron microscopy. *Thorax* 30:121–132, 1975.

66. Nicholson WJ, Perkel G, Selikoff IJ: Occupational exposure to asbestosis: population at risk and projected mortality, 1980–2030. *Am J Ind Med* 3:259–311, 1982.

67. Schwartz DA, Fuortes LJ, Galvin JR, et al. Asbestos-induced pleural fibrosis and impaired lung function. *Am Rev Respir Dis* 141:321–326, 1990.

68. Schwartz DA, Galvin JR, Yagla SJ, et al: Restrictive lung function and asbestos-induced pleural fibrosis. A quantitative approach. *J Clin Invest* 91:2685–2692, 1993.

69. Schwartz DA: New developments in asbestos-induced pleural disease. *Chest* 90:191–198, 1991.

70. Weiss W: Asbestos-related pleural plaques and lung cancer. *Chest* 103:1854–1859, 1993.

71. Nurminen M, Tossavainen A: Is there an association between pleural plaques and lung cancer without asbestosis? *Scand J Work Environ Health* 20:62–64, 1994.

72. Mintzer RA, Cugell DW: The association of asbestos-induced pleural disease and rounded atelectasis. *Chest* 81:457–460, 1982.

73. Murphy RL, Becklake MR, Brooks SM, et al: The diagnosis of nonmalignant diseases related to asbestos: official statement of the American Thoracic Society. *Am Rev Respir Dis* 134:363–368, 1986.

74. Griffith DE, Garcia JG, Dodson RF, Levin JL, Kronenberg RS: Airflow obstruction in non-smoking, asbestos- and mixed dust-exposed workers. *Lung* 141: 213–224, 1993.

75. Barnhart S, Hudson LD, Mason SE, et al: Total lung capacity: an insensitive measure of impairment in patients with asbestosis and chronic obstructive pulmonary disease? *Chest* 93:299–302, 1988.

76. Rom WN: Accelerated loss of lung function and alveolitis in a longitudinal study of non-smoking individuals with occupational exposure to asbestos. *Am J Ind Med* 21:835–844, 1992.

77. Schwartz DA, Galvin JR, Frees KL, et al: Clinical relevance of cellular mediators of inflammation in workers exposed to asbestos. *Am Rev Respir Dis* 148:68–74, 1993.

78. Coutts I, Gilson JC, Kerr IH, et al: Mortality in cases of asbestosis diagnosed by a pneumoconiosis medical panel. *Thorax* 42, 111–116, 1987.

79. Jones R, Diem JE, Hughes JM, et al: Progression of asbestos effects: a prospective longitudinal study of chest radiographs and lung function. *Br J Ind Med* 46:97–105, 1989.

80. Lapp NL, Parker JE: Coal workers' pneumoconiosis. In Epler GR (ed): *Clinics in Chest Medicine; Occupational Lung Diseases.* Philadelphia, WB Saunders, 1992, vol 13, pp 243–252.

81. Love RG, Miller BG: Longitudinal study of lung function in coal miners. *Thorax* 37:193–197, 1982.

82. Kleinerman J, Green F, Harley RA, et al: Pathology standards for coal workers' pneumoconiosis: report of the Pneumoconiosis Committee of the College of American Pathologists to the National Institute for Occupational Safety and Health. *Arch Pathol Lab Med* 103:375–429, 1979.

83. Attfield MD, Hodous TK: Pulmonary function of U.S. coal miners related to dust exposure estimates. *Am Rev Respir Dis* 145:605–609, 1992.

84. Musk AW, Cotes JE, Bevan C, et al: Relationship between type of simple coal workers' pneumoconiosis and lung function: a 9-year follow-up study of subjects with small rounded opacities. *Br J Ind Med* 38:313–320, 1981.

85. Lippman M, Eckert HL, Hahon W, et al: The presence of circulating antinuclear and rheumatoid factors in United States coal miners. *Ann Intern Med* 79:807–811, 1973.

86. Hardy HL, Tabershaw IR: Delayed chemical pneumonitis occurring in workers exposed to beryllium compounds. *J Ind Hyg Toxicol* 28:197–211, 1946.

87. Eisenbud M, Lisson J: Epidemiological aspects of beryllium-induced nonmalignant lung disease: a 30-year update. *J Occup Med* 25:196–202, 1983.

88. Kreiss K, Mroz Mm, Zhen B, et al: Epidemiology of beryllium sensitization and disease in nuclear workers. *Am Rev Respir Dis* 148:985–991, 1993.

89. Kreiss K, Wasserman S, Mroz MM, et al: Beryllium disease screening in the ceramics industry. Blood lymphocyte test performance and exposure-disease relations. *J Occup Med* 35:267–274, 1993.

90. Kriebel D, Brain JD, Sprince NL, et al: The pulmonary toxicity of beryllium. *Am Rev Respir Dis* 137:464–474, 1988.

91. Newman LS, Kreiss K, King TE, et al: Pathologic and immunologic alterations in early stages of beryllium disease: re-examination of disease definition and natural history. *Am Rev Respir Dis* 139:1479–1486, 1989.

92. Richeldi L, Sorrentino R, Saltini C: HLA-DPB1 glutamate 69: a genetic marker of beryllium disease. *Science* 262:242–243, 1993.

93. Newman LS: To Be2 + or not to be2 +: immunogenetics and occupational exposure (comment). *Science* 262: 197–198, 1993.

94. Hardy HL, Rabe EW, Lorch S: United States beryllium case registry (1952–1966). *J Occup Med* 9:271–276, 1967.

95. Mroz Mm, Kreiss K, Lezotte DC, et al: Reexamination of the blood lymphocyte transformation test in the diagnosis of chronic beryllium disease. *J Allergy Clin Immunol* 88:54–60, 1991.

96. Rossman MD, Kern JA, Elias JA, et al: Proliferative response of bronchoalveolar lymphocytes to beryllium: a test for chronic beryllium disease. *Ann Intern Med* 687–693, 1988.

97. De Vuyst P, Dumortier P, Schandene L, et al: Sarcoid-like lung granulomatosis induced by aluminum dusts. *Am Rev Respir Dis* 135:493–497, 1987.

98. Redline S, Barna BP, Tomashefski JF Jr, et al: Granulomatous disease associated with pulmonary deposition of titanium. *Br J Ind Med* 43:652–656, 1986.

99. Cugell DW: The hard metal diseases. In Epler GB (ed): *Clinics in Chest Medicine; Occupational Lung Diseases.* Philadelphia, WB Saunders, 1992, vol 13, pp 269–279.

100. Kusaka Y, Yokoyama K, Sera Y, et al: Respiratory diseases in hard metal workers: an occupational hygiene study in a factory. *Br J Ind Med* 43:474–485, 1986.

101. Demedts M, Gheysens B, Nagels J, et al. Cobalt lung

in diamond polishers. *Am Rev Respir Dis* 130:130–135, 1984.

102. Gheysens B, Auwerx J, Van den Eeckhout A, et al: Cobalt-induced bronchial asthma in diamond polishers. *Chest* 88:740–744, 1985.

103. Meyer-Bisch C, Pham QT, Mur JM, et al: Respiratory hazards in hard metal workers: a cross sectional study. *Br J Ind Med* 46:302–309, 1989.

104. Nam K, Gracey DR: Pulmonary talcosis from cosmetic talcum powder. *JAMA* 221:492–493, 1972.

105. Hopkins GB: Pulmonary angiothrombotic granulomatosis in drug offenders. *JAMA* 221:909–911, 1972.

106. Kleinfeld M, Messite J, Shapiro J, et al: Lung function changes in talc pneumoconiosis. *J Occup Med* 7:12–19, 1965.

107. Kennedy T, Rawlings W Jr, Baser M, et al: Pneumoconiosis in Georgia kaolin workers. *Am Rev Respir Dis* 127: 215–220, 1983.

108. Sakula A: Pneumoconiosis due to fuller's earth. *Thorax* 16:176–180, 1961.

109. Darris D, Cotton R: Mica pneumoconiosis. *Br J Ind Med* 40:22–27, 1983.

110. Kleinfeld M: Pleural calcification as a sign of silicatosis. *Am J Med Sci* 251:215–224, 1966.

111. Lockey JE, Wiese NJ: Health effects of synthetic vitreous fibers. *Clin Chest Med* 13:329–339, 1992.

112. Lemasters G, Lockey J, Rice C, et al: Pleural changes in workers manufacturing refractory ceramic fiber and products. Presented to British Occupational Hygiene Society, Seventh International Symposium on Inhaled Particles, Edinburgh, September 16–20, 1991.

113. Hughes JM, Jones RN, Glindmeyer HW, et al: Follow-up study of workers exposes to man-made mineral. *Br J Ind Med* 50:658–667, 1993.

114. Gaensler EA, Cadigan JB, Sasahara AA, et al: Graphite pneumoconiosis of electrotypers. *Am J Med* 41:864–882, 1966.

115. Watson AJ, Black J, Doig AT, et al: Pneumoconiosis in carbon electrode makers. *Br J Ind Med* 16:274–285, 1959.

116. Shaver CG, Riddell AR: Lung changes associated with the manufacture of alumina abrasives. *J Ind Hyg Toxicol* 29:145–157, 1947.

117. Mitchell J, Manning GB, Molyneux M, et al: Pulmonary fibrosis in workers exposed to finely powered aluminum. *Br J Ind Med* 18:10–20, 1961.

118. Kongerud J, Boe J, Soyseth V, et al: Aluminum potroom asthma: the Norwegian experience. *Eur Resp J* 7: 165–172, 1994.

119. Pimental JC: A granulomatous lung disease produced by Bakelite. *Am Rev Respir Dis* 108:1303–1310, 1973.

120. Soutar CA, Copland LH, Thornly PE, et al: Epidemiological study of respiratory disease in workers exposed to polyvinyl chloride dust. *Thorax* 35:644, 1980.

121. Morgan WKC: industrial bronchitis. *Br J Ind Med* 35: 285–291, 1978.

122. Oxman AD, Muir DCF, Shannon HS, et al: Occupational dust exposure and chronic obstructive pulmonary disease: a systemic overview of the evidence. *Am Rev Respir Dis* 148:38–48, 1993.

123. Becklake MR: Chronic airflow limitation: its relationship to work in dusty occupations. *Chest* 88:608–617, 1985.

124. Pham QT, Mur JM, Chan N, et al: Prognostic value of acetylcholine challenge test: a prospective study. *Br J Ind Med* 41:267–271, 1984.

125. Cockcroft A, Seal RME, Wagner JC, et al: Postmortem studies of emphysema in coalworkers and noncoalworkers. *Lancet* 2:600–603, 1980.

126. Samet JM (ed): *Epidemiology of Lung Cancer.* New York, Marcel Dekker, 1994.

127. Doll R, Mathews JD, Morgan LG: Cancers of the lung and nasal sinuses in nickel workers: a reassessment of the period of risk. *Br J Ind Med* 34:102–105, 1977.

128. Nylander LE, Dement JM: Carcinogenic effects of wood dust: review and discussion. *Am J Ind Med* 24:619–647, 1993.

129. Hernberg S, Westerholm P, Schultz-Larsen K, et al: Nasal and sinonasal cancer: connection with occupational exposures in Denmark, Finland and Sweden. *Scand J Work Environ Health* 9:315–325, 1983.

130. Roush GC, Meigs JW, Kelly J, et al: Sinonasal cancer and occupation: a case-control study. *Am J Epidemiol* 111:183–193, 1980.

131. Blair A, Saracci R, Steward PA, Hayes RB, Shy C: Epidemiologic evidence on the relationship between formaldehyde exposure and cancer. *Scand J Work Environ Health* 16:381–393, 1990.

132. Henderson BE, Loule E, Jang JS, et al: Risk factors associated with nasopharyngeal carcinoma. *N Engl J Med* 295; 20:1101–1106, 1976.

133. International Agency for Research in Cancer: *Monograph 15.* Lyon, IARC, 1977.

134. Smith AH, Handley MA, Wood R: Epidemiological evidence indicates asbestos causes laryngeal cancer. *J Occup Med* 32:499–507, 1990.

135. Eisen EA, Tolbert PE, Monson RR, Smith TJ: Mortality studies of machining fluid exposure in the automobile industry. *Am J Ind Med* 22:809–824, 1992.

136. Steenland K, Schnorr T, Beaumont J, et al: Incidence of laryngeal cancer and exposure to acid mists. *Br J Ind Med* 45:766–776, 1988.

137. Doll R, Hill AB: Lung cancer and other causes of death in relation to smoking: second report on mortality of British doctors. *Br Med J* 2:1071–1081, 1956.

138. Doll R, Peto R: The causes of cancer: quantitative estimates of avoidable risks of cancer in the United States today. *JNCI* 66:1192–1308, 1981.

139. Samet JM, Lerchen ML: Proportion of lung cancer caused by occupation: A critical review. In Gee JBL, Morgan WKC (eds): *Occupational Lung Disease.* New York, Raven Press, 1983.

140. Willett WC: Micronutrients and cancer risk. *Am J Clin Nutr* 59:1162S–1165S, 1994.

141. Omenn GS, Goodman GE, Thornquist MD, et al: The carotene and retinol efficacy trial (CARET) to prevent lung cancer in high-risk populations: pilot study with asbestos-exposed workers. *Cancer Epidemiology, Biomarkers & Prevention* 2:381–387, 1993.

142. Doll R: Mortality from lung cancer in asbestos workers. *Br J Ind Med* 12:81–86, 1955.

143. Berry G: Mortality of workers certified by pneumoconiosis medical panels as having asbestosis. *Br J Ind Med* 38:130–137, 1981.

144. Ives JC, Buffler PA, Greenberg SD: Environmental associations and histopathologic patterns of carcinoma of the lung: the challenge and dilemma in epidemiologic studies. *Am Rev Respir Dis* 128:195–209, 1983.

145. Kipen, HM, Lilis R, Suzuki Y, Valciukas JA, Selikoff IJ: Pulmonary fibrosis in asbestos insulation workers with lung cancer: a radiological and histopathological evaluation. *Br J Ind Med* 44:96–100, 1987.

146. Hillerdal G: Pleural plaques and risk for bronchial carcinoma and mesothelioma: a prospective study. *Chest* 105: 144–150, 1994.

147. Hughes JM, Weill H: Asbestos and man-made fibers. In Samet JM (ed): *Epidemiology of Lung Cancer*. New York, Marcel Dekker, 1994, pp 185–205.

148. Hammond EC, Selikoff IJ, Seidman H: Asbestos exposure, cigarette smoking, and death rates. *Ann NY Acad Sci* 33:473–490, 1979.

149. Blot WJ, Fraumeni JF: Arsenic and lung cancer. In Samet JM (ed): *Epidemiology of Lung Cancer*. New York, Marcel Dekker, 1994, pp 207–218.

150. McCallum RI, Wooley V, Petrie A: Lung cancer associated with chloromethyl methyl ether manufacture: an investigation at two factories in the United Kingdom. *Br J Ind Med* 40:384–389, 1983.

151. Wada S, Miyanishi M, Nishimoto Y, et al: Mustard gas as a cause of respiratory neoplasia in man. *Lancet* 1: 1161–1163, 1968.

152. Takahashi K, Ocubo T: A prospective cohort study of chromium plating workers in Japan. *Arch Environ Health* 45:107–111, 1990.

153. Dong MH, Redmond CK, Mazumdar S, Costantino JP: A multistage approach to the cohort analysis of lifetime lung cancer risk among steelworkers exposed to coke oven emissions. *Am J Epidemiol* 128:860–872, 1988.

154. Darby SC, Samet JM: Radon. In Samet JM (ed): *Epidemiology of Lung Cancer*. New York, Marcel Dekker, 1994, pp 219–243.

155. Reger RB, Morgan WK: Respiratory cancers in mining. *Occupational Medicine: State of the Art Reviews*. 8:185–204, 1993.

156. Wu W, Steenland K, Brown D, et al: Cohort and case-control analyses of workers exposed to vinyl chloride: an update. *J Occup Med* 31:518, 1989.

157. Mancuso TF: Mortality study of beryllium industry workers—occupational lung cancer. *Environ Res* 21: 48–55, 1980.

158. O'berg MT, Chen JL, Burke CA, et al: Epidemiologic study of workers exposed to acrylonitrile: an update. *J Occup Med* 27:835–840, 1985.

159. Sorahan T: Mortality from lung cancer among a cohort of nickel cadmium battery workers: 1946–84. *Br J Ind Med* 44:803–809, 1987.

160. Goldsmith DF: Silica exposure and pulmonary cancer. In Samet JM (ed): *Epidemiology of Lung Cancer*. New York, Marcel Dekker, 1994: pp 245–298.

161. Enterline PE: Carcinogenic effects of man-made vitreous fibers. *Annu Rev Pub Health* 12:459–480, 1991.

162. Coultas DB, Samet JM: Occupational Lung Cancer. In Epler GR (ed): *Clinics in Chest Medicine; Occupational Lung Diseases*. Philadelphia, WB Saunders, 1992, vol 13, pp 341–354.

163. Samet JM: Indoor radon and lung cancer—estimating the risks. *West J Med* 156:25–29, 1992.

164. Pershagen G, Akerblom G, Axelson O, et al: Residential radon exposure and lung cancer in Sweden. *N Engl J Med* 330:159–164, 1994.

165. Létoumeau EA, Krewski D, Choi NW, et al: Case control study of radon and lung cancer in Winnipeg, Manitoba, Canada. *Am J Epidemiol* 140:310–322, 1994.

166. Pershagen G: Passive Smoking and Lung Cancer. In Samet JM (ed). *Epidemiology of Lung Cancer*. New York, Marcel Dekker, 1994, pp 109–130.

167. Janerich DT, Thompson WD, Varela LR, et al: Lung cancer and exposure to tobacco smoke in the household. *N Engl J Med* 323:632–636, 1990.

168. Speizer FE, Samet JM: Air pollution and lung cancer. In Samet JM (ed): *Epidemiology of Lung Cancer*. New York, Marcel Dekker, 1994, pp 131–150.

169. Smith KR, Youcheng L: Indoor air pollution in developing countries. In Samet JM (ed): *Epidemiology of Lung Cancer*. New York, Marcel Dekker, 1994, pp 151–184.

170. Lilis R, Ribak J, Suzuki Y, et al: Non-malignant chest x-ray changes in patients with mesothelioma in a large cohort of asbestos insulation workers. *Br J Ind Med* 44: 402–406, 1987.

171. Antman DH: Natural history and epidemiology of malignant mesothelioma. *Chest* 103:373s–376s, 1993.

172. Schwartz J: Air pollution and the duration of acute respiratory symptoms. *Arch Environ Health* 47:116–122, 1992.

173. Pope CA: Respiratory disease associated with community air pollution and a steel mill, Utah valley. *Am J Public Health* 79:623–628, 1989.

174. Dockery DW, Pope AC 3d, Xu X, et al: An association between air pollution and mortality in six U.S. cities (see comments). *N Engl J Med* 329:1753–1759, 1993.

175. Schwartz J, Dockery DW: Increased mortality in Philadelphia associated with daily air pollution concentrations. *Am Rev Respir Dis* 145:600–604, 1992.

176. Gong JH: Health effects of air pollution. In Epler GR (ed): *Clinics in Chest Medicine; Occupational Lung Diseases*. Philadelphia, WB Saunders, 1992, vol 13, pp 201–214.

177. Samet JM, Utell MJ: Air pollution. In Bone RC (ed): *Pulmonary and Critical Care Medicine*. St. Louis, CV Mosby, 1994, vol 4, pp 1–15.

178. Hodgson MJ: Exposures in indoor air. In Rosenstock L, Cullen MR: *Textbook of Clinical Occupational and Environmental Medicine*. Philadelphia, WB Saunders, 1994, pp 866–875.

179. Gold DR: Indoor air pollution. In Epler GR (ed): *Clinics in Chest Medicine; Occupational Lung Diseases*. Philadelphia, WB Saunders, 1992, vol 13, pp 215–230.

180. Chilmonczyk BA, Salmun LM, Megathlin KN, et al: Association between exposure to environmental tobacco smoke and exacerbations of asthma in children. *N Engl J Med* 328:1665–1669, 1993.

# Chapter 15

# Lung Neoplasms

**Richard A. Matthay**
**Darryl C. Carter**

## LUNG CARCINOMA

LUNG CANCER IS the most common malignant neoplasm in men throughout the world (1–3). It constitutes 16% of all malignant tumors and accounts for 28% of all cancer deaths (35% in men and 19% in women) and about 6% of all deaths (1, 2, 4). In the United States, it is the leading cause of death from cancer in both men and women (1). While mortality due to solid tumors, such as stomach tumors and carcinoma of the uterine cervix, has been declining in this country, the incidence of deaths from lung cancer has continued to rise (Figs. 15.1 and 15.2) (1–4). An estimated 157,400 Americans will die of lung cancer in 1995—95,400 men and 62,000 women (1). Moreover, by the year 2000, the World Health Organization (WHO) states there will be 2,000,000 cases of lung cancer annually worldwide—resulting in enormous health costs (5, 6).

The average patient with carcinoma of the lung is a heavy cigarette smoker in the 6th or 7th decade of life. Other age groups are affected, but less than 5% of patients are under 40 years of age. In the past, lung cancer was a problem primarily confined to males. However, the incidence of this neoplasm has now increased more rapidly in women (1). Between 1953 and 1983, lung cancer deaths increased by 184% in men and by a staggering 360% in women. Also, lung cancer recently surpassed breast carcinoma as the leading cancer killer in women. The declining male:female ratio appears to parallel the well-documented increase in the number of women smokers (1, 7).

The economic costs of lung cancer are enormous (8). In the United States, lung cancer–associated medical costs are estimated to exceed $10 billion and represent 1.5% of the total national cost of illness. Twenty percent of the cost is for direct health care, while lost wages and productivity account for 80%. The potentially greater

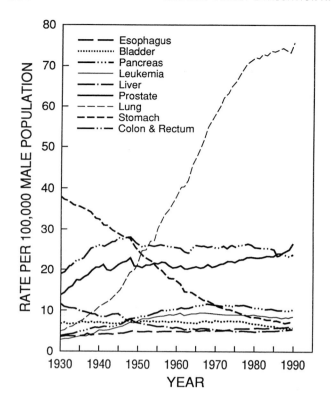

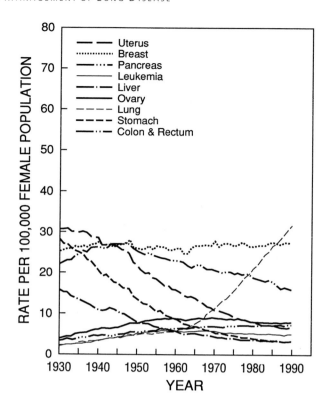

**FIGURE 15.1.** Age-adjusted cancer death rates for selected sites, males, United States, 1930–1990. Age-adjusted to the 1970 U.S. standard population. (Adapted with permission from Boring CC, Squire TS, Tong T, Montgomery S: Cancer statistics, 1994. *CA* 44:7–26, 1994.)

**FIGURE 15.2.** Age-adjusted cancer deaths for selected sites, females, United States, 1930–1990. Age-adjusted to the 1970 U.S. standard population. (Adapted with permission from Boring CC, Squire TS, Tong T, Montgomery S: Cancer statistics, 1994. *CA* 44:7–26, 1994.)

costs of other cigarette-related illnesses, such as heart disease and chronic obstructive lung disease, are not even taken into account in this figure.

### ETIOLOGY

#### Tobacco Smoking

A vast amount of statistical evidence has incriminated smoking of tobacco, especially cigarettes, as the main cause of the progressive rise in mortality from bronchial carcinoma (1, 4, 6, 9). Retrospective and a steadily increasing body of prospective data indicate that a dose-response relationship exists between cigarette smoking and lung cancer; the demographic distribution of this cancer correlates with long-term smoking habits; reduced lung cancer rates are found among ex-smokers; and lung cancer has been induced by the administration of tar or inhaled cigarette smoke in experimental animals (1, 7, 10).

For both men and women, the risk of developing lung cancer is related directly to total exposure to cigarette smoke as measured by the number of cigarettes

smoked, the duration of smoking in years, the age of initiation of smoking, the depth of inhalation, and the tar and nicotine levels in the cigarettes smoked (8). Worldwide prospective epidemiologic studies confirm these associations and indicate that in comparison with nonsmokers, average cigarette smokers have approximately a 9- to 10-fold increased risk of developing lung cancer, and heavy smokers at least a 10- to 25-fold increased risk (1, 7, 10, 11). In a review of 3070 new patients with lung cancer, the Edinburgh Lung Cancer Group found only 74 lifelong nonsmokers (2.4%), of whom 19 were men (0.6%) and 55 were women (1.8%) (12). Among smokers, the presence of airway obstruction is an additional risk factor for lung cancer, after adjustment for pack-years smoked (4).

In one of the more persuasive studies (13), all male doctors over 35 years of age in Britain were asked to state their smoking habits, and the proportion of these dying from carcinoma of the bronchus was determined during the later years. The risk of dying from carcinoma of the bronchus increased with the amount smoked and was highest for those who smoked cigarettes only. The risk for pipe smokers was considerably higher than for nonsmokers but was less than for cigarette smokers. An encouraging finding was that the risk decreased rapidly in those who stopped smoking, and it was halved in those who had stopped for 1 to 5 years. Moreover, data compiled in the United States indicate that the risk of lung cancer among ex-smokers declines progressively for 2 to 15 years following discontinuation of smoking, after which it equals that of lifelong nonsmokers (13).

The number of smokers in the United States is estimated to be more than 50 million (8). However, the percentage of white males still smoking has been decreasing steadily since 1964 when the Surgeon General of the United States issued the first major report linking smoking to lung cancer, and in 1982–1983, for the first time in over 50 years, new cases of lung cancer in adult white males dropped by 4%. In contrast, lung cancer cases in women are still increasing, since the smoking rate in women did not begin to decline until 1976. Brown and Kessler (14) have projected reductions in lung cancer mortality in the next century which depend primarily on the effectiveness of current efforts to reduce smoking prevalence. Figure 15.3 shows their projections of the United States age-adjusted lung cancer death rate with (*solid lines*) and without (*dashed lines*) additional successful interventions targeted at smoking prevention. In men, the higher current rate of lung cancer will plateau and begin to decline in the late 1990s, whereas in women, the rate will peak and start to decline after the year 2010.

An extremely controversial area is that of "passive smoking," or environmental tobacco smoke (ETS). Studies have shown that sidestream smoke actually has higher concentrations of carcinogens than mainstream smoke (15), and nonsmokers exposed to ETS may have measurable levels of carbon monoxide or urinary cotinine, an indication of significant smoke inhalation. Several studies have examined the risk of lung cancer developing in passive smokers, and the weight of evidence now shows that there is an increased, albeit small, risk of lung cancer in passive smokers (4, 16, 17). An average lifetime passive smoke exposure to a smoking spouse increases a nonsmoker's low risk by about 35% compared with the risk of 1000% (tenfold) for a lifetime of active smoking (4).

Lung cancer does, of course, exist in nonsmokers, but two features make it distinct: the considerably lower incidence of the disease in nonsmokers and a different histologic distribution among them (18). Thus, smoking is associated chiefly with squamous cell carcinoma and, to a lesser degree, with the small cell type (6, 18). In nonsmokers, the predominant cell type

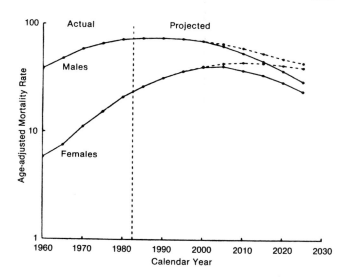

**FIGURE 15.3.** Actual (up to 1982) and projected age-adjusted lung cancer mortality rates for U.S. white men and women, 1960–2025. *Solid line* indicates projections based on current trends in smoking prevalence, per capita consumption, initiation, age, and cigarette tar content. *Dotted lines* represent projections assuming achievement of a reduction in overall smoking prevalence to 15% of U.S. adults in 1990, according to the National Cancer Institute Year 2000 Project. (This national goal in smoking cessation was not reached in 1990). (From Brown CC, Kessler LG: Projections of lung cancer mortality in the United States: 1986–2025. *JNCI* 80:43–51, 1988.)

is adenocarcinoma (17), although this tumor is more prevalent in smokers.

**Atmospheric Pollution**

Both in the United States and in the United Kingdom, mortality is higher in urban areas than in rural regions and increases with the degree of urbanization, even if allowance is made for differences in smoking habits (19). This fact suggests an etiologic role for atmospheric pollution in the development of lung carcinoma, yet such a role is difficult to elucidate. Various carcinogenic agents, such as 3,4-benzpyrene, 1:12-benzperylene, arsenious oxide, radioactive substances, nickel and chromium compounds, and noncombustible aliphatic hydrocarbons, are present in the atmosphere (20). There may be synergism between air pollutants such as these and tobacco smoke, for when extracts of filtered air pollutants and tobacco smoking condensate are applied to mouse skin, their carcinogenicity is at least additive (18).

**Occupational Factors (also see Chapter 14)**

Specific agents found in industrial exposure have been related to the development of bronchial carcinoma and are listed in Table 15.1 (4). The most

## Table 15.1
### Substances Encountered in Workplace Exposures Categorized as Causative for Bronchogenic Carcinoma

Arsenic
Asbestos
Bis(chloromethyl) ether and chloromethyl methyl ether
Chromium and certain chromium compounds (hexavalent chromium)
Ionizing radiation, gamma radiation x-rays
Manmade mineral fibers (certain kinds only)
Mustard gas
Nickel in nickel refining
Radon progency (decay products)
Soots, tars, mineral oils (polycyclic aromatic hydrocarbons)
Vinyl chloride

Adapted with permission from Beckett WS: Epidemiology and etiology of lung cancer. *Clin Chest Med* 14:1–15, 1993.

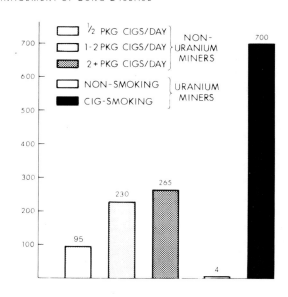

**Figure 15.4.** Lung cancer due to smoking and uranium exposure. (Adapted from Wright ES, Hammond EC: Radiation-induced carcinoma of the lung—the St. Lawrence tragedy. *J Thorac Cardiovasc Surg* 74:496, 1977.)

notorious ones are radioactive material, asbestos, chromates, nickel, mustard gas, isopropyl oil, hydrocarbons, arsenic, hematite, vinyl chloride, and bis(chloromethyl) ether (4, 10, 18–24).

*Radioactive Materials*

All types of radiation may be carcinogenic. The lung cancer risk is increased from 3 to 30 times, depending on the degree of exposure (19). The latent period (interval between beginning of exposure and onset of lung cancer) is more than 10 years, the mean value being 16 to 17 years. There is a strong association between exposure to uranium and development of bronchogenic carcinoma, particularly small cell carcinoma (6). It is well documented that the combination of smoking and uranium exposure markedly increases the risk of developing lung cancer (Fig. 15.4) (21–23).

*Asbestos*

Asbestos is now a universally recognized carcinogen and appears to be the most frequent occupational cause of human lung cancer (4, 18, 20, 25, 26). Among asbestos workers, 1 death of 5 is due to lung cancer, 1 of 10 to pleural or peritoneal mesotheliomas, and 1 of 10 to gastrointestinal carcinomas (20). The latent period is usually 20 years or more (20, 25).

There are differences in carcinogenic potential of the various types of asbestos. Men exposed to chrysotile asbestos have a respiratory tract cancer mortality 2 to 4 times higher than controls, while those exposed to a combination of chrysotile and crocidolite asbestos have a mortality rate 5.3 times higher than controls. For amosite asbestos, the death rate due to respiratory cancer is more than 10 times higher than in controls.

Tobacco is a critical cofactor (4, 6, 20, 26). Most cases

of lung cancer in occupationally exposed workers occur in smokers with asbestosis, and the distribution of cell types is about the same as that of smokers (6). Lung cancer in asbestos-exposed nonsmokers is uncommon (6).

Asbestos exposure is more than an occupational hazard confined to such industries as shipbuilding and manufacture and installation of brake lining and insulation (20, 25). Asbestos fibers (ferruginous bodies) have been found in the lungs of 100% of city dwellers in France, and the atmosphere in New York City contains $10 \times 10^{-9}$ g of asbestos per cubic meter of air, which corresponds to millions of submicroscopic fibrils (20). The significance of prolonged exposure to such concentrations of asbestos remains uncertain.

*Other Occupational Factors*

Workers engaged in the handling of chromates from chromium-containing iron ore have approximately a 4 to 15 times greater incidence of lung cancer than the general population (20). There is usually a long latent period, similar to the 20 years that commonly elapses between asbestos exposure and tumor occurrence (20). Nickel refinery workers were once noted to have a 3- to 5-fold increased lung cancer mortality and a 150-fold increased risk of nasal cancer. Nickel dust was the likely responsible carcinogen, although generally adopted changes in the refinery process made before World War II not only drastically reduced nickel dust levels but also reduced worker exposure to arsenic.

Arsenic is a known carcinogen that has been implicated in the development of lung cancer in individuals given arsenic-containing drugs or engaged in the manufacture and use of pesticides.

The mining of hematite (an iron ore containing ferric oxide and silica) is associated with an increased risk of lung cancer (20). In addition, a number of other industrial operations in which exposure to iron and silica is common may be responsible for a poorly quantified but increased risk of lung cancer. These include metal grinding, sandblasting, and iron and steel foundry work.

## Diet

Several epidemiologic studies have shown a relation between greater dietary intake of vegetables and modestly lower risk for lung and other cancers (4). Beta-carotene (a precursor to the class of retinoids, including retinol or vitamin A, which are found in many green, yellow, and orange fruits and vegetables) may be the substance associated with lower lung-cancer risk (4, 27). The protective effect is particularly evident in current or past cigarette smokers (4). A variety of studies in several countries have shown (a) low dietary intake of these fruits and vegetables is associated with an increased lung cancer risk (Fig. 15.5) and (b) a low serum level of beta-carotene is associated with risk for later development of lung cancer (4, 27, 28).

### Genetic Factors

A minority of heavy cigarette smokers (approximately one in eight) develops lung cancer, suggesting that other factors are important in determining risk (4). Family studies have shown repeatedly a slightly greater lung cancer risk, two- to threefold, in nonsmokers who are relatives of lung cancer patients, compared with nonsmokers who have no family history of lung cancer (29–31). Environmental factors are probably superimposed on genetic patterns that predispose to lung cancer (4). In fact, genetic factors may exert an influence on the development of lung cancer equal to that of cigarette smoking (18, 32–35).

The genetically determined ability to metabolize carcinogens may have a direct role in lung cancer risk (4). One such inherited variant in xenobiotic metabolism is the arylhydrocarbon hydroxylase system (4). The inducible enzyme aryl hydrocarbon hydroxylase (AHH) converts the polycyclic hydrocarbons of cigarette smoke into epoxides, compounds that are highly

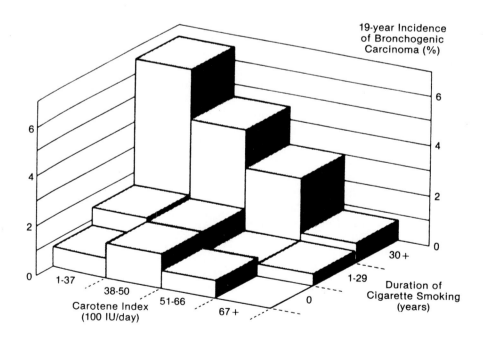

**FIGURE 15.5.** Association of an index of dietary beta-carotene and the duration of cigarette smoking with the 19-year index of cigarette smoking in the Western Electric study. Dietary index was based on questionnaires about food intake during the previous 28 days given to 2100 men aged 40 to 55 years at examinations separated by 1 year. Intake of preformed retinol (vitamin A) and other nutrients was not significantly associated with lung cancer risk. (From Shekelle RB, Liu S, Raynor WJ, et al: Dietary vitamin A and risk of cancer in the Western Electric Study. *Lancet* 2:1185–1190, 1981; with permission.)

carcinogenic (4, 21, 32, 33). The inducibility of AHH by polycyclic hydrocarbons appears to be controlled by a single gene. The degree of inducibility of this enzyme in lymphocytes from patients with and without lung cancer has been correlated with the presence or absence of lung cancer but also with cigarette smoking, independent of the presence of lung cancer (3, 36).

Moreover, several genetic changes have been associated with small cell and non–small cell carcinomas of the lung (4, 6, 34, 35). These include loss of DNA sequences on the short arm of chromosome 3 ("3p") or 11 ("11p") and amplification of a number of oncogenes (tumor-promoting genes), including the *myc* family (C-*myc*, N-*myc*, L-*myc*) and the *ras* family (K-*ras*, H-*ras*, N-*ras*). Such genetic markers, it should be emphasized, are not necessarily heritable and may represent markers for the effects of carcinogens such as those in tobacco (4).

It is likely, therefore, that the etiology of lung cancer is multifactorial, involving far more than a simple association with smoking. Undoubtedly, other environmental carcinogens have additive, even synergistic, effects, and certain genetic characteristics probably increase susceptibility to these environmental carcinogens (18, 34, 35, 37).

## PATHOLOGY

### Classification

A committee of pathologists convened by the World Health Organization (WHO) established the standard classification system for lung cancer (38). As new data become available on the natural history of treated and untreated lung cancer, this comprehensive system continues to be updated (6, 38, 39). According to this classification, the four major cell types of cancer and their approximate relative incidence include squamous cell carcinoma (30 to 32%), small cell carcinoma (20 to 25%), adenocarcinoma (33 to 35%), and large cell carcinoma (15 to 18%). Bronchoalveolar carcinomas (so-called alveolar cell carcinomas) are considered adenocarcinomas; as a group, they comprise 3 to 4% of all lung carcinomas (40, 41).

### Pathogenesis

Squamous cell bronchogenic carcinomas arise most commonly in segmental and subsegmental bronchi in response to repetitive carcinogenic stimuli, inflammation, or irritation (42). The mucosal lining is most susceptible to injury, particularly at the bifurcation of bronchial structures. Ciliary mechanisms and superficial columnar lining cells tend to shed or become denuded, a process abetted by the physiologically altered

air flow and reduced mucus flow rates at these sites. Carcinogenic agents are more likely to be deposited, absorbed, and retained in these zones. Basal (reserve) cells are stimulated to proliferate.

Hyperplasia of mucin-secreting columnar epithelial cells is followed, in some cases, by replacement of the bronchial lining by an orderly arrangement of metaplastic, stratified squamous epithelium. Metaplasia is a response to injury by either carcinogenic or noncarcinogenic agents. In the course of carcinogenesis, the basal half of the metaplastic epithelium may become disorganized. Cells lose their usual polarity and individual cells develop atypical, irregular, hyperchromatic nuclei. Abnormal mitoses may be identified, while the superficial layers of the mucosa retain a stratified, flattened, but unified pattern. These changes are termed atypical metaplasia or dysplasia (43). Eventually, the entire thickness of the mucosa may be replaced by proliferating neoplastic cells (carcinoma in situ).

Infiltrating neoplasms may develop at some unpredictable future time when the integrity of the basal membrane has been lost. This mechanism pertains particularly to bronchial squamous cell malignancies in experimental animals as well as in humans. Factors associated with these changes include smoking and occupational exposure to arsenic, uranium, chromium, asbestos, or other minerals (4, 10, 18). The pathogenesis of small cell carcinoma is not as well understood; but this tumor may also originate in the basal cells of the bronchial epithelium.

Multiple exogenous and endogenous factors are associated with adenocarcinomas, which probably arise from the mucin-secreting cells in the more peripheral bronchi (35, 36). Among the exogenous factors are asbestos, cadmium, chromium, beryllium, and pneumoconiotic dusts. Endogenous conditions include chronic interstitial pneumonitis and fibrosis, progressive systemic sclerosis (scleroderma), and scars associated with pulmonary infarction.

### Histology

#### Squamous Cell Carcinoma

Squamous cell carcinoma, also called epidermoid carcinoma (Figs. 7.20, 15.6, and 15.7), is the second most common bronchogenic carcinoma (6, 42, 43). These tumors are composed predominantly of flattened or polygonal neoplastic epithelial cells that tend to stratify, form intercellular bridges, and elaborate keratin on an individual cell basis or in the complex of an epithelial pearl. Based on the degree of differentiation, these tumors are divided into three subtypes: well differentiated, moderately well differentiated, and poorly differentiated. They usually arise from the bronchial mucosa and are frequently associated with adjoining foci of intraepithelial malignancy or dyspla-

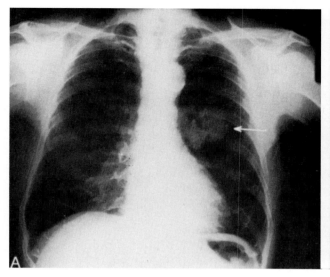

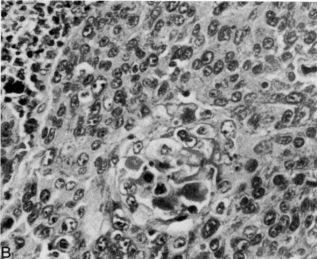

**FIGURE 15.6.** **A,** Squamous cell carcinoma. A posterior-anterior (PA) chest radiograph shows a 3-cm mass adjacent to the left hilum *(arrow)*. **B,** Squamous cell carcinoma histology. Squamous cell carcinomas are characterized by the presence of keratin in the cytoplasm of the malignant cell. The malignant cells are frequently connected by an extensive series of intercellular bridges and may form small "pearls" in which the squamous cells are arranged in small groups. In this figure, the cells at the periphery do not show differentiation, but the central portion contains some cells with markedly hyperchromatic nuclei and keratinized cytoplasm characteristic of squamous cell carcinoma.

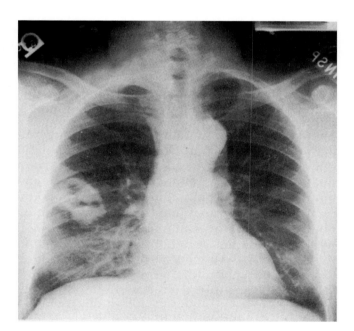

**FIGURE 15.7.** Squamous cell carcinoma. PA chest radiograph shows a large cavitating peripheral squamous cell carcinoma in the right hemithorax.

sia. In about two-thirds of cases, they present as a proximal or hilar lesion, and it is uncommon for them to metastasize early (6). The tumors tend to be bulky, to encroach on bronchial lumina, with the production of obstructing intraluminal granular or polypoid masses, and to invade cartilage and adjoining lymph nodes. One-half of differentiated squamous cell lung carcinomas are confined to the thorax at autopsy (44).

*Small Cell Carcinoma*

Small cell carcinomas (Fig. 15.8) have been divided by WHO into three groups: oat cell, intermediate, and combined (45). Oat cell (lymphocyte-like) carcinoma is composed of cells with round-to-oval nuclei. The nucleoli are always indistinct, and the cytoplasm is scanty. The intermediate (polygonal) cell type is the most common type and is characterized by cells with somewhat larger, more vesicular, fusiform or spindled nuclei. Nuclear chromatin retains a fine salt-and-pepper distribution, and the nucleoli are indistinct. The cytoplasm is minimal or appears absent. The third variant of small cell carcinoma is the combined type in which small cell carcinoma is combined with another cell type. The most important combined variant is the small cell and large cell variant, described by Radice and coworkers in 1982 (46), which is regarded as small cell carcinoma for treatment purposes. It lacks sensitiv-

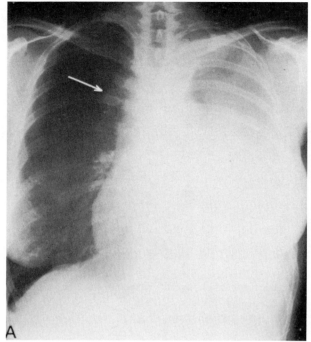
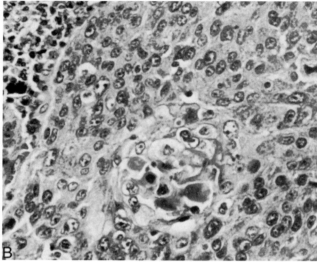

**FIGURE 15.8. A,** Small cell carcinoma. PA chest radiograph showing a large left pleural effusion opacifying the left hemithorax. Note the mediastinal adenopathy manifested on the chest radiograph by a density in the right paratracheal area *(arrow).* Pleural fluid analysis revealed malignant cells, and bronchoscopy revealed a large endobronchial mass identified as small cell carcinoma on biopsy. **B,** Histology of small cell carcinoma. The nucleus of small cell carcinoma is different from that of other types of lung cancer. It is characterized by the relatively even distribution of chromatin throughout the nucleus. There is no clearing of the chromatin, and nucleoli are never prominent. The cytoplasm of the cell varies from the small rim of cytoplasm seen in the oat cell variant (shown in this photomicrograph) to a moderate amount of eosinophilic cytoplasm seen in the polygonal variant. The subtyping of various types of small cell carcinoma has been shown to have a profound effect on prognosis or response to therapy.

ity to radiation and chemotherapy but retains the aggressiveness of the "pure" small cell carcinoma.

Although 75 to 80% of the small cell carcinomas present as proximal lesions, they may arise in any part of the tracheobronchial tree (38). They tend to lift the mucosa slightly to form a velvety, thickened lining; rapidly invade vascular channels, mediastinal lymph nodes, and soft tissue; and disseminate widely, often before pulmonary symptoms are recognized or provoked. In contrast to epidermoid carcinoma, the lumen is usually not filled with tumor. Instead, spread tends to occur through the submucosa and compromises the lumen in this way.

The tumor is usually extensive when discovered, with little or no chance of 5-year survival (6). The most common sites of metastatic involvement at initial presentation are listed in Table 15.2 (47).

### Adenocarcinoma

Adenocarcinoma, the most prevalent carcinoma of the lung in both sexes (6), forms acinar or glandular structures (Fig. 15.9) (42, 43, 48). Histologically, this tumor is divided broadly into well-differentiated, moderately well differentiated, poorly differentiated, and bronchioloalveolar types.

Fifty-five to 60% of adenocarcinomas are located in the periphery of lung, not obviously related to any bronchus. Peripheral adenocarcinomas are frequently circumscribed and subpleural with central pigmented fibrotic cores. Classic bronchioloalveolar carcinomas, whether single, multicentric, or lobar in type, tend to use existing alveolar septa as a framework for their growth and are not scar associated.

The liver, adrenals, bone, and central nervous system are frequent sites of metastases (6). In over half the cases studied at autopsy the brain is involved, and in 12% the brain was the sole site of metastasis (40).

### Large Cell Carcinoma

Large cell carcinoma, also called undifferentiated carcinoma, includes all tumors that show no evidence

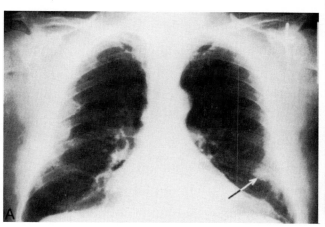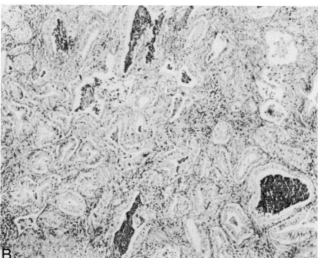

FIGURE 15.9. **A,** Adenocarcinoma. PA chest radiograph shows a 1.5-cm solitary lesion in the lingula *(arrow).* Note also rib fractures in the right hemithorax, a finding due to previous trauma. **B,** Histology of adenocarcinoma. Adenocarcinomas of the lung are characterized by gland formation in a fibrous background. Numerous glands are formed in this well-differentiated adenocarcinoma.

**TABLE 15.2**
**SITES OF METASTASES IN PATIENTS PRESENTING WITH SMALL CELL LUNG CANCER**

| Site | Percentage |
|---|---|
| Bone | 35 |
| Liver | 25 |
| Bone marrow | 20 |
| Brain | 10 |
| Extrathoracic lymph nodes | 5 |
| Subcutaneous masses | 5 |

Reproduced with permission from Johnson BE: Management of small cell lung cancer. *Clin Chest Med* 14:173–187, 1993.

of differentiation to small cell, squamous cell, or adenocarcinoma (Fig. 15.10) (42, 43). In general, these tumors are composed of pleomorphic cells with variably enlarged nuclei and prominent nucleoli with abundant cytoplasm. The tumors tend to form large, bulky, somewhat circumscribed and necrotic masses, are frequently subpleural in origin, invade locally, and disseminate widely. About 60% are in the periphery of the lung. The metastatic pattern of large cell carcinoma is similar to that of the adenocarcinomas, with cerebral metastases in over half the cases (6).

The giant cell variant of large cell carcinoma is composed of huge, multinucleated, bizarre cells that are frequently associated with an extensive inflammatory cell infiltrate (6). These tumors are usually large and peripheral, and are very aggressive, highly malignant, and most often found at a late stage (4, 6). These lesions show an ability to metastasize widely, curiously with a predilection for the small intestine (6, 49).

## CLINICAL MANIFESTATIONS

### Symptoms and Signs

Approximately 5% of patients with lung cancer are asymptomatic, and the tumor is discovered on routine radiographic examination of the chest (48). Other patients have one or more symptoms and signs related to the presence of the tumor, although the symptomatology may not be specific to lung cancer. Shields and Ritts have divided these symptoms and signs into the following categories: bronchopulmonary, extrapulmonary intrathoracic, extrathoracic metastatic, and extrathoracic nonmetastatic (48).

### Bronchopulmonary Symptoms

Irritation of the bronchus results in cough, which may be productive or nonproductive and is frequently described by the patient as being a "cigarette cough." Among 4000 patients with bronchial carcinoma, cough was present and considered severe in 40% (50). Ulceration of the tumor results in hemoptysis, which most often presents as episodic blood streaking of the sputum. Hemoptysis occurs in approximately 60% of patients; massive hemoptysis is rare (48).

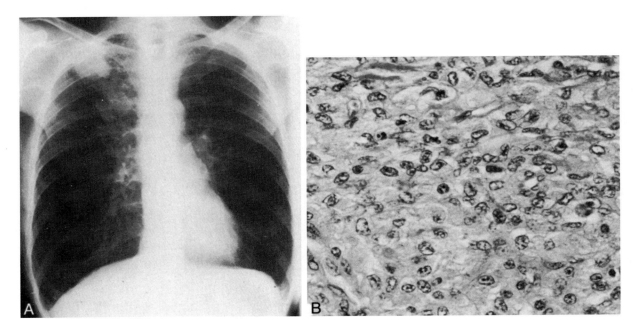

**Figure 15.10.** **A,** Large cell carcinoma. PA chest radiograph shows a right apical density adjacent to the pleura and chest wall and a proximal density adjacent to the right tracheal wall. **B,** Histology of large cell undifferentiated carcinoma. The cells of a large cell undifferentiated carcinoma are characterized by a moderate amount of cytoplasm, nuclei that are usually oval or round with some chromatin clearing, and the presence of one or several nucleoli, which may be markedly irregular in shape. These cells contain neither keratin nor mucin.

Airway obstruction, complete or partial, may lead to wheezing, dyspnea, and occasionally, stridor. The obstruction may lead to atelectasis with infection of the distal pulmonary parenchyma. The inflammatory process, obstructive pneumonitis, or abscess formation leads to febrile respiratory symptoms, which may be present in as many as one-third of patients (48). Unfortunately, the febrile episode may be misinterpreted by the physician, for it may be ameliorated by antibiotic therapy and thus lead to delay in diagnosis.

Vague chest pains, often described as a dull ache, occur in up to 50% of patients (48). This chest pain may be due to inflammatory involvement of the parietal pleura and chest wall.

*Extrapulmonary Intrathoracic Symptoms*

Approximately 15% of patients complain of symptoms due to growth of the tumor outside the lung into the pleura, chest wall, mediastinal structures, and contiguous nerves (38). Hoarseness, due to involvement of the left or rarely the right recurrent laryngeal nerve, and the superior vena caval syndrome both occur in approximately 5% of the patients with carcinoma of the lung (48). The latter syndrome is due to compression or invasion of the superior vena cava by neoplastic tissue from related lymph nodes or is sometimes due to direct invasion by a primary growth in the right upper lobe.

The neck is enlarged and the neck veins distended, which may prompt the patient to report that his or her collar is tight. The face may be suffused and one or both arms edematous. Distended venous collaterals may be observed on the anterior chest wall.

Pleural effusion of varying amounts occurs in 10% of patients and most commonly indicates obstruction to pulmonary lymph flow or metastatic involvement of the pleura (48). Partial obstruction of the esophagus by tumor in paraesophageal lymph nodes causes dysphagia in approximately 1% of patients with lung cancer, as does massive pleural effusion from metastatic involvement of the pleura. Involvement of the branches of the brachial plexus from tumors located in the superior sulcus can cause pain and weakness of the arm and shoulder. Horner's syndrome also may be present in the latter situation (48).

*Extrathoracic Metastatic Symptoms*

Symptoms due to metastatic spread of the tumor outside the thorax account for a small percentage of the presenting complaints of lung carcinoma patients (48). Neurologic symptoms due to intracranial metastases are present in 3 to 6%. These include hemiplegia, epilepsy, personality changes, confusion, speech defects, or only headache. Bone pain and pathologic fracture from metastatic involvement are noted on presentation in 1 to 2%. Rarely, jaundice, ascites, or an abdominal mass is a major complaint. Neck, muscle, or subcutaneous tissue masses are present infrequently.

*Extrathoracic Nonmetastatic Manifestations (Paraneoplastic Syndromes)*

Approximately 2% of patients with bronchial carcinoma seek medical advice for systemic symptoms and signs not related to metastatic spread of the tumor, the so-called paraneoplastic syndromes (Table 15.3) (6, 49, 50–53). These manifestations are not specific, and they may occur in association with malignant lesions other than bronchogenic carcinoma.

## Metabolic Manifestations

The majority of metabolic manifestations are the result of secretion of endocrine or endocrine-like substances by the tumor (Table 15.4). At times, these syndromes may be produced by tumors that are still resectable, and treatment of the primary tumor may result in complete or partial remission of the paraneoplastic syndrome. Most of the syndromes are found in association with small cell carcinoma (47, 48, 53).

*Cushing's Syndrome*

Approximately 50% of patients with paraneoplastic Cushing's syndrome have bronchogenic carcinoma, with small cell lung cancer and bronchial carcinoid being the most commonly associated tumor types (54). In patients with lung carcinoma, this syndrome differs from the classic syndrome (48, 53). In small cell carcinoma patients, for instance, it is characterized by reversal of the sex ratio, an older age incidence, the prominence of hypokalemic alkalosis, fewer physical stigmata of typical Cushing's syndrome, and a more rapid, fulminating course. This syndrome is clinically apparent in approximately 2 to 5% of patients with small cell carcinoma (47). Adrenocorticotropic hormone (ACTH) has been demonstrated in the tumor tissue and blood of many of these patients. This ectopic ACTH is indistinguishable from the normal hormone, although the tumors have physiologic autonomy, since dexamethasone fails to suppress the levels of ACTH end products in the urine. Excessive quantities of hydroxycorticosteroids (17-OHCS) are demonstrable in the urine. Treating the carcinoma is the most important therapy for patients with ectopic ACTH production.

*Antidiuretic Hormone*

The syndrome of inappropriate antidiuresis (SIAD) with excessive antidiuretic hormone secretion is associated with symptoms of water intoxication—anorexia, nausea, and vomiting accompanied by increasingly severe neurologic complications (53). SIAD is characterized by hyponatremia (serum sodium concentration

**TABLE 15.3**
**CLASSIFICATION OF EXTRAPULMONARY MANIFESTATIONS OF CARCINOMA OF THE LUNG**

Endocrine and metabolic
  Carcinoid syndrome
  Cachexia
  Antidiuretic hormone secretion
  Hypercalcemia
  Ectopic adrenocorticotropic hormone secretion
  Ectopic gonadotropic stimulating hormone secretion
  Gynecomastia
  Insulinlike activity
Neuromuscular
  Hoarseness
  Horner's syndrome
  Seizures
  Cranial nerve abnormalities
  Carcinomatous myopathy
  Peripheral neuropathies
  Eaton-Lambert syndrome
  Cortical-cerebellar degeneration
  Encephalomyelopathy
  Autonomic overactivity
  Dementia, psychosis
Skeletal
  Clubbing
  Pulmonary hypertrophic osteoarthropathy
  Monarticular arthritis
Dermatologic
  Acanthosis nigricans
  Scleroderma
  Dermatomyositis, polymyositis
Cardiovascular
  Migratory thrombophlebitis
  Nonbacterial verrucous endocarditis
  Arterial thrombosis
Hematologic
  Anemia
  Thrombocytosis
  Red cell aplasia
  Fibrinolytic purpura
  Nonspecific leukocytosis
  Polycythemia
  Gastrointestinal
  Jaundice
  Abnormal liver function tests
Renal
  Proteinuria
  Nephrotic syndrome

less than 135 mmol/liter), hyposmolality (plasma osmolality less than 280 mOsm/kg), and impaired water excretion in the absence of hypovolemia, hypotension, ineffective intravascular volume, or abnormalities of cardiac, renal, thyroid and adrenal function (55). Treating the carcinoma is the most important therapy for patients with paraneoplastic SIAD (56). Fluid restriction (less than 800 ml/day) to produce a negative water

**TABLE 15.4**
**TUMOR CELL MARKERS IN BRONCHOGENIC CARCINOMA**

Hormone production
  Adrenocorticotropic hormone (ACTH)
  Melanocyte-stimulating hormone (MSH)
  Human chorionic gonadotropin (HCG)
  Human placental lactogen (HPL)
  Human growth hormone (HGH)
  Parathyroid hormone (PTH)
  Calcitonin
  Antidiuretic hormone (ADH)
  Prolactin
  5-Hydroxytryptophan
  Estradiol
  Hypoglycemic factor
  Renin
  Insulin and glucagon
  Erythropoietin
  Gastrin
Fetoproteins
  α-Fetoprotein (AFP)
  Carcinoembryonic antigen (CEA)
Other compounds
  Placental alkaline phosphatase (PAP)
  Polyamines
  Histaminase
  L-Dopa decarboxylase

balance usually causes a modest rise in serum sodium (56). If hyponatremia persists, chronic daily furosemide with sodium chloride tablets, urea, mannitol, or glycerol has been used in outpatients with variable success. The prognosis is poor in these patients, since most have small cell carcinomas (48).

*Carcinoid Syndrome*

Carcinoid syndrome is a well-defined clinical entity characterized by cutaneous, cardiovascular, gastrointestinal, and respiratory manifestations (6, 48). Neurosecretory granules have been described in small cell tumors that are similar to those seen in carcinoid tumors and thought to be the source of this and other materials (57). Classically, the syndrome includes episodic signs and symptoms related to the release of various vasoactive amines. Flushing or edema, or both, of the face and upper body, hyperperistalsis and diarrhea, tachycardia, wheezing, pruritus, paresthesia, and vasomotor collapse may occur in varying combinations. Many vasoactive substances in addition to serotonin (5-hydroxytryptamine), which was originally thought to be the cause of the clinical features, have been shown to be produced by these tumors. These include 5-hydroxytryptophan, bradykinin and its precursor enzyme kallikrein, and various catecholamines (48).

Treatment of the manifestations of the carcinoid

syndrome, which is usually identified with small cell carcinoma, is only palliative. In addition to irradiation and cytotoxic chemotherapy, corticosteroids, phenothiazines, antihistamines, and kallikrein inhibitors have been used in the management of flushing, with varying degrees of success (48).

*Hypercalcemia*

Hypercalcemia may be caused by bony metastases (20% of cases) or excessive secretion by the tumor of parathyroid hormone–related protein (PTHRP), so-called humoral hypercalcemia of malignancy (80% of cases) (58). An accompanying hypophosphatemia is found frequently. Most of the lung tumors associated with hypercalcemia have been squamous cell in type (6, 48, 58–60). Clinically, the hypercalcemic patient may have somnolence and mental changes as well as anorexia, nausea, vomiting, and weight loss. In resectable cases, removal of the tumor has resulted in calcium blood levels returning to normal. Among treatments used to control hypercalcemia in patients with lung cancer are saline diuresis, calcitonin, plicamycin, etidronate, pamidronate, and gallium nitrate (58).

*Ectopic Gonadotropin*

Ectopic gonadotropin production has been found rarely in association with carcinoma of the lung. Most of these tumors have been large cell carcinomas. Usually the patient is a male with tender gynecomastia, often with hypertrophic osteoarthropathy, in whom production of gonadotropin has been documented (48, 53).

*Hypoglycemia*

Hypoglycemia, the result of increased insulin or insulin-like activity, has been described in association with squamous cell carcinoma and may be relieved after resection of the tumor (61).

**Neuromuscular Manifestations**

Carcinomatous neuromyopathies are the most frequent extrathoracic, nonmetastatic manifestations of carcinoma of the lung, occurring in approximately 15% of these patients (48). In one combined series of patients with such manifestations, 56% had small cell carcinoma, 22% squamous cell carcinoma, 16% large cell tumors, and 5% adenocarcinoma (62). Half of the patients had no other symptoms of the lung tumor, and in one-third, the neuromyopathy preceded by 1 year or more the symptoms or the diagnosis of the carcinoma (48). Thus, neuromyopathic complications are not related to metastases, and their pathogenesis is uncertain. The following main varieties occur.

1. *Mental abnormalities:* Progressive dementia, sometimes with depression, is the most common manifestation. Confusion, stupor, or emotional instability may occur.

2. *Cerebellar degeneration:* Manifested by ataxia, vertigo, and dysarthria.
3. *Sensory neuropathy:* This often starts with numbness and sometimes pain in the face and limbs, gradually progressing to loss of all forms of sensibility throughout the body, loss of reflexes, and occasionally deafness.
4. *Motor neuropathy:* Manifested by progressive wasting, weakness, and fasciculation.
5. *Polyneuritis:* Associated with mixed motor and sensory changes.
6. *Myopathy:* Manifested by atrophic pareses, especially of the muscles of the limb girdles and the proximal limbs, often accompanied by a smooth, red tongue.
7. *Polymyositis:* Characterized by weakness and marked fatigability of the proximal muscles of the extremities, particularly those of the pelvic girdle and thighs. Muscular wasting is prominent, and there is a primary degeneration of muscle fibers.
8. *Autonomic system abnormalities:* Those described include postural hypotension.

## Skeletal Manifestations

The most frequent peripheral sign of bronchial carcinoma is clubbing of the fingers, which at times is associated with generalized hypertrophic pulmonary osteoarthropathy (48). This clinical syndrome consists of swelling of the soft tissues of the terminal phalanges, with curvature of the nails, pain and swelling of the joints, and periostitis, with elevation of the periosteum and new bone formation. The mechanism of development of the tissue changes is not well known, although an increase in blood flow in the affected portions of the limbs has been reported. A prompt fall in the blood flow to normal levels occurs following successful treatment of the underlying condition. The cause of increased flow is unknown.

Both humoral and neurogenic factors have been implicated as the cause of the osteoarthropathy. Elevated levels of estrogen have been described, but the significance of this finding has been questioned. An efferent and afferent neurologic reflex has been postulated, with the afferent fibers running in the vagus or the intercostal nerves. This theory is supported by the observation that the osteoarthropathy may be reversed by cutting either the vagi or intercostal nerves without removal of the underlying disease (63, 64).

The incidence of hypertrophic pulmonary osteoarthropathy in patients with carcinoma of the lung has been reported to be from 2 to 12% (48). It occurs only rarely, if ever, in small cell tumors. Its occurrence is distributed equally among the other three major cell types (squamous, adenocarcinoma, and large cell).

The removal of the pulmonary lesion may give dramatic remission of the arthralgia and peripheral edema; however, osseous radiographic changes regress much more slowly. Recurrence of the pulmonary neoplasm does not necessarily indicate return of the symptoms of osteoarthropathy.

## Dermatologic Manifestations

The development of acanthosis nigricans may be associated with bronchial adenocarcinoma (48). Scleroderma, erythema gyratum, acquired ichthyosis, and nonspecific dermatoses also may occur in patients with bronchial carcinoma (48).

## Vascular Manifestations

Thrombophlebitis, recurrent or migratory, may be the first indication of the presence of bronchial tumor (6, 48). It occurs in approximately 0.3% of all patients with lung cancer (50). The incidence of operability is low in these individuals, and after resection the incidence of death from pulmonary embolism is high (48).

Nonbacterial, verrucous, marantic endocarditis, characterized by deposition of sterile fibrin plaques on the heart valves, and resultant arterial embolization, may occur (48). The mechanism by which these complications takes place is unknown.

## Hematologic Manifestations

Normocytic, normochromic anemia, red cell aplasia, fibrinolytic purpura, erythrocytosis, and nonspecific leukocytosis have all been reported in patients with bronchial carcinoma.

### PRODUCTION OF MARKERS BY BRONCHOGENIC CARCINOMA

Many biologic products are produced by malignancies or in association with malignant diseases (53). These products may be categorized as follows: hormones, antigens, enzymes, fetal proteins, and others. Table 15.4 shows some of the marker substances that have been found in patients with bronchogenic carcinoma. Although methods to measure tumor markers have become increasingly sensitive in clinical studies, the expectation that they will be useful in the diagnosis of lung neoplasia has failed to materialize fully, since elevation of markers in body fluids occurs in nonneoplastic states and some neoplasms fail to express the marker under study. Although none of the tumor markers studied so far has proven to be exclusively tumor specific, the search continues.

Carcinoembryonic antigen (CEA) was first studied as a marker for gastrointestinal neoplasms. Elevated serum levels of CEA (greater than 2.5 ng/ml) have been found in 60 to 86% of patients with bronchogenic carcinoma. Unfortunately, CEA blood levels are not useful for diagnosing lung cancer, since there is considerable overlap between healthy controls and lung cancer patients and because there are significant numbers of false-negative results among patients with widespread disease.

Among surgical patients, postoperative CEA values seem to correlate with survival whether or not the patient is rendered disease free (65–67). Unfortunately, early diagnosis of disease recurrence in lung cancer patients, which CEA levels may provide, is academic because of the lack of effective antitumor therapy. As further advances are made in the early diagnosis and management of cancer, however, tumor cell markers will probably play a valuable role. Moreover, occasionally when symptoms develop, it is difficult to be certain whether they are due to recurrent disease or to other pathologic processes. In such cases, rising CEA values may help in the differential diagnosis of the symptomatic lung cancer patient.

Among other potential lung cancer markers studied are three known markers of medullary thyroid carcinoma—histaminase, L-dopa decarboxylase, and calcitonin (68). Marker levels in mediastinal metastases reflected those in primary lung tumors in 80% of patients. However, in over 50% of patients, multiple hepatic metastases contained low to absent marker levels in spite of simultaneously high levels in chest lesions. Immunohistochemical studies of histaminase revealed that within each primary lung tumor, different cells contain different amounts of enzyme. Since marker contents vary among tumor cells, among primary tumors, and among metastases in individual patients, circulating levels of these markers cannot necessarily be expected to mirror tumor burden in patients with malignant lung tumors.

## DIAGNOSIS

### Screening Techniques for Early Diagnosis of Lung Cancer

Recently, emphasis has been placed on the role of screening high-risk patients (male smokers over the age of 45) for the early diagnosis of lung cancer, since the best chance for therapeutic cure is surgical removal of the small, localized tumor. Techniques include serial chest radiographs and sputum cytology. Five-year follow-up results from three large screening trials (69–73) indicate that (a) the prevalence rate of lung carcinoma increases in individuals over the age of 55, (b) there is an additive value of sputum cytology and chest radiographs in detecting central squamous cell carcinomas

and peripheral adenocarcinomas, and (c) screening patients with stage I tumors augments survival. However, survival was poor for patients with stage II and stage III tumors, and overall survival was not significantly improved by these screening modalities. Whether or not mass screening programs will ultimately have a beneficial impact on augmenting survival for lung cancer is not clear. At this time, there are no official recommendations that advocate screening high-risk patients for lung carcinoma, but the performance of chest radiographs and sputum cytology in long-term smokers over the age of 55 and in asbestos-exposed cigarette smokers may be reasonable.

### Chest Radiographic Features

Most lung cancers are detected by the standard chest radiograph. Although a small percentage of patients have a stage 0 lesion (endobronchial tumor and negative chest film), most will have a detectable lesion on chest radiograph. It is possible to visualize lesions as small as 3 mm, but generally lesions less than 5 to 6 mm in diameter are unlikely to be detected (69, 70). It is usually difficult to differentiate between benign and malignant lesions on a chest radiograph, yet certain radiographic signs may suggest malignancy (74, 75). Spiculation on poorly defined smooth margins of lesions are more indicative of a malignancy; however, a sharply defined smooth margin does not rule out malignancy (76–78). The presence of calcification within a lesion suggests a benign diagnosis when it is central, homogeneous, ring-like, or popcorn-like in distribution (79). Eccentric calcification may occur in bronchogenic carcinoma.

Certain radiographic patterns characterize the different cell types (76, 77, 80). Squamous cell carcinoma is centrally located two-thirds of the time but may arise in the lung periphery, often as a cavitating lesion (Fig. 15.7). In fact, it is the lung cancer cell type that cavitates most frequently. Small cell carcinoma is also a central lesion in most cases, often with central adenopathy at presentation (Fig. 15.8). It is peripheral in less than 20% of cases and does not cavitate. As stated, in 55 to 60% of cases adenocarcinoma is a peripheral lesion (Fig. 15.9). Frequently, there is associated pleural involvement, and in 50% of patients, hilar or mediastinal adenopathy is identified at initial presentation. Bronchoalveolar carcinoma, a subtype of adenocarcinoma, may have a variety of radiographic manifestations. Most commonly, it appears as a solitary peripheral nodule on the chest radiograph, but it may present as numerous small nodules resembling metastatic disease or as a consolidation with air bronchograms. Large cell carcinomas are more likely to be peripheral than central and are sharply defined, lobulated masses that occasionally cavitate (Fig. 15.10).

## Sputum Cytology

Sputum cytology may be particularly helpful in diagnosing central squamous cell and small cell carcinomas (81, 82). However, there are several potential problems in accurately interpreting sputum cytology specimens. Among these are an inexperienced cytologist, inadequate sample number (less than 3 or 4), inadequate specimen sample (without alveolar macrophages), purulent sputum causing degeneration of malignant cells prior to examination, and poor sample preparation (83). Accordingly, a negative sputum cytologic examination in a suspicious setting should never terminate further evaluation.

## Bronchoscopy

Flexible fiberoptic bronchoscopy is used widely for diagnosing both central airway and peripheral parenchymal lesions (84–88). For endobronchial lesions that are endoscopically visible, bronchial washings have a diagnostic yield of 79%, bronchial brushing 92%, and forceps biopsy 93% (84). Occasionally, in the setting of deeper submucosal lesions (e.g., small cell carcinoma), false-negative results occur because of an inability to grasp and bite tissue with biopsy forceps. Transbronchial needle aspiration in association with transbronchial biopsy may improve the diagnostic yield in these lesions (85). Bronchoscopy is less helpful in peripheral lesions, particularly lesions less than 2 cm in diameter (86, 87). For lesions less than 2 cm, the diagnostic yield is in the range of 20% or less; however, lesions larger than 4 cm may be diagnosed in 50 to 80% of cases (86–88).

Complications of fiberoptic bronchoscopy have been minimal. In one report, among 24,521 bronchoscopies performed by 192 bronchoscopists, mortality was only 0.1% (89), and there were no deaths in a series of 600 procedures performed by Zavala (90). Other potential complications include laryngospasm (0.13%), pneumothorax (0.1%), hypoxemia (0.3%), and significant hemorrhage (0.2%) (88–90).

## Needle Aspiration Biopsy

Transbronchial needle aspiration for both central and peripheral lesions was introduced for use with the fiberoptic bronchoscope by Wang and Terry (91). When used in conjunction with transbronchial biopsy, the diagnostic yield may be as high as 95% for central lesions and somewhat lower for peripheral lesions. Complications of this procedure are few and include minor bleeding or pneumothorax.

Percutaneous transthoracic thin-needle aspiration biopsy has proven to be a safe and reliable method for diagnosing nonendobronchial lung carcinomas (92, 93). A 95% or greater accuracy for diagnosing malignant lesions has been reported (93, 94). Computed tomography (CT) or fluoroscopy is used to guide most biopsies. A positive cytologic examination appears to be diagnostic for lung malignancy, since there have been only a few reported cases of false-positive results. However, because false-negative results may occur, a negative cytologic examination cannot be called a "benign lesion" unless the pathologist can provide a specific benign diagnosis such as "hamartoma." Twenty-nine percent of lesions initially diagnosed as negative on percutaneous needle aspiration were subsequently found to be malignant in one recent study (95). In most of these cases, the initial needle aspiration biopsy reading was nonspecifically benign (i.e., no specific benign diagnosis, such as hamartoma or granuloma, could be made). Also in this study, a specific benign diagnosis or granulomatous inflammation was associated with malignancy. Thus, serial follow-up chest radiographs must be obtained in patients with a specific benign diagnosis by transthoracic needle biopsy. When a high-risk patient has a nonspecific diagnosis by percutaneous needle biopsy, a further invasive diagnostic workup is necessary until either malignancy or a specific benign process has been diagnosed.

Pneumothorax, the major complication of transthoracic needle aspiration (93, 96), develops in 25 to 30% of patients and usually resolves spontaneously. The most important contributing factor for the development of a pneumothorax is the presence of chronic obstructive pulmonary disease (COPD) (93). In one study (97), there was a 46% incidence of pneumothorax in patients with COPD, compared with a 7% incidence in patients without COPD. The placement of a chest tube or small catheter connected to a Heimlich (one-way) valve may be required (93). Other infrequent complications include hemoptysis and transient parenchyma hemorrhage (93). Cardiac tamponade and fatal air embolism are rare complications. There have been only two reports of implantation of the needle tract with malignant cells (98, 99).

## Pleural Biopsy

Combined thoracentesis and pleural biopsy will provide up to a 90% yield in patients with carcinoma of the lung and malignant pleural involvement (100). Thoracoscopy, which involves introduction of either a flexible or a rigid bronchoscope into the pleural space with biopsy taken under direct vision, may augment the diagnostic yield in patients with pleural effusions (101).

**Table 15.5**
**TNM Definitions in the New International Staging System for Lung Cancer**

Primary Tumor (T)

TX  Tumor proven by the presence of malignant cells in bronchopulmonary secretions but not visualized roentgeno-graphically or bronchoscopically, or any tumor that cannot be assessed, as in a retreatment staging.

T0  No evidence of primary tumor.

TIS  Carcinoma in situ.

T1  A tumor that is 3.0 cm or less in greatest dimension, surrounded by lung or visceral pleura, and without evidence of invasion proximal to a lobar bronchus at bronchoscopy.[a]

T2  A tumor more than 3.0 cm in greatest dimension or a tumor of any size that either invades the visceral pleura or has associated atelectasis or obstructive pneumonitis extending to the hilar region. At bronchoscopy, the proximal extent of demonstrable tumor must be within a lobar bronchus or at least 2.0 cm distal to the carina. Any associated atelectasis or obstructive pneumonitis must involve less than an entire lung.

T3  A tumor of any size with direct extension into the chest wall (including superior sulcus tumors), diaphragm, or the mediastinal pleura or pericardium without involving the heart, great vessels, trachea, esophagus or vertebral body, or a tumor in the main bronchus within 2 cm of the carina without involving the carina.

T4  A tumor of any size with invasion of the mediastinum or involving heart, great vessels, trachea, esophagus, vertebral body or carina or presence of malignant pleural effusion.[b]

Nodal Involvement (N)

N0  No demonstrable metastasis to regional lymph nodes.

N1  Metastasis to lymph nodes in the peribronchial or the ipsilateral hilar region, or both, including direct extension.

N2  Metastasis to ipsilateral mediastinal lymph nodes and subcarinal lymph nodes.

N3  Metastasis to contralateral mediastinal lymph nodes, contralateral hilar lymph nodes, ipsilateral or contralateral scalene or supraclavicular lymph nodes.

Distant Metastasis (M)

M0  No (known) distant metastasis.

M1  Distant metastasis present—specify site(s).

From Mountain CF: A new international staging system for lung cancer. *Chest* 89 (Suppl):225S–233S, 1986.
[a] The uncommon superficial tumor of any size with its invasive component limited to the bronchial wall that may extend proximal to the main bronchus is classified as T1.
[b] Most pleural effusions associated with lung cancer are due to tumor. There are, however, a few patients in whom results of cytopathologic examination of pleural fluid (on more than one specimen) is negative for tumor; the fluid is nonbloody and is not an exudate. In such cases where these elements and clinical judgment dictate that the effusion is not related to the tumor, the patient should be staged T1, T2, or T3, excluding effusion *as a staging element*.

## Staging Classification

After the tissue diagnosis of lung carcinoma is made, the disease is staged to assess extent, to select correct therapy, and to determine prognosis (102). The most widely accepted staging system for non–small cell carcinoma is the tumor-node-metastasis (TNM) classification originally proposed in 1946 by Denoix (103). In 1986, the TNM classification was revised and updated (104). The details of each subset of the new system are given in Table 15.5, and stage groupings for TNM subsets are given in Table 15.6 The TNM system can be employed at any time from the initial clinical diagnosis to the time of autopsy (102, 104). The critical distinction is between clinical staging (TNM) made prior to the institution of any therapy and surgical-pathologic staging determined from histologic examination of resected specimens (102, 104). Figure 15.11 provides a general guide to the prognostic implications of each of the clinical stage groupings by showing the cumulative proportion of patients surviving 5

**Table 15.6**
**Stage Grouping of TNM Subsets in the New System of Lung Cancer Staging**

| Stage Grouping | | | |
|---|---|---|---|
| Occult carcinoma | TX | N0 | M0 |
| Stage 0 | TIS | Carcinoma in situ | Carcinoma in situ |
| Stage I | T1 | N0 | M0 |
| | T2 | N0 | M0 |
| Stage II | T1 | N1 | M0 |
| | T2 | N1 | M0 |
| Stage IIIa | T3 | N0 | M0 |
| | T3 | N1 | M0 |
| | T1–3 | N2 | M0 |
| Stage IIIb | Any T | N3 | M0 |
| | T4 | Any N | M0 |
| Stage IV | Any T | Any N | M1 |

From Mountain CF: A new international staging system for lung cancer. *Chest* 89(Suppl):225S–233S, 1986.

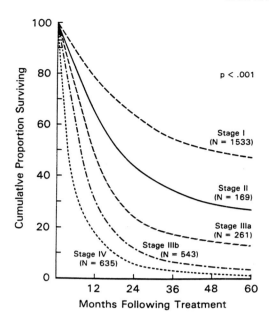

**FIGURE 15.11.** Cumulative proportion of patients surviving 5 years by clinical stage of disease using the new international TNM staging classification. (From Mountain CF: A new international staging system for lung cancer. *Chest* 89(Suppl):225S–233S, 1986.)

years by clinical stages of disease. Note that stage I (T1N0M0 or T2N0M0) patients without metastasis to regional lymph nodes have the best 5-year survival (50%). Stage II patients (T1N1M0 or T2N1M0) have a 5-year survival (30%) intermediate between stage I and stage III patients. Stage III is subdivided into two subgroups: stage IIIa, patients with potentially resectable lesions and approximately a 17% 5-year survival, and stage IIIb, patients with unresectable lesions and less than a 5% 5-year survival. Finally, stage IV patients with distant metastasis have a zero 5-year survival (104).

The uncommon superficial tumor of any size with its invasive component limited to the bronchial wall that may extend proximal to the main bronchus is classified as T1.

Most pleural effusions associated with lung cancer are due to tumor. There are, however, a few patients in whom results of cytopathologic examination of pleural fluid (on more than one specimen) is negative for tumor; the fluid is nonbloody and is not an exudate. In such cases where these elements and clinical judgment dictate that the effusion is not related to the tumor, the patient should be staged T1, T2, or T3, excluding effusion as a staging element.

The TNM classification has been less useful in staging small cell carcinoma because of the rapid extrathoracic spread of tumor (47, 105, 106). At the time of diag-

nosis, more than 85% of patients are stage III or stage IV, and even for those considered to be stage I or stage II, the prognosis is poor because of the frequent presence of undetected metastatic disease (105). The staging system most commonly used for small cell carcinoma is that of the Veterans Administration Lung Cancer Study Group, in which disease is simply classified as either limited or extensive (47, 105, 106). Limited disease refers to tumor confined to the ipsilateral hemithorax with or without superior vena caval obstruction or involvement of supraclavicular nodes. Extensive disease is defined as spread beyond the ipsilateral hemithorax and adjacent lymph nodes, recurrent disease after radiation to the primary tumor, or cytologically positive pleural effusion. With limited stage disease, complete response to therapy and prolonged survival are more likely, although fewer than one-third of patients fall into this category at the time of diagnosis.

### STAGING PROCEDURES

The staging process commences with a complete history and physical examination; attention is given to signs and symptoms related to central nervous system (CNS), bone, liver, chest wall, or mediastinal involvement (107). A full laboratory examination should include a complete blood count, liver function tests, and determination of calcium level. Hematologic abnormalities such as anemia, thrombocytopenia, or leukoerythroblastic peripheral blood may result from direct bone marrow involvement by the tumor. Hypercalcemia may be due to metastatic spread of tumor to bone or, more commonly, parathyroid-like hormone released by the malignancy (58–60). Abnormal liver function may reflect intrahepatic spread or extrahepatic obstruction.

### Thoracic Imaging Techniques (Also See Chapter 7)

The crucial element in staging is determining whether mediastinal involvement has occurred. Except in special cases, the presence or absence of mediastinal metastases will determine what surgery is performed. The conventional chest radiograph is only about 40% sensitive for detecting mediastinal lymph node involvement (108). Tomography may increase the yield, but the most sensitive technique is the chest CT scan, which is up to 95% sensitive for detecting malignant mediastinal disease (107, 109). Because of the excellent sensitivity of the CT scan, many thoracic surgeons now take patients directly to thoracotomy for tumor resection when the mediastinum appears to be without disease on chest CT. However, patients with enlarged mediastinal lymph nodes detected by CT scan require histologic examination of the nodes, because enlarged lymph nodes may be the result of an inflammatory, nonneoplastic process (110). Prior to thoracotomy, these patients should undergo further invasive staging procedures such as mediastinoscopy, percutaneous needle aspiration biopsy, or transbronchial needle aspiration (88, 93, 110).

Magnetic resonance imaging (MRI) has also been evaluated for imaging the mediastinum (78, 107, 111). However, because the sensitivity of MRI appears to be similar to that of CT, CT remains the initial procedure of choice for evaluating the mediastinum, and MRI is reserved for patients in whom CT results are equivocal. MRI is the procedure of choice for evaluating superior sulcus tumors (Fig. 7.20) and for assessing chest wall extension of lung cancer. Moreover, tumor invasion of the pericardium or heart (the latter indicating tumor unresectability) is best demonstrated with MRI (78). Gallium scanning has been used to evaluate both peripheral and mediastinal lesions, but this procedure is rarely used because its sensitivity is relatively poor (107).

### Invasive Staging Techniques

#### Bronchoscopy and Needle Aspiration Biopsy

Several procedures are available to stage the extent of disease after a primary tumor diagnosis has been established. Tumor proximity to carina is assessed, and tumors involving the carina or located within 1 to 2 cm of the carina are often considered to be nonoperable because of the technical difficulty of the surgical resection and a poorer prognosis with lesions in this location.

Transbronchoscopic needle aspiration biopsy has been used as a mediastinal staging technique (88, 91, 93). The sensitivity of this procedure varies, but a positive result indicates malignant involvement of peritracheal or subcarinal lymph nodes. Percutaneous needle aspiration biopsy has been used to diagnose enlarged mediastinal and hilar nodes as well as peripheral lesions (93).

#### Lymph Node Biopsy

Biopsy of lymph nodes in the supraclavicular fossa or in the mediastinal is necessary in some cases to obtain a tissue diagnosis and in others to assess the resectability of the tumor (48). Excision of lymph nodes in the scalene triangle should only be done in patients with carcinoma of the lung when these lymph nodes are palpable. The biopsy of nonpalpable lymph nodes is not indicated because the yield is 10% or less (112).

#### Mediastinoscopy and Mediastinotomy

Mediastinoscopy and mediastinotomy are two techniques used for direct exploration or sampling of tissues from the mediastinum (107, 113–115). In general,

only the superior aspects of the mediastinum can be fully evaluated by cervical mediastinoscopy because of the presence of large vessels, airways, and nerves. Lesions that involve the subcarinal and left anterior (periaortic) regions may be palpable, but biopsy specimens may be difficult to obtain. Anterior mediastinoscopy or mediastinotomy (Chamberlain procedure) is helpful for the latter situation (110, 113, 114). The procedure of choice depends largely on the site of the primary lesion, and selection may be guided by CT scan results.

The indication for mediastinoscopy in patients with carcinoma of the lung is to determine the presence or absence of metastatic tumor in the mediastinal nodes (Fig. 15.12). Such information may be of considerable prognostic significance and also may be helpful in planning the appropriate therapeutic approach. Contralateral positive lymph nodes (stage IIIb) are regarded as an absolute contraindication to thoracotomy. Contralateral spread is more likely to occur in patients with left lower lobe lesions (51). When ipsilateral mediastinal lymph nodes are involved (stage IIIa), opinion remains divided as to whether or not pulmonary resection with radical node dissection is recommended. Such a decision must be based on the extent of involvement.

Opinion is also divided as to whether or not mediastinoscopy should be performed in all patients with

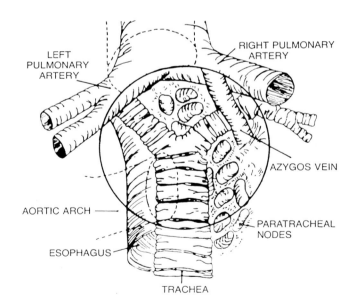

**FIGURE 15.12.** Representation of the view through a mediastinoscope at the level of the tracheal bifurcation with subcarinal lymph nodes and right pulmonary artery and azygous vein. (From Straus MJ: *Lung Cancer: Clinical Diagnosis and Treatment.* New York, Grune & Stratton, 1977, p 123.)

clinically resectable disease. Most surgeons believe it should be done only when a hilar mass or mediastinal lymph node enlargement is apparent either on the standard chest radiograph, on laminograms of the chest, or on chest CT. Also, mediastinoscopy should be done when a thoracotomy is not indicated because of the general condition of the patient and when all other simpler diagnostic methods have failed to give a positive histologic diagnosis of the tumor. Generally, mediastinoscopy is contraindicated in patients who have received mediastinal irradiation or who have had a tracheotomy. The highest positive yield is in patients with small cell tumors, the next highest with large cell carcinoma, and the least with squamous cell tumors (116). False-negative results are reported in only 4 to 6% of patients (116). Most often this is due to involvement of lymph nodes present in nonaccessible areas of the mediastinum.

Anterior mediastinotomy, a limited parasternal thoracotomy, provides a more direct approach to the mediastinal lymph nodes than mediastinoscopy. This approach is most popular for left-lung tumors when the major lymph node groups to be evaluated are in the subaortic anterior mediastinal areas. Neoplasms of the left upper lobe in particular may spread directly to the anterior mediastinal group or lymph nodes without involving the inferior tracheal bronchial, superior tracheal bronchial, or paratracheal nodal chain. Routine surgical mediastinoscopy does not sample the anterior mediastinal group (Figs. 15.12 and 15.13) (117).

*Thoracotomy for Diagnosis and Staging*

Historically, 5 to 20% of patients with bronchial carcinoma underwent surgery without a positive histologic or cytologic diagnosis. Today, due to widespread use of bronchoscopy and needle biopsy techniques, at least 95% of patients with lung cancer who undergo thoracotomy should have a histologic or cytologic diagnosis established prior to surgery. Thoracotomy should not be used for establishing the diagnosis when there appears to be no hope that the lesion is resectable; this is especially true in the elderly patient or one with limited functional pulmonary reserve (48).

A formal thoracotomy for diagnosis alone is usually not justified in patients with a superior sulcus tumor or superior vena caval syndrome. In the former situation, a tissue diagnosis may be obtained prior to institution of a therapeutic regimen by a bronchoscopy with fluoroscopic guidance, percutaneous needle aspiration biopsy, or one of three open surgical procedures: a posterior, an axillary, or a cervical approach. In patients with superior vena caval obstruction, tissue diagnosis may usually be obtained by bronchoscopy or mediastinotomy; however, mediastinoscopy could be

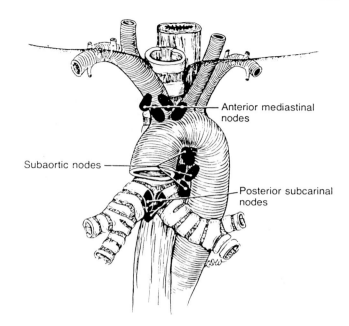

**FIGURE 15.13.** Diagrammatic representation of thoracic lymph nodes inaccessible to mediastinoscopy. The anterior mediastinal lymph nodes and subaortic lymph nodes may be reached by anterior mediastinotomy (Chamberlain procedure). (From Shields TW, Ritts RE: *Bronchial Carcinoma.* Springfield, IL, Charles C Thomas, 1974.)

hazardous, owing to increased pressure in large veins (48).

**Evaluation for Extrapulmonary Metastasis**

Prior to instituting therapy, particularly surgical resection for non–small cell lung cancer, it is important to assess whether disease has spread to extrathoracic organs (110). Metastases can be detected by CT scans or radionuclide scans of specific organs. A CT scan of the head is useful for detecting CNS spread and may reveal asymptomatic metastasis. CT scanning of the liver and adrenal glands may also detect metastatic lesions and is usually done at the time of the chest CT scan (110, 118). Bone scans and radionuclide liver-spleen scans are sensitive indicators of tumor spread; however, in asymptomatic patients with non–small cell carcinoma and normal laboratory tests, the routine use of these scans is unnecessary, and results may be potentially misleading (119, 120). Positive liver or bone scan findings may represent nonmalignant disease (e.g., old fracture, inflammation) and unnecessarily delay surgery while necessitating an invasive, costly further evaluation. The best screen for extrathoracic spread continues to be a thorough history and physical examination along with laboratory data, including calcium and alkaline phosphatase levels and liver function tests. Any abnormality should be followed by the appropriate radionuclide or CT scans (110).

As with non–small cell lung cancer, the radiographic staging of small cell tumors focuses on the presence or absence of extrathoracic disease. The approach remains the same as that for non–small cell tumors, but some clinicians recommend routine multiorgan (i.e., head, bone, liver, adrenal) scanning because of the frequent spread of disease. In addition, many investigators recommend routine bone marrow investigation with bone marrow aspiration and biopsy, because bone marrow involvement occurs in up to 50% of cases, even in the absence of peripheral blood abnormalities or a bone scan with positive findings. Certainly, patients who are considered for locoregional therapy (chest radiotherapy and/or surgical resection) or participation in clinical trials should undergo these additional staging studies to identify asymptomatic metastatic sites (47).

### Appropriate Investigation of a Solitary Peripheral Parenchymal Mass

A circumscribed, solitary, peripheral lung mass (the pulmonary coin lesion) in the asymptomatic patient frequently represents a relatively early primary carcinoma of the lung. However, it may be an inflammatory mass, a vascular lesion, a benign tumor, or even a solitary metastasis to the lung. On chest radiograph, the actual margins of the lesion may vary from ill-defined to sharply demarcated, and the size may vary, although in general no lesion greater than 3 cm in diameter should be included in this category (43, 121, 122). Table 15.7 shows some of the benign causes of the solitary pulmonary nodule.

The percentage of benign and malignant lesions in any given series of coin lesions varies with patient selection and the definition of such a lesion. In the general population, 5% of such masses discovered by a routine radiographic survey are carcinomas. However, in series in which resections have been performed, 50% of such masses in patients over 50 years of age are carcinomas (21, 48). Further, this percentage increases with advancing age of the patient group.

Of the malignant lesions, approximately 8 to 10% are metastatic (48). Less than 0.5% of all patients with coin lesions have metastatic disease in the lungs from an unknown, asymptomatic tumor elsewhere in the body (123). Consequently, in a patient with a coin lesion, any extensive radiographic examination for a possible primary tumor hidden in another organ system has little potential reward. As stated, investigation

**Table 15.7**
**Common Nonmalignant Lesions Presenting as Solitary Pulmonary Nodules**

Very common
  Granulomas
    Histoplasmoma, tuberculoma, coccidioidoma
    Cryptococcosis, blastomycosis, actinomycosis
    Unidentified granulomas
Common
  Lung abscess before evacuation into a bronchus
  Slowly resolving circumscribed pneumonia
  Lipoid pneumonia
  Hamartoma
Less common
  Bronchogenic cyst
  Pulmonary infarct
  Bronchial adenoma
  Arteriovenous fistula
  Enlarged pulmonary artery
  Infected, fluid-filled bulla
  Rheumatoid nodule

of a specific organ system is indicated only when the patient has a history of a previous malignant tumor or symptoms related to that system or when the routine laboratory studies reveal an abnormality that suggests the presence of a silent tumor (48, 110).

In the evaluation of a coin lesion, following a standard history, physical examination, and routine laboratory and radiographic studies of the chest, skin tests should be performed for *Mycobacterium tuberculosis* and other suspected infectious agents. Sputum smears for detection of acid-fast organisms and cytologic studies should be carried out. Chest CT should be done to confirm that the lesion is solitary and to assess for presence of calcification, and any available previous radiographs of the chest should be reviewed. When the lesion is found to have been present and unchanged for a period of 24 months or more or when any one of four specific types of calcification (central, ring-like, homogeneous, or popcorn-like) is seen, the lesion may be judged to be benign and may be observed radiographically at periodic intervals (46, 74, 104, 110). When acid-fast organisms are demonstrated in the sputum, the patient should receive appropriate antituberculous chemotherapy, and the lesion should be re-evaluated within 2 to 3 months. When none of these features is present, particularly when the patient is over 40 years of age, the lesion should be removed to permit diagnosis and treatment (48).

### Treatment

Lung cancer therapy varies depending on the cell type, the stage of the cancer, and multiple host factors such as age, general condition, and the presence of concomitant diseases, particularly chronic obstructive lung disease and coronary heart disease (110). Current modalities, used in various combinations, are surgical resection, radiation therapy, chemotherapy, immunotherapy, and laser therapy. Despite the aggressive application of these modalities, the 5-year survival of large groups of patients with lung cancer remains in the range of only 10% (124, 125). Obviously, improvement is needed in the management of this disease.

## Surgery

### Indications for Resection

Surgical resection of the tumor is the primary modality of therapy for non–small cell lung cancer (104, 110, 126–129). This remains true for all age groups, although surgical morbidity and mortality may be higher in older populations (129). The best long-term results have been obtained in patients who have true (i.e., pathologic staging) stage I disease and small primary tumors (T1N0M0) (104, 110, 126–129). Mountain (104) and Naruke et al. (127) have reported 68.5 and 75.5% 5-year survivals in this subgroup (Table 15.8) (110). Patients with stage I disease but tumors larger than 3 cm (T2N0M0) have a lower 5-year survival. The prognostic significance of the specific cell type (i.e., adenocarcinoma, squamous cell, or large cell) is debated. Some data suggest that with or without lymph node involvement, patients with adenocarcinoma do less

**TABLE 15.8**
**POSTSURGICAL SURVIVAL ACCORDING TO TNM CLASSIFICATION**

| TNM Subset | Mountain[a] | | Naruke[b] | |
|---|---|---|---|---|
| | No. Patients | 5-Year Survival (%) | No. Patients | 5-Year Survival (%) |
| T1N0M0 | 429 | 68.5 | 245 | 75.5 |
| T2N0M0 | 436 | 59.0 | 241 | 57.0 |
| T1N1M0 | 67 | 54.1 | 66 | 52.5 |
| T2N1M0 | 250 | 40.0 | 153 | 40.0 |
| T3N0M0 | 57 | 44.2 | 106 | 33.3 |
| T3N1M0 | 29 | 17.6 | 85 | 39.0 |
| ANY N2M0 | 168 | 28.8 | 368 | 15.1 |

Table reproduced with permission from Shields TW: Surgical therapy for carcinoma of the lung. *Clin Chest Med* 14:121–147, 1993.
[a] From Mountain CF: A new international staging system for lung cancer. *Chest* 89:225S–233S, 1986; with permission.
[b] From Naruke T, Goya T, Tsuchiya T, et al: Prognosis and survival in resected lung carcinoma based on the new international staging system. *J Thorac Cardiovasc Surg* 96:440–447, 1988; with permission.

well than those with squamous cell carcinoma (110). The usual surgical procedure is lobectomy, although patients with central lesions may require pneumonectomy. Procedures that spare pulmonary parenchyma (segmentectomy, wedge resection, or bronchial sleeve resection) have been used more frequently because of the common coexistence of chronic obstructive lung disease with lung cancer (110). Patients with stage II non–small cell tumors (T1N1M0, T2N1M0) also are considered eligible for complete resection, although they may require a more extensive surgical procedure, such as pneumonectomy, and have a poorer prognosis (Fig. 15.11 and Table 15.8).

The role of surgery in more extensive, stage III non–small cell carcinoma is controversial (104, 130). Some groups have claimed that patients with certain types of patterns, namely stage IIIa, may benefit from resectional surgery (Fig. 15.11) (104, 130). Among these stage IIIa patients are those who have solitary ipsilateral lymph node involvement (T1N2M0, T2N2M0) and those with direct extension into the chest wall but negative nodes (T3N0M0). An approximate 5-year survival rate of 35% has been observed in the latter group (110). However, when N1 and N2 disease is present in addition to chest wall involvement, the 5-year survival rate drops precipitously to less than half the aforementioned figure and in fact approaches zero (110).

The role of surgery in small cell carcinoma has been undergoing reevaluation (47, 110, 131). In general, surgery has not been shown to improve outcome because of the frequent presence of micro- or macroextrathoracic metastasis at the time of tumor diagnosis. However, there is renewed enthusiasm for operating on patients with limited-stage disease because removal of the primary tumor combined with chemotherapy may limit local chest relapse. Several prospective trials of primary surgery and surgery as an adjuvant to chemotherapy for small cell lung cancer are under way. As yet, surgical removal of small cell lung tumors has not been conclusively shown to favorably alter outcome (47, 110).

### Medical Contraindications to Resection

Almost all medical contraindications to resection of malignant lesions are related to either the lungs or the heart. Rarely does advanced age alone or the presence of other systemic disease preclude surgical resection. At times, the determination of what constitutes insufficient pulmonary reserve for tolerance of the required pulmonary resection is, at best, difficult to make. However, data suggest that in patients with borderline pulmonary reserve (preoperative forced expiratory volume in 1 second less than 2000 ml), the preoperative combination of simple spirometric analysis and quantitative perfusion lung scanning can permit an accurate assessment of postoperative lung function in most cases (also see Chapter 24) (107, 110, 132).

Cardiac contraindications include recent myocardial infarction, a changing pattern of angina pectoris, and uncontrolled or uncontrollable heart failure (110).

### General Summary of Surgical Therapy

Most authorities agree that surgical resection is the proper treatment of lung cancer whenever there is a reasonable chance of removing all the cancer with an acceptable risk of morbidity and mortality. Thus, stages I and II non–small cell lung cancers are usually resected. Small cell lung cancer requires chemotherapy, with or without radiation therapy, and perhaps removal of solitary peripheral lesions (47, 110). Some stage IIIa non–small cell lung cancers (Table 15.6) are resected if there is a reasonable probability that all the cancer can be removed (e.g., peripheral carcinomas with direct invasion of the chest wall without metastases to lymph nodes or T1 or T2 lesions with metastases to distal ipsilateral paratracheal lymph nodes) (110). Because the recurrence rate in such cases is high, postoperative radiation therapy or chemotherapy or a combination of both has been used, unfortunately with minimal success, in an effort to improve outcome (48, 125, 133, 134).

### Radiation Therapy

#### Curative

Radical radiation therapy (local dosage of 50 to 60 Gy) is capable of sterilizing carcinoma of the lung (135, 136). Thus, potential local control of a bronchial carcinoma may be accomplished. The various cell types respond differently to irradiation. Small cell carcinomas are moderately radiosensitive and may be eradicated by a dose of 35 to 40 Gy. Squamous cell tumors require a higher dose (50 to 55 Gy). Adenocarcinoma responds to similar dosage levels, but the response is sometimes said to be less favorable than that of squamous cell tumors. Large cell undifferentiated tumors respond least favorably of all. Response, of course, also depends on the size of the lesion as well as the presence of extraparenchymal intrathoracic spread of the tumor. The selection of radiation therapy as the curative modality is indicated in an occasional patient with stage I or stage II disease. This is either the patient in whom resection is contraindicated because of inadequate pulmonary or cardiac reserve or the patient who refuses the operation (48, 136–138). Patients who seem to benefit most from this approach are those with small peripheral lesions (T1N0M0), the same group with the best survival outcome from surgical resection. One special circumstance in which radiation may play a curative role is that of the superior sulcus tumor. Up to a 50% 5-year survival may be achieved in patients

treated with a combination of preoperative radiation and en bloc resection of the chest wall, including the involved lung, ribs, thoracic vertebrae, and brachial plexus (139).

Small cell carcinoma of the lung is extremely sensitive to radiation, but chemotherapy remains the treatment of choice because of the frequency of extrathoracic metastases at the time of therapy (47). However, local radiation has been combined with chemotherapy because of the high incidence of local chest relapse in patients receiving chemotherapy alone (140). The current treatment of choice for patients with limited-stage small cell carcinoma is combined chemotherapy and radiation therapy (47, 141). Patients with extensive disease may derive local benefit from chest irradiation, but survival does not appear to improve because of the involvement of extrathoracic organ by tumor (47).

The second role for radiation in small cell carcinoma is in treating cranial involvement (47). CNS spread occurs in more than 50% of patients at some time during the course of their disease and may provide a sanctuary from chemotherapeutic agents because of the blood-brain barrier. Cranial irradiation reduces the development of CNS metastases but has little effect on survival because of concomitant spread of disease to other sites (142). Thus, prophylactic cranial irradiation is reserved for patients who are judged to have a complete response to chemotherapy. Treatment is usually given 2 to 4 months after the beginning of chemotherapy.

#### Palliative Radiation Therapy

Most, if not all, patients with tumor spread beyond the confines of the ipsilateral hemithorax are candidates for radiotherapy, if only for the relief of distressing symptoms (47, 48, 125). When the tumor is obviously incurable, no attempt at long-term control is indicated, and the routine use of radiation therapy other than for control of symptoms cannot be defended from the present data in the literature. Longevity appears not to be increased, and unless irradiation is given with care, appreciable morbidity as well as shortened life span may occur (143).

In most cases, complications such as hemoptysis, superior vena caval obstruction, bone invasion, chest pain, and dyspnea can be controlled (47, 48, 125). Ventilation-perfusion relationships of the lung may improve rapidly after a course of radiation therapy (144).

#### Complications of Radiation Therapy

The primary complication of radiation therapy is an acute pneumonitis, usually occurring 1 to 3 months after radiation (145). Patients usually present with complaints of a nonproductive cough and dyspnea and

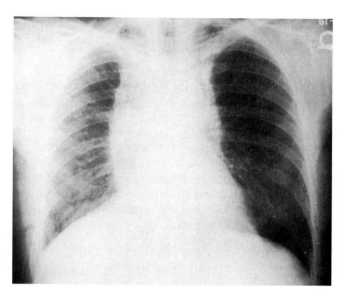

**FIGURE 15.14.** Radiation pneumonitis. PA chest radiograph illustrates profound radiation pneumonitis noted 3 months after irradiation (3500 rads) was completed to the central thorax for a squamous cell carcinoma invading the main carina. Note the well-demarcated, paramediastinal density and decreased lung volume in the right hemithorax.

on physical examination have evidence of either pulmonary consolidation or pleural inflammation. Typically, the chest radiograph shows a sharply demarcated alveolar or interstitial parenchymal infiltrate limited to the radiation port (Fig. 15.14). Significant pleural effusions are uncommon. These patients gradually improve over several weeks, with a minority progressing to severe respiratory insufficiency. It is unclear whether corticosteroids are beneficial in these cases. Other less common complications include esophagitis, pericarditis, and myelitis.

### Chemotherapy

*Non–Small Cell Carcinoma*

Although several trials are ongoing, chemotherapy does not appear to be of substantial benefit in patients with non–small cell lung cancer (125); in general, response rates are low and toxicity is high (2, 107). Single-drug agents have had response rates in the range of 10 to 20%, and combination regimens have offered only a slight improvement with significantly greater toxicity. Drugs that appear to have the best activity when used as single agents include cyclophosphamide, doxorubicin, methotrexate, cisplatin, vindesine, and VP-16. Combination regimens that produce the most consistent results include cyclophosphamide, doxorubicin, and cisplatin (CAP) and cyclophosphamide, doxorubicin, methotrexate, and procarbazine (CAMP), as

well as various other combinations of agents. Complete and partial response rates are at best in the range of 30 to 50%, and toxicity is high. Factors that appear to correlate best with response to chemotherapy are extent of disease and performance status. Whether a particular histologic subtype of tumor may respond better to chemotherapy has not been demonstrated consistently. Currently the most realistic recommendation is to use chemotherapy as part of a protocol in patients with a reasonably modest tumor burden and good performance (146). The role of chemotherapy as an adjuvant treatment in combination with radiation or surgery has not been established but is being studied (125).

*Small Cell Carcinoma*

Chemotherapy is the treatment of choice for small cell lung cancer (47). Survival has been increased from between 2 and 3 months in untreated patients to between 8 and 14 months and sometimes longer in patients treated with combination chemotherapy. A variety of drug regimens are effective, but the most active include cyclophosphamide in combination with adriamycin (doxorubicin) and vincristine (CAV) and etoposide and cisplatin (CP) (47). The other agents commonly used in the United States documented to have single agent activity against either previously untreated ( 20% response rate) or treated ( 10% response rate) are methotrexate, nitrogen mustard, carboplatin, teniposide, ifosfomide, lomustine, and hexamethylamine (47). Several studies have documented overall response rates in the range of 80 to 95% (147, 148). Complete response rates may be as high as 60% and the median survival approximately 10 to 14 months in patients with limited disease. Twenty percent of patients will achieve long-term disease-free survival (3 years or more).

Patients with extensive disease at initial treatment have a poorer initial response and long-term survival than those with limited disease (47, 141). In 25% of patients, complete response rates are achieved, and median survival ranges from 8 to 9 months. Long-term disease-free survival is achieved in only a minority of patients (1 to 3%).

As stated, combined-modality therapy using chemotherapy with radiation for the primary chest tumor is advocated (47, 140). This appears to improve the percentage of complete responses in patients with limited disease, diminish local tumor relapse, and increase overall survival. Among the newer approaches being tested are the use of non-cross-resistant chemotherapeutic agents to overcome tumor resistance, more aggressive "leukemia-style" induction and consolidation chemotherapy, autologous bone marrow transplantation with high-dose chemotherapy infusion, new drug development, and better in vitro cell cloning assays for prediction of chemotherapeutic efficiency (47, 146–148).

## Laser Therapy, Brachytherapy and Endobronchial Prostheses

Local approaches to the treatment of malignant endobronchial lesions have included laser therapy with or without hematoporphyrin derivative and brachytherapy with endobronchial radioisotopic implantation (149–151). These treatments have been used for in situ premalignant lesions as well as palliative therapy for advanced endobronchial disease. Although laser therapy may be curative for patients with in situ lesions, laser therapy and brachytherapy generally are palliative therapies and do not affect overall survival.

Many patients present with malignant large airway obstruction due to extrinsic compression from either tumor or enlarged lymph nodes. When surgical resection is not an option and radiotherapy has not adequately improved airway caliber, several endobronchial prosthetic devices (expandable metal wire, molded silicone, or combination of both) are now available as an alternative to disabling dyspnea (150).

## OTHER PULMONARY NEOPLASMS

### CARCINOID TUMOR (BRONCHIAL ADENOMA)

Bronchopulmonary carcinoid tumors constitute 1 to 4% of all primary lung neoplasms (151). These highly vascularized lesions arise in submucosal glands in the bronchial wall, grow slowly, invade locally, and occasionally metastasize to the lymph nodes, mediastinum, vertebra, and liver (6, 80, 152). The lesion usually appears as a polypoid or sessile mass protruding from the bronchial wall. It is red or pink and is covered by intact bronchial mucosa. Of these lesions, 90% are located in a major or segmental bronchus, but about 10% present as peripheral lesions. They are composed of small uniform cuboidal cells with fine granular homogeneous cytoplasm. The nuclei are round or oval and deeply staining. Usually the nucleus is in the center of the cell. Little pleomorphism is seen, and mitoses are usually absent. Argentaffin granules are rarely seen, in contrast to carcinoid tumors of the small intestine.

Carcinoid tumor occurs slightly more frequently in women (152). Most patients are in their thirties and have had symptoms for over 5 years when the tumor is first diagnosed. Signs and symptoms are secondary to bronchial obstruction or to the extreme vascularity of the tumor. Hemoptysis occurs in one-third of patients (153), but signs and symptoms secondary to pulmonary infection behind the obstructed bronchus are frequently noted. Occasionally, a patient is asymptomatic and the tumor is discovered after routine radiography of the chest.

Three types of chest radiographic abnormalities are seen in these patients with carcinoid tumor (152). Most frequently there appears to be a pneumonia or the sequela of such an infection, with poor bronchial drainage. A smooth, rounded hilar mass may be present, or rarely, a peripheral nodule is seen.

The diagnosis is usually made on the basis of the history of frequent hemoptysis or repeated bouts of pneumonia and observation of the characteristic tumor by the bronchoscope. Biopsy is usually inadvisable because of the severe hemorrhage that may result. Also, it may be difficult to make a definite histologic diagnosis from the small pieces of tissue obtained by bronchial biopsy. Cytologic study of sputum for bronchial washings is usually not diagnostic, since the mucous membrane over the tumor is usually intact. Operative removal is indicated, since this is the only means of preventing severe hemoptysis and preventing infection that can accompany these tumors. Moreover, early removal may prevent the late metastatic spread that occurs in a few instances (152). The 5-year survival rate after resection is over 90% (6).

### ATYPICAL CARCINOID TUMORS

In 1972, Arrigoni and coworkers (154) described an atypical carcinoid tumor that accounted for most but not all of the mortality for pulmonary carcinoids. Half of these lesions were large and peripherally located. Histologically, they are carcinoids with necrosis, numerous mitotic figures, and more anaplastic nuclei of the large cell type (154–156). A 41% survival rate has been reported (6).

### BRONCHIAL TUMORS OF THE SALIVARY GLAND TYPE

Neoplasms that are similar to those that arise in the major and minor salivary glands infrequently arise in bronchial submucosal glands. These include mucoepidermoid carcinoma, adenoid cystic carcinoma, and pleomorphic adenomas (157–159). All present as endobronchial or endotracheal masses. The mucoepidermoid carcinomas are divided into high and low grade, according to both size and histology. High-grade mucoepidermoid carcinomas are larger and invasive with both epidermoid and glandular elements that have more anaplastic nuclei, numerous mitotic figures, and foci of necrosis. Treatment is resection; survival is good for low-grade but very poor for high-grade lesions. Adenoid cystic carcinomas are characterized by cells that form a characteristic cylindromatous pattern of regular glands (157). Resection is the preferred treatment, if possible, and 5-year survival is good (85%), lower at 10 years (55%), and poor at 20 years (20%) (151, 157).

## PAPILLOMAS OF THE BRONCHUS

Papillomas are exceedingly rare lung tumors that are often associated with generalized papillomatosis of the upper respiratory tract (152). They are usually wart-like growths and have a well-developed connective tissue stroma (160). Bronchial papillomas in adults are often solitary growths but may be associated with papillomas elsewhere in the bronchial tree (80). Approximately 50% of the solitary adult tumors become malignant (80). They appear to be associated with human papilloma virus (160).

## MESODERMAL TUMORS OF THE BRONCHI AND LUNG

Mesodermal tumors of the lung as a group are rare and account for a small percentage of all pulmonary neoplasms (152). The following is a classification of these neoplasms (161).
1. *Benign parenchyma tumors*: hamartomas;
2. *Benign intrabronchial tumors*: chondroma, osteochondroma, lipoma, leiomyoma;
3. *Malignant intrabronchial tumors*: fibrosarcoma, leiomyosarcoma;
4. *Malignant parenchyma tumors*: sarcomas, lymphomas.

### Hamartoma

Hamartomas are the most common benign tumors of the lung (151). The characteristic feature of these tumors is that they are composed of disorganized elements of tissue normally present in the particular organ (80, 152, 162). In the lung, the term hamartoma is applied inappropriately to an interstitial mesenchymal tumor composed primarily of cartilage. Spicules of bone are frequently found in the cartilage. Deep septa of connective tissue extend from the periphery to the central portion of the nodule. Near the edge of the lesion, bronchial or alveolar epithelium is entrapped. No capsule is present, and the tumor does not invade the surrounding tissue. The cartilage found within the tumor is not related to the cartilage found normally in bronchi. However, 8 to 20% of the lesions arise within a major or segmental bronchus; the remainder are found in the periphery of the lung.

Most hamartomas are discovered on routine chest radiography (152). Characteristically, the lesion is round, has sharply defined margins, and varies in size from a few millimeters to 4 to 5 cm in diameter. As the lesion grows, it may become lobulated. On the chest

radiograph, it is most likely to be confused with a tuberculoma or metastatic lesion from a tumor elsewhere in the body. Calcification is evident on chest radiograph in 10% (151) and usually appears as small flecks throughout the lesion rather than in a ring form.

Definite diagnosis can be made only by histologic examination of the lesion (162–164). Rarely, adequate tissue can be obtained through the bronchoscope, but usually thoracotomy is required. The lesion does not start to grow and become large enough to be seen on radiographs until later in life.

Histologic confirmation is necessary to eliminate the possibility of a malignant lesion. Simple excision of the lesion is adequate, but usually a segmental resection of lobectomy is done, since in most cases the nature of the lesion is not clear until after its removal.

### Chondromas and Osteochondroma

Chondromas and osteochondromas are very rare neoplasms that arise in the trachea or a major bronchus in association with normal cartilaginous rings (152, 162, 165, 166). They are usually slow growing and may reach a large size, causing destruction of the pulmonary parenchyma. Histologically, the tumor is composed of hyaline or fibrous cartilage. It differs from a hamartoma in that it contains only cartilage. Endoscopic removal of the tumor is usually possible unless the base is sessile or the tumor is dumbbell-shaped. Bronchotomy is indicated in the latter two situations. If extensive lung destruction has occurred behind the tumor, pulmonary resection is indicated. All such tumors should be removed because of their tendency to undergo sarcomatous degeneration.

### Lipoma

Lipomas originate from fatty tissue normally present in fibrous tissue external to cartilaginous plates and to a lesser extent in connective tissue and muscular layers of the bronchi (152, 167, 168). Lipomas occur more frequently in men than in women, usually in the 5th or 6th decade of life. For some unexplained reason, they are seen much more frequently in the left bronchial tree (167, 168). They are usually soft and smooth and often lobulated. Removal of the tumor can usually be accomplished through the straight-tube bronchoscope with satisfactory results, unless bronchial obstruction has produced destruction of lung tissue.

### Leiomyoma

Nearly all of the smooth muscle tumors in the lung are well-differentiated metastases from leiomyosarcomas of the uterus. Leiomyoma is extremely rare (169, 170). In one series of 14 cases, 12 were in women. This tumor probably arises from the smooth muscle of the interstitium. Microscopically, sheets of smooth muscle predominate. Surgical removal is the treatment of choice.

### Fibrosarcoma (Malignant Fibrous Histiocytoma)

On histologic examination, this tumor is composed of elongated spindle-shaped cells, many of which are arranged in bands (171–173). A variable component of histiocytes is present. The tumor is relatively slow growing, and it metastasizes late. If complete removal of the primary tumor can be accomplished surgically, the prognosis is good (172, 173).

### Leiomyosarcoma

In a study of 20 patients with leiomyosarcoma, the age at presentation varied from 4 to 83 years, with 11 patients over 40 (174). The signs and symptoms were those of bronchial obstruction. The duration of symptoms varied from 1 month to 3½ years. Most of the tumors were encapsulated and on cut surface had a gray or white surface. Histologically, these neoplasms were composed of spindle-shaped cells with long nuclei and abundant cytoplasm with myofibrils. Mitotic figures are frequent. Palisading of nuclei was noted in most sections. Five of the patients had metastases at the time the cases were reported. Of the 11 patients in whom the tumor was resected, 9 were alive and well 6 years after operation. Radiation therapy in two patients had no effect on their disease.

### Sarcoma

Primary malignant tumors of mesenchymal tissue origin occur even less frequently than benign mesenchymal tumors (152, 170, 174). The highest incidence is during the 3rd decade of life, with no specific sex distribution (174). Most originate in the periphery of the lung. Cough, chest pain, dyspnea, and weight loss are the most frequent initial complaints. In general, they are slow-growing tumors with a good prognosis.

### Lymphoma

It is generally agreed that lymphogenous tumors usually have multicentric origins, and pulmonary involvement is a frequent finding (152). Solitary lymphoma occurs in the lung, but in the individual patient it is difficult to be sure there are no other sites of origin.

This tumor appears as a white, pale yellow, or grayish pink fleshy mass that has no capsule. Occasionally, there is a line of demarcation consisting of a compressed rim of normal lung tissue. Histologically, the tumor is composed of lymphocytes, lymphoblasts, or reticulum cells that infiltrate and replace the normal parenchyma. These cells may surround the bronchi

and blood vessels but do not invade. Usually, the diagnosis of solitary lymphoma is made after exploratory thoracotomy and workup reveals no extrapulmonary spread. Significant lymphadenopathy or hepatosplenomegaly or bone marrow involvement usually indicates lymphoma outside the chest, contraindicating surgical removal. Current techniques of radiation therapy and chemotherapy may further prolong life in patients with recurrence of lymphoma after surgery.

### REFERENCES

1. Wingo PA, Tong T, Bolden S: Cancer statistics 1995. *CA Cancer J Clin* 45:8–30, 1995.
2. Haskell CM, Holmes EC: Non–small cell lung cancer. *DM* 34:53–108, 1988.
3. Smoking and Health. *A Report of the Surgeon General.* Washington, DC, US Department of Health and Human Services, 1980.
4. Beckett WS: Epidemiology and etiology of lung cancer. *Clin Chest Med* 14:1–15, 1993.
5. Stjernsward J, Stanley K: A world-wide health problem. *Lung Cancer* 4(Suppl):11–24, 1988.
6. Yesner R: Pathogenesis and pathology [of lung cancer]. *Clin Chest Med* 14:17–30, 1993.
7. Stolley PD: Lung cancer: unwanted equality for women [Editorial]. *N Engl J Med* 297:886–887, 1977.
8. Loeb LA, Ernster VL, Warner KE, et al: Smoking and lung cancer: an overview. *Cancer Res* 44:5940–5948, 1984.
9. Wyndner EL, Graham EA: Tobacco smoking as a possible etiologic factor in bronchogenic carcinoma. A study of 684 proved cases. *JAMA* 143:329–338, 1950.
10. Morgan WKC, Andrews CE: Bronchogenic carcinoma. In Morgan WNC (ed): *Textbook of Pulmonary Diseases,* ed 2. Boston, Little, Brown & Co, 1974, p 755.
11. Gazdar AF, Carney DN, Minna JD: The biology of non-small cell lung cancer. *Semin Oncol* 10:3–19, 1983.
12. Capewell S, Sankaran R, Lam D, et al: Lung cancer in lifelong nonsmokers. Edinburgh Lung Cancer Group. *Thorax* 46:565–568, 1991.
13. Doll R, Hill AB: Mortality in relation to smoking: 10 years' observation of British doctors. *Br Med J* 1:1399–1410, 1964.
14. Brown CC, Kessler LG: Projections of lung cancer mortality in the United States. 1985–2025. *JNCI* 80:43–51, 1988.
15. Sandler DP, Everson RB, Wilcox AJ: Passive smoking in adulthood and cancer risk. *Am J Epidemiol* 121:37–48, 1985.
16. Matsukura S, Taminato T, Kitano N, et al: Effects of environmental tobacco smoke on urinary cotinine excretion in nonsmokers. Evidence for passive smoking. *N Engl J Med* 311:828–832, 1984.
17. Hirayama T: Non-smoking wives of heavy smokers have a higher risk of lung cancer: a study from Japan. *Br Med J* 282:183–185, 1981.
18. Holmes EC: Lung cancer. In Simmons DH (ed): *Current Pulmonology.* Boston, Houghton Mifflin, 1979, pp 239–250.

19. Brown LM, Pottern LM, Blot WJ: Lung cancer in relation to environmental pollutants emitted from industrial sources. *Environ Res* 34:250–261, 1984.

20. Chahinian AP, Chretien J: Present incidence of lung cancer: epidemiologic data and etiologic factors. In Israel L (ed): *Lung Cancer—Natural History, Prognosis, and Therapy.* New York, Academic Press, 1976, pp 1–22.

21. Frank AL: The epidemiology and etiology of lung cancer. *Clin Chest Med* 3:219–228, 1982.

22. Samet JM, Kutvirt DM, Waxweiler RJ, et al: Uranium mining and lung cancer in Navajo men. *N Engl J Med* 310:1481–1484, 1984.

23. Radford EP, Renard KGSC: Lung cancer in Swedish iron miners exposed to low doses of radon daughters. *N Engl J Med* 310:1485–1494, 1984.

24. Wright ES, Couves CM: Radiation-induced carcinoma of the lung—the St. Lawrence tragedy. *J Thorac Cardiovasc Surg* 74:495–498, 1977.

25. Selikoff IJ, Hammond EC: Asbestos-associated disease in United States shipyards. *CA* 28:87–89, 1978.

26. Craighead JE, Mossman BT: The pathogenesis of asbestos-related diseases. *N Engl J Med* 306:1446–1455, 1982.

27. Shekelle RB, Liu S, Raynor WJ, et al: Dietary vitamin A and risk of cancer in the Western Electric study. *Lancet* 2:1185–1190, 1981.

28. Samet JM, Skipper BJ, Humble CG, et al: Lung cancer risk and vitamin A consumption in New Mexico. *Am Rev Respir Dis* 131:198–202, 1985.

29. Sellers TA, Bailey-Wilson JE, Elston RC, et al: Evidence for mendelian inheritance in the pathogenesis of lung cancer. *JNCI* 82:1272–1279, 1990.

30. Tokuhata GK, Lilienfeld AM: Familial aggregation of lung cancer in humans. *JNCI* 30:289–312, 1963.

31. Kern JA, Filderman AE: Oncogenes and growth factors in human lung cancer. *Clin Chest Med* 14:31–41, 1993.

32. Kazazian, JH: A geneticist's view of lung disease. *Am Rev Respir Dis* 113:261–266, 1976.

33. Kellerman G, Shaw CR, Layten-Kellerman M: Aryl-hydrocarbon-hydroxylase inducibility in bronchogenic carcinoma. *N Engl J Med* 289:934–937, 1973.

34. Brauch H, Johnson B, Hovis J, et al: Molecular analysis of the short arm of chromosome 3 in small-cell and non–small cell carcinoma of the lung. *N Engl J Med* 317:1109–1113, 1987.

35. Rodenhuis S, Van de Wetering ML, Mooi WJ, et al: Mutational activation of the K-*ras* oncogene. A possible pathogentic factor in adenocarcinoma of the lung. *N Engl J Med* 317:929–935, 1987.

36. Karki NT, Pokela R, Nuutineu L, et al: Aryl hydrocarbon hydroxylase in lymphocytes and lung tissue from lung cancer patients and controls. *Int J Cancer* 39:565–570, 1987.

37. Cohen MH: Natural history of lung cancer. *Clin Chest Med* 3:229-241, 1982.

38. World Health Organization: The WHO histological typing of lung tumors. Second edition. *Am J Clin Pathol* 77:123–126, 1982.

39. Yesner R: Classification of lung cancer histology. *N Engl J Med* 312:652–653, 1985.

40. Cox JD, Yesner RA: Adenocarcinoma of the lung: recent results from the Veterans Administration Lung Group. *Am Rev Respir Dis* 120:1025–1029, 1979.

41. Matthews MJ, Mackay B, Lukeman J: The pathology of non–small cell carcinoma of the lung. *Semin Oncol* 10:34–55, 1983.

42. Matthews MJ: Problems in morphology and behavior of bronchopulmonary malignant disease. In Israel L (ed): *Lung Cancer—Natural History, Prognosis, and Therapy.* New York, Academic Press, 1976.

43. Matthews MJ: Morphologic classification of bronchogenic carcinoma. *Cancer Chemother Rep* 4(Suppl)229–230, 1973.

44. Yesner R, Carter D: Pathology of carcinoma of the lung: Changing Patterns. *Clin Chest Med* 3:257–289, 1982.

45. World Health Organization. In Shimosato Y, Subin L, Spencer H, et al (eds): *Histological Typing of Lung Tumours*, ed 2. Geneva, World Health Organization, 1981.

46. Radice PA, Matthew MJ, Ihde DK, et al: The clinical behavior of "mixed" small cell/large cell bronchogenic carcinoma compared to "pure" small cell subtypes. *Cancer* 50:2894–2902, 1982.

47. Johnson BE: Management of small cell lung cancer. *Clin Chest Med* 14:173–187, 1993.

48. Shields TW, Ritts RE: *Bronchial Carcinoma.* Springfield, IL, Charles C Thomas, 1974.

49. Razzak MA, Urschel HC Jr, Albers JE, et al: Pulmonary giant cell carcinoma. *Ann Thorac Surg* 21:540–545, 1976.

50. LeRoux BT: Bronchial carcinoma. *Thorax* 23:136–143, 1968.

51. Shields TW: Carcinoma of the lung. In Shields TW (ed): *General Thoracic Surgery.* Philadelphia, Lea & Febiger, 1972, pp 797–845.

52. Said SJ, Faloona GR: Elevated plasma and tissue levels of vasoactive intestinal polypeptide in the watery diarrhea syndrome due to pancreatic, bronchogenic and other tumors. *N Engl J Med* 293:155–160, 1975.

53. Merrill WW, Bondy PK: Production of biochemical marker substances by bronchogenic carcinomas. *Clin Chest Med* 3:307–320, 1982.

54. Patel AM, Bavila OG, Peters SG: Paraneoplastic syndromes associated with lung cancer. *Mayo Clin Proc* 68:278–287, 1993.

55. Kovacs L, Robertson GL: Syndromes of inappropriate antidiuresis. *Endocrinol Metab Clin North Am* 21:859–875, 1992.

56. List AF, Hainsworth SD, Davis BW, et al: The syndrome of inappropriate secretion of antidiuretic hormone (SIADH) in small-cell lung cancer. *J Clin Oncol* 4:1191–1198, 1986.

57. Bensch KG, Corrin B, Pariente R, et al: Oat-cell carcinoma of the lung. *Cancer* 22:1163–1172, 1968.

58. Gaich G, Burtis WJ: The diagnosis and treatment of malignancy associated hypercalcemia. *Endocrinologist* 1:371–378, 1991.

59. Bender RA, Hausen H: Hypercalcemia in bronchogenic carcinoma: a prospective study of 200 patients. *Ann Intern Med* 80:205–208, 1974.

60. Mundy GR, Ibbotson KJ, D'Soufa SM, et al: The hypercalcemia of cancer. Clinical implications and pathogenic mechanisms. *N Engl J Med* 310:1718–1727, 1984.

61. Daughtry DC, Chesney JG, Spear HC, et al: Unexplained systemic manifestations of malignant lung tumors. *Dis Chest* 52:632–639, 1967.

62. Morton DL, Itabashi HH, Grimes OF: Non-metastatic neurological complications of bronchogenic carcinoma. *J Thorac Cardiovasc Surg* 51:14–29, 1966.

63. Hollings HE, Brody RS, Boland HC: Pulmonary hypertrophic osteoarthropathy. *Lancet* 2:1269–1273, 1961.
64. Holman CW: Osteoarthropathy in lung cancer: disappearance after section of intercostal nerves. *J Thorac Cardiovasc Surg* 45:679–681, 1963.
65. Dent PB, McCulloch PB, Wesley-James O, et al: Measurement of carcinoembryonic antigen (CEA) in patients with bronchogenic carcinoma. *Cancer* 42(Suppl): 1481–1491, 1978.
66. Vincent RG, Chu TM, Lane WW, et al: Carcinoembryonic antigen as a monitor of successful surgical resection in 130 patients with carcinoma of the lung. *J Thorac Cardiovasc Surg* 75:734–739, 1978.
67. Concannon JP, Dalbow MH, Hodgson SE, et al: Prognostic value of preoperative carcinoembryonic antigen (CEA) plasma levels in patients with bronchogenic carcinoma. *Cancer* 42:1477–1483, 1978.
68. Baylin SB, Weisburger WR, Eggleston JC, et al: Variable content of histaminase, L-DOPA decarboxylase and calcitonin in small-cell carcinoma of the lung. *N Engl J Med* 299:105–110, 1978.
69. Frost SK, Ball WC, Levin ML, et al: Early lung cancer detection: results of the initial (prevalence) radiologic and cytologic screening in the Johns Hopkins Study. *Am Rev Respir Dis* 150:549–554, 1984.
70. Flehringer BJ, Melamed MR, Zaman MB, et al: Early cancer detection: results of the initial (prevalence) radiologic and cytologic screening in the Memorial Sloan Kettering Study. *Am Rev Respir Dis* 130:555–560, 1984.
71. Fontana RS, Sanderson DR, Taylor WF, et al: Early lung cancer detection: results of the initial (prevalence) radiologic and cytologic screening in the Mayo Clinic Study. *Am Rev Respir Dis* 130:561–565, 1984.
72. Melamed MR, Flehinger BJ, Zaman MB, et al: Detection of true stage 1 lung cancer in a screening program and its effect on survival. *Cancer* 47:1182–1187, 1981.
73. Melamed MR, Flehinger BJ: Should asymptomatic smokers have annual chest x-rays after age 55 years? *Debates in Medicine Yearbook* 3:123–124, 1990.
74. Heitzman ER: *The Lung: Radiologic-Pathologic Correlations.* St. Louis, CV Mosby, 1984.
75. Heitzman ER: Bronchogenic carcinoma: radiologic-pathologic correlations. *Semin Roentgenol* 12:165–174, 1977.
76. Filderman AE, Shaw C, Matthay RA: Lung cancer: Part I. Etiology, pathology, natural history, manifestations, and diagnosis. *Invest Radiol* 21:80–90, 1986.
77. Theros EG. 1976 Caldwell Lecture: Varying manifestations of peripheral pulmonary neoplasms: a radiologic-pathologic correlative study. *AJR* 128:893–914, 1977.
78. White CS, Templeton PA: Radiologic manifestations of bronchogenic cancer. *Clin Chest Med* 14:55–67, 1993.
79. O'Keefe ME Jr, Good CA, McDonald JR: Calcification in solitary nodules of the lung. *AJR* 77:1023–1033, 1957.
80. Spencer H: *Pathology of the Lung.* Philadelphia, WB Saunders, 1977, pp 773–859.
81. Savage P, Donovan WN, Dellinger RP: Sputum cytology in the management of patients with lung cancer. *South Med J* 777:840–842, 1984.
82. Mehta AC, Marty JJ, Lee FYW: Sputum cytology. *Clin Chest Med* 14:68–85, 1993.
83. Clee MD, Sinclair DJ: Assessment of factors influencing the result of sputum cytology in bronchial carcinoma. *Thorax* 36:143–146, 1981.
84. Martini N, McCormick PM: Assessment of endoscopically visible bronchial carcinomas. *Chest* 73:718–720, 1978.
85. Shure D, Fedullo PF: Transbronchial needle aspiration in the diagnosis of submucosal and peribronchial bronchogenic carcinoma. *Chest* 88:49–51, 1985.
86. Stringfield JT, Markowitz DJ, Bentz RR, et al: The effect of tumor size and location on diagnosis by fiberoptic bronchoscopy. *Chest* 72:474–476, 1977.
87. Wallace JM, Deutsch AL: Flexible fiberoptic bronchoscopy and percutaneous needle aspiration for evaluating the solitary nodule. *Chest* 81:655–671, 1982.
88. Arroliga AC, Matthay RA: The role of bronchoscopy in lung cancer. *Clin Chest Med* 14:87–98, 1993.
89. Credle WF, Smiddy JF, Eliott RC: Complications of fiberoptic bronchoscopy. *Am Rev Respir Dis* 109:67–72, 1974.
90. Zavala DC: Diagnostic fiberoptic bronchoscopy: techniques and results of biopsy in 600 patients. *Chest* 68: 12–19, 1975.
91. Wang KP, Terry PB: Transbronchial needle aspiration in the diagnosis and staging of bronchogenic carcinoma. *Am Rev Respir Dis* 127:344–347, 1983.
92. Westcott JL: Direct percutaneous needle aspiration of localized pulmonary lesions: results in 422 patients. *Radiology* 137:31–35, 1980.
93. Salazar AM, Westcott JL: The role of transthoracic needle biopsy for the diagnosis and staging of lung cancer. *Clin Chest Med* 14:99–110, 1993.
94. Khouri NF, Stitik FP, Erozan YS, et al: Transthoracic needle aspiration biopsy of benign and malignant lung lesions. *AJR* 144:281–288, 1985.
95. Calhoun P, Feldman PS, Armstrong P, et al: The clinical outcome of needle aspirations of the lung when cancer is not diagnosed. *Ann Thorac Surg* 41:592–596, 1986.
96. Poe RH, Kallay MC, Wicks CM, et al: Predicting risk of pneumothorax in needle biopsy of the lung. *Chest* 85: 232–235, 1984.
97. Fish GD, Stanley JH, Miller KS, et al: Post-biopsy pneumothorax: estimating the risk by chest radiography and pulmonary function tests. *Am J Roentgenol* 150:71–74, 1988.
98. Sinner WN, Zajicek J: Implantation metastasis after percutaneous transthoracic needle aspiration biopsy. *Acta Radiol [Diagn] (Stockh)* 17:473–480, 1976.
99. Muller NL, Bergin CJ, Miller RR, et al: Seeding of malignant cells into the needle tract after lung and pleural biopsy. *J Can Assoc Radiol* 37:192–194, 1986.
100. Salyer WR, Eggleston JC, Erozan YS: Efficacy of pleural needle biopsy and pleural fluid cytopathology in the diagnosis of malignant neoplasm involving the pleura. *Chest* 67:536–539, 1975.
101. Boutin C, Cargnino, Viallet JR: Thoracoscopy in the early diagnosis of malignant pleural effusions. *Endoscopy* 12:155–160, 1980.
102. Mountain CF: Lung cancer staging classification. *Clin Chest Med* 14:43–51, 1993.
103. Denoix PF: Enquete permanente dans les centres anti-cancereux. *Bull Inst Natl Hyg* 1:70–75, 1946.
104. Mountain CF: A new international staging system for lung cancer. *Chest* 89:225S–233S, 1986.
105. Hande KR, Des Prez RM: Current perspectives in small cell lung cancer. *Chest* 85:669–677, 1984.

106. Hansen HH, Dombernowsky P, Hirsch FR: Staging procedures and prognostic features in small cell anaplastic bronchogenic carcinoma. *Semin Oncol* 5:280–287, 1978.

107. Filderman AE, Shaw C, Matthay RA: Lung cancer: Part II. Staging and therapy. *Invest Radiol* 21:173–185, 1986.

108. Swett HA, Nagel JS, Sostman HD: Imaging methods in primary lung carcinoma. *Clin Chest Med* 3:331–351, 1982.

109. Inouye SK, Sox HC Jr: Standard and computed tomography in the evaluation of neoplasms of the chest. *Ann Intern Med* 105:906–924, 1986.

110. Shields TW: Surgical therapy for carcinoma of the lung. *Clin Chest Med* 14:121–147, 1993.

111. Webb WR, Jensen BG, Sollitto R: Bronchogenic carcinoma. Staging with MR compared with staging with CT and surgery. *Radiology* 156:117–124, 1985.

112. Brantigan JW, Brantigan CO, Brantigan OC: Biopsy of nonpalpable scalene lymph nodes in carcinoma of the lung. *Am Rev Respir Dis* 107:962–974, 1973.

113. Hashim SW, Baue AE, Geha AS: The role of mediastinoscopy and mediastinotomy in lung cancer. *Clin Chest Med* 3:353–359, 1982.

114. Nohl-Oser HC: Lymphatics of the lung. In Shields TW (ed): *General Thoracic Surgery*. Philadelphia, Lea & Febiger, 1972, pp 74–85.

115. Straus MJ: *Lung Cancer: Clinical Diagnosis and Treatment.* New York, Grune & Stratton, 1977, p 123.

116. Sarin CG, Nohl-Oser HG: Mediastinoscopy. *Thorax* 24:585–588, 1969.

117. Bowen TE, Zajtchuk R, Green DC, et al: Value of anterior mediastinotomy in bronchogenic carcinoma of the left upper lobe. *J Thorac Cardiovasc Surg* 76:269–271, 1978.

118. Sandler MA, Pearlberg JL, Madrazo BL, et al: Computed tomographic evaluation of the adrenal gland in the preoperative assessment of bronchogenic carcinoma. *Radiology* 145:733–736, 1982.

119. Hooper G, Beechler CR, Johnson MC: Radioisotope scanning in the initial staging of bronchogenic carcinoma. *Am Rev Respir Dis* 118:279–286, 1978.

120. Ramsdell JW, Peters RM, Taylor AT, et al: Multiorgan scans for staging lung cancer. Correlation with clinical evaluation. *J Thorac Cardiovasc Surg* 73:653–659, 1977.

121. Stoller JK, Ahmad M, Rice TW: Solitary pulmonary nodule. *Cleve Clin J Med* 55:68–74, 1988.

122. Lillington GA, Caskey CI: Evaluation and management of solitary and multiple pulmonary nodules. *Clin Chest Med* 14:111–119, 1993.

123. Steel JD: Solitary pulmonary nodule. *J Thorac Cardiovasc Surg* 46:21–39, 1963.

124. Geddes DM: Hypothesis: the natural history of lung cancer: review based on rates of tumor growth. *Br J Dis Chest* 73:1–17, 1979.

125. Murren JR, Buzaid AC: Chemotherapy and radiation for the treatment of non–small cell lung cancer: a critical review. *Clin Chest Med* 14:161–171, 1993.

126. Martini N, Beattie EJ Jr: Results of surgical treatment in stage I lung cancer. *J Thorac Cardiovasc Surg* 74:499–505, 1977.

127. Naruke T, Goya T, Tsuchiya T, et al: Prognosis and survival in resected lung carcinoma based on the new international staging system. *J Thorac Cardiovasc Surg* 96:440–447, 1988.

128. Shields TW: Surgical therapy for carcinoma of the lung. *Clin Chest Med* 3:369–387, 1982.

129. Yellin A, Benfield JR: Surgery for bronchogenic carcinoma in the elderly. *Am Rev Respir Dis* 131:197–198, 1985.

130. Martini N, Flehinger BJ, Zaman MB, et al: Prospective study of 445 lung carcinomas with mediastinal lymph node metastases. *J Thorac Cardiovasc Surg* 80:390–399, 1980.

131. Friess GG, McCracken JD, Troxell ML, et al: Effect of initial resection of small-cell carcinoma of the lung: a review of Southwestern Oncology Group Study 7628. *J Clin Oncol* 3:964–968, 1985.

132. Olsen GN, Block AJ, Tobias JA: Prediction of postpneumonectomy pulmonary function using quantitative macroaggregate lung scanning. *Chest* 66:13–16, 1984.

133. Lung Cancer Study Group: Effects of postoperative mediastinal radiation on completely resected stage II and stage III epidermoid cancer of the lung. *N Engl J Med* 315:1377–1381, 1986.

134. Lung Cancer Study Group: Surgical adjuvant therapy for stage II and III adenocarcinoma and large-cell undifferentiated carcinoma. *J Clin Oncol* 4:710–715, 1986.

135. Bloedern FG, Cowley RW, Cuccia CA, et al: Combined therapy: irradiation and surgery in the treatment of bronchogenic carcinoma. *Am J Roentgenol* 85:875–885, 1961.

136. Coy P, Kennelly GM: The role of curative radiotherapy in the treatment of lung cancer. *Cancer* 45:698–702, 1980.

137. Smart J, Hilton G: Radiotherapy of cancer of the lung: results in a selected group of cases. *Lancet* 270:880–881, 1956.

138. Cooper JD, Pearson G, Todd TRJ, et al: Radiotherapy alone for patients with operable carcinoma of the lung. *Chest* 87:289–292, 1985.

139. Hilaris BS, Luomanen RK, Beattie EJ: Integrated irradiation and surgery in the treatment of apical lung cancer. *Cancer* 27:1369–1373, 1971.

140. Hansen HH, Elliott JA: Patterns of failure in small cell lung cancer: implications for therapy. Recent results. *Cancer Res* 92:43–57, 1984.

141. Perry MC, Eaton WL, Propert KJ, et al: Chemotherapy with or without radiation therapy in limited small-cell carcinoma of the lung. *N Engl J Med* 316:912–918, 1987.

142. Rosen ST, Makuch RW, Lichter AS, et al: Role of prophylactic cranial irradiation in prevention of central nervous system metastases in small cell lung cancer. Potential benefit restricted to patients with complete response. *Am J Med* 74:615–624, 1983.

143. Roswit B, Patno ME, Rapp R, et al: The survival of patients with inoperable lung cancer: a large scale randomized study of radiation therapy versus placebo. *Radiology* 90:688–697, 1968.

144. Cox JD: Radiotherapeutic management of complications of carcinoma of the lung. *Clin Chest Med* 3:415–421, 1982.

145. Gross NJ: Pulmonary effects of radiation therapy. *Ann Intern Med* 86:81–92, 1977.

146. Souhami R: Chemotherapy in non–small cell bronchial carcinoma. *Thorax* 40:641–645, 1985.

147. Aisner J, Alberto P, Bitran J, et al: Role of chemotherapy in small cell lung cancer: a consensus report of the International Association for the Study of Lung Cancer Workshop. *Cancer Treat Rep* 67:37–43, 1983.

148. Ihde DC: Current status of therapy for small cell carcinoma of the lung. *Cancer* 54:2722–2728, 1984.

149. Hetzel MR, Nixon C, Edmonstone WM, et al: Laser therapy in 100 tracheobronchial tumors. *Thorax* 40:341–345, 1985.

150. Cortese DA, Edell ES: Role of phototherapy, laser therapy and prosthetic stents in the management of lung cancer. *Clin Chest Med* 14:149–159, 1993.

151. Arroliga AC, Carter D, Matthay RA: *Other Primary Neoplasms of the Lung in Pulmonary and Critical Care Medicine*, vol 1. Bone RC, Dantzker DR, George RB, Matthay RA, Reynolds HY (eds): St. Louis, Mosby-Year Book, 1993, pp H2-H6.

152. Andrews CE, Morgan WKC: Tumors of the lung other than bronchogenic carcinoma. In Morgan WKC (ed): *Textbook of Pulmonary Diseases*, ed 2. Boston, Little, Brown & Co, 1974, p 789.

153. Kee JL Jr: Bronchial adenoma. In Shaw RR, Paulson DL, Kee JS Jr (eds): *Treatment of Bronchial Neoplasms*. Springfield, IL, Charles C Thomas, 1955, pp 103–121.

154. Arrigoni MG, Woolner LB, Bernatz PE: Atypical carcinoid tumors of the lung. *J Thorac Cardiovasc Surg* 64:413–421, 1972.

155. Carter D, Yesner R: Carcinomas of the lung with neuroendocrine differentiation. *Semin Diagn Pathol* 2:235–255, 1985.

156. Mills SE, Cooper PH, Walker AN, et al: Atypical carcinoid of the lung: a clinicopathologic study of 17 cases. *Am J Surg Pathol* 6:643–654, 1982.

157. Reid JD: Adenoid cystic carcinoma of the trachea (cylindroma) of the bronchial trees. *Cancer* 5:685–694, 1952.

158. Turnball AD, Hu AG, Goodner JT, et al: Mucoepidermoid tumors of bronchial glands. *Cancer* 28:539–544, 1971.

159. Ashmore PG: Papilloma of the bronchus. *J Thorac Surg* 27:293–294, 1954.

160. Helmuth RA, Strate RW: Squamous carcinoma of the lung in a nonirradiated, nonsmoking patient with juvenile laryngotracheal papillomatosis. *Am J Surg Pathol* 11:643–650, 1987.

161. Liebow AA: Tumors of the lower respiratory tract. In Liebow AA (ed): *Atlas of Tumor Pathology*, Sec. V, Fasc. 17. Washington, DC, Armed Forces Institute of Pathology, 1952.

162. Bateson EM: So-called hamartoma of the lung—a true neoplasm of fibrous connective tissue of the bronchi. *Cancer* 31:1458–1467, 1973.

163. Hochberg LA, Schacter B: Benign tumors of the bronchus and lung. *Am J Surg* 89:425–438, 1955.

164. Pastlethwait RW, Hagerty RF, Trent JC: Endobronchial polypoid hamartochondroma. *Surgery* 24:732–738, 1948.

165. Sun CJ, Kroll M, Miller JE: Primary chondosarcoma of the lung. *Cancer* 50:1864–1866, 1982.

166. Chan K, Ma Fine G, Lewis J, et al: Benign mixed tumor of the trachea. *Cancer* 44:2260–2266, 1979.

167. Watts CF, Clagett OT, Mcdonald JR: Lipoma of the bronchus: discussion of benign neoplasms and a report of endobronchial lipoma. *J Thorac Surg* 15:132–144, 1946.

168. McCall RE, Harrison W: Intrabronchial lipoma: a case report. *J Thorac Surg* 29:317–322, 1955.

169. Agnos JW, Starkey GWB: Primary leiomyosarcoma and leiomyoma of the lung: review of the literature and report of two cases of leiomyosarcoma. *N Engl J Med* 258:12–17, 1958.

170. Guccion JG, Rosen SH: Bronchopulmonary leiomyosarcoma and fibrosarcoma. *Cancer* 30:836–847, 1972.

171. Misra DP, Sunderrajan EV, Rosenholt MJ, et al: Malignant fibrous histiocytoma in the lung masquerading as recurrent pulmonary thromboembolism. *Cancer* 51:538–541, 1983.

172. Lee JT, Shelburne JD, Linder J: Primary malignant fibrous histiocytoma of the lung: a clinicopathologic and ultrastructural study of five cases. *Cancer* 53:1124–1130, 1984.

173. Stuart AP: Fibrosarcoma: malignant tumor of fibroblasts. *Cancer* 1:30–63, 1948.

174. Noehren TH, McKee FW: Sarcoma of the lung. *Dis Chest* 25:663–678, 1954.

# Chapter 16

# Respiratory Tract Infections

**Michael S. Niederman**
**George A. Sarosi**

IN SPITE OF the sophistication and advances in modern medicine, respiratory tract infections remain a major source of morbidity, mortality, and economic cost in our society. The availability of new and potent antibiotics, the development of rapid and elegant diagnostic methods, the emergence of effective vaccines for certain infections, and the appreciation of the role of newly recognized organisms in causing disease have not reduced the scope of the problem presented by respiratory tract infections. In fact, the current ability of modern medicine to extend life and the application of novel life-sustaining therapies have created patient populations with specific impairments in their ability to resist infection and have thereby added to the problem of one specific infection, pneumonia. The patient at risk for pneumonia is always changing, and we now have individuals with novel forms of immunosuppressive illness, as the result of organ transplantation or infection with the HIV virus. Although our therapeutic armamentarium is ever-expanding, the organisms responsible for respiratory infections continue to adapt to the selective pressure of antibiotics. In the 1990s, we have multiply drug-resistant tuberculosis, penicillin-resistant pneumococci, β-lactamase–producing *Haemophilus influenzae*, and highly resistant Gram-negative enteric bacteria. The changing epidemiology and ecology of respiratory infections makes these illnesses an ongoing challenge.

## EPIDEMIOLOGY OF RESPIRATORY INFECTIONS

The common cold is a viral infection of the upper respiratory tract that accounts for 20% of all acute disabling conditions annually in the United States and for 40% of all acute respiratory conditions. Adults have more than 100 million disabling colds annually, leading to 250 million days of restricted activity and 30 million lost days of work, amounting to a staggering economic impact (1). Furthermore, more than 1 billion dollars are spent annually on over-the-counter cold remedies. In spite of these data, a preventative vaccine for the common cold is unlikely, since more than 200 different viruses lead to this type of infection. Similarly, the common cold is an unavoidable annual event for most adults, since even with four colds per year, it would take at least 50 years to contract an infection with every available cold virus and to develop immunity to each one.

Pneumonia, or infection of the lung parenchyma, is also common and occurs in as many as 4 million Americans annually. Pneumonia can occur in the community or in the hospital, and different types of individuals have varying susceptibilities to this infection.

It has been estimated that there are 1 million cases of community-acquired pneumonia requiring hospitalization each year, at an estimated cost of 4 billion dollars (2). Community-acquired infections may be viral, bacterial, or rarely fungal and parasitic. Nosocomial, or hospital-acquired pneumonia, occurs yearly in at least 275,000 individuals and is the most important hospital-acquired infection because it is associated with the highest mortality rate of nosocomial infections that contribute causally to death (3). Most nosocomial pneumonias are bacterial in origin, although hospital-acquired viral infections can also occur, particularly if personnel come to work carrying such an illness. In addition to direct patient care costs, pneumonia is responsible for over 50 million days of restricted activity from work and (in concert with influenza) is the sixth leading cause of death in this country, with a mortality rate of 13.4 per 100,000 (4, 5). In 1991 there were an estimated 129.6 million episodes of influenza, which accounted for over 450 million restricted-activity days (5).

Certain patient populations have an enhanced risk for pneumonia that reflects their disease-associated impairments in respiratory tract host defenses. Among the elderly, pneumonia is the fourth leading cause of death with a mortality rate of 169.7 per 100,000 (6). Similarly 80% of the excess deaths from influenza are in individuals above the age of 65 (5). This enhanced rate of dying from respiratory infection with advancing age has been recognized for a long time, and Sir William Osler called pneumonia the "friend of the aged" that allowed the elderly an escape from "those 'cold gradations of decay' that make the last state of all so distressing" (7).

Among the elderly, the risk of pneumonia varies with an individual's general health and is often reflected by his or her place of residence. Thus, pneumonia occurs in 25 to 44 per 1000 noninstitutionalized elderly individuals and in 68 to 114 per 1000 residents of chronic care institutions. At any one time, as many as 3.2% of all nursing home residents will have pneumonia (8). In the hospital, the elderly have a threefold greater incidence of pneumonia than younger patients, with 1.6% of all hospital admissions in the elderly being complicated by lung infection (8). In one study, patients over the age of 60 represented only 23% of all hospitalized patients, yet they accounted for 64% of all nosocomial infections (9). In the National Nosocomial Infection Surveillance (NNIS) study, 54% of more than 100,000 nosocomial infections were seen in patients over the age of 55. Pneumonia was more common in the elderly than in younger patients and accounted for 48% of all infection-related mortality in the elderly (10).

Among critically ill patients treated with mechanical ventilation, nosocomial pneumonia develops in 10 to 70% of all patients, depending on the type of illness that led to the need for mechanical ventilation. Patients who have had general surgery and require mechanical ventilation in an intensive care unit (ICU) have at least a 10% incidence of pneumonia; a general medical ICU population has a 20% incidence; and patients with the adult respiratory distress syndrome (ARDS) have a 70% incidence of secondary pneumonia (11). Particularly with ARDS, the mortality implications of this infection are striking. If ARDS is complicated by pneumonia, only 12% of patients survive; if the ARDS patient remains free of infection, survival rate is 67% (12). Recent data have shown that patients do not merely die with nosocomial pneumonia, but in fact they actually die because of nosocomial pneumonia, with half of all deaths being the direct effect of infection and not comorbid illness (13).

Other groups at increased risk for pneumonia include patients with cardiac disease, alcoholism, chronic obstructive lung disease, malnutrition, head injury, cystic fibrosis or bronchiectasis, splenic dysfunction, malignancy, cirrhosis, diabetes, renal failure, sickle cell disease, and any immunosuppressive therapy or disease state. Recognition of the increased risk of infection in all of these patient groups should prompt the use of available vaccines to prevent respiratory infection.

Bronchitis, infection of the large bronchi, can be caused by either viruses or bacteria. In children, more than 40% of episodes of acute bronchitis are viral, and the remainder are bacterial. Viral bronchitis in children may lead to transient or even persistent airway hyperreactivity and thereby may be a risk factor for subsequent adult asthma. Chronic bronchitis is an adult disease, characterized by a persistent inflammatory state of the large airways, generally caused by cigarette smoking, and found in 12.5 million Americans (5, 14, 15). Patients with this condition frequently have acute infectious bronchitis (viral or bacterial) superimposed on their chronic condition, with such exacerbations happening once every 20 to 36 weeks (16). Bronchiolitis is an acute infection, usually viral, of the small airways that occurs in children usually between the ages of 1 month and 1 year with an attack rate, in this age group, of 6 to 7 cases per 100 children per year (17).

In recent years, particularly with the application of immunosuppressive therapy for a variety of illnesses, with the emergence of the acquired immune deficiency syndrome (AIDS), and with an increasing number of institutionalized elderly individuals, tuberculosis and fungal and parasitic lung infections have emerged once again as important and common infections. Mycobacterial illnesses frequently complicate AIDS or occur in nursing homes, and fungal infections may emerge from a dormant state in patients living in endemic areas when a disease such as AIDS develops. Since 1985, the incidence of tuberculosis has been increasing, with a current case rate of 10.5 per 100,000. Certain populations are at increased risk for tuberculosis, particularly blacks, Hispanics, and immigrant populations. Minority groups now account for more than 71% of all tuberculosis cases in the United States, even though they represent only 26% of the population (5, 18). An additional concern today is the emergence of multiply drug-resistant disease, a phenomenon that is particularly common in certain areas of the country, such as large cities in the Northeast.

## DEFINITIONS

The respiratory tract can be anatomically divided into an upper and lower system, with the vocal cords serving as the dividing line between them. Infections of the upper respiratory tract include the common cold, sinusitis, pharyngitis, tonsillitis, and epiglottitis. Influenza is a viral infection that can involve the epithelial cells of both the upper and lower respiratory tract, and some patients have predominantly upper respiratory infectious symptoms while others have more marked lower airway signs and symptoms.

Infections of the lower respiratory tract can involve the airways, lung parenchyma, or pleural space. When infection involves the large airways, it is termed bronchitis, and symptoms are a reflection of this localization, with patients complaining of cough, sputum production, and often wheezing. If the infection involves smaller, more peripheral airways, it is termed bronchiolitis; this infection primarily involves children, but recently an adult version, possibly initiated by an infectious agent, has been recognized and is termed "bronchiolitis obliterans with organizing pneumonia." One chronic airways disease, bronchiectasis, is often a consequence of preceding respiratory infection and is frequently characterized by multiple episodes of infection in the areas of diseased airways. Bronchiectasis is characterized pathologically by abnormal and permanent dilation of subsegmental airways, which are inflamed and usually filled with secretions (19). It is these areas of stagnant secretions that frequently become infected. Similarly, chronic bronchitis, a disease caused usually by cigarette smoking, is often complicated by bouts of acute infectious bronchitis.

Pneumonia is an infection of the lung parenchyma itself, involving the alveolar space with microbial invasion. In the immunocompetent individual, this type of infection is accompanied by a brisk filling of the alveolar space with inflammatory cells and fluid. When this alveolar infection involves an entire anatomic lobe of the lung, it is termed "lobar pneumonia," and more than one lobe can be involved in some instances. When the alveolar process occurs in a distribution that is patchy and is adjacent to bronchi, without filling an entire lobe, it is termed a "bronchopneumonia." From a clinical perspective, pneumonias have been classified as being "typical" or "atypical," depending on their mode of clinical presentation. Although the "typical" pneumonia syndrome is characterized by sudden onset of fever, chills, pleuritic chest pain, and productive cough, this type of presentation can only be expected if the patient has an intact immune response system, and if the infection is due to a bacterial pathogen such as *Streptococcus pneumoniae*, *H. influenzae*, *Klebsiella pneumoniae*, *Staphylococcus aureus*, aerobic Gram-negative bacilli, and anaerobes. If a patient is infected by one of these organisms but has an impaired immune response, the classic pneumonia symptoms may be absent, as can be the case with the elderly and debilitated patient. The atypical pneumonia syndrome, characterized by preceding upper respiratory symptoms, fever without chills, nonproductive cough, headache, myalgias, and mild leukocytosis is often the result of infection with viruses, *Mycoplasma pneumoniae*, *Legionella* organisms and other unusual infectious agents (as in psittacosis and Q fever). In clinical practice, it is often very difficult to use this type of classification to predict the microbial etiology of pneumonia. In fact, clinical features may be at best only 40% accurate in distinguishing *M. pneumoniae*, pneumococcus, and other pathogens (20). Another classification system that is often applied to pneumonias is their place of origin, and thus the infection can be community-acquired or hospital-acquired (nosocomial). Patients who develop pneumonia while receiving immunosuppressive therapy or having abnormal immune systems are referred to as compromised hosts, and the infectious possibilities will vary with the localization of the immune defect.

When a parenchymal lung infection leads to necrosis and breakdown of lung tissue and a cavity is evident within the pneumonic area, the infection is termed a lung abscess. These infections are usually caused by anaerobes, but other etiologic agents include *S. aureus*, *K. pneumoniae*, *Escherichia coli*, and *Pseudomonas aeruginosa*. Empyema is an infection of the pleural space, characterized by grossly purulent material, and usually caused by anaerobes, Gram-negative bacilli, or *S. aureus*.

## BACTERIOLOGY OF THE RESPIRATORY TRACT

### THE NORMAL RESPIRATORY TRACT

Certain sites in the respiratory tract are sterile under normal conditions, and the isolation of a microorganism from these sites generally connotes infection; other sites may contain organisms because they are colonized but not infected. When organisms persist at a particular body site, without evidence of a host response or without adverse effects to the host, it is termed colonization. When organisms lead to a host response or adverse tissue effects, then an infection is present. Respiratory tract sites that are sterile in normal individuals include the paranasal sinuses and the lower respiratory tract. Although bacteria can colonize the proximal tracheobronchial tree of smokers and others with impaired host defenses, the more distal areas of the lung are normally sterile unless infection is present. On the other hand, the nasopharynx and oropharynx are normally colonized and have an endogenous microflora; it is the identity of these colonizing organisms that changes when disease is present.

*The Upper Airway*

The oropharynx is normally colonized by a mixture of aerobic and microaerophilic bacteria as well as by anaerobic organisms. The "normal" oral flora can include *S. mitis*, *Streptococcus salivarius*, *Staphylococcus epidermidis*, *Neisseria* species, pneumococcus, *Candida* species and lactobacilli. Colonizing anaerobes include *Veillonella* species, *Fusobacterium* species, anaerobic streptococci and micrococci, and certain *Bacteroides* species (17, 21). Conspicuously absent from this group of bacteria are the enteric Gram-negative bacilli. Multiple investigators have shown that normal individuals are not colonized by these Gram-negative bacteria, but patients with serious illness of any type may harbor these organisms in the oropharynx. The likelihood that a given individual will have upper airway colonization by these bacteria is directly related to the severity and duration of illness. Patients with "moderate" illness will harbor Gram-negative organisms in the oropharynx 35% of the time, while 73% of "moribund" individuals will be colonized (22). Most patients develop colonization of the oropharynx when they enter a hospital, usually by the third hospital day. Risk factors for upper airway colonization include alcoholism, endotracheal intubation, neutropenia, prior antibiotic use, azotemia, coma, hypotension, smoking, surgery, prior viral illness, and malnutrition (21–23).

The microbial ecology of the upper airway changes with infection, and the bacteriology of infection is different, depending on the site (Table 16.1). This tendency of specific organisms to cause infection at one airway site but not another can be described as a "tissue tropism," or preference, of certain organisms for certain epithelial locations. The reason for tissue tropisms is not fully known, but their existence would suggest that colonization and infection proceed in

**TABLE 16.1**
**Common Pathogens for Upper Respiratory Tract Infections**

Pharyngitis
  Group A streptococci
  Viruses
    Adenovirus
    Enteroviruses
    Influenza
    Epstein-Barr virus
    *Herpesvirus hominis*
Laryngitis
  Viruses
Common cold
  Viruses
    Rhinovirus
    Adenovirus
    Coronavirus
    Influenza
Sinusitis
  *Haemophilus influenzae*
  Pneumococcus
  Anaerobes
  Rhinovirus
Epiglottitis
  *H. influenzae*
  *Haemophilus parainfluenzae*
  *Staphylococcus aureus*
  Group A streptococcus
Croup
  Viruses
    Parainfluenza virus
    Respiratory syncytial virus
    Adenovirus
    *Mycoplasma pneumoniae*

unique ways for each mucosal site, making some sites more susceptible to the effects of a particular organism than are others.

*The Tracheobronchial Tree*

The lower respiratory tract is sterile in healthy individuals but may become colonized when illness is present (24). Smokers commonly will have *H. influenzae* recovered from tracheobronchial secretions, even when there is no evidence of an acute bronchitis. In patients with chronic bronchitis, tracheobronchial colonization is common and can include *H. influenzae*, viridans streptococci, *Moraxella catarrhalis*, and occasionally enteric Gram-negative bacteria (21). Gram-negative colonization becomes a particularly common event if the patient has one of a variety of acute or chronic illnesses, including ciliary dysfunction (cystic fibrosis and bronchiectasis), corticosteroid therapy, immunodeficiency, tracheostomy, prior antibiotic therapy, viral infection, malnutrition, and endotracheal intubation (21, 23). Most bacteria enter the lower airway via aspiration from a previously colonized oropharynx, and thus there is frequently congruence of organism identity at the two respiratory tract sites. Occasionally, organisms reach the lung hematogenously from nonrespiratory sites of infection. Inhalation is not a major route of bacterial entry to the lung, with the exception of certain organisms such as *Legionella pneumophila* and *Mycobacterium tuberculosis*. More recently, the intestinal tract has been identified as another important source of organism entry to the lung. Either by reflux or by passage along a nasogastric tube, gastric bacteria can pass to the oropharynx and then be aspirated into the lung (25). Also, in critically ill patients treated with an endotracheal tube or tracheostomy, certain organisms, such as *P. aeruginosa*, can enter the lower airway directly from environmental sources, and colonization can follow (26).

With infectious illness, as with the upper respiratory tract, the lower airway and lung parenchyma can also become infected with different organisms at different sites. These "tropisms" of specific organisms causing specific illnesses are summarized in Table 16.2.

## SPECIFIC INFECTIOUS SYNDROMES—CLINICAL FEATURES AND THERAPY

### THE UPPER RESPIRATORY TRACT (TABLE 16.1)

### The Common Cold

The common cold is a symptom complex caused by one of more than 200 viral agents. The most common viral etiologic agent is a rhinovirus, of which there are at least 100 types (27). Other common agents causing this infection are adenovirus, coronavirus, parainfluenza virus, respiratory syncytial virus and influenza A, B, and C viruses. Less common viral pathogens include enterovirus, Epstein-Barr, and herpes simplex viruses. Typical symptoms include nasal congestion and discharge, sneezing, sore throat, and cough. In contrast to some other viral illnesses, upper respiratory tract symptoms predominate, while systemic symptoms are mild or absent and fever is not usually high. Incubation period of the illness varies for each virus, but is generally 48 to 72 hours (28). The illness may last up to 1 week, but up to one-quarter of patients will be ill for up to 2 weeks. When symptoms persist, consideration must be given to the occurrence of a secondary bacterial infection such as sinusitis (in 0.5% of cases) or pharyngitis. Other complications can include bacterial otitis media (in 2% of cases) and persistent bronchospastic cough. Physical findings are generally confined to the upper respiratory tract and include nasal mucosal swelling and exudation and pharyngeal erythema.

**TABLE 16.2**
**COMMON PATHOGENS FOR LOWER RESPIRATORY TRACT INFECTIONS**

Bronchitis
  *Haemophilus influenzae*
  Pneumococcus
  *Branhamella catarrhalis*
  *Mycoplasma pneumoniae*
  Viruses
    Adenovirus
    Influenza
    Rhinovirus
    Respiratory syncytial virus
Bronchiolitis
  Viruses
    Respiratory syncytial virus
    Parainfluenza virus
    Adenovirus
    Rhinovirus
Pneumonia
  Pneumococcus
  *Legionella pneumophilia*
  *M. pneumoniae*
  *H. influenzae*
  Anaerobes
  *Staphylococcus aureus*
  Enteric Gram-negatives
  Viruses
    Influenza
    Respiratory syncytial virus
    Adenovirus
  *Chlamydia psittaci* (TWAR)
  *Pneumocystis carinii*
Bronchiectasis
  *Pseudomonas aeruginosa*
  *S. aureus*
  Mucoid *Escherichia coli*
  *H. influenzae*

Only a few viral "colds" will be accompanied by an exudative pharyngitis, most notably those caused by adenovirus.

Most adults develop two to four colds per year, while children may have six to eight such infections. Smokers have more frequent and more severe viral respiratory illnesses (29). Illness is more common in the fall and winter, helping to distinguish a cold from seasonal allergies, which are more common in the spring and early fall. The major route of viral transmission is person-to-person via the hand-nose-hand inoculation route, but there is some evidence that cold viruses can also be spread via droplet nuclei generated by sneezing (30).

Therapy is entirely symptomatic and supportive unless a secondary bacterial infection supervenes. Nasal decongestants, warm saline gargles, cough suppressants, and antipyretics are generally effective along with bed rest. Aspirin should be used cautiously in children and adolescents because of its association with Reye's syndrome, especially after influenza and varicella infection. Antibiotics should not be routinely administered unless bacterial infection is present. Therapy with vitamin C is unproven. Prevention of cold transmission can be achieved by careful hand washing after contact with an infected individual. Experimental prophylactic approaches have included the use of virucidal-impregnated tissues to wipe the nose of infected individuals and the application of intranasal interferon alpha-2 (31).

## Sinusitis

Infection of one or more of the paranasal sinuses can be a cryptogenic event (5% of cases) or can be associated with other conditions such as viral upper respiratory infection, allergic rhinitis, or mechanical obstruction of the sinuses. There are four different paranasal sinuses, which are ordinarily sterile, but they can fill with serous fluid when the ostia are obstructed as the result of inflammation or infection. The fluid-filled sinus can in turn become infected by viruses (especially rhinovirus), pneumococcus, *H. influenzae*, *M. catarrhalis*, or anaerobes. Most cases result from the common cold or from allergic rhinitis leading to ostial obstruction, but 10 to 15% of cases can arise from a dental abscess. The maxillary sinus is most frequently infected in both adults and children; the frontal sinus is the second most commonly infected site in adults (27).

If the maxillary or frontal sinuses are affected, the patient may note facial pain and tenderness to percussion over these areas. Purulent nasal discharge and low-grade fever are common symptoms. Infection of the ethmoid sinus can result in retro-orbital pain, tearing, and headache that worsens in the supine position. Sphenoidal sinusitis may lead to a vertex headache that is most severe at night.

A clinical diagnosis of sinusitis can be made with typical headache pain and other associated findings, particularly if they arise after a viral upper respiratory tract infection. Transillumination of the sinuses can lead to a diagnosis also. To perform this maneuver for the maxillary sinus, a light is placed over the orbital rim and transmission to the hard palate is observed. Opacity by this maneuver is highly related to bacterial infection, while bright transillumination makes sinus infection unlikely (32). Sinus radiographs may also confirm the diagnosis. In fact a four-view radiographic series is 72 to 96% as accurate for demonstrating maxillary sinusitis as is sinus aspiration and culture (33). When sinus radiographs are used to define the illness, certain clinical findings can be elicited that correlate highly with the presence of radiographic abnormalities. In a logistic regression model (33), patients were likely to have sinusitis if they had at least four of the following signs or symptoms: maxillary toothache, poor response of symptoms to nasal decongestants, a history of colored nasal discharge, purulent nasal secretions, and an abnormal transillumination of the sinuses. Sinus tenderness is only present in about half of all patients with sinusitis.

Bacteriologic studies have shown that sinusitis is caused by *H. influenzae*, pneumococcus, and anaerobes, with viruses (rhinovirus, influenza virus, parainfluenza virus) being found occasionally. Less common are *S. aureus*, Gram-negative bacteria, and fungi (32). Based on this spectrum, therapy is usually with an oral antimicrobial agent for 10 to 14 days. Some clinical improvement should be seen within 48 hours of therapy, but if the findings are not completely resolved by 2 weeks, then an additional week of therapy may be used. Appropriate therapy can be achieved with ampicillin, 2 g daily, or trimethoprim-sulfamethoxazole. Use of β-lactamase-resistant agents may also be appropriate if resistance to ampicillin is encountered. Adjunctive therapy can include analgesics and decongestants. When antibiotic therapy does not work, complications such as osteomyelitis, facial cellulitis, intracranial abscess, cavernous sinus thrombosis, and even meningitis must be considered.

## Epiglottitis

Acute swelling and inflammation of the epiglottis and aryepiglottic folds, caused by an infectious agent, can be a life-threatening illness, particularly in children. This infection does not descend into the lower airway and is usually bacterial, with *H. influenzae* type B being the most common etiologic pathogen (34–37). The seriousness of this infection is related to its potential to cause sudden upper airway obstruction and asphyxiation. The disease is more common in children than adults, with the incidence greatest between ages 2 and 4 and with a peak around age 3½. there is no seasonal predisposition. Adults can develop this illness with an incidence as high as 9.7 cases per million (34).

Patients with epiglottitis fall into one of three age ranges: less than age 2, children above the age of 2, and adults. Children above the age of 2 present with "classic" epiglottitis (36) with symptoms of sore throat or mild upper respiratory symptoms that can rapidly progress to high fever, drooling, dysphagia, and lethargy (38). The symptoms can be described as the "four D's" of dysphagia, dysphonia, dyspnea, and drooling (36). Generally, all patients have respiratory distress, and breathing can be noisy with signs of inspiratory stridor. Unlike the case with croup, there is not a prominent cough, stridor is lower pitched, and patients are generally older (the peak age for croup is 2 years).

When adults develop this disease, sore throat is the most common symptom, with less than one-half of the patients having respiratory distress and approximately one-quarter having drooling. Both infants (below age 2) and adults have a similar form of illness that is more a supraglottitis than an epiglottitis. In infants the illness is similar to croup but with a more severe clinical course. In adults, the infection is also primarily a supraglottitis, and the disease can be either gradual or accelerated (39). The most common pathogens in adults are type B *H. influenzae*, *S. aureus*, and *Klebsiella* species (36). In adults, abscess formation can be a complication, and the bacteriology of these lesions includes *S. aureus* and a variety of streptococci.

The diagnosis is usually made by recognition of typical signs and symptoms. An attempt at direct or indirect visualization of the epiglottis may reveal the presence of a swollen, cherry-red epiglottis projecting over the back of the tongue. The patient should never be examined with a tongue blade, as this may precipitate total airway obstruction. A lateral neck radiograph can confirm the diagnosis when the "thumb sign" of an enlarged epiglottis is seen, but this technique may be negative, even with life-threatening disease. In adults, the findings may be more subtle, with only mild erythema or even pale edema of the epiglottis. In one series, lateral neck radiographs were abnormal in 79% of affected adults (34). Recently, other radiographic signs of epiglottitis have been described. In one series, epiglottic width in relation to epiglottic height or in relation to the width of the third cervical vertebra have been described as sensitive and specific diagnostic findings (40). Other diseases to be considered in the differential diagnosis are angioedema, bacterial tracheitis, croup, foreign body aspiration, and peritonsillar abscess.

Management is directed at maintenance of a patent airway to minimize mortality. With the use of a prophylactic artificial airway, mortality in children has fallen below 1%. In adults, mortality was 7% in one series in which routine establishment of an artificial airway was not used. In that series, 15 of 56 patients had airway compromise and differed from less ill patients with a higher incidence of respiratory difficulty and positive blood cultures. All deaths were within 6 hours of hospital admission, indicating how rapidly progressive this illness may be. It is currently recommended that all affected children have an artificial airway established via orotracheal or nasotracheal intubation, usually under general anesthesia, and only if this

cannot be done is a tracheostomy needed. Routine intubation in adults is controversial, and management must be individualized, with careful observation being essential in the early hours of illness. In one series of 30 adults seen over a 10-year period, no patient required intubation or tracheostomy (39).

Other adjunctive measures include humidified oxygen and antibiotics. The pediatric illness is almost always caused by *H. influenzae*, and in adults, *H. influenzae* still is the predominant organism, being recovered in 56% of patients in one series (34). Blood cultures are positive, usually for *H. influenzae*, in up to 75% of children and 23% of adults. As mentioned, other possible infecting agents include pneumococcus, *S. aureus*, *H. parainfluenzae*, *Fusobacterium* spp., and group A streptococcus. With this bacteriologic spectrum in mind, therapy is usually with ampicillin (200 mg/kg/day in six divided doses) and chloramphenicol (50 mg/kg/day in four divided doses—if β-lactamase-resistant strains are suspected), or alternatively, a second- or third-generation cephalosporin or a β-lactamase-resistant agent combined with ampicillin. In adults, therapy with a second- or third-generation cephalosporin is preferable. The use of corticosteroids in conjunction with an antibiotic is of unproven benefit but may be helpful just prior to removal of an endotracheal tube to prevent laryngeal edema after extubation.

## Other Upper Respiratory Tract Infections

### Pharyngitis

Pharyngitis may occur with or without symptoms of the common cold. Etiologic agents may be viral or bacterial, with pharyngitis due to group A beta-hemolytic streptococci (GABHS) being potentially the most important to recognize and treat. In the first 2 years of life, infection by group A streptococci is uncommon, but the incidence rises between ages 5 and 10. In children, GABHS accounts for one-third of all cases of pharyngitis. In college-age students, one-quarter of cases are streptococcal, but viral pharyngitis is seen in 38% (41). In those over the age of 35, streptococcal infection is present in only 5% of those with pharyngitis (27). In children and adults, other common infecting agents besides streptococci include adenovirus, respiratory syncytial virus, rhinovirus, coronavirus, influenza and parainfluenza viruses, Epstein-Barr virus, herpesvirus hominis, and *M. pneumoniae*. Less common agents include *Neisseria gonorrhoeae* and *Neisseria meningitides*, *H. influenzae*, *Corynebacterium diphtheriae*, and anaerobes in a mixed pattern.

It may be difficult to distinguish the responsible pathogen from clinical features, but streptococcal pharyngitis onset may be sudden, with high fever, pharyngeal and uvular edema, yellowish pharyngeal exudate, along with red follicular lesions with yellow centers being found on the uvula. However, infections with the Epstein-Barr virus, herpesviruses, adenoviruses, and enteroviruses may also present with similar findings.

Streptococcal pharyngitis should be treated with penicillin VK, 500 mg every 6 hours for 10 days, or another antibiotic, such as erythromycin, if the patient is allergic. Therapy provides four benefits: reduction in illness duration, avoidance of spread to others, prevention of suppurative complications (such as peritonsillar and retropharyngeal abscess), and prevention of rheumatic fever (but probably not glomerulonephritis) (42).

*Croup*

Croup, or acute laryngotracheobronchitis, is a disease of young children usually between the ages of 3 months and 3 years, with a peak incidence in the second year of life. The etiology is usually viral, and this complication may occur in certain individuals while others infected with the same virus develop only a mild upper respiratory illness. Some children develop recurrent episodes whenever they acquire a viral upper respiratory infection, and in these instances the disease is termed "spasmodic croup." Parainfluenza virus type 1 is the most common cause, but the disease may also result from influenza viruses, respiratory syncytial virus, adenovirus, mycoplasma, and rhinoviruses (41). Patients with croup present with acute dyspnea following an upper respiratory illness. A barking cough is seen, followed by symptoms of hoarseness and stridor. The stridor may be accompanied by severe dyspnea, and the course may be fluctuating, with improvement in the daytime. Airway edema is less severe than with epiglottitis, and thus acute upper airway obstruction is less likely. Treatment is supportive with inhalation of moist cold air, racemic epinephrine, and possibly steroids, with the latter being controversial. Antibiotics are not needed unless the patient has secondary bacterial infection.

## AIRWAY INFECTIONS (TABLE 16.2)

### Bronchitis

*In the Previously Healthy Adult*

Bronchitis is acute infection and inflammation of the large conducting airways and may be viral or bacterial in origin. When this infection occurs in a previously normal host, the resulting acute bronchitis will present in a manner very similar to a mild form of pneumonia, and the responsible pathogens will be similar for both illnesses. In the presence of chronic respiratory disease or chronic inflammatory bronchitis, the manifestations and etiologic agents will differ from those seen with acute bronchitis in the normal host.

Acute bronchitis in the normal host may be due to viruses in at least 40% of cases and these include adenovirus, influenza A and B virus, coronavirus, rhinovirus, herpes simplex, respiratory syncytial virus, and parainfluenza virus. The role of bacteria in acute bronchitis is difficult to establish, particularly in those with chronic bronchitis, because it may be difficult to distinguish colonization from infection. Bacterial agents implicated include *H. influenzae*, both typable and nontypable strains, and pneumococcus. *M. pneumoniae* may account for 10% of infections. Newer agents identified as causing bronchitis are *M. catarrhalis* and *Chlamydia pneumoniae* (also called the TWAR agent) (43).

Patients with bronchitis have symptoms of cough, purulent sputum, low-grade fever, chest burning, and substernal discomfort. These lower respiratory symptoms usually follow a preceding upper respiratory infection. Hemoptysis can also occur, and acute bronchitis is the most common cause of this symptom. Dyspnea is generally mild, and the physical examination may demonstrate diffuse adventitious sounds such as crackles, rhonchi, and wheezes. Diagnosis is made by discovering appropriate clinical features in the absence of a lung infiltrate on chest film. Sputum Gram stain will show numerous polymorphonuclear cells and possibly bacterial pathogens. Therapy is supportive with cough suppressants, liquids, and antipyretics. Only if a bacterial etiology is likely are antibiotics indicated. Many patients with acute bronchitis will develop the frustrating complication of postinfectious bronchospasm. This is characterized by persistent dry cough and wheezing lasting 4 to 6 weeks after the acute infection subsides. Symptoms are treated with bronchodilators and sometimes corticosteroids, and only rarely will the airway reactivity persist and lead to chronic asthma. Some data indicate that children who have multiple episodes of acute viral bronchitis are at risk for developing adult chronic airways disease and asthma (44).

*In the Patient with Chronic Lung Disease*

Patients with chronic bronchitis and chronic lung disease frequently have episodes of acute bronchitis, but the clinical picture and bacteriology differ from those seen in the normal host. These episodes of acute airway infection occur every 20 to 78 weeks, with most studies reporting an exacerbation of chronic bronchitis due to acute infectious bronchitis every 20 to 36 weeks (16). With infection, patients may note increasing dyspnea, purulent sputum, wheezing, fever, and general malaise. The three cardinal symptoms of an exacerbation, dyspnea, increased sputum purulence, and increased sputum volume, can be counted and used to grade the severity of an exacerbation. Patients with all three symptoms have the most severe exacerbation, a type 1 exacerbation (45). It has been estimated that 80% of all exacerbations are accompanied by two or three of these cardinal symptoms (45).

Examination may reveal diffuse crackles, rhonchi, or wheezes, and the chest radiograph shows no acute infiltrate. Exacerbations in this setting may be viral or bacterial, with some investigators believing that viral causes are most common. It is very difficult to reach such a conclusion with any certainty, since patients with chronic bronchitis have bacterial colonization of the tracheobronchial tree in the absence of acute infection, and thus the recovery of bacterial pathogens from their sputum may represent either colonization or infection. However, in one study that used quantitative bacteriologic methods in patients with severe exacerbation, nearly half of all patients had bacteria present in concentrations equal to that seen in the presence of pneumonia (46). Common viral pathogens are adenovirus, influenza, rhinovirus, coronavirus, herpes simplex, and respiratory syncytial virus. The most common bacterial pathogens are *H. influenzae*, pneumococcus, and *M. catarrhalis*. Other recently recognized pathogens include *Chlamydia psittaci* and *M. pneumoniae* (43). *Moraxella* spp. are neisseria-like organisms that have only recently been recognized as pathogens, after being appreciated as simply part of the "normal" flora in the past (43, 47). *Moraxella* spp. are often resistant to $\beta$-lactamase antibiotics such as amoxicillin, because they can produce a $\beta$-lactamase, a phenomenon that is also present in 20 to 40% of all *H. influenzae* organisms. Most patients with *Moraxella* infections have abnormal host defenses, with up to 77% being smokers, and 84% having preexisting cardiopulmonary disease (47).

The role of antibiotics in treating acute bronchitic exacerbations of chronic bronchitis is controversial (15, 48). The benefits of such therapy are uncertain in many studies, possibly because many episodes are viral. However, the most recent studies do show some benefit, and thus most physicians would agree to use antibiotic therapy along with bronchodilators and, in some severely bronchospastic patients, corticosteroids (49). Antibiotics seem to lead to more frequent and more rapid clinical resolution of symptoms than if patients do not receive therapy, particularly if patients have two or three of the cardinal exacerbation symptoms (45). In addition, antibiotics can eradicate organisms and thus reduce the host inflammatory response to the presence of bacteria, thereby preventing inflammatory injury to the airway (15). In doing so, antibiotics may disrupt the "vicious cycle" of infection, inflammation, and further infection (48). In the past, amoxicillin, 500 mg three times a day for 10 days, or ampicillin were appropriate antibiotic choices, but now with the emergence of *M. catarrhalis* and $\beta$-lactamase-producing *H. influenzae* as pathogens, therapy with amoxicillin combined with a $\beta$-lactamase inhibitor (amoxicillin/clavulanate 500 mg every 8 hours), erythromycin (or one of the newer macrolides), a fluoroquinolone, trimethoprim-sulfamethoxazole, or tetracycline may be more appropriate.

In patients treated with chronic tracheostomy or mechanical ventilation, an illness termed febrile tracheobronchitis may develop (50). Clinically the disease is similar to nosocomial pneumonia with fever, leukocytosis, and purulent respiratory secretions. In some individuals, bacteremia may occur. Unlike with pneumonia, the patient has no new parenchymal lung infiltrate. The disease is diagnosed if the patient has a compatible clinical picture and no new parenchymal lung infiltrate. The etiology is usually enteric Gram-negative bacteria, particularly *P. aeruginosa* in the most seriously ill patients, and occasionally nontypable *H. influenzae*. Therapy is usually with systemic antibiotics directed against the responsible pathogen, but aerosolized antibiotics may be effective in patients without systemic toxicity.

**Bronchiolitis**

Bronchiolitis, an infection of the small airways, is primarily a viral infection of children, seen in the first year of life. Respiratory syncytial virus, parainfluenza virus type 3, influenza virus, adenovirus, and rhinovirus are the most common causes (17). Other infectious agents leading to bronchiolitis include *M. pneumoniae*, *L. pneumophila*, *Nocardia asteroides*, and *Pneumocystis carinii* (51). Children present with fever, tachypnea, wheezing, cough, and malaise. Therapy is supportive with hydration, oxygen, and possibly bronchodilators. Recently, aerosolized ribavirin has been advocated to treat respiratory syncytial virus, a common cause of bronchiolitis in the midwinter and spring.

An adult form of this infection has been recognized and termed "bronchiolitis obliterans with organizing pneumonia" (BOOP). Although bronchiolitis obliterans can result from any viral bronchiolitis, the adult disease may present in an indolent fashion, with cough and dyspnea and no evident acute infection. Because of distal atelectasis beyond the inflamed airways, segmental infiltrates may be seen, in what has been termed the "proliferative" form of bronchiolitis (51). BOOP may be of viral origin or may be the result of inhalational injury, drug effects, or inflammation from a noninfectious systemic illness such as rheumatoid arthritis (51, 52). Therapy is generally with corticosteroids.

**Influenza**

This acute respiratory infection results from an RNA virus of either type A or B, with the disease from type

A being generally more severe (53). Influenza A virus is the most important respiratory virus on a global scale, with the highest overall morbidity and mortality. The virus has two major surface glycoprotein antigens, the hemagglutinin (H) and neuraminidase (N), that can change yearly, and thus the disease appears in epidemics annually. Both antigenic drift and waning immunity make this infection a yearly threat, particularly to those who have underlying cardiac or respiratory illnesses, the elderly and pregnant women. The virus has an incubation period of 2 to 4 days and is spread via aerosol or mucosal contact with infected secretions. Epidemics occur yearly in the late fall and extend into the early spring. Influenza A can coexist with other viral infections including respiratory syncytial virus and parainfluenza virus, particularly in the elderly (54, 55).

The virus has its main site of infection in the respiratory mucosa, leading to desquamation of the respiratory mucosa with cellular degeneration, edema, and airway inflammation with mononuclear cells (56). Although up to half of the infections are subclinical, the typical illness lasts 3 days and is characterized by sudden onset of fever, chills, severe myalgia, malaise, and headache. As the major symptoms recede, respiratory symptoms dominate with dry cough and substernal burning which may persist for several weeks. Laboratory data and physical examination are not specific, and diagnosis is made by noting the presence of typical symptoms during the time of a known epidemic. Serologic evaluation, using hemagglutinating-inhibiting antibody or ELISA testing, and viral cultures can confirm the diagnosis. The illness can be more severe in smokers, the elderly, those less than age 1, pregnant women, and patients with chronic cardiorespiratory disease.

Influenza viruses can interfere with many aspects of respiratory host defenses and thus may be complicated by secondary bacterial pneumonia. The virus can interfere with mucociliary clearance, can promote tracheal bacterial colonization, and can interfere with the function of polymorphonuclear cells and macrophages. Respiratory complications include obliterative bronchiolitis, airway hyperreactivity, exacerbation of chronic bronchitis, primary viral pneumonia, and secondary bacterial pneumonia. When viral pneumonia develops, the disease follows the classic 3-day illness without a hiatus and is characterized by cough (dry or productive) and severe dyspnea. Chest radiograph reveals bilateral infiltrates, and mortality is high. Bacterial pneumonic superinfection has a lower mortality and follows the primary influenza illness with a hiatus of patient improvement for 3 to 4 days before the pneumonia begins. In this setting, pneumonia is usually lobar, and the most common pathogens are pneumococcus, *H. influenzae*, enteric Gram-negative organisms, and *S. aureus*. Other serious complications include myocarditis and pericarditis, seizures, neuritis, coma, transverse myelitis, toxic shock, and renal failure (53).

Therapy of influenza is mainly symptomatic with antipyretics, bed rest, and fluids. Amantadine can ameliorate the illness caused by influenza A if given within the first 24 to 48 hours. This medication may also be used prophylactically in high-risk individuals during an epidemic in doses of 100 mg twice a day until the epidemic passes or for 2 weeks, until vaccination can be given and become effective. Dosage must be reduced with renal insufficiency, and confusion may occur in 3 to 7% of treated individuals. Rimantadine, a derivative of amantadine, is also effective for the therapy and prevention of influenza A infection (57). Rimantidine can be given once daily because of its long half-life, and it has fewer central nervous system and other side effects than amantadine. Immunization should be given to all high-risk patients yearly with a vaccine prepared against the strains most likely to be epidemic. If an epidemic of influenza A develops in a closed environment (e.g., a nursing home) among nonimmunized patients, antiviral therapy should be given along with vaccination, and antiviral therapy is continued for 2 weeks, until the vaccine takes effect.

### Bronchiectasis

Bronchiectasis is another chronic airway disease that can be complicated by intermittent bouts of airway infection. In addition, the disease itself and its progression may be the result of airway infection. The disease is characterized pathologically by an abnormal and permanent dilation of subsegmental airways (19). In this condition, the airways are dilated and inflamed, and they become obstructed by thick secretions that may intermittently become infected. The actual shape of the abnormal airways has led to a classification system that characterizes the involvement as being either cylindrical, varicose, or saccular.

The causes of bronchiectasis are multiple, and in years past, it was most often the result of a preceding respiratory infection such as tuberculosis or a virulent bacterial, fungal, or viral illness. A localized process can lead to focal bronchiectasis, while a more extensive process or a systemic illness can lead to diffuse bronchiectasis. Some of the diseases that may be complicated by bronchiectasis include cystic fibrosis, rheumatoid arthritis, influenza, lung abscess, foreign body aspiration, hypoglobulinemia, immotile cilia syndrome, and allergic bronchopulmonary aspergillosis.

The major symptom of bronchiectasis is cough,

which is generally productive but may be dry. In severe disease, patients may expectorate more than 150 mL of sputum daily. Dyspnea and hemoptysis are also common, with massive hemoptysis at times of acute infection in some patients. The disease is accompanied by chronic bacterial colonization of the lower respiratory tract. When the quantity of sputum increases and the sputum becomes purulent, usually in association with fever and dyspnea, infection is present and requires antibiotics. In some settings, patients are given monthly antibiotics to prevent recurrent bouts of airway infection. The usual pathogens are bacterial and include pneumococcus and *H. influenzae*. Patients with cystic fibrosis may have *S. aureus*. In more advanced forms of bronchiectasis and cystic fibrosis, airway infection is with mucoid variants of *E. coli* or *P. aeruginosa*. Recovery of these mucoid variants should immediately prompt consideration of the diagnosis of bronchiectasis if it has not been previously recognized, because these organisms are not ordinarily found in the absence of chronic airway infection.

Some investigators (58) have found evidence for progression of the airway damage as a result of recurrent infection episodes. When airway infection occurs, it is accompanied by a brisk inflammatory response, with the release of neutrophilic proteases that can damage the airways and lead to more bronchiectasis. Observations such as these have prompted the suggestion that airway infection be treated promptly, and possibly in a prophylactic fashion, to limit disease progression. Episodes of airway infection are treated with antibiotics similar to those used in exacerbations of chronic bronchitis; it may not be necessary to treat every pathogen recovered from the sputum because some organisms may be colonizers and not infecting agents. One effective regimen is amoxicillin 500 to 1000 mg three times a day for 14 days. In cystic fibrosis, the use of aerosolized aminoglycosides in a prophylactic fashion may be effective in preventing acute episodes of airway infection. Other adjunctive therapies include chest physical therapy with percussion and postural drainage, bronchodilators, oxygen, pneumococcal vaccine, and yearly influenza vaccine. In cases of severe hemoptysis or localized recurrent infections due to bronchiectasis, surgical resection of the involved lung may be considered.

When bronchiectasis is suspected by history, it should be confirmed by computed tomography of the chest or bronchography. Routine chest radiographs (Fig. 16.1) may show areas of increased airway markings, atelectasis, dilated bronchi, "tram lines," or cavities. Physical examination may show clubbing, nasal polyposis, and adventitious breath sounds (rhonchi, rales, and wheezes). If the history is appropriate, a

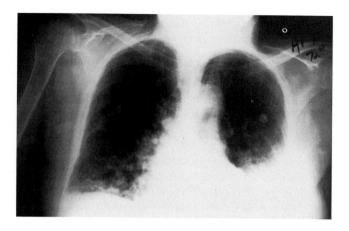

**FIGURE 16.1.** This patient had longstanding bronchiectasis with chronic increased markings in both lower lung zones. The typical increased markings of this disease are seen in the right lower lobe, while the left lower lobe had evidence of pneumonia due to *Pseudomonas aeruginosa*.

workup for hypogammaglobulinemia (immunoglobulin quantitation), immotile cilia syndrome (electron microscopy of nasal cilia), or cystic fibrosis (sweat chloride) may be indicated. Although cystic fibrosis is an inherited disease that usually appears in childhood, recognition in adolescence and longevity into adulthood are increasingly common.

## PARENCHYMAL LUNG INFECTIONS

### Pathogenesis of Pneumonia

Bacteria commonly enter the lower airway and do not lead to pneumonia because of the presence of an intact, elaborate, host defense system. When pneumonia does occur, it is the result of either an exceedingly virulent organism, a large inoculum, and/or an impaired host defense system. In the non-hospitalized person, bacteria reach the lung by one of four routes: inhalation from ambient air, hematogenous spread, direct inoculation from contiguous infected sites, or aspiration from a previously colonized upper airway. Critically ill patients in the hospital may acquire organisms from a colonized gastrointestinal tract (particularly if a nasogastric tube is present to direct bacteria from the stomach to the oropharynx), or bacteria may reach the lung directly down the endotracheal tube from a contaminated hospital environment (25, 26). Aspiration is the major route of acquisition for most forms of pneumonia, but in fact, very few individuals who do aspirate contaminated oropharyngeal secretions actually develop pneumonia. As many as 45% of normals and 70% of obtunded patients aspirate oral secretions, and the effectiveness of the normal respiratory tract defenses prevents most from becoming ill (59).

The upper airway is normally colonized, as mentioned above, and with increasing degrees of systemic illness, the flora becomes dominated by enteric Gram-negative bacteria. In healthy individuals, these organisms are unable to colonize the oropharynx because they are repelled by salivary proteases, lysozyme, and IgA (21). In addition, the "normal" flora of the oropharynx inhibits the growth of pathogens through a process termed "bacterial interference," whereby unfavorable growth conditions for pathogens are created. The absence of Gram-negative organisms in the oral flora of normals may also reflect the fact that these organisms have a poor ability to adhere, or bind, to the surface of normal upper airway epithelial cells. This process, bacterial adherence, is a bacterial-mucosal interaction in which organisms bind irreversibly to cell surfaces and form a nidus from which overt colonization may follow (21, 60) (Fig. 16.2). In many mucosal sites throughout the body, adherence is the first step leading to colonization. With systemic illnesses such as starvation, uremia, and surgical stress, salivary proteases are released into the oral cavity, and they act upon the mucosa to remove from it a glycoprotein, fibronectin, and thereby expose previously covered epithelial cell receptors for Gram-negative bacteria. An increase in oral mucosal cell receptivity for bacteria has

been observed in individuals with acute illness and has been correlated with the clinical finding of Gram-negative colonization of the oropharynx in such settings (21).

Once bacteria reach the lower airway, they encounter a variety of specific (organism-directed) and nonspecific defense mechanisms. The nonspecific physical barriers include cough, reflex bronchoconstriction, angulation of the airways (favoring impaction and subsequent transport upward), and the mucociliary escalator. Immune defenses in the lower airway include bronchus-associated lymphoid tissue, phagocytosis (by polymorphonuclear cells and macrophages), immunoglobulins A and G, complement, cytokines, surfactant, and cell-mediated immunity by T lymphocytes. Bacterial adherence also plays a role in colonization of the lower airway, and normal tracheal cells have the capacity to bind to Gram-negative bacteria such as *P. aeruginosa*. It is likely that when bacteria have prolonged contact with the tracheobronchial mucosa, as is the case when mucociliary clearance is reduced (bronchiectasis, cystic fibrosis, endotracheal intubation), then the potential interaction of organisms with the tracheobronchial mucosa will occur. In the lower airway, adherence would be a particularly useful way for bacteria to "stick" to the mucosa and resist the constant flow of air and secretions. In tracheostomized patients, colonization by Gram-negative organisms has been correlated with an increase in tracheal cell capacity to bind bacteria (61). In intubated patients, an increase in tracheal cell bacterial adherence has been correlated with the occurrence of ventilator-associated pneumonia (62).

Colonization of both the oropharynx and the tracheobronchial tree with Gram-negative bacteria is an important harbinger of pneumonia, particularly when it arises in an ill, hospitalized individual. In one study, 23% of ICU patients with Gram-negative bacteria in the oropharynx developed pneumonia, in contrast to only 3.3% of patients without this finding (63). Similarly, lower airway colonization by these organisms is a risk factor for pneumonia because bacteria have gained a foothold in the tracheobronchial tree from which they can propagate downward toward the alveoli. Many clinical features have been correlated with colonization, but a general principle is that colonization is a "marker" of a patient with systemic illness who has impairments in the host defense system at multiple sites throughout the respiratory tract. As mentioned, bacterial adherence is a cellular interaction that has been correlated with colonization, and it may represent one mechanism whereby systemic illness alters a specific cellular behavior, making the patient more receptive to invasion by bacteria. Thus, when a

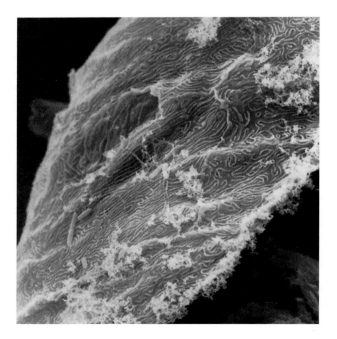

**FIGURE 16.2.** This scanning electron micrograph shows the bacterial adherence interaction between *Pseudomonas aeruginosa* and the surface of tracheal cells.

**TABLE 16.3**

**RISK FACTORS FOR AIRWAY COLONIZATION BY ENTERIC GRAM-NEGATIVE BACILLI**

Oropharyngeal colonization
    Underlying serious illness
    Prior antibiotic therapy
    Coma
    Diabetes
    Renal failure
    Malnutrition
    Hypotension
    Advanced age
    Recent surgery
    Underlying lung disease
    Cigarette smoking
Tracheobronchial colonization
    Advanced age
    Tracheostomy
    Malnutrition
    Endotracheal intubation
    Prior antibiotics
    Neurologic disease
    Bronchiectasis, cystic fibrosis
    Acute lung injury (ARDS)
    Chronic bronchitis
    Corticosteroid therapy
    Prolonged hospitalization
    Recent surgery

malnourished patient develops airway colonization by Gram-negative bacteria, one reason may be that an impaired nutritional status has made the patient's epithelial cells more receptive to binding by these organisms. Other clinical risk factors for colonization of either the oropharynx or tracheobronchial tree include antibiotic therapy, azotemia, diabetes, coma, hypotension, endotracheal intubation, corticosteroid therapy, smoking, chronic bronchitis, cystic fibrosis, and viral infection (Table 16.3).

When an organism of low virulence or a small inoculum enters the lung, containment is by phagocytosis and killing by the alveolar macrophage, and lung inflammation does not result. With more virulent insults, a complex inflammatory response is required for containment (64). This mechanism requires a variety of chemotactic factors (complement, alveolar macrophage cytokine products, and others) to attract polymorphonuclear cells to the alveolus and generate an inflammatory response to prevent the growth of any invading pathogens. Phagocytosis of bacteria by polymorphonuclear cells and macrophages can then occur, but this step requires opsonization by immunoglobulins, complement, or surfactant. In addition, effective phagocytosis by macrophages may require activation of these cells by T helper lymphocytes. Thus all the components of lower respiratory tract defenses can be integrated to deal with large inocula of bacteria or organisms of intrinsic virulence that reach them.

An understanding of the normal host defense system will allow the clinician to understand why pneumonia results in specific patient settings. In addition, with an understanding of any specific patient's immune function, a likely guess about the responsible pathogen is possible. Thus, if a previously healthy patient develops pneumonia, it will usually be with a pathogen of intrinsic virulence such as pneumococcus, *Legionella* species, or *M. pneumoniae*. Patients with certain specific host impairments may become infected by *H. influenzae*, *S. aureus*, tuberculosis, or Gram-negative bacteria.

Certain organisms are known to predominate in specific clinical settings, and these associations should always be considered when such a patient is encountered (Table 16.4). For example, alcoholics may develop pneumonia with *K. pneumoniae*; those with chronic bronchitis can be infected with *H. influenzae*; cystic fibrosis patients will be infected by *S. aureus* or *P. aeruginosa*; cardiac patients may develop pneumococcal infection; splenectomized patients become infected by encapsulated bacteria; the elderly have enteric Gram-negative bacteria causing pneumonia in 20 to 40% of all cases, and infection with *H. influenzae* and anaerobes is also common (65); postinfluenza patients may develop infection with *S. aureus*, *H. influenzae*, or pneumococcus; leukemics have Gram-negative and fungal pneumonias; and mechanically ventilated and tracheostomized patients often have Gram-negative pneumonias, particularly with *P. aeruginosa*. Similarly, if helper T lymphocyte function is impaired, as is the case with AIDS, then macrophage activation will be abnormal, and organisms usually contained by cell-mediated immunity will predominate.

When a patient is evaluated for the risk of developing pneumonia, several factors should be considered. First, the patient's primary medical status should be evaluated so that diseases associated with an increased risk of infection can be identified. These might include cardiac disease, advanced age, ARDS, or diabetes. In addition, other associated illnesses, in addition to the primary disease, should be recognized. For example, hypotension, cancer, stroke, head injury, sepsis, hypophosphatemia, hypoxia, and ethanol intake all have associated specific impairments in lower airway defenses. Another factor that may increase the risk of lung infection, and one that is frequently overlooked, is the therapeutic interventions that patients undergo while receiving medical care. Many medications can interfere with the lung's handling of bacteria, including oxygen, aspirin, digoxin, calcium channel blockers,

TABLE 16.4
PATHOGENS CAUSING PNEUMONIA IN SPECIFIC SETTINGS

| Setting | Pathogens |
| --- | --- |
| Elderly | Enteric Gram-negative bacilli, *Haemophilus influenzae*, pneumococcus |
| Cardiac disease | Pneumococcus, Gram-negative bacilli |
| Alcoholism | *Klebsiella pneumoniae, H. influenzae, M. tuberculosis*, pneumococcus |
| Cystic fibrosis | *Pseudomonas aeruginosa, Staphylococcus aureus* |
| Postinfluenza | Pneumococcus, *H. influenzae, S. aureus* |
| Mechanical ventilation, ARDS | *P. aeruginosa*, other enteric Gram-negative bacilli |
| Chronic bronchitis | *H. influenzae*, pneumococcus, *Branhamella catarrhalis* |
| Splenectomy | Pneumococcus, *H. influenzae*, staphylococcus |
| Neutropenia | *P. aeruginosa, Aspergillus*, Gram-negative bacilli |
| AIDS | *Pneumocystis carinii, Mycobacterium avium*, cytomegalovirus, *Salmonella, Cryptococcus* |

TABLE 16.5
HOST DEFENSES AND AGING FEATURES

| Defense Mechanism | Impairments Related to Age, Comorbid Illness or Drug Therapy |
| --- | --- |
| Upper airway | |
|   Nasal filtration | Bypassed by endotracheal tube, tracheostomy |
|   Oropharyngeal bacterial adherence | Severe coexisting illness, increased oral proteases, xerostomia with a fall in intraoral pH, malnutrition, viral illness, smoking, ? aging |
|   Bacterial interference | Prior antibiotic therapy, altered colonization patterns resulting from aging |
|   Epiglottis | Sedating medications, stroke, feeding tube, endotracheal tube, carcinoma of the upper airway |
| Lower airway | |
|   Cough | Sedating medications, stroke, neuromuscular illness, malnutrition, chronic bronchitis |
|   Mucociliary transport | Aging, cigarette smoking, chronic bronchitis, bronchiectasis, dehydration, vitamin A deficiency, decreased airway pH, airway inflammatory proteases, morphine, atropine, hyperoxia |
|   Immunoglobulins: IgG, IgA, IgM | Malnutrition, aging, vitamin deficiency ($B_6$, folate), zinc deficiency, malignancy |
|   Complement | Normal with aging |
|   Polymorphonuclear cells | Aging, hypothermia, cytotoxic therapy, diabetes, corticosteroids, ethanol, salicylates, malnutrition, hypophosphatemia |
|   T cells | Aging, zinc deficiency |
|   Tracheal cell adherence | Malnutrition, inflammatory proteases, viral illness, endotracheal intubation, ? zinc excess |
|   Alveolar macrophages | Viral illness, malnutrition, ? aging, corticosteroids, cytotoxic therapy, salicylates |

From Niederman MS, Fein AM: Pneumonia in the elderly. *Clin Geriatr Med* 2:247, 1986.

morphine, cimetidine, antacids, corticosteroids, antibiotics, and β-blockers. The last factor to be considered is the patient's nutritional status, since malnutrition can interfere with cell-mediated and humoral immunity in the lung, in addition to increasing epithelial cell receptivity for bacteria. Table 16.5 shows how many of these factors can interact with the respiratory host defenses in one population of patients, the elderly, thereby partially explaining the increased incidence of pneumonia in these individuals.

## Community-Acquired Pneumonia: General Clinical Features

The distinction between "typical" and "atypical" presentations of pneumonia has been referred to above. Although some clinicians have used this distinction in patterns of clinical presentation to predict the etiology of community-acquired pneumonia (CAP), in recent studies this approach does not work very well (20, 66). There are two reasons why clinical features correlate poorly with the etiology of pneumonia. First, certain pathogens, such as *Legionella* and *C. psittaci*, can have a clinical picture that overlaps both syndromes, with high fever, chills, prodromal symptoms, dry cough, leukocytosis, and relative bradycardia (66, 67). Secondly, if the host is not normal because of comorbid illness or advanced age, then the clinical features may be altered, even in the presence of a bacterial pathogen that should lead to the "typical" pneumonia syndrome. Thus in one study, clinical features were only 40% accurate in telling the difference between pneumococcal, mycoplasma, and other pneumonic infections (20). Similarly, in a study of 196 patients with CAP, multilobar disease, pleural effusion, lung collapse, and cavitation were sufficiently common in patients with pneumococcal pneumonia, Legionnaires' disease, mycoplasma and psittacosis, that the radiograph could not be used to determine etiology (68). Because it is usually impossible to recognize a specific pathogen by its clinical presentation or radiographic picture, a judicious use of epidemiology, laboratory data, and clinical findings is needed in approaching therapy, and often more than one potential pathogen is targeted for therapy. Recently, the American Thoracic Society has presented an approach to initial empiric therapy of CAP that is based on an assessment of disease severity, place of therapy, and advanced age (>60 years) and comorbid illness (66). In developing this approach, the use of clinical features to predict microbial pathogens was rejected as being unhelpful.

As mentioned, many patient populations present with bacterial pneumonia with unusual patterns and clinical features. When the elderly develop bacterial pneumonia, fever, rigors, and pleuritic chest pain are less common than in younger patients. In the elderly, pneumonia may present with such nonspecific findings as confusion, lethargy, worsening of an underlying chronic medical condition, or raised respiratory rate. Certain medications such as aspirin and corticosteroids can mask the expected features of pneumonia. Coexisting illness such as chronic obstructive pulmonary disease can interfere with expected physical findings, while congestive cardiac failure may be associated with lung infiltrates that mimic or hide pneumonia (65).

Pneumonia can be caused by a wide variety of pathogens, but the responsible agent will vary depending on the status of the patient's underlying host defenses, which often is reflected in the place of residence. Community-acquired infection has a specific etiologic agent identified in approximately 50% of cases. The exact incidence of viral pneumonia in the community setting is unclear, but these agents may account for up to one-third of all such pneumonias.

The most common bacterial pathogen for community-acquired infection is pneumococcus for all types of patients. The bacteriology varies for different populations, and one approach is to define likely pathogens on the basis of the severity of initial presentation, the need for hospitalization, and the presence of advanced age or comorbidity (66) (Fig. 16.3). In patients treated out of the hospital, with mild to moderate pneumonia, pathogens vary depending on the presence of advanced age or comorbidity. For those without advanced age or comorbidity, after pneumococcus, the most common pathogens are *M. pneumoniae*, respiratory viruses, *Chlamydia pneumoniae*, *H. influenzae*, and miscellaneous pathogens such as enteric Gram-negative bacteria, *Legionella* spp., anaerobes, and *S. aureus*. Unusual pathogens in this setting should be suspected if the patient has an unusual travel or exposure history. In these circumstances, pneumonia may be a presentation of tularemia (in hunters), plague (from exposure to small animals), anthrax (in wool sorters and tanners), cryptococcosis (from pigeon droppings), histoplasmosis (from river valleys or bat droppings), coccidioidomycosis (from travel to the southwestern United States), psittacosis (from infected birds), or parasitic infestation (from foreign travel to the tropics). If the patient has mild to moderate pneumonia but either advanced age, comorbidity, or both, then the most common pathogens are pneumococcus, respiratory viruses, *H. influenzae*, aerobic Gram-negative bacilli, *S. aureus*, and other miscellaneous organisms.

When the patient is hospitalized, a distinction is made between pneumonia treated out of the ICU and severe pneumonia, requiring admission to the ICU. As mentioned below, the bacteriology of severe CAP is predictable, but subtly different from that for CAP in general. Criteria for severe pneumonia include a respiratory rate above 30 to 35 per minute; respiratory failure, with a $PaO_2/FiO_2$ ratio less than 250 mm Hg; bilateral or multilobar infiltrates; increase in infiltrates by more than 50% within 48 hours; shock; need for vasopressors; oliguria; or acute renal failure (66). The mortality rate for severe CAP varies from 25 to 50% or higher, with the greatest death rates being found in populations that have the most patients treated with mechanical ventilation (66, 69). Other prognostic factors indicating a poor outcome for hospitalized patients with CAP include advanced age, the presence of comorbidity, hospitalization within the last year, altered mental status on presentation, fever above 101 F, BUN above 19.6 mg/dl, and extrapulmonary seeding of infection (66, 70).

If the patient is hospitalized but not in the ICU, then the likely pathogens are pneumococcus, *H. influenzae*, polymicrobial infection (including anaerobes), *Legion-*

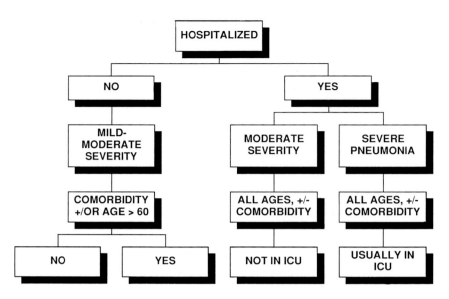

**FIGURE 16.3.** Shown here is an approach to stratifying patients with community-acquired pneumonia. Patients fall into one of four groups, each with its own likely pathogens and suggested therapy. The groups are defined by the need for hospitalization, severity of illness on initial presentation, and the presence of advanced age (>60 years) and/or comorbid illness.

ella spp., *S. aureus, C. pneumoniae,* viruses, and other miscellaneous pathogens. In patients with severe CAP requiring admission to the ICU, the most likely pathogens are pneumococcus, *Legionella* spp., and enteric Gram-negative bacteria (including *P. aeruginosa*). It is important to consider *Legionella* as a likely pathogen in patients with severe CAP, because many studies of this illness document the importance of this pathogen (69, 71). Other pathogens that can cause severe CAP include *M. pneumoniae,* respiratory viruses, and *H. influenzae.*

### Community-Acquired Pneumonia: Specific Illnesses

#### Streptococcus pneumoniae

This Gram-positive, lancet-shaped diplococcus is the most common cause of CAP and can be found in all age groups and all clinical settings. There are 84 different serotypes, each with a distinct antigenic polysaccharide capsule, but 85% of all infections are caused by one of 23 serotypes, which are now included in a vaccine. Type 3 pneumococcus is a particularly virulent serotype and is also one of the most commonly encountered (72). Infection is most common in the winter and early spring, which may relate to the finding that up to 70% of patients have a preceding viral illness (73). Spread is from person to person, but the organism commonly colonizes the oropharynx of patients before it leads to pneumonia. Carriage rates vary from 5% in childless adults to 60% in infants, and rates also vary

throughout the year. Pneumonia develops when colonizing organisms are aspirated into a lung that is unable to contain the aspirated inoculum. Infection is more common in the elderly; those with asplenia, multiple myeloma, congestive heart failure, alcoholism; after influenza; and in patients with chronic lung disease. In patients with AIDS, pneumococcal pneumonia with bacteremia is more common than in healthy populations of the same age.

Clinically, patients with an intact immune response present with the "typical" pneumonia syndrome of abrupt onset of illness accompanied by a toxic appearance, pleuritic chest pain, and rusty-colored sputum. In the past, a lobar pattern was most common, and patients with this finding will have consolidation by physical examination with bronchial breath sounds, egophony, dullness to percussion, and increased tactile fremitus (Fig. 16.4). More recently, it has been recognized that pneumococcus can cause bronchopneumonia, and in some series, this is the most common pattern (74). Bacteremia can occur in 15 to 25% of all patients and will increase the mortality rate of the illness (65, 72). In patients with AIDS, the incidence of bacteremia may exceed 50% but is not associated with an enhanced mortality rate. Laboratory data are not specific but will usually show leukocytosis and slight liver function abnormalities. With overwhelming infection, neutropenia may occur. In the absence of a positive blood culture, diagnosis is often empiric and epidemiologic, based on finding appropriate clinical

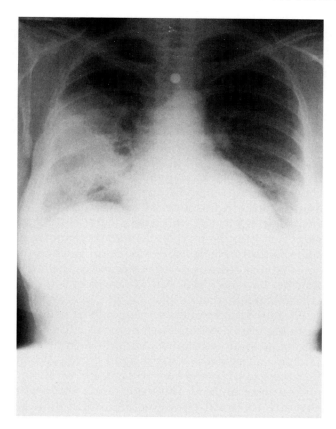

**FIGURE 16.4.** Pneumococcal pneumonia with lobar consolidation in the right lower lobe and a patchy bronchopneumonia in the left lower lobe.

features in a compatible setting. Sputum Gram stain may show pneumococci, but this finding can be absent in half of infected patients, while it may be present when there is oropharyngeal colonization without infection. Counterimmunoelectrophoresis can be applied to urine, serum, and sputum to detect pneumococcal antigen and may thus help establish the diagnosis.

Therapy is with penicillin G, or erythromycin if the patient is penicillin allergic. Uncomplicated cases can be treated with procaine penicillin G, 1.2 million units intramuscularly twice a day for 7 to 10 days. Intravenous therapy can be achieved with 6 to 12 million units daily, in divided doses given every 4 hours. Patients with serious complications or sepsis should be treated with 12 to 18 million units of penicillin G daily. If meningitis is present and the patient is penicillin allergic, then therapy can be effective with the use of chloramphenicol. Recently some strains resistant to penicillin have been isolated, a worrisome finding because of the widely held assumption that all pneumococci are penicillin sensitive. The incidence of resistant pneumococci

is rising, but resistance is of two types, defined by the MIC of penicillin against these organisms. Approximately 10% of strains in the United States are intermediately resistant to penicillin (and can still be treated with high-dose penicillin), while 1% are highly resistant, although the incidence of such resistance appears to be on the rise. These organisms can be treated with vancomycin.

With effective therapy, clinical improvement follows in 24 to 48 hours, but fever may persist for 5 to 7 days. Most patients are treated for 5 to 7 days, but patients with AIDS should be treated longer. Radiographic improvement may lag behind clinical response and only about 70% of patients have a normal radiograph after 2 months (75). Mortality is age related, with 4% below the age of 40 dying, and 26% dying if they are between ages 40 and 69 (65). More recent data have questioned these age-related mortality statistics and suggested that mortality could well be a function of coexisting diseases seen in the aged rather than the aging process itself. Diseases that can increase the mortality of pneumococcal infection are cardiac illness, pulmonary disease, cirrhosis, malignancy, and asplenia. Mortality is also greater with bacteremia, multilobar involvement, and extrapulmonary spread of infection. In patients with advanced illness, antibiotic therapy may be of no benefit because mortality in the first 36 hours of illness is unchanged by therapy (76). Extrapulmonary involvement may be seen with meningitis, arthritis, endocarditis, brain abscess, and pericarditis and should be suspected if the patient fails to improve in the expected time period. Although pleural effusion is common and may be seen in 25% of patients, empyema is rare.

Patients at risk for pneumococcal infection should be considered for prophylaxis with the currently available pneumococcal vaccine (76–78). This injection is active against 23 serotypes of pneumococcus that account for 85% of all cases. At the present time, the vaccine is not being utilized in many of the at-risk population for a variety of unsound reasons. There are no major side effects of immunization, and although the efficacy of vaccination has been questioned, the current consensus is that the vaccine is effective, particularly if given before the patient is ill enough to be unable to have an adequate immune response (78). In patients with an abnormal immune response, revaccination after 6 years may be advisable.

### Legionella pneumophila

This small, weakly staining, Gram-negative bacillus was first characterized after it led to an epidemic of pneumonia in Philadelphia in 1976 that was known as Legionnaires' disease. Since this initial recognition, it has become clear that *L. pneumophila* is not a new bacterium, but one that has only recently been recognized. It is one species of legionellae, of which 34 species have been identified. Legionellae have been isolated since as early as 1943, and retrospective serum analysis has shown that *L. pneumophila* has caused human disease since at least 1965 (79). At present, 12 different serogroups of the species *L. pneumophila* have been described, and these account for 90% of all cases of Legionnaires' disease, with serogroup 1 causing the most cases. The other species that commonly causes human illness is *Legionella micdadei*.

Infection by *Legionella* spp. can be in an epidemic fashion, and in the Philadelphia experience, more than 200 individuals were infected, with a mortality of at least 16%. The organism is water borne and can emanate from air conditioning equipment, drinking water, lakes and river banks, water faucets, and shower heads. When a water system becomes infected in an institution, endemic outbreaks may occur, as has been the case in some hospitals. In addition to these patterns, *Legionella* infection can be in the form of sporadic cases and may account for 7 to 15% of all cases of CAP (80, 81). In some studies, *Legionella* is the most common cause of CAP, a possible artifact of careful testing for this organism. *Legionella* has consistently emerged as a common pathogen in severe CAP. In a number of series (66, 69, 71), *Legionella* has been the second most commonly identified pathogen for severe CAP, leading some to advocate empiric *Legionella* therapy for any patient with severe CAP (66).

Infection is caused by inhalation of an infected aerosol generated by a contaminated water source. Person-to-person spread has not been documented, nor has infection via aspiration from a colonized oropharynx. It is also possible that infection can develop after subclinical aspiration of contaminated water. Incubation period is 2 to 10 days, and disease may occur in normal hosts, as some organisms have significant virulence. Other strains are less virulent and infect impaired hosts with risk factors for infection, including renal transplantation, dialysis, malignancy, smoking, chronic lung disease, diabetes, age greater than 50, male sex, and alcoholism. In hospitalized patients, the most important risk factor for nosocomial *Legionella* pneumonia is the use of corticosteroids (82). Once the organism is inhaled, it localizes intracellularly to the alveolar macrophage and multiplies, generating an inflammatory response that involves neutrophils, lymphocytes, and antibody. Since cell-mediated immunity is needed to contain infection, the disease can occur in compromised hosts and may relapse if not treated long enough.

Patients with *Legionella* pneumonia commonly have high fever, chills, headache, myalgias, and leukocytosis. Features that can suggest the diagnosis specifically are the presence of a pneumonia with preceding diarrhea, along with mental confusion, hyponatremia, relative bradycardia, and liver function abnormalities. Symptoms are rapidly progressive, and the patient may appear to be quite toxic. As mentioned, the presence of severe forms of CAP should automatically prompt consideration of *Legionella* spp. The patient may have purulent sputum, pleuritic chest pain, and dyspnea. The chest radiograph is not specific and may show bronchopneumonia, unilateral or bilateral disease, lobar consolidation, or rounded densities with cavitation. Up to 15% will have pleural effusion, but empyema is uncommon. Proteinuria is common, and some patients have developed glomerulonephritis and acute tubular necrosis. Myocarditis and cerebellar dysfunction have been reported as rare complications of *Legionella* pneumonia.

Diagnosis can be made serologically by detecting a serial rise in antibody titer to the organism. Using indirect immunofluorescence, a fourfold rise in titer, with samples collected 6 to 8 weeks apart during and after the illness, to 1:128 or greater is diagnostic, as is a single titer greater than 1:512. This method may not be useful clinically, since it may take up to 9 weeks to make a diagnosis. The organism can be identified in culture using special medium such as buffered charcoal–yeast extract. Direct fluorescent antibody staining of sputum or bronchoscopy specimens may lead to the diagnosis by detecting *Legionella* antigen, and an ELISA assay for urinary antigen has been used. The urinary antigen test can detect only *L. pneumophila* serotype 1 but has a high sensitivity and specificity for this organism, which causes more than 80% of clinically evident *Legionella* infections. In most clinical settings, the direct fluorescent antibody technique is available, and all appropriate clinical specimens should be tested with it, although it will not be positive in all cases. A DNA probe for the *Legionella* genome has also become available for use.

Once the diagnosis is suspected, therapy should be with erythromycin in doses of 500 to 1000 mg every 6 hours intravenously until fever is gone for 2 days. Then a daily dose of 2 g orally is continued for a total of 2 weeks in immunocompetent patients and for 3 weeks in immunocompromised patients. With severe infection, rifampin should be added in doses of 600 mg every 12 hours. Alternatives to erythromycin are trimethoprim/sulfamethoxazole and tetracycline, and clarithromycin has been reported to be effective when other agents have failed (83). Quinolone antibiotics, such as ciprofloxacin, may also be effective (83). With therapy, decline in fever may be slow, and high spikes in temperature may continue for 1 week after starting appropriate therapy. Mortality is less than 5% in normal hosts but may be as high as 25% in compromised hosts (80).

*Aspiration Pneumonia*

Pulmonary aspiration occurs in specific patient populations who are at risk of having material enter the lung because of impaired consciousness or altered respiratory tract anatomy. Aspiration can be in one of three forms: gastric acid or other toxic fluids may enter the lung and cause a chemical pneumonitis; inert substances such as water or solid particles can reach the lung and lead to drowning or airway obstruction, respectively; or pathogenic bacteria from the stomach or oropharynx can enter the lung and cause pneumonitis or lung abscess (84, 85). Risk factors for aspiration include uncontrolled seizures, stroke, drug intoxication, shock, acute neurologic illness, tracheoesophageal fistula, esophageal diverticulum or dysmotility, tracheostomy, intestinal obstruction, and nasogastric tube use. When aspiration occurs, it is generally in a dependent lung segment, and in a supine prone patient, this will be the superior segment of the lower lobe, or the posterior segment of the upper lobe, with the right side being affected more often than the left because of the relatively straighter takeoff of the right mainstem bronchus.

If gastric contents are aspirated and solid material obstructs the airway, patients may develop cough and atelectasis and later on may have secondary bacterial infection distal to the obstruction in the form of lung abscess, bronchiectasis, or even empyema. If gastric acid or other toxic material is aspirated, then a chemical pneumonitis results, which may be complicated by secondary infection. Acutely, patients who inhale gastric acid with a pH below 2.4 may have dyspnea, bronchospasm, hypotension, hypoxemia, frothy sputum, and pulmonary edema. When aspiration involves primarily bacteria, then acute infectious pneumonitis may follow. This process may be indolent and is characterized by fever and purulent sputum, followed by necrosis and possibly lung abscess 1 to 2 weeks later. When aspiration occurs out of the hospital, infection is usually with anaerobes that have colonized the mouth, including *Prevotella* (formerly *Bacteroides*) *melaninogenicus* and *Bacteroides fragilis*, *Fusobacterium* spp., peptococci, and peptostreptococci. Pneumococci and staphylococci may also be aspirated in this setting. In the hospital, aspiration is usually with both anaerobes and aerobes, usually *S. aureus* and enteric Gram-negative bacilli (86).

When aspiration is witnessed, the major therapy is to suction the airway, provide oxygen, and support the patient. The use of corticosteroids and prophylactic antibiotics is of no proven value. If an infiltrate is present, it should develop within 24 hours of the aspiration event, and then antibiotics are indicated. In cases of aspiration out of the hospital, penicillin G (up to 12 million units per day) or clindamycin (600 mg every 6 hours) can be used. Nosocomial aspiration is best treated with a second- or third-generation cephalosporin or a combination of clindamycin plus an agent active against enteric Gram-negative organisms. Failure to respond to therapy should prompt a search for continued aspiration conditions, airway obstruction by a foreign body, or lung abscess.

*Lung Abscess*

This is a necrotizing parenchymal lung infection generally caused by aspiration of anaerobic bacteria. When a lung abscess arises in this manner, it is termed a primary or simple abscess, and it follows the anatomic distribution of aspiration, discussed above. By definition, the radiograph will show a cavity of at least 2 cm. The cavity may contain an air-fluid level and may be associated with or preceded by a pneumonitis (Fig. 16.5). The cavities may be multiple, and generally average 4 to 5 cm (87). Empyema is often associated with lung abscess. The risk factors and microbiology of lung abscess are similar to those of out-of-hospital aspiration, and lung abscess is itself a complication of aspiration. Patients present with low-grade fever, weight loss, and cough with foul-smelling sputum. When lung abscess arises in the absence of a predisposing condition or in a patient without teeth (which can harbor the growth of anaerobes in the periodontal area), then lung cancer or another bronchial obstruction should be suspected. Even without these findings, many patients present with such an indolent course and with weight loss so that malignancy is part of the differential diagnosis. Therapy is with penicillin G or clindamycin, in the doses stated above, with some data to suggest that the latter is more effective (88). With therapy, the patient may improve within a week, with a decline in fever. However, it may take 1 month for the cavity to close and up to 2 months for the radiograph to clear, and therapy should be continued until the infection has cleared on chest film. Generally, therapy is intravenous until the patient is improving and then is continued orally for 4 to 8 weeks. Complications of lung abscess include empyema, bronchopleural fistula, and brain abscess.

If lung abscess arises unrelated to aspiration, other pathogens besides anaerobes should be considered. Cavitary pneumonias can result from infection with tuberculosis, fungi, *S. aureus*, *K. pneumoniae*, *P. aeruginosa*, and group A streptococci. Another clinical situation that may be confused with lung abscess is periemphysematous infection of lung bullae. In this setting,

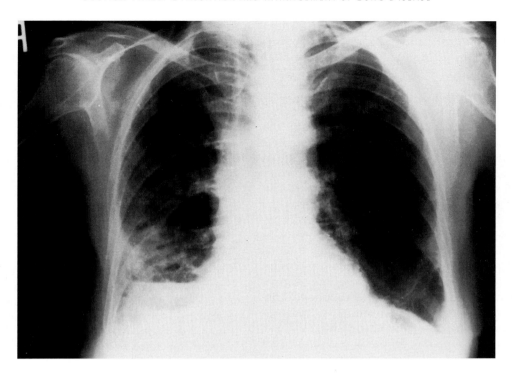

**FIGURE 16.5.** Aspiration pneumonia in the right lower lobe of an alcoholic with a seizure disorder. A patchy pneumonitis is evident in the right lower lobe along with two lung abscesses and a pleural effusion due to empyema. A thick-walled cavity is present in the right perihilar area, while an air-fluid level due to an abscess that has ruptured into the pleural space and caused an empyema is present in the lower lung zone.

pneumonia develops in a diseased lung with preexisting bullae due to emphysema. As these air sacs become infected, they fill with fluid and simulate a lung abscess. This type of infection can be distinguished from lung abscess if prior radiographs show bullae. In addition, the bullae are thin walled, in contrast to the thick and irregular walls of a true lung abscess (Fig. 16.6).

*Haemophilus influenzae*

This Gram-negative coccobacillary rod can occur in either a typable, encapsulated form or a nontypable, unencapsulated form; either can cause pneumonia. The nontypable organisms are also a common cause of bronchitis and a frequent colonizer in patients with COPD. The encapsulated organism can be one of seven types, but type B accounts for 95% of all invasive infections. Opsonizing IgG antibody is required to phagocytose the encapsulated organisms; this may not be the case for the unencapsulated bacteria. It has been suggested that since encapsulated organisms require a more elaborate host response, they are more virulent than unencapsulated organisms. However several studies have shown that in adults, infection with unencapsulated bacteria is more common than infection with encapsulated organisms and that opsonizing antibody is needed to control unencapsulated bacteria as

well (89). It is probably safe to assume that pneumonia from these bacteria can only result if there is some impairment in host defense, which may include both humoral immunity and local phagocytic dysfunction.

When pneumonia is present, the organism may be bacteremic in some patients, particularly in those with segmental pneumonias, as opposed to those with bronchopneumonia. It has been estimated (90) that 15% of cases are segmental, but that 70% of these patients have bacteremia, while only 25% of bronchopneumonia cases are bacteremic. The encapsulated type B organism is more common in patients with segmental pneumonia than in those with bronchopneumonia. Because pneumonia with *H. influenzae* represents a host defense failure, most patients have some underlying illness, and half may be alcoholics. In patients with chronic obstructive lung disease, bronchopneumonia is more common than segmental pneumonia.

Patients with segmental pneumonia present with a sudden onset of fever and pleuritic chest pain along with a sore throat. Those with bronchopneumonia will have a slightly lower fever, tachypnea, and constitutional symptoms. Multilobar, patchy bronchopneumonia is the most common radiographic pattern, and pleural reaction is also common, being seen in more

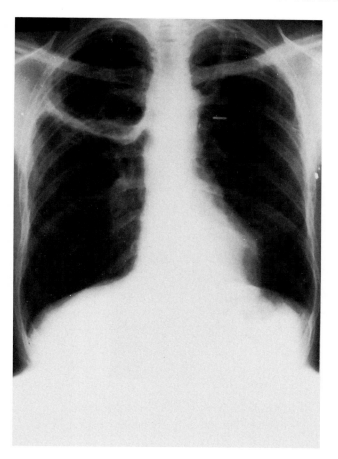

**FIGURE 16.6.** Periemphysematous bullous infection in a preexisting upper lobe bulla. Unlike a lung abscess, the location is the entire upper lobe, there is no air-fluid level, and the wall of the bulla are thin, unlike the thick and irregular walls of an abscess.

than half with segmental pneumonia and in approximately 20% with bronchopneumonia (Fig. 16.7). Overall, the adult mortality is 30%, a reflection of the type of impaired host who develops the illness. Complications include empyema, lung abscess, meningitis, arthritis, pericarditis, epiglottitis, and otitis media, particularly in children.

Therapy is usually with ampicillin, but recently resistance to this antibiotic has been reported in up to 20% of nontypable *H. influenzae* isolates and in up to 50% of type B organisms, as a result of bacterial production of β-lactamase enzymes. Other effective antibiotics are the third-generation cephalosporins, trimethoprim/sulfamethoxazole, and chloramphenicol (with some strains resistant to this agent as well). The newer macrolides, clarithromycin and azithromycin, also have activity against *H. influenzae*, as do the fluoroquinolones. A vaccine against type B organisms is available, but its use is limited, and it is best used in young children over the age of 2 to prevent invasive infection such as meningitis (77). Adults who are chronically colonized by *H. influenzae* achieve this condition in spite of the presence of antibodies to this organism, and it is thus unlikely that the vaccine will have utility in this type of adult population.

*Mycoplasma pneumoniae*

Although this organism closely resembles a bacterium, it lacks a cell wall and is surrounded by a three-layer membrane. Most of the respiratory infections caused by *M. pneumoniae* are minor and in the form of upper respiratory tract illness or bronchitis. Although pneumonia only occurs in 3 to 10% of all mycoplasma infections, this organism is still a common cause of pneumonia. In the general population, it may account for 20% of all pneumonia cases, and up to 50% in certain closed populations, such as college students (91). The disease is seen year-round, with a slight increase in the fall and winter. All age groups are affected, but it is more common in those less than 20 years of age.

Respiratory infection occurs after the organism is inhaled and then binds via neuraminic acid receptors to the airway epithelium. An inflammatory response with neutrophils, lymphocytes, and macrophages then follows, accompanied by the formation of IgM and then IgG antibody. Some of the observed pneumonitis may be mediated by the host response to the organism rather than by direct tissue injury by the mycoplasma. Up to 40% of infected individuals will have circulating immune complexes (92).

When pneumonia is present, it is usually in the form of an "atypical" pneumonia. Patients commonly have a dry cough, fever, chills, headache, and malaise after a 2- to 3-week incubation period. Up to half will have upper respiratory tract symptoms including sore throat and earache. Some of the patients with earache will have hemorrhagic or bullous myringitis. Pleural effusion is quite common, being seen in at least 20% of patients with pneumonia, although it may be small. Chest radiograph will show interstitial infiltrates, which are usually unilateral and in the lower lobe, but can be bilateral and multilobar, although the patient usually does not appear as ill as suggested by the radiographic picture. Rarely, patients will have a severe illness with respiratory failure or a necrotizing pneumonia, but most cases resolve in 7 to 10 days in an uncomplicated fashion (69).

Infection with *M. pneumoniae* is often characterized by its extrapulmonary manifestations. These include neurologic illness such as meningoencephalitis, meningitis, transverse myelitis, and cranial nerve palsies, which can be seen in 7% of hospitalized patients (91). The most common extrapulmonary finding is an IgM

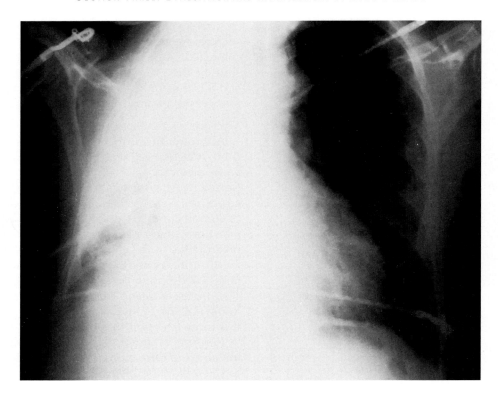

**FIGURE 16.7.**    This patient with advanced chronic bronchitis had bacteremic *Haemophilus influenzae* from this extensive segmental pneumonia. A dense pleural reaction accompanied the pneumonia.

autoantibody that is directed against the I antigen on the red blood cell and causes cold agglutination of the erythrocyte. Although up to 75% of patients may have this antibody and a positive Coombs' test, clinically significant autoimmune hemolytic anemia is uncommon. Other systemic complications include myocarditis, pericarditis, hepatitis, gastroenteritis, erythema multiforme, arthralgias, pancreatitis, generalized lymphadenopathy, and glomerulonephritis. The extrapulmonary manifestations may follow the respiratory symptoms by as long as 3 weeks.

Diagnosis is made by finding a compatible clinical picture and radiograph in a host with pneumonia and possibly some extrapulmonary findings. Confirmation can be made by isolating the organism in culture from respiratory tract secretions. Serologic diagnosis is made by finding a fourfold rise in specific antibody to *M. pneumoniae* by complement fixation test, although a single titer of 1:64 is suggestive of infection. If this finding is present with a cold agglutinin titer of 1:64, then the diagnosis is made. Once the diagnosis is made, therapy is given with erythromycin (2 g/day) or tetracycline, which can reduce the duration and severity of the illness. Therapy is given for 10 to 14 days, and alternative antibiotics include the newer macrolides, azithromycin or clarithromycin.

*Chlamydia Species*

Psittacosis is a pneumonia due to *C. psittaci*, an agent transmitted by inhaling infected excrement from avian species, although the infectious bird does not need to be ill to transmit disease. Patients commonly have headache, high fever, splenomegaly and dry cough, all of insidious onset after a 1- to 2-week incubation period (93). A macular rash similar to that of typhoid fever may also be seen, along with relative bradycardia. Other extrapulmonary involvement may occur, including hepatitis, encephalitis, hemolytic anemia, and renal failure. Diagnosis is on the basis of a compatible contact history and can be confirmed serologically. Treatment is with tetracycline (2 to 3 g/day) or chloramphenicol for 10 to 14 days.

Recently another *Chlamydia* species, *C. pneumoniae*, has been found to cause respiratory infection. This organism is not transmitted by birds and has been recognized and reported to be a relatively common cause of pneumonia. This organism has also been designated TWAR and can be seen in teenagers and adults. Antibody to TWAR has been found in 25 to 45% of adults, and the organism can cause up to 12% of pneumonias in a student population and 6% of pneumonias in an elderly population (94, 95). The disease has no specific

**TABLE 16.6**
**DIAGNOSTIC FEATURES OF THE ATYPICAL PNEUMONIAS**

| Key Characteristics | *Mycoplasma* Pneumonia | Legionnaires' Disease/LLO | Psittacosis | Q Fever | Tularemia | TWAR Agent *Chlamydia* |
|---|---|---|---|---|---|---|
| **Symptoms** | | | | | | |
| Mental confusion | ± | + | − | − | − | − |
| Prominent headache | − | − | + | + | − | − |
| Meningismus | − | − | + | − | − | − |
| Myalgias | + | + | + | + | − | ± |
| Ear pain | ± | − | − | − | − | − |
| Pleuritic pain | ± | + | − | − | − | − |
| Abdominal pain | − | + | − | − | − | − |
| Diarrhea | ± | + | − | − | − | − |
| **Signs** | | | | | | |
| Rash | ± (*E. multiforme*) | ± (Pretibial rash) | ± (Horder's spots) | − | − | − |
| Raynaud's phenomenon | ± | − | − | − | − | − |
| Nonexudative pharyngitis | + | − | + | − | ± | +[a] |
| Hemoptysis | − | + | + | − | − | − |
| Lobar consolidation | ± | ± | ± | ± | ± | − |
| Cardiac involvement | ± (Myocarditis/ heart block/ pericarditis) | − | ± (Myocarditis) | ± (Endocarditis) | − | − |
| Splenomegaly | − | − | + | − | − | − |
| Relative bradycardia | − | + | + | − | − | − |
| **Chest film** | | | | | | |
| Infiltrate | Patchy | Patchy/ consolidation[b] | Patchy/ consolidation | Perihilar pattern | "Ovoid bodies" | Single "circumscribed" lesions |
| Bilateral hilar adenopathy | − | − | − | − | + | − |
| Pleural effusion | ± (Small) | ± | − | − | + (Bloody) | ± |
| **Laboratory abnormalities** | | | | | | |
| WBC count | ↑/N | ↑ | ↓ | ↑/N | ↑/N | N[a] |
| Hyponatremia/ hypophosphatemia | − | + | − | − | − | − |
| Increase in SGOT/ SGPT | − | + | + | + | − | − |
| Cold agglutinins | + | − | − | − | − | − |
| Microscopic hematuria | − | + | − | − | − | − |
| **Diagnostic tests** | | | | | | |
| Direct isolation (culture) | ± | ± | ± | − | − | + |
| Serology (specific) | CF | IFA | CF | CF | TA | CF |
| Psittacosis CF titers | − | ↑ | ↑ | − | − | ↑ |
| *Legionella* IFA titers | − | ↑ | − | − | ↑ | − |

From Cotton EM, Strampfer MJ, Cunha BA: *Legionella* and mycoplasma pneumonia—a community hospital experience with atypical pneumonias. *Clin Chest Med* 8:443, 1987.
[a] Often associated with laryngitis.
[b] Asymmetric, rapidly progressive infiltrates are characteristic. *L. micdadei* pneumonia is suggested by a nodular infiltrate.

features but is commonly seen with laryngitis and pharyngitis. Patients have fever, chills, pleuritic chest pain, headache, and cough and occasionally can have respiratory failure. Therapy is with tetracycline (2 g/day), but erythromycin, as well as the newer macrolides, may also be effective; therapy should continue for 14 to 21 days.

Although all the agents of atypical pneumonia have not been thoroughly discussed, the clinical features of the most important infections are summarized in Table 16.6.

### Klebsiella pneumoniae

This enteric Gram-negative rod can cause both CAP and nosocomial pneumonia. When it arises out of the hospital, it can be an explosive illness with up to a 50% mortality, and it generally affects debilitated individuals (96). Known as Friedlander's pneumonia, after the physician who first observed this illness, patients are predominantly male and usually middle-aged or older, with alcoholism being the most common coexisting condition. Other patients at risk are diabetics, the elderly in nursing homes, those with malignancy, and patients with chronic cardiopulmonary or renal disease. The onset is sudden with productive cough, pleuritic chest pain, rigors, and prostration. Sputum may be thick and purulent with blood as well, or it may be thin with a "currant jelly" appearance. Patients appear toxic with high fever and tachycardia, and examination reveals signs of lobar consolidation. The radiographic finding that is most distinct is consolidation in the upper lobe with a fissure bulging downward because of the dense infiltrate. Lung abscess and bronchopneumonia may also occur. Other complications include pericarditis, meningitis, and empyema. Diagnosis is suspected by finding Gram-negative rods in the sputum in a patient with a compatible illness and risk factors. Therapy should be for 2 weeks, and usually two drugs that are active against the bacteria are used to avoid emerging resistance and to provide antibacterial synergy. There is some debate about the need for combination therapy, but if third-generation cephalosporins are used alone, resistance may emerge during therapy (97). Effective agents, in addition to third-generation cephalosporins include an aminoglycoside, an antipseudomonal penicillin, aztreonam, imipenem, or a fluoroquinolone.

### Staphylococcus aureus

*S. aureus* may account for up to 5% of CAPs but may also arise in the hospital. In the community setting, it is most common in the elderly and in residents of nursing homes. Pneumonia is also seen after influenza or in patients with chronic lung disease. Hematogenous pneumonia with this organism can be seen in drug addicts with right-sided endocarditis. Clinical features

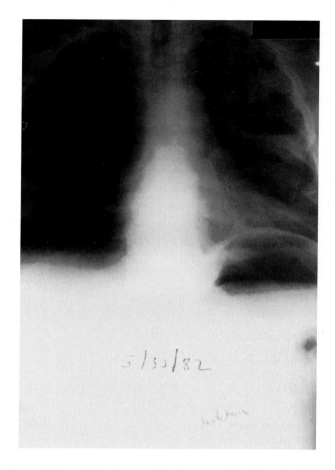

**FIGURE 16.8.** Multiple necrotizing lung cavities due to *Staphylococcus aureus*.

include sudden onset of fever, tachypnea, and cough with purulent sputum. The radiograph may show pleural effusion, cavitary bilateral infiltrates, lung abscess, or pneumatoceles (Fig. 16.8). Empyema is common, being found in 8 of 31 patients in one series (98). In that series, which included both CAP and nosocomial pneumonia, infiltrates were typically multilobar and bilateral and involved the lower lobes. Pleural effusion was common (48%), but abscess was infrequent (16%). Therapy is with an antistaphylococcal penicillin, a first-generation cephalosporin, or vancomycin; it should be continued for 4 to 6 weeks in complicated infections. Reinfection can occur, and a mortality rate of 32% was reported for all infected patients in one study (98). Strains resistant to methicillin have become increasingly common and require therapy with vancomycin. Extrapulmonary complications include endocarditis and meningitis.

### Viruses

The exact incidence of viral pneumonia is difficult to estimate because careful serologic testing for viruses

TABLE 16.7
CHARACTERISTICS OF COMMON RESPIRATORY VIRUSES CAUSING LOWER RESPIRATORY TRACT INFECTION

| Agent | Genetic Structure | Mode of Transmission | Epidemiology | Clinical Syndromes |
|---|---|---|---|---|
| Adenovirus group (41 serotypes) | Linear double-stranded DNA | Aerosol, direct person-to-person contact | Ubiquitous agent, no seasonal prevalence | Epidemic pneumonia in closed populations (e.g., military recruits), disseminated disease in immunosuppressed hosts |
| Coronavirus | Single-strand RNA | Presumed person-to-person contact | Commoner in winter and spring, clusters within families | Occasional pneumonia, exacerbation of asthma, bronchitis |
| Herpes group (CMV, HSV, VZV) | Double-stranded DNA | Venereal route, blood products, transplanted organs, aerosol (VZV) | Immunosuppressed host | Tracheobronchitis (HSV), interstitial pneumonitis |
| Influenza virus (types A, B) | Seven single RNA strands | Small particle aerosol | Peak prevalence in winter and early spring, highest attack rates at extreme ages of life | Tracheobronchitis, pneumonia with or without bacterial superinfection |
| Parainfluenza | Single-strand RNA | Direct person-to-person spread | Late fall to early winter peaks, severe infection commonest between 6 months and 6 years | Croup (serotypes 1–3), pneumonia and bronchitis (type 1–2) |
| Respiratory syncytial virus | Single-strand RNA | Self-inoculation with fomites | Outbreaks in winter and spring, most serious infection in 1st 2 years of life | Pneumonia and bronchitis (infants), bronchitis and pneumonia (adults) |

From Rose RM, Pinkston P, O'Donnell C, et al: Viral infections of the lower respiratory tract. *Clin Chest Med* 8:406, 1987.

is not done in most cases of lung infection. However, viral pneumonia probably accounts for 20% or more of all cases of CAP. The common agents causing lower respiratory infection may be spread by aerosol or via person-to-person contact through infected secretions (Table 16.7) and include adenovirus, influenza virus, herpes group viruses (which include cytomegalovirus), parainfluenza virus, and respiratory syncytial virus.

Viral lower respiratory infections are usually in the tracheobronchial tree or small airways, but primary pneumonia may also occur. The virus first localizes to the respiratory epithelial cell and causes destruction of the cilia and mucosal surface. The resulting loss of mucociliary function may then predispose the patient to a secondary bacterial pneumonia (99). If the infection reaches the alveoli, there may be hemorrhage, edema, and hyaline membrane formation, and the physiology of ARDS may follow. The initial host response to viral invasion is via the alveolar macrophage, which can have a variety of actions: it can phagocytose the virus; it can produce antiviral cytokines such as interferon gamma; and it can present the viral antigen to lymphocytes in the bronchus-associated lymphoid tissue. Lymphocytes can in turn lead to viral-specific antibody of the IgM, G, and A classes, activated T cells, and natural killer cells (99).

Viral lower respiratory tract involvement can be in the form of either an airway infection with a normal chest radiograph, a primary viral pneumonia, a bacterial superinfection, or a combined viral and bacterial pneumonia. As was discussed with influenza, primary viral pneumonia may be a severe illness with diffuse infiltrates and extensive parenchymal injury along with severe hypoxemia (Fig. 16.9). This pattern is often seen in those with underlying cardiopulmonary disease, immunosuppression, or pregnancy. However, many patients with primary viral pneumonia get only a mild "atypical" pneumonia with dry cough, fever, and a radiograph that is more severely affected than

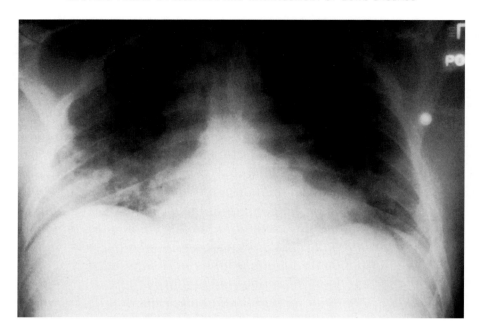

**FIGURE 16.9.**   Primary viral pneumonia due to varicella-zoster in a 35-year-old male with an extensive vesicular rash and a clinical syndrome of chickenpox.

the patient. When bacterial superinfection is present, the illness is biphasic, with initial improvement from the primary viral infection followed by sudden increase in fever along with purulent sputum and lobar consolidation. Another common complication of viral lower airway infection is bronchial hyperreactivity, and asthma and chronic airflow obstruction may occur.

The major clinical distinction between the many viral agents that can cause pneumonia is in the type of host who becomes infected and in the type of extrapulmonary manifestations that accompany the pneumonia. Immunocompromised hosts with AIDS, malignancy, and major organ transplantation are often infected by cytomegalovirus, varicella-zoster, and herpes simplex virus. Children are most affected by respiratory syncytial virus and parainfluenza virus, which can cause both airway and parenchymal lung infections. Children and military recruits develop pneumonia with adenovirus, while influenza pneumonia can develop in adults, particularly the debilitated elderly. Extrapulmonary signs may suggest a specific viral agent. Rash may be seen with varicella-zoster, cytomegalovirus, measles, and enterovirus infections (Fig. 16.9). Pharyngitis may accompany infection by adenovirus, influenza, and enterovirus. Hepatitis may be seen with cytomegalovirus and infectious mononucleosis (Epstein-Barr virus).

The diagnosis of viral illness can be clinical or it can be confirmed by specific laboratory methods. Viruses

can be isolated with special culture techniques if specimens are properly collected and prepared. Upper airway swabs, sputum, bronchial washes, rectal swabs, and tissue samples should be placed in viral transport media as early in the patient's illness as possible, while viral shedding is still prominent. These samples are then cultured on certain laboratory cell lines, and viral growth may be detected in 5 to 7 days. Viral illness can be rapidly diagnosed by using immunofluorescence or ELISA assays to test patient samples for viral antigens. Immunofluorescent tests are available for influenza, parainfluenza, respiratory syncytial virus, adenovirus, measles, rubella, coronavirus, and herpesvirus. ELISA assays are also available for most of these agents (100). Serology can be used retrospectively to diagnose a suspected viral infection, but this technique may be a "shot in the dark" if specific viruses are not suspected and sought directly. A new technique that shows promise is the use of genetic probes to detect specific viral DNA or RNA. Such methodology is now available for cytomegalovirus, varicella-zoster virus, herpes simplex, and adenovirus.

With the current interest and understanding of viral infections, some specific therapy with antiviral agents has become available. Pneumonia from herpes simplex and varicella-zoster can be treated with acyclovir or vidarabine, although acyclovir is preferable. Influenza A can be treated or prevented by the use of amantadine 200 mg orally per day. Ribavirin aerosol has been used to treat respiratory syncytial virus and influenza B. Some patients with cytomegalovirus infection have been successfully treated by the acyclovir analogue, DHPG (ganciclovir), and foscarnet may also have a role in the treatment of this infection.

## Hospital-Acquired Pneumonia

The epidemiology and pathogenesis of nosocomial pneumonia have been discussed above. When pneumonia arises in the hospitalized or institutionalized patient, the bacteriology shifts, and Gram-negative organisms are responsible for most cases. In addition to the enteric Gram-negative bacilli, other common causes of nosocomial pneumonia are *S. aureus, H. influenzae*, pneumococcus, aspiration with anaerobes, *Legionella* spp. in certain places, and viruses (in certain hosts or in settings of an epidemic among the staff) (64). It should be emphasized that nosocomial pneumonia is an opportunistic occurrence that preys upon the sickest patients in a hospital. In one study, nosocomial infections in general were seen in 2% of all hospitalized patients but in nearly one-quarter with an underlying fatal illness (101). In patients with ARDS, nearly 70% have secondary pneumonia, and this complication adversely affects survival (12, 102) (Fig. 16.10). The responsible pathogen is usually an enteric Gram-negative bacillus, particularly *P. aeruginosa* in the most ill

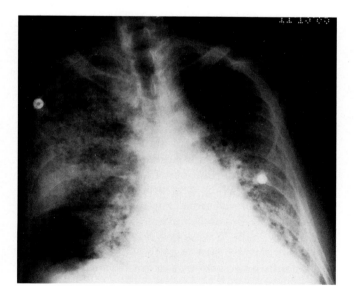

**FIGURE 16.10.** Adult respiratory distress syndrome with bilateral diffuse infiltrates and a complicating nosocomial pneumonia in the right upper lobe. Distinguishing pneumonia from the primary lung process is very difficult although asymmetry can be a clue, as it was in this case.

individuals, and it is the impairment of the host response to bacterial challenge, and not usually the intrinsic virulence of the organism, that leads to this infection. Much of the current research in this field is focused on prevention, and this approach arises out of a thorough understanding of pathogenesis.

There is still considerable difficulty in determining whether nosocomial pneumonia is present, because many noninfectious illnesses may present a similar clinical picture, particularly in the critically ill patient. An accepted definition of this infection is onset after 72 hours of hospitalization, with development of a new or progressive lung infiltrate on radiograph, plus two of the following: fever, leukocytosis, and purulent tracheobronchial secretions (103, 104). This diagnosis may be particularly difficult to make in the mechanically ventilated patient with coexisting ARDS or congestive heart failure because either illness is associated with lung infiltrates and the other clinical features of infection may be the result of tracheobronchitis and not pneumonia. Conversely, the elderly and the immunocompromised patient may have pneumonia in the absence of clear-cut signs and symptoms of infection, because of the absence of adequate inflammation. In these patients, fever and purulent sputum may not be present.

Risk factors for nosocomial pneumonia can be categorized as being one of four types: acute illness (such as ARDS, sepsis, hemorrhagic shock) with its attendant alterations in a variety of lower airway defense mechanisms; coexisting illnesses such as diabetes, smoking, chronic cardiac or pulmonary disease, recent intraabdominal surgery, advanced age, shock, intraabdominal infection, uremia, and other systemic illnesses; therapeutic interventions; and impaired nutritional status (102). The area of therapeutic interventions that predispose to pneumonia is particularly interesting, because an appreciation of these factors will prompt the physician to minimize therapies that increase the chance of developing infection. Such therapies include antacids, possibly $H_2$-blocking drugs, high oxygen concentrations, sedating drugs, corticosteroids, nasogastric tube use, broad-spectrum antibiotics, and endotracheal intubation (102).

The diagnosis of nosocomial pneumonia is hampered by the problems cited above. It is common practice to both underdiagnose and overdiagnose this illness in certain populations. For example, in patients with ARDS, one-third of all autopsy-proven cases of pneumonia had been unrecognized, while one-fifth of uninfected patients were treated for pneumonia (105). It is likely that this degree of misdiagnosis is common in other settings because of the imprecision of the clinical diagnosis of this illness. Some studies have reported that only one of three mechanically ventilated patients with a clinical diagnosis of pneumonia had microbiologic confirmation of the diagnosis (106). Although this estimate may be overly pessimistic, it is likely that pneumonia is overdiagnosed in mechanically ventilated patients. The use of sputum culture to diagnose pneumonia or identify the responsible pathogen is fraught with problems. Many hospitalized patients are colonized by potential pathogens, and thus their recovery from the lower airway does not always represent invasive infection.

In an effort to improve the accuracy of diagnosing nosocomial pneumonia, a number of invasive techniques have been developed (106). With these methods, lower respiratory secretions are sampled either bronchoscopically or via endotracheal suction, and the recovered material is cultured quantitatively. The bacteriologic results are then used to determine whether pneumonia is present on the basis of how many organisms are recovered. Invasive methods have involved the use of special "protected" brushes or bronchoalveolar lavage for the recovery of secretions for culture. Debate continues about the accuracy and clinical utility of invasive methods (106). Concern about invasive methods centers around the potential arbitrariness of thresholds selected to separate pneumonia from nonpneumonia. In addition, there are concerns about the reproducibility of the methods, the potential for these techniques to overlook early infection, and the limited value of the methods if the patient is on antibiotics at the time of testing.

Therapy is with antimicrobial agents directed at the likely pathogens, which fall into a "core" group of bacteria including *Klebsiella* spp., *Enterobacter* spp., *E. coli*, *Proteus* spp., *Serratia marcescens*, *H. influenzae*, and *S. aureus*. In some settings, pneumococcus has been observed as a common nosocomial pathogen (103, 104). Some patients with nosocomial pneumonia have infection with a polymicrobial flora, and up to 40% of nosocomial pneumonia in mechanically ventilated patients is polymicrobial (104). Patients with certain comorbidities or therapies can be at risk for other organisms in addition to the core bacteria. *S. aureus* (including its methicillin-resistant form) is more likely in patients who are in coma, as well as in those with head injury, renal failure, and recent influenza. *Legionella* spp. are more likely in patients receiving corticosteroids or cytotoxic chemotherapy, and *Aspergillus* spp. are more likely if patients have received antibiotics or corticosteroids (107). Patients with recent thoracoabdominal surgery or witnessed aspiration are at risk for anaerobic organisms. *P. aeruginosa* is a concern in patients who have severe nosocomial pneumonia and in those who

develop pneumonia in the setting of prolonged mechanical ventilation, prior broad-spectrum antibiotics, corticosteroid use, malnutrition, or chronic structural lung disease (such as bronchiectasis).

Therapy should be directed at the core bacteria for all patients, with modifications if specific other organisms are suspected or documented. The core organisms can be treated with a second-generation cephalosporin, a nonpseudomonal third-generation cephalosporin, a β-lactam/β-lactamase inhibitor combination, or a fluoroquinolone. If anaerobic organisms are likely, clindamycin or metronidazole should be added to one of these agents. If methicillin-resistant *S. aureus* is likely, vancomycin should be added. If *P. aeruginosa* is suspected, then dual antipseudomonal therapy should be initiated. The antipseudomonal antibiotics include the antipseudomonal penicillins (piperacillin, azlocillin, mezlocillin), certain third-generation cephalosporins (ceftazidime or cefoperazone), aztreonam, imipenem/cilastatin, ticarcillin/clavulanic acid, ciprofloxacin, and the aminoglycosides.

*Pseudomonas aeruginosa*

This aerobic Gram-negative bacillus is the most common cause of nosocomial pneumonia, accounting for up to 15% of all cases, and colonizes the airway of up to 40% of all mechanically ventilated patients (26). The bacteria reach the lung by aspiration, direct entry via the endotracheal tube, or hematogenously. Patients most at risk for infection are those with cystic fibrosis, bronchiectasis, burns, corticosteroid therapy, neutropenia, tracheostomy, and mechanical ventilation. A necrotizing pneumonia is common, with alveolar septal necrosis, microabscesses, and vascular thrombosis. In postoperative patients, the mortality from pseudomonal pneumonia is over 70% (108). The virulence of the organism can be enhanced by production of a slime layer in its surface capsule, endotoxin lipopolysaccharide, pili, exotoxins, and proteases. Exotoxin A, phospholipase, fibrinolysin, and elastase help to mediate the lung injury that accompanies infection. Patients with this infection may be quite toxic and have confusion, fever, chills, and productive cough, along with relative bradycardia, leukocytosis, and hemorrhagic pleural effusion. Bilateral bronchopneumonia, particularly in the lower lobes, nodular infiltrates, and cavitation may be seen (Fig. 16.11). With bacteremia in the neutropenic patient, a characteristic skin lesion, ecthyma gangrenosum, may be seen.

## Pneumonia in Special Settings

*The Immunocompromised Host*

Patients with specific immune impairments related to an underlying primary illness (often malignancy or HIV infection) or arising as a consequence of medical

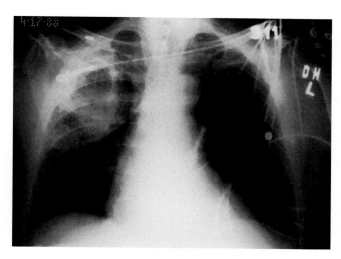

**FIGURE 16.11.** Nosocomial pneumonia due to *Pseudomonas aeruginosa* in a patient treated chronically with corticosteroids. Necrotization is evident with a cavity in the right upper lobe.

therapy (most typically chemotherapy or transplant-related immunosuppression) may develop respiratory infections; these individuals are referred to as immunocompromised hosts (ICH) (109). More recently, AIDS has led to a large and important population of ICH patients who may develop pneumonia. In any ICH, a new infiltrative pulmonary process may be infectious or noninfectious (such as an adverse drug reaction). Pneumonia may be a life-threatening infection in patients with malignancy or immunosuppressive therapy, and efforts at making a specific etiologic diagnosis are often necessary. As shown in Table 16.8, the spectrum of possible infections is broad and will vary with the nature of the immune deficit.

Often it is possible to narrow down the infectious possibilities with an understanding of the basic immune impairment (Table 16.8). Thus, patients who have had a splenectomy (including those with sickle cell anemia and autosplenectomy) are usually infected by encapsulated bacteria such as pneumococcus, staphylococci, *H. influenzae*, and *N. meningitides*. Patients with chemotherapy-induced neutropenia may be infected with *P. aeruginosa*, other Gram-negative bacteria, and *Aspergillus* species. Patients with abnormal T-lymphocyte function, such as those with certain lymphomas or AIDS, may be infected by bacteria such as *Listeria monocytogenes*, *Salmonella* species, *Legionella* spp., *Mycobacterium avium*, or *M. tuberculosis*; fungi such as *Cryptococcus neoformans*, *Histoplasma capsulatum*, or *Coccidioides immitis*; viruses such as cytomegalovirus and herpes simplex; or parasites such as *P. carinii*, *Toxoplasma gondii*, or *Cryptosporidium* spp. (110, 111). In the HIV-infected patient, the type of infection

that develops is directly related to the degree of immune dysfunction, as reflected by the patient's CD4 lymphocyte count. Those with little immune dysfunction and a CD4 count above 500/mm³ usually do not develop opportunistic infection, and their predominant pneumonia is bacterial, especially pneumococcal. As the CD4 count falls, the risk of opportunistic infection rises, and patients with a count above 200/mm³ are at particular risk for such infections as *P. carinii* (111).

Immunocompromised patients should have a careful clinical examination with attention to the skin, gastrointestinal tract, central nervous system, optic fundi, liver, and lungs. Respiratory symptoms may be minimal, with fever as the only finding, or the patient may have cough and dyspnea. Certain extrapulmonary findings in conjunction with a specific immune defect can suggest an etiologic agent. Skin lesions are common with infections caused by *P. aeruginosa*, *M. tuberculosis*, nocardia, varicella-zoster, herpes simplex, cryptococcus, and *Blastomyces*. The central nervous system may be affected by nocardia, pneumococcus, *H. influenzae*, *P. aeruginosa*, *M. tuberculosis*, *Legionella*, *Aspergillus*, *Cryptococcus*, *Toxoplasma*, varicella-zoster, and cytomegalovirus. Liver function abnormalities can be seen with cytomegalovirus, *Legionella*, and *Nocardia* infection, tuberculosis, histoplasmosis, toxoplasmosis, and *S. aureus* and *P. aeruginosa* infection. Diarrhea can occur with *Legionella*, *Cryptosporidium*, cytomegalovirus, or herpes simplex (109).

Patients who have received organ transplants represent an expanding population of ICH individuals. Infections in this population can be related to hospitalization, the presence of serious illness, and transplant immunosuppression. Within the first month of transplant, patients get the usual bacterial nosocomial pneumonias. In the period from 1 to 6 months after transplant, infection is related to immunosuppression and can be with cytomegalovirus, *P. carinii*, fungal agents, *L. monocytogenes*, and *Legionella* spp. After 6 months, these same pathogens may still lead to infection in patients who are heavily immunosuppressed, while chronic viral infection can develop in those less heavily immunosuppressed (112).

Chest radiography is often the way that the diagnosis of pneumonia is made, since many patients will have only fever and no respiratory complaints or findings. Focal lung lesions can be seen with bacterial, fungal, and mycobacterial illness. Diffuse infiltrates are seen with *P. carinii*, cytomegalovirus, *Legionella* infection, miliary tuberculosis, viral pneumonia, *Aspergillus*, and *Candida*. After a careful clinical examination, samples of sputum and blood should be collected and cultured for bacteria, fungi, *M. tuberculosis*, and viruses.

TABLE 16.8
TYPE OF IMMUNOLOGIC DEFECT AND ASSOCIATED MICROORGANISMS

| Defect or Factor | Microorganism | | | |
|---|---|---|---|---|
| | Bacteria | Fungi | Viruses | Parasites |
| Abnormal T lymphocyte function lymphoma, AIDS | Listeria monocytogenes Nocardia Salmonella (species other than S. typhi) Mycobacteria Legionella | Cryptococcus neoformans Histoplasma capsulatum Coccidioides immitis Candida Trichosporon | Cytomegalovirus Varicella-zoster Herpes simplex | Pneumocystis carinii Toxoplasma gondii Strongyloides stercoralis |
| Abnormal B lymphocyte function myeloma, primary and acquired deficiency | Streptococcus pneumoniae Haemophilus influenzae | | | |
| Neutropenia (<500 neutrophils/mm³): Myeloproliferative disease, lymphoma cytotoxic therapy, alcoholism, sickle cell disease | Pseudomonas aeruginosa Escherichia coli Klebsiella Serratia Aeromonas Other Gram-negative bacilli | Aspergillus Zygomycetes | | |
| Splenectomy | S. pneumoniae H. influenzae E. coli Staphylococcus aureus Neisseria meningitis | | | |
| Decreased serum complement | S. pneumoniae | | | |
| Primary, collagen vascular disease | H. influenzae Neisseria spp. | | | |
| Use of corticosteroid therapy equivalent to >20 mg of prednisone daily or cytotoxic therapy (or both) | S. aureus L. monocytogenes Mycobacteria P. aeruginosa Nocardia Other Gram-negative bacilli | Aspergillus Zygomycetes H. capsulatum C. neoformans C. immitis | Cytomegalovirus Varicella-zoster Herpes simplex | P. carinii T. gondii Strongyloides stercoralis |

From Rosenow EC, Wilson WR, Cockerill FR: Pulmonary disease in the immunocompromised host. *Mayo Clin Proc* 60:612, 1985.

Special stains for *M. tuberculosis, Legionella,* and *P. carinii* can be applied to respiratory tract secretions. Based on all available data, the patient usually is given empiric antibiotic therapy directed at the most likely pathogens. If improvement occurs, therapy is continued for 2 to 3 weeks. If there is no improvement, then an invasive procedure is performed. If the patient has an adequate platelet count, the procedure is either a transbronchial or an open lung biopsy. With inadequate platelets, bronchoalveolar lavage without biopsy can be performed, or transfusion and biopsy can be undertaken. The decision between bronchoscopic and surgical lung biopsy is made on the basis of how rapidly the patient is deteriorating and on the expected yield and risks of bronchoscopy. In all patients who are

immunocompromised, consideration must be given to drug-induced lung disease, malignant involvement of the lung, heart failure, and pulmonary hemorrhage, in addition to the possibility of opportunistic infection (109).

*Lung Infection in the Patient with AIDS*

Patients with AIDS have impairment of T cell function but also have humoral immune dysfunction. Thus, infections with bacteria, fungi, viruses, and parasites have all been seen in this population. The T cell deficiency can lead to pneumonia caused by *P. carinii,* cytomegalovirus, and *Mycobacterium, Legionella,* and *Nocardia* spp. (111). The humoral immune dysfunction has been responsible for infections by pneumococcus and *H. influenzae.* As mentioned, the degree of T lymphocyte depletion will determine which infections the patient is most likely to develop.

The most common pneumonia in immunosuppressed patients with HIV infection is that caused by *P. carinii*. This organism is probably a fungus that can exist in cyst form, containing sporozoites, or in free form as a trophozoite. The organism can be recognized by methenamine silver stain or by Giemsa stain, usually of lung tissue or bronchoalveolar lavage fluid. Infection may represent endogenous reactivation of latent infection present in early childhood. Most patients probably acquired *Pneumocystis* from natural sources prior to the onset of AIDS and contained it within the lung. Once AIDS develops, these latent stores of organism may become reactivated, but new primary infection or reinfection are also possible. Most patients present with a subacute course of fever, cough, dyspnea, and weight loss. Chest pain, malaise, fatigue, and night sweats may also occur, and some patients are even asymptomatic. Chest radiograph usually shows bilateral diffuse interstitial or alveolar infiltrates (Fig. 16.12). Asymmetric or focal infiltrates may occasionally be seen, as can predominantly upper lobe disease and solitary pulmonary nodules (113). Less common findings include pneumothorax and pleural effusion. Upper lobe disease and pneumothorax are more likely in patients who have received aerosolized pentamidine for prophylaxis of *P. carinii* infection.

The diagnosis of *Pneumocystis* may be elusive, since it may be the first presentation of AIDS for many individuals. Therefore, all patients with pneumonia, particularly one that is subacute, should be questioned for AIDS risk factors, and if present, *Pneumocystis* should be considered in the differential diagnosis. Findings that suggest the diagnosis are a compatible radiograph, leukopenia and lymphopenia, elevated serum LDH, oral candidiasis, and a widened alveolar-arterial oxygen tension gradient. When this infection arises in an AIDS patient, it is usually associated with a more prolonged course, lower fever, less tachypnea, and less hypoxemia than when it occurs in other immunocompromised patients, such as those with lymphoma. In AIDS patients, *Pneumocystis* may coexist with cytomegalovirus, toxoplasmosis, or mycobacterial illness. Diagnosis is usually made by bronchoalveolar lavage or transbronchial biopsy, and more recently, the induction of sputum for expectoration has led to the diagnosis in up to half of all patients.

With therapy, improvement is slower in the AIDS patient than in other ICHs with *Pneumocystis* infection. Fever may persist for 7 to 10 days, and overall survival from the infection is as high as 90%. Survival is more likely if the clinical manifestations are mild, the organism burden is not large, and if the infection is the first

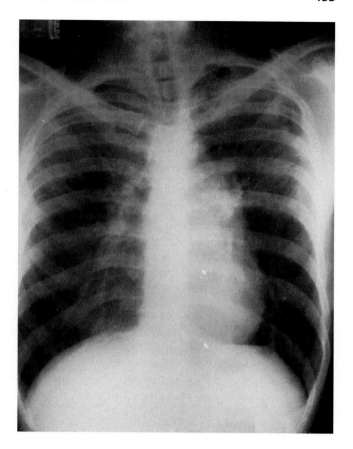

**FIGURE 16.12.** Diffuse bilateral interstitial infiltrates in a "ground glass" pattern in a 33-year-old intravenous drug abuser. This pattern is typical for *Pneumocystis carinii*.

episode of *P. carinii*. Therapy is begun with intravenous trimethoprim-sulfamethoxazole (15 to 20 mg/kg/day of trimethoprim and 75 to 100 mg/kg/day of sulfamethoxazole), but as many as half of all AIDS patients will not be able to tolerate therapy because of adverse reactions. These patients, as well as those who do not respond to trimethoprim-sulfamethoxazole, are then treated with pentamidine (4 mg/kg/day). Other effective agents are trimethoprim/dapsone, or for mild to moderate infections, atovaquone (750 mg orally three times daily). Trimetrexate and aerosolized pentamidine have been tried but are generally less effective than standard therapy (114, 115). Therapy with most regimens is continued for 21 days. If the illness leads to hypoxemia, with a room air arterial $P_{O_2}$ below 70 mm Hg, then corticosteroids should be added to ameliorate the host inflammatory response to the killing of organisms that accompanies therapy. Corticosteroids are given in a dose of prednisone 40 mg twice daily for 5 days, followed by 20 mg twice daily for 5 days, and then 20 mg once daily for 11 days (111). After recovery from pneumonia, patients should receive chemoprophylaxis against recurrent infection, which can be done with oral trimethoprim-sulfamethoxazole or aerosolized pentamidine.

### Approach to the Patient with Pneumonia

*History and Physical Examination*

Although it may be impossible to identify a specific etiologic agent on clinical grounds alone, a careful evaluation can help guide initial therapy. As shown in Figure 16.3, patients with CAP should have initial empiric therapy selected by assessing three factors: the need for hospitalization; advanced age (>60 years) or comorbid illness; and the severity of the patient's illness (66). Based on these assessments, a likely set of pathogens can be identified, and from this list, therapeutic choices follow. In a recent statement by the American Thoracic Society, an empiric approach utilizing these three determinations was endorsed; other approaches were discussed and found to have only limited value. For example, the use of clinical features to predict microbial etiology, the use of sputum Gram stain to guide initial therapy, and the routine use of extensive diagnostic testing were all regarded as not useful (66).

The initial history and physical examination can be used to define how ill the patient is and whether hospitalization will be needed (66). Indicators of severe pneumonia include a respiratory rate above 30/minute, diastolic hypotension (<60 mm Hg), systolic hypotension, oliguria, need for vasopressors, or the presence of respiratory failure. Examination can also reveal other findings indicating a poor prognosis, including altered mental status, high fever, or evidence of extrapulmonary spread of infection. Other historical information may help in determining the probable etiologic pathogen. Thus, patients should be specifically questioned about rash, diarrhea, headache, myalgias, change in mentation, and nausea. Travel history, pets, unusual occupations, and unusual hobbies can also help raise suspicion about certain of the less common infectious agents. If aspiration pneumonia is suspected, the patient should be asked about neurologic disease, esophageal disease, and alcohol use. In addition, an allergic history should be obtained before antimicrobial therapy is prescribed.

Physical examination can also help identify certain etiologic pathogens and disease complications. Respiratory examination can reveal consolidation, pleural effusion, and bronchopneumonia. Examination of the skin, fundi, liver, heart, and neurologic system can help point to specific etiologic diagnoses. In some patients, the examination may be the first clue to the presence of pneumonia. In the elderly, the most reliable physical finding for pneumonia, because of the abnormal inflammatory response in this population, is elevation of the respiratory rate above 25 per minute (116). Patients should also be evaluated for their ability to cough and expectorate sputum, so that individuals with impaired cough can receive physical therapy to aid in tracheobronchial toilet.

When a patient has nosocomial pneumonia, the same assessments of comorbidity and severity of illness should be made, and these factors can be used to guide initial therapy (103, 104). However, since many patients develop nosocomial pneumonia because of impaired host defenses, nosocomial pneumonia is commonly present in the absence of fever or other classic respiratory features of pneumonia.

*Chest Radiograph*

In many patients, the history and examination may suggest pneumonia, but the diagnosis is firmly established by finding a new parenchymal lung infiltrate. The infiltrate should be lobar, interstitial, nodular, cavitary or bronchopneumonic. Bilaterality, pleural effusion, and multiple lobe involvement should also be noted. Multilobar infiltrates, cavitation, and rapidly expanding infiltrates (>50% increase in 48 hours) all predict an increased mortality from CAP (66, 69). The location of the infiltrate can also be helpful: apical disease can suggest tuberculosis, disease in dependent segments is compatible with aspiration, and consolidation of the upper lobe suggests infection with *K. pneumoniae* or pneumococcus.

The chest film can also be used to follow the patient during therapy of pneumonia, to detect any complications. Cavitation and empyema should be suspected and sought if the patient develops a new or persistent fever during treatment. Serial radiographs can also be used to determine the duration of a pneumonia and whether it is resolving appropriately. When radiographs fail to show improvement, this may suggest an unusual or unsuspected organism (*M. tuberculosis* or fungus), an antibiotic-resistant organism, a noninfectious inflammatory disease (such as Wegener's granulomatosis), an impaired host (with a normally slow response to therapy), or an unsuspected malignancy (117). Before a pneumonia is termed unresolving, the natural course of radiographic improvement for each infection should be appreciated. Both pneumococcal and *Legionella* infections may have radiographic deterioration in up to half of all patients during the initial week of a successful course of therapy. In each of these infections, radiographic clearing will begin in the first 2 weeks of treatment, but the chest film may not be entirely normal for 3 to 6 months.

*Diagnostic Methods*

Many techniques are available to identify the etiologic agent in lower respiratory tract infection, including sputum Gram stain and culture, blood culture, transtracheal aspirate culture, bronchoscopic specimen culture (protected brush samples, bronchoalveolar lavage, transbronchial biopsy, bronchial wash), open lung biopsy, and immunologic methods (118). For most patients, collection of sputum is the primary diagnostic test, along with blood cultures (which are positive in no more than 15% of all cases of pneumonia) and a careful clinical evaluation. In spite of these assessments, many patients require empiric therapy, with modifications being made after the results of diagnostic testing become available. If there is no response or if a specific diagnosis is required (as in certain ICHs), then more-invasive tests are done.

Sputum samples are not always the source of reliable data. Culture of expectorated sputum may be of no help because the sample can be contaminated by oral flora as it passes through the oropharynx; the sample may not contain the responsible pathogen; or the sample may contain pathogens that are colonizing the patient but not causing the invasive infection. A sputum sample should be assessed for quality by microscopic examination. If there are fewer than 10 squamous epithelial cells and more than 25 neutrophils per low-power field, then the sample is probably a good representation of the lower airway's secretions. Samples with more than 25 squamous epithelial cells are too contaminated by oral secretions to be useful. The value of sputum Gram stain is widely debated (66). Although Gram's staining can show a dominant organism, the sensitivity and specificity vary widely depending on the criteria used to define a sample as "positive." Often the test is performed by individuals who cannot correlate the findings with the clinical picture, or else it is performed by clinicians with limited technical expertise. All of these practical considerations limit the utility of a sputum Gram stain. The difficulty with sputum Gram stain data is highlighted by finding false-positive rates of up to 88% and false-negative rates of 50% (118). With pneumococcal pneumonia, up to half of the sputum Gram stains will be negative. A high false-positive rate may result from the fact that many patients who have pneumonia also have airway colonization by enteric Gram-negative organisms. The exact role of these cultured organisms in causing any pneumonia in such a colonized patient is unclear. For example, up to 40% of the elderly are colonized by Gram-negative organisms, and up to 75% of hospitalized patients can harbor these organisms in their airway, even without pneumonia. Certain organisms can

be recovered on stain or culture of sputum whose presence alone is diagnostic, since these organisms never colonize without causing infection; they include *M. tuberculosis*, *P. carinii*, certain fungi, and *L. pneumophila*.

Of the noninvasive techniques, immunologic methods can be applied to many patients, with varying degrees of sensitivity and rapidity of receiving diagnostic information. Serologic titers for viral, fungal, *Legionella* and certain atypical agents can be diagnostic, but there is often a delay in receiving results, and often convalescent titers must be collected. Thus this method is of little use in the acute management of patients and is more helpful for epidemiologic studies. Immunologic staining of respiratory secretions for bacterial or viral antigens can be useful. Counterimmunoelectrophoresis can detect small amounts of pneumococcal antigen in the sputum, serum, or urine of up to half of the patients with pneumococcal pneumonia. Direct fluorescent antibody staining of sputum for *L. pneumophila* can be positive in 70% of cases (118). Genetic probes for the nucleic acids of *Legionella* and certain viruses are increasingly available.

Of the invasive techniques, open lung biopsy is generally reserved for the immunocompromised patient or for the patient with an unresolving pneumonia. The most commonly used invasive procedure is bronchoscopy, and it should only be used if its risks are less than the risks of empiric therapy or if empiric therapy is not successful. Transbronchial biopsy allows histologic examination and culture for mycobacteria, *Pneumocystis*, fungi, and viral agents. Bronchoscopy has its greatest utility in the ICH and (as mentioned) is controversial and of uncertain value in patients with suspected nosocomial pneumonia (119, 120). In patients with CAP, it should be reserved for the nonresponding patient. Bronchoalveolar lavage has been used in the ICH and has had a diagnostic yield of over 60% (119). By wedging the bronchoscope and instilling 210 ml of saline in 30-ml aliquots, the lavage fluid can be returned and collected for culture and staining. This method has detected ICHs with infections caused by *Pneumocystis*, viruses, fungi, and mycobacteria.

## Therapy of Pneumonia

Antibiotics represent the mainstay of pneumonia therapy and may be viewed as specific, in contrast to many of the other therapies, which are primarily supportive. Antibiotic therapy is organism directed, but if a specific pathogen is not identified, empiric therapy directed at the most likely pathogens is commonly used and will be selected after a careful epidemiologic assessment of the patient. The supportive measures that are not specific to any organism are adjunctive therapy and include supplemental oxygen, intravenous hydration, and measures to promote tracheobronchial toilet such as mucolytic and mucokinetic agents, bronchodilators, and bronchoscopy.

### Indications for Hospitalization of CAP Patients

Individuals who have moderate to severe illness generally require intravenous antibiotics, hydration, and supplemental oxygen (arterial oxygen tension less than 60 mm Hg on room air), and these therapies require admission to the hospital. In addition, those with serious coexisting illness or multiple risk factors for a poor outcome should also be treated in an inpatient setting. Risk factors for a complicated course of illness include the presence of coexisting diseases such as congestive heart failure, obstructive lung disease, diabetes, renal failure, hospitalization within the last year, and neurologic illness; age above 65 years; certain physical findings, such as tachypnea, hypotension, or high fever; hypoxemia or hypercarbia ($PaO_2$ less than 60 mm Hg or $PaCO_2$ above 50 mm Hg) on room air; and evidence of sepsis or end-organ dysfunction (66).

In addition to offering specific therapy that is unavailable to outpatients, hospitalization allows observation of the patient's course during therapy. Individuals with serious comorbidity may have deterioration of their underlying illness in response to infection, their pneumonia may progress rapidly, and on initial evaluation they may appear less ill than they actually are, because of an impaired host inflammatory response. Hospitalization is also able to provide specific therapy for patients who are in respiratory failure (severe hypoxemia or hypercarbia), as well as for those with an impaired cough reflex and copious sputum (so that they may receive adequate tracheobronchial toilet), those with atelectasis, and those with systemic sepsis.

### Antibiotic Therapy

If a specific pathogen is identified, then therapy should be as narrowly directed as possible, with the agents mentioned above for each organism. If no etiology can be established, then empiric therapy is required, with full appreciation of the pitfalls of this approach. With empiric regimens, multiple antibiotics are often required, not all likely pathogens can be covered, and some combination therapies are nephrotoxic.

Therapy for community-acquired infection is directed toward pneumococcus, *M. pneumoniae*, and *C. pneumoniae* if the patient has no host impairment (66). If the patient is elderly, has aspirated, is an alcoholic, or has serious coexisting illness, then in addition to these organisms, the empiric regimen must also cover enteric Gram-negative organisms, *H. influenzae*, *S. aureus*, and anaerobes. Hospitalized patients should be treated for pneumococcus, enteric Gram-negative organisms, *H. influenzae*, *S. aureus*, anaerobes, and possibly *Legionella*. Those with severe CAP should be treated for pneumococcus, *Legionella*, enteric Gram-negative organisms (including *P. aeruginosa*), and possibly *M. pneumoniae*, and *H. influenzae*.

When antibiotics are used, precautions are necessary in certain settings. With renal or hepatic failure, certain drugs will have their elimination interfered with, and dosage must be adjusted. Renally cleared drugs include the aminoglycosides, certain cephalosporins, quinolones, penicillins, and other $\beta$-lactams. Liver-excreted drugs include erythromycin, chloramphenicol, and nafcillin. In patients with a reduction in lean body mass and an increase in body fat, such as the elderly, there may be a rise in drug levels if they are given on a per-kilogram basis. With a reduction in serum albumin, the free concentration of certain drugs that are ordinarily highly protein bound may rise. Some drugs, particularly the penicillins, have a high sodium content, which should be considered if the patient has coexisting heart failure.

Some antibiotics penetrate poorly into bronchial secretions, and topical antibiotics may be indicated to increase antibiotic levels in the lung. This approach is not a standard one, but it has been used successfully to treat *P. aeruginosa* airway infections in patients with cystic fibrosis. It may also be indicated to treat patients with severe Gram-negative infections that have not responded to parenteral antibiotics. When topical therapy is given, it may be via direct intratracheal injection or aerosolization and should be preceded by bronchodilator treatment to avoid reflex bronchospasm. The drugs most commonly used in this manner are polymyxin and the aminoglycosides. Some evidence suggests that topical antibiotics can be used prophylactically in critically ill patients to prevent nosocomial pneumonia.

### Oxygenation and Mechanical Ventilation

Endotracheal intubation and mechanical ventilation are required in patients with refractory hypoxemia (arterial oxygen tension less than 60 mm Hg on maximal mask oxygen) or hypercarbic respiratory failure with acute respiratory acidosis, and in patients who cannot adequately clear secretions (to allow deep airway suctioning). When patients have severe hypoxemia and a unilateral pneumonia, their oxygenation can be improved by positioning them with the unaffected lung in a gravity-dependent position. This maneuver increases perfusion to the normal lung, relative to the diseased lung, and thereby minimizes ventilation-perfusion mismatches.

*Tracheobronchial Toilet*

Chest physiotherapy can be used to promote clearance of respiratory secretions. This therapy, which employs components of postural drainage, chest percussion, vibration, coughing, and forced expiratory breathing, is best used for patients with copious secretions (more than 30 ml/day) who have a reduced ability to cough. These physical methods may be no more effective than a good cough, but many patients are unable to provide this, and assistance may be required (121).

Agents that reduce the viscosity and consistency of sputum are termed mucolytic; those that increase mucociliary clearance are termed mucokinetic (122). Mucolytic therapy can be achieved with hydration, aerosolized saline, and inhaled *N*-acetylcysteine. The use of mucolytic agents is best reserved for patients with retained secretions who have developed atelectasis. Mucokinetic drugs are rarely used, but some agents that may be used for other purposes have mucokinetic effects. These include $\beta$-agonist bronchodilators and theophylline. Another technique that may be helpful for some patients with mucus plugging and retained secretions is bronchoscopy. If atelectasis is present without an air bronchogram, then there may be a large central airway plug and bronchoscopy can be used for suction removal under direct vision. Bronchoscopy can also be used in patients with unresolving pneumonia to evaluate for the presence of a tumor or aspirated foreign body. For patients with nosocomial pneumonia, secretions may also be mobilized by endotracheal suctioning. Another approach is to place the patient on an oscillating bed that rotates from side to side. Although it is unclear whether this approach can help pneumonia resolve more rapidly, there are data suggesting that this type of intervention can prevent pneumonia in high-risk patients, possibly by mobilizing secretions (123).

## Tuberculosis

*Epidemiology and Pathogenesis*

Tuberculosis may be a pulmonary disease, an extrapulmonary disease, or both and is caused by Koch's bacillus, *M. tuberculosis*. The organism is a nonmotile, acid-fast staining, Gram-positive rod with a high lipid content. It is an obligate aerobe, which is not pigmented (in contrast to some of the other mycobacterial species) and is normally contained by cell-mediated immunity. Patients with impaired cellular immune responses, such as the elderly, diabetics, patients treated with immunosuppressives, patients with renal failure, those with hematologic malignancy, and individuals with AIDS, are thus at increased risk of illness from this organism. Disease is spread from person to person

via inhalation of droplet nuclei produced by infected persons when they talk, cough, or sneeze. Casual contacts of infected persons are not usually infected, but those with prolonged and close contact, particularly in areas of poor ventilation, are most at risk. This mode of spread, which favors disease in crowded, small spaces, may contribute to the predominance of this illness among those of lower socioeconomic status and in persons living in underdeveloped nations.

In the United States, there were about 15 new cases per 100,000 population during the 1970s, and the incidence declined at a rate of 6.7% annually until 1985. Beginning in 1986, the incidence of new cases began to rise, which has been attributed to the frequent infection of AIDS patients with the tubercle bacillus (18, 124). In 1990, it was estimated that 4.3% of HIV-infected persons had tuberculosis infection (18). In addition, tuberculosis remains an important infection in many immigrants to this country, among the homeless, and in the elderly who are confined to nursing homes. Currently, more than two-thirds of TB cases occur in nonwhite racial and ethnic groups. One-quarter of all cases in the United States occur in the foreign born, but still one-third of cases occur in middle and upper-income groups (18). Among patients aged 25 to 44 years, most are nonwhites and Hispanics, while whites predominate in the elderly population of TB patients. One other recent change in tuberculosis epidemiology has been the emergence of organisms that are multiply resistant to traditional tuberculosis medications. Multidrug-resistant tuberculosis (MDR-TB) is a particular problem among HIV-infected individuals and those with a history of prior TB therapy. In New York City, as many as 23% of all previously untreated TB patients have primary drug resistance to at least one drug (125).

Most individuals who encounter the tubercle bacillus become infected with it, contain the organism within the lung by developing an adequate immune response, and thus do not develop clinical illness. Those with the clinical disease "tuberculosis" are either individuals who cannot contain the primary infection or persons who have reactivated a previously contained and dormant infection. Thus, much of the literature makes a distinction between "infection" and "disease" due to *M. tuberculosis*. Many people have had the infection, but fewer than 10% of infected individuals will develop the disease.

The initial infection with the organism, the primary infection, is usually in the middle or lower zones of the lung. Since these areas receive the most ventilation with each breath, it is not surprising that an airborne organism would localize in this fashion. Over the next few weeks, the organisms multiply and spread via lymphatics to the regional lymph nodes, particularly in the hilum. The combination of a primary peripheral lung lesion with an enlarged hilar lymph node is termed a Ghon complex. During this time, some organisms may disseminate via the bloodstream to extrapulmonary sites, where they are usually contained but may reactivate at a later date. The favored sites for secondary seeding and growth of these aerobic bacteria are ones with high tissue oxygen content such as the apex of the lung, the renal parenchyma, and the growing ends of long bones.

Within 3 to 6 weeks of primary infection, sensitized T lymphocytes release lymphokines that can attract monocytes and macrophages to the infected area in the lung to phagocytose the bacteria. Lymphocytes are also attracted, and during this time, the host develops immunity to reinfection, which becomes detectable by conversion of the tuberculin skin test to positive. Once the skin test becomes positive, the host usually can kill any other organisms that are inhaled, but it may not always be able to eliminate the organisms already within the lung and lung macrophages. Thus, most case of active tuberculosis are in patients with positive skin tests and are due to progressive primary disease or reactivation disease; they are less commonly due to reinfection after exposure to another infected patient with active disease. However, in the HIV-infected patient, superinfection with a resistant TB strain, during TB therapy for infection with another strain, has been reported (126).

The initial tissue response to infection involves mononuclear cells, which may crowd together, with their lipid-rich cytoplasm, and form a tubercle made up of cells that are described as epithelioid. The tubercle may contain multinucleated giant cells, called Langhans giant cells, and it is surrounded by fibroblasts, lymphocytes, and more monocytes to form a granuloma, which is characteristic of tuberculosis. This granulomatous reaction must be distinguished from other granulomatous tissue reactions such as those seen with sarcoidosis and fungal disease. When a host cannot contain the organism by this inflammatory response, the organism continues to multiply, and the center of the granuloma undergoes a process of liquefaction necrosis, termed caseation. The progression to this necrotizing process does not occur in most infected patients, only in those who cannot contain the organism. The caseous material is full of living organisms that can spread within the lung. The necrotic, caseating granuloma then becomes a tuberculous cavity, which may contain up to $10^9$ organisms (127). Without caseation, a granuloma has many fewer organisms. When large quantities of caseous material are spread along the bronchi from a cavity to another part of the lung, a

tuberculous pneumonia may develop. When granulomas finally do heal, they often develop calcification, particularly if caseation has occurred.

About 5% of patients with primary infection will not be able to contain the organism and will develop progressive primary disease within 2 years of infection. Rates of progressive primary disease may be higher with HIV infection, reaching 7 to 8% per year, and the onset of illness may be accelerated by the HIV coinfection. As primary infection usually involves the lower lung zones, the patient with progressive primary disease may manifest with lower lobe tuberculosis (Fig. 16.13). The failure to contain the organism may be related to the size of inoculum and the status of the host defense system. Patients at risk for progressive primary infection are the very young, the elderly, the malnourished, blacks, diabetics, alcoholics, and those with immunosuppressive medications or illnesses (including HIV infection). An additional 5% will develop disease more than 2 years after infection, which will

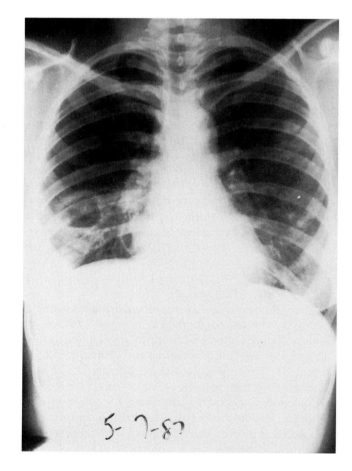

**FIGURE 16.13.** Lower lobe cavitary tuberculosis due to progressive primary disease in a 46-year-old black male diabetic.

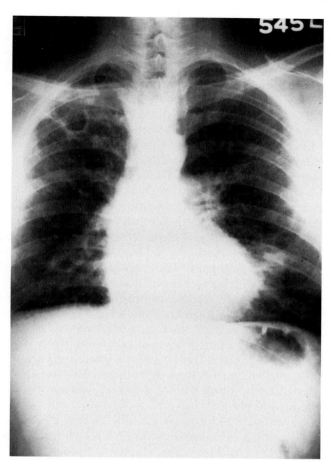

**FIGURE 16.14.** Reactivation tuberculosis with cavity formation and infiltrate in the upper lobe and endobronchial spread from an upper lobe cavity to the lower lobes.

be due to reactivation of live bacilli that had been contained and dormant within healed granulomas. This reactivation illness usually develops in sites where the organism was hematogenously disseminated during the primary infection. The lung apex is a common site for reactivation disease, particularly in the apical posterior segment (Fig. 16.14). Thus, based on this pathogenetic schema, lower lobe tuberculosis is usually a progressive primary disease, while upper lobe disease may represent reactivation. In either situation, the patient with tuberculous disease has been unable to contain the organism, whereas most people who are infected do not develop disease because they can contain the organism. For this reason, a deficit in host defense should be sought in all patients with active tuberculosis, and HIV testing should be considered in all patients with active tuberculosis. Extrapulmonary disease may occur as a result of progressive primary infection or with reactivation.

*Clinical Features*

With primary infection, most patients are asymptomatic or may have mild, nonspecific symptoms of a transient lower respiratory tract infection. When disease is present, symptoms are usually chronic and may cause respiratory symptoms as well as systemic manifestations. Many patients simply note malaise, headache, fever, night sweats, and weight loss. Some patients may have abdominal pain and anorexia. Pulmonary symptoms are common but not specific. Persistent cough may be present, with or without mucoid sputum, and occasionally hemoptysis is present. Hemoptysis can be the result of tuberculous pneumonia but is more commonly due to cavitary disease or rupture of an artery in an old tuberculous cavity (Rasmussen's aneurysm). Several late posttuberculous complications can cause hemoptysis, including bronchiectasis, broncholithiasis, or the presence of an aspergilloma in a prior tuberculous cavity. Another pulmonary symptom can be chest pain, particularly pleurisy-type pain, when a pleural effusion is present. Tuberculous effusions usually result when a small number of organisms from a subpleural granuloma, early in the course of the illness, rupture into the pleural cavity and the patient has a hypersensitivity response to this material. Because most of the pleural fluid is inflammatory, not many organisms are present, and culture of the pleural fluid yields the tubercle bacillus in no more than 20 to 40% of cases. Because the pleural response is a hypersensitivity one, it usually correlates with a positive tuberculin test. Much less commonly, a large inoculum of organisms can reach the pleural space and cause a tuberculous empyema. Dyspnea may occur as a result of extensive parenchymal disease, pneumothorax, or a large pleural effusion. Both the systemic and pulmonary symptoms are usually chronic, having been present for weeks to months prior to diagnosis, but occasionally an acute pneumonia presentation is seen, and acute respiratory failure may result (128). The elderly generally have less dramatic symptoms than do younger patients (129).

Extrapulmonary disease is seen in up to 16% of tuberculosis cases in the United States. However, in patients with AIDS, this pattern is much more common and may occur in 60 to 70% of all tuberculosis cases in this population (130, 131). When extrapulmonary involvement is present, the patient may present with a skin lesion that is slow to heal or a chronic draining cervical lymph node (scrofula, or cervical lymph node tuberculosis). When genital tuberculosis is present, men may have epididymal involvement with a slightly painful scrotal mass, while women may have pelvic pain or infertility. Renal tuberculosis is usually without symptoms, but patients will have "sterile" pyuria or hematuria on urinalysis. Tuberculous meningitis may cause dementia, coma, cranial nerve abnormalities (because the base of the brain is involved), focal neurologic deficits, or headache. Abdominal pain, fever, ascites, and anorexia can be manifestations of tuberculous peritonitis. Chest pain, fever, and dyspnea may result from pericardial involvement. Tuberculous involvement of the skeleton may cause bone pain or spine collapse with spinal cord compression. When the disease is fulminant and hematogenously disseminated, it is termed "miliary" because of the millet seed appearance of the multiple pulmonary lesions that are seen on chest radiograph. Miliary disease may occur with progressive primary infection or reactivation but is the result of bloodstream invasion and dissemination of large numbers of bacteria that overcome host defenses at multiple sites. Miliary tuberculosis may cause fever, malaise, cough, dyspnea, weight loss, anorexia, and headache. The lungs, liver, adrenals, kidneys, and spleen are often involved, and diagnosis may require lung or bone marrow biopsy, although organisms may be recovered from bronchoalveolar lavage or urine.

Physical findings are not specific, and patients may show signs of pneumonitis (rales), pleural effusion (dullness to percussion and reduced breath sounds), or specific extrapulmonary involvement. Laboratory data may reveal anemia, leukopenia, or severe leukocytosis. Hyponatremia and hypercalcemia are also common findings. Liver function tests may be abnormal with disseminated infection. Pleural fluid is usually an exudate with lymphocytosis, low glucose, and low pH. Spinal fluid may show low glucose, high protein, and lymphocytes if meningitis is present.

*Diagnosis*

The chest radiograph is an important clue to the presence of tuberculosis. Lower lobe involvement with infiltrates or cavitation may occur in progressive primary disease, but most patients have evidence of apical involvement, particularly in the posterior segments. Apical scarring may indicate prior infection, and a change in a previously stable upper lobe pattern may indicate reactivation. Cavitation is common with reactivation and may accompany a parenchymal, reticular upper lobe infiltrate (Fig. 16.14). Some patients will have extensive nodular lung involvement in conjunction with one or multiple cavities, and this pattern of extensive parenchymal infection is the result of endobronchial dissemination of bacteria from a caseating, cavitary lesion. Nodal enlargement in the hilum and mediastinum as well as nodal calcification can result from tuberculosis. Solitary nodules may occasionally represent a tuberculoma, and sometimes these lesions

can cavitate. Other radiographic findings can include a miliary pattern with bilateral diffuse small densities; or pleural effusion, with or without an evident parenchymal lesion. In one series (132), patients with primary tuberculosis had pulmonary consolidation in the lower lung zones or anteriorly in the upper lobe (50%), cavitation (29%), miliary disease (6%), or a normal radiograph (15%). Those with reactivation disease had a different pattern, with 91% having apical and posterior fibrous infiltrates, 45% having cavities, and 21% having bronchogenic spread of disease.

Clinical and radiographic features may be different when HIV infection is present. As mentioned, fewer HIV-infected patients than other infected individuals have only pulmonary disease. With lung involvement, HIV-infected patients with TB have lower lobe infiltrates and adenopathy and infrequently have cavitation. Even with bacteriologically confirmed pulmonary TB, HIV-infected persons can have a normal chest radiograph (124). In general, the more classic, typical, radiographic patterns are seen in HIV-infected persons who are early in their disease and are relatively intact immunologically. The severely immune-suppressed HIV patient tends to have more unusual TB manifestations, and infection with *M. avium intracellulare* is also frequently present.

A definitive diagnosis of tuberculosis disease is made by isolating the organism from a clinical specimen such as sputum, urine, a biopsy of involved tissue, pleural fluid, bone marrow aspirate, spinal fluid, ascites fluid, or bronchoscopic lavage. Sputum is best sampled by collecting the first sample produced in the early morning. In some patients, gastric aspirates can be collected and cultured, and these samples may contain organisms that have been expectorated and swallowed. Clinical specimens can be stained for organisms by the acid-fast method or with the rhodamine fluorochrome stain. Gastric aspirates may give a false-positive stain, as some gastric saprophytes are acid fast. If a patient has pulmonary involvement and sputum samples are negative, bronchoscopy should be performed with lavage, as the diagnostic yield may exceed 90%. Newer diagnostic modalities are becoming available, and they have the advantage of identifying a mycobacterial organism more rapidly than more traditional methods. With radiometric culture techniques and nucleic acid probes, organisms can be identified in a week or less, and fewer bacteria are needed than with traditional diagnostic methods (124).

Tuberculous infection (but not disease) is diagnosed by finding a positive skin test response to tuberculin antigen. The standard Mantoux test uses purified protein derivative (PPD) of tuberculin and a dose of 5 tuberculin units in 0.1 ml is administered intradermally.

The degree of induration at 48 to 72 hours is measured, and a positive test is defined in relation to the individual's relative risk of being infected with the tuberculosis bacterium (18, 133). A reaction of 5 mm or more is defined as positive for patients who are HIV positive or have HIV risk factors and are of unknown HIV status; close contacts of an active case; and those who have a chest radiograph consistent with old, healed tuberculosis. A reaction of 10 mm or more is defined as positive in patients who do not fall in any of the above categories but who are foreign born from high-prevalence countries; intravenous drug users; in minority or medically underserved groups; residents of a chronic care facility or correctional institution; and patients with medical conditions that increase the risk of tuberculosis. Such medical conditions include silicosis, gastrectomy, ileal bypass, chronic renal failure, diabetes mellitus, high-dose corticosteroids or immunosuppressive therapy or illness, and malnutrition. All other persons who do not fit into any of these groups are defined as positive only if the skin test reaction is 15 mm or more (130, 131, 133).

Over 90% of patients with tuberculous disease will have a positive skin test, and those that do not are either anergic due to overwhelming illness or are too early in the course of disease to have converted the skin test to positive. If a skin test reaction increases in size by 10 mm or more in a previously negative person less than age 35, a "conversion" is said to have occurred, and this indicates infection during the time between the two skin tests. For persons over the age of 35, an increase of 15 mm or more is needed to define a conversion, if the patient was previously negative (133). In some populations, particularly the elderly, a false-negative skin test can occur because of a "loss of immunologic memory." In such patients, a second skin test will be positive because the antigenic exposure of the first skin test "boosted" the immune response that had been present, but suppressed. When comparing the first and second skin test, one should not conclude that these patients have converted from a negative test to a positive one, but rather that they have had their false-negative result unmasked by the so-called "booster effect." It is important, in mass screening programs, to account for this phenomenon by giving a second skin test to all negative reactors 1 to 2 weeks after the first test, so that a boosted response will be recognized and not confused with a new conversion.

*Treatment*

Antituberculous therapy can be given to individuals with infection who are at high risk of developing active disease; this practice, which can prevent illness, is called prophylactic therapy. In addition, patients with active tuberculosis are treated with medications that are generally able to effectively cure the disease.

Prophylactic therapy is given with isoniazid 10 mg/kg/day (up to a maximum of 300 mg) for 6 to 9 months (130, 131). Those with AIDS may require prophylaxis longer than the usual 6 to 9 months (130, 131). Since any person with a positive PPD skin test has been infected with the tubercle bacillus and can develop disease, prophylactic therapy should be considered for all skin test reactors. However, isoniazid can cause hepatotoxicity, and the incidence of this complication rises with age, particularly above age 35. Thus, prophylactic therapy is only recommended for those whose risk of developing disease exceeds their risk of liver toxicity. A positive tuberculin test (as defined above) indicates the need for prophylaxis, regardless of age, if the patient falls into one of the following groups: (*a*) known or suspected HIV infection; (*b*) close contact of an active case; (*c*) recent convertor (defined above); (*d*) radiographic evidence of prior tuberculosis; (*e*) presence of a medical condition that increases the risk of TB (listed above). Prophylaxis is offered to other people only if they are under age 35 and fall into the following categories: (*a*) foreign born from a high-risk area; (*b*) medically underserved, low-income populations; (*c*) residents of long-term care facilities or correctional institutions; (*d*) patients with no risk factors, but a skin test of more than 15 mm.

Active tuberculosis, both pulmonary and extrapulmonary, should be treated with isoniazid 300 mg daily along with rifampin 600 mg daily for 9 months (134). This regimen combines the two most active antituberculous medications and is the most widely used today. Both drugs are bactericidal for the tubercle bacillus, and when used together, they can eliminate the organism rapidly and usually prevent relapse due to resistant bacteria. Rifampin is rapidly bactericidal to tubercle bacilli that exist in any of the three populations present in the body: actively growing extracellular organisms, slowly growing intracellular (in macrophages) organisms at acid pH, and slowly growing extracellular organisms. Isoniazid is bactericidal against the first two of these populations; streptomycin kills only actively growing extracellular bacteria; and pyrazinamide kills slowly growing intracellular bacteria. Two active drugs are needed for therapy because naturally occurring drug-resistant mutants are present in most patients. It has been estimated that 1 in $10^5$ organisms are resistant to isoniazid and 1 in $10^9$ are resistant to rifampin. Since an active tuberculous cavity has no more than $10^8$ to $10^9$ organisms, the combination therapy will effectively kill any naturally occurring drug-resistant mutants. More recently it has been suggested that if pyrazinamide (25 mg/kg) is given for the first

2 months with isoniazid and rifampin, therapy can be shortened to 6 months. If other drug combinations are used, therapy must be extended to 18 to 24 months, because the drugs are not as active. These regimens are used if the patient develops toxicity to one of the standard drugs or if drug-resistant disease is documented or suspected (as is common in certain immigrant populations). Ethambutol and streptomycin are commonly used in these extended regimens; second-line drugs include capreomycin, ethionamide, cyclo-serine, and PAS. Poorly compliant patients can be treated with intermittent regimens given under direct supervision three to five times per week.

The current concerns about MDR-TB have changed the initial approach to therapy in many parts of the country. When the possibility of resistance is entertained, patients are started on a four-drug regimen of isoniazid, rifampin, pyrazinamide, and ethambutol (135). If susceptibility patterns reveal that the organism is not drug resistant, then ethambutol is stopped, pyrazinamide is continued for a total of 2 months, and isoniazid is continued along with rifampin for a total of 6 months. In this way, short-course therapy can be achieved while still protecting for the possibility of resistant disease. If MDR-TB is identified, then therapy is continued with at least two active first-line drugs. These include INH, rifampin, pyrazinamide, ethambutol, and rifampin. If the organism is not sensitive to at least two of these agents, then second-line drugs should be used, but at least three will be required (125). Some patients with MDR-TB require multiple drugs for prolonged periods of time, and occasionally drug therapy must be supplemented with resectional surgery. To improve the outcome of therapy of MDR-TB in certain populations, directly observed therapy has been recommended (135).

### Mycobacteria Other Than Tuberculosis (MOTT)

MOTT are generally slow-growing mycobacteria that, unlike *M. tuberculosis*, are niacin negative (i.e., they metabolize and do not accumulate niacin) in the laboratory. Although some of the MOTT are niacin positive and some are rapid growers, most human disease is caused by species that do not fit this pattern. MOTT differ from the tubercle bacillus in several other important ways. They are not spread from person to person, and they are not always pathogens when isolated from human samples. In fact, most normal individuals can effectively resist infection by these organisms without tissue invasion occurring, while others may become colonized but not infected. MOTT can cause illnesses very similar to tuberculosis but usually only in abnormal hosts. Because of the similarities and

differences that these organisms and their manifestations have to the tubercle bacillus, they are sometimes called "atypical mycobacteria." In recent years, the incidence of infection by these organisms has risen, particularly in the AIDS population, where disseminated infection with *M. avium* complex (MAC) has occurred. There are multiple species of MOTT, many of which rarely cause human disease. The species that are potentially pathogenic in humans include MAC, *M. kansasii*, *M. fortuitum-chelonei*, *M. scrofulaceum*, *M. xenopi*, *M. szulgai*, *M. simiae*, *M. marinum*, *M. ulcerans*, and *M. haemophilum* (136).

The diseases caused by MOTT may cause findings in the lungs, the cervical lymph nodes (lymphadenitis), the skin (abscess or nonhealing ulcer), or occasionally systemically. The pulmonary disease may appear radiographically (Fig. 16.15) like tuberculosis but may differ in that cavities can be thin-walled with little surrounding infiltrate. In addition, bronchogenic spread is

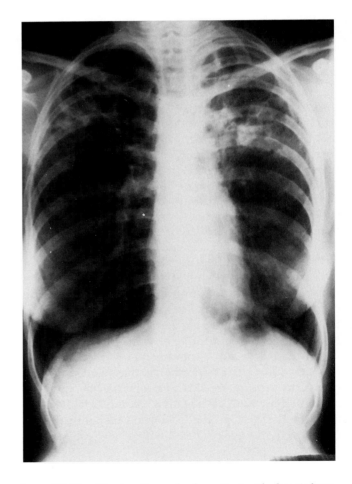

**Figure 16.15.** Chest radiograph of a patient with chronic bronchitis and slowly progressive cavitary disease in both upper lobes due to *M. avium* complex.

unusual, pleural disease is uncommon, and preexisting chronic pulmonary disease is often present (137). Symptoms are more slowly progressive than in tuberculosis but may include cough, dyspnea, weight loss, and occasionally hemoptysis and fever. The pulmonary disease is usually indolent, and when it occurs, it commonly affects older patients with chronic obstructive pulmonary disease. This pattern can occur with MAC, *M. kansasii*, or others of the MOTT group. Recently a much more virulent and disseminated form of disease, caused by MAC, has been found in AIDS patients (131). Up to one-quarter of AIDS patients may have disseminated MAC disease diagnosed antemortem, while half will have it at autopsy. Mortality from this infection is high, and symptoms are not specific and commonly include fever, weight loss, abdominal pain, malabsorption, and diarrhea. Pulmonary symptoms may also be present but not in every case. Patients may have generalized lymphadenopathy and hepatosplenomegaly. Diagnosis of disseminated MAC infection in the AIDS patient can be made by finding the organism in bone marrow, liver, urine, lymph nodes, or blood cultures.

In general, the diagnosis of MOTT infections is difficult, because simple isolation of the organisms from sputum is not sufficient to establish infection, since these bacteria may colonize diseased lungs yet not cause invasive infection. A diagnosis of pulmonary disease by MOTT is made by having a compatible clinical picture and radiograph in a patient with repeated isolation of organisms from sputum or with evidence of tissue invasion by organisms on biopsy. If cavitary disease is present, the diagnosis can be made by finding the organisms on two or more sputum samples, provided that other diagnoses have been excluded. If cavitary disease is absent, the diagnosis requires the above findings plus a failure to convert sputum samples to negative with either bronchial hygiene or 2 weeks of specific drug therapy (138). If the sputum is nondiagnostic, the diagnosis can also be established by finding the organisms in a biopsy specimen. Skin testing is not widely available or clinically useful in diseases caused by these bacteria. In the AIDS patient, the recovery of MAC organisms from blood or stool, in a patient with a compatible illness, will establish the diagnosis of disseminated infection. Once the diagnosis of MOTT infection is made, therapy is started with multiple antituberculous drugs, but the success rate, particularly in the AIDS patient, may be quite low, because the organisms are usually resistant to most available medications. Some newer agents that may be active against some of the MOTT organisms are clarithromycin, azithromycin, ciprofloxacin, ofloxacin, and rifabutin.

## FUNGAL LUNG DISEASE: NORMAL HOST

The dimorphic fungi *Histoplasma capsulatum*, *Blastomyces dermatitides*, *Coccidioides immitis*, *Paracoccidioides brasiliensis*, and *Sporothrix schenckii* are all soil growing organisms. With the exception of *Sporothrix*, they are sharply defined in their endemic areas. Again with the exception of *S. schenckii*, their primary mechanisms of infection are via the lungs; *S. schenckii* may also invade the host via the lungs, but the usual manifestation of the illness is lymphocutaneous. Moreover, most infections are asymptomatic, and only a certain percentage of infected individuals go on to develop clinically recognizable illness. Occasionally, following the acute illness, chronic or disseminated disease may develop.

After the infecting spores are inhaled, these organisms convert at body temperature to their pathogenic forms, which in all but *C. immitis* is a yeast. *C. immitis* at body temperature converts to giant spherules. While the yeast multiply by binary fission, giant spherules multiply by endosporulation.

The underlying state of immunity of the host will determine the extent and nature of human illness. Normal hosts are usually able to localize the illness to the lungs, and spontaneous recovery is the rule. However, when the disease occurs in patients who are immunocompromised either by another underlying illness or because of the administration of cytotoxic agents or glucocorticoids, dissemination to multiple organs is the rule.

### Histoplasmosis

The endemic area for *H. capsulatum* includes most of the midwestern and south-central United States, extending down to the Gulf Coast in Texas and to the St. Lawrence Valley in Canada (139). The organism occurs in microfoci in nature, and grows in soil enhanced by organic nitrogen, usually by droppings of birds or bats. In nature the organism grows as a mold, and when the sites are disturbed, an infecting aerosol is produced, leading to inhalation of the spores.

Following inhalation, the spores produce an area of pneumonitis in the lung after conversion to the yeast form. After spread to the hilar nodes, the organism gains access to the bloodstream and disseminates throughout the body. Cells of the reticuloendothelial (RE) system remove the organism from circulation, and once specific delayed hypersensitivity develops, the "armed" macrophages will destroy the organisms, leading to granuloma formation. Frequently, healing causes necrosis, which over the years may undergo calcification.

In abnormal hosts such as infants, the very elderly, or patients who are immunosuppressed by underlying disease or by administration of various agents, progressive disseminated disease frequently occurs (140). In these individuals adequate cell-mediated immunity fails to develop and the organism begins to replicate within cells of the RE system.

The vast majority of primary infections with *H. capsulatum* are either asymptomatic or minimally symptomatic. Only a small fraction of patients will ever visit a physician because of the onset of acute histoplasmosis. Those who are symptomatic usually have a "flu-like" illness, with arthralgias and myalgias as well as a nonproductive cough. Fever is usually low grade. Chest roentgenograms may be normal or show extensive bilateral nodular disease with hilar adenopathy. In addition, erythema nodosum may accompany the onset of clinical illness (141).

The primary infection in patients with altered lung anatomy, such as seen with centrilobular emphysema of smokers, looks different from that seen in normal hosts. In these patients the acute infection may surround these abnormal air spaces, giving the roentgenographic appearance of cavity formation. It is important to remember that the vast majority of these patients probably also recover spontaneously, and only in rare instances will the upper lobe disease become progressive and require treatment (142).

Symptoms of progressive upper-zone histoplasmosis are chronic illness with low-grade fever, weight loss, anorexia, and a cough productive of mucopurulent sputum. Because of the great similarity of the symptoms and the chest roentgenogram to tuberculosis, many of these patients are initially thought to have tuberculosis. (Fig. 16.16) (143). Among the other residuals following primary infection, the most common is the "coin lesion" caused by rounding off and hardening of the previous area of pneumonitis. The main significance of these lesions is that they frequently occur in patients otherwise at high risk for bronchogenic neoplasms.

An unusual complication of acute histoplasmosis is the development of mediastinal fibrosis, which is probably an abnormal host response rather than an unusual effect of the parasite (Fig. 16.17) (144).

In patients in whom the original dissemination of *Histoplasma* becomes progressive, a life-threatening illness occurs. As a rule, cell-mediated immunity is either weak or does not develop at all (140). In patients with the most severe form of immunodeficiency, such as those with AIDS or with Hodgkin's disease, progressive disseminated histoplasmosis (PDH) follows a fulminant course. Manifestations include fever, weight

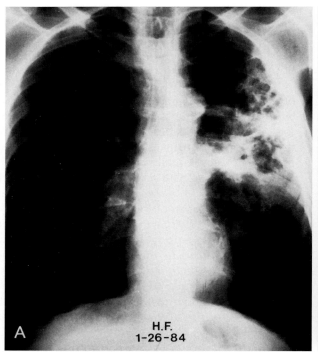
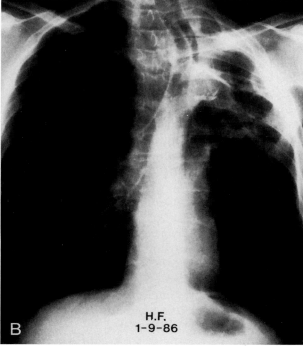

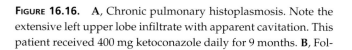

**Figure 16.16.** **A**, Chronic pulmonary histoplasmosis. Note the extensive left upper lobe infiltrate with apparent cavitation. This patient received 400 mg ketoconazole daily for 9 months. **B**, Fol-low-up chest roentgenogram shows clearing 15 months after completion of successful drug therapy. Note extensive retraction of the lobe with marked tracheal shift.

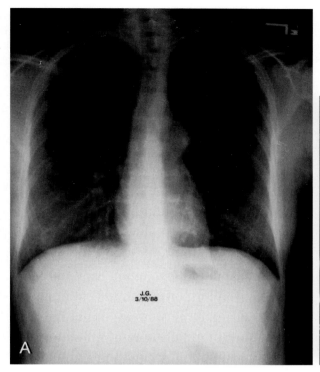

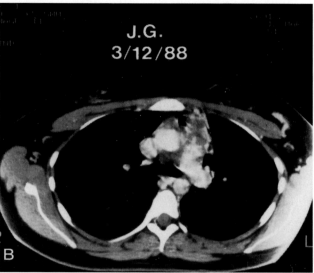

FIGURE **16.17.**   **A,** Chest roentgenogram of a 33-year-old woman with minimal respiratory symptoms. There is a large left-sided anterior mediastinal mass. **B,** Computed tomographic scan showing the full extent of the mass. Open biopsy showed healing granulomatous lesions. Histopathologic examination confirmed histoplasmosis.

loss, and hepatosplenomegaly as well as the appearance of severe bone marrow involvement with anemia, leukopenia, and thrombocytopenia. Histopathologic examination of affected tissues reveals complete absence of granulomata, and all one sees are macrophages containing multiple organisms (140, 145).

In patients in whom partial cell-mediated immunity still remains, PDH follows a much more subacute or chronic course. Histopathologically, the disease is characterized by the appearance of granulomata with a relative scarcity of organisms. Clinical symptoms in these patients are primarily those of a chronic illness; special areas of *Histoplasma* involvement include oropharyngeal, rectal, and genital ulcers as well as hepatosplenomegaly (140).

With the emergence of the AIDS epidemic, PDH became recognized as a frequent opportunistic infection in individuals infected by the human immunodeficiency virus (HIV). The nearly total deficiency of T lymphocyte–mediated immune function, which is the hallmark of AIDS, renders every HIV-positive individual uniquely susceptible to developing PDH. Two potential pathogenic mechanisms exist. First is the progression from primary infection. When immuno-

compromised individuals become infected with *H. capsulatum*, progressive dissemination will develop in most of them (146). Thus it is to be anticipated that when patients with AIDS become exposed to the fungus, the outcome will be the development of PDH.

The second mechanism is reactivation of previously dormant foci of infection. Following recovery from the primary infection, after development of specific cell-mediated immunity has successfully localized the fungus, healing with granuloma formation takes place. Resected specimens of such granulomas frequently show persisting organisms. Such dormant foci may reactivate when immunosuppressive treatment is given (147). During progression of HIV infection, most T cell–mediated immunity wanes, and when such an individual harboring dormant foci of histoplasmosis reaches the critical level of waning immunity, the fungus begins to multiply and PDH will develop. Most likely both mechanisms are operative in HIV-infected patients.

The second mechanism is probably the more important consideration for physicians who reside outside the usual endemic area for histoplasmosis. The first mechanism (as well as reactivation disease) is more likely to occur in the endemic area. As Wheat and co-workers have pointed out, the diagnosis of PDH should prompt one to evaluate the patient's HIV status (146).

In Houston, which is on the fringe of the endemic area, fully 5% of patients with AIDS have developed PDH (148). However, in more-endemic areas the risk is far greater. In Indianapolis almost 27% of HIV-infected patients developed PDH (149). Recent experiences from both the East Coast and the West Coast have documented a rapidly increasing incidence of PDH among HIV-infected individuals, most of whom resided in endemic areas for histoplasmosis prior to moving to either New York (150) or California. Remember that in addition to the central United States, both Central America and the Caribbean are endemic areas.

The clinical manifestation of PDH in AIDS is a severe febrile illness. Over half of the patients will not have had the diagnosis of AIDS established prior to the onset of PDH. Symptoms are those of a febrile illness with anorexia and weight loss. Physical examination is often normal, but hepatosplenomegaly may be present in up to one-third of patients. The chest roentgenogram may show diffuse interstitial changes with multiple small nodules but is often negative (Fig. 16.18)

(148). Pancytopenia is frequently present, but it is a nonspecific finding, since HIV-infected patients receiving zidovudine may have bone marrow suppression.

Rapid diagnosis is facilitated by remembering that any febrile individual at high risk for HIV infection may have PDH. Blood cultures and bone marrow examination and culture are the best tests (Fig. 16.19), and the fungus may be seen on examination of the buffy coat, where circulating phagocytes may be parasitized (151).

Isolation of the fungus from biologic material or visualization of the organism in histopathologic sections remains the gold standard. Proper handling of biologic specimens will yield a high frequency of positive cultures. Depending on inoculum size, a tentative diagnosis may be offered as early as 5 days, but usually this takes much longer, up to 4 to 6 weeks. When PDH is suspected, the best organ to sample is the bone marrow. Multiple blood cultures are frequently useful, especially when they are processed with the lysis-centrifugation system.

Skin testing for the diagnosis of histoplasmosis no longer has any role. While the skin test is still an outstanding epidemiologic tool, it simply cannot be used for the diagnosis of acute histoplasmosis.

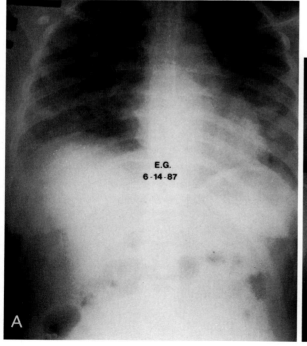

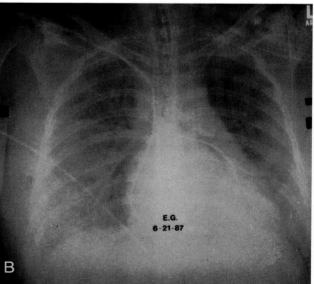

**FIGURE 16.18.** **A**, Admission chest radiograph of a 26-year-old, HIV-positive pregnant woman showing interstitial infiltrates bilaterally. The main complaint was shortness of breath and fever. Bronchial washings showed small, 2- to 4-$\mu$m round organisms thought to be *P. carinii*. **B**, One week later, in spite of aggressive therapy, infiltrates have progressed. Blood cultures obtained on the day of admission yielded *H. capsulatum*.

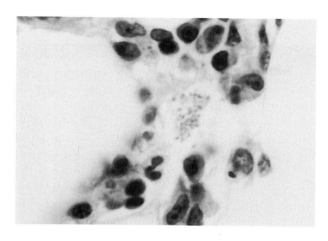

**FIGURE 16.19.** Bone marrow biopsy of an AIDS patient with progressive disseminated histoplasmosis. Note the large number of organisms inside a macrophage (hematoxylin and eosin stain × 1000).

In acute illness, serodiagnosis is the mainstay of diagnosis. Of the currently available serologic tests, complement fixation (CF) remains the best. Unfortunately, it suffers from the fact that it is seldom timely enough, since it frequently takes 2 weeks or more before a fourfold rise can be demonstrated. The immunodiffusion (ID) test, although highly specific, is relatively insensitive. In a recent outbreak, it was positive in only 50% of the proven cases (152). The best available test is the measurement of the *Histoplasma* polysaccharide antigen (153). The test is also helpful in following the course of treatment and detecting relapses (154).

Acute histoplasmosis, unless it results in significant interference with gas exchange, does not require treatment. Patients with severe, life-threatening, acute histoplasmosis will respond readily to intravenous administration of AMB (139).

Upper lobe cavitary disease, when progressive, will respond to 400 mg ketoconazole daily. The recently introduced oral triazole, itraconazole, is also highly effective and is much better tolerated than ketoconazole (155). The much lower price of ketoconazole, however, makes it the agent of choice. Treatment failures may occur with both oral agents, and in these patients, amphotericin B (AMB) in a total dose of 35 mg/kg is effective (156). PDH is best treated with full courses of AMB until the patient's clinical condition has stabilized. This stabilization occurs somewhere between 500 and 1000 mg of AMB. Following stabilization, our practice has been to switch to itraconazole. This form of combination therapy was worked out carefully in HIV-infected patients with PDH and is extremely effective. Itraconazole should be continued for life in HIV-infected patients. Although its use makes excellent sense, this form of combination therapy has not been tested in HIV-negative patients with PDH. Our practice has been to treat with AMB until stable, then follow up with at least 1 year of 400 mg/day itraconazole therapy.

Resected solitary pulmonary nodules containing *Histoplasma* need no treatment.

### Blastomycosis

The endemic area of blastomycosis overlaps that of histoplasmosis but extends farther north. Besides humans, dogs are frequently victims of the disease, and veterinary practitioners are usually quite knowledgeable about blastomycosis (157). Much less is known about the epidemiology of blastomycosis than about that of histoplasmosis. It appears that the organism exists in microfoci in nature, usually in areas well watered by streams (158). Disturbance of the mycelial growth results in the formation of the infecting aerosol, following which the infecting particles are inhaled into the lung. Once in the lung, conversion to the yeast phase takes place, and propagation begins by binary fission.

The portal of entry is the lung. In the original area of pneumonitis, the initial cellular exudate is primarily polymorphonuclear (PMN). Once delayed hypersensitivity develops, macrophages move in, but the PMN component of the infiltrate never disappears completely. The organism is frequently restricted to the lungs by the establishment of cell-mediated immunity, but in some instances blood-borne dissemination may occur. The organs most commonly involved are the skin, bone, prostate, and meninges (157).

Acute pulmonary blastomycosis may be a severe, febrile illness, with cough productive of mucopurulent sputum. Frequently it is accompanied by arthralgia and myalgia. Chest roentgenogram usually reveals single or multiple areas of pneumonitis. Pleural involvement is more common than in histoplasmosis. Acute blastomycosis is frequently self limited (159) (Fig. 16.20). Progressive pulmonary disease may occur, as well as dissemination outside the confines of the lung (Fig. 16.21). Frequently, the original pulmonary infiltrate may resolve spontaneously while the extrapulmonary components of the disseminated disease progresses at the same time. Recently a number of HIV-infected patients with blastomycosis have been described. The illness is usually rapidly progressive and is frequently widely disseminated, including frequent involvement of the meninges (160).

Visualization of the organism, either on histopathologic sections or in sputum, as well as culture of the organism, is the only means of diagnosing blastomycosis reliably. The simplest and most effective diagnostic

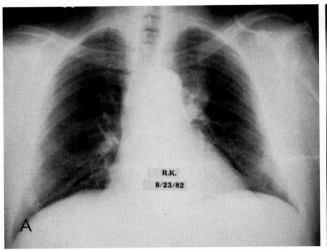
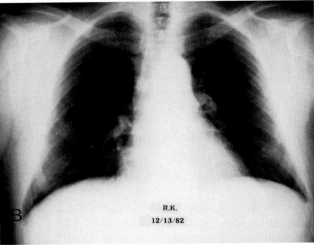

**Figure 16.20.** **A**, Active self-limited blastomycosis with left upper lobe infiltrate. Sputum digestion with 10% potassium hydroxide was positive for *B. dermatitidis*. **B**, Four months later, the infiltrate had diminished in size. Sputum examination no longer showed the fungus.

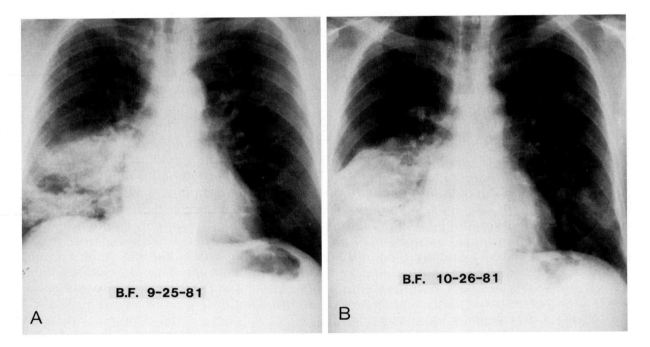

**Figure 16.21.** **A**, Extensive right lower lobe pneumonia due to *B. dermatitidis*. **B**, One month later, cultures are reported growing the fungus. Note worsening right lower lobe consolidation and spread of the infection to the left.

test is the examination of sputum (or aspirated pus) after digestion with 10% potassium hydroxide (KOH) (161). Under reduced light the characteristic large, double-refractile, thick-walled yeasts are readily identifiable. The daughter cell is attached by a broad neck. On histopathologic sections the organism is readily seen either by the periodic acid–Schiff (PAS) stain or by one of the silver stains. Culture identification is not difficult but may take time. A small inoculum usually takes up to 30 days before positive identification is possible. There is no commercially available skin test.

The serodiagnosis of blastomycosis is not well developed. Of the currently available serologic tests, complement fixation (CF) and immunodiffusion (ID) are more specific but far less sensitive; the recently introduced enzyme immunoassay (EIA) is far more sensitive but much less specific (162). At the present time a positive serodiagnostic test for blastomycosis does not establish the diagnosis of the disease. Nevertheless, a positive serologic test should serve as a strong indicator that the disease may be present.

In most instances, acute pulmonary blastomycosis resolves spontaneously (163). In rapidly progressive disease or in patients coinfected with HIV, especially when air exchange problems develop, AMB to a total of 2 g is the agent of choice (157). Similarly, meningeal involvement requires prompt intravenous AMB treatment. In more chronic or subacute forms of the illness, both pulmonary and disseminated, ketoconazole in a dose of 400 mg daily has proved to be an excellent drug (164, 165). Itraconazole is highly effective and is far less difficult to administer than ketoconazole (155).

## Coccidioidomycosis

The endemic area in the United States for coccidioidomycosis includes the southwestern states of Texas, New Mexico, Arizona, Nevada, and California. In addition, the disease is also found in Central and South America. The organism usually resides several inches below the surface, and following the brief rainy season, rapid growth occurs. Disruption of these microfoci results in the production of the infecting aerosol (166). Since much of the endemic area is dry, dusty desert, windborne outbreaks of coccidioidomycosis have been noted.

Although primary cutaneous inoculations may occur, the usual portal of entry for most patients is the lung. Following inhalation of the arthrospores, germination occurs in the alveoli, leading to the production of giant spherules. Following maturity of the giant spherule, it bursts and releases a large number of endospores that in turn lead to the formation of new giant spherules. Histopathologically, the inflammatory exudate involves PMNs as well as macrophages, and the PMN component seldom disappears completely even

after the development of cell-mediated immunity (166).

Following the successful development of cell-mediated immunity, the infection is contained. In certain high-risk groups this localization is not successful, leading to either progressive pulmonary or extrapulmonary disease. Diabetics, immunosuppressed individuals, members of the dark-skinned races, blacks especially, and men in general localize the disease poorly, and these "high-risk" groups provide most patients in whom progressive extrapulmonary spread occurs.

The primary infection is very similar to that seen in other soil-dwelling fungal infections. It usually is an influenza-like illness with a dry cough. Pleuritic chest pain is often severe. Arthralgias and myalgias are common. Erythema nodosum is a frequent accompaniment to these symptoms, leading to the characteristic "Valley fever" or "desert rheumatism." Chest roentgenogram may show single or multiple densities with involvement of the hilar nodes.

Resolution of the primary symptoms with clearing of the chest roentgenogram is the most common fate of acute infection. Occasionally, especially in members of the high-risk group, resolution is slow or incomplete, and progressive pulmonary or extrapulmonary illness may develop. Extrapulmonary spread involves the skin, bones, and visceral organs. In about one-third of these patients, the meninges are also involved. Dissemination, when it occurs, is usually a relatively early event. It is uncommon to see stable disease that leads to dissemination after 1 year. Coccidioidomycosis occurring in HIV-positive individuals produces a severe, relentlessly progressive disease with widespread dissemination (167, 168).

In an occasional patient, the pulmonary lesions may persist. The characteristic lesion is a thin-walled cavity (Fig. 16.22). Under observation, the vast majority of these cavities will close. Occasionally, however, the cavities grow and may reach the pleural surface where they may rupture, leading to a bronchopleural fistula (169). Rarely, progressive pulmonary coccidioidomycosis involves the upper zones, mimicking tuberculosis (170).

Although cultural identification is not difficult, extreme care must be taken when working with biologic material suspected of harboring *C. immitis*. In most laboratories, cultural identification no longer takes place, but cultures are processed for the presence of the characteristic exoantigen. In any event, clinicians suspecting coccidioidomycosis should alert the laboratory, to prevent laboratory-borne infections.

Although excellent skin test antigens exist, skin tests are seldom used to establish the diagnosis of coccidioi-

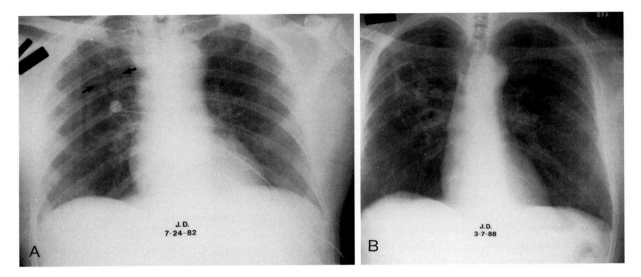

**FIGURE 16.22.**    **A**, Residual thin-walled cavity in right upper lobe (*arrows*). Sputum is positive for *C. immitis*. **B**, After almost 6 years and several courses of therapy with both amphotericin B and ketoconazole, the cavity still persists, and sputum is still intermittently positive for the organism. This patient declined surgery.

domycosis. In disseminated disease the skin test is frequently negative, while in endemic areas a positive skin test could easily have been acquired prior to the onset of the clinical illness in question.

Unlike the other fungal illnesses, serodiagnostic tests are not only diagnostic but frequently produce excellent prognostic information (171). Early on, determination of IgM antibodies, either by the tube precipitation or by the latex agglutination method, is extremely helpful. CF antibodies are readily measured, and a rising titer frequently signifies impending dissemination. The CF test is extremely useful in suspected meningitis, and any CF activity in cerebrospinal fluid (CSF) should be considered proof of disease (169).

Most recently, the more easily performed immunodiffusion test has replaced the time-honored but cumbersome tests for IgM and IgG antibody. Our practice is to screen patients with the immunodiffusion test and then follow up the positive test by CF testing performed at a reference laboratory for prognostic purposes.

Regrettably, coccidioidal infections are much more difficult to deal with than either histoplasmosis or blastomycosis. Some authorities recommend treating stable pulmonary disease in members of the high-risk group. It is thought that a brief course of 0.5 to 1.5 g of AMB might prevent subsequent dissemination. Even though this is common clinical practice, proof of efficacy is lacking. Disseminated disease, not involving the meninges, can usually be treated with large doses of AMB intravenously (169). Treatment courses of up to 3.5 g are not uncommon. Since AMB is far less effective in the treatment of coccidioidomycosis than it is in either histoplasmosis or blastomycosis, alternative treatments are needed. Ketoconazole, although originally thought to be effective, produces lasting benefit in less than a third of the patients (172). The recently introduced oral triazole Fluconazole appears to be a significant improvement over ketoconazole, both in reported lower toxicity and increased efficacy (173).

The treatment of coccidioidomycosis in HIV-infected patients has been difficult and generally not successful. Most patients are treated initially with AMB, until stabilization occurs. Fluconazole has been used successfully in several patients, especially those who are not critically ill initially, and it is especially helpful in meningeal coccidioidomycosis (174).

Coccidioidal meningitis requires both intravenous and intrathecal administration of AMB. Most authorities recommend long-term intrathecal therapy, even after all apparent disease activity has ceased in the central nervous system. Fluconazole is highly effective in the treatment of meningeal coccidioidomycosis and is now the treatment of choice for stable patients (174). In the event that surgery is attempted for an enlarging coccidioidal granuloma, some surgeons prefer to perform the surgery with pre- and postoperative administration of AMB. Although this is common practice, proof of efficacy is lacking.

### Paracoccidioidomycosis

*Paracoccidioides brasiliensis* is the most common dimorphic fungus in Latin America. The endemic area stretches from Mexico to Argentina. Occupational exposure to the soil is common, and males are most commonly affected. Interestingly, point source epidemics have not been reported, perhaps because of the rudimentary health care system in the endemic area.

As with all the other dimorphic fungi, the lung is probably the portal of entry. Inhalation of the infecting particles leads to the production of an area of pneumonitis, with granuloma formation occurring later. The organism may remain localized to the lung or may disseminate to the skin, mucous membranes, or organs with RE cells (175). Commonly, disseminated paracoccidioidomycosis occurs in younger patients in whom the major manifestations of the disease involve the RE system, leading to hepatosplenomegaly and hilar adenopathy. This form of the disease is referred to as the juvenile type. The adult form may present many years after the primary infection. Chronic pulmonary manifestations may still be present, and symptoms are those of low-grade chronic illness. Characteristic lesions involve the oropharynx, lips, and gums and frequently involve the skin, leading to ulcerations. Draining lymph nodes are frequent, and adrenal involvement may occur in up to half of the patients.

Recovery of the organism from culture or visualization in KOH-digested specimens is relatively easy. The characteristic "pilot wheel" appearance of the yeast is diagnostic in sputum or pus.

Ketoconazole in 200-mg doses is currently one of the drugs of choice (176). In cases that are difficult to treat, AMB or sulfadiazine may be used. Itraconazole is also highly effective at doses of 100 mg daily for 6 months (177).

## Sporotrichosis

By far the most common form of sporotrichosis is lymphocutaneous disease. Pulmonary involvement is rare, with perhaps less than 50 cases reported in the literature. The disease appears as a chronic pulmonary infection, indistinguishable by symptoms or by roentgen appearance from tuberculosis.

Diagnosis is usually by recovery of the fungus from sputum, although a serologic test is also available.

Although many authors recommend AMB as the initial treatment, it is far from certain that it is as effective as in the other fungal illnesses (178, 179). The other treatment modality is oral administration of saturated solution of potassium iodide. There have been numerous patients reported in whom drug therapy failed but resection of the involved tissues proved to be curative. The recently introduced oral agent itraconazole has shown considerable success in treating this infection (180).

## Cryptococcosis

The encapsulated yeast *Cryptococcus neoformans* is the one truly cosmopolitan fungus. The disease has been reported from all continents, and the fungus is easily recovered from pigeon droppings. Disturbance of the dried pigeon guano produces the infecting aerosol (181).

The portal of entry is the lung. Following inhalation the yeasts begin to germinate and form large capsules. This polysaccharide capsule is antiphagocytic. Histopathologic examination of tissue confirms the antiphagocytic nature of encapsulated cryptococci: large clumps of the yeast are surrounded by essentially no inflammatory exudate. In addition to the ability of the organism to resist phagocytosis and killing by PMNs, cell-mediated immunity also figures prominently into the normal host defenses for dealing with cryptococcal infection. Long before cytotoxic chemotherapy or glucocorticoid administration produced large numbers of immunocompromised hosts, the literature was replete with instances of cryptococcal disease complicating such naturally occurring immunocompromised states as Hodgkin's disease. To emphasize further the role of T cell–mediated protection against the cryptococcus, AIDS patients have an unusually high incidence of cryptococcal disease (182, 183).

Cryptococcal pulmonary disease in normal hosts is rapidly dealt with by the development of granulomatous inflammatory response and clearing of the infiltrate. It appears that the natural history of cryptococcal pulmonary disease in normal hosts is usually complete resolution.

Occasionally, however, even in immunologically competent hosts, the organism gains access to the bloodstream and establishes itself in extrapulmonary tissues, most commonly in the meninges. There is as yet no clear understanding of the remarkable tropism of cryptococci for the central nervous system.

Cryptococcal pulmonary infection in immunocompromised patients, on the other hand, is a severe, potentially life-threatening, and almost always disseminated illness. The general rule of thumb should be that anyone who is immunocompromised will develop disseminated disease following pulmonary infection by the fungus (184).

The acute pulmonary infection is relatively uncommon. Symptoms include acute onset of fever followed by chest pain and cough. Frequently, however, patients present with cryptococcal meningitis. In these instances, the inference is that an asymptomatic pulmonary infection preceded the obvious meningeal disease. Chest radiographic findings are variable but usually consist of patchy areas of consolidation involving the lower lung fields, often bilateral. Some lesions appear as nodules with associated areas of infiltration. Pleural effusions are uncommon.

The cornerstone of diagnosis in pulmonary cryptococcosis is the recovery of the fungus from respiratory secretions. A confounding variable is the frequent presence of cryptococci in patients with other, unrelated pulmonary diseases in whom *Cryptococcus* in respiratory secretions frequently represents colonization only.

Immunodiagnosis of cryptococcal disease is highly refined. Determination of cryptococcal antigen by the latex agglutination method is highly reproducible, and when the results are corrected for the possible presence of rheumatoid factor, false positives are remarkably infrequent.

The diagnosis of cryptococcal meningitis may be established by visualization of the large encapsulated yeasts on India ink preparation. Moreover, determination of the cryptococcal antigen on all cerebrospinal fluid samples will further hasten diagnosis. Cultural recovery of the organism is also relatively simple, and the organism grows in 3 to 5 days.

It is uncertain whether occasional isolates of *Cryptococcus* from sputum in patients with chronic pulmonary disease merit treatment. Established, acute cryptococcal disease in immunocompetent hosts can be observed with relative safety once the absence of central nervous system involvement has been documented by a negative lumbar puncture. In the unlikely event that treatment is deemed necessary, AMB 0.3 mg/kg/day should be administered along with 5-fluorocytosine (5FC), 150 mg/kg/day in four divided doses, for a total of 4 weeks. Meningeal disease should also be treated with a combination of AMB and 5FC in the same doses for a minimum of 4 weeks in nonimmunocompromised patients, and 6 weeks or longer in non–HIV-infected immunocompromised individuals (185).

Since the advent of the HIV endemic, cryptococcal meningitis increased in frequency 20-fold, to become the most common fungal complication of HIV infection. It usually occurs late during the course of the HIV infection. The best form of therapy for cryptococcal meningitis in these patients is not clear (186, 187). Our practice is to initiate therapy with AMB and 5FC 100 mg/kg/day until the patient is stable, then follow the therapy with lifelong administration of fluconazole, 200 mg daily (188).

## OPPORTUNISTIC FUNGAL INFECTIONS

The preceding subsections describe the normally pathogenic fungi which, although frequently infecting immunocompromised individuals, are also capable of infecting immunologically normal hosts. The following subsections deal with infections due to opportunistic fungi: *Aspergillus* species, *Mucorales*, and *Pseudallescheria boydii*.

### Aspergillosis

Members of the genus *Aspergillus* are widespread in nature. They are readily recoverable from decomposing organic matter, and the fungi are capable of withstanding extreme environmental conditions. Although well over 100 species of this genus have been identified in human illness, the vast majority of human illness is caused by *Aspergillus fumigatus*. Other *Aspergillus* species that occasionally cause human disease are *Aspergillus niger*, *Aspergillus terreus*, *Aspergillus flavus*, and *Aspergillus nidulans*. It is thought that initiation of the illness follows inhalation of spores from the fruiting head into the lungs.

*Aspergillus* causes a vast array of human illness, and thus a unitary hypothesis for its pathogenesis is difficult, if not impossible. A form of aspergillosis usually seen in asthmatics, allergic bronchopulmonary aspergillosis, is discussed in Chapter 10.

Aspergillomas, or fungus balls, occur in air spaces in the lungs. These air spaces may be the residua of healed tuberculosis, other fungal diseases, sarcoidosis, or tumor. The fungi grow within these epithelialized cavities as a mycelial mat, deriving their nourishment from the wall of the cavity. The most frequent symptom is hemoptysis, with occasional life-threatening result (189).

The other major form of aspergillosis involves granulocytopenic hosts. This illness is most frequently seen in patients with hematologic malignancies and leukemias who are undergoing intense, cytotoxic chemotherapy.

It appears that in these individuals the organism gains access to the lungs where, following multiplication in the alveolar spaces, the fungus invades blood vessels. The hallmark of this disease is the appearance of rapidly progressive, large pulmonary infiltrates accompanied by high fever and pleuritic chest pain. Frequently, a great deal of confusion exists because of the appearance of these infiltrates, closely mimicking pulmonary emboli with infarction. Indeed, histopathologically these lesions are pulmonary infarctions secondary to the growth of the organism within vascular channels. In the vast majority of the patients, invasive aspergillosis restricted to the lungs alone is capable of killing the host. Occasionally, however, apparent blood-borne dissemination takes place with dissemination of the organism. The most common sites of dissemination include the brain, the myocardium, and the thyroid gland (190).

Recent reports have described an admixture of the fungus ball and invasive aspergillosis. Most affected patients, in addition to underlying chronic lung disease, had mild immunosuppression, resulting from either diabetes or the administration of chronic glucocorticoid therapy. The disease appears as a chronic, low-grade infection in which most of the symptoms are those of the underlying lung disease. Radiographically there is an aspergilloma with a slowly progressive infiltrate surrounding it. Treatment with AMB appears to slow down the progression of the illness, but it is not yet certain whether the process can be arrested or cured (191). Itraconazole also appears to be effective (192).

Diagnosis of aspergillomas is relatively easy. The chest roentgenogram is characteristic, showing a round, freely movable density within a previously existing cavity. Sputum culture is frequently positive for the fungus, and serologic diagnosis is very helpful since the vast majority of patients with aspergillomas have positive serum precipitins against *Aspergillus*. One must remember, however, that precipitins are species specific, which accounts for the occasionally negative precipitin tests observed in patients with an obvious aspergilloma.

Disseminated aspergillosis or acute invasive aspergillosis is usually a difficult diagnosis. Although the disease is frequently suspected on clinical grounds alone, attempts to recover the organism from respiratory secretions or bronchoscopic material frequently fail. Occasionally, however, positive cultures can be obtained from respiratory secretions. Although these positive cultures do not definitely establish the etiology of the infection, they frequently serve to point one in the right direction.

Although aspergillosis was originally listed among the agents causing opportunistic infections complicating HIV infection, this fungus was removed soon after because of the paucity of reported patients. Recently, however, an increasing number of patients have been reported with various forms of aspergillosis complicating the late course of HIV infection. While most reported patients had the usual predisposing conditions to aspergillosis, such as drug-induced neutropenia or glucocorticoid administration, a sizable number of patients did not (193, 194). All previously reported forms of aspergillosis have been seen in HIV-infected individuals, and two new forms have been added. These new forms are obstructing endobronchial aspergillosis and pseudomembranous aspergillosis.

Most authorities consider the diagnosis of aspergillosis definite only when the organism is seen invading host tissues. This usually requires either bronchoscopic biopsy or open lung biopsy. Blood cultures are usually sterile.

Clinical and roentgenographic features of the infection are relatively nondiagnostic. The roentgenogram may show single or multiple areas of rapidly advancing pulmonary infiltrates, which do not cavitate until the granulocyte count begins to return toward normal.

Drug therapy is not indicated for the treatment of aspergillomas, since it universally fails. In patients with life-threatening hemoptysis, surgery is the only reasonable choice of therapy. Unfortunately, the majority of such patients have severely compromised pulmonary function, rendering surgery difficult if not impossible (189).

Treatment of acute invasive aspergillosis is frequently futile. AMB is the drug of choice, and the recommendation is that early and large doses of the agent be used. Our practice has been to aim at a minimum of 1 mg/kg/day for the acute phase of the illness and, after stabilization, to reduce the dose or switch to an alternate-day dosage regimen. Recently, especially in institutions dealing with large numbers of patients with hematologic malignancies, the custom has been to begin AMB treatment after 3 to 7 days of a febrile course not responding to routine antibiotic treatment (195). Although definite proof of the success of this regimen is still lacking, it appears to have significantly reduced the incidence of invasive aspergillosis at postmortem examination.

The recently introduced triazole, itraconazole, has been used in some patients with different forms of aspergillosis with good results. While it is uncertain whether rapidly progressive invasive disease is likely to improve, it appears that the more chronic indulin forms of aspergillosis infections can be treated with itraconazole and can be expected to respond (192).

## Mucormycosis

Members of the genus *Mucorales*, like *Aspergillus*, are widespread in nature. Although much less is known and understood about mucormycosis than of aspergillosis, it appears to be quite similar to aspergillosis. The organism has a high affinity for invasion of blood vessels and will frequently produce extensive tissue necrosis because of occlusion of blood vessels.

Clinical manifestations are very similar to those of aspergillosis, as is the chest roentgenogram, which usually shows multiple, large pulmonary infiltrates extending to the pleura, mimicking pulmonary embolization with infarction. The diagnosis requires identifying the invading broad, nonseptate fungus either in histopathologic material or by culture. There are no immunologic tests available. Blood culture and sputum culture are seldom, if ever, positive.

Treatment of mucormycosis is similar to that of aspergillosis and requires large doses of AMB. Early starting of the treatment is essential, and the best results have been in patients in whom treatment was started very early in the course of the illness.

## Pseudallescheriasis

The organism *Pseudallescheria boydii* is an occasionally identified saprophyte. Clinically and histopathologically the illness is indistinguishable from invasive aspergillosis. Cultural identification is extremely important because it appears that miconazole, rather than AMB, is the drug of choice in this illness.

▼

## References

1. Couch RB: The common cold: control? *J Infect Dis* 150: 167–173, 1984.
2. Dixon RE: Economic costs of respiratory tract infections in the United States. *Am J Med* 78(Suppl 6B):45–51, 1985.
3. Gross PA, Van Antwerpen C: Nosocomial infections and hospital deaths: a case-control study. *Am J Med* 75: 658–662, 1983.
4. Garibaldi RA: Epidemiology of community-acquired respiratory tract infections in adults: incidence, etiology, and impact. *Am J Med* 78(Suppl 6B):32–37, 1985.
5. *Lung Disease Data 1994.* New York, American Lung Association, 1994, pp 37–42.
6. Schneider EL: Infectious diseases in the elderly. *Ann Intern Med* 98:395–400, 1983.
7. Gleckman RA, Roth RM: Community-acquired bacterial pneumonia in the elderly. *Pharmacotherapy* 4:81–88, 1984.
8. Niederman MS: Nosocomial pneumonia in the elderly patient: chronic care facility and hospital considerations. *Clin Chest Med* 14:479–490, 1993.
9. Gross PA, Van Antwerpen C: Nosocomial infections and hospital deaths: a case-control study. *Am J Med* 75: 658–662, 1983.
10. Emori TG, Banerjee SN, Culver DH, et al: Nosocomial infections in elderly patients in the United States, 1986–1990. *Am J Med* 91(3):289S–293S, 1991.
11. Ashbaugh DG, Petty TL: Sepsis complicating the acute respiratory distress syndrome. *Surg Gynecol Obstet* 135: 865–869, 1972.
12. Seidenfeld JJ, Pohl DF, Bell RD, et al: Incidence, site, and outcome of infections in patients with the adult respiratory distress syndrome. *Am Rev Respir Dis* 134: 12–16, 1986.
13. Fagon JY, Chastre J, Hance A, et al: Nosocomial pneumonia in ventilated patients: a cohort study evaluating attributable mortality and hospital stay. *Am J Med* 94: 281–288, 1993.
14. Kronenberg RS: Chronic bronchitis: significant infection or social annoyance? *Semin Respir Infect* 3:1–4, 1988.
15. Niederman MS: Evaluating the difficult management issues in chronic bronchitis. *Contemp Intern Med* 5 (11): 8–16, 1993.

16. Ruben FL: Prophylactic treatment of chronic bronchitis. *Semin Respir Infect* 3:72–80, 1988.
17. Penn RL, George RB: Respiratory infections. In Matthay RA, Light RM, George RB (eds): *Chest Medicine*, ed 1. New York, Churchill Livingstone, 1983, pp 403–479.
18. American Thoracic Society: Contol of tuberculosis in the United States. *Am Rev Respir Dis* 146:1623–1633, 1992.
19. Barker AF, Bardana EJ: Bronchiectasis: update of an orphan disease. *Am Rev Respir Dis* 137:969–978, 1988.
20. Farr BM, Kaiser DL, Harrison BDW, Connolly CK: Prediction of microbial aetiology at admission to hospital for pneumonia from presenting clinical features. *Thorax* 44:1031–1035, 1989.
21. Niederman MS: Gram-negative colonization of the respiratory tract: pathogenesis and clinical consequences. *Semin Respir Infect* 5:173–184, 1990.
22. Johanson WG, Pierce AK, Sanford JP: Changing pharyngeal flora of hospitalized patients: emergence of Gram-negative bacilli. *N Engl J Med* 281:1137–1140, 1969.
23. Palmer LB: Bacterial colonization: pathogenesis and clinical significance. *Clin Chest Med* 8:455–466, 1987.
24. Laurenzi GA, Potter RT, Kass EH: Bacteriologic flora of the lower respiratory tract. *N Engl J Med* 265:1273–1278, 1961.
25. Pingleton SK, Hinthorn DR, Liu C: Enteral nutrition in patients receiving mechanical ventilation: multiple sources of tracheal colonization include the stomach. *Am J Med* 80:827–832, 1986.
26. Niederman MS, Mantovani R, Schoch P, et al: Patterns and routes of tracheobronchial colonization in mechanically ventilated patients: the role of nutritional status in colonization of the lower airway by *Pseudomonas* species. *Chest* 95:155–161, 1989.
27. Rabinowitz HK: Upper respiratory tract infections. *Prim Care* 17:793–809, 1990.
28. Gwaltney JM: The common cold: epidemiology and strategies for prevention. In Sande MA, Hudson LD, Root RK (eds): *Respiratory Infections*. New York, Churchill Livingstone, 1986, pp 139–147.
29. Blake GH, Abell TD, Stanley WG: Cigarette smoking and upper respiratory infection among recruits in basic combat training. *Ann Intern Med* 109:198–202, 1988.
30. Dick EC, Jennings LC, Mink KA: Aerosol transmission of colds. *J Infect Dis* 156:442–448, 1987.
31. Douglas RM, Moore BW, Miles HB, et al: Prophylactic efficacy of intranasal alpha 2-interferon against rhinovirus infections in the family setting. *N Engl J Med* 314: 65–70, 1986.
32. Evans FO, Syndor JB, Moore WEC, et al: Sinusitis of the maxillary antrum. *N Engl J Med* 293:735–739, 1975.
33. Williams JW, Simel DL: Does this patient have sinusitis? Diagnosing acute sinusitis by history and physical examination. *JAMA* 270:1242–1246, 1993.
34. MayoSmith MF, Hirsch PJ, Wodzinski SF, et al: Acute epiglottitis in adults: an eight-year experience in the state of Rhode Island. *N Engl J Med* 314:1133–1139, 1986.
35. Baker AS, Eavey RD: Adult supraglottitis (epiglottitis). *N Engl J Med* 314:1185–1186, 1986.
36. Loos GD: Pharyngitis, croup and epiglottitis. *Prim Care* 17:335–345, 1990.
37. Takala AK, Eskola J, van Alphen L: Spectrum of invasive *Haemophilus influenzae* type b disease in adults. *Arch Intern Med* 150:2573–2576, 1990.

38. Ashcraft CK, Steele RW: Epiglottitis: a pediatric emergency. *J Respir Dis* 9(7):48–60, 1988.

39. Wolf M, Strauss B, Kronenberg J, Leventon G: Conservative management of adult epiglottitis. *Laryngoscope* 100:183–185, 1990.

40. Rothrock SG, Pignatiello GA, Howard RA: Radiologic diagnosis of epiglottitis: Objective criteria for all ages. *Ann Emerg Med* 19:978–982, 1990.

41. Hall CB, McBride JT: Upper respiratory tract infections: the common cold, pharyngitis, croup, bacterial tracheitis and epiglottitis. In Pennington JE (ed): *Respiratory Infections: Diagnosis and Management*. New York, Raven Press, 1988, pp 97–118.

42. Centor RM, Meier FA: Throat cultures and rapid tests for diagnosis of group A streptococcal pharyngitis. *Ann Intern Med* 105:892–899, 1986.

43. Wallace RJ Jr: Newer oral antimicrobials and newer etiologic agents of acute bronchitis and acute exacerbations of chronic bronchitis. *Semin Respir Infect* 3:49–54, 1988.

44. Schroeckenstein DC, Busse WW: Viral bronchitis in childhood: relationship to asthma and obstructive lung disease. *Semin Respir Infect* 3:40–48, 1988.

45. Anthonisen NR, Manfreda J, Warren CPW, et al: Antibiotic therapy in exacerbations of chronic obstructive pulmonary disease. *Ann Intern Med* 106:196–204, 1987.

46. Fagon JY, Chastre J, Trouillet JL, et al: Characterization of distal bronchial microflora during acute exacerbation of chronic bronchitis: use of the protected specimen brush technique in 54 mechanically ventilated patients. *Am Rev Respir Dis* 142:1004–1008, 1990.

47. Karnad A, Alvarez S, Berk SL: *Branhamella catarrhalis* pneumonia in patients with immunoglobulin abnormalities. *South Med J* 79:1360–1362, 1986.

48. Murphy TF, Sethi S: Bacterial infection in chronic obstructive pulmonary disease. *Am Rev Respir Dis* 146:1067–1083, 1992.

49. Nicotra MB, Rivera M: Chronic bronchitis: when and how to treat. *Semin Respir Infect* 3:61–71, 1988.

50. Niederman MS, Ferranti RD, Ziegler A, et al: Respiratory infection complicating long-term tracheostomy: the implication of persistent Gram-negative tracheobronchial colonization. *Chest* 85:39–44, 1984.

51. King TE Jr: Overview of bronchiolitis. *Clin Chest Med* 14:607–610, 1993.

52. Epler GR, Colby TV, McLoud TC, et al: Bronchiolitis obliterans organizing pneumonia . *N Engl J Med* 312:152–158, 1985.

53. Nicholson KG: Clinical features of influenza. *Semin Respir Infect* 7:26–37, 1992.

54. Mathur U, Bentley DW, Hall CB: Concurrent respiratory syncytial virus and influenza A infections in the institutionalized elderly and chronically ill. *Ann Intern Med* 93:49–52, 1980.

55. Gross PA, Rodstein M LaMontagne JR, et al: Epidemiology of acute respiratory illness during an influenza outbreak in a nursing home: a prospective study. *Arch Intern Med* 148:559–561, 1988.

56. Hayden FG, Gwaltney JM: Viral infections. In Murray JF, Nadel JA (eds): *Textbook of Respiratory Medicine*. Philadelphia, WB Saunders, 1988, pp 769–778.

57. Van Voris LP, Newell PM: Antivirals for the chemoprophylaxis and treatment of influenza. *Semin Respir Infect* 7:61–70, 1992.

58. Stockley RA: Bronchiectasis—new therapeutic approaches based on pathogenesis. *Clin Chest Med* 8:481–494, 1987.

59. Huxley EJ, Viroslav J, Gray WR, et al: Pharyngeal aspiration in normal subjects and patients with depressed consciousness. *Am J Med* 64:565–568, 1978.

60. Beachey EH: Bacterial adherence: adhesin-receptor interactions mediating the attachment of bacteria to mucosal surfaces. *J Infect Dis* 143:325–345, 1981.

61. Niederman MS, Merrill WW, Ferranti RD, et al: Nutritional status and bacterial binding in the lower respiratory tract in patients with chronic tracheostomy. *Ann Intern Med* 100:795–800, 1984.

62. Todd TRJ, Franklin A, Mankinen-Irvin P, et al: Augmented bacterial adherence to tracheal epithelial cells is associated with Gram-negative pneumonia in an intensive care unit population. *Am Rev Respir Dis* 140:1585–1589, 1989.

63. Johanson WG Jr, Pierce AK, Sanford JP, et al: Nosocomial respiratory infections with Gram-negative bacilli: the significance of colonization of the respiratory tract. *Ann Intern Med* 77:701–706, 1972.

64. Toews GB: Nosocomial pneumonia. *Clin Chest Med* 8:467–479, 1987.

65. Fein AM, Feinsilver SH, Niederman MS: Atypical manifestations of pneumonia in the elderly. *Clin Chest Med* 12:319–336, 1991.

66. Niederman MS, Bass JB, Campbell GD, et al: Guidelines for the initial management of adults with community-acquired pneumonia: diagnosis, assessment of severity, and initial antimicrobial therapy. *Am Rev Respir Dis* 148:1418–1426, 1993.

67. Wollschlager CM, Khan FA, Khan A: Utility of radiography and clinical features in the diagnosis of community-acquired pneumonia. *Clin Chest Med* 8:393–404, 1987.

68. MacFarlane JT, Miller AC, Smith WH, et al: Comparative radiographic features of community-acquired Legionnaires' disease, pneumococcal pneumonia, mycoplasma pneumonia, and psittacosis. *Thorax* 39:28–33, 1984.

69. Torres A, Serra-Batlles J, Ferrer A, et al: Severe community-acquired pneumonia. Epidemiology and prognostic factors. *Am Rev Respir Dis* 144:312–318, 1991.

70. Farr BM, Sloman AJ, Fisch MJ: Predicting death in patients hospitalized for community-acquired pneumonia. *Ann Intern Med* 115:428–436, 1991.

71. Pachon J, Prados MD, Capote F, Cuello JA, Garnacho J, Verano A: Severe community-acquired pneumonia. Etiology, prognosis, and treatment. *Am Rev Respir Dis* 142:369–373, 1990.

72. Mufson MA: Pneumococcal infections. *JAMA* 246:1942–1948, 1981.

73. Johnson CC, Finegold SM: Pyogenic bacterial pneumonia, lung abscess, and empyema. In Murray JF, Nadel JA (eds): *Textbook of Respiratory Medicine*. Philadelphia, WB Saunders, 1988, pp 803–841.

74. Ort S, Ryan JL, Barden G, et al: Pneumococcal pneumonia in hospitalized patients: clinical and radiological presentations. *JAMA* 249:214–218, 1983.

75. Jay SJ, Johanson WG, Pierce AK: The radiographic resolution of *Streptococcus pneumoniae* pneumonia. *N Engl J Med* 293:798–801, 1975.

76. Austrian R: A reassessment of pneumococcal vaccine. *N Engl J Med* 310:651–653, 1984.

77. Niederman MS: Strategies for the prevention of pneumonia. *Clin Chest Med* 8:543–556, 1987.

78. LaForce FM, Eickhoff TC: Pneumococcal vaccine: an emerging consensus. *Ann Intern Med* 108:757–759, 1988.

79. Brenner DJ: Classification of the legionellae. *Semin Respir Infect* 4:190–205, 1987.

80. Davis GS, Winn WC: Legionnaires' disease: respiratory infections caused by *Legionella* bacteria. *Clin Chest Med* 8:419–439, 1987.

81. Yu VL, Kroboth FJ, Shonnard J: Legionnaires' disease: new clinical perspective from a prospective pneumonia study. *Am J Med* 73:357–361, 1982.

82. Carratala J, Gudiol F, Pallares R, Dorca J, Verdaguer R, Ariza J, et al: Risk factors for nosocomial *Legionella pneumophila* pneumonia. *Am J Respir Crit Care Med* 149:625–629, 1994.

83. Muder RR, Yu VL: Legionella. In Niederman MS, Sarosi GA, Glassroth J (eds): *Respiratory Infections: A Scientific Basis For Management*, ed 1. Philadelphia, WB Saunders, 1994, pp 319–330.

84. Bartlett JG, Gorbach SL: The triple threat of aspiration pneumonia. *Chest* 68:560–566, 1975.

85. Wynne JW, Modell JH: Respiratory aspiration of stomach contents. *Ann Intern Med* 87:466–474, 1977.

86. Mier L, Dreyfuss D, Darchy B, Lanore JJ, Djedaini K, Weber P, et al: Is penicillin G an adequate initial treatment for aspiration pneumonia? A prospective evaluation using a protected specimen brush and quantitative cultures. *Intensive Care Med* 19:279–284, 1993.

87. Bartlett JG, Finegold SM: Anaerobic infections of the lung and pleural space. *Am Rev Respir Dis* 110:56–77, 1974.

88. Levison ME, Mangura CT, Lorber B, et al: Clindamycin compared with penicillin for the treatment of anaerobic lung abscess. *Ann Intern Med* 98:466–471, 1983.

89. Musher DM, Kubitschek KR, Crennan J, et al: Pneumonia and acute febrile tracheobronchitis due to *Haemophilus influenzae*. *Ann Intern Med* 99:444–450, 1983.

90. Smith AL: *Haemophilus influenzae* pneumonia. In Pennington JE (ed): *Respiratory Infections: Diagnosis and Management*. New York, Raven Press, 1988, pp 364–380.

91. Cassell GH, Cole BC: Mycoplasmas as agents of human disease. *N Engl J Med* 304:80–89, 1981.

92. Tuazon CU, Murray HW: Atypical pneumonias. In Pennington JE (ed): *Respiratory Infections: Diagnosis and Management*. New York, Raven Press, 1988, pp 341–363.

93. Cotton EM, Strampfer MJ, Cunha BA: *Legionella* and mycoplasma pneumonia—a community hospital experience with atypical pneumonias. *Clin Chest Med* 8:441–453, 1987.

94. Grayston JT, Kuo CC, Wang SP, et al: A new *Chlamydia psittaci* strain, TWAR, isolated in acute respiratory tract infections. *N Engl J Med* 315:161–168, 1986.

95. Marrie TJ, Grayston JT, Wang SP, et al: Pneumonia associated with the TWAR strain of *Chlamydia*. *Ann Intern Med* 106:507–511, 1987.

96. Pierce AK, Sanford JP: Aerobic Gram-negative bacillary pneumonias. *Am Rev Respir Dis* 110:647–658, 1974.

97. Meyer KS, Urban C, Eagan JA, Berger BJ, Rahal JJ: Nosocomial outbreak of *Klebsiella* infection resistant to late-generation cephalosporins. *Ann Intern Med* 119:353–358, 1993.

98. Kaye MG, Fox MJ, Bartlett JG, Braman SS, Glassroth J: The clinical spectrum of *Staphylococcus aureus* pulmonary infection. *Chest* 97:788–792, 1990.

99. Rose RM, Pinkston P, O'Donnell C, et al: Viral infections of the lower respiratory tract. *Clin Chest Med* 8:405–418, 1987.

100. Sullivan CJ, Jordan MC: Diagnosis of viral pneumonia. *Semin Respir Infect* 3:148–161, 1988.

101. Britt MR, Schleupner CJ, Matsumiya S: Severity of underlying disease as a predictor of nosocomial infection. *JAMA* 239:1047–1051, 1978.

102. Niederman MS, Fein AM: Sepsis syndrome, the adult respiratory distress syndrome, and nosocomial pneumonia: a common clinical sequence. *Clin Chest Med* 11:633–656, 1990.

103. Mandell LA, Marrie TJ, Niederman MS: Initial antimicrobial treatment of hospital acquired pneumonia in adults: a conference report. *Can J Infect Dis* 4:317–321, 1993.

104. Niederman MS: An approach to empiric therapy of nosocomial pneumonia. *Med Clin North Am*, 1994, in press.

105. Andrews CP, Coalson JJ, Johanson WG Jr: Diagnosis of nosocomial bacterial pneumonia in acute diffuse lung injury. *Chest* 80:254–258, 1981.

106. Niederman MS, Torres A, Summer W: Invasive diagnostic testing is not needed routinely to manage suspected VAP. *Am J Respir Crit Care Med*, 1994, in press.

107. Rodrigues J, Niederman MS, Fein AM, Pai PB: Nonresolving pneumonia in steroid-treated patients with obstructive lung disease. *Am J Med* 93:29–34, 1992.

108. Stevens RM, Teres D, Skillman JJ, et al: Pneumonia in an intensive care unit: a 30-month experience. *Arch Intern Med* 134:106–111, 1974.

109. Rosenow EC, Wilson WR, Cockerill FR: Pulmonary disease in the immunocompromised host. *Mayo Clin Proc* 60:473–487, 1985.

110. Rankin JA, Collman R, Daniele RP: Acquired immune deficiency syndrome and the lung. *Chest* 94:155–164, 1988.

111. Gallant JE, Chaisson RE: Respiratory infections in persons infected with human immunodeficiency virus. In Niederman MS, Sarosi GA, Glassroth J (eds): *Respiratory Infections: A Scientific Basis For Management*, ed 1, Philadelphia, WB Saunders, 1994, pp 199–215.

112. Hibberd PL, Rubin RH: Renal transplantation and related infections. *Semin Respir Infect* 8:216–224, 1993.

113. Levine SJ, White DA: *Pneumocystis carinii*. *Clin Chest Med* 9:395–423, 1988.

114. Conte JE, Hollander H, Golden JA: Inhaled or reduced-dose intravenous pentamidine for *Pneumocystis carinii* pneumonia: a pilot study. *Ann Intern Med* 107:495–498, 1987.

115. Allegra CJ, Chabner BA, Tuazon CU, et al: Trimetrexate for the treatment of *Pneumocystis carinii* pneumonia in patients with the acquired immunodeficiency syndrome. *N Engl J Med* 317:978–985, 1987.

116. McFadden JP, Price RC, Eastwood HD, et al: Raised respiratory rate in elderly patients: a valuable physical sign. *Br Med J* 1:626–627, 1982.

117. Fein AM, Feinsilver SH, Niederman MS, et al: When pneumonia doesn't get better. *Clin Chest Med* 8:529–541, 1987.

118. Tobin MJ: Diagnosis of pneumonia: techniques and problems. *Clin Chest Med* 8:513–527, 1987.

119. Stover DE, Zaman MB, Hajdu SI, et al: Bronchoalveolar

lavage in the diagnosis of diffuse pulmonary infiltrates in the immunosuppressed host. *Ann Intern Med* 101:1–7, 1984.

120. Chastre J, Fagon JY, Bornet M, et al: Diagnosis of nosocomial bacterial pneumonia in intubated patients undergoing ventilation: comparison of the usefulness of bronchoalveolar lavage and the protected specimen brush. *Am J Med* 85:499–506, 1988.

121. Graham WGB, Bradley DA: Efficacy of chest physiotherapy and intermittent positive-pressure breathing in the resolution of pneumonia. *N Engl J Med* 299:624–627, 1978.

122. Wanner A, Rao A: Clinical indications for and effects of bland, mucolytic and antimicrobial aerosols. *Am Rev Respir Dis* 122:79–87, 1980.

123. deBoisblanc BP, Castro M, Everret B, et al: Effect of air-supported, continuous, postural oscillation on the risk of early ICU pneumonia in nontraumatic critical illness. *Chest* 103:1543–1547, 1993.

124. Glassroth J: Tuberculosis. In Niederman MS, Sarosi GA, Glassroth J (eds): *Respiratory Infections: A Scientific Basis For Management*, ed 1. Philadelphia, WB Saunders, 1994, pp 449–458.

125. Hirschtick RE, Glassroth J: Multidrug-resistant tuberculosis: epidemiology, treatment, and prevention. *Clin Pulmonary Med* 1:78–83, 1994.

126. Small PM, Shafer RW, Hopewell PC, et al: Exogenous reinfection with multidrug-resistant *Mycobacterium tuberculosis* in patients with advanced HIV infection. *N Engl J Med* 328:1137–1144, 1993.

127. Bates JH: Transmission and pathogenesis of tuberculosis. *Clin Chest Med* 1:167–174, 1980.

128. Levy H, Kallenbach JM, Feldman C, et al: Acute respiratory failure in active tuberculosis. *Crit Care Med* 15:221–225, 1987.

129. Alvarez S, Shell C, Berk SL: Pulmonary tuberculosis in elderly men. *Am J Med* 82:602–606, 1987.

130. American Thoracic Society: Treatment of tuberculosis and tuberculosis infection in adults and children. *Am Rev Respir Dis* 134:355–363, 1986.

131. American Thoracic Society: Mycobacteriosis and the acquired immunodeficiency syndrome. *Am Rev Respir Dis* 136:492–496, 1987.

132. Woodring JH, Vandiviere HM, Fried AM, et al: Update: the radiographic features of pulmonary tuberculosis. *AJR* 497–506, 1986.

133. American Thoracic Society: Diagnostic standards and classification of tuberculosis. *Am Rev Respir Dis* 142:725–735, 1990.

134. Grosset J: Bacteriologic basis of short-course chemotherapy for tuberculosis. *Clin Chest Med* 1:231–241, 1980.

135. Nardell EA: Beyond four drugs: public health policy and the treatment of the individual patient with tuberculosis. *Am Rev Respir Dis* 148:2–5, 1993.

136. Woods GL, Washington JA: Mycobacteria other than *Mycobacterium tuberculosis*: review of microbiologic and clinical aspects. *Rev Infect Dis* 9:275–294, 1987.

137. Tellis CJ, Bombenger: Pulmonary disease caused by nontuberculous mycobacteria. In Pennington JE (ed): *Respiratory Infections: Diagnosis and Management*. New York, Raven Press, 1988, pp 544–569.

138. American Thoracic Society: Diagnosis and treatment of disease caused by nontuberculous mycobacteria. *Am Rev Respir Dis* 142:940–953, 1990.

139. Goodwin RA, DesPrez RM: Histoplasmosis: state of the art. *Am Rev Respir Dis* 117:929–956, 1978.

140. Goodwin RA, Shapiro JL, Thurman GH, et al: Disseminated histoplasmosis: clinical and pathologic correlations. *Medicine* 59:1–33, 1980.

141. Goodwin RA, Loyd JE, DesPrez RM: Histoplasmosis in normal hosts. *Medicine* 60:231–266, 1981.

142. Davies SF, Sarosi GA: Acute cavitary histoplasmosis. *Chest* 73:103–105, 1978.

143. Goodwin RA, Owens FT, Snell JD, et al: Chronic pulmonary histoplasmosis. *Medicine* 55:413–452, 1976.

144. Loyd JE, Tillman BF, Atkinson JB, DesPrez RM: Mediastinal fibrosis complicating histoplasmosis. *Medicine* 67:295–310, 1988.

145. Davies SF, McKenna RW, Sarosi GA: Trephine biopsy of the bone marrow in disseminated histoplasmosis. *Am J Med* 67:617–622, 1979.

146. Wheat LJ, Slama TG, Norton JA, et al: Risk factors for disseminated or fatal histoplasmosis. *Ann Intern Med* 96:159–163, 1982.

147. Davies SF, Khan M, Sarosi GA: Disseminated histoplasmosis in immunologically suppressed patients. *Am J Med* 64:94–100, 1978.

148. Johnson PC, Khardori N, Najjar AF, et al: Progressive disseminated histoplasmosis in patients with acquired immunodeficiency syndrome. *Am J Med* 85:152–158, 1988.

149. Wheat LJ, Connolly-Stringfield PA, Baker RL, et al: Disseminated histoplasmosis in the acquired immune deficiency syndrome: Clinical findings, diagnosis and review of the literature. *Medicine (Baltimore)* 69:361–374, 1990.

150. Mandell W, Goldberg DM, Neu HC: Histoplasmosis in patients with the acquired immune deficiency syndrome. *Am J Med* 81:974–978, 1986.

151. Sarosi GA, Johnson PC: Disseminated histoplasmosis in patients infected with human immunodeficiency virus. *Clin Infect Dis* 14(Suppl)1:60–67, 1992.

152. Davies SF: Serodiagnosis of histoplasmosis. *Semin Respir Infect* 1:9–15, 1986.

153. Wheat LJ, Kohler RB, Tewari RP: Diagnosis of disseminated histoplasmosis by detection of *Histoplasma capsulatum* antigen in serum and urine specimens. *N Engl J Med* 314:83–88, 1986.

154. Wheat LJ, Connolly-Stringfield P, Kohler RB, Frame PT, Gupta MR: *Histoplasma capsulatum* polysaccharide antigen detection in diagnosis and management of disseminated histoplasmosis in patients with acquired immunodeficiency syndrome. *Am J Med* 87:396–400, 1989.

155. Dismukes WE, Bradsher RW Jr, Cloud GC, et al: Itraconazole therapy for blastomycosis and histoplasmosis: NIAID Mycosis Study Group. *Am J Med* 93:489–497, 1992.

156. Parker JD, Sarosi GA, Doto IL, Bailey RE, Tosh FE: Treatment of chronic pulmonary histoplasmosis. A National Communicable Disease Center Cooperative Mycoses Study. *N Engl J Med* 283:225–229, 1970.

157. Sarosi GA, Davies SF: Blastomycosis: state of the art. *Am Rev Respir Dis* 120:911–938, 1979.

158. Klein BS, Vergeront JM, Weeks RJ, et al: Isolation of *Blastomyces dermatitidis* in soil associated with a large outbreak of blastomycosis in Wisconsin. *N Engl J Med* 314:529–534, 1986.

159. Sarosi GA, Hammerman KJ, Tosh FE, Kronenberg RS:

Clinical features of acute pulmonary blastomycosis. *N Engl J Med* 290:540–543, 1974.

160. Pappas PG, Pottage JC, Powderly WG, et al: Blastomycosis in patients with the acquired immunodeficiency syndrome. *Ann Intern Med* 116:847–853, 1992.

161. Sanders JS, Sarosi GA, Nollet DJ, Thompson JI: Exfoliative cytology in the rapid diagnosis of pulmonary blastomycosis. *Chest* 72:193–196, 1977.

162. Klein BS, Vergeront JM, Kaufman L, et al: Serological tests for blastomycosis: assessments during a large point source outbreak in Wisconsin. *J Infect Dis* 155:262–268, 1987.

163. Sarosi GA, Davies SF, Phillips JR: Self-limited blastomycosis: a report of 39 cases. *Semin Respir Infect* 1:40–44, 1986.

164. National Institute of Allergy and Infectious Diseases Mycoses Study Group: Treatment of blastomycosis and histoplasmosis with ketoconazole. *Ann Intern Med* 103:861–872, 1985.

165. Bradsher RW, Rice DC, Abernathy RS: Ketoconazole therapy for endemic blastomycosis. *Ann Intern Med* 103:872–879, 1985.

166. Drutz DJ, Catanzaro A: Coccidioidomycosis: state of the art. Part I. *Am Rev Respir Dis* 117:559–585, 1978.

167. Bronnimann DA, Adam RD, Galgiani JN, et al: Coccidioidomycosis in the acquired immunodeficiency syndrome. *Ann Intern Med* 106:372–379, 1987.

168. Ampel NM, Dols CL, Galgiani JN: Coccidioidomycosis during human immunodeficiency virus infection. Results of a prospective study in a coccidioidal endemic area. *Am J Med* 94:235–240, 1993.

169. Drutz DJ, Catanzaro A: Coccidioidomycosis: state of the art. Part II. *Am Rev Respir Dis* 117:727–771, 1978.

170. Sarosi GA, Parker JD, Doto IL, Tosh FE: Chronic pulmonary coccidioidomycosis. *N Engl J Med* 283:325–329, 1970.

171. Smith CD, Saito MT, Beard RR, et al: Serologic tests in the diagnosis and prognosis of coccidioidomycosis. *Am J Hyg* 52:1–21, 1950.

172. Galgiani JN, Stevens DA, Graybill JR, et al: Ketoconazole therapy of progressive coccidioidomycosis. *Am J Med* 84:603–610, 1988.

173. Graybill JR, Stevens DA, Galgiani JN, Dismukes WE, Cloud GA, NIAID Mycoses Study Group: Itraconazole treatment of coccidioidomycosis. *Am J Med* 89:282–290, 1990.

174. Galgiani JN, Catanzaro A, Cloud GA, et al: Fluconazole therapy for coccidioidal meningitis. *Ann Intern Med* 119:28–35, 1993.

175. Restrepo A, Robledo M, Giraldo R, et al: The gamut of paracoccidioidomycosis. *Am J Med* 61:33–42, 1976.

176. Cuce LC, Wroclawski EL, Sampaio SAP: Treatment of paracoccidioidomycosis with ketoconazole. *Rev Inst Med Trop Sao Paulo* 23(2):82–85, 1981.

177. Restrepo A, Gomez I, Robledo J, Patino MN, Canole: Itraconazole in the treatment of paracoccidioidomycosis: a preliminary report. *Rev Infect Dis* 9(Suppl 1):551–553, 1987.

178. Gerding DN: Treatment of pulmonary sporotrichosis. *Semin Respir Infect* 1:61–65, 1986.

179. Pluss JL, Opal SM: Pulmonary sporotrichosis: review of treatment and outcome. *Medicine* 65:143–153, 1986.

180. Sharkey-Mathis PK, Kauffman CA, Graybill JR, et al: Treatment of sporotrichosis with itraconazole: NIAID Mycoses Study Group. *Am J Med* 95:279–285, 1993.

181. Powell KE, Dahl BA, Weeks RJ, Tosh FD: Airborne *Cryptococcus neoformans*: particles from pigeon excreta compatible with alveolar deposition. *J Infect Dis* 125:412–415, 1972.

182. Kovacs JA, Kovacs AA, Polis M, et al: *Cryptococcus* in the acquired immunodeficiency syndrome. *Ann Intern Med* 103:533–538, 1985.

183. Zuger A, Louie E, Holzman RS, et al: Cryptococcal disease in patients with the acquired immunodeficiency syndrome. *Ann Intern Med* 104:234–240, 1986.

184. Kerkering TM, Duma RD, Shadmy S: The evolution of pulmonary cryptococcosis. *Ann Intern Med* 94:611–616, 1981.

185. Dismukes WE, Cloud G, Gallis HA, et al: Treatment of cryptococcal meningitis with combination amphotericin B and flucytosine for four as compared with six weeks. *N Engl J Med* 317:334–341, 1987.

186. Saag MS, Powderly WG, Cloud GA, et al: Comparison of amphotericin B with fluconazole in the treatment of acute AIDS associated cryptococcal meningitis. *N Engl J Med* 326:83–89, 1992.

187. Larsen RA, Leal MAE, Chan LS: Fluconazole compared with amphotericin B plus flucytosine for cryptococcal meningitis in AIDS: a randomized trial. *Ann Intern Med* 113:183–187, 1990.

188. Powderly WG, Saag MS, Cloud GA, et al: A controlled trial of fluconazole or amphotericin B to prevent relapse of cryptococcal meningitis in patients with the acquired immunodeficiency syndrome. *N Engl J Med* 326:793–798, 1992.

189. Varkey B, Rose HD: Pulmonary aspergilloma–a rational approach to treatment. *Am J Med* 61:626–631, 1976.

190. Young RC, Bennett JE, Vogal CL, et al: Aspergillosis: the spectrum of the disease in 98 patients. *Medicine* 49:147–173, 1970.

191. Binder RE, Faling LJ, Pugatch RD, et al: Chronic necrotizing pulmonary aspergillosis: a discrete clinical entity. *Medicine* 60:109–124, 1982.

192. Denning DW, Tucker RM, Hanson LH, Stevens DA: Treatment of invasive aspergillosis with itraconazole. *Am J Med* 86:791–800, 1989.

193. Denning DW, Follansbee SE, Scolaro M, Norris S, Edelstein H, Stevens DA: Pulmonary aspergillosis in the acquired immunodeficiency syndrome. *N Engl J Med* 324:654–662, 1991.

194. Minamoto GY, Barlam TF, Vander Els NJ: Invasive aspergillosis in patients with AIDS. *Clin Infect Dis* 14:66–74, 1992.

195. Pizzo PA, Robichaud KJ, Gill FA, Witebsky FG: Empiric antibiotic and antifungal therapy for cancer patients with prolonged fever and granulocytopenia. *Am J Med* 72:101–111, 1982.

# Chapter 17

# Infectious and Noninfectious Pulmonary Complications in Patients Infected with the Human Immunodeficiency Virus

**Scott Sasse**
**Françoise Kramer**

OVER 15 MILLION PEOPLE worldwide have been infected with the human immunodeficiency virus (HIV) as of December 1993, according to the World Health Organization. In the United States, estimates of the number of people infected with HIV exceed one million, and more than 330,000 cases of AIDS have been reported to the Centers for Disease Control (1). In patients with AIDS, the lungs are the principal target organ for development of infectious diseases. The lungs are also a common site of noninfectious complications in HIV-infected patients (2).

The CD4 count (absolute number of CD4 + lymphocytes) serves as an indicator of immune function in HIV-infected persons. Many opportunistic infections of the lung, such as *Pneumocystis carinii* pneumonia (PCP) and *Mycobacterium avium* complex do not occur until the CD4 count drops to below 200 or 250 cells/$mm^3$. Patients with higher CD4 counts are, however, at increased risk for development of other infectious diseases of the lung (such as tuberculosis and bacterial pneumonia). The development of noninfectious complications of the lung is less dependent upon the CD4 count or severity of HIV disease (3).

This chapter is organized into two main sections; infectious and noninfectious pulmonary complications. The infectious section covers PCP, bacterial pneumonia, mycobacterial diseases, and viral and fungal infections of the lung. The noninfectious section covers the pulmonary manifestations of Kaposi's sarcoma (KS) and non-Hodgkin's lymphoma as well as the interstitial pneumonitides that occur in HIV-infected individuals. Within each section, primary emphasis is given to those diseases which are most prevalent in the HIV-infected patient (i.e., PCP and KS).

## PNEUMOCYSTIS CARINII PNEUMONIA

The first cases of PCP in patients with an acquired immunodeficiency state were published in 1981 (4, 5). Since 1981, the number of cases of PCP has increased to an estimated 20,000 to 60,000 cases per year in the U.S. (6). Prior to the advent of effective prophylaxis, PCP was the most common respiratory complication as well as the most frequent life-threatening opportunistic infection in patients infected with HIV (2, 7). It was estimated that up to 75% of all HIV-infected patients would develop PCP within their lifetimes (8). With prophylaxis, the incidence of PCP has probably decreased. However, in 1991, PCP was still the AIDS-defining illness in 20,000 cases reported to the Centers for Disease Control.

### Microbiology and Epidemiology

The life cycle of *Pneumocystis carinii* is still poorly understood because the organism cannot be propagated in vitro using cell culture lines. Animal models have been developed in rats, rabbits, mice, guinea pigs, and ferrets in which the animals spontaneously develop PCP after the administration of steroids. The organism exists in a cystic form (containing up to eight intracystic bodies or sporozoites) and in an extracystic form (trophozoite) (9).

The taxonomy of *Pneumocystis carinii* is still debated. The organism was originally classified as a eucaryotic protozoan on the basis of its amoeboid appearance, its filopodia, and its sensitivity to antiprotozoal drugs (i.e., pentamidine and sulfonamides). However, its staining characteristics (methenamine silver) and ribosomal RNA sequencing suggest links to the fungi (9, 10).

There are two theories relating to the transmission of PCP. First, it has been hypothesized that the *Pneumocystis carinii* infection results from reactivation of a previously dormant infection acquired during childhood. Evidence for this theory is based upon the fact that most healthy children by the age of four have antibodies to *Pneumocystis carinii* (11, 12). The second theory is that the organism is transmitted among susceptible individuals by the airborne route. There are two lines of evidence to support airborne transmission: (*a*) in animal studies, susceptible animals that share the same airspace can become infected (13, 14) and (*b*) clustering of PCP cases occurs in persons with close contact (15, 16).

### Clinical Presentation and Laboratory Testing

The usual clinical presentation is one of gradually increasing fatigue, fevers, chills, sweats, dyspnea, nonproductive cough, and chest pressure. The mean duration of symptoms prior to diagnosis is usually weeks (17). On physical examination, tachypnea is present, and rales can be heard upon chest auscultation in up to one-third of patients (18).

Most patients have CD4 counts in the range of 50 to 75 cells/mm$^3$ at the time of diagnosis of their first episode of PCP (3, 19), and more than 90% of PCP episodes occur when the CD4 count is below 200 cells/mm$^3$ (20). Routine laboratory testing is usually remarkable only for the findings of an acute pneumonia. PCP rarely occurs without an elevation of the LDH (2, 21). Two other nonspecific laboratory values that are elevated are the ACE level and the ESR (22). Arterial blood gas analysis usually reveals a respiratory alkalosis with a widened alveolar-to-arterial oxygen pressure difference (17).

### Radiologic Imaging

Typical chest radiographic findings are those of diffuse bilateral interstitial infiltrates without a pleural effusion. As the disease progresses, alveolar infiltrates may also develop (23, 24). Although abnormal chest radiographs have been reported in up to 90% of patients, normal chest radiographs can occur (25–27). Many other less common chest radiographic findings have been reported including focal infiltrates, nodules, cystic lesions, pleural effusions, and pneumothoraces (26, 28–31). Atypical radiographic findings are more commonly found in patients who either have other underlying lung disease, have had previous episodes of PCP, or are receiving inhalation prophylaxis. Upper lobe disease is more common in patients receiving inhaled pentamidine prophylaxis (32–34).

Gallium lung scanning has been used as a diagnostic radiographic procedure for PCP with some success (35). A high sensitivity and specificity for PCP have been reported with a grading system in which lung uptake of gallium is graded relative to its uptake in the soft tissues and liver (35, 36). Technetium-DTPA is another nuclear imaging test with reported high sensitivity for PCP (37). Chest computerized tomography (CT) is usually not helpful unless it is used to visualize a suspected concurrent or alternate disease in the chest.

### Diagnostic Procedures

Various indirect and direct diagnostic procedures have been used to confirm the diagnosis of PCP in an HIV-infected patient who is clinically and radiologically suspected of having PCP. Indirect methods include pulmonary function tests and exercise testing.

Direct methods include expectorated or induced sputum, transtracheal aspiration, nonbronchoscopically guided bronchoalveolar lavage (BAL), bronchoscopically guided BAL, transbronchial biopsies during bronchoscopy, percutaneous needle aspiration, and open lung biopsy.

Of the indirect procedures, pulmonary function testing reveals a reduction in the diffusing capacity for carbon monoxide (DLco) (38, 39). Typically, there is also a reduction in the vital capacity and total lung capacity (40, 41). The main value of exercise testing is in its ability to exclude PCP in patients clinically suspected of having PCP. During exercise testing with pulse oximetry or arterial blood gas determinations, a normal exercise test without desaturation or widening of the alveolar-to-arterial oxygen pressure gradient essentially rules out the diagnosis of PCP (38, 42).

Of the direct procedures, the yield from induced sputum ranges from 25 to 85%, depending on the center and method of specimen staining (43–46). Bronchoscopically guided BAL is the principal method of diagnosis. It has a sensitivity of 86 to 97% (47, 48). Two additional sampling techniques that may further improve the yield from BAL are multiple lobe BAL and upper lobe BAL (49, 50). Transbronchial biopsies obtained during bronchoscopy have a sensitivity and specificity similar to those of BAL alone (51). When both BAL and transbronchial biopsies are performed during fiberoptic bronchoscopy, the sensitivity approaches 100% (51). Nonbronchoscopically guided BAL, in which a catheter is inserted blindly into a distal airway, is also associated with a sensitivity and specificity above 90% (52, 53). Percutaneous needle aspiration, which has a sensitivity of 90%, is associated with an unacceptably high rate (44%) of iatrogenic pneumothorax (54). Open lung biopsy, which theoretically should have the greatest yield, is rarely necessary because of the high yield from induced sputum and bronchoscopy with or without transbronchial biopsies. Open lung biopsy should be reserved for undiagnosed patients in whom bronchoscopically guided transbronchial biopsies are contraindicated, such as patients with bleeding disorders or those requiring mechanical ventilation with high airway pressures (55, 56).

### Diagnostic Algorithm

A frequently used diagnostic algorithm is to first obtain an induced sputum, which if nondiagnostic can be followed by a bronchoscopically guided BAL with or without transbronchial biopsies. Empiric treatment for suspected PCP should not be withheld while awaiting bronchoscopy, as large numbers of Pneumocystis carinii cysts and trophozoites remain in lung tissues

and pulmonary secretions for weeks to months after the initiation of therapy (57, 58).

Prior to bronchoscopy, the risks of bleeding and pneumothorax should be weighed against the increased yield from transbronchial biopsies. Estimates of the incidence of pneumothorax requiring a chest tube after transbronchial biopsies in patients suspected of having PCP are up to 5% (53, 59). Transbronchial biopsies should be more strongly considered in patients receiving prophylaxis or in those who have unusual chest radiographic findings, as the Pneumocystis carinii burden may be lower in these patients. Some investigators recommend performing an initial bronchoscopically guided BAL alone, which if nondiagnostic would then lead to a second bronchoscopy with transbronchial biopsies.

### Specimen Staining

The methenamine silver stain, which requires overnight preparation, is used to visualize the cyst walls. The Wright-Giemsa or Diff-Quik stains, which require less than 2 hours of preparation, can be used to visualize the trophozoites (extracystic form) or sporozoites within the cysts. The toluidine blue O stain is also commonly used to stain the cyst walls. Direct and indirect immunofluorescent staining using monoclonal antibodies are also now available with sensitivities greater than those obtained with traditional staining techniques (44).

### Treatment

In patients clinically suspected of having PCP, there are two possible first-line antibiotic regimens from which to choose: trimethoprim-sulfamethoxazole (TMP/SMX) and parenteral pentamidine isethionate. The usual dose of TMP/SMX is 15 to 20 mg/kg/day orally or parenterally at 6- or 8-hour intervals daily. The usual dose of pentamidine is 4 mg/kg/day parenterally once daily. The recommended length of therapy for both medications is 14 to 21 days. Both medications have similar efficacy, although one study suggested improved survival from TMP/SMX (60). TMP/SMX also has an added benefit in that its antibacterial properties are beneficial in patients with concurrent or misdiagnosed bacterial pneumonia.

Both medications are associated with significant and potentially life-threatening side effects. In numerous studies, approximately 50% of the patients in whom therapy was initiated with one medication were forced to change to an alternate therapy (61). For TMP/SMX, the side effects include rash, neutropenia, elevation of liver function tests, nausea and vomiting, anemia, elevation of creatinine, and hyponatremia. The most common reasons for a change in therapy are neutropenia (15 to 28%) and severe rash (15 to 33%) (17, 62, 63).

For pentamidine, the side effects include elevated creatinine levels, elevated liver function test values, hyponatremia, neutropenia, and anemia. Pancreatitis and hypoglycemia occur, because of the detrimental effect of pentamidine on the pancreatic islet cells. Hypotension can also occur, but it can be minimized by adequate hydration and by infusion of pentamidine over 1 or 2 hours (60, 64).

Response to therapy should be evaluated on the basis of clinical parameters such as fever, dyspnea, and cough as well as LDH and arterial blood gas values and chest radiographic changes. It is common for patients who ultimately recover from PCP to deteriorate during the initial 2 to 3 days of treatment. With this in mind, it has been recommended that alternate medications should not be started until the patient has received at least 5 to 7 days of therapy (2). Combination therapy with TMP/SMX and pentamidine together is not superior to the use of either medication alone.

A number of other medications are presently in use as second-line agents or are undergoing testing. These include TMP/dapsone, clindamycin/primaquine, reduced-dose TMP/SMX, atovaquone, aerosolized pentamidine, trimetrexate with leucovorin rescue, eflornithine (DFMO), and piritrexim.

## Corticosteroids as Adjunctive Therapy

Several studies have now been completed that examine whether corticosteroids are beneficial as adjunctive therapy in the treatment of PCP (65–68). A consensus conference convened in May 1990 to address this issue concluded that "adjunctive corticosteroid therapy can clearly reduce the likelihood of death, respiratory failure or deterioration of oxygenation in patients with moderate to severe PCP" (69). Moderate-to-severe PCP was defined by an arterial $P_{O_2}$ below 80 mm Hg on room air or an alveolar-to-arterial oxygen pressure difference above 35 mm Hg. The corticosteroid regimen recommended is a tapering schedule that begins with oral prednisone at 40 mg twice daily (or its equivalent) for 5 days. It was also recommended that corticosteroids be initiated when antipneumocystis therapy is started. No benefit from the addition of corticosteroids was found when the corticosteroids were added more than 72 hours after the start of antipneumocystis therapy. At the above doses, life-threatening side effects were not seen, although an increase in oral thrush and mucocutaneous herpes was reported. No conclusions were reached regarding the use of corticosteroids in patients with mild disease.

## Prognosis

Survival studies over the past decade have shown a trend toward decreasing mortality from PCP (70).

The possible explanations for this improvement are earlier recognition and treatment of PCP, the use of corticosteroids, the increased use of antiretroviral therapy, and prophylaxis for PCP. The mortality rate for cases of moderate-to-severe PCP (i.e., ideal alveolar minus arterial $P_{O_2}$ > 35 mm Hg), despite the use of corticosteroids, approaches 30%. The mortality rate for cases of mild-to-moderate PCP (ideal alveolar minus arterial $P_{O_2}$ < 35 mm Hg), is less than 5% (57, 69).

A number of prognostic indicators have been studied, which can be used to predict the outcome of an acute episode of PCP. Poor prognostic indicators include a high initial LDH level, increasing LDH level during treatment, a low CD4 count, a wide alveolar-minus-arterial oxygen pressure gradient, and more than 5% PMNs on BAL. Other indicators of poor outcome include the severity of chest radiographic findings, a recurrent episode of PCP, a low serum albumin level, and respiratory failure (21, 57, 71, 72).

## Mechanical Ventilation

The mortality rate of patients requiring mechanical ventilation has decreased from rates of 85 to 100% early in the AIDS epidemic to 50% or less in recent years (72–74). For mechanically ventilated patients, a low serum albumin level, an arterial pH below 7.35, and a positive end-expiratory pressure above 10 cm water after 96 hours in the ICU are associated with an increased mortality rate (72, 75). Continuous positive airway pressure (CPAP) has been used with some success to delay or avoid intubation in selected patients (76).

## Prophylaxis

Without prophylaxis, patients with CD4 counts below 200 cells/mm$^3$ have a risk of developing PCP that is 8.4% at 6 months, 18.4% at 12 months, and 33% at 36 months (20). The medications best tested for prophylaxis are TMP/SMX (TMP 160 mg and SMX 800 mg) once daily or aerosolized pentamidine 300 mg every 4 weeks. A United States Public Health Service consensus statement published in 1993 recommended TMP/SMX as the first-line medication for prophylaxis, although up to 30% of patients develop side effects that require substitution of another medication. The second-line medication recommended is nebulized pentamidine (77). Other medications such as dapsone, intermittent parenteral pentamidine, oral dapsone-pyrimethamine, oral clindamycin-primaquine, and oral atovaquone are presently undergoing testing.

## Special Circumstances

### Pneumothorax

Pneumothorax with bronchopleural fistula is a life-threatening condition in patients infected with HIV.

The pneumothorax may be due to an acute episode of PCP, may be associated with aerosolized pentamidine prophylaxis, or may be related to a chronic form of PCP in which lung cavitation and honeycombing can occur (78–81). The persistent air leak will rarely heal on its own and may require surgical or thoracoscopically guided closure, which may or may not be successful. HIV-infected patients who present with pneumothoraces should be suspected of having PCP.

## Occupational Exposure Associated with Nebulization Therapy

Health care workers are commonly exposed to the respiratory secretions of HIV-infected patients in two settings: (*a*) administration of aerosolized pentamidine (for prophylaxis or treatment of PCP) and (*b*) sputum induction with an ultrasonic nebulizer. In both settings, there is potential risk for exposure to *Mycobacterium tuberculosis* from patients who have either undiagnosed or inadequately treated tuberculosis. Transmission of *M. tuberculosis* to health care workers has been reported in association with both of these procedures (82).

Aerosolized pentamidine administration can lead to both significant ambient air concentrations of the drug and significant urinary pentamidine levels in health care workers (83, 84); the long-term effects of which are unknown. Ocular irritation, perioral numbness, and bronchospasm have also been reported in health care workers administering pentamidine (85, 86). Careful screening for tuberculosis in patients receiving aerosolized pentamidine, as well as physical measures that decrease the exposure of health care workers to respiratory secretions (such as adequate ventilation and the use of isolation hoods), are now required.

## OTHER PARASITIC INFECTIONS

*Toxoplasma gondii* is an opportunistic organism that causes focal brain lesions in patients with AIDS. Pulmonary toxoplasmosis is rare and is diagnosed by demonstrating *T. gondii* organisms in lung tissue or BAL (87). *Cryptosporidium* species can cause severe diarrheal illnesses in HIV-infected patients. Few cases of pulmonary cryptosporidiosis have been reported (88).

## BACTERIAL PNEUMONIA

Up to 10% of all pneumonias in HIV-infected patients are due to community-acquired bacteria (89). The most common pathogens are the encapsulated organisms *Streptococcus pneumoniae* and *Haemophilus influenzae*. Other reported bacterial organisms include group B streptococci, *Staphylococcus aureus*, *Moraxella catarrhalis*, *Mycoplasma pneumoniae*, and *Rhodococcus equi*. Simultaneous infections with bacteria and *P. carinii* can also occur (74).

The clinical presentation of acute bacterial pneumonia in HIV-infected patients is similar to that in the seronegative population. Patients present with productive cough, fever, and pleuritic chest pain (90). Bacteremia is frequently present. Chest radiographs commonly reveal diffuse infiltrates with *H. influenzae* infection and lobar infiltrates with *S. pneumoniae* infection. Signs and symptoms in patients with bacterial pneumonia are usually more acute than those in patients with PCP alone.

The treatment of bacterial pneumonia in HIV-infected patients is the same as for patients without HIV infection. Empiric therapy with trimethoprim/sulfamethoxazole or a second-generation cephalosporin is a reasonable initial choice, pending results of sputum and blood cultures. The pneumococcal vaccine is recommended by the Centers for Disease Control for primary prevention of pneumococcal pneumonia in HIV-infected patients, although its efficacy in this population has not been proven (91).

## TUBERCULOSIS

### Epidemiology

The HIV pandemic has been associated with a worldwide increase in tuberculosis. In early 1992, the World Health Organization estimated that 1.7 billion people (one-third of the world population) were infected with *M. tuberculosis* (92). Coinfections with HIV and tuberculosis were estimated to affect 4 million persons, 95% of whom were from developing countries, particularly in Africa and Southeast Asia (93). The HIV seroprevalence among tuberculous patients in sub-Saharan Africa has ranged between 20 and 67% (94).

In the United States, the annual number of tuberculosis cases rose from 22,201 in 1985 to 26,673 in 1992, a 20.1% increase (95). This resurgence of tuberculosis has been strongly linked to the HIV epidemic (95, 96). Coinfections with HIV and tuberculosis have been most frequent among foreign-born Haitians and Cubans, 25- to 44-year-old African Americans and Hispanics, the homeless, and intravenous drug users (97–99). The HIV seroprevalence in tuberculosis clinics around the country has ranged from 0% (Honolulu) to 46.3% (New York City), with a median rate of 3.4% (97).

### Pathogenesis

Almost all cases of tuberculosis are acquired through the pulmonary route after inhalation of droplet nuclei infected with *M. tuberculosis*. An intact cell-mediated immunity is crucial to contain the infection.

Out of 100 immunocompetent individuals newly infected with *M. tuberculosis*, only 10% will develop the clinical disease "tuberculosis." The remaining 90% will mount an adequate immune response, and their tuberculous infection will stay clinically silent. A distinction is therefore made between infection and disease due to *M. tuberculosis*, with infection being 10 times more frequent than disease in nonimmunosuppressed people. In 5% of infected persons, the host defenses do not control the infection, and clinically apparent tuberculosis develops within 2 years (primary tuberculosis). The remaining 5% will develop tuberculosis later in life, when their immunity wanes because of age, drugs, or immunosuppressive illnesses (reactivation tuberculosis).

Lymphocytes bearing the CD4+ marker (also called T4 lymphocytes) and macrophages play a key role in the cell-mediated immune response against *M. tuberculosis*. HIV specifically infects the CD4+ cells and macrophages, resulting in a truncated and dysfunctional cell-mediated immune response. The reduced host resistance of HIV-infected persons allows the development of progressive primary pulmonary tuberculosis, hematogenous dissemination of *M. tuberculosis* to extrapulmonary sites, and reactivation of previous tuberculous infection (98). After close contact with a tuberculous patient, 37% of HIV-infected persons develop disease within 5 months (100). The risk of reactivation of tuberculosis in HIV-infected patients is 8 to 10% per year (101, 102).

### Tuberculin Skin Test

The Centers for Disease Control recommends that all HIV-infected persons receive a tuberculin skin test (Mantoux test with five tuberculin units of purified protein derivative [PPD]-tuberculin) (103). A tuberculin skin test resulting in 5 mm of induration or more is considered positive and indicative of tuberculous infection in individuals coinfected with HIV. A negative tuberculin skin test, however, does not rule out tuberculous infection. The responsiveness to delayed-type hypersensitivity skin test antigens declines as the HIV infection progresses, as the number of CD4 cells decreases, and as the cell-mediated immunity wanes. In one study of patients with known tuberculosis, tuberculin skin tests were found to be positive in 64% of HIV-infected patients with more than 100 CD4 cells/mm$^3$ but in none of 13 patients with fewer than 100 CD4 cells/mm$^3$ (104). Delayed-type hypersensitivity skin testing with *Candida*, mumps, or tetanus toxoid antigens as controls has been advocated at the time of PPD testing (105). A negative tuberculin skin test with a positive control makes tuberculous infection unlikely. A negative PPD with negative controls (anergy)

does not exclude tuberculosis, and further diagnostic evaluation should be undertaken in all suspect cases.

### Multidrug-Resistant Tuberculosis

In the United States, a rise in resistant tuberculosis has paralleled the overall increase in tuberculosis since the mid-1980s (106). Historically, most patients with resistant tuberculosis acquired resistant *M. tuberculosis* organisms through ineffective courses of treatment (often because of erratic compliance with therapy). Since 1990, several outbreaks of multidrug-resistant tuberculosis have occurred in institutional facilities. *M. tuberculosis* organisms resistant to isoniazid, rifampin, and up to seven antimycobacterial agents were transmitted to contacts in New York and Florida hospitals as well as in New York state prisons (107–109). During these epidemics, more than 200 patients were newly infected with multidrug-resistant tuberculosis, 96% of whom were coinfected with the HIV virus. Death occurred within 4 to 16 weeks after diagnosis of tuberculosis in 72 to 89% of the outbreak cases (106). The fact that many HIV-infected individuals develop active tuberculosis soon after being infected with *M. tuberculosis* contributed to the rapid nosocomial spread of multidrug-resistant tuberculosis among HIV-infected persons. Other factors that facilitated these outbreaks include delayed diagnosis of tuberculosis, delayed recognition of drug resistance resulting in prolonged ineffective therapy, failure to observe recommended isolation precautions, and lack of appropriate negative-pressure ventilation in isolation rooms (106).

### Clinical Features

Tuberculosis, although often an early manifestation of HIV disease, can occur during any stage of HIV infection. *M. tuberculosis* is more virulent than other HIV-related opportunistic pathogens (e.g., *Pneumocystis carinii* or cytomegalovirus) and tends to cause disease earlier in the natural history of HIV infection.

Pulmonary involvement occurs in 70 to 100% of HIV-infected patients with tuberculosis (96, 110, 111). Symptoms include weight loss, fever, night sweats, cough, and dyspnea. These symptoms, however, can be caused by other HIV-associated pulmonary processes. The physical findings are also indistinguishable from those of other HIV-related conditions.

One of the most striking features of tuberculosis in HIV-infected patients is the high frequency of extrapulmonary involvement, often with concomitant pulmonary tuberculosis (110). The most frequent forms of extrapulmonary disease are lymphadenitis and mycobacteremia, occurring in up to 30 and 40% of cases, respectively (112, 113). Other sites of extrapulmonary tuberculosis include the bone marrow, the genitourinary tract, and the central nervous system (114). Intra-abdominal lymphadenopathy and hepatic, splenic, or pancreatic abscesses can often be demonstrated by computed tomography (115).

Many reports suggest that the clinical and radiographic manifestations of tuberculosis vary with the severity of HIV-induced immunodeficiency. In patients with less-advanced HIV infection (when cell-mediated immunity is only partially compromised), extrapulmonary tuberculosis is uncommon, tuberculin skin tests are usually positive, and the chest roentgenogram findings are often suggestive of reactivation tuberculosis with upper lobe infiltrates and cavitations (111, 116). In contrast, patients with tuberculosis and advanced HIV infection or AIDS tend to have frequent extrapulmonary disease, negative tuberculin skin tests, and chest roentgenogram changes typical of primary tuberculosis, with hilar adenopathy and interstitial or miliary infiltrates (114, 117, 118). In one study, 35% of HIV-infected patients with tuberculosis and 200 CD4 cells/mm$^3$ or more had extrapulmonary tuberculosis; mycobacteremia was present in 4% of these patients, and mediastinal adenopathy was present in 14%. On the other hand, 63% of HIV-infected patients with tuberculosis and fewer than 200 CD4 cells/mm$^3$ had extrapulmonary tuberculosis; 40% of these patients had mycobacteremia, and 34% had mediastinal adenopathy (104). Pleural effusions are quite common in HIV-infected patients with tuberculosis and have been reported in 11 to 29% of cases (93, 113, 119).

Hilar adenopathy, pleural effusions, and cavitation are most helpful in suggesting a diagnosis of tuberculosis, as they are rare findings in PCP or cytomegalovirus pneumonitis. Kaposi's sarcoma and lymphoma can present with hilar adenopathy and pleural effusion; however, extrapulmonary evidence of these diseases is usually present. Fungal infections such as coccidioidomycosis, histoplasmosis, and cryptococcosis can present with chest roentgenogram findings similar to those of tuberculosis, but diffuse infiltrates are more typical, extrapulmonary manifestations are common, and serologic tests help in the differential diagnosis. Ninety-eight percent of patients with cavitary tuberculosis have a positive acid-fast smear, which helps to make an early diagnosis. A miliary pattern on chest roentgenogram suggests tuberculosis, but other interstitial processes such as PCP, cytomegalovirus pneumonitis, fungal infections, and noninfectious pneumonitis should be considered. Upper lobe infiltrates, although frequent in tuberculosis, can also be found in patients developing PCP while receiving prophylaxis with aerosolized pentamidine.

## Diagnosis

The diagnosis of tuberculosis relies upon the isolation and identification of *M. tuberculosis* on culture. Acid-fast smears of sputum are positive in 31 to 82% of HIV-infected persons with tuberculosis; sputum cultures are positive in 88 to 100% of cases (96, 110, 111). When the acid-fast smears of sputum are negative or cannot be obtained, bronchoscopy yields a rapid presumptive diagnosis of tuberculosis in 34% of cases (120). Acid-fast bacilli can be seen in the BAL, the transbronchial biopsy, or postbronchoscopy sputum, and granulomata can be found on transbronchial biopsy.

Aspiration biopsy of tuberculous lymphadenopathy reveals acid-fast organisms in 67 to 90% of HIV-infected patients (113, 119, 121). Blood cultures prepared by the lysis-centrifugation system are positive in up to 40% of patients with HIV infection and tuberculosis (104, 113). Acid-fast smears of stools are positive in 40% of cases, probably representing organisms swallowed in sputum.

Newer techniques for rapid diagnosis of tuberculosis are now in use or under investigation. Radiometric culture methods (Bactec) combined with an *M. tuberculosis*–specific DNA probe (Gen-Probe) permit the identification of *M. tuberculosis* in 1 to 3 weeks. Amplification of mycobacterial DNA by polymerase chain reaction is another promising technique for rapid and specific diagnosis of tuberculosis (122).

## Treatment

In response to the increase in drug-resistant tuberculosis in the United States, the Centers for Disease Control has recommended a four-drug regimen including isoniazid (INH), rifampin (RIF), pyrazinamide (PZA), and ethambutol (EMB) as the initial empiric treatment of tuberculosis in all patients, including those infected with HIV (106). This four-drug regimen should be continued for 2 months, at which time the treatment can be altered according to drug-susceptibility results. Patients who are not immunosuppressed and have susceptible organisms can be treated with INH and RIF for another 4 months, a total of 6 months of treatment. Patients who are HIV-infected and have susceptible *M. tuberculosis* organisms should receive INH and RIF for an additional 7 months (a total of 9 months) or for 6 months after cultures have converted to negative, whichever is longer. A prolonged treatment of tuberculosis is advocated in patients infected with HIV because the efficacy of a 6-month regimen remains unproven in this population.

HIV-infected patients with either INH or RIF resistance should be treated with INH or RIF (whichever has activity against the resistant organism), PZA, and

EMB for 18 months or for 12 months after cultures have converted to negative, whichever is longer (98).

Multidrug-resistant tuberculosis in patients with HIV infection should be treated empirically with six drugs until the drug susceptibility results are available. If the resistance pattern of a source case is known or once the drug susceptibilities of the patient's isolate are available, four effective agents should be used for at least 24 months. Antituberculous medications that can be used in the treatment of multidrug-resistant tuberculosis include amikacin, kanamycin, streptomycin, and capreomycin as injectable agents and ethionamide, cycloserine, aminosalicylic acid, and ofloxacin or ciprofloxacin as oral agents. Medications of potential but unproven utility include clofazamine and amoxicillin-clavulanate (98, 123).

### Prophylaxis

Prophylaxis with INH, 300 mg/day for 12 months is recommended for all HIV-infected patients with a positive tuberculin skin test, regardless of age, unless specifically contraindicated (124). Anergic HIV-infected patients who have (*a*) close contacts with contagious tuberculous patients, (*b*) a previously untreated positive tuberculin skin test, (*c*) chest roentgenographic changes suggesting previous untreated tuberculosis, or (*d*) a history of inadequately treated tuberculosis should receive INH prophylaxis as well. Other anergic patients infected with HIV who should be considered for prophylaxis include intravenous drug users, the homeless, and foreign-born persons from countries with a high endemicity of tuberculosis.

Patients exposed to drug-resistant tuberculosis should receive prophylaxis according to the drug susceptibility pattern of the source case. In the case of INH resistance (but RIF susceptibility), prophylaxis should be initiated with RIF, with or without EMB, for 12 months (125). HIV-infected patients exposed to multidrug-resistant tuberculosis should be given 12 months of prophylaxis with 2 agents to which the organism is susceptible. Possible regimens include PZA (25 to 30 mg/kg/day) plus EMB (15 to 25 mg/kg/day) and PZA plus either ofloxacin (400 mg twice daily) or ciprofloxacin (750 mg twice daily) (126).

### Prognosis

When diagnosed and treated promptly, drug-susceptible tuberculosis has a favorable prognosis in patients with HIV infection. In one study, conversion of sputum cultures to negative occurred after a median of 10 weeks, and treatment failures or relapses occurred in only 6% of cases (110). Nevertheless, the mortality rate remains high because of other HIV-related complications.

The outcome of patients with HIV infection and multidrug-resistant tuberculosis has been poor. One hopes that the new recommendations of using at least 4 drugs with in vitro activity against the mycobacteria will improve the prognosis of HIV-infected patients with drug-resistant tuberculosis.

## THE *MYCOBACTERIUM AVIUM* COMPLEX

The *M. avium* complex (MAC) includes two species of nonchromogenic mycobacteria classified within Runyon's group III: *M. avium* and *Mycobacterium intracellulare*. MAC organisms are ubiquitous in the environment and are commonly isolated from water, soil, dust, and aerosol droplets (127). Although human exposure to MAC is frequent, disease due to these mycobacteria was less common prior to the AIDS epidemic (128). Most cases presented as progressive lung disease resembling tuberculosis in elderly males with underlying chronic pulmonary diseases. Cervical lymphadenitis in children was another infrequent manifestation of MAC infection, and disseminated MAC was rare, even among immunosuppressed patients (129).

HIV-infected patients with advanced disease and CD4 lymphocyte counts below 100 cells/mm$^3$ have a unique predisposition for MAC infection (130, 131). Disseminated MAC is found in 43% of patients with a diagnosis of AIDS for 2 years and in 50% of AIDS patients at autopsy (132, 133). It appears that most AIDS patients will eventually be infected with MAC as they survive other HIV-related opportunistic infections or malignancies.

Colonization of the respiratory or GI tracts with MAC organisms is not uncommon in patients with AIDS and is a risk factor for disseminated MAC (134). Current knowledge suggests that the intestinal tract is a more common site of dissemination than is the respiratory tract.

### Clinical Features

Typically, in patients with AIDS, MAC infection disseminates widely and causes a wasting syndrome. Patients present with fevers, night sweats, weakness, anorexia, and weight loss, often of many weeks duration. Other frequent symptoms include diarrhea, nausea, vomiting, and abdominal pain. Hepatosplenomegaly is commonly found on physical examination, but peripheral lymphadenopathy is unusual. Pancytopenia and specifically anemia reflect bone marrow involvement, while a markedly elevated alkaline phosphatase level (often without comparable elevations in hepatic transaminases) indicates hepatic infiltration (130, 131,

135, 136). Numerous large mesenteric and retroperitoneal lymph nodes can be demonstrated by abdominal computed tomography (137).

MAC occasionally causes focal infections in patients with AIDS. These include peripheral lymphadenitis, pneumonitis, endophthalmitis, and cutaneous or visceral abscesses. Patients with localized disease tend to have somewhat higher CD4 lymphocyte counts than do patients with disseminated disease (138). Symptoms of pulmonary disease due to MAC are nonspecific and consist of productive cough, dyspnea, fever, and sweats; hemoptysis is rare. Chest roentgenographic studies show interstitial infiltrates in 50%, alveolar infiltrates in 20%, and apical scarring, cavitation, and upper lobe infiltrates in 15% of patients (119). Pleural effusions are rare.

### Diagnosis

Disseminated MAC infection is usually diagnosed by blood culture. Only one or two cultures suffice, as most patients have a high-grade bacteremia. Culture methods include the lysis-centrifugation system and the radiometric liquid broth system. When these two methods are combined, they result in a positive culture within 5 to 7 days; conventional techniques may require 2 to 3 weeks. Once mycobacteria are isolated, DNA probes can rapidly differentiate MAC from *M. tuberculosis*. Biopsies of the bone marrow, liver, or lymph nodes have a high yield of positive cultures as well, but such procedures are usually not necessary to confirm the diagnosis of disseminated MAC. The demonstration of acid-fast bacilli on smear or biopsy does not suffice to make a diagnosis of MAC because these organisms may be *M. tuberculosis* or other mycobacteria.

The diagnosis of MAC pulmonary disease in HIV-infected patients is made by (*a*) demonstrating MAC organisms on serial sputum cultures in a symptomatic patient with an abnormal chest roentgenogram and (*b*) excluding other causes of pneumonitis, especially tuberculosis. Any HIV-infected patient who presents with pneumonia and whose sputum shows acid-fast bacilli on smear should receive empirical treatment for tuberculosis pending identification of these organisms.

### Treatment

The optimal therapy for disseminated MAC has yet to be determined. However, based on currently available data, it is recommended that at least two agents be used to treat MAC. Every regimen should include either clarithromycin or azithromycin as first-line drugs. Most investigators suggest using ethambutol as a second agent and clofazimine, rifabutin, rifampin, ciprofloxacin, or amikacin as third or fourth agents

(138). These recommendations also apply for the treatment of focal symptomatic MAC infection.

### Prophylaxis

All HIV-infected patients with fewer than 100 CD4 lymphocytes/mm$^3$ should receive prophylaxis against MAC. Rifabutin, 300 mg orally once a day, is the recommended regimen, because it reduces the frequency of disseminated MAC infection in patients with AIDS (138, 139).

## OTHER MYCOBACTERIAL INFECTIONS

Disseminated infections with mycobacteria other than *M. tuberculosis* or MAC occasionally occur in HIV-infected patients. *M. kansasii* infection usually presents as a pulmonary disease with or without concomitant extrapulmonary involvement. Chest radiographs show diffuse interstitial involvement, focal upper lobe disease and/or thin-walled cavities. In one study, patients treated with isoniazid, rifampin, and ethambutol responded well to therapy (140), unlike the poor response noted in an earlier report (141). Other atypical mycobacteria can cause disseminated disease in HIV-infected patients. Infections with *M. fortuitum, M. chelonei, M. gordonae, M. zenopi, M. haemophilum, M. flavescens, M. malmoense, M. asiaticum, M. scrofulaceum, M. szulgae,* and *M. genavense* have been reported.

## VIRAL INFECTIONS

The only viruses that are uniquely pathogenic in the setting of HIV-induced immunosuppression are the herpesviruses—namely cytomegalovirus (CMV), herpes simplex virus (HSV), and varicella-zoster virus (VZV). Herpesviruses share the capacity to remain latent in tissue after a primary infection and have the ability to reactivate if their host's immune response declines. Most HIV-infected patients have been exposed to herpesviruses and can present with clinical illnesses due to resurgent herpetic activity. Pneumonia, however, is not a frequent manifestation of infection with the herpesviruses in HIV-infected patients. CMV is the organism most commonly described as a cause of viral pneumonia in patients with HIV infection; HSV and VZV are rarely implicated as causes of lower respiratory tract infection in this population.

### CYTOMEGALOVIRUS INFECTION

CMV is a ubiquitous human herpesvirus. By 40 years of age, 50 to 95% of the general population are infected with CMV. CMV infection is usually asymptomatic in immunocompetent individuals. By contrast, in immunosuppressed patients such as those with bone marrow or organ transplant recipients, as well as patients with HIV infection, CMV can be the cause of several end-organ diseases. Retinitis, esophagitis, colitis, pneumonitis, and encephalitis are the most common clinical manifestations of CMV infection in patients with AIDS (142, 143). By the time HIV-infected patients develop CMV end-organ disease, most are severely immunosuppressed and have CD4 cell counts below 50 cells/mm$^3$. Reactivation of latent CMV probably accounts for most clinical illnesses; however new CMV infections can occur through blood transfusions or sexual contacts.

### Clinical Features

The importance of CMV as a cause of pulmonary disease in AIDS is controversial. Although CMV is frequently isolated from pulmonary secretions or lung tissue in AIDS patients with pneumonia, a pathogenic role of CMV in the disease process is usually not evident. CMV is commonly isolated from the respiratory secretions of patients with concomitant PCP or *S. pneumoniae* pneumonia. In such instances, patients recover with treatment of the copathogens and without specific anti-CMV therapy (144, 145). CMV is the sole pathogen in only 4% of all episodes of pneumonitis in HIV-infected patients and may be the cause of invasive CMV pneumonia in those instances (74). Symptoms of CMV pneumonia in AIDS patients include dyspnea and dry cough. Chest radiographic studies show interstitial infiltrates similar to those seen in patients with PCP.

### Diagnosis

A diagnosis of CMV pneumonia in patients with AIDS is enhanced by several findings: (*a*) positive CMV cultures from respiratory secretions or lung tissue, (*b*) cytologic or histopathologic demonstration of pathognomonic cells with intranuclear inclusion bodies, (*c*) detection of CMV antigen or nucleic acid in tissue and, (*d*) absence of other pathogenic organisms (2, 146). A clinical response to anti-CMV therapy confirms the diagnosis.

### Treatment

Therapy with ganciclovir 5 mg/kg twice daily should be considered in HIV-infected patients with documented CMV pneumonia. A treatment course of 14 days is recommended, although the ideal length of therapy for CMV pneumonitis in this patient population has not been established. Treatment with foscarnet, another antiviral agent effective in the treatment of CMV retinitis in AIDS patients, is a possible alternative in patients intolerant to, or not responding to, ganciclovir therapy. The indication for suppressive therapy to prevent relapse of CMV pneumonia is yet to be established.

### OTHER VIRAL PNEUMONITIDES

Infrequently, HIV-infected patients present with pneumonia due to HSV or VZV (74). A diagnosis of HSV pneumonia should be made using the criteria recommended for the diagnosis of CMV pneumonia, as asymptomatic HSV shedding is frequent in the oropharyngeal secretions of patients with HIV infection. The recommended treatment is acyclovir 5 mg/kg every 8 hours for 10 to 14 days.

VZV pneumonia is usually easy to diagnose because it occurs in the setting of varicella or disseminated herpes zoster and cutaneous manifestations are prominent (147). The treatment of choice is acyclovir 10 mg/kg every 8 hours for 10 to 14 days. Foscarnet should be considered for the treatment of HSV and VZV pneumonia in patients with acyclovir resistance.

## FUNGAL INFECTIONS

HIV-infected patients are susceptible to several fungal infections of diverse manifestations and severity. Cutaneous mycoses (dermatophytoses) such as seborrheic dermatitis, tinea corporis, or onychomycosis tend to occur early in the course of HIV infection. Although not life threatening, such disorders can cause significant discomfort and morbidity. Infections with *Candida* species are frequent in HIV-infected individuals and often indicate decreasing immunity. Mucocutaneous and esophageal candidiasis account for most clinical presentations. Invasive pulmonary candidal disease on rare occasions may occur as a late or terminal manifestation of HIV infection (2). Cryptococcosis is the most common disseminated fungal disease found in HIV-infected patients worldwide. Histoplasmosis, coccidioidomycosis, blastomycosis, and penicilliosis occur in areas where the causative organisms are endemic (148, 149). Finally, pulmonary aspergillosis is usually diagnosed in the later stages of HIV infection, often in the presence of neutropenia (150).

### CRYPTOCOCCOSIS

The yeastlike fungus *Cryptococcus neoformans* is distributed worldwide in the environment and can be isolated from soil, fruits, and other sources in nature. Although pigeons are not infected with *C. neoformans*, their feces harbor a high concentration of this organism (151). Human infection probably results from the inhalation of the aerosolized yeast, although a clear-cut exposure-disease association does not exist. Cryptococcosis was a relatively rare disease prior to the AIDS epidemic, occurring in patients with lymphoreticular malignancies or sarcoidosis or in patients receiving corticosteroids (152). In HIV-infected patients, cryptococcosis is the fourth most common serious infection (after PCP, CMV, and mycobacterial diseases), affecting up to 13% of patients (153). *C. neoformans* is a pathogen of relatively low virulence, and severe immunosuppression is required for cryptococcal disease to occur. Most HIV-infected patients with cryptococcosis have CD4 cell counts below $100/mm^3$ (3).

### Clinical Features

Cryptococcosis in patients with HIV infection presents as a meningitis in 85% of cases (154). Concomitant or isolated pneumonia occurs in up to 50% of patients (155). Symptoms of pulmonary cryptococcal disease include fever, shortness of breath, pleuritic chest pain, and productive cough (156–158). Chest roentgenographic findings most often consist of diffuse or focal interstitial infiltrates (156, 159). Nodular infiltrates, intrathoracic adenopathy, focal alveolar consolidation, cavitation, or isolated pleural effusion are less common findings (156–158, 160).

### Diagnosis

The definitive diagnosis of cryptococcosis relies upon the isolation of *C. neoformans* from body fluids or tissue. A positive sputum culture indicates disease, even in the absence of radiographic changes (2). The serum cryptococcal antigen is a very sensitive test that is positive in 75 to 99% of patients with AIDS-related cryptococcosis (153, 154, 161).

### Treatment

The optimal treatment regimen for cryptococcal disease in HIV-infected patients is still a matter of debate. Some investigators recommend an initial induction course of amphotericin B alone (0.7 to 0.8 mg/kg/day) or amphotericin B (0.3 to 0.5 mg/kg/day) combined with 5-flucytosine (100 mg/kg/day in four divided doses) for a period of 2 weeks or until the patient's condition stabilizes. Treatment can then be continued with fluconazole 400 mg orally, daily for 8 to 10 weeks. Patients presenting with a mild episode of cryptococcosis can be treated with fluconazole from the onset (162). Other therapeutic approaches under investigation include the combination of fluconazole and 5-flucytosine as well as the use of itraconazole. Daily maintenance therapy with fluconazole 200 mg per day is very effective in preventing relapse of cryptococcal disease in HIV-infected patients (163).

### HISTOPLASMOSIS

*Histoplasma capsulatum* is a dimorphic fungus that grows in nature in the mycelial form but converts in the infected host to its pathogenic yeast form. *H. capsulatum* is endemic in the central and south-central states of the United States, southern Mexico, Central America, South America, and the Caribbean. The fungus thrives in soil fertilized by bat or bird droppings and sporulates under favorable climatic conditions. Human exposure occurs via inhalation of the infecting spores. Most infections with *H. capsulatum* are asymptomatic in the immunocompetent host. Pulmonary symptoms occur in only 10% of cases, and disseminated histoplasmosis affects only one out of a thousand infected individuals (164, 165). In contrast, histoplasmosis presents as a disseminated disease in HIV-infected patients (166). In areas of high endemicity, disseminated histoplasmosis has been reported to be the second or third most frequent opportunistic infection in patients infected with HIV. Evidence suggests that both newly acquired infection with *H capsulatum* as well as reactivation of latent foci of infection lead to dissemination in patients with HIV infection (167).

### Clinical Features

Symptoms of disseminated histoplasmosis in HIV-infected patients include fevers, chills, and weight loss, often lasting for weeks. Cough and dyspnea are present in 50% of patients, and diarrhea occurs in 20% of patients (167, 168). Hepatosplenomegaly and lymphadenopathy are observed in one-third of cases, while mucosal and skin lesions are less common (169). Pancytopenia occurs in half of the cases, and the LDH is usually elevated (170, 171). Diffuse interstitial infiltrates are the most common chest radiographic abnormalities (169). Occasional patients will present with a fulminant illness manifested by hypotension, acute renal failure, adult respiratory distress syndrome, disseminated intravascular coagulation, and encephalopathy (166, 168).

### Diagnosis

The recovery of *H. capsulatum* on culture or the visualization of the organism in histopathologic material is necessary for the diagnosis of histoplasmosis. Blood cultures using the lysis-centrifugation method are positive in 90% of cases (166). Cultures of bone marrow have a positive yield in three-fourths of patients (170). *H. capsulatum* is also frequently recovered in material obtained from BAL, washings, brushings, or transbronchial biopsies (169, 172). A rapid diagnosis is possible in more than a third of patients when *H. capsulatum* organisms are identified in a smear of peripheral blood or bone marrow (167, 169). The *H. capsulatum* polysaccharide antigen (HPA) appears to be an excellent marker for early diagnosis; however, it is only available through a single research laboratory (166).

## Treatment

Amphotericin B is very effective in the treatment of histoplasmosis in HIV-infected patients and is the drug of choice in patients with severe disease. An acute treatment course of 2 g of amphotericin B has been recommended in such cases (173). Itraconazole at a dose of 200 mg orally, 3 times a day for 3 days, then twice a day for 12 weeks is very effective as primary therapy in patients with mild-to-moderate disease (167). Itraconazole has also become the treatment of choice for suppression of potential relapse of histoplasmosis in patients who have received successful acute therapy. Maintenance therapy with itraconazole 200 mg orally twice a day prevented relapse of histoplasmosis in 95% of patients over a median follow-up period of 109 weeks (174). The efficacy of high doses of fluconazole in the treatment of histoplasmosis is under investigation. Ketoconazole has not shown efficacy in HIV-infected patients with histoplasmosis (166).

### COCCIDIOIDOMYCOSIS

The fungus *Coccidioides immitis* is a soil organism endemic to the semiarid regions of the southwestern United States, northern Mexico, and some areas of Central and South America. *C. immitis* grows in nature as a mycelium that produces highly infective arthrospores. Once inhaled and deposited in the pulmonary alveoli, the infecting particles transform into their parasitic form, the spherules. Most immunocompetent individuals infected with *C. immitis* are either asymptomatic or present with a self-limited pulmonary disease. Dissemination occurs in less than 1% of cases and involves the meninges, the bone, the skin, or lymph nodes (175). In HIV-infected patients, coccidioidomycosis can present either as a primary progressive infection or as reactivated disease. A diagnosis of AIDS, a CD4 cell count below 250 cells/mm³, or residing in an endemic area are risk factors for developing coccidioidomycosis (176).

### Clinical Features

Most HIV-infected patients with coccidioidomycosis present with fever and pulmonary symptoms such as cough and dyspnea (176, 177). Both focal and diffuse pulmonary disease can occur. Other sites of involvement include the meninges, the skin, the lymph nodes, and the liver (176). Chest radiographic findings consist of focal alveolar infiltrates, diffuse interstitial infiltrates, and less commonly nodules, hilar lymphadenopathy, or pleural effusions (176).

### Diagnosis

The diagnosis of coccidioidomycosis is made by demonstrating the organisms on stain or culture from an infected site. Bronchoscopy, with BAL and transbronchial biopsy, is usually helpful in making a diagnosis. Cultures of the blood and bone marrow are frequently positive in disseminated disease. The tube precipitin immunodiffusion or the complement fixation serologic tests are positive in 90% of patients with active coccidioidomycosis (176, 178). Coccidioidin or spherulin skin testing are not helpful because they are positive in less than 20% of patients with active disease (176, 178).

### Treatment

Amphotericin B is the treatment of choice in HIV-infected patients with life-threatening coccidioidomycosis. Less severe forms of the disease may be treated with fluconazole at 400 to 1200 mg per day or itraconazole at 400 mg per day (179). Both of these agents have also been used for maintenance therapy.

### ASPERGILLOSIS

Invasive aspergillosis in patients with AIDS is not a frequent opportunistic infection. Major risk factors include neutropenia, treatment with corticosteroids, and advanced HIV infection. Other possible risk factors are marijuana smoking, use of broad-spectrum antibiotics, alcohol abuse, and PCP (150). Pulmonary involvement is most frequent; however, cerebral involvement and aspergillosis of the sinuses, ears, larynx, muscles, and heart can occur. Symptoms of pulmonary aspergillosis in patients with AIDS include cough, fever, night sweats, chest pain, dyspnea, and hemoptysis (150). Radiologic findings consist of unilateral or bilateral thin-walled cavities of the upper lobes, nodular infiltrates, or (in neutropenic patients) diffuse lower lobe infiltrates. Bronchial obstruction can occur when invasive aspergillosis arises in the bronchi. The diagnosis of pulmonary aspergillosis is made by isolating and demonstrating the organisms in tissue. Bronchoscopy with BAL and biopsy is the initial procedure of choice. Positive sputum cultures for *Aspergillus* species in a patient with a normal chest radiograph probably indicate colonization. Positive sputum cultures in the appropriate clinical setting, however, suggest invasive aspergillosis. Treatment remains difficult, although both amphotericin B and itraconazole have been effective in treating invasive pulmonary aspergillosis (150).

## NONINFECTIOUS COMPLICATIONS

Malignancies and interstitial lung diseases are the most common noninfectious complications of the chest to which HIV-infected patients are susceptible. The most common malignancies are Kaposi's sarcoma and non-Hodgkin's lymphoma; the most common interstitial lung diseases are lymphocytic interstitial pneumonitis and nonspecific interstitial pneumonitis. Other less frequent pulmonary complications include primary lung cancers, pulmonary edema secondary to an AIDS cardiomyopathy, pulmonary hypertension, radiation pneumonitis, and lymphocytic alveolitis.

## KAPOSI'S SARCOMA

### Background

Kaposi's sarcoma (KS) is the most common malignancy in HIV-infected individuals and was the initial presenting illness in more than 300 of the first 1000 patients diagnosed with AIDS (180–182). Since the early 1980s, however, the incidence of KS has decreased, and many investigators now no longer consider KS in HIV-infected patients to be a true malignancy. Instead, it is classified as a proliferative hyperplasia secondary to poor control and regulation of growth factors (183–185). KS occurs almost exclusively (more than 93% of cases) in homosexual or bisexual men (186). The strong male predominance, the inconsistency of cytogenetic abnormalities, and the fact that KS can regress spontaneously are points used to argue that KS is not a true malignancy (180). The development of KS does not directly depend upon the CD4 count. It occurs at a constant rate in patients who are at least 1 to 2 years post–HIV infection, and the incidence does not increase as immune function declines (187). Lung or pleural involvement at autopsy is present in up to one-half of all patients with known KS (188–190).

### Histology and Pathology

The characteristic histology of KS is that of spindle-shaped cells separated by elongated spaces containing extravasated red blood cells. Fibroblasts, inflammatory cells, and endothelial cells are also present in the KS lesion, and there is frequently evidence of angiogenesis (191–193). In the lung, KS lesions are commonly found involving the airways, blood vessels, or pleura (189).

### Clinical Presentation

KS typically presents as purplish skin or mucosal lesions that often disseminate to lymph nodes and viscera (180). Pulmonary or pleural involvement is found clinically in up to one-third of cases (194–196). The most common symptoms of patients with KS involving the lungs are dyspnea, fever, and nonproductive cough. Less commonly, hemoptysis, pleuritic chest pain, and hoarseness occur (194, 197–199). Chest auscultation is usually normal, although crackles are occasionally heard. Chest radiographs typically reveal nodular infiltrates, areas of focal consolidation, or pleural

effusions (196, 198, 200–202). Radiologically detected adenopathy may or may not be present. Gallium scanning usually reveals no uptake in the lung, which is in contrast to the uptake seen in PCP (203, 204).

Pleural effusions, which are frequently bilateral, are present in up to 60% of patients with KS involvement of the chest (189, 199). In an autopsy study of AIDS patients with KS and pleural effusions, the visceral pleura was found to be the main site of involvement (189).

### Diagnosis

The diagnosis of pulmonary KS is usually made by demonstrating characteristic endobronchial lesions during bronchoscopy. When present, endobronchial lesions are usually flat or slightly raised but can on occasion lead to bronchial obstruction (196, 199, 205–207). The lesions are bright red, without the violaceous hue that is seen in cutaneous skin lesions (200, 206). Endobronchial or transbronchial biopsies have a poor diagnostic yield. A segment of tissue larger than that provided by the bronchoscopic forceps is usually needed by the pathologist for recognition of the characteristic architecture of KS (189, 200, 201, 206). Because of the poor yield and risk of hemorrhage, some investigators avoid biopsies altogether in patients with characteristic endobronchial lesions (201, 206). Since a single diagnostic malignant cell type is not present, cytology specimens are uniformly nondiagnostic (208). Open lung biopsy is on rare occasions necessary to make the diagnosis of pulmonary KS (188, 194).

Pulmonary function tests and arterial blood gas determinations are not specific for KS, although decreases in the $D_{LCO}$ and the $FEV_1/FVC$ ratio have been reported (189). Exercise testing is highly variable (189, 209, 210). The LDH is frequently normal or only mildly elevated (211), and there is a report of elevated ACE levels in pulmonary KS (212). Most pleural effusions are serosanguinous and exudative. Pleural fluid analysis with pleural biopsies are usually nondiagnostic (199).

### Treatment and Prognosis

Treatment modalities for pulmonary KS include chemotherapy, radiotherapy and biologic response modifiers (alpha interferon, TNF-α) (213). In one study of 20 patients with pulmonary KS, combination chemotherapy with doxorubicin, bleomycin, and vincristine or bleomycin and vincristine, resulted in a response rate of 80 to 100%. The median survival for the responders was 10 months; the nonresponders lived a median of 6 months (214). Radiation therapy has been used as a palliative modality in pulmonary KS as well as a treatment for upper airway obstruction or hemoptysis (189, 215). Alpha interferon and TNF-$\alpha$ have been used with some success in selected patients with KS (216, 217). The survival rate in patients diagnosed with pulmonary KS varies from months to years. The presence of a pleural effusion or CD4 counts below 100 predict poor survival (199, 214).

## NON-HODGKIN'S LYMPHOMA

Non-Hodgkin's lymphoma (NHL) is the second most common malignancy affecting patients infected with HIV (218). NHL is diagnosed in 4 to 10% of all AIDS patients, and it is 60 times more likely to occur in an HIV-infected individual than in the general population (219, 220). Of all cases of NHL in the United States, 8 to 27% occur in HIV-infected individuals (221). The NHL that occurs in HIV-infected patients is usually a high-grade B cell tumor, which can be polyclonal or monoclonal (222).

### Pathogenesis

Unlike KS, NHL does not occur in any specific subgroup of HIV-infected patients (223). It has been hypothesized that this malignant B-cell proliferation is secondary to poor T-cell surveillance or possibly an as-yet undiscovered cofactor.

### Clinical Presentation

HIV-infected patients with NHL present with symptoms of fever, weight loss, and sweats (B symptoms). Disseminated disease and extranodal involvement are more frequent in the HIV-infected patient than in the immunocompetent patient (224, 225). One-third to one-half of patients develop thoracic involvement (226, 227).

### Radiologic Presentation

Bilateral nodular densities and interstitial infiltrates are the most common radiologic presentations of patients with AIDS-related lymphomatous involvement of the chest (226, 228, 229). Pleural effusions were present in 72% of cases in one series (230).

### Diagnosis

The diagnostic yield from bronchoscopy with transbronchial biopsies is very poor (228, 229, 231). However, the yield from cytology and histologic specimens obtained by thoracentesis with pleural biopsy can be greater than 35% (228, 230, 232). Patients without pleural effusions may require a thoracoscopic or an open lung biopsy for definitive diagnosis (229, 230).

### Treatment and Prognostic Indicators

The primary treatment modality is chemotherapy. Doxorubicin, vincristine, and/or bleomycin have been used with some success (220, 233). Unfortunately, chemotherapy is associated with increased toxicity in patients with AIDS. The median survival in one study of 63 patients with NHL was 6 months (234). The stage of lymphoma, CD4 count, and performance status of the patients can be used to predict survival (223, 224, 233).

## PRIMARY LUNG CANCER

Epidemiologic studies have not shown an increased risk of bronchogenic cancer in patients infected with HIV (235). However, HIV-infected patients with lung cancer have been found to be younger and have a shorter survival time than non-HIV-infected patients with primary lung cancer (236, 237). In a study of 19 HIV-infected patients with bronchogenic lung cancer, the predominant cell type was adenocarcinoma, and there were no 1-year survivors (236).

## LYMPHOID INTERSTITIAL PNEUMONITIS

In the non-HIV-infected patient, lymphoid interstitial pneumonitis (LIP) is a benign pneumonitis associated with a hyperglobulinemia and dysproteinemia (238–240). It is seen in patients with connective tissue disorders such as systemic lupus erythematosus, Sjögren's syndrome, and myasthenia gravis.

In the HIV-infected population, LIP is primarily a disease of children. LIP affects up to 50% of children infected perinatally with HIV and is a criterion for the Centers for Disease Control definition of AIDS in children under age 13. Rarely, LIP occurs in HIV-infected adults (241–243). LIP, in both HIV-infected and non-HIV-infected individuals, is characterized histologically by a diffuse infiltration of the alveolar septa by lymphocytes, plasma cells, plasmacytoid lymphocytes, and immunoblasts (244–246).

The clinical presentation of LIP is chronic progressive dyspnea, cough, and fever (245, 247–250). Weight loss and fatigue are also frequently present. In children with LIP, clubbing is common. Chest radiographs usually demonstrate bilateral interstitial or nodular infiltrates (251). There is a polyclonal gammmopathy and a lymphocytosis present on laboratory analysis (245, 247, 252). Arterial blood gas analysis reveals a normal-to-widened alveolar-to-arterial oxygen pressure gradient, and pulmonary function testing shows a restrictive pattern with a decreased $D_{LCO}$ (248, 252, 253).

## Diagnosis

BAL fluid usually reveals a nonspecific lymphocytosis, and transbronchial biopsies can on occasion yield the diagnosis (249, 254). Open lung biopsies are usually required for definitive diagnosis.

## Prognosis and Treatment

LIP can regress spontaneously or gradually progress over months to years, leading to respiratory insufficiency (247, 248, 253). In patients requiring treatment, positive responses have been reported with corticosteroids or zidovudine antiretroviral therapy alone (247, 254, 255).

### NONSPECIFIC INTERSTITIAL PNEUMONITIS

Nonspecific interstitial pneumonitis refers to a pneumonitis of HIV-infected patients in whom no infectious or neoplastic process can be identified, despite appropriate evaluation (257–259). The clinical presentation is usually dyspnea, cough, and/or fever. Chest radiographs can be normal or show bilateral reticulonodular or interstitial infiltrates. Histologically, there is a mononuclear cell interstitial infiltration of the lung. The etiology of nonspecific interstitial pneumonitis is unknown, although a dysfunctional immune response related to the HIV infection has been postulated. The disorder may resolve spontaneously or recur at varying time intervals.

### LYMPHOCYTIC ALVEOLITIS

A lymphocytic alveolitis has been reported in association with HIV infection. It is characterized by a BAL fluid that has increased levels of T suppressor/natural killer lymphocytes and can occur at any time in the course of the HIV infection (260, 261). The clinical significance of this alveolitis is unknown.

### PRIMARY PULMONARY HYPERTENSION

Primary pulmonary hypertension has been noted rarely in HIV-infected patients. Plexogenic arteriopathy is the most commonly reported pathologic diagnosis. The most common clinical presentation is dyspnea with signs of right heart failure (262, 263).

▼

## REFERENCES

1. WHO: AIDS Data as of 12/31/93. *Weekly Epidemiol Record* 2:5–8, 1994.
2. Murray JF, Mills J: Pulmonary infectious complications of human immunodeficiency virus infection. *Am Rev Respir Dis* 141:1356–1372, 1990.
3. Masur H, Ognibene FP, Yarchoan R, et al: CD4 counts as predictor of opportunistic pneumonia in human immunodeficiency virus (HIV) infection. *Ann Intern Med* 111:223–231, 1989.
4. Gottlieb MS, Schroff R, Schanker HM, et al: *Pneumocystis carinii* pneumonia and mucosal candidiasis in previously healthy homosexual men. *N Engl J Med* 305: 1425–1431, 1981.
5. Masur H, Michelis MA, Greene JB, et al: An outbreak of community-acquired *Pneumocystis carinii* pneumonia. *N Engl J Med* 305:1431–1438, 1981.
6. Masur H: Prevention and treatment of *Pneumocystis pneumonia. N Engl J Med* 327:1853–1860, 1992.
7. Weinberger SE: Recent advances in pulmonary medicine. *N Engl J Med* 328:1462–1470, 1993.
8. Hay JW, Osmond DH, Jacobson MA: Projecting the medical costs of AIDS and ARC in the United States. *J Acquir Immune Defic Syndr* 1:466–4485, 1985
9. Walzer PD: *Pneumocystis carinii*. In Mandell GL, Douglas RG, Bennett JE, et al (eds): *Principles and Practice of Infectious Diseases*. New York, Churchill Livingstone, 1990, pp 2103–2110.
10. Leoung GS, Hopewell PC: *Pneumocystis carinii* pneumonia: Epidemiology, microbiology, and pathophysiology. In Cohen PT, Sande MA, Volberding PA, et al (eds): *The AIDS Knowledge Base*. Waltham, Massachusetts, The Medical Publishing Group, 1990, pp 1–3.
11. Pfier LL, Hughes WT, Stagno S: *Pneumocystis carinii* infection: evidence for high prevalence in normal and immunosuppressed children. *Pediatrics* 61:35–41, 1978.
12. Hofman B, Odum N, Platz P, et al: Humoral responses to *Pneumocystis carinii* in patients with acquired immunodeficiency syndrome and in immunocompromised homosexual men. *J Infect Dis* 152;838–840, 1985.
13. Hughes WT. Natural mode of acquisition for de novo infection with *Pneumocystis carinii*. *J Infect Dis* 145: 842–848, 1982.
14. Hughes WT, Bartley DL, Smith BM: A natural source of infection due to *Pneumocystis carinii*. *J Infect Dis* 147: 595, 1983.
15. Watanabe JM, Chinchinian H, Weitz C, et al: *Pneumocystis carinii* pneumonia in a family. *JAMA* 193:685–686, 1965.
16. Goesch TR, Gotz G, Stellbrinck KH, et al: Possible transfer of *Pneumocystis carinii* between immunodeficient patients. *Lancet* 336:627, 1990.
17. Kovacs JA, Himenez JX, Macher AM: *Pneumocystis carinii* pneumonia: a comparison between patients with acquired immunodeficiency syndrome and patients with other immunodeficiencies. *Ann Intern Med* 100:633–671, 1984.
18. Hopewell PC: *Pneumocystis carinii* pneumonia. Diagnosis. *J Infect Dis* 157:1115–1119, 1988.
19. Lidman C, Berglund O, Tynell E, et al: CD4+ cells and CD4+ percent as risk markers for *Pneumocystis carinii* pneumonia (PCP): implications for primary PCP prophylaxis. *Scand J Infect Dis* 24:157–160, 1992.
20. Phair J, Munoz A, Detels R, et al: The risk of *Pneumocystis carinii* pneumonia among infected with human immunodeficiency virus type 1. *N Engl J Med* 322: 161–165, 1990.
21. Zaman MK, White DA: Serum lactate dehydrogenase

levels and *Pneumocystis carinii* pneumonia: diagnostic and prognostic significance. *Am Rev Respir Dis* 137: 796–800, 1988.

22. Brooks KR, Ong R, Spector RS, Greenbaum DM: Acute respiratory failure due to *Pneumocystis carinii* pneumonia. *Crit Care Clin* 9:31–48, 1993.

23. Delorenzo LJ, Huang CT, Maguire GP, et al: Roentgenographic patterns of *Pneumocystis carinii* pneumonia in 104 patients with AIDS. *Chest* 91:323–327, 1987.

24. Scott WW, Kuhlman JE: Focal pulmonary lesions in patients with AIDS: percutaneous transthoracic needle biopsy. *Radiology* 180;419–421, 1991.

25. Heron CW, Hine AL, Pozniak AL, et al: Radiologic features in patients with pulmonary manifestations of the acquired immune deficiency syndrome. *Clin Radiol* 36: 583–588, 1985.

26. Chaffey MH, Klein JS, Gamsu G, et al: Radiologic distribution of *Pneumocystis carinii* in patients with AIDS treated with prophylactic inhaled pentamidine. *Radiology* 175;715–719, 1990.

27. Israel HI, Gottlieb JE, Schulman ES. Hypoxemia with normal chest roentgenogram due to *Pneumocystis carinii* pneumonia. Diagnostic errors due to low suspicion of AIDS. *Chest* 92:857–859, 1987.

28. Bleiweiss, IJ, Jagirdar JS, Klein MJ, et al: Granulomatous *Pneumocystis carinii* pneumonia in three patients with the acquired immune deficiency syndrome. *Chest* 94: 580–583, 1988.

29. Sandhu JS, Goodman PC. Pulmonary cysts associated with *Pneumocystis carinii* pneumonia in patients with AIDS. *Radiology* 173: 33–35, 1989.

30. Jules-Elysee KM, Stover DM, Aaman MB, et al: Aerosolized pentamidine: effect on diagnosis and presentation of *Pneumocystis carinii* pneumonia. *Ann Intern Med* 112: 750–757, 1990.

31. Sherman M, Levin D, Breidlbart D.: *Pneumocystis carinii* pneumonia with spontaneous pneumothorax. A report of three cases. *Chest* 90:609–619, 1986.

32. Edelstein H, McCabe RE: Atypical presentations of *Pneumocystis carinii* pneumonia in patients receiving inhaled pentamidine prophylaxis. *Chest* 98:1366–1369, 1990.

33. Travis WD, Pittaluga S, Lipschik GY: Atypical pathological manifestations of *Pneumocystis carinii* pneumonia in the acquired immune deficiency syndrome. Review of 123 lung biopsies from 76 patients with emphasis on cysts, vascular invasion, vasculitis and granulomas. *Am J Surg Pathol* 14:615–625, 1990.

34. Shin MS, Veal CF, Jessup JG: Apical P*neumocystis carinii* pneumonia in AIDS patients not receiving inhaled pentamidine prophylaxis. *Chest* 100:1462–1464, 1991.

35. Golden JA, Sollitto RA: The radiology of pulmonary disease. *Clinics Chest Med* 9:481–495, 1988.

36. Coleman DL, Hattner RS, Luce JM, et al: Correlation between gallium lung scans and fiberoptic bronchoscopy in patient with suspected *Pneumocystis carinii* pneumonia and the acquired immunodeficiency syndrome. *Am Rev Respir Dis* 130:1166–1169, 1984.

37. Rosso J, Guillon JM, Parrot A, et al: Technetium-99-DTPA aerosol and gallium-67 scanning in pulmonary complications of human immunodeficiency virus infection. *J Nucl Med* 33:81–87, 1992.

38. Stover DE, Greeno RA, Galgiardi AJ. The use of a simple exercise test for the diagnosis of *Pneumocystis carinii*

pneumonia in patients with AIDS. *Am Rev Respir Dis* 139:1343–1346, 1989.

39. Coleman DL, Dodek PM, Golden JA, et al: Correlation between serial pulmonary function tests and fiberoptic bronchoscopy in patients with *Pneumocystis carinii* pneumonia and the acquired immunodeficiency syndrome. *Am Rev Respir Dis* 129:491–493, 1984.

40. Hopewell PC, Luce JM. Pulmonary involvement in the acquired immunodeficiency syndrome. *Chest* 87: 104–112, 1985.

41. Mitchell DM, Fleming J, Pinching AJ, et al: Pulmonary function in human immunodeficiency virus infection. A prospective 18-month study of serial lung function in 474 patients. *Am Rev Respir Dis* 146:745–751, 1992.

42. Chouaid C, Maillard D, Housset B, et al: Cost effectiveness of noninvasive oxygen saturation measurement during exercise for the diagnosis of *Pneumocystis* pneumonia. *Am Rev Respir Dis* 147:1360–1363, 1993.

43. Zaman MK, Wooten OJ, Suprahmanya B, et al: Rapid noninvasive diagnosis of *Pneumocystis carinii* from induced liquefied sputum. *Ann Intern Med* 109:107–110, 1988.

44. Kovacs JA, Ng VL, Masur H, et al: Diagnosis of *Pneumocystis carinii* pneumonia: improved detection in sputum with use of monoclonal antibodies. *N Engl J Med* 318: 589–593, 1988.

45. Keigh TR, Hume C, Gazzard B, et al: Sputum induction for diagnosis of *Pneumocystis carinii* pneumonia. *Lancet* 2:205–206, 1989.

46. O'Brien RF, Quinn JL, Miyahara BT, et al: Diagnosis of *Pneumocystis carinii* pneumonia by induced sputum in a city with moderate incidence of AIDS. *Chest* 95:136–138, 1989.

47. Broaddus C, Dake MD, Stulbarg MS, et al: Bronchoalveolar lavage and transbronchial biopsy for the diagnosis of pulmonary infections in the acquired immunodeficiency syndrome. *Ann Intern Med* 102:747–752, 1985.

48. Golden JA, Hollander H, Stulbarg MS, et al: Bronchoalveolar lavage as the exclusive diagnostic modality for *Pneumocystis carinii* pneumonia. A prospective study among patients with acquired immunodeficiency syndrome. *Chest* 90:18–22, 1986.

49. Meduri Gu, Stover DE, Greeno RA, et al: Bilateral bronchoalveolar lavage in the diagnosis of opportunistic pulmonary infections. *Chest* 100:1272–1276, 1991.

50. Baughman RP, Dohn MN, Frame PT. Preference of *Pneumocystis carinii* for the upper lobes. *Chest* 100:1275, 1991.

51. Stover DE, Zaman MB, Hajdu SI, et al: Bronchoalveolar lavage in the diagnosis of diffuse pulmonary infiltrates in the immunosuppressed host. *Ann Intern Med* 101:1–7, 1984.

52. Martin WR, Ablertson TE, Siegel B. Tracheal catheters in patients with acquired immunodeficiency syndrome for the diagnosis of *Pneumocystis carinii* pneumonia. *Chest* 98:29–32, 1990.

53. Caughey G, Wong H, Gamsu G, et al: Nonbronchoscopic bronchoalveolar lavage for the diagnosis of *Pneumocystis carinii* pneumonia in the acquired immunodeficiency syndrome. *Chest* 88:659–662, 1985.

54. Wallace JM, Batra P, Gong H: Percutaneous needle lung aspiration in patients with AIDS. *Am Rev Respir Dis* 131: 389–392, 1985.

55. Fitzgerald W, Bevelaqua FA, Garay SM, et al: The role

of open lung biopsy in patients with the acquired immunodeficiency syndrome. *Chest* 91:659–661, 1987.

56. Bonfils-Roberts EA, Nickodem A, Nealon TF, et al: Retrospective analysis of the efficacy of open lung biopsy in acquired immunodeficiency syndrome. *Ann Thorac Surg* 49:115–117, 1990.

57. Brenner M, Ognibene FP, Lack EE, et al: Prognostic factors and life expectancy of patients with acquired immunodeficiency syndrome and *Pneumocystis carinii* pneumonia. *Am Rev Respir Dis* 136:1199–1206, 1987.

58. Shelhamer JH, Ognibene FP, Macher AM, et al: Persistence of *Pneumocystis carinii* in lung tissue of acquired immunodeficiency syndrome patients treated for pneumocystis pneumonia. *Am Rev Respir Dis* 130:1661–1665, 1984.

59. Harcup C, Baier HJ, Pitchenik AE: Evaluation of patients with the acquired immunodeficiency syndrome by fiberoptic bronchoscopy. *Endoscopy* 17:217–220, 1985.

60. Sattler FR, Cowan R, Nielsen DM, et al: Trimethoprim-sulfamethoxazole compared with pentamidine for treatment of *Pneumocystis carinii* pneumonia in the acquired immunodeficiency syndrome. A prospective, noncrossover study. *Ann Intern Med* 109:280–287, 1988.

61. Haverkos HW: Assessment of therapy for *Pneumocystis carinii* pneumonia: PCP therapy project group. *Am J Med* 76:501–508, 1984.

62. Wharton Jm, Coleman DL, Wofsy CB, et al : Trimethoprim-sulfamethoxazole or pentamidine for *Pneumocystis carinii* pneumonia in the acquired immunodeficiency syndrome. A prospective trial. *Ann Intern Med* 105:37–44, 1986.

63. Gordin FM, Simon GL, Wofsy CB, et al: Adverse reactions to trimethoprim-sulfamethoxazole in patients with the acquired immunodeficiency syndrome. *Ann Intern Med* 100:495–499, 1984.

64. Waskin H, Stehr-Green JK, Helmick CJ, et al: Risk factors for hypoglycemia associated with pentamidine therapy for *Pneumocystis* pneumonia. *JAMA* 260:345–347, 1988.

65. Montaner JSG, Lawson LM, Levitt N, et al: Corticosteroids prevent early deterioration in patients with moderately severe *Pneumocystis carinii* pneumonia and the acquired immunodeficiency syndrome (AIDS). *Ann Intern Med* 113:14–20, 1990.

66. Clement M, Edison R, Turner J, et al: Corticosteroids as adjunctive therapy in severe *Pneumocystis carinii* pneumonia: a prospective placebo-controlled trial. *Am Rev Respir Dis* 139(Suppl):A250, 1990.

67. Bozzette SA, Sattler FR, Chiu J, et al: A controlled trial of early adjunctive treatment with corticosteroids for *Pneumocystis carinii* pneumonia in the acquired immunodeficiency syndrome. *N Engl J Med* 323:1444–1450, 1990.

68. Gagnon S, Boota AM, Fischl MA, et al: Corticosteroids as adjunctive therapy for severe *Pneumocystis carinii* pneumonia in the acquired immunodeficiency syndrome: a double-blind, placebo controlled trial. *N Engl J Med* 323:1444–1450, 1990.

69. The National Institutes of Health—University of California Expert Panel for Corticosteroids as Adjunctive Therapy for *Pneumocystis* Pneumonia: Consensus statement on the use of corticosteroids as adjunctive therapy for *Pneumocystis* pneumonia in the acquired immunodeficiency syndrome. *N Engl J Med* 323:1500–1504, 1990.

70. Rosen MJ, De Palo VA. Outcome of intensive care for patients with AIDS. *Crit Care Clin* 9:107–114, 1993.

71. Mason GR, Hashimoto CH, Dickman PS, et al: Prognostic implications of bronchoalveolar lavage neutrophilia in patients with *Pneumocystis carinii* pneumonia and AIDS. *Am Rev Respir Dis* 139:1336–1342, 1989.

72. Wachter RM, Russi MB, Bloch DA, et al: *Pneumocystis carinii* pneumonia and respiratory failure in AIDS. *Am Rev Respir Dis* 143:251–256, 1991.

73. Wachter RM, Luce JM, Turner J, et al: Intensive care of patients with the acquired immunodeficiency syndrome: outcome and changing patterns of utilization. *Am Rev Respir Dis* 134:891–896, 1986.

74. Murray JF, Felton CP, Garay SM, et al: Pulmonary complications of the acquired immunodeficiency syndrome: a report of a National Heart Lung and Blood institute workshop. *N Engl J Med* 310:1682–1688, 1984.

75. Peruzzi WT, Shapiro BA, Noskin GA, et al: Concurrent bacterial lung infection in patients with AIDS, PCP and respiratory failure. *Chest* 101:1399–1403, 1992.

76. Gregg RW, Friedman BC, Williams JF, et al: Continuous positive airway pressure by face mask in *Pneumocystis carinii* pneumonia. *Crit Care Med* 18:21–24, 1990.

77. U.S. Public Health Service: Recommendations for prophylaxis against *Pneumocystis carinii* pneumonia for persons infected with human immunodeficiency virus. *J Acquir Immune Defic Syndr* 6:46–55, 1993.

78. Wasserman K, Pothoff G, Kirn E, et al: Chronic *Pneumocystis carinii* pneumonia in AIDS. *Chest* 104:667–672, 1993.

79. Feuerestein IM, Archer A, Pluda JM, et al: Thin-walled cavities, cysts and pneumothorax in *Pneumocystis* pneumonia: further observations with histopathological correlation. *Thorac Radiol* 174:697–702, 1990.

80. Chechani V, Zaman MK, Finch JP: Chronic cavitary *Pneumocystis carinii* pneumonia in a patient with AIDS. *Chest* 95:1347–1348, 1989.

81. Sepkowitz KA, Telzak EE, Gold JM, et al: Pneumothorax in AIDS. *Ann Intern Med* 114:455–459, 1991.

82. Centers for Disease Control. *Mycobacterium tuberculosis* transmission in a health clinic, Florida, 1988. *MMWR* 38:256–258, 1989.

83. Montgomery AB, Corkery KJ, Brunette ER: Occupational exposure to aerosolized pentamidine. *Chest* 89:386–388, 1990.

84. Smaldone GC, Vinciguerra C, Marchese J: Detection of inhaled pentamidine in health care workers. *N Engl J Med* 325:891–892, 1991.

85. Green S, Nathwani D, Christie P, et al: Aerosolized pentamidine. *Lancet* 1:1284, 1989.

86. Doll DC: Aerosolized pentamidine. *Lancet* 1:1284–1285, 1989.

87. Mendelson MH, Finkel LJ, Meyers BR, et al: Pulmonary toxoplasmosis in AIDS. *Scand J Infect Dis* 19:703–706, 1987.

88. Ma P, Villanueva TG, Kaufman D, et al: Respiratory cryptosporidiosis in the acquired immune deficiency syndrome. *JAMA* 252:1298–1301, 1984.

89. Polsky B, Gold JWM, Whimbey E, et al: Bacterial pneumonia in patients with acquired immunodeficiency syndrome. *Ann Intern Med* 104:38–41, 1986.

90. Witt DJ, Craven DE, McCabe WR: Bacterial infections

in adult patients with the acquired immune deficiency syndrome (AIDS) and AIDS-related complex. *Am J Med* 82:900–906, 1987.

91. Simberkoff MS, El Sadr W, Schiffman G, et al: *Streptococcus pneumoniae* infections and bacteremia in patients with acquired immunodeficiency syndrome, with report of pneumococcal vaccine failure. *Am Rev Respir Dis* 130:1174–1176, 1984.

92. Sudre P, ten Dam G, Kochi A: Tuberculosis: a global overview of the situation today. *Bull WHO* 70(2):149–159, 1992.

93. Raviglione MC, Narain JP, Kochi A: HIV-associated tuberculosis in developing countries: clinical features, diagnosis, and treatment. *Bull WHO* 70(4):515–526, 1992.

94. De Cock KM, Soro B, Coulibaly IM, et al: Tuberculosis and HIV infection in sub-Saharan Africa. *JAMA* 268:1581–1587, 1992.

95. Centers for Disease Control: Tuberculosis morbidity—United States, 1992. *MMWR* 42:696–697,703–704, 1993.

96. Barnes PF, Bloch AB, Davison PT, et al: Tuberculosis in patients with human immunodeficiency virus infection. *N Engl J Med* 324:1645–1650, 1991.

97. Onorato IM, McCray E, Field Services Branch: Prevalence of human immunodeficiency virus infection among patients attending tuberculosis clinics in the United States. *J Infect Dis* 165:87–92, 1992.

98. Barnes PF, Le HQ, Davidson PT: Tuberculosis in patients with HIV infection. *Med Clin North Am* 77(6):1369–1390, 1993.

99. Handwerger S, Mildvan D, Senie R, et al: Tuberculosis and the acquired immunodeficiency syndrome at a New York City hospital: 1978–1985. *Chest* 91:176–180, 1987.

100. Daley CL, Small PM, Schecter GF, et al: An outbreak of tuberculosis with accelerated progression among persons infected with the human immunodeficiency virus. An analysis using restriction-fragment-length-polymorphisms. *N Engl J Med* 326:231–235, 1992.

101. Narain JP, Raviglione MC, Kochi A: HIV-associated tuberculosis in developing countries: epidemiology and strategies for prevention. *WHO/TB/92* 164:1–23, 1992.

102. Selwyn PA, Sckell BM, Alcabes P, et al: High risk of active tuberculosis in HIV-infected drug users with cutaneous anergy. *JAMA* 268:504–509, 1992.

103. Centers for Disease Control: Tuberculosis and human immunodeficiency virus infection: Recommendations of the Advisory Committee for the Elimination of Tuberculosis (ACET). *MMWR* 38:236–250, 1989.

104. Jones BE, Young SMM, Antoniskis D, et al: Relationship of the manifestations of tuberculosis to CD4 cell counts in patients with human immunodeficiency virus infection. *Am Rev Respir Dis* 148:1292–1297, 1993.

105. Centers for Disease Control: Purified protein derivative (PPD) — Tuberculin anergy and HIV infection: guidelines for anergy testing and management of anergic persons at risk of tuberculosis. *MMWR* 40:27–33, 1991.

106. Centers for Disease Control: Initial therapy for tuberculosis in the era of multidrug resistance: Recommendations of the Advisory Council for the Elimination of Tuberculosis. *MMWR* 42(RR-7):1–8, 1993.

107. Centers for Disease Control: Nosocomial transmission of multidrug-resistant tuberculosis among HIV-infected persons—Florida and New York, 1988–1991. *MMWR* 40(34):585–591, 1991.

108. Fischl MA, Daikos GL, Uttamchandani RB, et al: Clinical presentation and outcome of patients with HIV infection and tuberculosis caused by multiple-drug-resistant bacilli. *Ann Intern Med* 117:184–190, 1992.

109. Centers for Disease Control: Transmission of multidrug-resistant tuberculosis among immunocompromised persons in a correctional system—New York. *MMWR* 41:507, 1991.

110. Small PM, Schecter GF, Goodman PC, et AL: Treatment of tuberculosis in patients with advanced human immunodeficiency infection. *N Engl J Med* 324:289–294, 1991.

111. Theuer CP, Hopewell PC, Elias D, et al: Human immunodeficiency virus infection in tuberculosis patients. *J Infect Dis* 162:8–12, 1990.

112. Chaisson RE, Schecter GF, Theuer CP, et al: Tuberculosis in patients with the acquired immunodeficiency syndrome: clinical features, response to therapy, and survival. *Am Rev Respir Dis* 136:570–574, 1987.

113. Kramer F, Modilevsky T, Waliany AR, et al: Delayed diagnosis of tuberculosis in patients with human immunodeficiency virus infection. *Am J Med* 89:451–456, 1990.

114. Sunderam G, McDonald RJ, Maniatis T, et al: Tuberculosis as a manifestation of the acquired immunodeficiency syndrome (AIDS). *JAMA* 256:362–366, 1986.

115. Radin DR: Intraabdominal *Mycobacterium tuberculosis* vs *Mycobacterium avium intracellulare* infection in patients with AIDS: distinction based on CT findings. *AJR* 156:487–491, 1991.

116. Pitchenik AE, Burr J, Suarez M, et al: Human T-cell lymphotropic virus-III (HTLV-III) seropositivity and related disease among 71 consecutive patients in whom tuberculosis was diagnosed. A prospective study. *Am Rev Respir Dis* 135:875–879, 1987.

117. Pitchenik AE. Tuberculosis control and the AIDS epidemic in developing countries. *Ann Intern Med* 113:89–91, 1990.

118. Pitchenik AE, Rubinson HA. The radiographic appearance of tuberculosis in patients with the acquired immune deficiency syndrome (AIDS) and pre-AIDS. *Am Rev Respir Dis* 131:393–396, 1985.

119. Modilevsky T, Sattler FR, Barnes PF. Mycobacterial disease in patients with human immunodeficiency virus infection. *Arch Intern Med* 149:2201–2205, 1989.

120. Kennedy DJ, Lewis WP, Barnes PF: Yield of bronchoscopy for the diagnosis of tuberculosis in patients with human immunodeficiency infection. *Chest* 102:1040–1044, 1992.

121. Hewlett D Jr, Duncanson FP, Jagadha V, et al: Lymphadenopathy in an inner-city population consisting principally of intravenous drug abusers with suspected acquired immunodeficiency syndrome. *Am Rev Respir Dis* 137:1275–1279, 1988.

122. Barnes PF, Barrows SA: Tuberculosis in the 1990s. *Ann Intern Med* 119:400–410, 1993.

123. Iseman MD: Treatment of multidrug-resistant tuberculosis. *N Engl J Med* 329:784–791, 1993.

124. Centers for Disease Control: The use of preventive therapy for tuberculosis infection in the United States: recommendations of the Advisory Committee for Elimination of Tuberculosis. *MMWR* 39:9–12, 1990.

125. American Thoracic Society: Treatment of tuberculosis and tuberculosis infection in adults and children. *Am Rev Respir Dis* 134:355–363, 1986.

126. Centers for Disease Control: National action plan to

combat multidrug-resistant tuberculosis; meeting the challenge of multidrug-resistant tuberculosis: summary of a conference; management of persons exposed to multidrug-resistant tuberculosis. *MMWR* 41(RR 41): 1–71, 1992.

127. Kirschner RA, Parker BC, Falkingham JO III: Epidemiology of infection with nontuberculous mycobacteria. *Am Rev Respir Dis* 145:271–275, 1992.

128. Edwards LB, Acquaviva FA, Livesay VT, et al: An atlas of sensitivity to tuberculin, PPD-B and histoplasmin in the United States. *Am Rev Respir Dis* 19:1–132, 1969.

129. Wolinsky E: Nontuberculous mycobacteria and associated diseases. *Am Rev Respir Dis* 119:107–159, 1979.

130. Horsburgh CR Jr: *Mycobacterium avium* complex infection in the acquired immunodeficiency syndrome. *N Engl J Med* 19:1332–1337.

131. Chaisson RE, Moore RD, Richman DD, et al: Incidence and natural history of *Mycobacterium avium* complex infections in patients with advanced human immunodeficiency virus disease treated with zidovudine. *Am Rev Respir Dis* 148:285–289, 1992.

132. Nightingale SD, Byrd LT, Southern PM, et al: Incidence of *Mycobacterium avium* complex bacteremia in human immunodeficiency virus-positive patients. *J Infect Dis* 165:1082–1085, 1992.

133. Wallace JM, Hannah JB: *Mycobacterium avium* complex infection in patients with the acquired immunodeficiency syndrome: a clinicopathologic study. *Chest* 93: 926–932, 1988.

134. Horsburgh CR, Metchock BG, McGowan JE Jr, et al: Clinical implications of recovery of *Mycobacterium avium* complex from the stool or respiratory tract of HIV-infected individuals. *AIDS* 6:512–514, 1992.

135. Inderlied CB, Kemper CA, Bermudez LE: The *Mycobacterium avium* complex. *Clin Microbiol Rev* 6:266–310, 1993.

136. Havlik JA Jr, Horsburgh CR Jr, Metchock B, et al: Disseminated *Mycobacterium avium* complex infection: clinical identification and epidemiologic trends. *J Infect Dis* 165:577–580, 1992.

137. Nyberg DA, Federle MP, Jeffrey RB, et al: Abdominal CT findings of disseminated *Mycobacterium avium-intracellulare* in AIDS. *Am J Radiol* 145:297–299, 1985.

138. Masur H and the Public Health Service Task Force on Prophylaxis and Therapy for *Mycobacterium avium* Complex: Recommendations on prophylaxis and therapy for disseminated *Mycobacterium avium* complex disease in patients infected with the human immunodeficiency virus. *N Engl J Med* 329:898–904, 1993.

139. Nightingale SD, Cameron W, Gordin FM, et al: Two controlled trials of rifabutin prophylaxis against *Mycobacterium avium* complex infection in AIDS. *N Engl J Med* 329:828–833, 1993.

140. Levine B, Chaisson RE: *Mycobacterium kansasii*: a cause of treatable pulmonary disease associated with advanced human immunodeficiency virus (HIV) infection. *Ann Intern Med* 114:861–868, 1991.

141. Hirasuna JD: Disseminated *Mycobacterium kansasii* infection in the acquired immunodeficiency syndrome (AIDS). *Ann Intern Med* 107:784, 1987.

142. Jacobson MA, Mills J: Serious cytomegalovirus disease in the acquired immunodeficiency syndrome (AIDS). *Ann Intern Med* 108:585–594, 1988.

143. Schooley RT: Cytomegalovirus in the setting of infection with human immunodeficiency virus. *Rev Infect Dis* 12: S811–S819, 1990.

144. Millar AB, Patou G, Miller RF, et al: Cytomegalovirus in the lungs of patients with AIDS. *Am Rev Respir Dis* 141:1474–1477, 1990.

145. Bower M, Barton SE, Nelson MR, et al: The significance of the detection of cytomegalovirus in the bronchoalveolar lavage fluid in AIDS patients with pneumonia. *AIDS* 4:317–320, 1990.

146. Drew Wl, Buhles W, Erlich KS: Management of herpes virus infections (CMV, HSV, VZV). In Sande MA (ed): *The Medical Management of AIDS*, ed 3. Philadelphia, WB Saunders, 1992, pp 359–382.

147. Cohen PR, Beltrani VP, Grossman ME: Disseminated herpes zoster in patients with human immunodeficiency virus infection. *Am J Med* 84:1076–1080, 1988.

148. Pappas PG, Pottage JC, Powderly WG, et al: Blastomycosis in patients with the acquired immunodeficiency syndrome. *Ann Intern Med* 116:847–853, 1992.

149. Supparatpinyo K, Chiewchanvit S, Hirunsri P, et al: *Penicillium marneffei* infection in patients infected with human immunodeficiency virus. *Clin Infect Dis* 14: 871–874, 1992.

150. Denning DW, Follansbee SE, Scolaro M, et al: Pulmonary aspergillosis in the acquired immunodeficiency syndrome. *N Engl J Med* 324:654–662, 1991.

151. Littman ML, Walter JE: Cryptococcosis: current status. *Am J Med* 45:922–932, 1968.

152. Diamond RD: *Cryptococcus neoformans*. In Mandel GL (ed): *Principles and Practice of Infectious Diseases*. New York, Churchill Livingstone, 1990.

153. Zuger A, Louie E, Holzman RS, et al: Cryptococcal disease in patients with the acquired immunodeficiency syndrome. *Ann Intern Med* 104:234–240, 1986.

154. Chuck SL, Sande M: Infections with *Cryptococcus neoformans* in the acquired immunodeficiency syndrome. *N Engl J Med* 321:794–799, 1989.

155. Gal AA, Koss MN, Hawkins J, et al: The pathology of pulmonary cryptococcal infections in the acquired immunodeficiency syndrome. *Arch Pathol Lab Med* 110: 502–507, 1986.

156. Cameron ML, Bartless J, Gallis HA, et al: Manifestations of pulmonary cryptococcosis in patients with acquired immunodeficiency syndrome. *Rev Infect Dis* 13:64–67, 1991.

157. Chechani V, Kamholz S: Pulmonary manifestations of disseminated cryptococcosis in patients with AIDS. *Chest* 98:1060–1066, 1989.

158. Wasser L, Talavera W. Pulmonary cryptococcosis in AIDS. *Chest* 92:692–695, 1987.

159. Clark RA, Greer DL, Valainis GT, et al: *Cryptococcus neoformans* pulmonary infection in HIV-1-infected patients. *J Acquir Immune Defic Syndr* 3:480–484, 1990.

160. Miller WT Jr, Edelman J, Miller WT: Cryptococcal pulmonary infection in patients with AIDS: radiographic appearance. *Radiology* 175:725–728, 1990.

161. Kovacs JA, Kovacs AA, Polis M, et al: Cryptococcosis in the acquired immunodeficiency syndrome. *Ann Intern Med* 103:533–538, 1985.

162. Stansell JD, Sande MA: Cryptococcal infection in AIDS. In Sande MA (ed): *The Medical Management of AIDS*, ed 3. Philadelphia, WB Saunders, 1992.

163. Bozette SA, Larsen RA, Chiu J, et al: A placebo-controlled trial of maintenance therapy with fluconazole

after treatment of cryptococcal meningitis in the acquired immunodeficiency syndrome. *N Engl J Med* 324: 580–584, 1991.

164. Medoff G, Kobayashi GS: Systemic fungal infections: an overview. *Hosp Pract* 26:41–52, 1991.

165. Wheat LJ, Slama TG, Norton JA, et al: Risk factors for disseminated or fatal histoplasmosis. *Ann Intern Med* 96:159–163, 1982.

166. Wheat LJ, Connolly-Stringfield PA, Baker RL, et al: Disseminated histoplasmosis in AIDS: clinical findings, diagnosis and treatment, and review of the literature. *Medicine* 69:361–374, 1990.

167. McKinsey DS, Driks MR: Histoplasmosis in HIV Disease. *AIDS Read* 3:203–209, 1993.

168. Johnson PC, Khardori N, Najjar A, et al: Progressive disseminated histoplasmosis in patients with AIDS. *Am J Med* 85:152–158, 1988.

169. Sarosi GA, Johnson PC: Disseminated histoplasmosis in patients infected with human immunodeficiency virus. *Clin Infect Dis* 14(Suppl 1):S60–S67, 1992.

170. Kurtin PK, Mc Kinsey DS, Gupta MR, et al: Histoplasmosis in patients with AIDS: hematologic and bone marrow manifestations. *Am J Clin Pathol* 93:367–372, 1990.

171. McKinsey DS: Histoplasmosis in patients with human immunodeficiency virus infection. *J Mycol Med* 2(Suppl 1):23–34, 1992.

172. Salzman SH, Smith RL, Aranda CP: Histoplasmosis in patients at risk for the acquired immunodeficiency syndrome in a nonendemic setting. *Chest* 93:916–921, 1988.

173. McKinsey DS, Gupta MR, Riddler SA, et al: Long-term amphotericin B therapy for disseminated histoplasmosis in patients with the acquired immunodeficiency syndrome (AIDS). *Ann Intern Med* 111:655–659, 1989.

174. Wheat LJ, Hafner RE, Wulfsohn M, et al: Prevention of relapse of histoplasmosis with itraconazole in patients with the acquired immunodeficiency syndrome. *Ann Intern Med* 118:610–616, 1993.

175. Stevens DA: *Coccidioides immitis.* In Mandell GL (ed). *Principles and Practice of Infectious Diseases,* ed 3. New York. Churchill Livingstone, 1990.

176. Fish DG, Ampel NM, Galgiani JN, et al: Coccidioidomycosis during human immunodeficiency virus infection. A review of 77 patients. *Medicine* 69:384–391, 1990.

177. Bronnimann DA, Adam RD, Galgiani JN, et al: Coccidioidomycosis in the acquired immunodeficiency syndrome. *Ann Intern Med* 106:372–379, 1987.

178. Galgiani JN, Ampel NM: Coccidioidomycosis in human immunodeficiency virus-infected patients. *J Infect Dis* 162:1165–1169, 1990.

179. Denning DW: Invasive aspergillosis, coccidioidomycosis and penicilliosis. In: *Management of Emerging Fungal Infections in AIDS.* Symposium from the University of Alabama School of Medicine. Bayside, New York, Reiss Consultants, 1993.

180. Ensoli, B, Barillari, G, Gallo, RC. Pathogenesis of AIDS-associated Kaposi's sarcoma. *Hematol/Oncol Clin North Am* 5;281–285, 1991.

181. Jaffe H, Bregman K, Selik RM: The first 100 cases of acquired immunodeficiency syndrome in the United States. *J Infect Dis* 148:339–345, 1983.

182. Des Jarlais DC, Stoneburner R, Thomas P, Friedman SR. Declines in proportion of Kaposi's sarcoma among cases of AIDS in multiple risk groups in New York City. *Lancet* 2:1024–1025, 1987.

183. Auerbach HE, Brooks JJ. Kaposi's sarcoma: observation and a hypothesis. *Lab Invest* 52:44–46, 1985.

184. Brooks JJ: Kaposi's sarcoma: a reversible hyperplasia. *Lancet* 2:1309–1311, 1986.

185. Costa J, Rabson AS: Generalized Kaposi's sarcoma is not a neoplasm. *Lancet* 1:58, 1983.

186. Beral V, Peterman TA, Berkelman RL: Kaposi's sarcoma among persons with AIDS: a sexually transmitted infection? *Lancet* 1:123, 1990.

187. Rabkin CS, Biggar RJ, Horm JW: Increasing incidence of cancers associated with the human immunodeficiency virus epidemic. *Int J Cancer* 5:692–696, 1991.

188. Niedt GW, Schinella RA. Acquired immunodeficiency syndrome: a clinicopathologic study of 56 autopsies. *Arch Pathol Lab Med* 109:727–734, 1985.

189. Meduri GU, Stover DE, Lee M, Myskowski PL, Caravelli JF, Zaman MB. Pulmonary Kaposi's sarcoma in the acquired immune deficiency syndrome. *Am J Med* 81: 11–18, 1986.

190. Lemlich G, Schwam L, Lebohl M. Kaposi's sarcoma and acquired immunodeficiency syndrome. Postmortem findings in twenty four cases. *J Am Acad Dermatol* 16: 319–325, 1987.

191. Friedman-Kien AE. Disseminated Kaposi's sarcoma syndrome in young homosexual men. *J Am Acad Derm* 5:468–471, 1981.

192. Gotlieb GJ, Ackerman AB: Kaposi's sarcoma: an extensively disseminated form in young homosexual men. *Hum Pathol* 13:882–892, 1982.

193. McNutt NS, Fletcher V, Conant MA: Early lesion of Kaposi's sarcoma in homosexual men. An ultrastructural comparison with other vascular proliferations in the skin. *Am J Pathol* 111:62–77, 1983.

194. Ognibene FP, Steis RG, Macher AM, et al: Kaposi's sarcoma causing pulmonary infiltrates and respiratory failure in the acquired immunodeficiency syndrome. *Ann Intern Med* 102:471–475, 1985.

195. Stover DE, White DA, Romano PA: Diagnosis of pulmonary disease in acquired immune deficiency syndrome (AIDS): role of bronchoscopy and bronchoalveolar lavage. *Am Rev Respir Dis* 130:659–662, 1984.

196. Zibrak JD, Silvestri RC, Costello P: Bronchoscopic and radiologic features of Kaposi's sarcoma involving the respiratory system. *Chest* 90:476–479, 1986.

197. Fouret PJ, Touboul JL, Mayaud CM, et al: Pulmonary Kaposi's sarcoma in patients with acquired immune deficiency syndrome: a clinicopathological study. *Thorax* 42:262–268, 1987.

198. Gill PS, Akil B, Colletti P, et al: Pulmonary Kaposi's sarcoma: clinical findings and results of therapy. *Am J Med* 87:57–61, 1989.

199. O'Brien RF, Cohn DL: Serosanguinous pleural effusions in AIDS-associated Kaposi's sarcoma. *Chest* 96: 460–466, 1989.

200. Garay SM, Belenko M, Fazzini E, et al: Pulmonary manifestations of Kaposi's sarcoma. *Chest* 91:39–43, 1987.

201. Kaplan LD, Hopewell PC, Jaffe H, et al: Kaposi's sarcoma involving the lung in patients with the acquired immunodeficiency syndrome. *J Acquir Immune Defic Syndr* 1:23–30, 1988.

202. Sivit Cj, Schwartz AM, Rockoff SD: Kaposi's sarcoma

of the lung in AIDS: radiologic-pathologic analysis. *Am J Radiol* 148:25–28, 1987.

203. Kramer EL, Sanger JH, Garay SM: Gallium-67 scans of the chest in patients with acquired immunodeficiency syndrome. *J Nucl Med* 28:1107–1114, 1987.

204. Woolfenden JM, Carrasquillo JA, Larson SM: Acquired immunodeficiency syndrome: Ga-67 citrate imaging. *Radiology* 162:383–387, 1987.

205. Au JP, Krauthammer M, Lau KY: Kaposi's sarcoma presenting with endobronchial lesions. *Heart Lung* 15:411–413, 1986.

206. Pitchenik AE, Fischl MA, Saldana MJ: Kaposi's sarcoma of the tracheobronchial tree: clinical, bronchoscopic, and pathologic features. *Chest* 87:122–124, 1985.

207. Nathan S, Vaghaiwalla R, Mohsenifar Z: Use of ND: YAG laser in endobronchial Kaposi's sarcoma. *Chest* 98:1299–1300, 1990.

208. White DA, Matthay RA: Noninfectious pulmonary complications of infection with the human immunodeficiency virus. *Am Rev Respir Dis* 140:1763–1787, 1989.

209. Stover DE, White DA, Romano PA, Gellene RA, Robeson WA: Spectrum of pulmonary diseases associated with the acquired immune deficiency syndrome. *Am J Med* 78:429–437, 1985.

210. Stover DE, Greeno RA, Gagliardi AJ: The use of a simple exercise test for the diagnosis of *Pneumocystis carinii* pneumonia in patients with AIDS. *Am Rev Respir Dis* 139:1343–1346, 1989.

211. Zaman MK, White DA: Serum lactate dehydrogenase levels and *Pneumocystis carinii* pneumonia. *Am Rev Respir Dis* 19:796–800, 1988.

212. Alcalay J, Grossman E, Sandbank M, et al: Increased levels of angiotensin-converting enzyme activity in Kaposi's sarcoma. *J Am Acad Dermatol* 19:911–912, 1988.

213. Northfelt DW, Kahn JO, Volberding PA: Treatment of AIDS-related Kaposi's sarcoma. *Hematol/Oncol Clin* 5:297–310, 1991.

214. Gil PS, Akil B, Colletti P, Rarick M, et al: Pulmonary Kaposi's sarcoma: clinical findings and results of therapy. *Am J Med* 87:57–61, 1989.

215. Nobler MP: Pulmonary irradiation for Kaposi's sarcoma in AIDS. *Am J Clin Oncol* 8:441, 1985.

216. Krown SE, Myskowski PL, Paredes J: Management of Kaposi's sarcoma in HIV-infected patients. *Med Clin North Am* 76:235–252, 1992.

217. Kahn JO, Kaplan LD, Volberding PA, et al: Intralesional recombinant tumor necrosis factor-alpha for AIDS-associated Kaposi's sarcoma: a randomized, double blind trial. *J Acquir Immune Defic Syndr* 2:217, 1989.

218. Kaplan MH, Susin M, Pahwa SG, et al: Neoplastic complications of HTLV-III infection. Lymphomas and solid tumors. *Am J Med* 82:389–396, 1987.

219. Beral V, Peterman T, Berkelman R, et al: AIDS-associated non-Hodgkin's lymphoma. *Lancet* 337:805–809, 1991.

220. Rapheal BG, Knowles DM: Acquired immunodeficiency syndrome–associated non-Hodgkin's lymphoma. *Semin Oncol* 17:361–366, 1990.

221. Gail MH, Pluda JM, Rabkin CS: Projections of the incidence of non-Hodgkin's lymphoma to acquired immunodeficiency syndrome. *JNCI* 83:695–701, 1991.

222. Meeker TC, Shiranizu B, Kaplan L, et al: Evidence for molecular subtypes of HIV-associated lymphoma: division into peripheral monoclonal, polyclonal and central nervous system lymphoma. *AIDS* 5:669–674, 1991.

223. Levine AM: Epidemiology, clinical characteristics, and management of AIDS-related lymphoma. *Hematol/Oncol Clin North Am* 5:331–342, 1991.

224. Kaplan LD, Abrams DI, Feigal E, et al: AIDS-associated non-Hodgkin's lymphoma in San Francisco. *JAMA* 261:719–724, 1989.

225. Knowles DM, Chamulak GA, Subar M, et al: Lymphoid neoplasia associated with acquired immunodeficiency syndrome (AIDS). *Ann Intern Med* 108:744–753, 1988.

226. Sider L, Weiss AJ, Smith MD, et al: Varied appearance of AIDS-related lymphoma in the chest. *Radiology* 171:629–632, 1989.

227. Loureiro C, Gill PS, Meyer PR, et al: Autopsy findings in AIDS-related lymphoma. *Cancer* 62:735–739, 1988.

228. Marchevsky A, Rosen MJ, Chrystal G, et al: Pulmonary complications of the acquired immunodeficiency syndrome: a clinicopathologic study of 70 cases *Hum Pathol* 16:659–670, 1985.

229. Polish LB, Cohn DL, Ryder JW, et al: Pulmonary non-Hodgkin's lymphoma in AIDS. *Chest* 96:1321–1326, 1989.

230. Sider L, Horton ES. Pleural effusion as a presentation of AIDS-related lymphoma. *Invest Radiol* 24:150–153, 1989.

231. Poelzleitner D, Huebsch P, Mayerhofer S, et al: Primary pulmonary lymphoma in a patient with acquired immune deficiency syndrome. *Thorax* 44:438–439, 1989.

232. Walts AE, Shintaku IP, Said JW: Diagnosis of malignant lymphoma in effusions from patients with AIDS by gene rearrangement. *Am J Clin Pathol* 94:170–175, 1990.

233. Levine AM: AIDS-associated lymphoma. *Med Clin North Am* 76:253–268, 1992.

234. Lowenthal DA, Straus DJ, Campbell SW, et al: AIDS-related lymphoid neoplasia: the Memorial Hospital experience. *Cancer* 61:2325–2337, 1988.

235. Biggar RJ, Burnett W, Mikl J, et al: Cancer among New York men at risk of acquired immunodeficiency syndrome. *Int J Cancer* 43:979–985, 1989.

236. Sridhar KS, Flores MR, Raub WA, et al: Lung cancer in patients with human immunodeficiency virus infection compared with historic control subjects. *Chest* 102:1704–1708, 1992.

237. Tenholder MF, Jackson HD: Bronchogenic carcinoma in patients seropositive for human immunodeficiency virus. *Chest* 104:1049–1053, 1993.

238. Liebow AA, Carrington CB: Diffuse pulmonary lymphoreticular infiltrates associated with dysproteinemia. *Med Clin North Am* 57:809–843, 1992.

239. Montes M, Tomasi TB, Noehren TH, et al: Lymphoid interstitial pneumonia with monoclonal gammopathy. *Am Rev Respir Dis* 98:277–280, 1968.

240. Strimlan CV, Rosenow EC, Weiland LH, et al: Lymphocytic interstitial pneumonitis. *Ann Intern Med* 78:429–437, 1978.

241. Jason J, Stehr-Green J, Holman R, et al: Human immunodeficiency virus infection in hemophilic children. *Pediatrics* 82:565–570, 1988.

242. Pizzo PA, Eddy J, Faloon J: Acquired immune deficiency syndrome in children. *Am J Med* 85(Suppl 2A):195–202, 1988.

243. Scott GB, Hutto C, Makuch RW, et al: Survival in children with perinatally acquired human immunodeficiency virus type I infection. *N Engl J Med* 321:1791–1796, 1989.

244. Joshi VV, Oleske JM, Minnefor AB, et al: Pathology of

suspected acquired immune deficiency syndrome in children: a study of eight cases. *Pediatr Pathol* 2:71–87, 1984.

245. Joshi VV, Oleske JM, Minnefor AB, et al: Pathologic pulmonary findings in children with the acquired immunodeficiency syndrome: A study of 10 cases. *Human Pathol* 16:241–246, 1985.

246. Morris JC, Rosen MJ, Marchevsky A, et al: Lymphocytic interstitial pneumonia in patients at risk for the acquired immune deficiency syndrome. *Chest* 91:63–67, 1987.

247. Andiman WA, Martin K, Rubinstein A, et al: Opportunistic lymphoproliferations associated with Epstein-Barr viral DNA in infants and children with AIDS. *Lancet* 2: 1390–1393, 1985.

248. Grieco MH, Chinoy-Acharya P: Lymphocytic interstitial pneumonia associated with the acquired immune deficiency syndrome. *Am Rev Respir Dis* 131:952–955, 1985.

249. Resnick L, Pitchenik AE, Fisher E, et al: Detection of HTLV -III/LAV-specific IgG and antigen in bronchoalveolar lavage fluid from two patients with lymphocytic interstitial pneumonitis associated with AIDS-related complex. *Am J Med* 82:553–556, 1987.

250. Ziza JM, Brun-Vezinet F, Venet A, et al: Lymphadenopathy-associated virus isolated with lymphoid interstitial pneumonitis. *N Engl J Med* 313:183, 1985.

251. Oldham SAA, Castillo M, Jacobson FL, et al: HIV-associated lymphocytic interstitial pneumonia: radiologic manifestations and pathologic correlations. *Radiology* 170:83–87, 1989.

252. Rubinstein A, Morecki R, Silverman B, et al: Pulmonary disease in children with acquired immune deficiency syndrome and AIDS-related complex. *J Pediatr* 108: 498–503, 1986.

253. Solal-Celigny P, Couderc LJ, Herman D, et al: Lymphoid interstitial pneumonitis in acquired immunodeficiency syndrome–related complex. *Am Rev Respir Dis* 131:956–960, 1985.

254. Bach MC: Zidovudine for lymphocytic interstitial pneumonia associated with AIDS. *Lancet* 2:655–661, 1987.

255. Rubinstein A, Berstein LJ, Charytan M, et al: Corticosteroid treatment for pulmonary lymphoid hyperplasia in children with the acquired immunodeficiency syndrome. *Pediatr Pulmonol* 4:13–17, 1988.

256. Principi N, Marchislo P, Massironi E, et al: Effect of zidovudine in HIV-infected children with lymphocyte interstitial pneumonitis. *AIDS* 5:468–469, 1991.

257. Ramaswamy G, Jagadha V, Tchertoff V: Diffuse alveolar damage and interstitial fibrosis in acquired immunodeficiency patients without concurrent pulmonary infection. *Arch Pathol Lab Med* 109:408–412, 1985.

258. Ognibene FP, Masur H, Rogers P, et al: Nonspecific interstitial pneumonitis without evidence of *Pneumocystis carinii* in asymptomatic patients infected with human immunodeficiency virus. *Ann Intern Med* 109:874–879, 1988.

259. Suffredini AF, Ognibene FP, Lack EE, et al: Nonspecific interstitial pneumonitis: a common cause of pulmonary disease in the acquired immunodeficiency syndrome. *Ann Intern Med* 107:7–13, 1987.

260. Longworth DL, Spech TJ, Ahmad M, et al: Lymphocytic alveolitis in primary HIV infection. *Cleve Clin J Med* 57: 379–382, 1990.

261. Guillon JM, Autran B, Denis M, et al: Human immunodeficiency virus-related lymphocytic alveolitis. *Chest* 94: 1264–1270, 1988.

262. Coplan NL, Shimony RY, Ioachim HL, et al: Primary pulmonary hypertension associated with human immunodeficiency viral infection. *Am J Med* 89:96–99, 1990.

263. Polos PG, Wolfe D, Harley RA, et al: Pulmonary hypertension and immunodeficiency virus infection. Two reports and a review of the literature. *Chest* 101:474–478, 1992.

# Chapter 18

# Diseases of the Pleura, Mediastinum, Chest Wall, and Diaphragm

## Richard W. Light

## DISEASES OF THE PLEURA

THE PLEURAL SPACE is not really a space but rather a potential space between the lung and chest wall. It is a crucial feature of the breathing apparatus, since it serves as a coupling system between the lung and chest wall. There is normally a very thin layer of fluid (from 2 to 10 $\mu$m thick) between the two pleural surfaces. The pleural space and the fluid within it are not under static conditions. During each respiratory cycle the pleural pressures and the geometry of the pleural space fluctuate widely. Fluid constantly enters and leaves the pleural space. In this section are discussed the anatomy and physiology of the pleural space, as well as the etiology, diagnosis, and treatment of various diseases that affect it.

### ANATOMY OF THE PLEURAL SPACE

The serous membrane covering the lung parenchyma is called the *visceral pleura*. The remainder of the lining of the pleural cavity is designated the *parietal pleura*. The parietal pleura includes the diaphragmatic pleura, the mediastinal pleura, and the costal pleura, which cover the diaphragm, mediastinum, and thoracic skeleton, respectively. The visceral pleura and the parietal pleura meet at the lung root.

The parietal pleura receives its blood supply from the systemic capillaries. The visceral pleura is supplied predominantly by branches of the bronchial artery in humans and in large animals with thick visceral pleura such as sheep or horses (1). The lymphatic vessels in the parietal pleura are in direct communication with the pleural space by means of stomas (2). These stomas are the only route through which cells and large particles can leave the pleural space and are the primary route through which liquid exits the pleural space. Although there are abundant lymphatics in the visceral pleural, these lymphatics do not appear to participate in the removal of particulate matter from the pleural space.

## PHYSIOLOGY OF THE PLEURAL SPACE

Fluid can enter the pleural space from the capillaries in the parietal or visceral pleura or from the interstitial spaces or lymphatics in either pleural surface. The passage of protein-free liquid across the pleural membranes is dependent on the hydrostatic and oncotic pressures across them (Fig. 18.1). When the capillaries in the parietal pleura are considered, it can be seen that the net hydrostatic pressure favoring the movement of fluid from these capillaries to the pleural space is the systemic capillary pressure (28 cm $H_2O$) minus the negative pleural pressure ($-5$ cm $H_2O$), or 33 cm $H_2O$. Opposing this is the oncotic pressure in the blood (30 cm $H_2O$) minus the oncotic pressure in the pleural fluid (4 cm $H_2O$), or 26 cm $H_2O$. The resulting net pressure differences of 7 cm $H_2O$ (33 − 26) favors movement of fluid from the parietal pleura into the pleural space.

The only difference between the visceral and the parietal pleura in the scheme outlined in Figure 18.1 is that the capillaries of the visceral pleura have a slightly lower hydrostatic pressure because they drain into the low-pressure pulmonary veins. The net force across the visceral pleura is 2 cm $H_2O$, again favoring the formation of pleural fluid.

In recent years it has become apparent that the origin of much pleural fluid is the interstitial spaces of the lung. The pleural membranes are leaky to both liquid and protein (3). The pleural pressure is lower than the interstitial pressure, and this pressure difference produces a gradient for fluid to move from the interstitium to the pleural space (4). When the acute respiratory distress syndrome is induced in sheep with the intravenous injection of oleic acid, 20% of the edema fluid exits the lung via the pleural space (5). When high-pressure pulmonary edema is induced in sheep with fluid overload, again about 20% of the edema fluid is cleared via the pleural space (6). In the clinical situation, patients with heart failure are much more likely to have pleural effusions if there is radiologic evidence of pulmonary edema (7).

The rate of pleural fluid formation in normal animals with thick pleura is approximately 0.01 ml/kg/hour or 15 ml per 24 hours for a 60-kg individual. There is a small amount of protein in this fluid. Normally, the pleural space is maintained nearly fluid free because the filtered fluid is removed from the pleural space by the pleural lymphatics, which can remove over 0.20 ml/kg/hour (8). Pleural fluid will accumulate, producing a pleural effusion when the rate of pleural fluid formation exceeds the capacity of the lymphatics in the parietal pleura to remove the fluid.

## PLEURAL EFFUSIONS

### Pathophysiology

Pleural fluid will accumulate when the rate of pleural fluid formation is greater than the rate of pleural fluid removal by the lymphatics. Pleural fluid will continue to accumulate until another equilibrium is reached. Pleural effusions have classically been divided into transudative and exudative pleural effusions. A transudative pleural effusion occurs when alterations in the systemic factors that influence pleural fluid movement result in a pleural effusion. Examples are increased pulmonary interstitial fluid and elevated visceral pleural capillary pressure with left heart failure, elevated parietal pleural capillary pressure with right heart failure, and decreased serum oncotic pressure with the nephrotic syndrome. In contrast, exudative pleural effusions occur when local factors are altered in such a way that pleural fluid accumulates. Inflammation of the lung or the pleura leading to increased flux of fluid from the capillaries of the lung or the pleura into the pleural space is the most common cause of exudative pleural effusions. However, exudative effusions can also occur with decreased lymphatic flow or with a more negative pleural pressure, as with atelectasis.

### Clinical Manifestations

The symptoms of a patient with a pleural effusion are to a large extent dictated by the underlying process

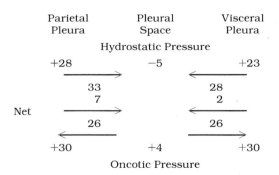

| Parietal Pleura | Pleural Space | Visceral Pleura |
|---|---|---|
| | Hydrostatic Pressure | |
| +28 | −5 | +23 |
| 33 → | | ← 28 |
| 7 → | | ← 2 |
| Net | | |
| 26 | | 26 |
| ← | | → |
| +30 | +4 | +30 |
| | Oncotic Pressure | |

**FIGURE 18.1.** Diagrammatic representation of the pressures involved in the formation and absorption of pleural fluid.

causing the effusion. Many patients have no symptoms referable to the effusion. When symptoms are related to the effusion, they arise either from inflammation of the pleura or from compromise of pulmonary mechanics. Pleuritic chest pain is the usual symptom of pleural inflammation. Since there are pain fibers only in the parietal pleura, pleuritic chest pain indicates inflammation of the parietal pleura. Some patients with pleural effusion experience dull, aching chest pain. This symptom is particularly common if the underlying process directly involves the parietal pleura, as with metastatic tumor or lung abscess. Irritation of the pleural surfaces may also result in a dry, nonproductive cough.

A pleural effusion acts as a space-occupying process in the thoracic cavity and therefore reduces all subdivisions of lung volumes. However, the increase in lung volumes after a therapeutic thoracentesis is much less than the volume of fluid removed (9). With larger effusions, dyspnea results from lung compression. Even though an entire lung may be compressed when the pleural effusion occupies a complete hemithorax, blood gases usually remain nearly normal, owing to a reflex reduction in perfusion to the unventilated lung.

Physical examination of a patient with pleural effusion reveals decreased or absent tactile fremitus, dullness to percussion, and diminished breath sounds over the site of the effusion. Bronchial breath sounds and egophony are frequently present immediately above the effusion.

### Radiographic Appearance

Since pleural fluid is more dense than the lung, the fluid tends to go to the lowermost parts of the thoracic cavity as the lung floats in the fluid. In contrast, with pneumothorax the air is lighter than the lung, so it tends to rise to the uppermost part of the thoracic cavity. The other factor governing the radiologic appearance of a pleural effusion is the inherent tendency of the lung to maintain its usual shape at all stages of collapse.

The first fluid accumulates in the lowest portion of the thoracic cavity, which is the posterior costophrenic angle. Therefore, the earliest radiologic sign of a pleural effusion is blunting of the posterior costophrenic angle on the lateral chest radiograph. As more fluid accumulates, it spills out into the costophrenic sinuses laterally and anteriorly. At this time the lateral costophrenic angle on the posteroanterior radiograph is obliterated. Blunting of the posterior and lateral costophrenic angles also occurs as a result of previous inflammation or chronic obstructive pulmonary disease (COPD). Pleural fluid can be differentiated from these entities by obtaining lateral decubitus radiographs. If

a posteroanterior radiograph is obtained with the patient lying on the affected side, free pleural fluid will gravitate inferiorly and a pleural fluid line (see Fig. 6.2) will be visible. If the film is obtained with the patient lying on the contralateral side, the angle will clear if the blunting is caused by fluid. Alternatively, if the blunting is not due to fluid, neither a pleural fluid line nor clearing of the blunted angle will be observed.

Pleural fluid is said to be *loculated* when it does not shift freely in the pleural space as the patient's position is changed. Loculated pleural effusions occur when there are adhesions between the visceral and parietal pleurae. Such adhesions result from marked inflammation of the pleura. It follows that loculated pleural effusions are more common with pyothorax or hemothorax. At times the differentiation of loculated pleural fluid from pleural thickening or parenchymal disease is quite difficult. Both ultrasound and computed tomography have proved useful in making this differentiation (10).

### Approach to the Patient with Pleural Effusion

There are many different diseases that can be associated with pleural effusion (Table 18.1). When a pleural effusion is discovered, two questions need to be answered: (*a*) Is the effusion a transudate (i.e., is it due to systemic factors) or is it an exudate (i.e., is it due to disease of the pleura itself)? (*b*) If the effusion is an exudate, what is the disease responsible for its production? Answers to these two questions can only be obtained by examining the pleural fluid.

Nearly every patient with a pleural effusion should have a diagnostic thoracentesis. No difficulty should be encountered in obtaining fluid if the pleural fluid is more than 10 mm in thickness on the lateral decubitus roentgenogram. The performance of the diagnostic thoracentesis, the separation of transudates from exudates, and the utility of various diagnostic tests on the pleural fluid are discussed in Chapter 6.

### Therapeutic Thoracentesis

When a patient is found to have a moderate or large pleural effusion, the immediate reaction of most physicians is to remove all the pleural fluid. However, there is little evidence that patients benefit from this procedure. In one study in which a mean of 1740 ml of pleural fluid was removed, the vital capacity improved by only 410 ml (9). Additionally, serial therapeutic thoracenteses may lead to protein depletion. If 2000 ml of pleural fluid with a protein content of 5 g/100 ml is removed, there will be a net protein loss of 100 g. The pleural effusion will reaccumulate if nothing is done to alter the basic pathophysiology that caused it in the first place; therefore, it is much better to determine the

TABLE **18.1**
DIFFERENTIAL DIAGNOSIS OF PLEURAL EFFUSION

TRANSUDATIVE PLEURAL EFFUSIONS
Congestive heart failure
Cirrhosis
Pericardial disease
Nephrotic syndrome
Myxedema
Peritoneal dialysis
Pulmonary embolization
EXUDATIVE PLEURAL EFFUSIONS
Infectious diseases
    Bacterial infections
    Tuberculosis
    Fungal infections
    Viral infections
    Parasitic infections
Neoplastic diseases
    Metastatic disease
    Mesotheliomas
Collagen vascular diseases
    Systemic lupus erythematosus
    Rheumatoid pleuritis
Pulmonary embolization
Gastrointestinal diseases
    Acute pancreatitis
    Pancreatic pseudocyst
    Esophageal perforations
    Intraabdominal abscess
    After abdominal surgery
Chylothorax
    Traumatic
    Nontraumatic
Drug hypersensitivity
    Nitrofurantoin
    Methysergide
    Dantrolene
Miscellaneous diseases
    Asbestos exposure
    Meigs' syndrome
    Pulmonary and lymph node myomatosis
    Uremia
    Post-cardiac injury syndrome
    Trapped lung
    Yellow nail syndrome
    Sarcoidosis
    Urinary tract obstruction
    Iatrogenic injury
    Hemothorax

original cause of the pleural effusion and to treat it accordingly than merely to remove the fluid that is present.

At times it is diagnostically important to remove as much pleural fluid as possible so that one can determine whether there are any abnormalities in the underlying lung. In view of the large decreases in pleural pressures that occur in some patients during the removal of large amounts of pleural fluid, thoracentesis should be limited to 1000 ml unless pleural pressures are monitored (11). If pleural pressures are monitored, the thoracentesis can be safely continued as long as the pleural pressure remains above $-20$ cm $H_2O$ (11).

## TRANSUDATIVE PLEURAL EFFUSIONS

### Congestive Heart Failure

Congestive heart failure is probably responsible for more pleural effusions than any other disease entity. The accumulation of pleural fluid can be secondary to increases in the hydrostatic pressures in either the systemic or the pulmonary circulation. Clinically, however, pleural effusion due to congestive heart failure usually occurs only when the pulmonary wedge pressure is elevated (7). It is thought that the origin of the increased pleural fluid is the interstitial spaces of the lung. The pleural effusion is usually bilateral, but if it is unilateral it is most commonly on the right (12). A large unilateral effusion is uncommon in uncomplicated congestive heart failure and suggests malignancy, pulmonary emboli, or other complicating disease.

The diagnosis is usually suggested by the clinical picture of congestive heart failure. With appropriate treatment of the heart failure the effusion will resolve rapidly in most cases. When the patient is first evaluated a thoracentesis is indicated if the effusions are not bilateral and comparable in size, if the patient has pleuritic chest pain, or if the patient is febrile. If the pleural effusion persists after treatment, a diagnostic thoracentesis should be performed. In congestive heart failure, the pleural fluid is a transudate and its characteristics change very little with diuresis (13).

### Cirrhosis

The incidence of pleural effusion with cirrhosis varies from 0.5 to 10%. The predominant mechanism leading to a pleural effusion in a patient with cirrhosis and ascites appears to be the movement of the ascitic fluid from the peritoneal cavity through a diaphragmatic defect into the pleural space (14). The decreased plasma oncotic pressure is only a secondary factor.

The clinical picture is of cirrhosis and ascites. The effusions are most common on the right side but may be bilateral or left-sided. At times the effusions may be very large, occupying almost an entire hemithorax. These large effusions may induce respiratory symptoms. Therapeutic thoracentesis is of virtually no use, since the fluid reaccumulates very rapidly and the thoracentesis further depletes the patient's protein stores.

Some patients with very large effusions and respiratory symptoms may benefit from pleurodesis effected by chest tube placement followed by instillation of talc slurry (15) into the pleural space as described later in this chapter. If one does elect to attempt a pleurodesis, the patient should be observed carefully in an intensive care unit, since deaths from electrolyte imbalance have been reported following this procedure (16).

### Other Causes of Transudative Pleural Effusions

*Pericardial Disease*

The incidence of pleural effusion in patients with pericardial disease is about 30% (17). Most of the effusions are left-sided or bilateral and are small to moderate in size. The pleural effusion is usually transudative and results from either elevated capillary pressures or pericardial inflammation.

*Nephrotic Syndrome*

Patients with the nephrotic syndrome commonly have an associated pleural effusion. The mechanism responsible for the effusion is probably the decreased plasma oncotic pressure secondary to the hypoproteinemia. The fluid is a typical transudate. Treatment is aimed at the nephrotic syndrome in an attempt to increase the serum proteins.

*Myxedema*

A pleural effusion sometimes occurs as a complication of myxedema. Most patients with myxedema and pleural effusion have a concomitant pericardial effusion, in which case the pleural effusion is a transudate. The rare isolated pleural effusion seen in conjunction with myxedema can be either a transudate or an exudate (18).

*Peritoneal Dialysis*

Approximately 10% of patients on continuous ambulatory peritoneal dialysis will develop a pleural effusion. The mechanism is probably the same as that with cirrhosis and ascites. The peritoneal dialysis increases the intraabdominal pressure, and the dialysate flows from the peritoneal cavity into the pleural cavity through pores in the diaphragm. The pleural fluid in such instances is similar to the dialysate. The treatment of choice is chemical pleurodesis combined with a short period of small-volume, intermittent peritoneal dialysis (19).

### EXUDATIVE PLEURAL EFFUSIONS

### Parapneumonic Effusion

Any pleural effusion associated with bacterial pneumonia, lung abscess, or bronchiectasis is a parapneumonic effusion. Parapneumonic effusions are common, since more than 1 million cases of pneumonia occur annually in the United States and 40% of these have an associated parapneumonic effusion (20). The amount of fluid varies from a few milliliters, in which case the fluid is usually not detected, to several liters. The character of the fluid varies from a clear, straw-colored fluid with a few hundred white blood cells per cubic millimeter to frank pus.

When managing a patient with a parapneumonic effusion, the key therapeutic decision to make is whether or not a chest tube should be inserted into the pleural space for drainage. If a patient is going to require a chest tube, it is best to insert it as early as possible, since drainage becomes progressively more difficult with time. Alternatively, one would prefer to institute tube thoracostomy only when it is necessary because the procedure is painful, with some morbidity. Parapneumonic effusions that require tube thoracostomy are designated *complicated parapneumonic effusions*.

*Natural History of Parapneumonic Effusions*

The evolution of a parapneumonic effusion can be divided into three stages (21). The first stage is the *exudative* stage, in which a focus of parenchymal infection leads to increased pulmonary interstitial fluid which traverses the visceral pleura and results in the accumulation of pleural fluid. In this stage the pleural fluid is characterized by a relatively low lactate dehydrogenase (LDH) level and a normal glucose and pH.

The second stage is the *fibropurulent* stage, which is characterized by the invasion of the pleural fluid by bacteria. As this stage progresses, the pleural fluid becomes increasingly cloudy and viscous since it contains large amounts of fibrin, cellular debris, and white blood cells. In this stage, there is a progressive tendency toward loculation of the fluid and the formation of limiting membranes. Although the loculation prevents extension of the pleural infection, it makes drainage of the pleural space difficult.

The third stage is the *organization* stage, in which fibroblasts grow into the exudate from both the visceral and parietal pleural surfaces to produce an inelastic membrane called the *pleural peel*. This peel encases the lung and renders it virtually functionless. At this stage the exudate is very thick, and if the patient has remained untreated the fluid may drain spontaneously through the chest wall (*empyema necessitatis*) or into the lung, in which case a bronchopleural fistula will be produced.

*Initial Management of Patients with Parapneumonic Effusion*

When a patient with acute bacterial pneumonia is initially evaluated, the physician should determine whether or not a parapneumonic effusion is present.

If the posterior costophrenic angles are not blunted on the lateral chest radiograph, one can assume that there is not a clinically significant pleural effusion unless the chest radiograph reveals loculated fluid elsewhere in the chest. If the posterior costophrenic angles are blunted or if the diaphragm is obscured by the infiltrate, then a lateral decubitus chest roentgenogram should be obtained with the suspicious side down. The amount of pleural fluid can be semiquantitated on the decubitus film by measuring the distance between the inside of the chest wall and the bottom of the lung. If this measurement is less than 10 mm, it can be assumed that the effusion is not clinically significant and thoracentesis is not indicated (20).

If the thickness of the fluid is greater than 10 mm on the decubitus x-ray film, a diagnostic thoracentesis should be performed, since it is impossible without fluid examination to separate effusions that are complicated from those that are not. With the diagnostic thoracentesis, 30 to 50 ml of pleural fluid is withdrawn into a heparinized syringe. The fluid is examined grossly for color, turbidity, and odor. Aliquots are sent for determination of glucose, LDH, protein, and amylase levels; pH; and total and differential WBC counts of the pleural fluid. It is important to send pleural fluid for anaerobic as well as aerobic cultures, since more than one-third of culture-positive parapneumonic effusions will contain anaerobic organisms (22).

If upon examination of the pleural fluid, any *one* of the following four conditions is met, chest tubes should be inserted immediately (20):

1. Gross pus is obtained on thoracentesis;
2. The Gram stain of the pleural fluid is positive for organisms;
3. The pleural fluid glucose level is less than 40 mg/100 ml;
4. The pleural fluid pH is below 7.00.

The use of the pleural fluid pH and glucose level as guides to the placement of chest tubes only pertains to parapneumonic effusions. Pleural effusions from other causes (e.g., malignancy, tuberculosis, or rheumatoid disease) may have a low pleural fluid pH or glucose level, and the placement of chest tubes in these conditions should not be dictated by the pleural fluid pH or glucose level. To use the pleural fluid pH measurement, the pleural fluid must be collected anaerobically and placed on ice during its transfer to the laboratory. The pH must be determined with a blood gas analyzer; paper pH strips are not sufficiently accurate.

If, upon the initial evaluation of the pleural fluid, the pH is above 7.20, the LDH level is below 1000 IU/liter, the glucose level is above 60 mg/100 ml, and the Gram stain is negative, the parapneumonic effusion is in stage 1 and no further diagnostic or therapeutic measures need be directed toward the effusion. In particular, serial therapeutic thoracenteses are not necessary.

Patients who have an initial pleural fluid pH between 7.00 and 7.20 or an LDH level above 1000 IU/liter and who do not meet any of the previously mentioned criteria for the placement of chest tubes present a special problem. Since some of these patients will need chest tubes while others will not, each case should be considered individually. If the patient has a very large effusion and the pH is close to 7.00, the patient probably should have chest tubes inserted. In contrast, if the effusion is small and the pH is close to 7.20, the patient probably will not require tube thoracostomy. In borderline cases, serial thoracenteses at 12- to 24-hour intervals are useful. If the pleural fluid pH and glucose level tend to increase and the pleural fluid LDH tends to fall with serial thoracenteses, the patient is handling the parapneumonic effusion, and tube thoracostomy probably will not be necessary. In contrast, if the pleural fluid pH and glucose level fall and the LDH level increases, tube thoracostomy drainage of the pleural space should be instituted (20).

The initial antibiotic therapy for patients with parapneumonic effusions should be based on the Gram stain of the sputum. Since the antibiotic levels in the pleural fluid are comparable with those in the serum, the dose of antibiotic need not be increased in patients with parapneumonic effusions (23).

*Tube Thoracostomy for Complicated Parapneumonic Effusions*

The goal of tube thoracostomy in patients with complicated parapneumonic effusions is to completely drain the pleural space and to reexpand the underlying lung. Although in the past large-diameter thoracostomy tubes were recommended, it appears that small tubes are equally effective if they are placed in the appropriate position (24, 25). The tube should be positioned in the most dependent part of the fluid accumulation, which most commonly is the posterior costophrenic sulcus.

The adequacy of pleural drainage should be assessed daily by evaluation of the patient's clinical status, chest radiographs, ultrasonsography, and chest tube drainage measurements. Adequate drainage is characterized by defervescence and general clinical improvement in conjunction with radiologic improvement. The chest tubes should be left in place until the drainage ceases to be purulent and the amount of drainage decreases to less than 50 ml/day. At that time the chest tubes should be removed and the patient observed for recurrence of toxicity. Chest tubes that cease to function should be removed expeditiously, since they are serving no useful purpose and can serve as conduits for pleural infection.

*Failure of Tube Thoracostomy*

In some patients, closed drainage is unsuccessful because the lung does not reexpand to fill the pleural cavity, or loculi of infected pleural fluid remain. Failure of closed drainage is usually due to a delay in the institution of the drainage. With the delay, the pleural fluid becomes loculated and a thick peel forms over the visceral pleura, which prevents the lung from reexpanding. The four alternatives available when tube thoracostomy fails are intrapleural injection of thrombolytic agents; mechanical breakdown of the loculations via thoracoscopy; decortication; or an open drainage procedure.

Unsuccessful drainage is frequently due to the presence of pleural fluid loculations caused by the presence of limiting membranes composed of fibrin. If a thrombolytic agent is injected intrapleurally, it can destroy these fibrin membranes and facilitate drainage of the pleural space. Either streptokinase 250,000 units (26) or urokinase 100,000 units (27) diluted in 100 ml saline appears to be efficacious. It is recommended that patients who do not respond adequately to tube thoracostomy within 24 hours be given a trial of intrapleural thrombolytic therapy. After the injection, the tube is clamped for approximately 1 hour to allow the fibrinolytic agent to attack the fibrin membranes. The treatment can be repeated daily for 10 to 14 days if it appears to be effective as evidenced by increased drainage following injection.

*Decortication* is the removal of the inflammatory peel that covers the visceral pleura of the affected lung. This procedure allows the underlying lung to reexpand and obliterate the pleural space. In contrast to the relatively minor open drainage procedure, decortication is major surgery and should never be performed on a seriously ill patient. However, in relatively healthy patients, decortication is the treatment of choice when closed drainage fails, since it allows the patient to return to a normal life much sooner than does open drainage.

Some thoracic surgeons recommend decortication in all cases in which a thick pleural peel remains after either closed or open drainage of a pleural infection. However, since the pleural peel frequently improves substantially in the months after the drainage, it is recommended that decortication be delayed for at least 6 months if the infection has been controlled and the lung reexpanded. After this time, decortication should be performed only if the patient has limited exercise capacity and if close evaluation of the patient's pulmonary status suggests that the procedure will improve pulmonary function.

An alternative to decortication is *thoracoscopy with mechanical lysis of adhesions.* Indeed, this procedure has been advocated in all patients who are not responding satisfactorily to tube thoracostomy (28). The procedure is performed under general anesthesia and all loculations are broken down with the thoracoscope. If at the time of thoracoscopy the patient is found to have a very thick pleural peel with a large amount of debris and entrapment of the lung, the thoracoscopy incision can be enlarged to allow for decortication (28).

With *open thoracotomy drainage,* a short segment of one or more ribs at the most dependent part of the cavity is removed and a large drainage tube is inserted into the pocket. A colostomy bag can be placed over the opening in the chest to capture the drainage. The pleural cavity gradually (over months) heals from within via the formation of granulation tissue. The advantages that open drainage has over closed drainage are that the drainage is more complete with the larger opening and the patient is freed from the chest tube.

**Tuberculous Pleural Effusions**

In many parts of the world, the most common cause of an exudative pleural effusion is tuberculosis. However, in the United States the annual incidence of tuberculous pleural effusion is only about 1000 cases. Approximately one in every 30 cases of tuberculosis is tuberculous pleuritis, and this ratio has remained constant with the advent of AIDS (29).

*Pathogenesis*

The exudative pleural effusion associated with pleural tuberculosis appears to be predominantly a manifestation of delayed hypersensitivity to tuberculous protein. Frequently it is difficult to demonstrate the tubercle bacillus in either the pleural fluid or the pleural tissue. It is probable that granulomatous pleuritis results any time a patient with a positive tuberculin purified protein derivative (PPD) skin test gets tubercle bacillus protein into the pleural space. It should be emphasized that many patients with tuberculous pleuritis have a negative PPD test when first seen. The possible explanations for the negative PPD test in these individuals are that there are circulating adherent cells that suppress the delayed hypersensitivity reaction to the PPD in the skin or that the specifically sensitized lymphocytes are sequestered in the pleural space (30).

*Clinical Manifestations*

A pleural effusion as a manifestation of tuberculosis has been likened to a primary chancre as a manifestation of syphilis. Both are self-limited and of little immediate concern, but both may lead to serious disease at a later date. Most cases of tuberculous effusion will resolve spontaneously without treatment, but active tuberculosis will subsequently develop in a large percentage of patients. Patiala (31) followed 2816 members of the Finnish armed forces who developed pleural effusion during World War II before antituberculous drugs were available. Over 40% of these individuals developed active tuberculosis during the 7-year follow-up period. Accordingly, when managing a patient with a pleural effusion, it is the physician's obligation either to treat the patient for tuberculous pleuritis or to exclude this diagnosis.

At the onset of tuberculous pleuritis, most patients have symptoms of an upper respiratory tract infection, and many also have pleuritic chest pain. Most but not all patients also have a temperature elevation not uncommonly in the 103 to 105 F range. Subsequently the patient develops a chronic illness characterized by anorexia, weight loss, and a low-grade fever. Without treatment most patients will recover completely only to develop active tuberculosis at another site later. Most patients with tuberculous pleuritis do not have radiologically evident parenchymal infiltrates. In those without parenchymal infiltrates, the effusion is almost always unilateral.

*Diagnosis*

The diagnosis of tuberculous pleuritis should be considered in every patient with an exudative pleural effusion. The diagnosis of tuberculous pleuritis depends on the demonstration of tubercle bacilli in the sputum, pleural fluid, or pleura or of granulomas in the pleura. As mentioned earlier, a negative PPD test when the patient is first seen certainly does not rule out the diagnosis. Although the sputum is usually negative for tubercle bacilli unless there are parenchymal infiltrates, it should be analyzed for the tubercle bacillus.

Pleural fluid analysis in tuberculous pleuritis is useful. The fluid is invariably an exudate. Frequently the pleural fluid protein is over 5.0 g/100 ml, and this finding is very suggestive of tuberculous pleuritis. In most cases, the differential white cell count reveals more than 80% lymphocytes, but if symptoms have been present less than 1 week, neutrophils at times predominate. A pleural effusion that contains more than 10% eosinophils at the time of the initial thoracentesis is seldom if ever tuberculous. The pleural fluid glucose level may be reduced with tuberculous pleuritis, but the majority of patients have a pleural fluid glucose level above 60 mg/dl (21). Cultures of the pleural fluid for tubercle bacilli are positive in less than 20% of cases (32).

Two biochemical tests are useful in establishing the diagnosis of tuberculous pleuritis (32). Adenosine deaminase (ADA) is the enzyme that catalyzes the conversion of adenosine to inosine and is found predominantly in T lymphocytes. Pleural fluid ADA levels above 70 IU/liter are essentially diagnostic for tuberculous pleuritis, while levels below 40 IU/liter essentially rule out the diagnosis. High pleural fluid levels of gamma interferon above 2.5 IU/ml also appear to be highly suggestive of tuberculous pleuritis.

Pleural biopsy has its greatest utility in establishing the diagnosis of tuberculous pleuritis. The demonstration of granuloma in the parietal pleura is highly suggestive of tuberculous pleuritis. Caseous necrosis or acid-fast bacilli need not be demonstrated. Although other disease entities including fungus diseases, sarcoidosis, and rheumatoid pleuritis can at times produce granulomatous pleuritis, more than 95% of patients with granulomatous pleuritis have tuberculosis. In approximately 60% of patients with tuberculous pleuritis, the initial pleural biopsy will reveal granulomas. If the pleural biopsy is repeated twice, the proportion increases to roughly 85%. When culture of a biopsy specimen is combined with microscopic examination, the diagnosis of tuberculosis can be made more than 90% of the time (33).

In some patients with exudative pleural effusions, no diagnosis is reached despite several biopsies and cultures. We recommend the following approach to antituberculous chemotherapy in such individuals: (*a*) if the patient has a positive PPD test or is anergic, he or she should be treated; or (*b*) if the patient has a negative PPD test he or she should have a second skin test in 6 weeks and be treated then if the skin test is positive.

*Treatment*

Adequate therapy for tuberculous pleuritis is a 9-month course of 300 mg isoniazid and 600 mg of rifampin daily if the organisms are sensitive to these medications (21). However, if the patient is from an area where the likelihood of isoniazid or rifampin resistance is not low, the initial therapy should consist of four drugs (34). With treatment, patients generally become afebrile within about 2 weeks, and the pleural effusion resolves within 6 weeks. Repeated pleural fluid aspiration has not been shown to be beneficial in preventing chronic pleural thickening. The administration of corticosteroids will rapidly relieve the patient's symptoms of pleuritic chest pain, malaise, and fever and does not seem to lead to dissemination of the tuberculosis. Markedly symptomatic patients should be started on prednisone 40 mg/day and then gradually tapered over several weeks.

## Actinomycosis

Over 50% of patients with thoracic actinomycosis have pleural involvement. The characteristic chest radiographic finding is a localized lung lesion extending to the chest wall with pleural thickening or effusion. The presence of chest wall abscesses or draining sinus tracts suggests the diagnosis, as do bone changes consisting of periosteal proliferation or bone destruction. The definitive diagnosis is established with the demonstration of *Actinomyces israelii* by anaerobic cultures. The appropriate treatment is high doses of penicillin or another suitable antimicrobial agent for prolonged periods.

## Nocardiosis

Pleural effusions develop in nearly 50% of patients with pulmonary nocardiosis. When pleural involvement does occur, grossly purulent pleural fluid and draining sinuses are common. The diagnosis is established by demonstrating the organism on aerobic culture. Since the organism is slow-growing, cultures should be maintained for 4 weeks to exclude the diagnosis. Frequently with pleural nocardiosis, tuberculosis is wrongly diagnosed because the organisms are acid-fast. The drug treatment of choice is the combination of trimethoprim and sulfamethoxazole (Bactrim), two tablets twice a day for at least 2 months.

## Fungal Diseases of the Pleura

### Aspergillosis

Pleural aspergillosis usually occurs in one of two settings. Pleural aspergillosis may complicate lobectomy or pneumonectomy, in which situation a bronchopleural fistula is almost always present. Once the diagnosis is established, a chest tube should be inserted, and the pleural space should be irrigated daily with amphotericin B 25 mg or nystatin 75,000 units. The diagnosis of pleural aspergillosis should also be suspected in any patient with a history of artificial pneumothorax therapy for tuberculosis who has signs and symptoms of a chronic infection. The optimal treatment for pleural aspergillosis in this situation is surgical removal of the involved pleura and resection of the involved lobe or the entire ipsilateral lung if necessary (35).

### Blastomycosis

Approximately 10% of patients with blastomycosis will have a pleural effusion. The clinical picture with pleural blastomycosis is identical to that with pleural tuberculosis. The diagnosis is established by demonstrating the organism in the pleural fluid or histologic sections. The treatment of choice is amphotericin B.

### Coccidioidomycosis

Pleural effusions of two types occur in association with coccidioidomycosis. The incidence of pleural effusion with symptomatic primary coccidioidomycosis is about 7%, and 50% of the patients with pleural effusion will also have a coexisting parenchymal infiltrate. Most patients are febrile and have pleuritic chest pain, and nearly 50% have either erythema nodosum or erythema multiforme. The pleural effusion is a lymphocyte-predominant exudate. Pleural fluid cultures are positive in about 20%, while cultures of pleural biopsy specimens are almost always positive. Most patients with primary coccidioidal pleural effusion require no systemic antifungal therapy. Only patients with a negative skin test or other evidence of dissemination need be treated with antifungal therapy (36).

Hydropneumothoraces develop in 1 to 5% of patients with chronic cavitary coccidioidomycosis. These patients should undergo tube thoracostomy immediately to drain the air and fluid from the pleural space. Most patients will require a thoracotomy with a partial or total lobectomy, and most will require some degree of decortication. The administration of antifungal drugs does not appear to be required (37).

### Cryptococcosis

Pleural involvement with cryptococcosis appears to result from extension of a primary subpleural cryptococcal nodule into the pleural space. The majority of patients who have a cryptococcal pleural effusion are immunosuppressed and many have AIDS (38). The pleural fluid usually is a lymphocyte-predominant exudate. Immunosuppressed patients should be treated with a combination of amphotericin B (0.4 mg/kg) and 5-fluorocytosine (150 mg/kg) daily for 6 weeks, as should patients with cryptococcal antigen in either their blood or their cerebrospinal fluid. If none of these criteria are met, then the patient probably does not need to be treated. However, if the effusion increases in size, if the LDH levels in the effusion tend to increase, or if antigens appear in the blood or cerebrospinal fluid, treatment should be initiated (32).

### Histoplasmosis

On rare occasions patients with histoplasmosis will have a lymphocyte-predominant exudative pleural effusion. The pleural biopsy will reveal noncaseating granulomas. No systemic treatment is necessary unless the patient is immunosuppressed or the effusion persists for more than 4 weeks.

## Viral Diseases of the Pleura

Viral infections are probably responsible for a sizable percentage of undiagnosed exudative pleural effusions. However, the diagnosis is rarely established because it depends on isolation of the virus or the demonstration of a significant increase in the antibodies to the virus. The incidence of pleural effusion with primary atypical pneumonia is as high as 20% (39).

## Parasitic Diseases of the Pleura

### Amebiasis

Pleural involvement with the parasite *Entamoeba histolytica* is almost invariably secondary to a liver abscess. Most patients present with fever and right upper quadrant tenderness. Right-sided pleuritic chest pain is common and it is frequently referred to the right shoulder as a manifestation of diaphragmatic irritation. Thoracentesis can yield either "chocolate-sauce" fluid or a serous exudate that develops in response to the diaphragmatic irritation. The expectoration of "chocolate-sauce" sputum is nearly pathognomonic and indicates that a bronchohepatic fistula has developed. The discovery of "chocolate sauce" in either the sputum or the pleural space serves as an indication for therapy with metronidazole, 750 mg 3 times a day for 5 to 10 days. Tube thoracostomy should be performed if "chocolate sauce" is found on thoracentesis.

### Paragonimiasis

This diagnosis should be suspected in patients with undiagnosed pleural effusion who have recently been in the Orient, since the Oriental lung fluke, *Paragonimus westermani*, at times produces pleural disease. Patients with pleural paragonimiasis present with a chronic illness. The pleural fluid in patients with pleural paragonimiasis is quite characteristic in that it is an exudate with a glucose level less than 10 mg/dl, an LDH level above 1000 IU/liter, a pH below 7.10, and a differential revealing a high percentage of eosinophils (40). The pleural fluid findings are virtually pathognomonic, but the diagnosis is established by demonstrating the typical operculated eggs in the sputum, pleural fluid, or stool. The treatment of choice is bithionol, 30 to 50 mg/kg, on alternate days for 14 days. At times thoracotomy with decortication is necessary for resolution of the process.

### Echinococcosis

Pleural disease from *Echinococcus granulosus* usually results from rupture of either a pulmonary or a hepatic hydatid cyst into the pleural space. When the cyst ruptures the patient experiences the abrupt onset of chest pain, fever, and systemic toxicity. Diagnosis is dependent on the demonstration of hooklets from scolices in the sputum or pleural fluid. The treatment of choice is surgical excision of the cyst combined with tube drainage of the pleural space. After surgery, patients should be treated with albendazole 400 mg twice a day for several weeks (41).

## Pleural Effusions Secondary to Neoplasms

### Pathogenesis

Neoplasms are responsible for a high percentage of pleural effusions. Along with congestive heart failure, they account for the majority of pleural effusions in patients over the age of 50 years. Pleural effusions associated with neoplasms arise through at least five different mechanisms:

1. The pleural surfaces may be involved by the tumor, which leads to increased permeability of the pleural membranes.
2. The neoplasm may obstruct the lymphatics or veins draining the pleural space, leading to the accumulation of pleural fluid.
3. An endobronchial tumor may completely obstruct a bronchus, leading to atelectasis and decreasing the pleural pressure.
4. A pneumonitis distal to a partially obstructed bronchus may lead to a parapneumonic effusion.
5. The hypoproteinemia associated with a neoplasm may be responsible for the effusion.

Pleural effusions in patients with known malignancy may not be related to the malignancy itself; these patients may also develop heart failure, pulmonary emboli, pneumonia, or tuberculosis, any of which may be responsible for the effusion. It should be noted that not all patients with metastases to the pleura develop pleural effusions. Meyer (42) reviewed 52 cases of metastatic carcinoma to the pleura and found that only 14 of these patients had had recognized pleural effusions during their lifetime. He found that the development of an effusion is closely related to neoplastic infiltration of the mediastinal lymph nodes and that in all types of tumors the visceral pleura is involved much sooner and more extensively than is the parietal pleura. Pleural involvement with most bronchogenic tumors arises from pulmonary arterial emboli, while pleural involvement with nonbronchogenic tumors usually represents tertiary spread from established hepatic metastases.

Bronchogenic carcinomas in men and breast carcinomas in women are the leading types of tumors causing neoplastic effusions. The lymphomas and leukemias are the third leading type of malignancy with secondary effusions. However, many other tumors, predominantly carcinomas, are associated with metastases to the pleura and pleural effusions.

### Diagnosis

The diagnosis of a malignant effusion should be considered in all patients with exudative pleural effusions. The diagnosis is established by demonstrating malignant cells by cytopathologic studies or by pleural biopsy. Although there is nothing absolutely characteristic about the pleural fluid secondary to malignancy, several generalizations can be made.

The pleural fluid is almost always an exudate. A grossly bloody pleural fluid is suggestive of malignancy, but nearly 50% of malignant effusions have pleural fluid RBC counts of less than 10,000. The pleural fluid WBC count is usually between 500 and 25,000 and the differential can be characterized by a predominance of polymorphonuclear leukocytes, small lymphocytes, or other mononuclear cells. The pleural fluid glucose level is usually similar to the corresponding serum level, but occasionally is less than 50 mg/100 ml. The pleural fluid amylase level is elevated in approximately 10% of malignant pleural effusions. In such cases the primary tumor is usually not in the pancreas and the amylase has a salivary rather than a pancreatic isoenzyme pattern. The pleural fluid pH may be normal or markedly reduced. A low pleural fluid pH usually occurs in conjunction with a low pleural fluid glucose, and this combination indicates a poor prognosis because it is due to a large tumor burden in the pleural space. Pleural fluid carcinoembryonic antigen (CEA) levels are above 10 ng/ml in about one-third of patients with malignant pleural effusions, but since these are usually the effusions with the positive cytology, the routine use of this test is not recommended (43).

The diagnosis of a malignant pleural effusion is most commonly established by cytologic examination of the pleural fluid. When specimens from three separate thoracenteses are submitted for cytologic examination, the diagnosis can be established in nearly 90% of individuals who have pleural metastases (44). Needle biopsy of the pleura will be diagnostic for malignancy about 40% of the time.

At times no diagnosis will be obtained despite at least two cytologies on the pleural fluid and at least one pleural biopsy. How aggressive should one be in attempting to establish the diagnosis of malignancy in these patients? Only about 20% of such patients have pleural malignancy, and almost all who do have a pleural malignancy will have a clinical picture suggestive of malignancy (45). Accordingly, if the patient is symptomatic from the effusion and the symptoms are tending to increase, thoracoscopy or thoracotomy with pleural biopsy should be performed. If thoracoscopy is performed, talc should be insufflated at the time of the procedure to effect a pleurodesis (46).

In a patient with a known neoplasm and pleural effusion, the key questions are whether the pleural effusion is secondary to the malignancy and, if so, by what mechanism. Again, cytopathologic study and pleural biopsy can demonstrate direct involvement of the pleura. The chest x-ray is useful in delineating the responsible mechanisms. If the mediastinum is shifted toward the contralateral side, the pleural surfaces are probably involved. If the mediastinum is shifted toward the ipsilateral side and the bronchi are not outlined by air on the routine chest radiograph, total bronchial obstruction with resulting atelectasis and effusion is the probable explanation. A parapneumonic effusion is suggested by a high white cell count, predominantly neutrophils, in the pleural fluid. Protein analysis of peripheral blood demonstrates hypoproteinemia. A mediastinal mass on the chest x-ray film suggests lymphatic obstruction.

*Treatment*

The proper therapy for a pleural effusion associated with malignancy depends on the mechanism responsible for it. If an endobronchial tumor is responsible for complete bronchial obstruction, laser therapy should be directed toward the obstruction. If pneumonitis behind a partial obstruction is present, appropriate antibiotics and postural drainage in combination with laser therapy should be given. If the pleural effusion is due to lymphatic blockage in the mediastinum, radiotherapy to the mediastinum may be effective in controlling the effusion, particularly with lymphomas.

When the effusion is due to pleural metastases, consideration should be given to obliterating the pleural space with a pleurodesis. Patients who are subjected to this procedure should meet the following two criteria. First, the patient should have the quality of his or her life diminished by dyspnea. Second, a therapeutic thoracentesis should cause improvement in the patient's dyspnea. Many patients with malignant pleural effusions do not meet the above two criteria and therefore are not candidates for pleurodesis.

If the above two conditions are met, a pleurodesis should be attempted. With chemical pleurodesis an irritant (e.g., talc) is injected into the pleural space, which creates intense pleural inflammation and leads to fusion of the visceral and parietal pleurae. Many different agents have been used as pleural sclerosants, but talc (5 g) plus thymol iodide (3 g) is probably the agent of choice, given its low cost and high efficacy in both humans (47) and animals (48). Other reasonable alternatives for pleural sclerosants include the tetracycline derivatives (minocycline or doxycycline) and bleomycin. It should be remembered that pleurodesis is less likely to be successful if the pleural fluid glucose level is below 60 mg/dl or if the pleural fluid pH is less than 7.3 (49).

The following procedure is recommended for pleurodesis. A chest tube is inserted into the pleural space to drain the fluid. As soon as the underlying lung has reexpanded, a slurry consisting of 20 ml 1% xylocaine, 50 ml saline, 5 g of sterile asbestos-free talc, and 3 g of thymol iodine powder is thoroughly mixed up. Then without leaving time for the talc to settle out, the suspension is injected through the chest tube into the pleural space. After the injection the chest tube is clamped for the next 60 to 90 minutes. There appears to be no need to place the patient into various positions after the injection (50). The chest tube is then unclamped and negative pressure is applied through the chest tube for 48 to 72 hours or until the drainage becomes less than 15 ml/hour. At this time the chest tube is removed. The intense inflammation induced by the talc results in fusion of the visceral and parietal pleural surfaces when they are brought into close approximation by the negative pressure of the chest tubes. Pleurodesis performed in this manner is effective in obliterating the pleural space and controlling the pleural effusion about 90% of the time (47).

An alternative to pleurodesis is the implantation of a pleuroperitoneal shunt (51). The shunt, which can be placed with local anesthesia, consists of two catheters connected by a pump chamber containing two one-way valves. Fluid flows from the pleural space to the pump chamber and then from the pump chamber to the peritoneal cavity. The patient pumps on the reservoir daily to move fluid from the pleural space to the peritoneal space.

Patients who have primary tumors that are responsive to systemic chemotherapy, such as small cell carcinoma of the lung, breast carcinoma, and lymphoma, should be given chemotherapy to treat the primary disease.

## Mesothelioma

Malignant mesothelioma is an unusual disease that is highly malignant and has been shown to be associated with exposure to asbestos. It is thought that asbestos exposure is responsible for most mesotheliomas, but no history of asbestos exposure can be obtained in approximately one-third of patients with mesothelioma (52). Mesotheliomas are thought to arise from the cells that line the pleural cavity.

Once the tumor is present, it spreads rapidly along the pleural surfaces. Eventually, the entire visceral and parietal pleural surfaces become infiltrated by a continuous layer of tumor, encasing the entire lung. Metastases to regional lymph nodes are common, but distant metastases are rare. Histologically, diffuse mesotheliomas frequently contain large amounts of fibrous tissue. The predominant cellular type may be either mesenchymal or epithelial, and the majority of these tumors have both cell types.

Most patients with malignant mesothelioma present with either chest pain or dyspnea. The chest pain is nonpleuritic, aching, and frequently referred to the upper abdomen or shoulder. When the patient initially presents, the chest film almost invariably reveals a unilateral pleural effusion. The prognosis of patients with mesothelioma is poor, with a median survival time of slightly more than 12 months after diagnosis (53).

It is difficult to definitely establish the diagnosis of malignant mesothelioma. Although cytologic smears, needle biopsies, and sections from cell blocks of pleural fluid can establish the diagnosis of malignancy, they usually cannot distinguish between a metastatic adenocarcinoma and a mesothelioma. Thoracoscopy is probably the best procedure with which to establish the diagnosis of mesothelioma (54). At thoracostomy a small portion of the specimen should be placed in glutaraldehyde for electron microscopy in any patient suspected of having mesothelioma (52). In addition, attempts should be made to create a pleurodesis using insufflated talc at the time of thoracoscopy.

Three techniques are available that help establish the diagnosis of mesothelioma with greater certainty. Most adenocarcinomas are positive with the periodic acid–Schiff (PAS) stain after diastase digestion, while all mesotheliomas are negative. Electron microscopy is also useful in differentiating mesothelioma from metastatic adenocarcinoma in that mesotheliomas are characterized by long, lush microvilli. Lastly, with immunohistochemical studies, mesotheliomas have a high rate of positivity for keratin and hyaluronidase-sensitive colloidal iron, while adenocarcinomas are uniformly positive for CEA and keratin and generally positive for PAS-D and mucicarmine (55).

There is no satisfactory treatment for malignant mesothelioma, and it is unclear whether any of the available treatments prolong life (56). If the patient appears to have resectable disease, surgery should probably be performed. Chemical pleurodesis should be attempted if the patient is dyspneic from a large pleural effusion, and sufficient analgesics, including opiates when necessary, should be given to alleviate the pain.

## Localized Benign Pleural Mesothelioma

Benign fibrous mesotheliomas are localized pleural tumors with an excellent prognosis. Their occurrence does not appear to be related to previous asbestos exposure. These tumors appear radiologically as solitary, sharply defined, discrete masses located at the periphery of the lung or related to a fissure. The most frequent symptoms are cough, chest pain, and dyspnea, but approximately 50% of patients are asymptomatic. Hypertrophic pulmonary osteoarthropathy occurs in approximately 20% of patients with benign mesotheliomas, and in such instances the tumor is usually greater than

7 cm in diameter. The association of hypertrophic osteoarthropathy and a large intrathoracic mass should strongly suggest the possibility of a localized pleural mesothelioma. Symptomatic hypoglycemia occurs in about 4% of patients with benign mesothelioma. The treatment is surgical excision and the prognosis is excellent (57).

## Pleural Effusions Secondary to Collagen Vascular Disease

### Systemic Lupus Erythematosus

The pleura is frequently involved in systemic lupus erythematosus. Pleurisy without effusion is more common than pleurisy with effusion. In one series of patients observed for prolonged periods, 72% had pleuritic chest pain and 40% had pleural effusions some time during their course (58). The effusions are frequently bilateral but may be unilateral and change from one side to the other. Pericardial effusions are frequently present concomitantly with the pleural effusions.

The diagnosis of systemic lupus erythematosus should be considered in all patients with undiagnosed pleurisy or pleural effusion. The pleural fluid is typically a serous exudate, and the differential may reveal predominantly lymphocytes, neutrophils, or mesothelial cells. The pleural fluid in the majority of cases is characterized by an antinuclear antibody (ANA) titer of 1:160 or greater and a pleural fluid to serum ANA ratio of 1 or more (59). In contrast to the pleural fluid associated with rheumatoid pleuritis, the pleural fluid with lupus pleuritis has a normal pH and glucose level and the LDH is below 500 IU/liter (60).

Usually no treatment other than analgesia is necessary for the patient with lupus pleuritis, since the effusion is small and resolves spontaneously. However, in those few patients in whom the pleuritis is prolonged and severe or in whom the effusion is massive, corticosteroids in moderately large doses may bring dramatic relief. Corticosteroids should be given when a pericardial effusion is present.

### Rheumatoid Pleuritis

Approximately 20% of patients with rheumatoid arthritis will at some time have pleuritic chest pain and about 4% will have a pleural effusion. The pleuritic chest pain may occur before, be coincident with, or occur after the onset of arthritis. The pleural effusion usually occurs after the onset of the arthritis, frequently in conjunction with an arthritic flare-up. Most rheumatoid pleural effusions occur in men, and the majority of patients with rheumatoid effusions also have subcutaneous rheumatoid nodules. The effusion may be on either side and is sometimes bilateral. It is usually small to moderate in size and only occasionally does it produce symptoms, including fever and pleuritic chest pain (60).

The diagnosis is suggested by the clinical picture of rheumatoid arthritis and the presence of a pleural effusion. The pleural fluid with rheumatoid pleuritis is very distinctive in that it is characterized by a glucose level less than 30 mg/100 ml, an LDH level above 700 IU/liter, a pH less than 7.20, low levels of complement, and the presence of immune complexes (60). The other condition that is likely to yield similar pleural fluid findings is a complicated parapneumonic effusion. Since patients with rheumatoid disease tend to have a high incidence of complicated parapneumonic effusion, the differentiation of the two entities is important and is dependent on the Gram stain and culture of the pleural fluid.

The optimal therapy for rheumatoid pleural effusions remains unclear. Although the majority of such effusions resolve spontaneously over several months, in some the effusion persists, leading to the development of a thick peel covering the visceral pleura and producing a severe restrictive ventilatory defect. There is no treatment that has been shown to alter the course of rheumatoid pleuritis.

### Other Collagen Vascular Diseases

An eosinophilic pleural effusion with a very high LDH level, a low glucose level, and a low pH may occur with the Churg-Strauss syndrome, which is characterized by hypereosinophilia and systemic vasculitis in the patient with asthma. Patients with Wegener's granulomatosis, familial Mediterranean fever, and immunoblastic lymphadenopathy also at times get pleural effusions. The effusions in these situations rarely dominate the clinical picture (21).

## Pleural Effusions Secondary to Pulmonary Embolization

The diagnosis of pulmonary embolization should be considered in every patient with an undiagnosed pleural effusion. Nearly 50% of patients with pulmonary emboli have a pleural effusion. There are two separate mechanisms by which pulmonary emboli can produce pleural effusion. First, the vascular obstruction associated with the emboli can lead to elevated intravascular pressures in the lung or pleura, which can produce a transudative pleural effusion. Second, the ischemia and release of the vasoactive amines secondary to the embolus can increase the permeability of the capillaries in the lung, leading to an increased amount of interstitial fluid and an exudative pleural effusion.

Most pleural effusions associated with pulmonary emboli are small, occupying less than 15% of the hemithorax, and the majority are unilateral. If parenchymal infiltrates are present, the pleural effusions tend to be larger but they rarely occupy more than 50% of the hemithorax (61). The pleural fluid may be either a transudate or an exudate depending on which of the two mechanisms is responsible for its formation. With exudative pleural effusions, the pleural fluid has a red cell count below 10,000/mm³ in nearly one-third of cases. The diagnosis is established by demonstrating mismatching of perfusion and ventilation on lung scans or obstruction of the pulmonary vasculature on pulmonary angiography. If the patient has a large pleural effusion, a therapeutic thoracentesis should be performed before the lung scans are obtained, because the presence of large amounts of pleural fluid makes interpretation of the lung scans difficult.

The treatment of choice for the patient with pleural effusions secondary to pulmonary embolization is adequate anticoagulation (see Chapter 13). The presence of blood in the pleural fluid does not serve as a contraindication for anticoagulation. Tube thoracostomy for a bloody pleural effusion secondary to pulmonary emboli should be performed only if the hematocrit of the pleural fluid is above 20%.

## Pleural Effusions Secondary to Gastrointestinal Conditions

### Acute Pancreatitis

Between 5 and 20% of patients with acute pancreatitis have an associated pleural effusion (52). The mechanism responsible for the pleural effusion associated with pancreatitis appears to be inflammation of the diaphragmatic pleura secondary to the transdiaphragmatic transfer of pancreatic enzymes. The clinical picture is usually dominated by abdominal symptoms; however, at times respiratory symptoms consisting of pleuritic chest pain and dyspnea may predominate. In addition to the small to moderate-sized pleural effusion, the chest radiograph may reveal an elevated diaphragm and basilar infiltrates. The diagnosis is confirmed with demonstration of an elevated pleural fluid amylase level. Patients with pancreatitis and a pleural effusion should be treated for their pancreatitis in the usual manner.

### Chronic Pancreatic Pleural Effusion

Patients with a pancreatic pseudocyst at times develop a large chronic pleural effusion. The pathogenesis of the large pleural effusion is a sinus tract that runs from the pancreas to the pleural space. The clinical picture is usually dominated by chest symptoms, and most patients do not have abdominal symptoms because the pancreaticopleural fistula decompresses the pseudocyst. The pleural effusion is usually massive

and recurs rapidly after thoracentesis. It most commonly is left-sided but it may be right-sided or bilateral. The diagnosis is supported by a markedly elevated pleural fluid amylase level. This is an important diagnosis to consider, because most patients with this entity look like they have malignancy. Accordingly, the pleural fluid amylase level should be measured in all patients with large chronic pleural effusions. The diagnosis is established with CT scan of the abdomen. Treatment consists of total parenteral nutrition plus drainage of the pleural space. Some patients also require surgical drainage of the pancreas or decortication (63).

### Esophageal Perforations

Most esophageal perforations are associated with either a pleural effusion or a hydropneumothorax. Since the mortality associated with this condition approaches 100% if it remains undiagnosed for several days, it should be considered in every patient with a pleural effusion who appears acutely ill. Esophageal perforations occur in three different settings: (*a*) as a complication of endoscopy, esophageal dilation, or thoracic surgery; (*b*) spontaneously when there is a sudden explosive rise in intraabdominal pressure, usually in association with vomiting; and (*c*) as a complication of esophageal carcinoma.

The clinical picture associated with esophageal rupture is impressive and is highly suggestive of the diagnosis. Pain is the most striking symptom and is characteristically excruciating, unremitting, and unrelieved by opiates. Thirst is a prominent symptom, and most patients show at least some degree of circulatory collapse. A pathognomonic triad of physical signs consists of rapid respiration, abdominal rigidity, and subcutaneous emphysema in the suprasternal notch. The chest radiograph usually reveals a pleural effusion or hydropneumothorax.

The diagnosis is not difficult if it is considered. The pleural fluid amylase level is usually very high (greater than 2500 units). The amylase in this condition has a salivary origin, and the high pleural fluid amylase level is due to the saliva leaking from the esophagus into the pleural space (64). The pleural fluid pH is usually low (below 7.00) owing to the mediastinal and pleural infection. Both Gram stains and cultures of the pleural fluid usually reveal organisms. If there is any doubt as to the diagnosis, it can be substantiated by having the patient swallow methylene blue, in which case the pleural fluid will turn blue if there is an esophageal perforation. Immediate thoracotomy with drainage of the mediastinum and pleural space is indicated once the diagnosis is made. A delay of only several hours is associated with a much higher mortality than if treatment is initiated promptly. The tear in the esophagus should be repaired and high doses of systemic broad-spectrum antibiotics should be administered (65).

### Intraabdominal Abscess

Pleural effusions frequently occur with intraabdominal abscesses. The incidence of pleural effusion is approximately 80% with subphrenic, 40% with pancreatic, 33% with splenic, and 20% with intrahepatic abscess. The possibility of intraabdominal abscess should be considered in any patient with an undiagnosed exudative pleural effusion containing predominantly polymorphonuclear leukocytes, particularly when there are no pulmonary parenchymal infiltrates. The diagnosis of intraabdominal abscess is best established with abdominal CT scanning. The appropriate treatment is drainage of the abscess combined with parenteral antibiotics (16).

## Pleural Effusions Due to Drug Reactions

Pleural effusions have been reported to occur as a complication of the administration of six different drugs, namely nitrofurantoin, methysergide, dantrolene, bromocriptine, procarbazine, and amiodarone (16). In addition, many other drugs may cause drug-induced lupus erythematosus, which frequently has an associated pleural effusion.

### Nitrofurantoin

The administration of nitrofurantoin is occasionally associated with the development of a syndrome characterized by chills, fever, and cough, soon followed by dyspnea, malaise, and pleuritic chest pain. The chest x-ray is characterized by bilateral interstitial infiltrates, and a pleural effusion is present in about 25% of the cases. This diagnosis should be suspected in any patient taking nitrofurantoin who has a pleural effusion associated with bilateral pulmonary infiltrates. If the drug is discontinued, the symptoms and radiologic abnormalities resolve within a few days.

### Methysergide

The administration of methysergide for migraine headaches can be complicated by the development of pleuritis with effusion without parenchymal infiltrates. The pleural effusions are bilateral in nearly 50% of the patients. They develop within 3 weeks to 3 years after starting the drug. Discontinuation of the drug early in the course results in complete resolution. However, if the pleuritis has been present for several months, pleural thickening may remain after the drug is discontinued.

### Dantrolene

Dantrolene sodium is a long-acting skeletal muscle relaxant used in treating patients with spastic neurologic disorders. It is structurally similar to nitrofurantoin. Its administration is at times associated with the development of sterile exudative pleural effusions without parenchymal infiltrates. Patients with this syndrome have both peripheral and pleural eosinophilia. The syndrome only develops after at least 2 months of therapy with dantrolene and may be complicated by the presence of pericardial effusion. The pleural effusion and eosinophilia typically take several months to resolve after the drug is discontinued.

### Bromocriptine

The long-term administration of bromocriptine mesylate, a dopamine receptor agonist, which is sometimes used in the long-term treatment of Parkinson's disease, can lead to pleuropulmonary changes. Patients who have taken the drug for more than 6 months many develop pleural thickening and/or a pleural effusion. The natural history of pleuropulmonary disease during bromocriptine therapy is unclear, as the disease progresses only in some of the patients who continue taking the drug (21).

### Procarbazine

There have been two detailed case reports in which pleuropulmonary reactions consisting of chills, cough, dyspnea, and bilateral pulmonary infiltrates with pleural effusion occurred after treatment with procarbazine. In both cases symptoms redeveloped within hours of rechallenge (21).

### Amiodarone

Amiodarone is a new antiarrhythmic that may produce severe pulmonary toxicity. Pleural effusions occur as a complication of amiodarone administration, but pulmonary infiltrates are much more common. Most cases with pleural effusion have concomitant parenchymal involvement (21).

## Postsurgical Procedures

### Abdominal Surgery

Nearly 50% of patients who have undergone abdominal surgery will develop a pleural effusion postoperatively (66). The incidence of pleural effusion is higher after upper abdominal surgery, in patients with postoperative atelectasis, and in patients with free abdominal fluid at surgery. Most of the effusions are exudates and are thought to be due to diaphragmatic irritation or atelectasis. Nevertheless, a diagnostic thoracentesis should be performed if the effusion is more than minimal in size to rule out a complicated parapneumonic effusion. Pleural effusions developing several days after abdominal surgery suggest either pulmonary embolization or subphrenic abscess.

### Endoscopic Variceal Sclerotherapy

Small pleural effusions complicate this procedure approximately 50% of the time. The effusion is thought to result from extravasation of the sclerosant into the esophageal mucosa, which results in an intense inflammatory reaction in the mediastinum and pleura. If the effusion persists for more than 24 to 48 hours and is accompanied by fever, or if the effusion occupies more than 25% of the hemithorax, a thoracentesis should be done to rule out an infection or an esophagopleural fistula (67).

### Post–Cardiac Injury Syndrome

The post–cardiac injury (Dressler's) syndrome is characterized by pericarditis with effusion, pleuritis, and pneumonitis following myocardial infarction, cardiac surgery, or cardiac trauma (68). This syndrome occurs between 1 and 12 weeks following the initiating event and complicates about 1% of myocardial infarctions. The pleural effusions may be either unilateral or bilateral and are usually small to moderate in size. The pleural fluid is an exudate that is often bloody. The diagnosis is established by excluding other causes of pleural effusion in the patient with a recent history of myocardial insult. The treatment of choice is salicylates if the patient is not excessively symptomatic, since the syndrome is self limiting. If the patient is distressed, corticosteroids are rapidly effective in relieving symptoms.

### Coronary Artery Bypass Surgery

The incidence of pleural effusion after coronary artery bypass surgery exceeds 50%. The incidence of effusion is higher after internal mammary artery grafting than after saphenous vein grafting alone. Most of the effusions are left-sided and small. With time the effusion gradually disappears. However, at 30 days postoperatively, the prevalence of pleural effusion still exceeds 30% when patients are examined with ultrasound. If the effusion is moderate-sized or larger, or if the effusion remains more than minimal and the patient has pleural symptoms, a diagnostic thoracentesis should be performed (69).

### Exudative Pleural Effusions Due to Other Diseases

### Asbestosis

Asbestos exposure that may have been brief, intermittent, and in the immediate or distant past may lead to a pleural effusion. Epler and coworkers (70) reviewed the medical histories of 1135 asbestos workers whom they had observed for several years and found that 35 of the workers (3%) had pleural effusions for which there was no other explanation. The heavier the asbestos exposure, the more likely the patient is to develop a pleural effusion. The pleural effusion sometimes develops within 5 years of the initial exposure but sometimes may not develop until more than 30 years after the initial exposure (71). Most patients with

pleural effusions caused by asbestos are asymptomatic. The pleural fluid is an exudate and frequently has more than 10% eosinophils.

The diagnosis of benign pleural effusion caused by asbestos is one of exclusion and requires the following: (*a*) a history of exposure to asbestos; (*b*) exclusion of other causes, notably infection, pulmonary embolism, and malignancy; and (*c*) a follow-up of at least 3 years to verify that the effusion is benign. There is no known treatment for pleural effusion caused by asbestos.

### Meigs' Syndrome

By definition, Meigs' syndrome is the presence of a pleural effusion and ascites in association with an ovarian tumor that is solid, benign, and characteristically a fibroma. Resection of the tumor must effect resolution of the ascites and pleural effusion with no recurrence. The basic abnormality with Meigs' syndrome appears to be fluid loss from the benign tumor into the peritoneum (72). At laparotomy, these tumors are frequently noted to be oozing serous fluid. The effusion is usually on the right side but may be bilateral or left-sided. The size of the pleural effusion is largely independent of the amount of ascites. The pleural fluid may be either a transudate or an exudate. The diagnosis is made at laparotomy with the demonstration of the benign tumor and is confirmed when the ascites and pleural fluid disappear postoperatively. Although Meigs' syndrome is uncommon, it is important to remember it so that patients with a pelvic mass, pleural effusion, and ascites are not labeled as having disseminated ovarian malignancy without histologic proof.

### Pulmonary and Lymph Node Myomatosis

This rare condition (73) is characterized by the widespread proliferation of smooth muscles in the lymph nodes and lungs, resulting in a honeycomb lung and frequently a chylothorax. Almost all the cases have been in females, and most of the patients present with dyspnea, which is usually due to chylothorax. The chylothorax results from obstruction of the lymphatics by the smooth muscle proliferation. Diagnosis is made by lung biopsy. Treatment in general is unsatisfactory, and most patients die within 10 years of onset. There is some evidence that the smooth muscle proliferation is hormonally dependent. It is therefore recommended patients be treated with medroxyprogesterone intramuscularly at a dose of 400 to 800 mg per month for at least 1 year. Other therapies that can be tried if the medroxyprogesterone fails are oophorectomy or tamoxifen (73).

### Uremia

A fibrinous pleurisy occasionally occurs in the course of uremia (74). The pathogenesis of the pleuritis is probably similar to that of the pericarditis seen with uremia. More than half of the patients with uremic pleuritis also have uremic pericarditis. The blood urea nitrogen concentration has borne little relationship to the occurrence of the pleuritis. The pleural fluid with uremic pleuritis is an exudate, which is frequently bloody with many eosinophils. The diagnosis is made by excluding other causes of exudative pleural effusions in patients with uremia. In approximately 80% of patients, the effusions will resolve over a 4- to 6- week period with hemodialysis. In the remainder, pleurodesis such as that done for malignant pleural effusions should be considered.

*Trapped Lung*

As a result of inflammation, a fibrous peel may form over the visceral pleura. The peel can prevent the underlying lung from expanding and lead to a chronic decrease in the pleural pressure. From Figure 18.1 it is easily seen how a more negative pleural pressure could lead to pleural fluid accumulation. The effusion usually becomes evident several months after the initial insult, which can be pneumonitis, thoracic surgery, pneumothorax, trauma, or any other condition producing intense inflammation of the pleura. The pleural fluid with trapped lung usually meets the criteria for an exudate. The diagnosis of trapped lung is best made by measuring the pleural pressures as fluid is withdrawn during a therapeutic thoracentesis (11). If the pleural pressure drops more than 2 cm $H_2O$ for each 100 ml of pleural fluid withdrawn, the patient in all probability has a trapped lung. If the patient is asymptomatic, no therapy is necessary. If the patient is symptomatic from the effusion, a decortication should be considered.

*Yellow Nail Syndrome*

Pleural effusions are frequently associated with congenital abnormalities of the lymphatics. The most common syndrome is characterized by yellow nails, lymphedema, and chronic pleural effusion (75). Often the pleural effusion does not appear until the patient reaches middle age. Examination of the pleural fluid reveals an exudate that is not chylous. The diagnosis can be made by examining the fingernails. When the patient is symptomatic from a large effusion, pleurodesis with talc or a tetracycline derivative should be considered.

*Sarcoidosis*

The incidence of pleural effusion with sarcoidosis is probably between 1 and 2%. The pleural effusions are usually small, and the pleural fluid is an exudate with predominantly small lymphocytes. The pleural biopsy with sarcoid pleural effusion may reveal noncaseating granulomas. The pleural effusion secondary to sarcoidosis may resolve spontaneously, or corticosteroid therapy may be required for its resolution. It is important to rule out the diagnosis of tuberculous pleuritis in patients with known sarcoid and an exudative pleural effusion (76).

*Urinary Tract Obstruction*

Obstruction of the urinary tract with its associated retroperitoneal urine collection can lead to a pleural effusion. It is believed that the urine moves directly retroperitoneally into the pleural space. The diagnosis is established by the demonstration that the pleural fluid creatinine level is higher than the serum creatinine level. The pleural effusion will rapidly disappear when the urinary tract obstruction is relieved (77).

**Chylothorax and Pseudochylothorax**

Pleural fluid is occasionally found to be milky or at least turbid. When this cloudiness persists after centrifugation, it is almost always due to a high lipid content in the pleural fluid. Two different situations bring about the accumulation of high levels of lipid in the pleural liquid. In the first, chyle enters the pleural space as a result of disruption of the thoracic duct, producing a *chylothorax* or a *chylous* effusion. In the second, large amounts of cholesterol or lecithin-globulin complexes accumulate in a longstanding pleural effusion to produce a *pseudochylothorax* or a *chyliform* pleural effusion.

Chylothoraces can be traumatic or nontraumatic in origin. The most common traumatic cause is a cardiovascular surgical procedure, but penetrating injuries or nonpenetrating injuries in which the spine is hyperextended can lead to chylothorax. Tumors, most commonly lymphomas, are the most common cause of nontraumatic chylothorax. Other diseases associated with chylothorax include pulmonary lymphangiomyomatosis (discussed earlier in this chapter), abnormalities of the lymphatic vessels such as intestinal lymphangiectasis, filariasis, lymph node enlargement, lymphangitis of the thoracic duct, and tuberous sclerosis (21). If no etiology can be found for the chylothorax, it is labeled as idiopathic. Before attaching this label, however, lymphoma should be excluded.

Patients with chylothorax present with large pleural effusions. Pleuritic chest pain is very rare because chyle is not irritating to the pleura. The pleural fluid with chylothorax is distinctive in that it looks like milk and has no odor. At times the pleural fluid may be blood-tinged or frankly bloody. Chemical analysis of the pleural fluid usually reveals triglyceride levels above 110 mg/dl. Triglyceride levels below 50 mg/dl rule out the diagnosis. If doubt remains as to whether a patient has a chylothorax, lipoprotein analysis of the pleural fluid should be obtained. The demonstration of chylomicrons in the pleural fluid by lipoprotein analysis establishes the diagnosis of chylothorax.

The primary danger to the patient with chylothorax is malnutrition and a compromised immunologic status caused by the removal of large amounts of protein, fat, electrolytes, and lymphocytes with repeated thoracenteses or chest tube drainage. Therefore, it is important to undertake definitive treatment for the chylothorax before the patient becomes too cachectic to tolerate the treatment. Most patients with traumatic or idiopathic chylothorax should originally be treated with a pleuroperitoneal shunt (78). The shunt takes the chyle with its nutrients and leukocytes from the pleural space to the peritoneal cavity, where it is absorbed. This treatment keeps the patient from becoming malnourished and allows the thoracic duct time to heal, which it will do spontaneously in the majority of patients. If the chylothorax persists for more than 4 weeks, consideration should be given to surgical exploration with ligation of the thoracic duct (21). Patients with nontraumatic chylothorax can also be treated with the pleuroperitoneal shunt, and this is probably the treatment of choice if the patient's life expectancy is limited. If the patient has mediastinal lymphoma, the chylothorax will usually resolve after radiotherapy or effective chemotherapy. If the patient has benign disease, consideration should be given to chemical pleurodesis with talc (79) or surgical exploration with ligation of the thoracic duct.

The diagnosis of pseudochylothorax is usually easy. The patient has usually had a pleural effusion for 5 years or longer, and the pleura is thickened or calcified. Chemical analysis of the pleural fluid usually reveals cholesterol crystals or pleural fluid cholesterol levels above 250 mg/dl. If the patient's exercise capacity is limited by shortness of breath, a therapeutic thoracentesis should be performed because some patients will improve markedly. If the patient is symptomatic and the underlying lung is believed to be functional, a decortication should be considered (80).

### Hemothorax

A hemothorax is said to be present when the hematocrit in the pleural fluid is greater than 50% of the peripheral hematocrit. Most hemothoraces are due to trauma. A spontaneous hemothorax occasionally occurs with malignancy when the vasculature is invaded by the tumor. Among other causes, hemothoraces can occur as a result of a leaking aortic aneurysm or pulmonary arteriovenous malformations, as a complication of overzealous anticoagulation for pulmonary emboli, or as a complication of splenoportography. There are several other rare causes of hemothorax, and at times the etiology of the hemothorax remains unknown despite exploratory thoracotomy.

One would think that the diagnosis of a hemothorax is simple. However, frequently pleural fluid will appear to be pure blood when in fact the hematocrit of the fluid is less than 5%. Accordingly, when bloody pleural fluid is obtained on thoracentesis, a hematocrit should be obtained. The diagnosis of hemothorax should be made only when the pleural fluid hematocrit is above 20%. At times it may be difficult to determine whether the bloody fluid obtained is venous or arterial blood or pleural fluid. However, blood that has been present in the pleural space for more than a few minutes will not clot, while both venous and arterial blood will clot.

Patients with traumatic hemothoraces should be initially managed by inserting a chest tube (81). Not only can the blood be removed by the chest tube, diminishing the likelihood of a subsequent fibrothorax, but the drainage from the chest tube will allow an assessment of persistent bleeding and will serve as a guide as to whether a thoracotomy is necessary for control of the bleeding. If persistent bleeding is not observed but the hemothorax cannot be completely evacuated with the chest tube, thoracotomy is not recommended, since the majority of such cases will spontaneously absorb the clotted blood over the subsequent weeks to months (81). However, one must be constantly alert to the possibility of pleural infection in such patients (81).

### Pleural Diseases Not Associated with Effusion

*Fibrothorax*

A dense layer of fibrous tissue may be deposited over the pleural surface when there is intense inflammation in the pleural space, most commonly following empyema or hemothorax. The fibrous tissue creates a cast for the lung and renders it immobile and essentially unavailable for air exchange. On physical examination the affected side is fixed and does not move with respiration. Breath sounds are absent and the percussion note is dull. The treatment of fibrothorax is to remove the fibrous peel from the visceral pleura in an operation called a decortication. If the underlying lung is intact, decortication may result in spectacular improvement in the subjective feeling and in the pulmonary functions of the patient. This improvement can occur even if the fibrothorax has been present 10 or more years.

*Pleural Thickening Associated with Asbestos Exposure*

The pleura of patients exposed to asbestos may develop plaques or diffuse thickening. The pleural disease is thought to be the result of short, submicroscopic asbestos fibers entering the pleural space. Then the small asbestos fibers lodge in the pleural lymphatics and in conjunction with appropriate inflammatory cells create inflammation that eventually leads to plaque formation or diffuse fibrosis (80). Pleural calcification usually occurs only 20 or more years after the initial exposure to asbestos. Patients with pleural thickening or calcification are usually asymptomatic. The pleural involvement with asbestos exposure is usually bilateral, but if it is unilateral the left hemithorax is more frequently involved. The detection of pleural thickening or calcification is significant only as an indication of previous exposure to asbestos. However, since it is known that heavy asbestos exposure is associated with a markedly higher incidence of bronchogenic carcinomas and mesotheliomas, the presence of these abnormalities should alert the clinician to these possibilities.

## Pneumothorax

Pneumothorax is the presence of gas in the pleural space. A *spontaneous* pneumothorax is one that occurs without antecedent trauma to the thorax. These pneumothoraces can be subdivided into *primary* spontaneous pneumothorax, for which there is no underlying predisposing disease, and *secondary* spontaneous pneumothorax, for which there is an underlying disease such as cystic fibrosis or emphysema that is known to be associated with the development of pneumothorax. A *traumatic* pneumothorax occurs as a result of penetrating or nonpenetrating chest injuries. An iatrogenic pneumothorax occurs as an intended, unavoidable, or inadvertent consequence of a diagnostic or therapeutic maneuver. A *tension* pneumothorax is a pneumothorax in which the pressure in the pleural space is positive throughout the respiratory cycle.

### Pathogenesis

The pressure in the pleural space is negative in reference to the atmospheric pressure and the alveolar pressure. Therefore, if there is a communication either between the alveoli and the pleural space or between the outside of the thoracic cavity and the pleural space, air will continue to enter the pleural space until the pleural pressure becomes atmospheric. The increase in the pleural pressure will result in both a hyperexpanded hemithorax and a collapsed lung. Occasionally, when the communication is between the alveoli and the pleural space, a ''ball-valve'' effect is present, resulting in a one-way flow of air into the pleural space. Since the alveolar pressure becomes very positive with respect to atmospheric pressure during expiration, especially when there is coughing, the pleural pressure may become quite positive, producing a tension pneumothorax.

### Primary Spontaneous Pneumothorax

Approximately 8600 individuals in the United States develop a primary spontaneous pneumothorax each year (21). Tall, thin individuals appear to be more susceptible to this entity. Primary spontaneous pneumothoraces are usually due to the rupture of apical pleural blebs. These are small cystic spaces, seldom exceeding 1 to 2 cm in diameter, which lie within or immediately under the visceral pleura. The main symptoms associated with a spontaneous pneumothorax are chest pain and dyspnea. The symptoms start abruptly in about two-thirds of the cases and insidiously in the remainder. In the majority of cases the symptoms start while the patient is sedentary. The diagnosis is established with the demonstration of a visceral pleural line on the chest radiograph.

The recommended initial treatment for primary spontaneous pneumothorax is simple aspiration (82). A 16-gauge needle with an internal polyethylene catheter is inserted into the second anterior intercostal space at the midclavicular line after local anesthesia. After the needle is inserted, it is extracted from the cannula. Then a three-way stopcock and a 60-ml syringe are attached to the catheter and air is manually withdrawn until no more can be aspirated. If the total volume of air aspirated exceeds 4 liters and no resistance has been felt, it can be assumed that no expansion has occurred and a chest tube should be inserted (82).

The recurrence rate for primary spontaneous pneumothorax is between 30 and 50% over 5 years (82). If a patient has a chest tube on the initial occurrence or an ipsilateral recurrence he or she should have a sclerosing agent injected into the pleural space in an attempt to prevent a recurrence. The intrapleural injection of tetracycline will decrease the recurrence rate by about 50% (83), but tetracycline is no longer available. Alternatives include minocycline (4 to 5 mg/kg), doxycycline (5 to 10 mg/kg) (82), or 5 g talc in slurry (79). Intrapleural bleomycin should not be used because it does not produce pleurodesis in a normal pleural space (84). If there is a subsequent recurrence, thoracoscopy or open thoracotomy with pleural abrasion should be performed, since in this situation the likelihood of another recurrence exceeds 80%.

### Secondary Spontaneous Pneumothorax

COPD is responsible for more secondary spontaneous pneumothoraces than is any other disease. The occurrence of a pneumothorax in these patients is more life-threatening than it is in a normal individual on account of their limited pulmonary reserve. Owing to the diminished breath sounds and lung hyperinflation of these patients, the diagnosis, both by physical examination and radiographically, is much more difficult than it is in the normal individual. The possibility of a pneumothorax should be considered in all patients with an exacerbation of their COPD, and the chest radiograph should be closely examined for a pleural line. Since small pneumothoraces can lead to marked respiratory embarrassment, all patients should be treated with tube thoracostomy. We routinely instill talc slurry or a tetracycline derivative into the pleural space of such patients in an attempt to prevent a recurrence. If after 7 days of tube thoracostomy the lung remains collapsed or a bronchopleural fistula persists, thoracoscopy is indicated. At thoracoscopy the blebs should be ligated and pleurodesis should be attempted using pleural scarification or the insufflation of talc (85).

Secondary spontaneous pneumothoraces complicate about 1% of parenchymal tuberculosis cases. Such cases should be treated with tube thoracostomy. Frequently multiple tubes are necessary for long periods to effect resolution of the process. Bacterial pneumonia, particularly that due to *Staphylococcus aureus*, may be complicated by pneumothorax. In this situation there is usually a complicating empyema. Such cases should have two chest tubes inserted: one high to drain the air and the other one low to drain the pus. Secondary spontaneous pneumothoraces have also been reported in association with AIDS and *Pneumocystis carinii* pneumonia, asthma, cystic fibrosis, scleroderma, histiocytosis X, tuberous sclerosis, interstitial pneumonitis, sarcoidosis, pulmonary embolization, rheumatoid disease, hydatid disease, silicosis, metastatic malignancy, and primary carcinoma of the lung.

*Tension Pneumothorax*

A tension pneumothorax is present when the intrapleural pressure exceeds the atmospheric pressure throughout expiration and often during inspiration as well. The positive pleural pressure is life threatening, not only because ventilation is severely compromised, but also because the positive pressure is transmitted to the mediastinum, resulting in decreased venous return to the heart and reduced cardiac output. In addition, patients with tension pneumothorax are usually markedly hypoxemic. With a tension pneumothorax, the positive pressure in the pleural space is sustained by a "ball-valve" mechanism during most of inspiration as well as during expiration. Strong inspiratory efforts promote the entry of air into the pleural space, but the check valve prevents its egress, so the pressure continues to increase in the pleural space.

Tension pneumothorax most commonly develops in patients who are receiving positive-pressure mechanical ventilation or during cardiopulmonary resuscitation. Occasionally a tension pneumothorax will evolve during the course of a spontaneous pneumothorax. Patients with tension pneumothorax are acutely ill with dyspnea, tachycardia, and tachypnea. The neck veins are distended and the decreased venous return results in a thready pulse and hypotension. The trachea is deviated toward the side contralateral to the pneumothorax. With tension pneumothorax, the ipsilateral diaphragm is depressed, the involved hemithorax is enlarged, and the mediastinum is shifted to the contralateral side, but all three of these changes also occur to a lesser degree with nontension pneumothorax.

The treatment of a tension pneumothorax is a medical emergency. If the tension in the pleural space is not relieved, the patient is likely to die from inadequate cardiac output or marked hypoxemia. If the diagnosis is suspected, a large-bore needle should be inserted into the pleural space through the second anterior intercostal space. If large amounts of gas come forth through the needle after its insertion, the diagnosis is confirmed. Observation of this phenomenon is facilitated by attaching the needle to a syringe containing sterile saline. If this procedure confirms the presence of a tension pneumothorax, the needle should be left in place until a thoracostomy tube can be inserted. In contrast, if air passes from the atmosphere into the pleural space, a tension pneumothorax is not present and the needle should be immediately withdrawn.

## DISEASES OF THE MEDIASTINUM

The mediastinum is the region between the pleural sacs. It is bounded laterally by the mediastinal pleura and extends from the thoracic inlet superiorly to the diaphragm inferiorly and from the sternum anteriorly to the spine posteriorly. The mediastinum contains the heart; the thoracic aorta and its proximal branches; the venae cavae; the azygos and proximal innominate veins; the thoracic duct; the lymph nodes and lymphatics; the esophagus; the trachea; the thymus; and the vagus, phrenic, posterior intercostal, and sympathetic nerves. Anatomically the mediastinum is divided into three compartments (Fig. 18.2). The anatomical boundaries, the normal contents, and the lesions that occur in the three compartments are shown in Table 18.2.

### MEDIASTINAL MASSES

Mediastinal masses may be discovered as a result of routine chest radiographs or in the evaluation of symptoms suggestive of mediastinal disease. Regardless, the differential diagnosis involves an abnormal shadow in the mediastinum on a radiograph. Since a given mediastinal lesion tends to be located in one mediastinal compartment, the first step in evaluating a mediastinal lesion is to place it in one of three mediastinal compartments. The lesions that tend to appear in

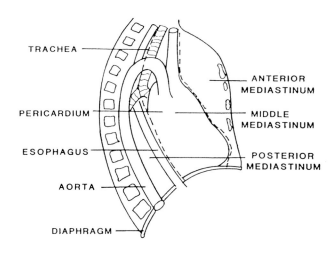

**FIGURE 18.2.** Subdivisions of the mediastinum. The *dashed lines* separate the middle mediastinum from the anterior and the posterior mediastinum.

the various compartments are tabulated in Table 18.2, and the following discussion of mediastinal masses is organized according to the three compartments. It should be emphasized that the locations tabulated in Table 18.2 are those in which the various masses are most likely to occur. For example, lymph node involvement in lymphoma occurs almost as frequently in the anterior as in the middle compartment. Aortic aneurysms may be situated in any of the three compartments.

It is evident from Table 18.2 that there are many different abnormalities that can produce abnormal mediastinal shadows. The relative incidence of the more common primary mediastinal tumors and cysts is outlined in Table 18.3. This table was compiled by combining nine series of adult patients and five series of pediatric patients (86). The incidence is heavily dependent on the patient's age. Thymomas are the most common abnormality in adults but are rare in children. Neurogenic tumors occur very frequently in children, while pleuropericardial cysts and endocrine (thyroid, parathyroid) tumors are very uncommon.

It should be emphasized that the majority of abnormal mediastinal shadows do not represent primary mediastinal cysts or tumors. In a review of 782 cases of mediastinal masses, Lyons and coworkers (87) found that neoplasms accounted for the most mediastinal masses (41.6%), followed closely by inflammatory diseases (35.7%) such as sarcoidosis, histoplasmosis, and tuberculosis and then by vascular abnormalities (10.6%), hernias, diverticula, and achalasia (5.4%), cysts (2.8%), and miscellaneous disorders (3.9%).

The diagnostic approach to disorders of the mediastinum may be divided into imaging techniques (computed tomography, magnetic resonance imaging, radionuclide studies, and barium studies) and

**TABLE 18.2**

**THE ANATOMICAL BOUNDARIES, THE NORMAL CONTENTS, AND THE LESIONS THAT OCCUR PREDOMINANTLY IN THE THREE DIFFERENT MEDIASTINAL COMPARTMENTS**

| | **Anterior Compartment** | **Middle Compartment** | **Posterior Compartment** |
|---|---|---|---|
| Anatomical boundaries | Manubrium and sternum anteriorly; pericardium, aorta, and brachiocephalic vessels posteriorly | Anterior mediastinum anteriorly; posterior mediastinum posteriorly | Pericardium and trachea anteriorly; vertebral column posteriorly |
| Contents | Thymus gland, anterior mediastinal lymph nodes, internal mammary arteries and veins | Pericardium, heart, ascending and transverse arch of aorta, superior and inferior venae cavae, brachiocephalic arteries and veins, phrenic nerves, trachea and main bronchi and their contiguous lymph nodes, pulmonary arteries and veins | Descending thoracic aorta, esophagus, thoracic duct, azygous and hemiazygos veins, sympathetic chains, and the posterior group of mediastinal lymph nodes |
| Common abnormalities | Thymoma, lymphomas, teratomatous neoplasms, thyroid masses, parathyroid masses, mesenchymal tumors, giant lymph node hyperplasia, hernia through foramen of Morgagni | Metastatic lymph node enlargement, granulomatous lymph node enlargement, pleuropericardial cysts, bronchogenic cysts, masses of vascular origin | Neurogenic tumors, meningocele, meningomyelocele, gastroenteric cysts, esophageal diverticula, hernia through foramen of Bochdalek, extramedullary hematopoiesis |

**Table 18.3**
**Relative Frequency of Various Primary Mediastinal Tumors and Cysts in Adults and Children**

| Tumor or Cyst | Adults | | Children | |
|---|---|---|---|---|
| | Number | % | Number | % |
| Neurogenic tumor | 384 | 21 | 135 | 39 |
| Thymoma | 387 | 21 | 0 | 0 |
| Lymphoma | 242 | 13 | 68 | 19 |
| Teratomatous neoplasm | 201 | 11 | 42 | 12 |
| Primary carcinoma | 65 | 4 | 16 | 5 |
| Mesenchymal tumor | 134 | 7 | 35 | 10 |
| Endocrine tumor | 115 | 6 | 0 | 0 |
| Pleuropericardial cysts | 126 | 7 | 0 | 0 |
| Bronchogenic cysts | 126 | 7 | 28 | 8 |
| Enteric cysts | 57 | 3 | 24 | 7 |
| | 1832 | 100 | 349 | 100 |

From Jones KW, Pietra GG, Sabiston DC Jr: Primary neoplasms and cysts of the mediastinum. In Fishman AP (ed): *Pulmonary Diseases and Disorders.* New York, McGraw-Hill, 1980. With permission of McGraw-Hill Book Co.

procedures for obtaining tissue samples (needle aspiration and biopsy and mediastinoscopy). Computed tomographic (CT) imaging of the mediastinum is the most valuable imaging technique. The accurate cross-sectional information provided by CT can be very useful when a mediastinal mass cannot be accurately delineated by conventional radiographic methods, as illustrated in Figure 18.3. With thoracic CT, normal variations and benign neoplasms such as fat and fluid-filled cysts can be distinguished from other processes, and the site of origin of masses can be better identified. Magnetic resonance imaging (MRI) is usually reserved for clarifying problems encountered on CT or to examine patients who cannot tolerate IV administration of contrast material (88). At times barium studies of the gastrointestinal tract are indicated since hernias, diverticula, and achalasia are readily diagnosed in this manner.

In many patients with mediastinal masses, a definitive diagnosis can be obtained with radiologically guided percutaneous needle biopsy of the mass. In a recent series of 95 patients, the diagnosis of malignancy was established with greater than 90% sensitivity and 100% specificity (89). Fine-needle aspiration techniques usually suffice for carcinomatous lesions, but a cutting-needle biopsy should be performed whenever possible when lymphoma, thymoma, or neural masses are suspected to obtain larger specimens for more accurate histologic diagnosis. At times mediastinoscopy (90) or anterior mediastinotomy (91) is necessary to establish the diagnosis.

### Mediastinal Masses Located Primarily in the Anterior Compartment

*Thymoma*

Thymic tumors are the most common tumors in the anterior mediastinum and account for about 20% of all primary mediastinal tumors. About 25% are malignant and are invasive by direct extension rather than by distant metastasis. The differentiation between benign and malignant tumors must be made at surgery, since they cannot be distinguished histologically.

The peak incidence of thymomas is between the ages of 40 and 60; they are rare in children. Benign tumors are usually discovered on routine chest radiography since they are asymptomatic. Malignant thymomas produce symptoms by invading contiguous structures. Substernal chest pain and dyspnea are the most frequent symptoms.

There are several paraneoplastic syndromes that occur in patients with thymomas (92). The most common is myasthenia gravis. Approximately 40% of patients with thymic tumors have myasthenia gravis, while 10% of patients with myasthenia have thymomas. Since thymectomy will lead to improvement of the myasthenia gravis in approximately two-thirds of patients with myasthenia and thymoma, mediastinal CT is indicated in all patients with myasthenia gravis. Thymectomy should also be strongly considered for difficult patients with myasthenia gravis even if they do not have a thymoma (92). Thymomas have also been linked to the occurrence of agammaglobulinemia, aregenerative anemia, Cushing's disease, idiopathic granulomatous myocarditis, and many other diseases (92).

Radiologically, thymomas present as irregular tumors on one or both sides of the superior mediastinal shadow (Fig. 18.4). At times they are visible only in the lateral views, where they appear as a rounded or elongated shadow in the anterior part of the upper mediastinum. The upper pole of a thymoma can usually be seen clearly in the posterior-anterior (PA) film, and this differentiates it from retrosternal goiter.

All thymomas should be treated surgically. Irradiation is subordinate to surgery in the treatment of thymomas, although palliation by radiation can be obtained when complete removal of the tumor is not possible. It also appears that patients with unresectable disease may benefit from chemotherapy (92).

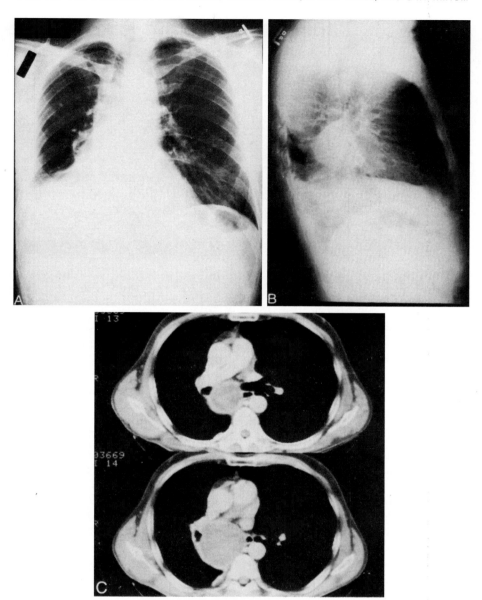

**FIGURE 18.3.** The value of CT scanning of the mediastinum in delineating mediastinal masses. Posteroanterior (**A**) and lateral (**B**) radiographs of a patient, demonstrating a mediastinal mass or a right lower lobe mass. Mediastinal CT scan (**C**) reveals that the mass is in the middle and posterior mediastinum and is separate from the right lower lobe. The patient had a bronchogenic cyst.

*Lymphomatous Tumors*

Lymphomas as a group are the second most common kind of tumor in the anterior mediastinum and are the third most frequently encountered kind of primary neoplasm of the entire mediastinum after neurogenic tumors and thymomas (93). Any of the several types of lymphatic tumors may arise in the mediastinal nodes, but Hodgkin's disease and lymphocytic lymphoma are seen most frequently. Lymph node enlarge-ment with lymphomas is most common in the anterior mediastinum but occurs frequently in the middle mediastinum and sometimes in the posterior mediastinum (Fig. 18.5).

Patients with lymphomatous involvement of the mediastinum rarely present with isolated asymptomatic mediastinal disease. Usually they also have enlargement of peripheral lymph nodes, hepatospleno-megaly, constitutional symptoms, or cutaneous or

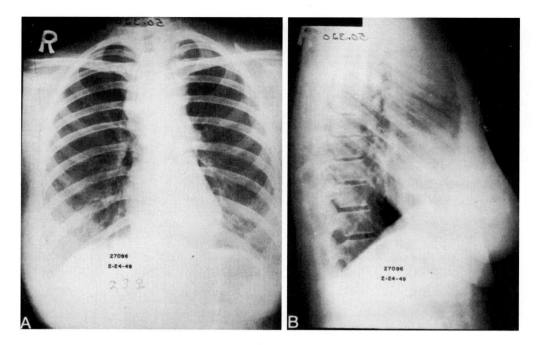

**Figure 18.4.** Thymoma. Posteroanterior (**A**) and lateral (**B**) radiographs from a 23-year-old woman with a malignant thymoma. On the posteroanterior view, the superior mediastinum is widened, while on the lateral view, the retrosternal air space is obliterated.

retroperitoneal disease. The mediastinal lymph node enlargement secondary to lymphoma is usually bilateral but asymmetric. In most cases, the mass has a nodular contour that suggests lymph node enlargement. If the diagnosis cannot be made by biopsy of a peripheral or scalene node, then mediastinoscopy is recommended. Although the treatment in the past has included attempted surgical excision, radiotherapy and chemotherapy now appear to be the treatments of choice (94).

*Germ Cell Tumors*

These neoplasms, which include teratoma, seminoma, embryonal cell carcinoma, and choriocarcinoma, constitute the third most common tumors (following thymomas and lymphomas) occurring in the anterior mediastinum. These tumors develop from embryonal tissues originating within the branchial clefts. *Dermoid cysts* are germ cell tumors that consist of only epidermis and its appendages, while *teratomas* contain ectodermal, mesodermal, and endodermal derivatives. Although they presumably are present from birth, in the majority of cases they are discovered only in adolescence or early adulthood. About 20% of mediastinal teratomatous neoplasms are malignant, with malignancy much more common in male patients. More than

90% of these neoplasms are located in the anterior mediastinum, but a few are located in the middle or posterior mediastinum (95). Adenocarcinoma is the most common malignancy found in these tissues, but seminomas, choriocarcinomas, and embryonal carcinomas are also found. Mixed histologic patterns are common.

It is unusual for symptoms to be associated with these tumors if they are benign, but symptoms are common with malignant tumors (95). Tumors that grow large may give rise to shortness of breath, cough, or a sensation of pressure in the retrosternal area. Rarely, a cystic tumor becomes infected and spills its contents into the mediastinum or pleural cavity.

Radiographically, the majority of teratodermoid tumors are in the anterior mediastinum close to the origin of the major vessels from the heart. Benign lesions tend to be oval and smooth in contour, while malignant lesions tend to be lobulated. In rare cases a bone or tooth is visible radiographically in the mass, and this establishes the diagnosis.

Measurement of serum tumor markers, $\beta$-subunit human chorionic gonadotropin (HCG), $\alpha$-fetoprotein (AFT), and lactate dehydrogenase is indispensable in the management of mediastinal germ cell tumors. Patients with benign teratoma are marker negative; a significant elevation of HCG or AFT implies a malignant

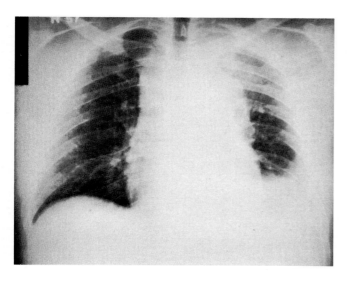

**FIGURE 18.5.** Mediastinal lymphoma. Posteroanterior radiograph from a patient with lymphocytic lymphoma demonstrating marked widening of the entire mediastinum.

component of the tumor (95). The AFT is elevated in approximately 80% of malignant nonseminomatous germ cell tumors, while the HCG is elevated in 30%. Between 50 and 70% of patients with mediastinal testicular germ cell tumors will have elevated HCG or AFP. The diagnosis of malignant germ cell tumors can be made with fine-needle aspiration or cutting-needle biopsy of the mass.

Benign teratomatous tumors should be removed surgically, since they have a tendency toward malignant transformation and infection is common in cystic lesions. The management of malignant teratomatous tumors is in transition. Although in the past megavoltage radiotherapy to the mediastinum was considered to be the treatment of choice, it now appears that cisplatin-based chemotherapy is at least as effective (95). Two-year survival with seminoma is now approaching 90% (96). Cisplatin-based chemotherapy is now considered to be the principal mode of therapy in mediastinal nonseminomatous germ cell tumors (95). If the patient's serum tumor marker levels normalize, complete resection of persistent roentgenographic abnormalities by an experienced thoracic surgeon is crucial to remove residual teratoma. The 2-year survival rate with nonseminomatous germ cell tumors now exceeds 50% (96).

*Thyroid Masses*

Intrathoracic goiter (Fig. 18.6) is the fourth most frequently seen anterior mediastinal mass, despite the fact that fewer than 3% of goiters at thyroidectomy extend into the thorax (87). Most intrathoracic thyroid masses

arise from a lower pole or from the isthmus of the thyroid and extend into the anterior mediastinum in front of the trachea. Patients are usually asymptomatic, but if the trachea becomes compressed, stridor and respiratory distress may occur. More than half the patients will have associated thyromegaly with a nodular goiter, but hyperthyroidism is uncommon. The diagnosis may be made noninvasively with a CT scan of the mediastinum that demonstrates the thyroidal origin of the mass (97). The treatment should be surgical if symptoms are present and in most other cases (97). However, if the $^{131}$I scan is positive and the patient is asymptomatic, observation may be the treatment of choice if the patient is a poor surgical candidate.

*Parathyroid Masses*

Parathyroid tumors are a rare cause of anterior mediastinal masses. They are usually small, encapsulated, benign lesions situated in the upper or middle portion of the anterior mediastinum. Since most of these tumors produce parathormone, the presence of signs and symptoms of hyperparathyroidism allows one to make the diagnosis preoperatively. It is difficult to identify the tumor preoperatively, but CT will demonstrate the lesion about 50% of the time, as will MRI (98). The treatment of choice is surgical excision.

*Mesenchymal Tumors*

The mesenchymal tumors (lipomas, fibromas, leiomyomas, lymphangiomas, hemangiomas, and mesotheliomas) account for fewer than 5% of mediastinal masses. Each tumor type has its malignant counterpart, and malignant changes occur in about 50% of these tumors (93). The majority of these tumors occur in the anterior mediastinum, with the exception of fibrosarcoma, which occurs primarily in the posterior mediastinum. The recommended treatment for all these tumors is surgical removal. In spite of treatment, malignant mesenchymal tumors are almost universally fatal (93).

*Giant Lymph Node Hyperplasia*

This unusual condition, also known as Castleman's disease, usually presents as a solitary mass in the anterior mediastinum, but sometimes it can occur in the middle or posterior mediastinum. A distinctive microscopic appearance is present, with lymphoid follicles scattered widely throughout the mass instead of being confined to the peripheral cortical zones as in normal lymph nodes (99). Radiographically there is a solitary mass up to 10 cm in diameter with a smooth or lobulated contour. Giant lymph node hyperplasia is a benign condition, and surgical excision results in permanent cure (99).

*Hernia through Foramen of Morgagni*

The foramina of Morgagni are small triangular deficiencies in the diaphragm between the muscle fibers

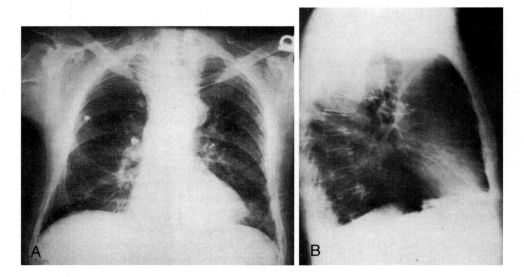

**FIGURE 18.6.** Intrathoracic goiter. Posteroanterior (**A**) and lateral (**B**) radiographs from a patient with intrathoracic goiter. The goiter is evident as a right paratracheal mass in the posteroanter- ior view and as an anterior superior mediastinal mass in the lateral view.

originating from the xiphisternum and the seventh rib. They are a few centimeters from the midline on each side. When the foramina of Morgagni are larger than normal, abdominal contents may herniate into the thorax. This herniation is into the anterior mediastinum and is usually right-sided, since the left foramen is protected by the pericardium. The diagnosis is easily established with thoracic CT. To avoid the possibility of obstruction, these hernias should be repaired surgically if they are large or if the bowel has herniated (99).

## Mediastinal Masses Occurring Predominantly in the Middle Compartment

### Lymph Node Involvement in Granulomatous Mediastinitis

Granulomatous inflammation of the mediastinal lymph nodes (Fig. 18.7) is the most common cause of a middle mediastinal mass. This entity is discussed later in this chapter.

### Metastatic Lymph Node Enlargement

Nearly 90% of tumors that develop in the middle mediastinum are malignant (93). Metastatic disease from the lungs, upper gastrointestinal tract, prostate, or kidney is the most common middle mediastinal neoplasm (Fig. 18.8). With metastatic disease, the bronchopulmonary nodes as well as the mediastinal nodes are almost invariably enlarged. When the primary lesion is in the lung, node enlargement is usually unilateral. The majority of patients with metastatic disease to the mediastinum are symptomatic with weight loss, retrosternal pain, fever, cough, or dyspnea. Symptoms secondary to involvement of other mediastinal structures, including the superior vena cava, the phrenic nerve, and the recurrent laryngeal nerve, are common. Treatment is dependent on the site of the primary tumor, but the prognosis is in general dismal, except possibly for patients with small cell undifferentiated bronchogenic carcinoma.

### Pleuropericardial Cysts

Pleuropericardial cysts have a developmental origin and appear to result from sequestration of part of the pleuroperitoneal cavity by the developing diaphragm. They rarely cause symptoms and are usually discovered on screening chest radiographs. Their most common location by far is anteriorly in the right cardiophrenic angle (100). They may also occur in the left cardiophrenic angle, in the hilar region, and in the anterior mediastinum. Pleuropericardial cysts contain crystal-clear fluid and are at times called "spring water cysts" because of their contents. The diagnosis is strongly suggested by the CT and ultrasound. Aspiration of the lesion with demonstration of the clear fluid will establish the diagnosis. Once the diagnosis is established, resection is unnecessary since these cysts virtually never produce symptoms (100).

### Bronchogenic Cysts

Bronchogenic cysts represent pinched-off buds of the primitive foregut or trachea and are lined with

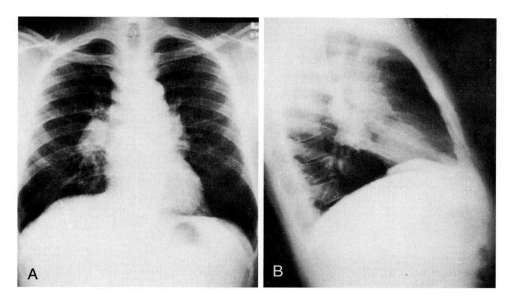

FIGURE **18.7.** Mediastinal sarcoidosis. Posteroanterior (**A**) and lateral (**B**) radiographs from a 54-year-old patient with mediastinal sarcoidosis. Note that the lymph node enlargement is relatively symmetrical and involves both the bronchopulmonary and mediastinal lymph nodes.

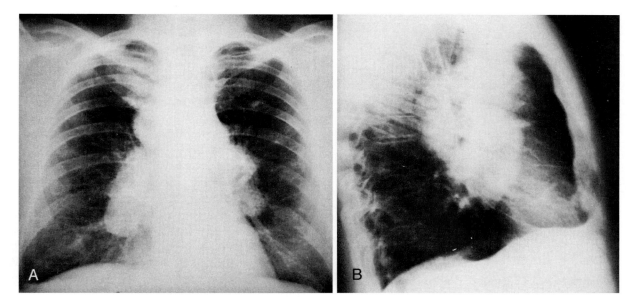

FIGURE **18.8.** Metastatic lymph node enlargement. Posteroanterior (**A**) and lateral (**B**) radiographs from a patient with metastatic kidney carcinoma, demonstrating marked enlargement of both the mediastinal and bronchopulmonary nodes.

pseudostratified columnar epithelium. They occur paratracheally or adjacent to the main carina and project into the posterior part of the middle mediastinum. Because they contain fluid, they have a relatively uniform density, a smooth border, and a round or teardrop configuration (as do pleuropericardial cysts). Bronchogenic cysts frequently become symptomatic, and for this reason surgical removal is recommended (101).

*Mediastinal Masses of Vascular Origin*

Mediastinal masses of vascular origin are most frequently found in the middle mediastinum. However, it is important to consider this diagnosis with all medi-

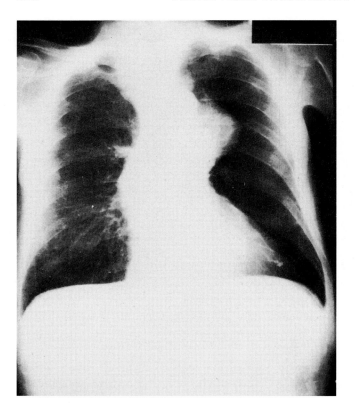

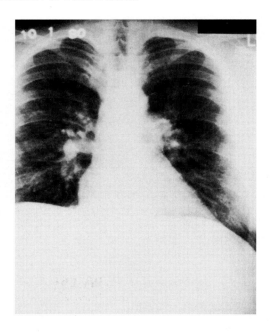

**FIGURE 18.10.** Enlarged pulmonary arteries. Posteroanterior radiograph from a 37-year-old man with primary pulmonary hypertension, demonstrating markedly enlarged pulmonary arteries that could be confused with a mediastinal mass.

**FIGURE 18.9.** Aneurysm of ascending aorta. Posteroanterior radiograph demonstrating a mass in the superior left mediastinum. At aortography the mass proved to be an aneurysm of the ascending aorta. This case illustrates how deceiving vascular masses may be at times. In fact, this patient underwent needle aspiration of the mass before the correct diagnosis was established.

astinal masses, since invasive procedures such as needle aspiration or mediastinoscopy may have disastrous consequences if the lesion is vascular (Figs. 18.9 and 18.10). CT with contrast effectively demonstrates the vascular nature of the apparent mass.

## Mediastinal Masses Situated Predominantly in the Posterior Compartment

### Neurogenic Tumors

Neurogenic tumors are the most common primary tumors in the mediastinum (93). They are characteristically situated in the posterior mediastinum because they arise from the paravertebral sympathetic nerve trunk and the spinal nerves. Approximately 20% of neural tumors are malignant.

Neurogenic tumors may be divided into three groups: (*a*) tumors that arise from peripheral nerves (neurofibroma, neurofibrosarcoma, and neurilemoma); (*b*) tumors that arise from sympathetic ganglia (ganglioneuroma, neuroblastoma, and sympathicoblastoma); and (*c*) tumors that arise from paraganglionic cells (pheochromocytoma and chemodectoma). Chemodectoma is the only neurogenic tumor that shows no strong tendency to be located in the posterior mediastinum.

The highest incidence of neurogenic neoplasms is in the younger age group, but they may develop at any age. In von Recklinghausen's disease, mediastinal neurofibromas are associated with neurofibromas elsewhere in the body. The majority of patients with neurogenic tumors are asymptomatic, the tumors being discovered only on screening radiographs. When symptoms are present, the most common is pain, presumably resulting from bony erosion. Radiographically, the tumors typically appear as round, dense, well-demarcated, solid-appearing masses in the posterior mediastinum in close association with a vertebral body. At times the ribs or vertebrae are eroded, with either benign or malignant lesions. A neurofibroma that originates in a nerve root within the spinal canal may be shaped like a dumbbell or hourglass, part being inside and part outside the spinal canal, with enlargement of the intervertebral foramen. Neurogenic tumors should be surgically removed because of their propensity to undergo malignant change (102).

*Meningocele and Meningomyelocele*

These are rare anomalies of the spinal canal in which the leptomeninges herniate through an intervertebral foramen. They are therefore located in the posterior mediastinum and are difficult to distinguish from neurogenic tumors. A meningocele contains only cerebrospinal fluid; a meningomyelocele contains nerve elements also. Myelography may be diagnostic; treatment is by excision.

*Diseases of the Esophagus*

The esophageal diseases described below produce masses in the posterior mediastinum.

*Gastroenteric Cysts.* These cysts are identical to bronchogenic cysts except that they are lined with esophageal, gastric, or small intestinal mucosa. They are located adjacent to the esophagus at any level in the posterior mediastinum. Most are found in infants less than 1 year of age, in whom they produce symptoms from tracheal or esophageal compression. Since most are attached to the esophagus, the diagnosis is strongly suggested by a barium swallow that discloses a localized defect, covered with intact mucosa, in the esophageal lumen. Treatment is by surgical excision (100).

*Esophageal Diverticula.* Zenker's diverticulum originates between the transverse and oblique fibers of the inferior pharyngeal constrictor muscle (99). It may become large enough to be visible on a plain radiograph of the superior mediastinum. Frequently there is an air-fluid level. The diagnosis can be made with a barium swallow, and treatment is surgical. Diverticula arising from the lower third of the esophagus are almost always congenital. They present as round, cyst-like structures to the right of the midline and just above the diaphragm (99). An air-fluid level is present in most cases. The diagnosis is established with a barium swallow, and surgical treatment is definitive.

*Hiatal Hernia.* In patients with hiatal hernia, the chest radiograph often shows abnormalities behind the heart and slightly to the right of the midline. Many times an air-fluid level is present. A barium swallow should be obtained in all patients with radiographic abnormalities in this area to rule out hiatal hernia (99).

*Dilation.* When the esophagus becomes dilated, it is apparent as a shadow projecting entirely to the right side of the mediastinum. Depending on the underlying cause of the dilation, an air-fluid level may be present or the entire esophagus may contain air. The diagnosis is made with a barium swallow.

*Hernia through the Foramen of Bochdalek*

The Bochdalek hernia is the most common congenital diaphragmatic hernia, and at times it presents as a posterior mediastinal mass. Although any portion of the diaphragm may be absent, most defects are posterolateral on the left side and result from failure of the fetal pleuroperitoneal membrane to fuse. Since the defects are congenital, herniation is identified most frequently in children and only occasionally in adults. Any intraabdominal organ may herniate through these foramina. A definitive diagnosis can be established with CT. Only symptomatic hernias require surgical intervention (103).

*Diseases of the Thoracic Spine*

A wide variety of primary neoplasms of bone and cartilage may involve the thoracic spine and posterior rib cage. The majority of these lesions do not produce an extraosseous mass, but occasionally the major radiographic finding is a posterior mediastinal mass. Tuberculous and nontuberculous spondylitis are often associated with a paraspinal mass. This is most commonly manifested as a bilateral fusiform mass in the paravertebral zone, with its maximal diameter at the point of major bone destruction. Fractures of thoracic vertebral bodies may result in extraosseous hemorrhage and the development of unilateral or bilateral paraspinal masses (99).

*Extramedullary Hematopoiesis*

This is a rare entity but should be kept in mind in any case of a paravertebral mass in a patient with severe anemia. Characteristically, extramedullary hematopoiesis is manifested as multiple paravertebral masses, smooth or lobulated in contour and of homogeneous density, either unilaterally or bilaterally. A presumptive diagnosis can usually be made on the basis of the radiographic appearance in patients with severe anemia and splenomegaly.

## MEDIASTINITIS

### Acute Mediastinitis

Most cases of acute mediastinitis are either due to esophageal perforation or occur after median sternotomy for cardiac surgery. The diagnosis and management of patients with esophageal perforation has been discussed earlier in this chapter. Rupture or perforation of the trachea or bronchi can also lead to acute mediastinitis. Occasionally, acute mediastinitis results from direct extension of infection from adjacent soft tissues. Prognosis in acute mediastinitis is inversely related to how long it takes to establish the diagnosis. Therapy in all cases consists of immediate surgical drainage in conjunction with high doses of systemic broad-spectrum antibiotics.

*Mediastinitis after Cardiac Surgery*

The incidence of mediastinitis following median sternotomy is approximately 1% (104). The incidence is much higher in patients who have a postoperative hemorrhage with the formation of a mediastinal hematoma. Most commonly the mediastinitis becomes manifest between 4 and 30 days postoperatively and usually within 2 weeks of the original procedure. The most common presentation of patients with mediastinitis is wound drainage. Some will have a widened mediastinum on the chest radiograph; at times the patients may present with occult sepsis. The primary diagnostic procedure has been mediastinal needle aspiration, although computed tomography, indium-111 leukocyte scanning, and epicardial pacer wire cultures also appear to be useful (105). Treatment requires immediate drainage, debridement, and parenteral antibiotic therapy. Mortality is in the range of 20%, but it may be decreased with the use of omental transposition (104).

### Granulomatous Mediastinitis and Fibrosing Mediastinitis

These two conditions represent separate ends of a spectrum of chronic granulomatous inflammation of the mediastinum. The mediastinal lymph nodes participate in the primary phase of certain granulomatous infections of the lung. Tuberculosis and histoplasmosis are the most common causes of mediastinal granulomatous disease, but it can also be due to sarcoidosis (Fig. 18.7), silicosis, and other fungal diseases. In the vast majority of patients, the primary infections are relatively asymptomatic and the adenitis subsides spontaneously over a period of weeks to months without untoward incident. However, in some instances there may be considerable periadenitis, and eventually a mediastinal granuloma is formed when a cluster of caseating lymph nodes breaks down into a single mass, which then heals by fibrous encapsulation. The diameter of these mediastinal granulomas ranges from 4 to 10 cm. The thickness of the fibrous capsule rather than the size of the mass is the major determinant of structural and functional damage to contiguous organs. The reason that inflammation and fibrosis progress in some individuals but not in others is unknown (99).

In the spectrum from active granulomatous mediastinitis to burned-out mediastinal fibrosis, the former tends to be asymptomatic and to be discovered incidentally on chest roentgenography, while the latter is symptomatic either from a localized mass effect or as a result of the fibrotic process invading or compressing mediastinal structures. Clinical presentations include (*a*) the superior vena cava syndrome; (*b*) traction diverticula, disturbances of esophageal motility, or dysphagia from esophageal involvement; (*c*) obstruction of the trachea or major bronchi; (*d*) obstruction of the pulmonary artery or proximal pulmonary veins; or (*e*) involvement of the mediastinal nerves producing hoarseness due to compression of the recurrent laryngeal nerve, diaphragmatic paralysis due to phrenic nerve involvement, or Horner's syndrome from involvement of autonomic ganglions or nerves.

Although most cases of mediastinal fibrosis are thought to represent end stages of chronic granulomatous mediastinitis, there appear to be a few other situations in which this entity occurs. A small percentage of patients have an associated similar fibrotic process elsewhere, such as retroperitoneal fibrosis, pseudotumor of the orbit, Riedel's struma of the thyroid, or ligneous perityphlitis of the cecum, and the term *multifocal fibrosclerosis* has been proposed (106). In more than 40 cases, sclerosing mediastinitis has occurred during treatment with methysergide, an antiseritonin drug used for the relief of migraine headaches. In all cases but one, regression occurred when the drug was withdrawn (107).

In most instances surgical exploration is necessary to distinguish between benign and malignant causes for most of these clinical manifestations. Occasionally, dense calcification within the mass allows a definite diagnosis without operation. The chest radiograph with granulomatous mediastinitis usually demonstrates a localized mass, usually in the right paratracheal area. Subsequently with the development of fibrosing mediastinitis, there is generalized widening of the superior portion of the mediastinum. CT may be helpful in demonstrating areas of impingement on mediastinal structures or other abnormalities not evident on plain radiographs (108). MRI is superior in assessing vascular patency without the need for contrast media (99).

Specific therapy for granulomatous mediastinitis or mediastinal fibrosis is generally not indicated. Antituberculous therapy should be initiated if smears or cultures are positive for tuberculosis. If histoplasmosis is demonstrated, amphotericin B need not be administered. Corticosteroids may be useful in the treatment of mediastinal fibrosis (109). At the time of exploration for diagnosis, some surgeons advise removal of as much of the inflammatory or fibrous mass as possible, but the efficacy of this practice has not been demonstrated by a controlled clinical trial. Surgery to relieve the obstruction of an airway or a blood vessel is difficult technically, but at times is successful (110).

### MEDIASTINAL EMPHYSEMA

Mediastinal emphysema (pneumomediastinum) is the presence of gas in the interstices of the mediastinum. The primary causes are (*a*) alveolar rupture with dissection of air into the mediastinum; (*b*) perforation or rupture of the esophagus, trachea, or main bronchi;

and (c) dissection of air from the neck or the abdomen into the mediastinum.

If there is a local increase in alveolar pressure, the alveolus may rupture. Air then enters the interstitial space of the lungs, and, if air dissects along interstitial spaces to the hilum and mediastinum, mediastinal emphysema is produced (111). If the air dissects peripherally and the visceral pleura ruptures, a pneumothorax is produced. With mediastinal emphysema, a pneumothorax can also be produced if the mediastinal pleura ruptures.

To produce the local increase in alveolar pressure, there usually needs to be airway disease plus some maneuver such as coughing, vomiting, sneezing, mechanical ventilation, or repeated Valsalva maneuvers to increase alveolar pressure. It follows that mediastinal emphysema is seen in asthmatics and in patients with diabetic ketoacidosis with hyperventilation and pernicious vomiting, and may also occur during childbirth (repeated Valsalva maneuvers), mechanical ventilation, scuba diving, and rapid ascents in airplanes. Pneumomediastinum has been reported in an individual who inhaled cocaine while his partner was applying positive ventilatory pressure (112).

The symptoms associated with pneumomediastinum range from none to severe. Typically, there is severe substernal chest pain with or without radiation into the neck and arms. The pain may be aggravated by respiration or swallowing. Physical examination usually reveals subcutaneous emphysema in the suprasternal notch. *Hamman's sign,* a crunching or clicking noise synchronous with the heart beat and best heard in the left lateral decubitus position, is present in about 50% of cases. The diagnosis is confirmed by the radiographic demonstration of gas within the mediastinal tissues. In the posteroanterior projection, the mediastinal pleura is displaced laterally, creating a longitudinal line shadow parallel to the heart border and separated from the heart by gas (99).

Usually no treatment is required, but the mediastinal air will be absorbed faster if the patient inspires high concentrations of oxygen. On rare occasions the mediastinal air can compress the veins in the mediastinum, impeding venous return and leading to hypotension. In such cases surgical decompression of the mediastinum should be performed, usually through needle aspiration or mediastinotomy just above the suprasternal notch (113).

## DISEASES OF THE CHEST WALL

### KYPHOSCOLIOSIS

Kyphoscoliosis is a combination of excessive anteroposterior and lateral curvature of the thoracic spine.

The abnormal curvature may be predominantly lateral (scoliosis) or posterior (kyphosis). Abnormalities of curvature are common, occurring in about 3% of the population. However, deformity of a sufficient degree to lead to symptoms and signs referable to the heart and lungs is rare, occurring in less than 3% of those with abnormal curvature.

### Etiology

About 85% of the cases of scoliosis are idiopathic, that is, of no clear origin. Idiopathic scoliosis is classified into one of three types—infantile, juvenile, or adolescent—depending on the age at onset (114). Most cases fall into the adolescent class, in which the onset is between ages 10 and 14. In these patients the curvature increases rapidly in the fast-growth period. The ratio of females to males is 4:1. The second category of kyphoscoliosis is congenital. These cases are related either to abnormalities of the thoracic spine, such as hemivertebrae, or to various hereditary diseases in which deformity of the thoracic spine constitutes only a part of the clinical picture—neurofibromatosis, muscular dystrophy, Friedreich's ataxia, and several others. The third category is neuromuscular, in which kyphoscoliosis develops in response to asymmetrical neuromuscular diseases such as poliomyelitis.

### Pathophysiology

The major pathophysiologic effects of severe kyphoscoliosis are restrictive lung disease and ventilation-perfusion imbalances that result in chronic alveolar hypoventilation, hypoxic vasoconstriction, and eventually pulmonary arterial hypertension and cor pulmonale. Pathologic studies of the lungs of patients with kyphoscoliosis and cor pulmonale reveal severe muscular hypertrophy of the pulmonary arteries (115). The genesis of the pulmonary artery hypertension is thought to be chronic hypoxia secondary to regional inhomogeneity of ventilation and perfusion. Arterial hypoxemia may be present in some adolescents with severe kyphoscoliosis, but it becomes more prevalent as the age of the patient increases (116). Older patients with kyphoscoliosis also tend to develop an elevated $Paco_2$. This elevation is thought to be related to the combination of the increased work of breathing secondary to the skeletal abnormality and the decreased functional capacity of the inspiratory muscles. Indeed, the $Pao_2$ and the $Paco_2$ are much more closely correlated with the maximal transdiaphragmatic pressure than with the forced vital capacity or the degree of scoliosis (117).

As would be expected from the deformity of the chest wall, pulmonary function tests reveal a decreased vital capacity and total lung capacity and an increase in residual volume. Flow is reduced only in proportion to the reduction in vital capacity. In addition, the inspiratory muscle function is markedly impaired in patients with severe kyphoscoliosis, presumably from the mechanical disadvantages from the thoracoabdominal deformity.

In general, the degree of scoliosis correlates with the severity of the cardiopulmonary disease. The degree of scoliosis is best quantitated by using the Cobb method to calculate the angle of curvature (Fig. 18.11). In subjects with an angle of curvature less than 60, there is seldom severe ventilatory impairment or significant alteration of blood gases. Individuals with curvatures between 60 and 90 have an increasing frequency of severe ventilatory abnormalities, and most patients with curvatures exceeding 90 develop marked ventilatory abnormalities.

It should be emphasized that there are other factors in addition to the degree of scoliosis that are correlated with the reduction in the vital capacity. Patients with a greater number of vertebrae involved with the scoliosis, with a more cephalad location of the curve, and with loss of the normal thoracic kyphosis will have a

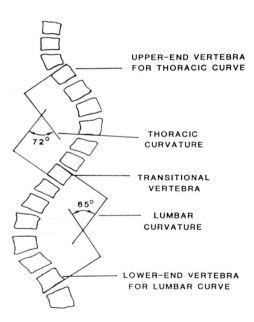

**FIGURE 18.11.** Cobb method of measuring scoliosis curves. First the ''end vertebrae'' of the curve are identified. These are the vertebrae that have the maximum tilting toward the curve to be measured. Then horizontal lines are drawn at the superior border of the superior end vertebra and at the inferior border of the inferior end vertebra. Then perpendicular lines are erected from each of the horizontal lines. The angle between the intersecting perpendicular lines is the angle of curvature.

greater reduction in the FVC for a given degree of scoliosis (118). Patients with kyphoscoliosis have a reduced work capacity. In a recent study of 79 patients with a mean Cobb angle of 45 ±18.5, the mean work capacity was 86% of predicted. The work capacity correlated better with the vital capacity than with the angle of scoliosis (119).

## Clinical Picture

Patients with severe spinal deformity generally present with increasing exertional dyspnea and exercise intolerance. Eventually they may develop a rapidly deteriorating course characterized by recurrent respiratory infections, hypoxia, hypercapnia, and the development of pulmonary hypertension and right heart failure. There may be associated polycythemia secondary to hypoxemia. Respiratory failure rarely appears before the fourth decade. Some adults with severe kyphoscoliosis remain asymptomatic.

## Treatment

Much effort has been devoted to restoring the normal curvature of the spine by either internal or external devices. In general, these manipulations result in more improvement in the cosmetic appearance of the patients than in their pulmonary function. However, one report of 15 teenagers studied 1 year after corrective therapy demonstrated that the maximal inspiratory pressure increased by 14 cm $H_2O$ and the peak expiratory flow rate increased by 32% (120). The earlier corrective actions are undertaken, the better the results. Once cardiorespiratory failure has developed, there is a high mortality from operative intervention.

It appears that patients with kyphoscoliosis and recurrent episodes of respiratory failure benefit from chronic nocturnal mechanical ventilation. Studies with substantial follow-up have demonstrated that chronic nocturnal ventilation with either custom-made cuirass or positive-pressure ventilators can significantly diminish the symptoms of dyspnea on exertion and the signs of cor pulmonale. In addition, the arterial $P_{CO_2}$ falls markedly, the arterial $P_{O_2}$ increases, and the pulmonary artery pressures fall (121). Therefore, consideration of nocturnal ventilation should be given to all patients with kyphoscoliosis and recurrent respiratory failure. Recent studies have suggested that nasal continuous positive airway pressure (CPAP) with the machines used for treating sleep-disordered breathing is probably the initial therapy of choice (122, 123).

## ANKYLOSING SPONDYLITIS

Ankylosing spondylitis is an inherited arthritic condition that ultimately immobilizes the spine. Ankylosis of the posterior intervertebral, costovertebral, and sacroiliac joints and ossification of the spinal ligaments and the margins of the intervertebral disks result in fixation of the thoracic cage. Accordingly, ventilation becomes almost entirely dependent on diaphragmatic movement. Since the diaphragm is the major contributor to ventilation normally, the fixation of the chest wall results in only minimal disability, and respiratory symptoms are uncommon. In the most severely affected, the vital capacity may be reduced by up to 50%, with an accompanying increase in the residual volume. Blood gases remain nearly normal and the lungs are usually normal at autopsy, although some patients develop upper-lobe fibrosis (124).

## PECTUS EXCAVATUM (FUNNEL CHEST)

In this congenital condition, the lower portion of the sternum is displaced posteriorly. The anterior ribs are markedly bowed, which results in a depressed panel in the anterior chest. The intrathoracic structures may be displaced laterally, and this may cause the heart to appear enlarged when actually it is not. Symptoms referable to this condition are mainly due to psychological embarrassment from the deformity. Respiratory symptoms are uncommon and pulmonary function tests are nearly normal. The general consensus is that surgical correction is seldom indicated, and then only to prevent psychological upset resulting from the cosmetic deformity (115).

## PECTUS CARINATUM (PIGEON BREAST)

This condition is the reverse of pectus excavatum, with the sternum protruding anteriorly. The most common cause of acquired pectus carinatum is congenital atrial or ventricular septal defects. Approximately 50% of individuals with these cardiac defects have a pigeon breast. Severe prolonged childhood asthma is also associated with pectus carinatum. The deformity itself does not cause pulmonary symptoms. Surgery is for cosmetic purposes only (115).

## FRACTURES OF SINGLE RIBS

Trauma to the chest is responsible for most rib fractures. Nevertheless, minimal stress can result in fracture of a single rib if the rib is diseased. Ribs affected with bone cysts or metastatic neoplasms may fracture during stresses so slight that they have been unrecognized by the patient. An apparently normal rib may be fractured with modest stress such as from coughing or a passionate embrace. Cough fractures of the ribs occur more often in women than in men and almost invariably involve the sixth to ninth ribs, most often the seventh, and usually in the posterior axillary line.

Typically the patient with a fractured rib will complain of severe, well-localized chest pain with deep breathing, coughing, stooping, and lifting. Physical examination usually reveals point tenderness over the fractured rib. Chest radiographs may demonstrate the fracture; however, with nondisplaced fractures, the chest x-ray film frequently is positive only after 3 to 6 weeks, when callus formation is established. Therefore, the diagnosis should be made on the basis of the history and physical examination.

The treatment of fractured ribs has two goals: to alleviate the chest pain and to prevent secondary disease. The chest pain is probably best treated with systemic analgesics, although these must be administered carefully to patients with chronic obstructive pulmonary disease. Local relief may be provided by a local anesthetic injected at the fracture site or by an intercostal nerve block. Chest strapping to immobilize the ribs may be used, but in general it is not recommended because it is not very effective. The pain and tenderness tend to improve markedly within 10 days regardless of treatment, although some pain on inspiration or cough may persist for up to 6 months.

## FRACTURES OF MULTIPLE RIBS

When multiple rib fractures are present, the chest wall may become unstable; this condition is designated *flail chest*. During inspiration when the thorax normally expands in all directions, the negative intrapleural pressure will cause the unstable portion of the chest wall to draw in. Similarly, on expiration the unstable portion of the chest wall will move outward with the positive pleural pressure. Frequently the flail chest is not apparent within the first few hours of the injury on account of splinting. Flail chest generally results from fractures of three or more ribs in at least two locations. The major result of flail chest is to diminish the effectiveness of ventilation. The pain from the rib fractures with the resultant splinting of the chest wall further impairs ventilation. The major determinant of survival of patients with flail chest is the extent of the associated injuries.

The management of patients with flail chest is difficult and requires a great deal of skill and judgment. Patients with minimal degrees of instability require no ventilatory assistance but should be observed carefully for the development of atelectasis or pulmonary infections related to the rib fractures. In patients with larger degrees of chest wall instability, mechanical ventilation must be considered. Hypoxia can usually be managed with increased concentrations of inspired oxygen.

However, if a $PaO_2$ of 60 mm Hg cannot be maintained or if the $PaCO_2$ starts to increase, intubation and mechanical ventilation should be initiated (125). The mechanical ventilation provides internal fixation of the unstable chest wall. For optimal care, the patient should not be permitted to make an inspiratory effort, since the resulting negative intrapleural pressure would result in retraction of the mobile panel. Although one would expect that controlled ventilation would be necessary until the chest wall becomes fixed, mechanical ventilation can usually be discontinued within 14 days (125). This is probably related to the recovery of the underlying lung from its acute injuries. Patients who survive flail chest usually show little residual defect (126).

## Diseases of the Diaphragm

### Unilateral Paralysis of the Diaphragm

Diaphragmatic paralysis results from interruption of the nerve supply (the phrenic nerve) to the diaphragm. The most common cause is nerve invasion from malignancy, usually a bronchogenic carcinoma. The second most common category of diaphragmatic paralysis is that for which no etiology can be detected. An increasingly common cause is open heart surgery. Injury to the phrenic nerve occurs in approximately 20% of open heart surgery patients and is attributed to cold or stretching of the nerve. Benign causes of diaphragmatic paralysis include poliomyelitis, herpes zoster, Huntington's chorea, injuries or diseases of the cervical vertebrae, diphtheria, lead poisoning, tetanus antitoxin, measles, pulmonary infarction, pneumonia, mediastinitis, and pericarditis (127).

The diagnosis of unilateral paralysis of the diaphragm is suggested by finding an elevated hemidiaphragm on the chest roentgenogram. With diaphragmatic paralysis, the negative pleural pressure tends to pull the paralyzed diaphragm upward. Normally, the right diaphragmatic dome is on a plane approximately half an interspace above the left. In a review of 500 normal subjects by Felson (128), the right diaphragm was more than 3 cm higher than the left in 2%. However, the left diaphragm was at the same height or higher than the right in 9%. Confirmation of diaphragmatic paralysis is best established with the "sniff test." In this test the diaphragm is observed fluoroscopically as the patient sniffs. The normal diaphragm will move downward during the sniff maneuver as the diaphragmatic muscles contract. A paralyzed diaphragm will move paradoxically upward because of the negative pleural pressure (115).

Patients with a paralyzed diaphragm may be asymptomatic or may complain of dyspnea on effort. Pulmonary function testing reveals that the vital capacity and the total lung capacity are reduced by about 25%. In addition, the maximal transdiaphragmatic pressure is reduced by about 50% and the maximal inspiratory pressure is reduced by about 40% (129).

The management of patients with diaphragmatic paralysis depends on the likely diagnosis. For example, a hilar mass in conjunction with diaphragmatic paralysis suggests bronchogenic carcinoma and serves as an indication for bronchoscopy. In asymptomatic patients with normal chest roentgenograms save for the diaphragmatic paralysis, no invasive procedures are probably warranted. In one report of 142 such patients, the diaphragmatic paralysis persisted in more than 90%, but over a mean follow-up period of nearly 10 years, only 4% developed intrathoracic malignancy (130).

### Bilateral Paralysis or Paresis of the Diaphragm

The presence of bilateral diaphragmatic paralysis or severe paresis almost always causes severe morbidity in adults. The most common causes include high spinal cord injury, thoracic trauma (including cardiac surgery), multiple sclerosis, anterior horn cell disease, and muscular dystrophy.

Most patients with severe diaphragmatic weakness will present with hypercapnic respiratory failure, frequently complicated by cor pulmonale and right ventricular failure, atelectasis, and pneumonia. Most will have dyspnea at rest that is worse in the supine position. Anxiety, insomnia, and excessive daytime somnolence are common, as is morning headache. The chest roentgenogram usually shows elevation of both hemidiaphragms, and the respiratory excursion of the diaphragm is usually minimal or absent.

The degree of diaphragmatic weakness is best quantitated by measuring transdiaphragmatic pressures. Probably the best measure is the transdiaphragmatic pressure generated during a sniff maneuver. Normally, this pressure is greater than 98 cm $H_2O$, but in patients with diaphragmatic weakness the pressure may be less than 20 cm $H_2O$. The transdiaphragmatic pressures generated during the sniff maneuver appear to be more reproducible than the maximal transdiaphragmatic pressure at total lung capacity or functional residual capacity. In patients with severe diaphragmatic weakness, the forced vital capacity diminishes from the seated to the supine position. A decrease of more than 30% is suggestive of severe diaphragmatic weakness (131). The maximal inspiratory pressure at the mouth is also reduced proportional to the diaphragmatic weakness (131).

The clinical course of patients with bilateral diaphragmatic weakness (and accordingly the treatment) depends on the underlying disease. There can be recovery of diaphragmatic function when the nerve injury is not permanent. A good example of such recovery is that which occurs in patients who have bilateral diaphragmatic paralysis after cardiac surgery (132). In such patients it may take 6 or more months for recovery to occur. In such cases nasal intermittent positive airway pressure at night may be helpful until recovery (132). Most patients with progressive neuromuscular disease eventually require mechanical ventilation to maintain adequate ventilation.

**Diaphragmatic Pacing**

This is one alternative that can be considered in patients in whom the primary problem is above the anterior horn cell and the phrenic nerve is intact—for example, a patient with a high cervical spinal cord lesion. Before pacing is seriously considered, one must document the functional integrity of the phrenic nerve. This can be done by measuring the velocity of conduction of an electrical pulse delivered percutaneously in the neck and recorded as the diaphragm action potential. This is best done by recording the diaphragmatic electromyelogram with an esophageal electrode and measuring the transdiaphragmatic pressure (133).

Once the functional integrity of the phrenic nerve has been demonstrated, consideration can be given to implanting a permanent diaphragmatic pacer. There are three different systems currently available and each costs approximately $30,000. If continuous ventilation is required, bilateral pacers must be implanted, since one can stimulate a phrenic nerve continuously only for about 12 hours. It should be emphasized that even in centers with much experience with diaphragmatic pacing, the outcome is not always successful. In one series of 81 patients in whom diaphragmatic pacers were implanted, only 38 (47%) were fully successful in that no other method of ventilatory support was needed (134).

EVENTRATION

Eventration is a congenital anomaly resulting from faulty muscular development of part or all of one or both diaphragms. The eventrated diaphragm consists of a thin membranous sheet attached peripherally to normal muscle at points of origin from the rib cage. Radiologically, eventration cannot be distinguished from diaphragmatic paralysis. However, a previously normal chest x-ray will rule out eventration. If the eventration is complete, consideration should be given to diaphragmatic plication. With this procedure the redundant fibrous tissue is folded on itself and stitched laterally to the chest wall so that the dome becomes almost flat.

HICCUP

A hiccup is an involuntary spasm of the inspiratory muscles followed by an abrupt closure of the glottis, which is responsible for the characteristic sound. Hiccups are usually precipitated by irritation of the diaphragm. This is most commonly due to gastric distention or inflammation following rapid or excessive eating or drinking. Hiccups also occur in other conditions in which the vagus nerve is stimulated, such as inferior wall myocardial infarction, peritonitis, pleurisy, pericarditis, and mediastinitis. Hiccups may be troublesome in uremia, in which instance they are thought to have a central origin.

Although hiccups usually are of short duration and resolve spontaneously, long-continued hiccups can be a serious symptom and a manifestation of important disease. Engleman's treatment with granulated sugar is very effective and consists of having the patient swallow, dry, 1 teaspoon of ordinary white granulated sugar (135). If this does not work, the stomach can be decompressed with a nasogastric tube in conjunction with pharyngeal irritation. The next step is to administer chlorpromazine, 25 to 50 mg intravenously. If this works, the drug should be administered orally 10 to 20 mg every 4 to 6 hours for 10 days. An alternative drug is quinidine, 200 mg 4 times a day orally. If the hiccups are pernicious and distressing to the patient, a phrenic nerve injection followed by a phrenic nerve crush should be considered (136).

▼

## REFERENCES

1. Albertine KH, Wiener-Kronish JP, Roos RJ, Staub NC: Structure, blood supply, and lymphatic vessels of the sheep's visceral pleura. *Am J Anat* 165:277–294, 1982.
2. Albertine KH, Wiener-Kronish JP, Staub NC: The structure of the parietal pleura and its relationship to pleural liquid dynamics in sheep. *Anat Rec* 208:401–409, 1984.
3. Negrini D, Townsley MI, Taylor AE: Hydraulic conductivity of the canine parietal pleura in vivo. *J Appl Physiol* 69:438–442, 1990.
4. Bhattacharya J, Gropper MA, Staub NC: Interstitial fluid pressure gradient measured by micropuncture in excised dog lung. *J Appl Physiol* 56:271–277, 1984.
5. Wiener-Kronish JP, Broaddus VC, Albertine KH, Gropper MA, Matthay MA, Staub NC: Relationship of pleural effusions to increased permeability pulmonary edema in anesthetized sheep. *J Clin Invest* 82:1422–1429, 1988.
6. Broaddus VC, Wiener-Kronish JP, Staub NC: Clearance

of lung edema into the pleural space of volume-loaded, anesthetized sheep. *J Appl Physiol* 68:2623–2630, 1990.

7. Wiener-Kronish JP, Matthay MA, Callen PW et al: Relationship of pleural effusions to pulmonary hemodynamics in patients with congestive heart failure. *Am Rev Respir Dis* 132:1253–1256, 1985.

8. Broaddus C, Staub NC: Pleural liquid and protein turnover in health and disease. *Semin Respir Med* 9:7–12, 1987.

9. Light RW, Stansbury DW, Brown SE: The relationship between pleural pressures and changes in pulmonary function following therapeutic thoracentesis. *Am Rev Respir Dis* 133:658–661, 1986.

10. McLoud TC, Flower CD: Imaging the pleura: sonography, CT, and MR imaging. *AJR* 156:1145–1153, 1991.

11. Light RW, Jenkinson SG, Minh VD, George RB: Observations on pleural fluid pressures as fluid is withdrawn during thoracentesis. *Am Rev Respir Dis* 121:799–804, 1980.

12. Weiss JM, Spodick DH: Laterality of pleural effusions in chronic congestive heart failure. *Am J Cardiol* 53:951, 1984.

13. Shinto RA, Light RW: The effects of diuresis upon the characteristics of pleural fluid in patients with congestive heart failure. *Am Rev Respir Dis* 137:458S, 1988.

14. Lieberman FL, Hidemura R, Peters RL, Reynolds TB: Pathogenesis and treatment of hydrothorax complicating cirrhosis with ascites. *Ann Intern Med* 64:341–351, 1966.

15. Milanez JRC, Vargas FS, Filomeno LTB, Fernandez A, Jatene A, Light RW: Intrapleural talc for the prevention of recurrence in benign or undiagnosed pleural effusions. *Chest* 106;1771–1775, 1994.

16. Runyon BA, Greenblatt M, Ming RHC: Hepatic hydrothorax is a relative contraindication to chest tube insertion. *Am J Gastroenterol* 83:333–334, 1986.

17. Weiss JM, Spodick DH: Association of left pleural effusion with pericardial disease. *N Engl J Med* 308:696–697, 1983.

18. Gottehrer A, Roa J, Stanford GG, et al: Hypothyroidism and pleural effusions. *Chest* 98:1130–1132, 1990.

19. Chow CC, Sung JY, Cheung CK, et al: Massive hydrothorax in continuous ambulatory peritoneal dialysis: diagnosis, management and review of the literature. *N Z Med J* 27:475–477, 1988.

20. Light RW, Girard WM, Jenkinson SG, George RB: Parapneumonic effusions. *Am J Med* 69:507–511, 1980.

21. Light RW: *Pleural Diseases,* ed 2. Philadelphia, Lea & Febiger, 1990.

22. Brook I, Frazier EH: Aerobic and anaerobic microbiology of empyema. A retrospective review in two military hospitals. *Chest* 103:1502–1507, 1993.

23. Morgenroth A, Pleuffer HP, Seelmann R, Schweisfurth H: Pleural penetration of ciprofloxacin in patients with empyema thoracis. *Chest* 100:406–409, 1991.

24. Kerr A, Vasudevan VP, Powell S, Ligenza C: Percutaneous catheter drainage for acute empyema. Improved cure rate using CAT scan, fluoroscopy, and pigtail drainage catheters. *NY State J Med* 91:4–7, 1991.

25. Silverman SG, Mueller PR, Saini S, Hahn PF, Simeone JF, Forman BH, Steiner E, Ferrucci JT: Thoracic empyema: management with image-guided catheter drainage. *Radiology* 169:5–9, 1988.

26. Henke CA, Leatherman JW: Intrapleurally administered streptokinase in the treatment of acute loculated nonpurulent parapneumonic effusions. *Am Rev Respir Dis* 145:680–684, 1992.

27. Lee KS, Im JG, Kim YH, Hwang SH, Bae WK, Lee BH. Treatment of thoracic multiloculated empyemas with intracavitary urokinase: a prospective study. *Radiology* 179:771–775, 1991.

28. Moores DWO: Management of acute empyema [Editorial]. *Chest* 102:1316–1317, 1992.

29. Mehta JB, Dutt A, Harvill L, Mathews KM: Epidemiology of extrapulmonary tuberculosis. *Chest* 99: 1134–1138, 1991.

30. Rossi GA, Balbi B, Manca FP: Tuberculous pleural effusions: evidence for selective presence of PPD-specific T-lymphocytes at site of inflammation in the early phase of the infection. *Am Rev Respir Dis* 136:575–579, 1987.

31. Patiala J: Initial tuberculous pleuritis in the Finnish armed forces in 1939–1945 with special reference to eventual post-pleuritic tuberculosis. *Acta Tuberc Scand Suppl* 36:1–57, 1957.

32. Light RW: Pleural diseases. *Dis Mon* 28:266–331, 1992.

33. Levine H, Metzger W, Lacera D, Kay L: Diagnosis of tuberculous pleurisy by culture of pleural biopsy specimen. *Arch Intern Med* 126:269–271, 1970.

34. Mahmoudi A, Iseman MD: Pitfalls in the care of patients with tuberculosis. *JAMA* 270:65–68, 1993.

35. Hillerdal G: Pulmonary aspergillus infection invading the pleura. *Thorax* 36:745–751, 1981.

36. Lonky SA, Catanzaro A, Moser KM, Einstein H: Acute coccidioidal pleural effusion. *Am Rev Respir Dis* 114: 681–688, 1976.

37. Cunningham RT, Einstein H: Coccidioidal pulmonary cavities with rupture. *J Thorac Cardiovasc Surg* 84: 172–177, 1982.

38. Conces DJ Jr, Vix VA, Tarver RD: Pleural cryptococcosis. *J Thorac Imaging* 5:84–86, 1990.

39. Fine NL, Smith LR, Sheedy PF: Frequency of pleural effusions in mycoplasma and viral pneumonias. *N Engl J Med* 282:790–793, 1970.

40. Johnson RJ, Johnson JR: Paragonimiasis in Indochinese refugees. *Am Rev Respir Dis* 128:534–538, 1983.

41. Wen H, New RRC, Craig PS: Diagnosis and treatment of human hydatidosis. *Br J Clin Pharmacol* 35:565–574, 1993.

42. Meyer P: Metastatic carcinoma of the pleura. *Thorax* 21: 437–443, 1966.

43. Marel M, Stastny B, Melinova L, Svandova E, Light RW: Diagnosis of pleural effusions—experience with clinical studies 1986–1990. *Chest* 1995 (in press).

44. Light RW, Erozan Y, Ball WC Jr: Cells in pleural fluid. *Arch Intern Med* 132:854–860, 1973.

45. Poe RW, Israel RH, Utell MJ, Hall WJ, Greenblatt DW, Kallan MC: Sensitivity, specificity, and predictive values of closed pleural biopsy. *Arch Intern Med* 144: 325–328, 1984.

46. Hartman DL, Gaither JM, Kesler KA, Mylet DM, Brown JW, Mathur PN: Comparison of insufflated talc under thoracoscopic guidance with standard tetracycline and bleomycin pleurodesis for control of malignant pleural effusions. *J Thorac Cardiovasc Surg* 105:743–748.

47. Webb WR, Ozmen V, Moulder PV, Shabahang B, Breaux J: Iodized talc pleurodesis for the treatment of pleural effusions. *J Thorac Cardiovasc Surg* 103:881–885, 1992.

48. Light RW, Vargas FS, Sassoon CSH, Gruer SE, Wang NS: Induction of a pleurodesis by the intrapleural injection of talc slurry in rabbits. *Chest* 104:161S, 1993.

49. Rodriguez-Panadero F, Lopez-Mejias J: Survival time of patients with pleural metastatic carcinoma predicted by glucose and pH studies. *Chest* 95:320–324, 1989.

50. Vargas FS, Teixeira LR, Coelho IJC, Braga GA, Terra-Filho M, Light RW: Distribution of pleural injectate: effect of volume of injectate and animal rotation. *Chest* 106:2146–2149, 1994.

51. Little AG, Kadowaki MH, Ferguson MK, et al: Pleuroperitoneal shunting: alternative therapy for pleural effusions. *Ann Surg* 208:443–450, 1988.

52. Antman KH: Natural history and epidemiology of malignant mesothelioma. *Chest* 103(suppl 4):373S–376S, 1993.

53. De Pangher Manzini V, Brollo A, Franceschi S, De Matthaeis M, Talamini R, Bianchi C: Prognostic factors of malignant mesothelioma of the pleura. *Cancer* 72:410–417, 1993.

54. Boutin C, Rey F: Thoracoscopy in pleural malignant mesothelioma: a prospective study of 188 consecutive patients. Part 1: Diagnosis. *Cancer* 72:389–393, 1993.

55. Lucas JS, Tuttle SE: Diagnostic histochemical and immunohistochemical studies in malignant mesothelioma. *J Surg Oncol* 35:30–34, 1987.

56. Ruffie PA: Pleural mesothelioma. *Curr Opin Oncol* 3:328–334, 1991.

57. Briselli M, Mark EJ, Dickersin GR: Solitary fibrous tumors of the pleura: eight new cases and review of 360 cases in the literature. *Cancer* 47:2678–2689, 1981.

58. Winslow WA, Ploss LN, Loitman B: Pleuritis in systemic lupus erythematosus: its importance as an early manifestation in diagnosis. *Ann Intern Med* 49:70–88, 1958.

59. Good JT Jr, King TE, Antony VB, Sahn SA: Lupus pleuritis: clinical features and pleural fluid characteristics with special reference to pleural fluid antinuclear antibodies. *Chest* 84:714–718, 1983.

60. Halla JT, Schrohenloher RE, Volanakis JE: Immune complexes and other laboratory features of pleural effusions. A comparison of rheumatoid arthritis, systemic lupus erythematosus and other disease. *Ann Intern Med* 92:748–752, 1980.

61. Bynum LJ, Wilson JE: Radiographic features of pleural effusions in pulmonary embolism. *Am Rev Respir Dis* 117:829–834, 1978.

62. Kaye M: Pleuropulmonary complications of pancreatitis. *Thorax* 23:297–306, 1968.

63. Rockey DC, Cello JP: Pancreaticopleural fistula. Report of 7 patients and review of the literature. *Medicine* 69:332–344, 1990.

64. Sherr HP, Light RW, Merson MH, et al: Origin of pleural fluid amylase in esophageal rupture. *Ann Intern Med* 76:985–986, 1972.

65. Graeber GM, Niezgoda JA, Albus RA, Burton NA, Collins GJ, Lough FC, Zajtchuk R: A comparison of patients with endoscopic esophageal perforations and patients with Boerhaave's syndrome. *Chest* 92:995–998, 1987.

66. Light RW, George RB: Incidence and significance of pleural effusion after abdominal surgery. *Chest* 69:621–626, 1976.

67. Edling JE, Bacon BR: Pleuropulmonary complications of endoscopic variceal sclerotherapy. *Chest* 99:1252–1257, 1991.

68. Stelzner TJ, King TE Jr, Antony VB, Sahn SA: The pleuropulmonary manifestations of postcardiac injury syndrome. *Chest* 84:383–388, 1983.

69. Vargas FS, Cukier A, Hueb W, Terra-Filho M, Carcia HL, Teixeira LR, Light RW: Relationship between pleural effusion and pericardial involvement after myocardial revascularization. *Chest* 105:1749–1752, 1994.

70. Epler GR, McLoud TC, Gaensler EA: Prevalence and incidence of benign asbestos pleural effusion in a working population. *JAMA* 247:617–622, 1982.

71. Hillerdal G, Ozesmi M: Benign asbestos pleural effusion: 73 exudates in 60 patients. *Eur J Respir Dis* 71:113–121, 1987.

72. Lemming R: Meigs' syndrome and pathogenesis of pleurisy and polyserositis. *Acta Med Scand* 168:197–204, 1960.

73. Taylor JR, Ryu J, Colby TV, Raffin TA: Lymphangioleiomyomatosis: clinical course in 32 patients. *N Engl J Med* 323:1254–1260, 1990.

74. Berger HW, Rammohan G, Neff MS, Buhain W: Uremic pleural effusion: study in 14 patients on chronic dialysis. *Ann Intern Med* 82:362–364, 1975.

75. Nordkild P, Kromann-Andersen H, Stuve-Christensen E: Yellow nail syndrome—the triad of yellow nails, lymphedema and pleural effusions. *Acta Med Scand* 219:221–227, 1986.

76. Nicholls AJ, Friend JAR, Legge JS: Sarcoid pleural effusion: three cases and review of the literature. *Thorax* 35:277–281, 1980.

77. Baron RL, Stark DD, McClennan BL, et al: Intrathoracic extension of retroperitoneal urine collections. *AJR* 137:37–41, 1981.

78. Murphy MC, Newman BM, Rodgers BM: Pleuroperitoneal shunts in the management of persistent chylothorax. *Ann Thorac Surg* 48:195–200, 1989.

79. Milanez JRC, Vargas FS, Filomeno LTB, Fernandez A, Jatene A, Light RW: Intrapleural talc for the prevention of recurrent pneumothorax. *Chest* 106:1162–1165, 1994.

80. Hillerdal G: The pathogenesis of pleural plaques and pulmonary asbestosis: possibilities and impossibilities. *Eur J Respir Dis* 61:129–138, 1980.

81. Wilson JM, Boren CH Jr, Peterson SR, Thomas AN: Traumatic hemothorax: is decortication necessary? *J Thorac Cardiovasc Surg* 77:489–495, 1979.

82. Light RW: Management of spontaneous pneumothorax. *Am Rev Respir Dis* 148:245–248, 1993.

83. Light RW, O'Hara VS, Moritz TE, McElhinney AJ, Butz R, Haakenson CM, Read RC, Sassoon CS, Eastridge CE, Berger R, Fontenelle LJ, Bell RH, Jenkinson SG, Shure D, Merrill W, Hoover E, Campbell SC: Intrapleural tetracycline for the prevention of recurrent spontaneous pneumothorax. *JAMA* 264:2224–2230, 1990.

84. Vargas FS, Wang N-S, Lee HM, Gruer SE, Sassoon CSH, Light RW: Effectiveness of bleomycin in comparison to tetracycline as pleural sclerosing agent in rabbits. *Chest* 104:1582–1584, 1993.

85. Cannon WB, Vierra MA, Cannon A: Thoracoscopy for spontaneous pneumothorax. *Ann Thorac Surg* 56:686–687, 1993.

86. Jones KW, Pietra GG, Sabiston DC Jr: Primary neoplasms and cysts of the mediastinum. In Fishman AP (ed): *Pulmonary Diseases and Disorders.* New York, McGraw-Hill, 1980, p 1490.

87. Lyons HA, Calvy GL, Sammons BP: The diagnosis and

classification of mediastinal masses. A study of 782 cases. *Ann Intern Med* 51:897–932, 1959.

88. Brown LR, Aughenbaugh GL: Masses of the anterior mediastinum: CT and MR imaging. *AJR* 157:1171–1180, 1991.

89. Morrissey B, Adams H, Gibbs AR, Crane MD: Percutaneous needle biopsy of the mediastinum: review of 94 procedures. *Thorax* 48:632–637, 1993.

90. Widstrom A, Schnurer L: The value of mediastinoscopy—experience of 374 cases. *J Otolaryngol* 7:103–109, 1978.

91. Best LA, Munichor M, Ben-Shakhar M, et al: The contribution of anterior mediastinotomy in the diagnosis and evaluation of diseases of the mediastinum and lung. *Ann Thorac Surg* 43:78–81, 1987.

92. Morgenthaler TI, Brown LR, Colby TV, Harper CM Jr, Coles DT: Thymoma. *Mayo Clin Proc* 68:1110–1123, 1993.

93. Wychulis AR, Payne WS, Clagett OF, Woolner LB: Surgical treatment of mediastinal tumors. A 40 year experience. *J Thorac Cardiovasc Surg* 62:379–392, 1971.

94. Vaeth JM, Moskowitz SA, Green JP: Mediastinal Hodgkin's disease. *Am J Roentgenol* 126:123–126, 1976.

95. Nichols CR: Mediastinal germ cell tumors. Clinical features and biologic correlate. *Chest* 99:472–479, 1991.

96. Lemarie E, Assouline PS, Diot P, Regnard JF, Levasseru P, Droz JP, Ruffie P: Primary mediastinal germ cell tumors. *Chest* 102:1477–1483, 1992.

97. Wax MK, Briant TDR: The management of substernal goiter. *J Otolaryngol* 21:165–170, 1992.

98. Hoffman OA, Gillespie DJ, Aughenbaugh GL, Brown LR: Primary mediastinal neoplasms (other than thymoma). *Mayo Clin Proc* 68:880–891, 1993.

99. Fraser RG, Paré JAP, Paré PD, Fraser RS, Genereux GP: Diseases of the mediastinum. In *Diagnosis of Diseases of the Chest*, ed 3. Philadelphia, WB Saunders, 1991, pp 2794–2920.

100. Salyer DC, Salyer WR, Eggleston JC: Benign developmental cysts of the mediastinum. *Arch Pathol Lab Med* 101:136–139, 1977.

101. St-Georges R, Deslauriers J, Duranceau A, Waillancourt R, Deschamps C, Beauchamp G, Page A, Brisson J: Clinical spectrum of bronchogenic cysts of the mediastinum and lung in the adult. *Ann Thorac Surg* 52:6–13, 1991.

102. Gale AW, Jelihovsky T, Grant AF, et al: Neurogenic tumors of the mediastinum. *Ann Thorac Surg* 17:434–443, 1974.

103. Shin MS, Mulligan SA, Baxley WA, Ho KJ: Bochdalek hernia of diaphragm in the adult. Diagnosis by computed tomography. *Chest* 92:1098–1101, 1987.

104. Kutsal A, Ibrisim E, Catav Z, Tasdemir O, Bayazit K: Mediastinitis after open heart surgery. *J Cardiovasc Surg* 32:38–41, 1991.

105. Borwdie DA, Bernsetein RW, Agnew R, Damle A, Fischer M, Balz J: Diagnosis of poststernotomy infection: comparison of three means of assessment. *Ann Thorac Surg* 51:290–292, 1991.

106. Comings DE, Skubi KB, Van Eyes J, Motulsky AG: Familial multifocal fibrosclerosis. Findings suggesting that retroperitoneal fibrosis, mediastinal fibrosis, sclerosing cholangitis, Riedel's thyroiditis, and pseudotumor of the orbit may be different manifestations of a single disease. *Ann Intern Med* 66:884–892, 1967.

107. DuPont HL, Varco RL, Winchell CP: Chronic fibrous mediastinitis simulating pulmonic stenosis, associated with inflammatory pseudotumor of the orbit. *Am J Med* 44:447–452, 1968.

108. Loyd JE, Tillman BF, Atkinson JB, Des Prez RM: Mediastinal fibrosis complicating histoplasmosis. *Medicine* 67: 295–310, 1988.

109. Field C, Arnold W, Gloster ES, et al: Steroid therapy as treatment for idiopathic fibrosis of the retroperitoneum and mediastinum. *Pediatrics* 78:936–938, 1986.

110. Dunn EJ, Ulicny KS Jr, Wright CB, Gottesman L: Surgical implications of sclerosing mediastinitis. *Chest* 97: 338–346, 1990.

111. Macklin MT, Macklin CC: Malignant interstitial emphysema of the lungs and mediastinum as an important occult complication in many respiratory diseases and other conditions: an interpretation of the clinical literature in the light of laboratory experiment. *Medicine* 23: 281–352, 1944.

112. Adrouny A, Magnusson P: Pneumopericardium from cocaine inhalation. *N Engl J Med* 313:48–49, 1985.

113. Maunder RJ, Pierson DJ, Hudson LD: Subcutaneous and mediastinal emphysema. *Arch Intern Med* 144: 1447–1453, 1984.

114. Bergofsky EH, Turino GM, Fishman AP: Cardiorespiratory failure in kyphoscoliosis. *Medicine* 38:263–317, 1959.

115. Fraser RG, Paré JAP, Paré PD, Fraser RS, Genereux GP: Diseases of the diaphragm and chest wall. In *Diagnosis of Diseases of the Chest*, ed 3. Philadelphia, WB Saunders, 1991, pp 2921–2973.

116. Kafer, ER: Idiopathic scoliosis. Gas exchange and the age dependence of arterial blood gases. *J Clin Invest* 58: 825–833, 1976.

117. Lisboa C, Moreno R, Fava M, et al: Inspiratory muscle function in patients with severe kyphoscoliosis. *Am Rev Respir Dis* 132:48–52, 1985.

118. Kearon C, Viviani G, Kirkley A, Killian KJ: Factors determining pulmonary function in adolescent idiopathic thoracic scoliosis. *Am Rev Respir Dis* 148:288–294, 1993.

119. Kearon C, Viviani GR, Killian KJ: Factors influencing work capacity in adolescent idiopathic thoracic scoliosis. *Am Rev Respir Dis* 148:295–303, 1993.

120. Cooper D, Rojas J, Mellins R, et al: Respiratory mechanics in adolescents with idiopathic scoliosis. *Am Rev Respir Dis* 130:16–22, 1984.

121. Hoeppner V, Cockcroft D, Dosman J, Cotton D: Nighttime ventilation improves respiratory failure in secondary kyphoscoliosis. *Am Rev Respir Dis* 129:240–243, 1984.

122. Hill NS: Noninvasive ventilation. Does it work, for whom, and how? *Am Rev Respir Dis* 147:1050–1055, 1993.

123. Leger P, Bedicam JM, Cornette A, Reybet-Degat O, Langevin B, Polu JM, et al: Nasal intermittent positive pressure ventilation. *Chest* 105:100–105, 1994.

124. Gacad G, Hamosh P: The lung in ankylosing spondylitis. *Am Rev Respir Dis* 107:286–289, 1973.

125. Shackford SR, Virgilio RW, Peters RM: Selective use of ventilator therapy in flail chest injury. *J Thorac Cardiovasc Surg* 81:194–201, 1981.

126. Christensson P, Gisselsson L, Lecerof H, et al: Early and late results of controlled ventilation in flail chest. *Chest* 75:456–460, 1979.

127. Riley EA: Idiopathic diaphragmatic paralysis. A report of eight cases. *Am J Med* 32:404–416, 1962.

128. Felson B: *Chest Roentgenology.* Philadelphia, WB Saunders, 1973.
129. Lisboa C, Paré PD, Pertuze J, et al: Inspiratory muscle function in unilateral diaphragmatic paralysis. *Am Rev Respir Dis* 134:488–492, 1986.
130. Piehler JM, Pairolero PC, Gracey DR, Bernatz PE: Unexplained diaphragmatic paralysis: a harbinger of malignant disease? *J Thorac Cardiovasc Surg* 84:861–864, 1982.
131. Mier-Jedrzejowica A, Brophy C, Moxham J, Green M: Assessment of diaphragm weakness. *Am Rev Respir Dis* 137:877–883, 1988.
132. Efthimious J, Butler J, Benson MK, Westaby S: Bilateral diaphragm paralysis after cardiac surgery with topical hypothermia. *Thorax* 46:351–354, 1991.
133. Moxham J, Shneerson JM: Diaphragmatic pacing. *Am Rev Respir Dis* 148:533–536, 1993.
134. Glenn WW, Phelps ML, Elefteriades JA, et al: Twenty years of experience in phrenic nerve stimulation to pace the diaphragm. *PACE* 9:780–784, 1986.
135. Engleman EG, Lankton J, Lankton B: Granulated sugar as treatment for hiccups in conscious patients. *N Engl J Med* 285:1489, 1971.
136. Williamson BWA, MacIntyre IMC: Management of intractable hiccup. *Br Med J* 2:501–503, 1977.

# Chapter 19

# Lung Transplantation

**Jay I. Peters**
**Stephanie M. Levine**

For only a decade has lung transplantation been a therapeutic option for patients with end-stage pulmonary parenchymal or vascular disease. Although Hardy performed the first human lung transplant in 1963, the patient survived only 18 days (1). From 1963 until 1980, 37 more lung transplants were attempted; however, the longest survival was only 10 months (2, 3). Early attempts at lung transplantation were unsuccessful because of the development of rejection or infection in the transplant recipients (2, 3). Most of these patients would not be considered good candidates for lung transplantation by today's standards. Many had systemic diseases, were acutely ill, were ventilator dependent, or were receiving chronic high-dose corticosteroids.

Since that time, research has led to improved surgical techniques, markedly improved immunosuppressive therapy with cyclosporine A (4), and standardization of selection criteria for trannsplant recipients. Pulmonologists must understand the surgical procedures available to their patients, the selection criteria for transplantation, the immunosuppressive regimens, and the management of complications that commonly occur in transplant recipients. This chapter reviews each of these topics.

## INDICATIONS AND SURGICAL OPTIONS

Any patient with end-stage pulmonary or cardiopulmonary disease with the capacity for rehabilitation can be considered for transplantation. Obviously, many patients will not be suitable candidates, and the patients most likely to survive the early postoperative transplant period are those who, although terminally ill, maintain an active lifestyle and an acceptable nutritional status. The patient should have untreatable end-stage pulmonary disease, no other significant medical illness, and a limited life expectancy. The candidate should be ambulatory with rehabilitation potential. Patients must be psychologically stable, committed to the idea of transplantation, and willing to comply with the

**TABLE 19.1**
**GENERAL RECIPIENT SELECTION GUIDELINES**

Untreatable end-stage pulmonary disease of any etiology
No other significant medical diseases
Substantial limitation of daily activity
Limited life expectancy
Ambulatory with rehabilitation potential
Acceptable nutritional status
Satisfactory psychosocial profile and emotional support
  system

Modified from Official ATS Statement—June 1992. Lung transplantation: report of the ATS Workshop on Lung Transplantation. *Am Rev Respir Dis* 147:772–776, 1993.

rigorous medical protocols required for successful lung transplantation. These general guidelines have been accepted by the American Thoracic Society (5) and are outlined in Table 19.1.

### Indications for Single Lung Transplantation

In 1983, the Toronto Group reported the first long-term survival of a single lung transplant (SLT) in a patient with idiopathic pulmonary fibrosis. Restrictive parenchymal lung disease is ideal for SLT. The transplanted lung possesses normal compliance and vascular resistance and allows preferential ventilation and perfusion to the transplanted organ. SLTs have been performed for idiopathic pulmonary and familial pulmonary fibrosis, drug- or toxin-induced lung disease, occupational lung disease, sarcoidosis, limited scleroderma, and many other disorders resulting in end-stage fibrotic lung disease.

SLT has also been used successfully in patients with pulmonary vascular disease. A single lung allograft with normal pulmonary vasculature can accommodate the entire right ventricular output without elevation of pulmonary artery pressure (6). The right ventricle has been shown to be extremely resilient, and SLTs have been done in patients with right ventricular ejection fractions below 20%. The right ventricle shows significant improvement in function postoperatively. Patients with Eisenmenger's syndrome (a cardiac abnormality resulting in pulmonary hypertension) and a repairable cardiac anomaly are also candidates for SLT.

Initially, there was concern that patients with obstructive lung disease might develop severe ventilation-perfusion mismatch after SLT. These disorders are characterized by increased lung compliance and destruction of the vascular bed. Perfusion could be diverted to the transplanted lung while ventilation remained in the native emphysematous lung. Early attempts at SLTs in patients with emphysema resulted

in hyperinflation of the native lung with compression of the transplanted lung. Fortunately, careful management of mechanical ventilation and control of postoperative infections and rejection has resulted in successful SLTs in patients with obstructive lung disease. Although the patients have continued airway obstruction on pulmonary function testing, there is no significant ventilation-perfusion mismatch (7). This has allowed SLTs to be performed in patients with chronic obstructive lung disease (COPD) and in patients with $\alpha_1$-antitrypsin deficiency.

The advantages of SLT include reduced surgical morbidity, shortened hospitalization, and often the avoidance of cardiopulmonary bypass with anticoagulation. This procedure also optimizes the use of donor organs, which are in critical shortage.

### Indications for Double Lung Transplantation

Patients with suppurative pulmonary lung disease are not candidates for SLTs. Once immunosuppressed, the native lung would infect the transplanted lung or lead to systemic infection. Initially, patients with cystic fibrosis or bronchiectasis underwent heart-lung transplantation. Double lung transplantation (DLT) avoids concurrent or asynchronous rejection of the heart (8) and may avoid the accelerated coronary artery disease seen with heart transplantation (9). In patients with acceptable right ventricular function, DLT is the procedure of choice. Initially, this procedure involved anastomosis at the level of the trachea; however, the rate of ischemic airway complications was prohibitive. Now transplant surgeons perform "bilateral" or "sequential" SLT, since the anastomosis occurs at each mainstem bronchus.

The best procedure for severe obstructive lung disease (single versus bilateral) remains to be determined. In young patients with emphysema and a longer post-transplant life expectancy or in patients with extensive bilateral bullae, DLT may be preferable. Similarly, patients with pulmonary hypertension with reduced right ventricular function are the most difficult to manage in the intraoperative and postoperative periods (10). Some centers, therefore, prefer bilateral SLT for pulmonary hypertension in an attempt to distribute blood flow equally to both lungs.

### Indications for Heart-Lung Transplantation

Heart-lung transplantation remains the primary procedure for patients with combined end-stage lung disease and heart disease (e.g., emphysema with cardiomyopathy or coronary artery disease). Patients with Eisenmenger's syndrome and irreparable cardiac lesions also require heart-lung transplantation (HLT). Patients with end-stage parenchymal disease and good

**Table 19.2**
**Transplantation Procedures by Disease State**

| Transplant Procedure | Disease State |
| --- | --- |
| Single lung | Restrictive fibrotic lung disease, COPD (emphysema, $\alpha_1$-antitrypsin deficiency), pulmonary hypertension |
| Double lung | Suppurative lung disease (cystic fibrosis, bronchiectasis), some patients with COPD, pulmonary hypertension |
| Heart-lung | End-stage cardiac and pulmonary disease |

Modified from Official ATS Statement—June 1992. Lung transplantation: report of the ATS Workshop on Lung Transplantation. *Am Rev Respir Dis* 147:772–776, 1993.

cardiac function (e.g., cystic fibrosis) may also participate in the "domino" procedure in which their heart is donated to a new recipient. Most transplant centers require that patients be less than 50 years of age for HLT. There is approximately a 25% risk of major morbidity in the postoperative period with HLT (11, 12). Opportunistic infections and bronchiolitis obliterans are major causes of mortality after this procedure. Despite the increased incidence of complications, HLT remains the only appropriate option for some patients with combined end-stage cardiac and pulmonary disease. A summary of transplantation procedures by disease state is outlined in Table 19.2.

## Recipient Selection Criteria

Although most transplant centers agree on major criteria for lung transplantation, there is some variation between different transplant programs. As a program develops experience with certain patient populations, there may be a slight relaxation in their selection criteria. This allows the potential recipient to be considered an adequate candidate at one center, even though that person may have been rejected at another center.

### Age

Most transplant centers set the maximum age limit at 60 years of age. Although this is somewhat arbitrary, numerous patients with end-stage pulmonary disease are young to middle-aged, and there is a relative lack of available donors. If the patient is an excellent candidate in all aspects except age, most centers will be flexible within 1 or 2 years of the upper age limit. Once accepted by a program, patients will usually not be dropped if they go beyond the age limit while awaiting lung transplantation. Most centers set the maximum age for DLT at 50 to 55 years. Most centers require

patients to be below the age of 50 for consideration for an HLT. In all candidates over the age of 40 to 50, the risk of coronary artery disease is significant, and screening for coronary disease is important.

### Systemic or Multisystem Disease

Transplantation should not be offered to patients with systemic diseases that affect the lung. Collagen vascular diseases such as systemic lupus erythematosus, polymyositis, destructive rheumatoid arthritis, and systemic vasculitides all preclude the maximum benefit from lung transplantation.

Patients with diabetes mellitus, poorly controlled hypertension, or neurologic disease are also not appropriate candidates for lung transplants. Gastrointestinal disease is very common posttransplantation, and active peptic ulcer disease is a relative contraindication. Occasionally, selected patients with limited scleroderma and well-controlled reflux esophagitis are considered acceptable candidates.

Patients with a history of malignancy should demonstrate a multiyear disease-free interval. Even then, there is some worry that immunosuppressive therapy may increase the risk of relapse or induce a second malignancy (13). Patients with a prior malignancy should be restaged before they become transplant candidates.

Patients with active sites of infection are also not considered good transplant candidates. Treated tuberculosis and fungal disease pose a particular problem, since these infections are difficult to manage if they recur while the patient is on immunosuppression. Many centers will not consider transplanting a patient that is chronically colonized with a resistant organism (*Pseudomonas cepacia*, methicillin-resistant *Staphylococcus*, atypical *Mycobacterium*, or *Aspergillus*). Some centers try to eradicate these organism in the pretransplant period and are willing to accept the added risk.

Abnormal hepatic function is another contraindication to lung transplantation, particularly in view of the hepatotoxicity of the immunosuppressive drugs. Even among patients with passive congestion from cor pulmonale, those with a bilirubin above 2.5 mg/ml despite maximal therapy with diuretics tend to be at high risk for complications posttransplantation, including infection, hepatic encephalopathy, bleeding diathesis, and cyclosporine nephrotoxicity (11, 14–16). Some centers accept patients with mild hepatic dysfunction if there is no evidence of cirrhosis or esophageal varices; however, many require a liver biopsy to rule out active hepatitis.

Transplant candidates require adequate renal reserve, since most patients will develop some degree of cyclosporine nephrotoxicity in the posttransplantation period (17). Transplant programs require a serum creatinine level below 1.5 mg/dl and a creatinine clearance above 50 ml/min. A patient with severe pulmonary hypertension and poor renal perfusion may be a candidate if the creatinine clearance exceeds 35 ml/min and intrinsic renal disease is excluded (13). Improvement in cardiac output may result in a dramatic improvement in renal function after transplantation in this group of patients.

### Corticosteroids

Initial data implicated corticosteroids as a cause of tracheal or bronchial dehiscence (14). At most centers, patients were required to be completely tapered off corticosteroids. This eliminated a large number of patients with chronic obstructive lung disease and pulmonary fibrosis. More recently, low-dose pretransplant corticosteroid therapy has proved to be acceptable in patients who can not be completely weaned off corticosteroids (10, 19, 20). Most transplant programs will consider patients who can be chronically maintained on 15 mg/day of prednisone or less.

### Psychosocial Criteria

The patient must be well motivated and emotionally stable to withstand the extreme stress of the pretransplant and perioperative period. Drug abuse or alcoholism are considered contraindications because these patients are a high risk for noncompliance. Patients who continue to smoke despite end-stage pulmonary disease are not candidates for lung transplantation. Most transplant centers require a patient to abstain from cigarette smoking for 6 months to 2 years before consideration for lung transplantation. A history of significant psychiatric illness is also a contraindication, although many patients will present with reactive depression or anxiety in the terminal phase of their pulmonary illness. Prior to transplantation, a thorough psychiatric evaluation is required to exclude an underlying psychiatric illness. The importance of a support system cannot be overemphasized. The support person (usually a family member) should live with the transplant recipient to provide emotional support and help provide care when necessary.

Thus, the emotional and the overall physical condition of a candidate for lung transplantation must be good. The general contraindications to lung transplantation are listed in Table 19.3.

### LIFE EXPECTANCY AND TIMING OF TRANSPLANTATION

Patients who meet all criteria for lung transplantation are usually placed on the active waiting list when their life expectancy is less than 18 to 24 months. This

**TABLE 19.3**
**CONTRAINDICATIONS TO LUNG TRANSPLANTATION**

Age greater than 60 years
Significant disease of other organ system
Active extrapulmonary infection
Poor nutritional status (cachexia, obesity)
Current cigarette smoking
Significant psychosocial problems, substance abuse, or history of medical noncompliance

Modified from Official ATS Statement—June 1992. Lung transplantation: report of the ATS Workshop on Lung Transplantation. *Am Rev Respir Dis* 147:772–776, 1993.

period of time has been referred to as the "transplant window," when the patient is ill enough to require transplantation and healthy enough to assure a reasonable chance for success (14). Data from the United Network for Organ Sharing show that the mean waiting period ranges from 8 to 12 months. Approximately 12% of patients for lung transplants and 47% of patients for heart-lung transplants wait for more than 1 year (21). Therefore, guidelines for the timing of transplantation are difficult to determine but must be based on the natural history of each disease process.

### Cystic Fibrosis

Despite the improvement in life expectancy for cystic fibrosis, most patients still die from respiratory failure and cor pulmonale. A recent study followed almost 700 patients with cystic fibrosis over 12 years to determine whether the risk from respiratory failure could be predicted 1 or 2 years in advance (22). The study concluded that patients with an $FEV_1$ less than 30% predicted, a partial pressure of oxygen below 55 mm Hg, or a partial pressure of carbon dioxide above 50 mm Hg had a 2-year mortality of 50%. Female patients and patients under the age of 18 years old had a more progressive course and might be considered for lung transplantation at an earlier stage.

### Primary Pulmonary Hypertension

The median survival of patients with primary pulmonary hypertension is 2.8 years after diagnosis. The National Heart, Blood, and Lung Patient Registry has followed approximately 200 patients 3 to 7 years to characterize variables associated with poor survival (23). Median survival decreased from 58.6 months (for patients in New York Heart Association class I or II) to 31.5 months (for patients in functional class III) to 6 months (for patients in functional class IV). An increase in mean pulmonary artery pressure from less than 55 mm Hg to more than 85 mm Hg was associated with a decrease in mean survival from 48 months to 12 months. A decrease in cardiac index of 4.0 liters/minute/m² to 2.0 liters/minute/m² was associated with a decrease in median survival from 43 months to 17 months. The presence of Raynaud's phenomena also predicted a poor prognosis, with a median survival of less than 1 year. Over 80% of patients were discharged on some drug therapy, usually a combination of vasodilators, anticoagulants, and diuretics. Patients with significantly elevated pulmonary artery pressures (PA means above 85 mm Hg), depressed cardiac index (below 2.0 liters/minute/m²), or Raynaud's should be considered for transplantation at the time of their initial diagnosis. Others should be followed closely and reassessed for transplantation at 6-month intervals. Referral to a transplant center is usually made when the patient reaches New York Heart Association class III.

### Idiopathic Pulmonary Fibrosis

Prospective longitudinal studies show that the mean survival in patients with usual interstitial pneumonia (idiopathic pulmonary fibrosis) is 5.6 years after diagnosis (24). Although 10% of patients respond to therapy and 15% remain stable, this pattern is seen with only mild or moderate disease (24). Most patients have a progressive downhill course despite therapy. In one prospective randomized trial comparing prednisolone with cyclophosphamide and prednisolone, only the initial total lung capacity (TLC) and forced vital capacity (FVC) were associated with time to "failure." Patients with a TLC below 60% of predicted did poorly regardless of the initial regimen and had a 50% 1-year survival (25). A diffusion capacity (DLCO) below 40% of predicted has also been used by some transplant centers as a criterion for referral. For patients with a TLC between 60 and 79%, increasing exercise desaturation, oxygen requirements, and rate of decline should be used as clinical guides for consideration of lung transplantation.

### Chronic Obstructive Lung Disease

The variability in the natural course of COPD makes it especially difficult to predict when patients should be referred for lung transplantation. The National Institute of Health's Intermittent Positive-Pressure Breathing (IPPB) Trial demonstrated that patients less than 65 years old with an FEV$_1$ below 30% of predicted had a 3-year survival rate of 80% (26). This study excluded patients with hypoxemia. Nevertheless, this study confirmed prior reports that the postbronchodilator FEV$_1$ was the best predictor of survival. Another study reviewed two community-based populations with COPD during a 7- to 15-year study period (27).

Again, the best predictor of survival was the percentage of predicted FEV$_1$ after the administration of bronchodilators. The presence or absence of cor pulmonale further improved the prediction of subsequent mortality. Cor pulmonale was clinically determined by history and physical examination, radiographic findings, and electrocardiogram. Poor nutritional status (assessed by serum albumin) and DLCO also showed some statistical significance. This study showed an overall 1-year survival of 65% when the postbronchodilator FEV$_1$ fell below 30% of predicted. Patients with cor pulmonale and an FEV$_1$ below 30% of predicted had a 2-year survival of 50% and a 3-year survival of only 20%. Both studies showed wide individual variability, and the decision to transplant these patients is frequently based on the progression of disease.

The functional status of the patient and the rate of change in exercise tolerance are especially useful predictors for future decline. Other useful indicators include the number and duration of hospitalizations, frequency of exacerbations, increases in supplemental oxygen requirement, and increasing right ventricular dysfunction.

## DONOR SELECTION

Most potential donors are brain dead as a result of head trauma or a primary noninfectious central nervous system event. The ideal donor should be less than 65 years of age for lung transplant procedures and less than 45 years of age for HLT. Serial chest radiographs should be grossly clear prior to consideration for lung donation. When donation is being considered for HLT or DLT, both lungs must meet criteria for donation. However, for SLT, unilateral lung injury secondary to trauma does not automatically exclude the contralateral lung from consideration for donation (28). The physiologic capacity of the potential donor graft is further accessed by gas exchange capability. Typically, a PaO$_2$ above 300 mm Hg on an FIO$_2$ of 1.0 and 5 cm H$_2$O of positive end-expiratory pressure (PEEP) is required. Oxygenation not meeting the above criterion could indicate potential ventilation/perfusion mismatch following surgery.

Most lung transplant centers require a Gram's stain of a tracheal aspirate and/or bronchoscopy to be performed on all potential donor candidates, to minimize the possibility of transmitting infectious agents from an infected donor organ. Fiberoptic bronchoscopy is often a routine part of the organ harvest, to access blood, purulent secretions, or foreign bodies in the tracheobronchial tree that are not apparent on chest radiograph. If bronchoscopic examination is abnormal, the organ should be excluded from consideration for donation.

The donor evaluation process is completed by obtaining serologic tests for HIV, hepatitis B, and cytomegalovirus (CMV). The patient is not a donor candidate if hepatitis B surface antigen or HIV antibody is present.

Certain donor-recipient compatibility tests should be met following availability of an acceptable donor organ. Unlike other solid-organ donations, SLT, HLT, and DLT are ABO matched only and not HLA matched. Currently, lung graft preservation time is limited to approximately 4 hours, and this short time precludes HLA typing prior to transplantation. Furthermore, retrospective analysis of HLA compatibility of SLT donors and recipients does not appear to correlate with subsequent episodes of rejection or mortality (29).

Some transplant centers perform donor and recipient CMV serology matching. In other words, a CMV-negative recipient receives lungs only from a CMV-negative donor, if possible. A CMV-positive recipient can receive organs from either a CMV-negative or a CMV-positive donor. There is an increased incidence of posttransplant CMV pneumonia in those patients who are CMV negative prior to transplantation and who receive lungs from a CMV-positive donor (30).

Size matching of the donor and the recipient is done differently at different institutions. Some centers measure the chest circumference of the transplant recipient and match it to the corresponding donor chest wall circumference within 3 inches in either direction (10). Other groups estimate the size match by determining the lung capacities of the donor and recipient with a height and sex nomogram (31). Some institutions perform size matching by estimating chest wall size by plain radiograph or by using a combination of measurements of body weight and chest wall circumference plus horizontal thoracic length (32). Regardless of the method of size matching used, the donor lung size approximates that of the recipient soon after transplantation (31, 33).

## SURGICAL TECHNIQUE: SINGLE LUNG TRANSPLANTATION

The donor lung is usually removed at the time of cardiac harvest via a median sternotomy incision. The pulmonary veins with a residual 5-mm cuff of left atrium are detached from the heart. The pulmonary artery is transected from the main pulmonary trunk, and the mainstem bronchus is transected between two staple lines (10). The donor lung graft is preserved in

Euro-Collins solution (a crystalloid solution with intracellular electrolyte composition) at 4 C during transportation to the recipient site and is usually stored in a partially inflated position.

The recipient surgery is performed through a posterolateral thoracotomy incision. Initially the donor pulmonary vein is anastomosed end to end to the recipient's left atrium. The technical details of the bronchial anastomosis vary among institutions. The lungs are the only solid organs that are transplanted without a complete vascular anastomosis (i.e., the bronchial circulation of the recipient and donor lungs are not anastomosed). Because of this lack of revascularization of the bronchial circulation, anastomotic complications including bronchial dehiscence, bronchial stenosis, and bronchial infection remain a major complication in lung transplantation. Some transplant centers perform an end-to-end anastomosis and wrap a piece of omentum with an intact vascular pedicle around the anastomosis to help in bronchial revascularization. Other institutions use the telescoping technique when performing the bronchial anastomosis. In the telescoping technique, the recipient and donor bronchi are overlapped by approximately one cartilaginous ring. This allows the intact bronchial circulation of the recipient to better supply the donor bronchus. The use of the telescoping technique has significantly reduced the incidence of anastomotic complications (20). The end-to-end anastomotic technique, even when used in conjunction with the omental wrap, has continued to result in reported cases of bronchial infection, stenosis, and dehiscence. SLT surgery is completed by performing an end-to-end anastomosis of the donor and recipient pulmonary arteries.

An interesting issue to consider when performing SLT is which side to transplant. This choice is based on a number of factors. For example, if the recipient's pleural space has been previously invaded by open lung biopsy or pneumothorax requiring chemical or surgical pleurodesis, the contralateral hemithorax should be chosen. If preoperative quantitative ventilation and perfusion scanning shows one lung functioning significantly better than the other lung, the less functional lung should be transplanted. Assuming that the lungs function equally and the recipient has had no prior surgery, the left side has traditionally been chosen for transplantation. Technically, the surgery is easier to perform on the left side, since it is easier to clamp the left atrium proximal to the left pulmonary vein and it is possible to leave a larger donor atrial cuff and longer recipient bronchus (10).

Some cardiothoracic surgeons prefer the right side for transplantation in obstructive lung disease (10). It is believed that left SLTs in obstructive patients allow the right native hyperinflated lung to compress the transplanted left lung because the right lung is limited inferiorly by the liver. Therefore, if a right graft is used, the native left lung can expand inferiorly without compressing the right lung graft (10). This concept is apparent on chest radiographs. Radiographically, the transplanted left lung is apparently compressed by the native hyperinflated right lung. This compression is less dramatic when the transplant is placed on the right side. Despite the radiographic differences, the results of pulmonary function testing, exercise oximetry, and $\dot{V}/\dot{Q}$ lung scanning do not support a functional difference between the right and left graft position for the treatment of obstructive lung diseases (34).

## The Postoperative Period

### General Postoperative Management

Following lung transplant surgery, patients remain intubated and require mechanical ventilation. Most patients are ventilated on a volume control mode, although some transplant centers have changed to pressure control ventilation in recent years. Airway pressures should be maintained as low as possible to avoid barotrauma and anastomotic dehiscence. Most institutions use routine pharmacologic sedation and paralysis. Patients are generally maintained with tidal volumes of 6 to 10 ml/kg following surgery. At some institutions, 5 to 10 cm $H_2O$ of PEEP is applied immediately after lung expansion in the operating room and continued for 24 to 72 hours following transplantation (10). Uncomplicated lung transplant recipients are extubated within the first 24 to 72 hours following transplantation. Both postural drainage and chest physiotherapy can be routinely employed without concern about mechanical complications at the anastomosis.

Certain patient populations require special ventilator management. In patients undergoing SLT for pulmonary hypertension, reperfusion pulmonary edema is often severe because nearly all perfusion is going to the newly implanted lung. Often prolonged sedation and paralysis for up to 3 to 7 days is required following surgery. This patient population should have aggressive diuresis, and they may require higher levels of PEEP for longer periods of time. Some transplant centers have recommended that patients with significant pulmonary hypertension be kept in bed for the first few days following surgery with the transplant side up to increase blood flow to the native lung, which is not as severely affected by the pulmonary reimplantation response.

In patients with obstructive lung disease, problems can be encountered if the delivered tidal volume or required levels of PEEP are high. Occasionally, significant hyperinflation of the native lung can result, which can compromise the newly transplanted lung. To avoid this problem, most transplant centers avoid PEEP when performing SLT for obstructive disease. Several reports have described the use of selective independent ventilation with a double-lumen tube to prevent this possible complication (40).

Since many patients are nutritionally depleted prior to transplantation because of their underlying disease, postoperative nutritional needs are important. Ideally, immediate nutritional alimentation should be begun. Parenteral nutrition is recommended particularly in patients undergoing omentopexy whose abdominal cavities have been entered. In addition, pain medications administered postoperatively can contribute to a paralytic ileus. Patients with cystic fibrosis can have a meconium ileus equivalent postoperatively, and in these patients, supplementation of pancreatic enzymes should be begun prior to surgery and continued postoperatively (41, 42). Some transplant centers routinely add N-acetylcysteine to enteral feedings in cystic fibrosis patients to prevent the formation of a meconium ileus equivalent (42).

Antibiotics are routinely administered for the first 48 to 72 hours following transplantation. Routine antibiotic regimens vary between centers but include a broad-spectrum Gram-negative agent. Several centers routinely use antifungal agents such as amphotericin B or itraconazole postoperatively. Empiric anaerobic coverage has been advocated by some centers. Gram stains and cultures of donor and recipient sputa may be used to choose appropriate antibiotics when available. Ganciclovir is administered for CMV prophylaxis in most transplant programs if either the patient or the donor are CMV positive prior to surgery.

Induction immunosuppression is begun with cyclosporine 5 to 6 mg/kg intravenously preoperatively then 5 to 6 mg/kg/day, adjusting the dose to maintain whole blood trough levels of 100 to 200 ng/ml as determined by high-pressure liquid chromatography. Conversion to an oral regimen requires increasing the cyclosporine dose approximately 3 times (i.e., 10 to 15 mg/kg/day). Azathioprine is begun at 1 to 2 mg/kg/day intravenously and then converted to an equivalent oral dose. Corticosteroids are administered as intravenous methylprednisolone 0.5 to 1 g in the operating room (usually given at the time of reperfusion), then 1 to 3 mg/kg/day for the subsequent 3 days, followed by 1 mg/kg/day, then converted to an equivalent oral dose. Many centers use lympholytic medications such as antilymphocyte globulin at 10 to 15 mg/kg/day intravenously or Orthoclone (OKT3) 5 mg/day for the first 5 to 10 days following transplantation.

## POSTOPERATIVE PROBLEMS

Perhaps the most significant and ubiquitous problem following lung transplantation is the development of the pulmonary reimplantation response (PRR). It is estimated that up to 80% of patients will experience some degree of reimplantation injury (43). To varying degrees, the PRR can persist for hours to days following lung transplant surgery. Clinically, the PRR is characterized by new radiographic alveolar and/or interstitial infiltrates, a decrease in pulmonary compliance, and disrupted gas exchange. Thirteen of 14 patients were found to develop a PRR in a series of patients undergoing SLT at Toronto (44). Radiographic findings in these patients included a perihilar haze in three patients, patchy alveolar consolidations in three patients, and dense perihilar and basilar alveolar consolidations with air bronchograms in seven patients (Fig. 19.1). The PRR worsened or stabilized in all patients over the subsequent 2 to 4 days and then began to resolve.

Although the mechanism for the PRR has not been completely delineated, several contributing factors have been postulated including the disruption of lymphatics, bronchial vasculature, and/or nerves as well as lung injury occurring either during preservation of the graft or following reperfusion. The PRR is thought to be a form of membrane permeability edema that to various degrees develops in all lung transplant recipients in whom warm ischemia persists for more than 30 minutes or cold ischemia persists for more than 2

hours (35, 45). Animal studies have suggested that the severity of the PRR is related to the ischemic time and may relate to the production of toxic oxygen free radicals (35).

In general, the PRR appears in the immediate postoperative period, whereas rejection and infection are more common after the first 24 hours. However, since the timing of these disorders may vary, differentiation may be difficult. The PRR can be minimized by the avoidance of prolonged ischemic times, the optimization of organ preservation, the appropriate use of postoperative hemodynamic monitoring, and the timely use of diuretics, inotropic agents, and antibiotics or augmented immunosuppression if other diagnoses are suspected.

## MANAGEMENT AFTER THE POSTOPERATIVE PERIOD

After discharge, follow-up is performed in the outpatient clinic. A sample follow-up schedule is weekly for the first 2 months, biweekly for the next month, and monthly thereafter. After 3 months of uncomplicated posttransplant observation, patients often return home and resume follow-up with their referring pulmonologists.

Weekly studies include a cyclosporine level, a CBC to monitor the leukocyte count on azathioprine, blood chemistries to follow creatinine while on cyclosporine and to follow liver function tests while on azathioprine, a chest radiograph, routine spirometry, and exercise oximetry. In addition, patients bring in their home spirometric measurements at each visit. Some institutions perform surveillance bronchoscopy on a routine schedule, while other institutions reserve this procedure for clinical deterioration.

The most efficient and effective way to monitor the patient following transplantation to detect early rejection, infection, or anastomotic complications remains controversial. Early in the transplant experience, quantitative ventilation and perfusion to the lung graft was examined as an indicator of graft rejection. Early acute rejection was often heralded by a decrease in perfusion to the lung graft (32). Subsequently, quantitative ventilation-perfusion lung scanning was found to be neither sensitive nor specific for graft complications.

Likewise, chest radiographs have been shown to be neither specific nor sensitive for early detection of infection or rejection (41, 44–46). Seventy-four percent of cases of rejection or infection in HLT recipients were associated with abnormal chest radiographs in the first month following transplantation. However, after the first posttransplant month, only 23% of rejection episodes were associated with an abnormal chest radiograph (45).

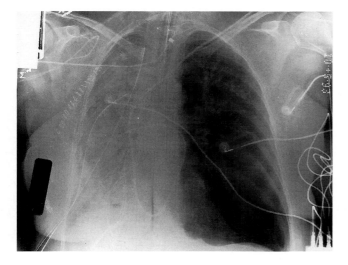

**FIGURE 19.1.** Anteroposterior portable chest radiograph of a 50-year-old woman with chronic obstructive lung disease taken 6 hours after a right single lung transplant procedure. Note the alveolar infiltrates caused by the pulmonary reimplantation response.

Close monitoring of pulmonary function has also been studied as a way of detecting graft complications (47, 48). At most transplant centers, patients are given home spirometers and instructed to document their $FEV_1$ and FVC twice a day. Patients are instructed to notify their local physician or the transplant center if the $FEV_1$ or FVC declines by 10 to 15% on two subsequent measurements. If this decline is confirmed in the PFT laboratory, transbronchial biopsy is indicated, because this degree of deterioration in pulmonary function has been associated with either rejection or infection (47, 48). A study of HLT recipients comparing pulmonary function, chest radiographs, and transbronchial biopsies found pulmonary function testing to have 86% sensitivity in detecting rejection in the first 3 months following transplantation and 75% sensitivity subsequently. The sensitivity for detecting infection was 75%. Although pulmonary function testing was not able to distinguish between rejection and infection, pulmonary function testing did have an 84% specificity for detecting complications in the lung graft. This study also reinforced prior data showing chest radiographs to be sensitive early following transplantation but subsequently having only 19% sensitivity for rejection (44). Desaturation of more than 4% or a drop below an absolute oxygen saturation of 90% on constant workload cycle exercise oximetry has also been suggested as an indicator of a complication in the lung graft (49).

## OUTCOME

SLT for obstructive lung disease results in residual mild-to-moderate obstructive pulmonary dysfunction secondary to the remaining native lung. SLT recipients with underlying restrictive lung disease have a residual mild restrictive defect (50–53). SLT recipients with pulmonary vascular disease maintain their normal pulmonary function and develop normal hemodynamics following transplantation (54). DLT, BLT, or HLT performed for any indication results in improved spirometry following surgery (55, 56). Pulmonary function continues to improve over 3 to 6 months following lung transplant surgery.

Most ventilation and perfusion go to the transplanted lung following SLT for obstructive or restrictive lung disease (55). SLT for pulmonary hypertension results in nearly equal division of ventilation between the transplanted and native lung, with nearly all perfusion going to the new lung graft (51, 56). This ventilation-perfusion imbalance (increased dead space ventilation) results in normal gas exchange under baseline conditions but can pose a problem during episodes of graft complications (57). Following DLT, BLT, or HLT,

ventilation and perfusion are divided between the lungs.

All of the different lung transplant procedures result in normal gas exchange following transplantation. Exercise testing uniformly results in reduced maximum exercise capacities with no evidence of ventilatory limitation or arterial oxygen desaturation. There is no significant difference in exercise capacities in patients undergoing SLT versus DLT, BLT, or HLT, despite the differences in spirometry for the SLT procedure (50–52, 58). Proposed reasons for the reduced exercise capacity following transplantation include deconditioning, myopathy secondary to immunosuppressive medications, chronic anemia, and limited pulmonary vascular capacities in the case of SLT. Despite the reduced exercise capacities, all stable patients are able to carry out activities of daily living without compromise.

Although 1- and 2-year survival rates of lung transplant recipients are 60 to 70%, somewhat lower than those achieved with heart or liver transplantation, significant progress has been made in the last 10 years. Some lung transplant recipients are surviving 5 years or more and maintaining a normal functional status. Mortality in the early postoperative period has been caused primarily by technical and cardiac complications of surgery. Mortality beyond the first month has been primarily related to rejection and infections.

## COMPLICATIONS FOLLOWING LUNG TRANSPLANTATION

### AIRWAY COMPLICATIONS

Airway problems, a significant cause of morbidity and mortality following early attempts at lung transplantation, developed in 20 to 50% of transplant recipients (35, 36, 38). Airway complications can be divided into early and late time periods. Early complications typically develop in the first 1 to 2 months following transplantation and are characterized by anastomotic infection and/or partial or complete anastomotic dehiscence. Subsequently, anastomotic strictures can develop, which significantly compromise the function of the transplanted lung or lungs. Several theoretical causes of airway complications following lung transplantation have been postulated including ischemia at the site of the anastomosis, infection of the anastomosis, poor organ preservation, pneumonia, graft rejection, early corticosteroid administration, and an excessively long donor bronchus. As stated previously, the lung is the only solid organ that is transplanted without complete revascularization of the systemic blood supply. Therefore, oxygenation of the new lung graft or grafts depends upon collateral blood flow from the pulmonary to the bronchial circulation.

Airway complications have been reduced with the development of the omental wrap and the telescoping anastomotic technique (10). Experimental work in an animal model has been done on direct bronchial revascularization to decrease airway complications following transplantation (59, 60).

Different lung transplant procedures are associated with varying incidences of airway complications. HLT, SLT, and bilateral sequential lung transplantations have fewer anastomotic complications than en bloc DLT (38, 61). Bronchial circulation is preserved via collateral tracheal blood supply from the donor coronary and pulmonary arteries following HLT. SLT results in most perfusion going to the transplanted lung graft in addition to a shorter anastomosis (55). Bilateral sequential SLT results in two separate short anastomoses (38). En bloc DLT, in contrast, results in a substantially greater amount of poorly vascularized bronchial tree and a higher airway complication rate.

Both animal and human studies suggested that early corticosteroid administration following lung transplant procedures was associated with a higher incidence of airway complications, but recent clinical studies have found no correlation between early corticosteroid use and airway complications or infections (20, 62, 63).

Clinically, bronchial stenosis can present with cough, shortness of breath, dyspnea on exertion, and worsening obstruction on pulmonary function testing. A characteristic flow volume loop with an inspiratory and expiratory concave pattern has been noted (64). Radiographically, bronchial strictures may be seen on posteroanterior chest radiographs and can be clearly visualized by CT and/or bronchoscopy. Partial or complete bronchial dehiscence can present with mediastinal emphysema on chest radiograph or air adjacent to the bronchial anastomosis on CT (46).

Many transplant centers advocate early routine surveillance bronchoscopy to evaluate the anastomosis and aid in early detection of complications. Anastomotic ischemia warrants close bronchoscopic observation. If an anastomotic infection is diagnosed, appropriate antibiotics should be initiated. There have been several cases of *Aspergillus* tracheobronchitis involving the anastomosis described in HLT patients and more recently in SLT patients (65). These have been successfully treated with amphotericin B followed by itraconazole.

Anastomotic strictures should be treated with balloon dilation, wire or silastic stent placement, or surgery (66). Partial anastomotic dehiscence is managed conservatively. Complete dehiscence requires surgical revision of the anastomosis or retransplantation.

## GRAFT REJECTION

Any solid organ transplanted into a genetically nonidentical recipient is an allograft and provokes an immunologic response called rejection. Rejection results from the activation, differentiation, and proliferation of effector T cells directed against the donor organ cells. The transplanted organ is rejected primarily because of differences between the donor and the recipient cell-surface molecules that are encoded by genes in the major histocompatibility complex (MHC). The MHC molecules allow the immune system to discriminate between "self" and "nonself." The human MHC was discovered in the mid-1950s, when leukoagglutinating antibodies were found in the sera of multiparous women and was designated the human leukocyte antigen (HLA) complex.

Traditionally, graft rejection has been classified according to the time of onset and defined by the histopathologic pattern as hyperacute, acute, or chronic rejection.

## HYPERACUTE AND ACUTE REJECTION

Hyperacute rejection occurs when preexisting alloantibodies bind to the vascular endothelium of the donor lung, activate complement, and cause widespread thrombosis of the vessels within the transplanted lung. Alloantibodies may be present in the donor's serum prior to transplantation through blood transfusions, pregnancy, or previous transplantation. Hyperacute rejection has been virtually eliminated by ABO blood group matching between the recipient and the donor and by pretransplantation screening of the recipients for panel-reactive antibodies (PRA). This panel uses a large group of antigens within the general donor population, and reactivity is measured between the panel and the serum of a prospective transplant recipient. Even though a recipient's serum shows no panel-reactive antibodies, antibodies against donor alloantigens not represented in the screening panel could be present and cause hyperacute rejection. Fortunately, hyperacute rejection is uncommon, and only one pathologically proven case has been documented following lung transplantation (67).

Acute rejection is a common immunologic response that usually occurs between 10 and 50 days after lung transplantation, and many patients experience two to three episodes within the first month. Acute rejection is usually not seen after the first year posttransplantation (68).

The clinical features of acute rejection include cough, dyspnea, malaise, fever, and adventitious lung sounds (rales, wheezes). The chest radiograph is usually abnormal during rejection in the first month post-transplantation but is abnormal in only 25% of cases after the first month (69). The most common radiographic pattern has been a perihilar or lower lobe infiltrate, often associated with a small pleural effusion (70).

Hypoxemia and a deterioration in pulmonary function studies frequently occur in the setting of acute rejection. Although pulmonary function abruptly improves in the early postoperative period, PFT values continue to improve for 1 to 3 months. Once lung function has stabilized, the coefficient of variation for most PFT parameters remains below 5% (44). Thus, a decline of 10% or more in FVC or $FEV_1$ and a 10 to 15% decline in $FEF_{25\%-75\%}$ are significant changes and may signal either acute rejection or infection (44).

Clinical criteria alone can not differentiate acute rejection from infection. Transbronchial biopsy (TBB) with bronchoalveolar lavage (BAL) has emerged as the primary procedure in separating these entities. TBB has a positive predictive value of 69 to 83% in lung transplant patients with clinical deterioration (71, 72). The sensitivity for diagnosing rejection has ranged from 70 to 95%, and the specificity from 90 to 100% (72–74). A minimum of five transbronchial specimens containing pulmonary parenchyma should be obtained for histologic evaluation; however, 10 to 18 biopsies may be required to reach the 95% confidence level for the detection of rejection (74).

Histologically, acute rejection is characterized by both perivascular mononuclear infiltrates and a lymphocytic bronchitis or bronchiolitis (75) (Fig. 19.2).

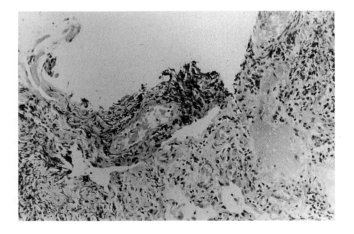

**FIGURE 19.2.** Transbronchial biopsy specimen revealing perivascular lymphocytic infiltration and necrosis around a small pulmonary artery, consistent with acute rejection

**TABLE 19.4**
**HISTOLOGIC GRADING SYSTEM FOR ACUTE PULMONARY REJECTION**

| Grade | Description |
| --- | --- |
| Normal | No significant abnormality |
| Minimal acute rejection (A1) | Infrequent perivascular infiltrates |
| Mild acute rejection (A2) | Frequent perivascular infiltrates around venules and arterioles |
| Moderate acute rejection (A3) | Dense perivascular infiltrates with extension into alveolar septa |
| Severe acute rejection (A4) | Diffuse perivascular, interstitial, and air-space infiltrates; alveolar pneumocyte damage; possibly parenchymal necrosis, infarction, or necrotizing vasculitis |

Adapted from Yousem SA, Berry GJ, Brunt EM, Chamberlain D, Hruban RH, Sibley RK: A working formulation for the standardization of nomenclature in the diagnosis of heart and lung rejection: Lung Rejection Study Group. *J Heart Transplant* 8:593–601, 1990.

As rejection progresses, the perivascular lymphocytic infiltrate surrounding the venules and arterioles becomes dense and extends into the perivascular and peribronchiolar alveolar septa. With severe rejection, this process spills into the alveolar space and is usually associated with parenchymal necrosis, hyaline membranes, and a necrotizing vasculitis. A histologic grading system for acute pulmonary rejection is illustrated in Table 19.4. Altugh rejection and infection frequently coexist, a definitive diagnosis of acute rejection cannot be made in the setting of an active infection. Perivascular and interstitial infiltrates may occur with infections, particularly CMV and *Pneumocystis* pneumonia, as well as with acute rejection. Because of the problem in differentiating these disorders, the clinician may have to initiate antimicrobials as well as increase immunosuppression in some cases.

Standard therapy for acute pulmonary rejection is high-dose corticosteroids. Methylprednisolone, 10 mg/kg/day for 3 days, is a common regimen and usually leads to a dramatic improvement in the patient's condition within 24 hours if the diagnosis is correct. The maintenance immunosuppressive regimen should also be optimized, and frequently the dose of azathioprine is increased to 1.5–2 mg/kg/day and the prednisone escalated to 1 mg/kg/day with a taper over several weeks. Some centers titrate azathioprine to maintain a total neutrophil count between 4500 and 6000 cells/mm³. Adjusting the immunosuppressive regimen is particularly important with severe episodes of rejection or when rejection occurs late in the post-transplant period (69).

## OBLITERATIVE BRONCHIOLITIS

Obliterative bronchiolitis (OB) following transplantation is defined clinically by an obstructive and restrictive pulmonary function defect and histologically by obliteration of terminal bronchioles. In the early HLT experience, 50% of recipients developed OB, a major cause of morbidity and mortality (76–78). With the use of increased immunosuppression including corticosteroids and cyclosporine and with the addition of azathioprine, the incidence of OB decreased to approximately 15 to 25% (79). Furthermore, with augmented immunosuppression, the progression of disease has been slowed (76). Initially, it was thought that SLT and DLT procedures would result in a lower incidence of OB than HLT procedures; however, when followed over time, it is apparent that the incidence of OB in SLT and DLT recipients is comparable to that currently seen in HLT patients (45, 80). Many large transplant centers are reporting a 20 to 40% incidence of OB in SLT recipients (38, 61, 81). OB remains a major problem in lung transplantation and one of the leading causes of late mortality. Although the etiology of OB remains unclear, several possible causes have been proposed including uncontrolled acute rejection (77, 82,) and early CMV infection (83).

Clinically, OB has been reported any time following the second month posttransplantation, but the typical onset is 8 to 12 months after surgery (81). The onset of OB may he heralded by an upper respiratory tract infection and can be mistakenly treated as such. Other patients present without clinical symptoms but with a gradual obstructive dysfunction on pulmonary function testing (84).

Typically, chest radiographs are not helpful in the diagnosis of OB because most patients have radiographs that are unchanged from their baseline posttransplant film (84). Some investigators have described central bronchiectasis as an occasional radiographic finding suggesting a diagnosis of OB (85). High-resolution CT in OB may reveal peripheral bronchiectasis, patchy consolidation, and decreased peripheral vascular markings, which investigators feel may aid in the early diagnosis of OB (86, 87).

TBB is used to confirm the diagnosis of OB (Fig. 19.3). In addition to revealing histologic changes of OB, bronchoscopy is important in excluding other possible diagnoses such as acute rejection, infection, or airway complications as contributing causes of deteriorating pulmonary function. Unfortunately, it may be difficult

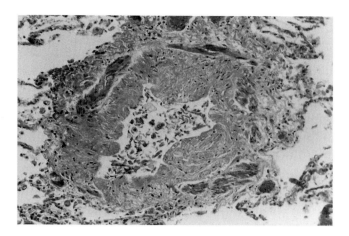

**FIGURE 19.3.** Transbronchial biopsy specimen revealing obliterative bronchiolitis.

to obtain diagnostic specimens of the terminal bronchioles by TBB. The sensitivity for detection of OB by TBB ranges from 5 to 100% (69, 88). Since some patients are unable to tolerate open lung biopsy, OB is sometimes a diagnosis of exclusion in a patient presenting with progressive obstruction on pulmonary function testing with an otherwise normal TBB.

If OB has been diagnosed histologically or clinically by exclusion of alternate diagnoses, treatment is begun with high-dose methylprednisolone followed by a tapering course of oral corticosteroids. Lympholytic agents such as ALG or OKT3 can be considered if there is no clinical response to steroid treatment. Therapy may stabilize the pulmonary function but uncommonly results in significant improvement. The use of corticosteroids has been associated with a 65% response rate, while antilymphocytic agents resulted in a response in 81% of patients. Although relapses may be less likely with lympholytic therapy, relapses still occur in over 50% of patients (89). Unfortunately, infection frequently complicates intensive immunosuppression for OB and may result in death. Methotrexate, total lymphoid irradiation, and newer immunosuppressive agents such as FK506 have been used in refractory cases of OB. Since most cases of OB can only be stabilized, early diagnosis and treatment are necessary for preservation of lung function.

## INFECTIOUS COMPLICATIONS

Infection is the leading cause of morbidity and mortality in recipients of lung or heart-lung transplantation (91, 92). The act of surgically removing the donor lung, leaving it without a blood supply for several hours, and then reimplanting it without reestablishing the lymphatic drainage or nerve supply dramatically diminishes the defense mechanisms of the lung. Mucosal ischemia impairs mucociliary clearance, and the anastomosis impairs the movement of mucus up the trachea. These factors, along with immunosuppression, explain why 30 to 80% of transplant recipients develop major infections within the first 4 months following transplantation (93). Pneumonia accounts for 50 to 80% of infections and is the leading cause of death in these patients (91, 92).

Bacterial pneumonia is the first life-threatening infection to occur in the early postoperative period. The risk of pneumonia in the first 2 postoperative weeks has been reported to be as high as 35% (94). With the use of broad-spectrum antibiotic prophylaxis (usually an antipseudomonal cephalosporin and clindamycin) and routine culturing of the trachea of the donor at the time of harvest, the incidence of bacterial pneumonia has been significantly reduced. If the cultures remain negative, prophylactic antibiotics are discontinued after 3 to 4 days.

The diagnosis of early bacterial pneumonia may be difficult because ischemic-reperfusion injury, pulmonary edema, rejection, and atelectasis may all present with similar clinical features. Gram-negative organisms are frequently found in the tracheal aspirate, and differentiating colonization from infection may require invasive procedures or semiquantitative bacterial cultures.

Atypical pneumonias, including *Pneumocystis carinii* pneumonia (PCP), *Legionella*, mycobacteria, and *Nocardia*, occur in 2 to 9% of lung and heart-lung transplant recipients (96, 97). The technique of BAL must be standardized, and the fluid must be processed in a way to ensure maximum sensitivity and specificity in all tests performed.

In transplant centers where trimethoprim-sulfamethoxazole prophylaxis is routinely used during the first year posttransplant and reinitiated when immunosuppression is augmented, the incidence of *Pneumocystis carinii* pneumonitis is less than 1% (97–99). Nevertheless, lung transplant recipients have a fivefold higher prevalence of PCP pneumonia than comparably immunosuppressed recipients of a cardiac allograft, and PCP must be considered in patients who are poorly compliant with their medications or intolerant to trimethoprim-sulfamethoxazole (99).

Bacterial infections may also present outside the transplanted lung. Wound infections, line sepsis, and intraabdominal abscess are not uncommon and may be difficult to detect in patients on large doses of corticosteroids (95).

Among transplant recipients, viral infections are a major cause of mortality and morbidity. The DNA herpesviruses, such as CMV and herpes simplex virus, account for most of the infections in these patients. CMV is the most common cause of infections in the interval between 30 to 60 days postoperatively (94). Predisposing factors for CMV infection include receipt of blood products or organs from a CMV-positive donor, CMV seropositivity of the recipient before transplantation, the use of an antilymphocyte agent (ALG, ATG, OKT3), and high-intensity immunosuppressive therapy.

CMV causes a wide spectrum of disease that ranges from asymptomatic infection (shedding of virus in urine or bronchoalveolar secretions) to widespread dissemination with fulminant pneumonitis. While only 4 to 20% of kidney, liver, or cardiac allograft recipients develop CMV pneumonia, the prevalence rate among lung or heart-lung allograft recipients may be as high as 50% (30, 82, 100–102).

CMV pneumonia typically presents insidiously, with nonproductive cough, fever, malaise, hypoxemia, and a mild interstitial or alveolar infiltrate. Sputum smears and cultures are rarely diagnostic for CMV pneumonia. Fiberoptic bronchoscopy with TBB and BAL diagnose 60 to 90% of patients with CMV pneumonia (93, 97).

The microscopic hallmark of CMV infection is the large (cytomegalic) 250-nm cell containing a large, central, basophilic intranuclear inclusion. The inclusion is referred to as an "owl's eye" because it is separated from the nuclear membrane by a halo. These inclusions are well seen on hematoxylin-eosin or Papanicolaou stain (Fig. 19.4). Cytologic identification of CMV inclusion cells is very specific (98%) but lacks sensitivity

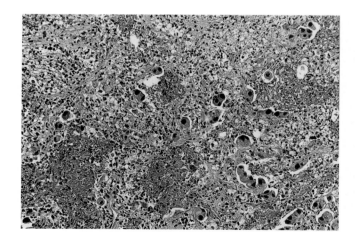

**FIGURE 19.4.** A photomicrograph revealing "owl's eye" intranuclear inclusions of cytomegalovirus in the lung graft.

(21%) for the presence of infection (103). Biopsy specimens of the lung parenchyma contain CMV inclusion cells with a surrounding lymphocytic/mononuclear cell interstitial pneumonitis.

Ganciclovir, an acrylic guanine analogue, is currently the mainstay of therapy for invasive CMV disease. Initial doses of 5 mg/kg twice daily for 2 to 4 weeks reduce mortality from 60 to 80% to 15 to 20% in symptomatic CMV pneumonitis (103). If CMV relapses, ganciclovir, 5 mg/kg/day may be required for 2 to 4 months. Some patients develop bone marrow toxicity on ganciclovir and require therapy with foscarnet. Major toxic reactions associated with foscarnet include renal failure and severe electrolyte disturbances. CMV-specific IgG or polyclonal IgG in combination with ganciclovir is associated with an improved survival among bone marrow transplant recipients with CMV pneumonitis (101). Because of the cost of immunoglobulin and the lack of data in solid organ transplant recipients, IgG preparations are often reserved for life-threatening episodes of CMV infection. With any severe CMV infection, a reduction in the level of immunosuppression is recommended.

Prophylaxis against CMV infection has become a major strategy in many transplant centers. The easiest way to reduce CMV infections is to match CMV-negative recipients with CMV-negative donors whenever possible. Limited studies suggest that CMV hyperimmune globulin may prevent or ameliorate serious CMV infections in high-risk patients after renal, liver, or heart transplantation (105, 106). Preemptive therapy with ganciclovir reduced CMV-related morbidity and mortality in asymptomatic bone marrow patients with positive cultures from BAL fluid (107). However, indications for prophylactic treatment with ganciclovir or hyperimmune globulin in the prevention of CMV pneumonia need to be established in specific groups of transplant recipients.

Fungal infections are more common in lung and heart-lung transplant recipients than in those with other solid organ transplants. The overall incidence of invasive fungal infections with lung or heart-lung transplantation ranges from 10 to 22% (95, 108). Most fungal infections are caused by *Candida* or *Aspergillus* species, and over 80% of fungal infections occur within the first 2 months (108). The overall mortality of fungal infections in heart-lung and lung transplant recipients is reported between 40 and 70% (95, 108).

*Aspergillus* species (*A. fumigatus, A. flavus, A. terreus,* and *A. niger*) may present as an indolent progressive pneumonia or as an acute fulminant infection that rapidly disseminates. *Aspergillus* exhibits a propensity to invade blood vessels and may present as an infarct or

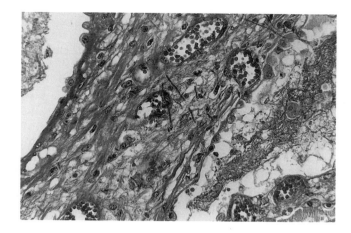

**FIGURE 19.5.** A photomicrograph revealing *Aspergillus* organisms in the lung graft.

with hemoptysis. The radiographic features of pulmonary aspergillosis include focal lobar or bronchopneumonic infiltrates or single or multiple nodules that tend to cavitate.

Definitive diagnosis of invasive aspergillosis requires identification of organisms within tissue. These organisms appear as septated hyphae that branch at acute angles and are visible on the hematoxylin-eosin and methenamine-silver stains (Fig. 19.5). Even with documented cases of invasive aspergillosis, cultures are positive in less than 50% of cases (93, 109). Another form of *Aspergillus* infection recently recognized is *Aspergillus* tracheobronchitis (65, 110). These patients develop ulcerative tracheobronchitis that usually starts distal to the anastomosis and may result in progressive narrowing of the airway.

Improved survival has been achieved with the early initiation of high-dose amphotericin (1 mg/kg/day) and the reduction of immunosuppressive therapy (111–113). Surgical resection as well as medical therapy may be required to maximize cure rates in patients with invasive aspergillosis, especially those with persistent signs of infections or necrotic tissue (109). Oral itraconazole (400 mg/day) compares favorably with amphotericin in uncontrolled studies (65, 114). For life-threatening *Aspergillus* infections, amphotericin B remains the agent of choice.

*Candida* species cause a variety of syndromes, including mucocutaneous, line sepsis, wound infections, and pulmonary involvement associated with widespread dissemination. A heavy growth of *Candida* in the donor tracheal culture has been associated with the occurrence of dissemination in the recipient (115). This has led to some programs initiating low-dose amphotericin (0.3 mg/kg/day) for the first 14 postoperative days (94); other centers have tried another azole, fluconazole (116). Although amphotericin B remains the therapy of choice for life-threatening invasive candidiasis, fluconazole has emerged as an effective alternative for infections caused by *Candida albicans*.

Less common cause of fungal infections in lung transplant recipients include *Cryptococcus neoformans* and the dimorphic fungi (*Coccidioides, Histoplasma, Blastomyces*). Amphotericin B is the initial choice for therapy for serious infections with all these invasive mycoses. The dose, duration of therapy, and alternative therapy differ depending on the organism (113).

*Mycobacterium tuberculosis* (117), atypical mycobacteria (117, 119), *Nocardia* (120–122), *Legionella* (96), and *Pneumocystis carinii* pneumonia (98, 99) may all occur in lung transplant recipients, and the diagnosis and therapy of these organisms have recently been reviewed.

## LYMPHOPROLIFERATIVE DISORDERS

Posttransplant lymphoproliferative disorders (PTLD), although rare, are a reported complication of immunosuppression following lung transplantation (127). Lymphomas comprise the majority (22%) of posttransplant malignancies in solid organ transplant recipients. The B-cell non-Hodgkin's lymphomas are the most frequent form of posttransplant lymphoma and have been associated with Epstein-Barr virus activity either serologically or by identification of viral DNA in tissue. The incidence of PTLD following heart-lung and lung transplantation has been reported to be between 4.6 and 9.4% (46, 124–126); however, patients who have negative EBV serology prior to transplantation may be at a significantly higher risk for developing posttransplant lymphomas.

## IMMUNOSUPPRESSION

One of the most important factors in the successful evolution of lung transplantation has been advances in the area of immunosuppression. Currently, most transplant centers use a maintenance immunosuppressive regimen including cyclosporine, corticosteroids, and azathioprine. Cytolytic agents such as antilymphocyte globulin or OKT3 are used for induction and/or treatment of rejection (127). A typical maintenance immunosuppressive regimen consists of cyclosporine (5 mg/kg twice daily with dose adjusted to serum levels), azathioprine 1 to 2 mg/kg/day adjusted to maintain a leukocyte count above 4500/mm$^3$, and prednisone approximately 0.5 mg/kg/day for the first 3 months tapered over the next 3 months to 15 mg/day

then to 5 mg/day or 15 mg on alternate days by the 12th posttransplant month.

Unfortunately, immunosuppressive medications have numerous toxicities. Cyclosporine, an 11–amino acid polypeptide derived from the fungus *Tolypocladium inflatum*, was introduced into clinical transplantation in 1981, and has markedly increased survival in all forms of solid organ transplantation (128). Cyclosporine is highly selective in its ability to inhibit activation of T cells (129) without causing myelosuppression. Although the exact site and mechanism of action of cyclosporine remain unknown, the drug inhibits the ability of helper T cells to respond to antigenic or regulatory stimuli. The current theory is that cyclosporine inhibits messenger RNA transcription of the *IL-2* gene of activated helper T cells (128).

Nephrotoxicity is the major clinical toxic manifestation of cyclosporine use and occurs in 25 to 75% of patients receiving the drug (130). The acute renal toxicity is usually dose related and typically reversible. Cyclosporine can decrease renal blood flow by causing afferent arteriolar vasoconstriction resulting in decreased glomerular filtration (131). Interstitial fibrosis, tubular changes, and vascular abnormalities can result with chronic use. Several other potentially nephrotoxic agents that can compound the nephrotoxicity of cyclosporine include amphotericin B, aminoglycoside antibiotics, trimethoprim-sulfamethoxazole (even at low doses), and furosemide (43). The renal toxicity due to cyclosporine may resolve with a reduction in the dose or discontinuation of the drug, although this improvement is not universal. Recent studies report the concurrent administration of calcium channel blockers diminishes the vasoconstrictive effects of cyclosporine (132). These agents affect the P450 system, allowing reduction in the cyclosporine dose.

A second serious complication of cyclosporine immunosuppression is systemic hypertension, which develops in approximately 25% of lung transplant recipients. The most likely etiology of hypertension related to cyclosporine use is a defect in renal sodium excretion (43). Many patients respond to sodium restriction and/or a reduction in cyclosporine dose, although approximately one-third of patients require antihypertensive medications to achieve adequate blood pressure control. Hypercholesterolemia is also commonly reported and can develop in up to 75% of transplant recipients.

Numerous less common side effects of cyclosporine can develop. The spectrum of neurologic toxicity includes tremors, paresthesias, headaches, confusion, depression, somnolence, and seizures. Hypertrichosis is a common side effect of cyclosporine therapy and may resolve with a reduction of the dose. Gingival hyperplasia can develop and usually responds to improvement in dental hygiene. Cyclosporine is known to cause an increase in photosensitivity and has been implicated in the increased risk of squamous and occasionally basal cell skin carcinomas. All patients undergoing cyclosporine immunosuppression should be cautioned and advised to use sun screen. Several electrolyte deficiencies have been reported with cyclosporine use including hypomagnesemia in up to 50% of lung transplant patients (43) and hyperkalemia in 10 to 15% of transplant recipients. Cholestatic hepatotoxicity has also been reported (128).

Corticosteroids are the original drugs used in solid organ transplantation (133). Corticosteroids decrease inflammation, block antigen recognition, and block neutrophil chemotaxis (134). Both B-cell and T-cell messenger RNA transcription and lymphokine production are altered by corticosteroids. IL-2 production is prevented by blocking macrophage release of IL-1. The corticosteroid side effects seen in other patient populations on chronic corticosteroid use occur in lung transplant recipients as well (135), including hyperglycemia, hypercholesterolemia, osteoporosis, cataracts, myopathy, exacerbation of peptic ulcer disease, Cushing's syndrome, and mood changes. Many of these side effects are improved with a reduction in corticosteroid dosage.

Azathioprine is metabolized to 6-mercaptopurine, which inhibits nucleic acid synthesis and suppresses mitosis and proliferation of lymphocytes (73, 133). Bone marrow toxicity and suppression are the most common toxic effects of azathioprine, and it is important to adjust the dose to maintain a leukocyte count above 4500/mm$^3$. Miscellaneous side effects related to azathioprine include pancreatitis, hepatitis, cholestatic jaundice, and an increased risk of malignancy (135).

Antilymphocyte globulin (ALG) or antithymocyte globulin (ATG) are polyclonal IgGs produced by immunization of animals (e.g., horses) with human lymphoid cells. Their immunosuppressive effects are via opsonization and cytolysis of T cell lymphocytes (136). Toxicity of these compounds is due to lympholytic cytokine release and is most severe with the initial dose (135). Toxicities include fever, chills, nausea, and vomiting. Premedication with antihistamines and antipyretic agents can alleviate these effects. In addition, arthralgias, myalgias, leukopenia, thrombocytopenias, rash, and serum sickness have been described with administration of ALG (135).

OKT3 is a murine antibody directed against the CD3 receptor on all mature T lymphocytes (127). OKT3 results in immunosuppression because of opsonization of lymphocytes. The initial administration of OKT3 can

be complicated by severe fever, chills, headache, dyspnea, nausea, vomiting, diarrhea, leukopenia, and hypotension (135). These effects can be alleviated by adequate premedication. Aseptic meningitis has also been described. Severe pulmonary edema has been reported following the first two doses and usually occurs in the setting of fluid overload (137).

Ongoing research in the field of immunosuppressive therapy, as well as improvements in the prevention and treatment of infections and better graft preservation, has made lung transplantation a therapeutic option for the treatment of end-stage lung disease.

▼

## REFERENCES

1. Hardy JD, Webb WR, Dalton ML, Walker GR: Lung homotransplantation in man; report of the initial case. *JAMA* 186:1065–1074, 1963.
2. Derom F, Barbier F, Ringoir S, et al: Ten-month survival after lung homotransplantation in man. *J Thorac Cardiovasc Surg* 61:835–846, 1971.
3. Nelems JM, Rebuck AS, Cooper JD, et al: Human lung transplantation. *Chest* 78:569–573, 1980.
4. Borel JF, Feurer C, Gubler HB, Stahelin H: Biological effect of cyclosporine A: a new antilymphocyte agent. *Agents Actions* 6:465–475, 1976.
5. Offical ATS Statement—June 1992. Lung transplantation: report of the ATS Workshop on Lung Transplantation. *Am Rev Respir Dis* 147:772–776, 1993.
6. Mal H, Andreassian B, Fabrice P, et al: Unilateral lung transplantation in end-stage pulmonary emphysema. *Am Rev Respir Dis* 140:797–802, 1989.
7. Veith FJ, Montefusco CM: Long-term fate of lung autografts charged with providing total pulmonary function. 2. Hemodynamic, functional and angiographic studies. *Ann Surg* 190:654–656, 1979.
8. Griffith BP, Hardesty RL, Trento A, et al: Asynchronous rejection of heart and lungs following cardio-pulmonary transplantation. *Ann Thorac Surg* 40:488, 1985.
9. Dawkins KD, Jamieson SW, Hunt SA, et al: Long-term results, hemodynamics and complications after combined heart-lung transplantation. *Circulation* 71:919–926, 1985.
10. Calhoon JH, Grover FL, Gibbons WJ, et al: Single lung transplantation—alternative indications and technique. *J Thorac Cardiovasc Surg* 101(5):816–825, 1991.
11. Harjula A, Baldwin JC, Oyer PE, et al: Recipient selection for heart-lung transplantation. *Scand J Thor Cardiovasc Surg* 22:193–196, 1988.
12. Tuna I, Jamison SW: Human heart and lung transplantation. *Adv Surg* 22:251–276, 1989.
13. Penn I, Brunson ME: Cancers after cyclosporin therapy. *Transplant Proc* 20(Suppl):885–892, 1988.
14. Marshall SE, Kramer MR, Lewiston NJ, Starnes VA, Theodore J: Selection and evaluation of recipients for heart-lung transplantation. *Chest* 98:1488–1494, 1990.
15. Jamieson SW, Stinson EB, Oyer PE, Reitz BA, Baldwin

J, Modry D, et al: Heart-lung transplantation for irreversible pulmonary hypertension. *Ann Thorac Surg* 38: 554–562, 1984.

16. Kramer MR, Tiroke A, Mrshall SE, Starnes VA, Lewiston NJ, Theodore J: The clinical significance of hyperbilirubinemia in patients with pulmonary hypertension undergoing heart-lung transplant [Abstract]. *J Heart Transplant* 9:79A, 1990.

17. Myers BD, Ross J, Newton L, Luetscher J, Perlroth M: Cyclosporine-associated chronic nephropathy. *N Engl J Med* 311:699–705, 1984.

18. Morgan E, Lima O, Goldberg M, et al: Improved bronchial healing in canine left lung reimplantation using omental pedical wrap. *J Thorac Cardiovasc Surg* 85: 134–139, 1983.

19. Lima O, Cooper JD, Peters WJ, et al: Effects of methylprednisolone and azathioprine on bronchial healing following lung autotransplantation. *J Thorac Cardiovasc Surg* 82:211–215, 1981.

20. Bryan CL, Anzueto A, Levine SM, et al: Corticosteroid therapy does not potentiate bronchial anastomotic complications in single lung transplantation (SLT) [Abstract]. *Am Rev Respir Dis* 143(4):A461, 1991.

21. United Network for Organ Sharing: Annual report for January 1, 1990–June 30, 1991. Richmond, VA, UNOS, 1991, pp 19–26.

22. Kerem E, Reisman J, Corey M, Canny GJ, Levison H: Prediction of mortality in patients with cystic fibrosis. *N Engl J Med* 326:1187–1191, 1992.

23. D'Alonzo GE, Barst RJ, Ayres SM, et al: Survival in patients with primary pulmonary hypertension. *Ann Intern Med* 115:343–349, 1991.

24. Carrington CB, Gaensler EA, Coutu RE, Fitzgerald MX, Gupta RG: Natural history and treated course of usual and desquamative interstitial pneumonia. *N Engl J Med* 298:801–809, 1978.

25. Johnson MA, Kwan S, Snell NJC, et al: Randomised controlled trial comparing prednisolone alone with cyclophosphamide and low dose prednisolone in combination in cryptogenic fibrosing alveolitis. *Thorax* 44: 280–288, 1989.

26. Anthonisen NR: Prognosis in chronic obstructive pulmonary disease: results from multicenter clinical trails. *Am Rev Respir Dis* 140:S95–S99, 1989.

27. Traver GA, Cline MG, Burrows B: Predictors of mortality in chronic obstructive pulmonary disease. *Am Rev Respir Dis* 119:895–902, 1979.

28. Puskas JD, Winton TL, Miller JD, Scavuzzo M, Patterson GA: Unilateral donor lung dysfunction does not preclude successful contralateral single lung transplantation. *J Thorac Cardiovasc Surg* 103(5):1015–1017, 1992; discussion May 1017–1018, 1992.

29. Mohar DE, Bryan CL, Jenkinson SG, et al: HLA matching as a predictor of OB or death in SLT [Abstract]. *Chest* 104(2):157S, 1993.

30. Calhoon JH, Nichols L, Davis R, et al: Single lung transplantation—factors in postoperative cytomegalovirus infection. *J Thorac Cardiovasc Surg* 103(1):21–25, 1992.

31. Otulana BA, Mist BA, Scott JP, et al: The effect of recipient lung size on lung physiology after heart-lung transplantation. *Transplantation* 48(4):625, 1989.

32. The Toronto Lung Transplant Group: Experience with single-lung transplantation for pulmonary fibrosis. *JAMA* 259(15):2258, 1988.

33. Lloyd KS, Holland VA, Noon GP, Lawrence EC: Pulmonary function after heart-lung transplantation using larger donor organs. *Am Rev Respir Dis* 142:1026, 1990.

34. Levine SM, Anzueto A, Gibbons WJ, et al: Graft position and pulmonary function after single lung transplantation for obstructive lung disease. *Chest* 103(2):444–448, 1993.

35. Bryan CL, Cohen DJ, Gibbons WJ, et al: Lung transplantation: the reimplantation response. *Crit Care Rep* 2:217, 1991.

36. Bryan CL, Cohen DJ, Dew JA, et al: Glutathione decreases the pulmonary reimplantation response in canine lung autotransplants. *Chest* 100(6):1694–1702, 1991.

37. Smiley RM, Navedo AT, Kirby T, Schulman LL: Postoperative independent lung ventilation in a single-lung transplant recipient. *Anesthesiology* 74(6):1144, 1991.

38. de Hoyos AL, Patterson GA, Maurer JR, et al: Pulmonary transplantation: early and late results. *J Thorac Cardiovasc Surg* 103:295–306, 1992.

39. de Leval MR, Smyth R, Whitehead B, et al: Heart and lung transplantation for terminal cystic fibrosis: a 4-year experience. *J Thorac Cardiovasc Surg* 101:633–642, 1991.

40. Bierman MI, Stein KL, Stuart RS, Dauber JH: Critical care management of lung transplant recipients. *J Intensive Care Med* 6:135, 1991.

41. Herman SJ, Rappaport DC, Weisbrod GL, et al: Single-lung transplantation: imaging features. *Radiology* 170: 89–93, 1989.

42. Siegelman SS, Sinha SBP, Veith FT: Pulmonary reimplantation response. *Ann Surg* 177:30, 1973.

43. Maurer JR: Therapeutic challenges following lung transplantation. *Clin Chest Med* 11(2):279–291, 1990.

44. Otulana BA, Higenbottam T, Scott J, et al: Lung function associated with histologically diagnosed acute lung rejection and pulmonary infection in heart-lung transplant patients. *Am Rev Respir Dis* 14:329, 1990.

45. Millet B, Higenbottam TW, Flower CDR, et al: The radiographic appearances of infection and acute rejection of the lung after heart-lung transplantation. *Am Rev Respir Dis* 140:62–67, 1989.

46. Herman SJ: Radiologic assessment after lung transplantation. *Clin Chest Med* 11(2):333–347, 1990.

47. Otulana BA, Higenbottam TW, Scott JP, et al: Pulmonary function monitoring allows diagnosis of rejection in heart-lung transplant recipients. *Transplant Proc* 21(1):2583, 1989.

48. Otulana BA, Higenbottam T, Ferrari L, et al: The use of home spirometry in detecting acute lung rejection and infection following heart-lung transplantation. *Chest* 97(2):353, 1990.

49. Bryan CL, Levine SM, Anzueto A, et al: Exercise oximetry surveillance in single lung transplant recipients [Abstract]. *Am Rev Respir Dis* 145(4):A702, 1992.

50. Williams TJ, Patterson GA, McClean PA, Zamel N, Maurer JR: Maximal exercise testing in single and double lung transplant recipients. *Am Rev Respir Dis* 145: 101–105, 1992.

51. Miyoshi S, Trulock EP, Schaefers H-J, Hsieh CM, Patterson GA, Cooper JD: Cardiopulmonary exercise testing after single and double lung transplantation. *Chest* 97: 1130–1136, 1990.

52. Gibbons SJ, Levine SM, Bryan CL, et al: Cardiopulmonary exercise responses after single lung transplantation for severe obstructive lung disease. *Chest* 100: 106–111, 1991.

53. Grossman RF, Frost A, Zamel N, et al: Results of single-lung transplantation for bilateral pulmonary fibrosis. *N Engl J Med* 322:727–733, 1990.

54. Levine SM, Gibbons WJ, Bryan CL, et al: Single lung transplantation for primary pulmonary hypertension. *Chest* 98:1107–1115, 1990.

55. Patterson GA, Maurer JR, Williams TJ, Cardoso PG, Scavuzzo M, Todd TR, and the Toronto Lung Transplant Group: Comparison of outcomes of double and single lung transplantation for obstructive lung disease. *J Thorac Cardiovasc Surg* 101:623–632, 1991.

56. Theodore J, Jamieson SW, Burke CM, et al: Physiologic aspects of human heart-lung transplantation. Pulmonary function status of the post-transplanted lung. *Chest* 86(3):349–357, 1984.

57. Levine SM, Jenkinson SG, Bryan CL, et al: Ventilation-perfusion inequalities during graft rejection in patients undergoing single lung transplantation for primary pulmonary hypertension. *Chest* 101:401–405, 1992.

58. Levy RD, Ernst P, Levine SM, et al: Exercise performance after lung transplantation. *J Heart Lung Transplant* 12(1):27–33, 1993.

59. Laks H, Louie HW, Haas GS, et al: New technique of vascularization of the trachea and bronchus for lung transplantation. *J Heart Lung Transplant* 10(2):280–287, 1991.

60. Nazari S, Prati U, Berti A, et al: Successful bronchial revascularization in experimental single lung transplantation. *Eur J Cardiothorac Surg* 4:561–567, 1990.

61. Maurer JR, Morrison D, Winton TL, et al: Late pulmonary complications of isolated lung transplantation. *Transplant Proc* 23(1):1224–1225, 1991.

62. Miller JD, DeHoyos A: An evaluation of the role of omentopexy and of early perioperative corticosteroid administration in clinical lung transplantation. *J Thorac Cardiovasc Surg* 105:247–252, 1993.

63. Schafers H-J, Wagner TOF, Demertzis S, et al: Preoperative corticosteroids. A contraindication to lung transplantation? *Chest* 102:1522–1525, 1992.

64. Anzueto A, Levine SM, Tillis WP, Calhoon JH, Bryan CL: The use of the flow-volume loop in the diagnosis of bronchial stenosis after single lung transplantation. *Chest* 105:934–936, 1994.

65. Kramer MR, Denning DW, Marshall SE, et al: Ulcerative tracheobronchitis after lung transplantation. *Am Rev Respir Dis* 144:552–556, 1991.

66. Keller C, Frost A: Fiberoptic bronchoplasty. Description of a simple adjunct technique for the management of bronchial stenosis following lung transplantation. *Chest* 102(4):995–998, 1992.

67. DeHoyos A, Mauer JR: Complications following lung transplantation. *Semin Thorac Cardiovasc Surg* 4(2):132–146, 1992.

68. Lawrence EC: Diagnosis and management of lung allograft rejection. *Clin Chest Med* 11:269–277, 1990.

69. Trulock EP: Management of lung transplant rejection. *Chest* 103:1566–1576, 1993.

70. Bergin CJ, Castellino RA, Blank N, Berry FJ, Sibley RK, Starnes VA: Acute lung rejection after heart-lung transplantation: correlation of findings on chest radiographs with lung biopsy results. *AJR* 155:23–27, 1990.

71. Starnes VA, Theodore J, Oyer PE, et al: Pulmonary infiltrates after heart-lung transplantation: evaluation by serial transbronchial lung biopsies. *J Thorac Cardiovasc Surg* 98:945–950, 1989.

72. Trulock EP, Ettinger NA, Brunt EM, Pasque MK, Kaiser LR, Cooper JD: The role of transbronchial lung biopsy in the treatment of lung transplant recipients: an analysis of 200 consecutive procedures. *Chest* 10:1049–1054, 1992.

73. Higenbottam T, Stewart S, Penketh A, Wallwork J: Transbronchial lung biopsy for the diagnosis of rejection in heart-lung transplant patients. *Transplantation* 46:532–539, 1988.

74. Scott JP, Fradet G, Smyth RL, Mullins P, Pratt A, Clelland CA: Prospective study of transbronchial biopsies in the management of heart-lung and single lung transplant patients. *J Heart Lung Transplant* 10:626–637, 1991.

75. Yousem SA, Berry GJ, Brunt EM, Chamberlain D, Hruban RH, Sibley RK: A working formulation for the standardization of nomenclature in the diagnosis of heart and lung rejection: Lung Rejection Study Group. *J Heart Transplant* 8:593–601, 1990.

76. Glanville AR, Baldwin JC, Burke CM, et al: Obliterative bronchiolitis after heart-lung transplantation: apparent arrest by augmented immunosuppression. *Ann Intern Med* 107:300–304, 1987.

77. Burke CM, Glanville AR, Theodore J, et al: Lung immunogenicity, rejection, and obliterative bronchiolitis. *Chest* 92(3):547–549, 1987.

78. McCarthy PM, Starnes VA, Theodore J, et al: Improved survival after heart-lung transplantation. *J Thorac Cardiovasc Surg* 99:54–60, 1990.

79. Scott JP, Sharples L, Mullins, P, et al: Further studies on the natural history of obliterative bronchiolitis following heart-lung transplantation. *Transplant Proc* 23(1):1201–1202, 1991.

80. LoCicero J III, Robinson PG, Fisher M: Chronic rejection in single-lung transplantation manifested by obliterative bronchiolitis. *J Thorac Cardiovasc Surg* 99:1059–1062, 1990.

81. Anzueto A, Levine SM, Bryan CL, et al: Obliterative bronchiolitis in single lung transplant recipients. *Am Rev Respir Dis* [Abstract]. 145(4):A700, 1992.

82. Griffith BP, Paradis IL, Zeevi A, et al: Immunologically mediated disease of the airways after pulmonary transplantation. *Ann Surg* 208(3):371–378, 1988.

83. Kennan RJ, Lega ME, Drummer JS, et al: Cytomegalovirus: serologic status and postoperative infection correlated with risk of developing chronic rejection after pulmonary transplantation. *Transplantation* 51(2):433–438, 1991.

84. Burke CM, Theodore J, Dawkins KD, et al: Post-transplant obliterative bronchiolitis and other late lung sequelae in human heart-lung transplantation. *Chest* 86(6):824–829, 1984.

85. Skeens JL, Fuhrman CR, Yousem SA: Bronchiolitis obliterans in heart-lung transplantation patients: radiologic findings in 11 patients. *AJR* 153:253–256, 1989.

86. Halvorsen RA Jr, DuCret RP, Kuni CC, et al: Obliterative bronchiolitis following lung transplantation diagnostic utility of aerosol ventilation lung scanning and high resolution CT. *Clin Nucl Med* 16(4):256–258, 1991.

87. Morrish WF, Herman SJ, Weisbrod GL, et al: Bronchiolitis obliterans after lung transplantation: findings at chest radiography and high-resolution CT. *Radiology* 179:487–490, 1991.

88. Yousem SA, Paradis IL, Dauber JH, Griffith BP: Efficacy

of transbronchial lung biopsy in the diagnosis of bronchiolitis obliterans in heart-lung transplant recipients. *Transplantation* 47:893–895, 1989.

89. Paradis IL, Duncan SR, Dauber JH, et al: Effect of augmented immunosuppression on human chronic lung allograft rejection [Abstract]. *Am Rev Respir Dis* 145(4;pt2): A705, 1992.

90. Westerman JH, Egan JM: Utility of invasive monitoring following lung transplantation [Abstract]. *Chest* 100(2): 655, 1991.

91. Brooks RG, Hofflin JM, Jamieson SW, et al: Infectious complications in heart-lung transplant recipients. *Am J Med* 79:412, 1985.

92. Egan TM, Kaiser LR, Cooper JD: Lung transplantation. *Curr Probl Surg* 26:675–751, 1989.

93. Lynch JP III, Chauncey JB III, Gyetko M: Pulmonary and infectious complications in organ transplant recipients. In Tenholder MF (ed): *Approach to Pulmonary Infections in the Immunocompromised Host.* Mount Kisco, NY, Futura Publishing, 1991, pp 229–276.

94. Dauber JH, Paradis IL, Dummer JS: Infectious complications in pulmonary allograft recipients. *Clin Chest Med* 11:291–308, 1990.

95. Peters JI, Levine SM, Anzueto A, et al: Infectious complications iin single lung transplant recipients [Abstract]. *Am Rev Respir Dis* 147(4):A601, 1993.

96. Ampel NM, Wing EJ: *Legionella* infection in transplant patients. *Semin Respir Infect* 5:30–37, 1990.

97. Ettinger NA, Trulock EP: Pulmonary considerations of organ transplantation. *Am Rev Respir Dis* 143:1386–1405, 144:213–223, 433–454, 1991.

98. Davey RT, Masur H: Recent advances in the diagnosis, treatment, and prevention of *Pneumocystis carinii* pneumonia. *Antimicrob Agents Chemother* 34:499–504, 1990.

99. Dummer JS: *Pneumocystis carinii* infections in transplant recipients. *Semin Respir Infect* 5:50–57, 1990.

100. Ettinger NA, Bailey TC, Trulock EP, et al: Cytomegalovirus infection and pneumonitis. *Am Rev Respir Dis* 147: 1017–1023, 1993.

101. Snydman DR: Cytomegalovirus infection in solid organ transplantation. Prospects for prevention. *Transplant Rev* 4:59–67, 1990.

102. Maurer JR, Tullis E, Scavuzzo M, et al: Cytomegalovirus infection in isolated lung transplantation. *J Heart Lung Transplant* 10:647–649, 1991.

103. Paradis H, Grgurick WF, Drummer JS, et al: Rapid detection of cytomegalovirus pneumonia by evaluation of bronchoalveolar cells. *Am Rev Respir Dis* 138:697–702, 1988.

104. Ho M: Human cytomegalovirus infections in immunosuppressed patients. In Ho M (ed): *Cytomegalovirus: Biology and Infection,* 2nd ed. New York, Plenum, 1991, pp 249–300.

105. Saliba F, Arulnaden JL, Gugenheim J, et al: CMV hyperimmune prophylaxis after liver transplantation: a prospective randomized controlled study. *Transplant Proc* 21:2260–2262, 1989.

106. Havel M, Teufelsbauer H, Lackovics A, et al: Cytomegalovirus hyperimmunoglobulin prophylaxis in the prevention of cytomegalovirus infection in immunosuppressed heart transplant patients. *Transplant Proc* 22: 1805–1806, 1990.

107. Ho M: Cell-mediated immunity to cytomegalovirus infection. In Ho M (ed): *Cytomegalovirus: Biology and Infection,* 2nd ed. New York, Plenum, 1991, pp 127–143.

108. Paya CV: Fungal infections in solid-organ transplantation. *Clin Infect Dis* 16:677–688, 1993.

109. Denning DW, Stevens DA: Antifungal and surgical treatment of invasive aspergillosis: review of 2,121 published cases. *Rev Infect Dis* 12:1147–1201, 1990.

110. Levine SM, Peters JI, Anzueto A, et al: *Aspergillus* infection in single lung transplant recipients [Abstract]. *Am Rev Respir Dis* 147(4):A599, 1993.

111. Saral R: *Candida* and *Aspergillus* infection in immunocompromised patients: an overview. *Rev Infect Dis* 13: 487–492, 1991.

112. Wajszczuk CP, Dummer JS, Ho M, et al: Fungal infections in liver transplant recipients. *Transplantation* 40: 347–353, 1985.

113. Zeluff BJ: Fungal pneumonia in transplant recipients. *Semin Respir Med* 13:216–233, 1992.

114. Denning D, et al: Treatment of invasive aspergillosis with itraconazole. *Am J Med* 86:791–800, 1989.

115. Zenati M, Dowling RD, Dummer S, et al: Influence of the donor lung on development of early infections in lung transplant recipients. *J Heart Transplant* 9:502–509, 1990.

116. Conti DJ, Tolkoff-Rubin NE, Baker GP, el al: Successful treatment of invasive fungal infection with fluconazole in organ transplant recipients. *Transplantation* 48: 692–695, 1989.

117. Sinnott JV IV, Emmanual PJ: Mycobacterial infections in the transplant patient. *Semin Respir Infect* 5:65–73, 1990.

118. Novick RJ, Moreno-Cabral CE, Stinson EB, et al: Nontuberculous mycobacterial infections in heart transplant recipients: a seventeen-year experience. *J Heart Transplant* 9:357–363, 1990.

119. Shelhamer JH, Toews GB, Masur H, et al: Respiratory disease in the immunosuppressed patient. *Ann Intern Med* 117:415–431, 1992.

120. Rolfe M, Strieter RM, Lynch JP III: Nocardiosis. *Semin Respir Med* 13:216–233, 1992.

121. Wilson JP, Turner HR, Kirchner KA, et al: Nocardial infections in renal transplant recipients. *Medicine* (Baltimore) 68:38–57, 1989.

122. Lynch JP III, Rolfe MW: Today's approach to managing and preventing nocardiosis. *J Respir Dis* 14:112–121, 1993.

123. Fairley JW, Hunt BJ, Glover GW, et al: Unusual lymphoproliferative oropharyngeal lesions in heart and heart-lung transplant recipients. *J Laryngol Otol* 104(9): 720–724, 1990.

124. Nalesnik MA, Makowka L, Starzl TE: The diagnosis and treatment of lymphoproliferative disorders. *Curr Probl Surg* 25:371–472, 1988.

125. Randhawa PS, Yousem SA, Paradis IL, et al: The clinical spectrum, pathology, and clonal analysis of Epstein-Barr virus-associated lymphoproliferative disorders in heart-lung transplant recipients. *Am J Clin Pathol* 92: 177–185, 1989.

126. Yousem SA, Randhawa P, Locker J, et al: Posttransplant lymphoproliferative disorders in heart-lung transplant recipients: primary presentation in the allograft. *Hum Pathol* 20:361–369, 1989.

127. Goldstein G: An overview of Orthoclone OKT3. *Transplant Proc* 18(4):927–930, 1986.

128. Kahan BD: Cyclosporine. *Med Intell* 321(25):1725–1737, 1989.

129. Borel JF: Cyclosporine: historical perspectives. *Transplant Proc* 15:3–13, 1983.

130. Vine W, Bowers LD: Cyclosporine: structure, pharmacokinetics, and therapeutic drug monitoring. *CRC Crit Rev Clin Lab Sci* 25:275–311, 1988.

131. Kaskel FJ, Devarajan P, Arbeit LA, et al: Effects of cyclosporine on renal hemodynamics and autoregulation in rats. *Transplant Proc* 20(3):603–609, 1988.

132. Mihatsch M, Thiel G, Ryffel B: Cyclosporin nephrotoxicity. *Adv Nephrol* 17:303, 1988.

133. Bach JF, Strom TB: *The Mode of Action of Immunosuppressive Drugs,* ed 8. New York, Elsevier, 1985.

134. Strom TB: The immunopharmacology of graft rejection. *Transplant Proc* 19(1):128–129, 1987.

135. Cameron DE, Traill TA: Complications of immunosuppressive therapy. In Baumgartner WA, Reitz BA, Achuff SC (eds): *Heart and Heart-Lung Transplantation.* Philadelphia, WB Saunders, 1990, pp 237–247.

136. Shumway SJ: Basic immunologic concepts involved in organ transplantation. In Baumgartner WA, Reitz BA, Achuff SC (eds): *Heart and Heart-Lung Transplantation.* Philadelphia, WB Saunders, 1990, pp 15–24.

137. Ortho Multicenter Transplant Study Group: A randomized clinical trial of OKT3 monoclonal antibody for acute rejection of cadaveric renal transplants. *N Engl J Med* 313:337–342, 1985.

# THE CRITICALLY ILL PATIENT

# Chapter 20

# General Principles of Managing the Patient with Respiratory Insufficiency

## Michael A. Matthay

THIS CHAPTER REVIEWS the assessment of respiratory failure in severely ill patients and describes the major elements of supportive care and monitoring available in intensive care units.

## ASSESSMENT OF SEVERE RESPIRATORY DYSFUNCTION

This section considers the clinical and laboratory evaluation of patients with acute respiratory failure.

### CLINICAL EVALUATION

The course of acute respiratory failure may evolve slowly over a period of days, or rapidly, in minutes to a few hours. The clinical manifestations and the ways in which they are perceived by the patient will vary depending on the nature of the process itself and on its course. In most instances, the symptomatic hallmark of acute respiratory failure is dyspnea. However, the presence of this symptom, as with any subjective manifestation of disease, requires that the patient be sufficiently alert to be aware of the sensation and be able to convey that awareness to observers. Thus, for example, patients who have taken overdoses of sedative-hypnotic drugs or narcotic agents, even if awake, may not be dyspneic in the presence of marked gas exchange abnormalities. Also, dyspnea tends to be more intense when it develops rapidly. When respiratory failure develops more slowly, dyspnea may appear at first only with exertion or with assumption of the supine position (orthopnea), but as the process becomes more severe the dyspnea becomes constant and may even be present at rest. Patients with chronic airways obstruction commonly have chronic dyspnea; in these patients, minor changes from the baseline level of dyspnea may represent a major worsening of gas exchange. Progressive hypoxemia, hypercarbia, or both may blunt the sensation of dyspnea and occasionally result in a misleading symptomatic assessment. In spite of its frequency as a symptom, dyspnea is poorly defined and difficult to quantify and correlates very poorly with the severity of respiratory failure (2). For these reasons, more objective assessments are important in evaluating dyspneic patients. Other symptoms such as cough, sputum production, and chest pain are important manifestations of processes that may be associated with respiratory failure but are less helpful than dyspnea as indicators of respiratory dysfunction.

In addition to the symptoms that are frequently directly associated with respiratory or cardiac disease, other, less specific, subjective manifestations may be important. Patients with progressive hypoxemia or hypercarbia may have alterations in mental function, including headache, visual disturbances, memory loss, confusion, insomnia, hallucinations, and even transient loss of consciousness.

The physical examination may also provide important information in patients with respiratory failure. Perhaps the most important evaluation rests on a general assessment of the severity of illness based on the patient's appearance, including the degree of apparent respiratory distress and the patient's mental status. Both of these assessments help guide the initial approach to management by indicating the degree of cooperation that can be anticipated. Cyanosis, especially central cyanosis, is helpful as an indication of hypoxemia but it may not be detectable. The respiratory rate, although influenced by a large number of factors, may serve as an indicator of the severity of respiratory distress, and measuring the respiratory rate also can be used as a monitoring technique to judge the response to therapy. As described for the symptom of dyspnea, however, tachypnea may not be present in patients whose ventilatory drive is blunted. The degree of respiratory failure may be estimated by noting the patient's ability to speak. Severely distressed patients will be able to speak only a few words at a time. As the respiratory failure becomes less severe, longer phrases and sentences are possible. Stridorous breathing is an important finding that suggests severe upper airway obstruction. An inability to phonate may be associated with marked obstruction at the larynx or above. Retraction of the sternum and supraclavicular, suprasternal, and intercostal spaces constitutes evidence of respiratory distress and increased resistance to lung inflation, generally caused by airways obstruction or an infiltrative process. These findings have been correlated with the severity of airways obstruction in patients with asthma (3) and with pneumonia in children (4). The decrease in arterial systolic blood pressure that occurs with inspiration (pulsus paradoxus) also correlates

with the severity of airways obstruction, especially in asthma (5). Changes in the magnitude of the pulsus paradoxus can also be used to evaluate the response to therapy.

Examination of the lungs does not provide sufficient information concerning the severity of respiratory dysfunction but may be helpful in determining the cause of respiratory failure. The findings associated with specific processes are discussed in Chapter 5, but several points are worth making. First, although wheezing is the characteristic feature of severe airways obstruction, the absence of wheezing may be even more important. In patients with very severe airways obstruction, air flow may be so reduced as to be inadequate to produce the turbulence required for wheezing. Second, unilateral absence of breath sounds in a patient with respiratory distress may be associated with pneumothorax or mucous plugging of a main bronchus. Physical findings suggesting pneumothorax are especially important in a mechanically ventilated patient because of the greater likelihood of a tension pneumothorax. Subcutaneous emphysema and a systolic "crunch" heard with systole (Hamman's sign) indicate pneumomediastinum with or without pneumothorax. Digital clubbing in a person with respiratory failure suggests a chronic process. This finding may be helpful, for example, in distinguishing chronic interstitial fibrosis (in which clubbing is common) from a diffuse infiltrative process caused by an acute infection or left ventricular failure. It is important to search for evidence of heart failure, although in patients who are critically ill the physical examination may not suggest left ventricular failure when it is present (6). Right ventricular failure usually implies a chronic pulmonary process, usually with longstanding hypoxemia. On the other hand, left ventricular failure with consequent pulmonary edema may be the cause of the respiratory failure, either alone or superimposed on lung disease.

## GENERAL LABORATORY EVALUATION

Routine hematologic and blood chemistry studies have limited relevance in assessing patients with respiratory failure, although clues to the acuity or chronicity of the process may be provided. An elevated hemoglobin level with a high hematocrit implies the presence of chronic hypoxemia, which leads to secondary polycythemia.

Hypercarbia may be inferred to be chronic if the plasma bicarbonate concentration is increased. Renal compensation for respiratory acidosis requires several days to occur; hence, increases in bicarbonate concentration do not result from acute respiratory failure of short duration (7). Patients who have longstanding elevations in arterial carbon dioxide tension ($Pa_{CO_2}$) are also likely to be hypochloremic and hypokalemic. These abnormalities tend to be more marked in patients who have been taking diuretics or adrenal corticosteroids. Hypokalemia and hypophosphatemia may be associated with weakness of the respiratory muscles, which on occasion can lead to respiratory failure or can complicate underlying lung disease (8, 9). These electrolyte abnormalities can also cause difficulties in weaning a patient from mechanical ventilation.

As with the physical examination of the chest, the chest radiograph cannot assist in quantifying the severity of respiratory dysfunction. It is, however, often very valuable in determining the etiology of the respiratory disorder, and it is an essential component of the initial evaluation. Likewise, the electrocardiogram is essential to detect arrhythmias, myocardial ischemia or infarction, and cardiac chamber enlargement.

## ARTERIAL BLOOD GASES

The single most useful test in evaluating the severity of respiratory dysfunction is the measurement of arterial blood gas tensions ($Pa_{O_2}$, $Pa_{CO_2}$) and pH. This provides an indication of the status of integrated cardio-respiratory function and acid-base balance. Although these measurements are not specific for the kind of abnormality present, they provide valuable physiologic information in patients with severe dysfunction. This section focuses on the interpretation of arterial blood gas and pH values in the assessment of severely ill patients and discusses how these interpretations can be used to infer the pathophysiology of respiratory failure and to guide the general approach to treatment.

### Hypoxemia

The mechanisms by which clinically significant reductions in $Pa_{O_2}$ are produced include alveolar hypoventilation ($Pa_{CO_2}$ greater than 40 mm Hg), mismatching of ventilation to perfusion, and right-to-left intrapulmonary or intracardiac shunting of blood. It is important to identify the physiologic basis for hypoxemia to provide insight into the pathologic process causing the hypoxemia. If the hypoxemia is caused purely by hypoventilation, this implies that the lung itself is normal and that the only necessary therapeutic goal is improved ventilation. This type of hypoxemia is characterized by a normal alveolar-to-arterial $Po_2$ difference ($Pa_{O_2} - Pa_{O_2}$). The $Pa_{O_2} - Pa_{O_2}$ can be determined by using the alveolar gas equation to calculate $Pa_{O_2}$ and measuring $Pa_{O_2}$. In young patients breathing room air, the difference should not be greater than 10 mm Hg and may increase to 16 mm Hg in

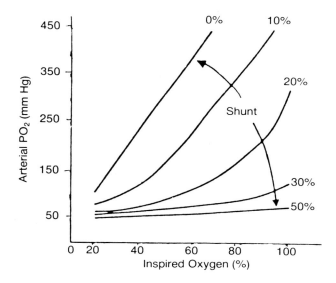

**FIGURE 20.1.** The relationship between inspired oxygen concentration and arterial $Po_2$ for lungs with varying degrees of shunt. The increase in $Po_2$ is small for lungs with large shunts. (From Dantzker DR: Gas exchange in ARDS. *Clin Chest Med* 3:57–62, 1982.)

older persons (10). With an increased fractional concentration of oxygen in inspired gas ($Fi_{O_2}$) sufficient to cause a $Pa_{O_2}$ of 200 mm Hg or greater, the $Pa_{O_2} - Pa_{O_2}$ should not exceed 40 mm Hg.

The distinction between ventilation-perfusion mismatching and shunting can be made by measuring the response to administration of 100% $O_2$. The $Pa_{O_2}$ will increase normally to values of nearly 600 mm Hg if the hypoxemia is due purely to mismatching; with a shunt, the increase may be markedly reduced depending on the magnitude of the shunt flow (Fig. 20.1). The approach to treatment of acute respiratory failure varies considerably depending on whether the hypoxemia is caused primarily by shunting or by ventilation-perfusion mismatching. With ventilation-perfusion mismatching, relatively small amounts of supplemental oxygen can increase the $Pa_{O_2}$ sufficiently, whereas with shunting mechanical ventilation is much more likely to be necessary.

### Hypercapnia

Alveolar hypoventilation is the only mechanism by which hypercapnia occurs. The amount of alveolar ventilation necessary to eliminate $CO_2$ and maintain a normal $Pa_{CO_2}$ varies depending on carbon dioxide production. Also, alveolar ventilation will in turn be influenced by the amount of wasted ventilation, as discussed in Chapter 4. Thus, alveolar hypoventilation can occur because of increased production of $CO_2$, a decrease in minute ventilation, or an increase in wasted ventilation, or a combination of all three mechanisms.

The relationship between $Pa_{CO_2}$ and plasma bicarbonate concentrations ($[HCO_3^-]$) determine the arterial pH as shown in the Henderson-Hasselbalch equation. The relationship between $Pa_{CO_2}$ and arterial pH varies, however, depending on the time during which the $Pa_{CO_2}$ has increased. Thus, by examining the relationships among $Pa_{CO_2}$, arterial pH, and $[HCO_3^-]$, the acuity or chronicity of the carbon dioxide elevation can usually be determined (Fig. 20.2). Acute increases in $Pa_{CO_2}$ are accompanied by only small increases in $[HCO_3^-]$, and arterial pH changes in a nearly linear fashion with $Pa_{CO_2}$. For every 1 mm Hg change in $Pa_{CO_2}$ the pH changes by approximately 0.008 in the opposite direction (11). An acute rise in $Pa_{CO_2}$ from 40 to 60 mm Hg would be expected to cause a decrease in arterial pH to 7.25. Over a period of 1 to 3 days, however, renal conservation of bicarbonate causes the $[HCO_3^-]$ to increase and buffer the pH change. Thus, for a given change in $Pa_{CO_2}$, the change in pH is much less than when the change occurs slowly. Obviously, the therapeutic implications of an acute versus a chronic change in $Pa_{CO_2}$ make this an important distinction.

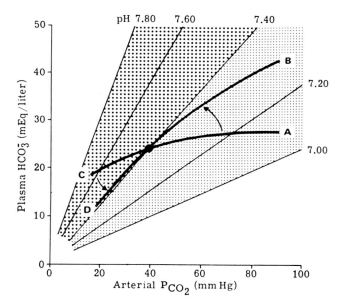

**FIGURE 20.2.** Effects of acute and chronic variations in $Pa_{CO_2}$ on plasma $HCO_3^-$ and pH. The line connecting points *A* and *C* represents the effects of an acute change in $Pa_{CO_2}$ to a value above or below 40 mm Hg. Renal compensation over time results in a shift of the relationship to that represented by the line connecting points *B* and *D*, as indicated by the *arrows*. (From Murray JF: *The Normal Lung.* Philadelphia, WB Saunders, 1976, p 215.)

## ACID-BASE ABNORMALITIES

In addition to respiratory acidosis, other acid-base disorders such as metabolic acidosis, metabolic alkalosis, and respiratory alkalosis are important problems in some patients with acute respiratory dysfunction. One of the several causes of metabolic acidosis is an imbalance between oxygen delivery and metabolic oxygen needs, which can lead to anaerobic metabolism and lactic acid production. In patients with severe respiratory disorders, such as severe asthma, this imbalance may occur because the work of breathing increases the demand for oxygen in the presence of hypoxia caused by the lung disease. Metabolic acidosis in this setting is a particularly ominous finding, suggesting that rapid deterioration is imminent and that prompt therapeutic interventions are necessary (12).

Both respiratory and metabolic alkalosis have important nonrespiratory effects in critically ill patients. Alkalosis predisposes to arrhythmias, decreases cardiac output, and reduces the threshold for seizures (13). Hypocapnia per se with or without alkalosis reduces cerebral blood flow and may depress the level of consciousness (14). For these reasons, alkalosis should be recognized as an important acid-base disturbance, and corrective measures should be taken.

## MEASUREMENTS OF LUNG FUNCTION

The lung function studies that can be used in severely ill patients are rather limited. Depending on the nature and severity of the illness and the patient's ability to cooperate, one may measure vital capacity (VC), timed forced expiratory volume ($FEV_1$), peak expiratory flow rate (PEFR), and maximal inspiratory pressure (MIP). The VC is the maximal volume of air that can be exhaled after maximal inspiration and provides an indication of the patient's ventilatory capability. Because the VC is influenced by the respiratory neuromuscular system, the chest wall, the elastic properties of the lung, and the caliber of the airways, it cannot be used to identify specific abnormalities. Nevertheless, it is particularly helpful in assessing and observing patients with neuromuscular illness and in evaluating patients being ventilated mechanically to determine if it is feasible to consider weaning from the ventilator. The minimal acceptable VC in most instances is 10 to 15 ml/kg body weight. This value must, however, be interpreted in light of the patient's clinical condition.

Measurement of MIP provides some of the same information as the VC and it is influenced by most of the same factors. However, the ability to generate an acceptable inspiratory pressure, less than $-20$ cm $H_2O$, does not necessarily imply that the VC will be acceptable.

The timed forced expiratory volume, which is usually expressed as the $FEV_1$ over the forced vital capacity (FVC), is used to measure the severity of airways obstruction in patients with asthma or chronic airways obstruction. The measurement may not be possible in severely obstructed patients who have marked tachypnea; the maneuver may even transiently worsen airways obstruction. However, the $FEV_1$ provides the best objective indicator of the degree of airways obstruction and, when measured serially, the response to therapy. Absolute $FEV_1$ values below 0.75 liter or less than 25% of the predicted value are commonly associated with increased $Paco_2$ values (15).

Measurement of the peak expiratory flow rate (PEFR) provides information similar to that from the $FEV_1$ in patients with airways obstruction. The PEFR has the distinct advantage, however, of not requiring a full inhalation followed by a full forced exhalation. It is measured by having the patient slowly inhale and then blow a short forced puff through the flowmeter, a maneuver similar to a cough. Values below 60 liters/minute indicate severe obstruction.

### CALCULATIONS OF RESPIRATORY VARIABLES

A number of equations and calculations are helpful in the assessment of respiratory function. The use of these equations is discussed later in the chapter in the section that considers specific cases of acute respiratory failure. Descriptions of the physiologic principles involved with the equations were presented in the preceding section. Representative normal values for selected cardiorespiratory variables are listed in Table 20.1.

### EQUATIONS RELATED TO ARTERIAL CARBON DIOXIDE TENSION

$Paco_2$ is related directly to carbon dioxide production ($Vco_2$ in milliliters per minute—$\dot{V}co_2$) and inversely to alveolar ventilation ($V_A$, in liters per minute—$\dot{V}_A$) as follows:

$$Paco_2 = K \times \dot{V}co_2/\dot{V}_A$$

where K is a constant.

The $\dot{V}_A$ is the difference between the tidal volume ($V_T$ in liters) and the wasted or dead-space ventilation ($V_D$) multiplied by the respiratory rate ($F$, in breaths per minute):

$$\dot{V}_A = (V_T - V_D) \times F$$

Total minute ventilation ($V_E$ in liters per minute—$\dot{V}_E$) is the product of $V_T$ and $F$:

$$\dot{V}_E = V_T \times F$$

**TABLE 20.1**

**REPRESENTATIVE NORMAL VALUES FOR SELECTED RESPIRATORY AND HEMODYNAMIC VARIABLES**

| Variable | Normal |
|---|---|
| $Pao_2$ | 95 mm Hg |
| $Paco_2$ | 40 mm Hg |
| pH (arterial) | 7.40 |
| $PAo_2 - Pao_2$ | <10–15 mm Hg |
| $O_2$ saturation | 98–100% |
| $Cao_2$ | 19.8 ml/100 ml |
| $P\bar{v}o_2$ | 40 mm Hg |
| $Vo_2$ | 240 ml/min |
| $Vco_2$ | 192 ml/min |
| R | 0.8 |
| Respiratory rate | 12 |
| $V_E$ | 6 liters/min |
| $V_D$ | 150 ml |
| $V_T$ | 450 ml |
| $V_D/V_T$ | 0.33 |
| $Q_t$ | 5 liters/min |
| $Q_s/Q_t$ | 7% |
| PVR | 50–150 dyn·s/cm$^5$ |
| SVR | 800–1200 dyn·s/cm$^5$ |

Modified from Matthay MA, Hopewell P: Critical care for acute respiratory disease. In Baum GL, Wolinski EL (eds): *Textbook of Pulmonary Diseases*, 5th ed. Boston, Little, Brown, 1994, p 1166.

From these three equations, it can be seen that the factors determining the $Paco_2$ are $V_T$, $V_D$, $F$, and $\dot{V}co_2$.

The volume of dead-space or wasted ventilation can be calculated from a modification of the Bohr equation.

$$V_D = (Paco_2 - Peco_2 \times V_T)/Paco_2$$

where $Peco_2$ is the partial pressure of carbon dioxide in mixed expired air. The $V_D$ so derived is commonly expressed as a fraction of $V_T$. Normal values for the $V_D/V_T$ are 0.30 to 0.35.

### EQUATIONS RELATED TO OXYGENATION

The partial pressure of oxygen in the alveolus ($Pao_2$) can be calculated from the alveolar gas equation as follows:

$$(Pao_2) = Fio_2 (P_b - 47 \text{ mm Hg}) - Paco_2/R$$

where R is the respiratory exchange ratio ($Vco_2/Vo_2$), $P_b$ is barometric pressure, and 47 is the partial pressure of water vapor in millimeters of mercury in fully saturated air at body temperature. The value of R is usually assumed to be 0.8. Having calculated the $Pao_2$, the $PAo_2 - Pao_2$ can then be determined, enabling a more quantitative assessment of the degree of hypoxemia and the mechanisms responsible for it. For example, a normal $P_{AO_2} - P_{ao_2}$ indicates that hypoxemia is secondary to alveolar hypoventilation alone. On the other hand, an increased $P_{AO_2} - P_{ao_2}$ indicates either an intrapulmonary or intracardiac right-to-left shunt or mismatching of ventilation and perfusion.

Oxygen consumption ($V_{O_2}$, in liters per minute $\dot{V}_{O_2}$) can be estimated fairly accurately from the relationship.

$$\dot{V}_{O_2} = (F_{IO_2} - F_{EO_2}) \times \dot{V}_E$$

where $F_{EO_2}$ is the fractional concentration of oxygen in expired air.

## TREATMENT MODALITIES

### SUPPLEMENTAL OXYGEN

The administration of supplemental oxygen is frequently necessary in patients with any cardiorespiratory disorder that results in hypoxemia or in which hypoxemia may be expected. The decision to use an external device rather than an endotracheal tube depends on the quantity of oxygen needed and the potential consequences of failure to provide oxygen should the external device be malpositioned. Generally speaking, it is not prudent to rely on external oxygen delivery devices for patients with hypoxemia sufficient to require an $F_{IO_2}$ of 0.7 or greater or those who could be expected to suffer serious consequences should the device not be positioned properly.

There are a variety of types of external oxygen delivery systems that can be used to provide supplemental oxygen. The choice of a particular device depends on at least four factors: (*a*) the amount of oxygen needed; (*b*) the need for precise control of the $F_{IO_2}$; (*c*) the need for humidification; and (*d*) the patient's comfort. Nasal prongs are the simplest and most comfortable delivery device. However, the $F_{IO_2}$ provided cannot be quantitated reliably and humidification is poor. Open face masks or face tents provide a high flow of well-humidified gas with a moderately reliable $F_{IO_2}$ usually set by a Venturi device in a humidifier-mixer. Tight-fitting face masks provide higher concentrations of oxygen, and the same sort of tight mask fitted with a nonbreathing valve and a reservoir bag can be used to provide even higher concentrations of oxygen, perhaps up to an $F_{IO_2}$ of 0.8 to 0.9 for short periods. One version of this system incorporates a valve for providing positive end-expiratory pressure (PEEP) (16). However, such devices are generally uncomfortable, and the oxygen may be poorly humidified. The $F_{IO_2}$ is controlled much more precisely by the Venturi mask, which uses a calibrated Venturi device in the delivery line to provide

high flows of gas containing 24, 28, 35, or 40% oxygen (17). This sort of mask is used for patients with chronic airways obstruction and chronic hypercapnia in whom uncontrolled high oxygen concentrations may cause further alveolar hypoventilation.

### VENTILATORY ASSIST DEVICES

A variety of devices have been used to provide temporary ventilatory assistance without resorting to an endotracheal airway and mechanical ventilation. These devices are generally of limited usefulness in the acute setting; however, under proper circumstances, some may be helpful. The devices of this sort that are used most frequently are simple pressure-limited ventilators used to provide intermittent positive-pressure ventilation via a mouthpiece. These devices only transiently increase alveolar ventilation and are of little value for this purpose (18). External negative-pressure devices, such as the cuirass ventilator, which fits over the chest wall and augments ventilation by lowering the pressure around the chest, causing it to expand, may be of value in patients with chronic neuromuscular diseases even in the presence of acute deterioration (19). Other ventilatory assist devices include the rocking bed and surgically implanted phrenic nerve pacemakers; however, these are of little applicability in acute respiratory failure.

### AIRWAY MANAGEMENT

Definitive, unambiguous indications for endotracheal intubation that apply to all situations are difficult to define. Often, however, the decision to proceed to endotracheal intubation is based on more subjective criteria and observation of the patient's course over time. Regardless of the situation, the potential reversibility of the patient's underlying disorder must be considered to determine if endotracheal intubation is required.

Endotracheal tubes may be passed through either the mouth or the nose. The oral route has the advantage of accepting a larger-diameter tube and is easier to use under emergency circumstances. Because direct laryngoscopy is required, sedation and often muscle-relaxing agents are needed in awake patients. Semielective tube placement in a spontaneously ventilating patient may be accomplished via the nose without direct visualization of the vocal cords; however, direct visualization may be necessary to guide the tube into the larynx. Topical anesthesia is necessary, but systemic agents are not usually required. In difficult situations, such as when the neck is immobilized, placement of either an oral or nasal tube may be accomplished over a fiberoptic bronchoscope. In any case, intubation should be done only by physicians experienced with the procedure who are familiar with the pharmacologic agents that may be necessary, such as intravenous anesthetics and muscle-relaxing agents. A recent prospective study of 297 endotracheal intubations in critically ill patients indicated that mortality associated with emergent endotracheal intubations is highest in patients who are hemodynamically unstable and receiving vasopressor therapy before intubation (20).

Nasal endotracheal tubes are generally more comfortable for the patient and are more acceptable for long-term management. In addition, oral hygiene can be better maintained. Nasal tubes have the disadvantage of being more difficult to suction through than are oral tubes, because usually they are smaller in diameter. The effective lumen may be further narrowed by compression or kinking within the nose or nasopharynx. In addition it may be difficult or impossible to perform fiberoptic bronchoscopy through a nasal tube because of its smaller diameter.

Immediately after the tube is placed, the lungs should be auscultated to determine if air is entering both hemithoraces. Because of the relatively obtuse angle of the right main bronchus, positioning of the tip of the tube in the right main airway is quite common (Fig. 20.3). If the tube seems to be in good position by auscultation, it should be taped securely in place. The position should then be confirmed by a chest radiograph.

All endotracheal tubes should be fitted with a bonded high-volume, low-pressure cuff that will occlude the trachea around the tube, enabling positive-pressure ventilation and preventing aspiration of oropharyngeal contents. Care should be taken to avoid overinflating the cuff. An overinflated cuff (more than 20 mm Hg) may cause pressure necrosis of the adjacent tracheal mucosa and predispose to development of a tracheoesophageal fistula or subsequent tracheal stenosis (21, 22).

Nasal or, occasionally, oral endotracheal tubes can be left in place for long periods of time in patients who continue to require mechanical ventilation or airway protection. There is no absolute time limit for endotracheal intubation beyond which tracheostomy is indicated (21, 22). Tracheostomy may be necessary, however, because of complications such as infection or soft tissue necrosis in the upper air passages, including the nose. Occasionally, tracheostomy facilitates removal of secretions more effectively than an endotracheal tube. In addition, patients may find a tracheostomy more comfortable and may be able to eat and talk with a tracheostomy tube in place (22).

Because endotracheal and tracheostomy tubes bypass the normal humidifying mechanisms in the upper airway, all inspired gas must be fully humidified. Pulmonary secretions should be removed with a suction catheter at regular intervals, as determined by the volume of secretions present. Sterile technique must be used for suctioning. Likewise, all gas delivery circuits in direct communication with the airway should be

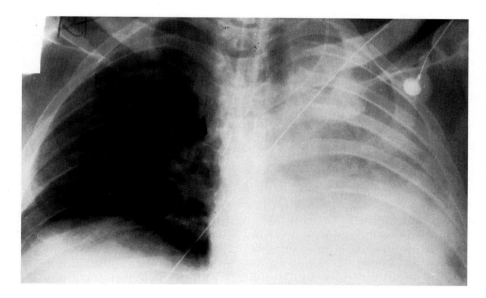

**Figure 20.3.** An anterior-posterior chest radiograph of a recently intubated patient. Note that the tip of the endotracheal tube is in the right mainstem bronchus, resulting in atelectasis of the left lung.

sterile when connected and should be changed at least at 48-hour intervals (23).

Remember that once an endotracheal or tracheostomy tube is in place, complete responsibility for the airway rests with the individuals caring for the patient. The patient can no longer humidify inspired air, cough effectively, or defend the lower airways against airborne microorganisms. Perhaps more important, the patient cannot call for help or unblock the tube should it become obstructed. For all of these reasons, in addition to the gravity of the illness for which the tube was placed, patients with an artificial airway should nearly always be managed in a critical care unit.

## MECHANICAL VENTILATION

Through the use of mechanical ventilation, patients who have severe derangements of gas exchange may be supported until the underlying process has resolved. Thus, nearly always, mechanical ventilation is a temporary life support technique, although in some situations the need for ventilatory support may not be temporary but lifelong. This is especially true for patients with chronic, progressive neuromuscular diseases that preclude effective spontaneous ventilation.

The general clinical situations in which mechanical ventilation is most commonly used include hypoxemia, usually due to intrapulmonary shunting of blood wherein external devices cannot provide a sufficiently high $FIO_2$, and progressive alveolar hypoventilation with respiratory acidosis. Other indications include prophylactic mechanical ventilation in patients in whom respiratory support is needed following cardiac, thoracic, or upper abdominal surgery and in patients who are barely maintaining adequate gas exchange at the cost of expending energy with a high work of breathing. Finally, mechanical ventilation is necessary in patients who require general anesthesia or heavy sedation to allow diagnostic or therapeutic interventions.

## FEATURES OF MECHANICAL VENTILATORS

The most common feature used to categorize mechanical ventilators is the mechanism determining the point at which the changeover from the inspiratory phase to the expiratory phase takes place. This point may be determined by the volume of gas delivered (volume cycled), the airway pressure achieved (pressure cycled), or the elapsed time of inspiration (time cycled). Both time-cycled and pressure-cycled ventilators have the disadvantage of not necessarily delivering a constant tidal volume. For this reason, volume-cycled ventilators are most commonly used. Many

ventilators, however, have options that allow the machine to be pressure or time cycled in addition to a volume-cycling mode.

To be of optimum usefulness in providing adequate ventilatory support in patients with different types of respiratory disorders, mechanical ventilators must have certain essential features. The most important of these is the capacity to deliver a wide range of tidal volumes (100 to 2000 ml) with an adjustable respiratory frequency between 5 and 60 per minute and an accurate, adjustable $FIO_2$ (0.21 to 1.0). Also, controls for adjusting the inspiration-expiration ratio (or the inspiratory flow rate) and the inspiratory pressure limit are important. The device should be capable of operating in an assist (patient-triggered) mode, a controlled (machine-triggered) mode, and an assist-control combination mode. The ventilator must be equipped with devices that monitor exhaled tidal volume, inspiratory pressure, and $FIO_2$ and have battery-operated alarms that signal loss of exhaled tidal volume, excessive inspiratory pressure, and reduction in $FIO_2$. In addition, the temperature of the inspired gas must be monitored.

Although not essential to their basic operation, it is desirable that ventilators have built-in controls for adjusting PEEP, for allowing intermittent mandatory ventilation (IMV), and for providing continuous positive airway pressure (CPAP) in spontaneously breathing patients.

## TYPES OF VENTILATORY SUPPORT

There are two basic modes of ventilatory support that are usually employed in the management of patients with respiratory failure. These are intermittent positive-pressure ventilation (IPPV) and IMV. The airway pressure patterns that characterize these modes are shown in Figure 20.4. The obvious difference is that there is no allowance for spontaneous ventilation with IPPV, whereas with IMV a portion of respiration is spontaneous. The use of one or the other of these two modes is often a matter of the physician's personal preference; however, some guidelines can be provided. The use of IPPV is clearly indicated in patients who have no spontaneous ventilation. In addition, in patients who have severe pain with respiration or an unstable chest wall IPPV should be used. Also, for patients whose work of breathing is substantial, IMV is of limited value.

On the other hand, IMV may offer an advantage in maintaining the condition of the respiratory muscles. For this reason, IMV may be more useful in patients who have acute respiratory failure without preexisting deconditioned muscles (24). In addition, some patients may find IMV more comfortable than IPPV. IMV may

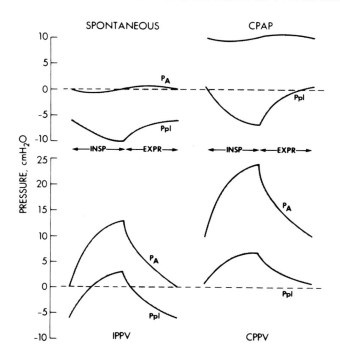

**FIGURE 20.4.** Schematic representations of airway and pleural pressures with spontaneous respiration, spontaneous respiration with continuous positive airway pressure (CPAP), intermittent positive-pressure ventilation (IPPV), and continuous positive-pressure ventilation (CPPV). Note that with CPAP and CPPV, the pressure gradient between the airway and the pleural space is increased compared with spontaneous respiration and IPPV, respectively. (From Hinshaw HC, Murray JF: Treatment of respiratory failure. In Hinshaw HC, Murray JF [eds]: *Diseases of the Chest.* Philadelphia, WB Saunders, 1980, p 989.)

also be useful for patients who develop significant reductions of cardiac output with mechanical ventilation, especially with PEEP, in that it may allow greater amounts of PEEP to be used. In patients who are not capable of synchronizing their inspiratory efforts with the ventilator, IMV may enable adequate ventilation without the need for sedation or muscle-relaxing agents. It may also be a useful weaning technique in some situations.

In addition to IMV, it is also possible to provide a patient with a certain pressure-limited support ventilation in between the regular cycling of the ventilator at the preset rate and tidal volume. This mode is called pressure support. When patients exert negative pleural pressure, they receive a tidal volume generated by a preset pressure level (perhaps 10 to 20 cm $H_2O$), which therefore relieves them of some of the work of breathing. This mode of ventilation may be useful in weaning some patients from mechanical ventilation, but

its superiority over current T-piece or CPAP or standard IMV weaning remains to be demonstrated (25).

It is also possible to provide patients with a certain pressure-limited support ventilation in between the regular cycling of the ventilator at the preset rate and tidal volume. This mode is called *pressure support.* When patients exert negative pleural pressure, they receive a tidal volume generated by preset pressure levels (perhaps 20 cm $H_2O$), which therefore relieves them of some of the work of breathing. This mode of ventilation is often used along with IMV once a patient's respiratory failure has stabilized. Some authorities believe that pressure-support is useful for weaning some patients from mechanical ventilation, but its superiority over current T-piece on standard IMV weaning has not been demonstrated (25). In fact, a recent study showed no difference in patient comfort or progress in weaning between IMV alone and IMV plus pressure support (26).

### POSITIVE END-EXPIRATORY PRESSURE

PEEP may be added to IPPV to produce continuous positive-pressure ventilation (CPPV), or it may be added to IMV. In addition, it can be used in spontaneously ventilating patients to produce CPAP. By increasing the distending pressure across the walls of the airways and alveoli, PEEP increases the volume of gas in the lung (27). This effect is most beneficial in disorders characterized by pulmonary edema (usually noncardiogenic) with consequent loss of functioning gas exchange units because of fluid filing or atelectasis. PEEP tends to increase the functional residual capacity by reexpanding collapsed units and allowing more gas exchange, thereby reducing intrapulmonary shunting of blood and improving $PaO_2$.

PEEP generally is not beneficial and in fact may be harmful in patients with other types of respiratory failure, especially those caused by airway obstruction in which the lung is already overinflated. In such cases further increases in lung volume may be hazardous. This caution applies not only to CPPV but also to IMV with PEEP and to CPAP. Levels of PEEP that are commonly used range from 3 to 20 cm $H_2O$. Higher levels are occasionally used with IMV, but the indications for and the value of high levels of PEEP have not been clearly defined.

Because PEEP increases intrathoracic pressure, return of blood from the venous circulation to the right ventricle may be impaired, and as a consequence, cardiac output may be reduced (28). Even though $PaO_2$ may be increased by PEEP, this apparently beneficial effect may be offset by the fall in cardiac output with a consequent decrease in systemic oxygen transport (28). Application of PEEP may cause generalized overdistention of the lungs in patients with airway obstruction or focal overdistention in patients with infiltrative processes. Such overdistention sets the stage for pneumothorax, the second major complication of PEEP. Finally, when infiltrative processes are unevenly distributed, PEEP may decrease blood flow to the more normal alveoli and increase flow to the fluid-filled or collapsed alveoli. This will be manifested as a decrease in $Pao_2$ when PEEP is applied (27).

### EMERGENCIES IN THE VENTILATED PATIENT

Patients who are being mechanically ventilated are subject to many potentially disastrous events that can occur suddenly and may be related either to the underlying disorder or to malfunction of the ventilator or artificial airway. Because such occurrences may be rapidly fatal, personnel caring for critically ill patients must develop a routine for assessment and management of these situations.

The most frequent indication that a problem has developed is that the patient is no longer being ventilated. This may be manifested by patient distress, by sounding of the high-pressure limit or low tidal volume alarm, or by sudden hemodynamic changes in the patient. The problems that should be suspected when the high-pressure limit is exceeded include obstruction of the endotracheal or tracheostomy tube by kinking, mucus, or blood clot, obstruction in the patient's airways, or pneumothorax. Occasionally, migration of the tip of the tube into a mainstream bronchus (usually the right) (Fig. 20.3) will cause the high-pressure limit to be exceeded, but this is usually not so dramatic an occurrence. When the high-pressure limit is exceeded and the patient is not being ventilated adequately, the first step is to disconnect the patient from the ventilator and begin hand ventilation with an anesthesia bag using an $FIO_2$ of 1.0. At nearly the same time as bagging begins, the artificial airway should be checked for position and for evidence of external obstruction such as kinking between the ventilator tubing connection and the nose, mouth, or hypopharynx. If there is no external obstruction, the tube position seems correct, and compression of the bag is still difficult, the next step should be to pass a suction catheter through the tube to check its patency and to remove mucous plugs or blood clots that may be causing the problem. Assuming the suction catheter can be passed, failure of these maneuvers to relieve the apparent obstruction indicates that the problem is within the thorax and may be caused by major airway obstruction that was not

removed by suctioning, sudden severe peripheral airways obstruction, or pneumothorax. These can usually be distinguished from one another by a rapid physical examination of the chest. Tracheal obstruction is manifested by no, or markedly reduced, entry of air into the lungs. Main bronchial obstruction is indicated by the absence of entry of air into the lung distal to the obstruction, causing a rocking motion of the chest with the affected side not expanding with inspiration and the unobstructed side being overinflated. Peripheral airways obstruction may be suspected from the patient's history and is usually indicated by wheezing, although with severe bronchoconstriction there may be little air movement and thus little or no wheezing. Nearly always, a pneumothorax that occurs in a patient being ventilated mechanically quickly becomes a tension pneumothorax. This is signaled not only by difficulty with ventilation but also by a reduction in systemic arterial blood pressure and an increase in central venous pressure. In addition, examination of the chest shows no entry of air on the affected side, but in contrast to the findings of mainstem bronchial obstruction, the affected side is hyperinflated and hyperresonant to percussion. If the clinical situation allows, a chest roentgenogram (Fig. 20.5) will allow a definitive diagnosis; often, however, there is not sufficient time and a presumption of pneumothorax must be acted on.

Management of each of these situations is obviously different. Vigorous chest physical therapy and suctioning of the airway will usually remove obstructing

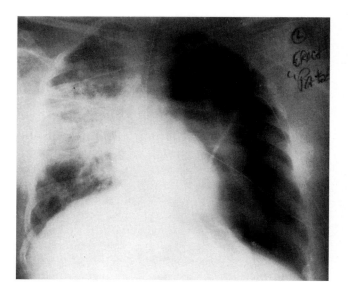

**FIGURE 20.5.** Anterior-posterior chest radiograph showing a large left pneumothorax in a patient who was being mechanically ventilated for the adult respiratory distress syndrome.

mucous plugs or clots. Occasionally, emergency fiberoptic bronchoscopy may be necessary. A tension pneumothorax requires prompt intervention to reduce the intrathoracic pressure. In an emergency situation, a 14-gauge needle can be placed in the second anterior intercostal space. This will relieve the tension, with prompt restoration of the hemodynamic status and the ability to ventilate the patient. After the needle is inserted, a chest tube should always be placed. Even if the diagnosis of pneumothorax was mistaken, a chest tube must be placed because of the high probability of lung puncture with the needle.

When inadequate ventilation is noted and the high-pressure limit is not being exceeded, the possible problems to be considered are (*a*) leaks in the ventilator tubing or around the cuff of the artificial airway, (*b*) ventilator malfunction, or (*c*) a tracheoesophageal fistula. Again, the first step is to disconnect the ventilator and begin manual ventilation using an $FIO_2$ of 1.0. At the same time, the position of the tube and the inflation of the cuff should be checked. If the external pilot balloon is deflated, more air should be added. Leaks around the cuff may be indicated by air escaping from the mouth with each ventilator inflation. The leaks may be caused by breaks in the cuff itself or in the external pilot balloon. Occasionally, an endotracheal tube may have migrated too high in the airway with the cuff at the level of the vocal cords or higher, causing air to leak around the cuff. If the cuff itself is leaking, the tube must be replaced. With some kinds of tubes, the outer balloon may be replaced without changing the tube. Leaks may also be caused by enlargement of the trachea at the site of the cuff because of the pressure on the tracheal wall. If this is the origin of the leak, the problem may be solved by adding air to the cuff within the trachea. If air is added, care should be taken in general to not exceed a measured intracuff pressure of 20 to 25 mm Hg, especially in patients with systemic hypotension (20, 21).

Tracheal dilation is often the precursor of a much more serious problem, formation of a tracheoesophageal fistula. This can usually be prevented by maintaining the intracuff pressures below 20 to 25 mm Hg (20). When a fistula does develop, however, it is often catastrophic. Patients with fistulas can sometimes be managed temporarily by placing the tube at a lower level in the trachea with the cuff below the fistula. Definitive management is surgical correction of the fistula.

## Weaning from Mechanical Ventilation

Patients who are being mechanically ventilated should be frequently evaluated to determine if their lung function has sufficiently improved to enable weaning from the ventilator and subsequent removal of the endotracheal tube. Both the technique of weaning and the rapidity of the process may vary considerably depending on the nature of the underlying disorder that caused the need for mechanical ventilation. There are, however, some basic criteria that are generally applicable in determining if it is feasible to initiate weaning (29). First, the patient should be awake and reasonably alert. Second, the underlying medical problem that necessitated mechanical ventilation must be improving. For example, hemodynamic abnormalities associated with sepsis or cardiac failure must be stabilized before weaning can begin. Lung function should be adequate as indicated by the ability of the patient to generate a VC of more than 10 ml/kg body weight and a maximum inspiratory pressure of less (more negative) than −20 cm $H_2O$, and in general the patient should not require $FIO_2$ above 0.6. Additional criteria that may be useful include a resting minute ventilation of less than 10 liters, the ability to double this volume voluntarily, a $PAO_2 − PaO_2$ below 350 mm Hg, and a $VD/VT$ below 0.55 (29). Remember, however, that some patients with severe chronic airways obstruction cannot meet these criteria but can be extubated after they tolerate a more extended weaning trial with acceptable blood gases and stable vital signs.

The techniques used in weaning include progressive lengthening of periods of spontaneous ventilation with the endotracheal tube attached to a T-piece or a similar arrangement with CPAP. Weaning by IMV can be accomplished with a progressive reduction in the number of breaths delivered by the ventilator. Patients whose lungs were previously normal and who have required only a short period of mechanical ventilation can usually be quickly weaned and extubated. The process is often much longer in patients who have required an extended period of ventilatory support.

A recent clinical study has demonstrated that successful weaning from mechanical ventilation depends on more than simply the respiratory status of the patient (30). In adult medical and surgical patients who have been ventilated for 48 hours or more, there is a high prevalence of significant neurologic abnormalities that contribute to a delay in weaning patients with respiratory failure from mechanical ventilation. A diminished level of consciousness is the most common cause of impaired neurologic status that leads to unsuccessful weaning. The decrease in mental status is often attributable to sepsis, liver failure, or some other metabolic problem as opposed to a primary neurologic disease. A summary of the primary factors that limited weaning from mechanical ventilation in this study demonstrated that pulmonary abnormalities accounted for the primary reason for failure to wean from

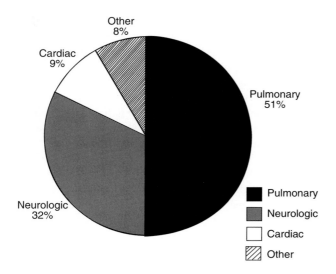

**FIGURE 20.6.** The primary factors that limit weaning from mechanical ventilation in the 90 evaluations completed: the relative contribution of pulmonary and neurologic factors. (From Kelly BJ, Matthay MA: Prevalence and severity of neurologic dysfunction in critically ill patients. *Chest* 104:1818–1824, 1993, with permission.)

mechanical ventilation in 51% of patients, neurologic abnormalities in 32% of patients, cardiac dysfunction in 9%, and the rest were contributed by other miscellaneous causes (Fig. 20.6) (30).

Thus, clinical evaluation and treatment for patients with difficulty in weaning from mechanical ventilation must consider both pulmonary and nonpulmonary factors that contribute to the need for continued mechanical ventilation.

## RESPIRATORY MONITORING

This section considers a wide range of techniques for monitoring the respiratory status of critically ill patients with respiratory failure. Recently, there has been increasing interest in developing noninvasive methods for monitoring important physiologic variables with the goal of reducing the risk and expense of invasive measurements whenever possible.

Respiratory monitoring should always include the measurement of respiratory rate and, depending on the patient's clinical condition, measurement of the arterial pH, $PaO_2$, and $PaCO_2$. The respiratory rate can be measured and recorded automatically in nonintubated, spontaneously ventilating patients with impedance devices to which alarms can be attached. In patients who are intubated and spontaneously breathing, respiratory rates and tidal volume can be monitored

with a pneumotachograph. Other approaches include the use of a respiratory inductance plethysmograph (RIP) to monitor lung volume by recording the inductance change in wire coils applied to the abdomen and rib cage. RIP has been used to measure tidal volume in both normal subjects and those with respiratory disease (31). This method may be useful for the early detection of respiratory failure in patients in critical care units, but further study of its sensitivity and clinical value is needed.

Because respiratory muscle fatigue has been recognized as an important contributing factor in many patients with acute respiratory failure, attempts have been made to monitor respiratory muscle function (32, 33). In one study, investigators demonstrated that a fall in the ratio of high- to low-frequency power over the diaphragm often preceded clinical manifestations of impending respiratory failure in recently weaned patients. The change in the power ratio preceded the development of tachypnea, altered breathing patterns (respiratory alternans and abdominal paradox), and the increase in $PaCO_2$ (Fig. 20.7) (34). It is possible that monitoring respiratory muscle EMG signals may become clinically useful to follow patients with early respiratory failure or to aid in assessing patients during weaning with spontaneous breathing trials on a T-piece or CPAP.

In patients who are mechanically ventilated, it is mandatory to monitor the respiratory rate, exhaled tidal volume, and airway pressure. An acute decrease in airway pressure indicates a leak in the system or a disconnection of the ventilator tubing from the endotracheal tube. Therefore, a low-pressure alarm system is essential. Acute increases in airway pressure may indicate simply the need for suctioning the endotracheal tube or a change in chest wall compliance because the patient is agitated or in pain. On the other hand, acute increases in airway pressure may herald a more serious problem such as pneumothorax, lobar atelectasis, malposition of the endotracheal tube in the right mainstem bronchus, or acute bronchospasm. Patients with severe airway obstruction will have elevated peak airway pressures during gas flow but normal plateau pressures (measured by occluding outflow on the ventilator momentarily) during no flow (35). The effects of inhaled bronchodilator therapy can be followed sequentially in patients with an increase in the peak-plateau pressure difference (greater than 10 cm $H_2O$).

The interrupter technique has been adapted to determine the mechanical properties of the respiratory system in patients. Flow, volume, and tracheal pressure have been measured through a series of brief (1.5-second) interruptions of expiratory flow in patients to

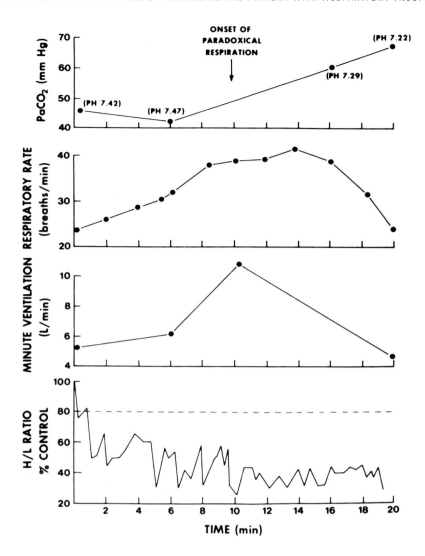

**FIGURE 20.7.** Sequence of changes in a patient during a 20-minute attempt to discontinue mechanical ventilation. The initial change was a fall in the ratio of high- to low-frequency power of the respiratory muscles as detected by surface electromyography. After the change in high:low ratio, there was a progressive rise in respiratory rate and an initial respiratory alkalosis. After the onset of paradoxic respiration, minute ventilation progressively decreased, and hypercapnia and respiratory acidosis developed. Thus, the fall in high:low ratio may be a useful predictor of diaphragmatic fatigue that precedes clinical evidence of impending respiratory failure. (From Cohen CA, Zagelbaum G, Gross D, et al: Clinical manifestations of inspiratory muscle fatigue. *Am J Med* 73:308–316, 1982.)

determine passive flow resistances as well as elastance of the total respiratory system. This method is yet another approach to assess respiratory compliance. The limitations of the method are that lung volume cannot be directly assessed and the chest wall needs to be relaxed (36).

Another approach to measuring mechanical function and work of breathing has been developed. The work of breathing can be estimated by simultaneous recording of pressure changes and flow over time.

Work (expressed in kg-m) is obtained by integration of power (pressure times flow in kg/m/second) over time. Work can be analyzed as either total respiratory work (lung and chest wall) by using transthoracic pressure differences (airway opening minus atmosphere) or only work done to move the lungs and produce air flow by using transpulmonary pressures (airway-esophageal balloon pressures). The inspiratory work of breathing during assisted mechanical ventilation has been measured, and evidence has been presented that even with the assist control mode of ventilation, patients may exert considerable respiratory muscle work (37).

There are a number of additional monitoring techniques, but their clinical value is uncertain. Breath-by-breath measurements of respiratory system compliance and both volume-pressure and volume-flow relationships can be made. Also, mass spectrometer systems are available to measure $F_{IO_2}$ and exhaled carbon dioxide and oxygen. These measurements of exhaled gases, especially the $P_{ECO_2}$, may provide an early indicator of changes in alveolar ventilation, but their utility in a critical care unit has not been clearly demonstrated. In some patients with respiratory failure, however, measurement of expired gas $P_{ECO_2}$ concentration is useful for calculation of the dead-space fraction. Measurements of the dead space fraction can be used to assess the physiologic basis for respiratory failure. Physiologic dead space may be elevated in patients with pulmonary vascular disease, chronic obstructive lung disease, necrotizing pneumonitis, or the adult respiratory distress syndrome. A dead space fraction greater than 0.55 often correlates with major difficulty in weaning a patient from mechanical ventilation because the required minute ventilation and work of breathing are excessive.

Measurement of $CO_2$ production can also be useful in determining an etiology for persistent hypercapnic respiratory failure. For example, elevated $CO_2$ production has been associated with excessive caloric and carbohydrate nutritional therapy, thus making it difficult for the patient to be weaned from mechanical ventilation (29).

Arterial oxygen and carbon dioxide tensions can be most accurately monitored with direct arterial blood gas sampling. Indwelling catheter electrodes are now available for continuous intraarterial measurement of $Pa_{O_2}$, $Pa_{CO_2}$, and pH. They have some technical limitations, and their superiority over more conventional periodic blood sampling from an indwelling arterial line has not been proved. In addition, there is a fiberoptic pulmonary artery catheter for continuous measurement of oxyhemoglobin saturation in the mixed venous blood. The clinical value of these devices remains to be definitively established (38).

Transcutaneous $P_{O_2}$ and $P_{CO_2}$ measurements are noninvasive methods that use heated skin electrodes and provide indirect reflections of $Pa_{O_2}$ and $Pa_{CO_2}$. They have been useful in infants but are not as clinically valuable in adults. A more useful noninvasive approach is pulse oximetry, which measures oxygen saturation in arterialized blood in a fingertip (39). Pulse oximetry is an advance from the prior technique of using ear oximetry, which required preparation of the site and calibration. Pulse oximetry, unlike transcutaneous $P_{O_2}$ and $P_{CO_2}$ measurements, does not require skin preparation or rotation to a new site. Under conditions of poor perfusion from local vasoconstriction or a low cardiac output, both methods may become inaccurate (40). The pulse oximeter can be very useful, particularly when weaning patients from mechanical ventilation, evaluating oxygen saturation during sleep, and performing procedures such as bronchoscopy and gastroscopy. Monitoring of pulmonary and systemic hemodynamics may be important in some patients with acute respiratory failure (see Chapter 23) (41).

▼

## REFERENCES

1. Matthay MA, Hopewell PC: Critical care for acute respiratory failure. In Wolinsky E, Baum G (eds): *Textbook of Pulmonary Disease, ed 5.* Boston, Little, Brown, 1994, pp 1161–1214.
2. Wasserman K: Exercise testing in the dyspneic patient. The chairman's postconference reflections. *Am Rev Respir Dis* 129(Suppl):1–2, 1984.
3. McFadden ER, Kiser R, De Groot WJ: Acute bronchial asthma: relations between clinical and physiologic manifestations. *N Engl J Med* 288:221–225, 1973.
4. Leventhal JM: Clinical predictors of pneumonia as a guide to ordering chest roentgenograms. *Clin Pediatr* 21: 730–734, 1982.
5. Rebuck AS, Pengelly LD: Development of pulsus paradoxus in the presence of airways obstruction. *N Engl J Med* 288:66–69, 1973.
6. Connors AF Jr, McCaffree DR, Gray BA: Evaluation of right-heart catheterization in the critically ill patient without acute myocardial infarction. *N Engl J Med* 308: 263–267, 1983.
7. Brackett NC Jr, Wingo CF, Muren O, Solano JT: Acid-base response to chronic hypercapnia in man. *N Engl J Med* 280:124–130, 1969.
8. Sperelakis N: Pathophysiology of skeletal muscle and effect of some hormones. In Roussos C, Macklem PT (eds): *The Thorax.* New York, Marcel Dekker, 1985, pp 115–140.
9. Newman JH, Neff Ta, Zipporin P: Acute respiratory failure associated with hypophosphatemia. *N Engl J Med* 296:1101–1103, 1977.
10. Mellemgaard K: The alveolar-arterial oxygen difference: its size and components in normal man. *Acta Physiol Scand* 67:10–20, 1967.
11. Brackett NC Jr, Cohen JJ, Schwartz WB: Carbon dioxide titration curve of normal man. Effect of increasing degrees of acute hypercapnia on acid-base equilibrium. *N Engl J Med* 272:6–12, 1965.
12. Appel D, Rubenstein R, Schrager K, Williams MH Jr: Lactic acidosis in severe asthma. *Am J Med* 75:580–584, 1983.
13. Kilburn KH: Shock, seizures and coma with alkalosis during mechanical ventilation. *Ann Intern Med* 66: 977–984, 1966.
14. Ketty SS, Schmidt CF: The effects of altered arterial tensions of carbon dioxide and oxygen on cerebral blood

flow and cerebral oxygen consumption of normal young men. *J Clin Invest* 27:484–492, 1948.

15. Rebuck AS, Read J: Assessment and management of severe asthma. *Am J Med* 51:788–798, 1971.

16. Branson RD, Hurst JM, DeHaven CB Jr: Mask CPAP: state of the art. *Respir Care* 30:846–857, 1985.

17. O'Donohue WJ Jr, Baker JP: Controlled low-flow oxygen in the management of acute respiratory failure. *Chest* 63:818–821, 1973.

18. Fouts JB, Brashear RE: Intermittent positive-pressure breathing, a critical appraisal. *Postgrad Med* 59:103–107, 1976.

19. Rochester DF, Martin LL: Respiratory muscle rest. In Roussos C, Macklem PT (eds): *The Thorax.* New York, Marcel Dekker, 1985, pp 1303–1328.

20. Schwartz DE, Matthay MA, Cohen NH: Death and other complications of emergency airway management in critically ill patients. *Anesthesiology* 82:367–376, 1995.

21. Stauffer JL, Silvestri RC: Complications of endotracheal intubation, tracheostomy and artificial airways. *Respir Care* 27:417–434, 1982.

22. Heffner J, Miller KS, Sahn SA: Tracheostomy in the intensive care unit. *Chest* 90:269–274 (pt I) and 430–436 (pt II), 1986.

23. Lareau SC, Ryan KJ, Diener CF: The relationship between frequency of ventilator circuit changes and infectious hazard. *Am Rev Respir Dis* 118:493–496, 1978.

24. Luce JM, Pierson DJ, Hudson LD: Intermittent mandatory ventilation. *Chest* 76:678–684, 1981.

25. MacIntyre NR: Respiratory function during pressure support ventilation. *Chest* 89:677–683, 1986.

26. Knebel AR, Janson-Bjerklie, Malley JD, Wilson AG Marini JJ: Comparison of breathing comfort during weaning with two ventilatory modes. *Am J Respir Crit Care Med* 149:14–18, 1994.

27. Weisman IM, Rinaldo JE, Rogers RM: Positive end-expiratory pressure in adult respiratory failure. *N Engl J Med* 307:1381–1382, 1982.

28. Fewell JE, Abendschein DR, Carlson CJ, et al: Mechanism of decreased right and left ventricular end-diastolic volumes during continuous positive-pressure ventilation in dogs. *Circ Res* 47:467–472, 1980.

29. Pierson DJ: Weaning from mechanical ventilation in acute respiratory failure: concepts, indications, and techniques. *Respir Care* 28:646–662, 1983.

30. Kelly BJ, Matthay MA: Prevalence and severity of neurologic dysfunction in critically ill patients. *Chest* 104:1818/1824, 1993.

31. Sackner JD, Nixon AJ, Davis B, et al: Noninvasive measurement of ventilation during exercise using a respiratory inductive plethysmograph. *Am Rev Respir Dis* 122:867–871, 1981.

32. Dantzker DR, Tobin MJ: Monitoring respiratory muscle function. *Respir Care* 30:422–431, 1985.

33. Roussos CS, Macklem PT: Diaphragmatic fatigue in man. *J Appl Physiol* 43:189–197, 1977.

34. Cohen CA, Zagelbaum G, Gross D, et al: Clinical manifestations of inspiratory muscle fatigue. *Am J Med* 73:308–316, 1982.

35. Bone RC: Monitoring ventilatory mechanics in acute respiratory failure. *Respir Care* 28:597–604, 1983.

36. Gottfried SB, Higgs BD, Rossi A, et al: Interrupter technique for measurement of respiratory mechanics in anesthetized humans. *J Appl Physiol* 59:647–652, 1985.

37. Marini JJ, Rodriguez RM, Lamb V: Bedside elimination of the inspiratory work of breathing during mechanical ventilation. *Chest* 89:56–63, 1986.

38. Boutros AR, Lee C: Value of continuous monitoring of mixed venous blood oxygen saturation in the management of critically ill patients. *Crit Care Med* 14:132–135, 1986.

39. Fanconi S, Doherty P, Edmonds J, Barker G: Pulse oximetry in pediatric intensive care comparison with measure saturations and transcutaneous oxygen tension. *J Pediatr* 107:362–366, 1985.

40. Barker SJ, Tremper KK, Gamel DM: A clinical comparison of transcutaneous $P_{O_2}$ and pulse oximetry in the operating room. *Anesth Analg* 65:805–808, 1986.

41. Matthay MA, Chatterjee K: Bedside pulmonary artery catheterization. *Ann Intern Med* 109:826–834, 1988.

# Chapter 21

# Acute Hypercapnic Respiratory Failure:
## Neuromuscular and Obstructive Diseases

## Michael A. Matthay

NEUROMUSCULAR ETIOLOGIES OF RESPIRATORY
    FAILURE
DRUG OVERDOSES
CHEST WALL ABNORMALITIES AS A CAUSE OF
    ACUTE RESPIRATORY FAILURE

UPPER AIRWAY OBSTRUCTION
CHRONIC OBSTRUCTIVE AIRWAYS DISEASE
RESPIRATORY FAILURE IN ASTHMA

THIS CHAPTER CONSIDERS the causes of acute respiratory failure that are primarily associated with inadequate alveolar ventilation, which often results in arterial hypercapnia and acute respiratory acidosis. These patients usually have abnormal oxygenation because of ventilation and perfusion mismatch in the lung. However, the primary cause of respiratory failure is usually associated with inadequate alveolar ventilation and carbon dioxide excretion, either from (*a*) inadequate central ventilatory drive, (*b*) insufficient neuromuscular transmission of the respiratory drive, or (*c*) lung disease with obstructive airway disease and the need for a high work of breathing.

## NEUROMUSCULAR ETIOLOGIES OF RESPIRATORY FAILURE

There are numerous causes of acute respiratory failure from neuromuscular disorders. These include the Guillain-Barré syndrome, myasthenia gravis, botulism, poliomyelitis, heavy metal intoxication, organic phosphate poisoning, and, rarely, administration of aminoglycoside antibiotics. Severe electrolyte disorders such as hypokalemia and hypophosphatemia may also be associated with sufficient muscle weakness to cause or worsen acute respiratory failure. Recent data

indicate that respiratory failure may be worsened by the use of neuromuscular blocking agents in critically ill patients (1). There are, of course, a variety of congenital and acquired neuromuscular diseases that may be associated with progressive respiratory failure. Acute respiratory failure may also follow injury to the spinal cord, if the lesion is at a high enough level to affect function of the phrenic nerve (2).

Acute respiratory failure is the most life-threatening complication of the Guillain-Barré syndrome. In most large series, approximately 20 to 30% of patients with Guillain-Barré syndrome require mechanical ventilation (3, 4). The average duration of mechanical ventilation is 4 to 6 weeks, but the range is quite variable (7 to 93 days in one series) (42). Characteristically, patients who require mechanical ventilation have a forced vital capacity below 4 to 5 ml/kg body weight, are progressively unable to handle oral secretions, have a poor cough, and develop hypoventilation. In addition, lobar atelectasis and pneumonia may occur (3, 5). The basic pathophysiology stems from a combination of inadequate neuromuscular strength leading to alveolar hypoventilation, low tidal volume breathing, and diffuse atelectasis. While this form of acute respiratory failure can be classified as primarily hypercapnic respiratory failure, it is frequently accompanied by a widened alveolar-arterial oxygen gradient secondary to atelectasis and pneumonia.

Patients who develop Guillain-Barré syndrome should be closely monitored with frequent measurements of vital capacity, arterial blood gases, and careful clinical evaluation of their ability to cough and protect the airway. Initial monitoring in a critical care unit is usually desirable so that immediate respiratory support can be provided if the patient's respiratory status deteriorates. Treatment for Guillain-Barré syndrome has been mainly supportive, with mechanical ventilation, intravenous fluids, and nutritional support. In addition, the use of prophylactic subcutaneous heparin is recommended (3). Careful attention to psychosocial issues is very important in managing Guillain-Barré patients in the intensive care unit (5, 6).

A prospective controlled study of 245 patients reported that plasmapheresis was superior to conventional, supportive therapy in hastening recovery of muscle strength (7). If plasmapheresis was started before the patient required mechanical ventilation, the median time on the ventilator was 9 days, versus 23 days in the control group. There was less clear-cut benefit of plasmapheresis in shortening the duration of mechanical ventilation if the patient already required ventilation. Although the study was not blinded, the basic beneficial effects of plasmapheresis in this syndrome seem to have been well established (8). Presumably, plasmapheresis removes a circulating factor from the plasma that is important in the pathogenesis of acute paralysis.

Myasthenia gravis may result in acute respiratory failure at any time during the clinical course of the disease. Some patients present with acute respiratory failure, others develop respiratory failure at some point during the course of their illness, while other patients may develop the need for mechanical ventilation following thymectomy. The muscle weakness caused by the disease results in a decrease in vital capacity and consequent inadequate alveolar ventilation with the associated risks of atelectasis and secondary pneumonia. Frequent monitoring of the vital capacity is useful but should not substitute for clinical evaluation of the patient's weakness, ability to protect the airway, and the trend in arterial blood gases. In trying to assess the need for postoperative mechanical ventilation in patients undergoing thymectomy, investigators in one study found that four risk factors were particularly helpful in predicting the need for mechanical ventilation: duration of myasthenia gravis, history of chronic respiratory disease, pyridostigmine dosage above 750 mg/day, and a preoperative vital capacity of less than 2.9 liters (9). Management of patients who require mechanical ventilation with myasthenia gravis is primarily supportive unless the respiratory failure is complicated by secondary pneumonia. Treatment with both anticholinesterase agents are useful for improving muscle strength. Corticosteroids and plasmapheresis have been effective in treating acute exacerbations in many patients with myasthenia gravis (10, 11).

The other causes of acute neuromuscular failure (Table 21.1) require supportive treatment similar to that described for Guillain-Barré syndrome and

## TABLE 21.1
### CLINICAL DESCRIPTION OF RESPIRATORY FAILURE IN DERANGEMENTS OF THE THORAX

| Category | Respiratory Failure | | Clinical Course | Secretions, Atelectasis, Pneumonia[a] |
| | Incidence | Severity[a] | | |
|---|---|---|---|---|
| Mechanical | | | | |
| Scoliosis | Common | +++ | Slow | NL+ |
| Obesity-hypoventilation | Common | +++ | Periodic | NL or ↑ |
| Fibrothorax | Common | +++ | Slow | NL |
| Thoracoplasty | Common | +++ | Slow | NL or ↑ |
| Ankylosing spondylitis | Rare | + | Slow | NL |
| Neuromuscular | | | | |
| Postpoliomyelitis | Common | +++ | Slow | ↑ |
| Amyotrophic lateral sclerosis | Common | +++ | Fast | ↑ |
| Muscular dystrophies | Common | + | Slow | ↑ |
| Spinal cord injury | Common | ++ | Slow | ↑ |
| Multiple sclerosis | Uncommon | + | Slow | ↑ |
| Myasthenia gravis | Common | +++ | Periodic | ↑ |

From Bergofsky EH: Respiratory failure in disorders of the thoracic cage. *Am Rev Respir Dis* 119:643, 1979.
[a] +, dyspnea on exertion; ++, dyspnea, mild hypoxemia, and hypercapnia only; +++, severe hypoventilation; NL, normal lungs; ↑, increased incidence.

myasthenia gravis. With patients who have a neuromuscular etiology for their acute respiratory failure, weaning from mechanical ventilation must be done gradually.

Unilateral or bilateral impairment of diaphragm function may also lead to acute respiratory failure (13). The diaphragm is the principal muscle of inspiration, being almost totally responsible for inspiration during quiet breathing. Weakness or paralysis of both hemidiaphragms is most likely to be associated with chronic neuromuscular disease, but it may also occur as an isolated abnormality and with spinal cord trauma. In addition, the phrenic nerves may be interrupted inadvertently during surgical procedures in the neck or thorax such as coronary artery bypass (13). Clinically, paradoxical or inward movement of the abdominal wall during spontaneous inspiration in the supine posture may be overlooked, and it is therefore necessary to use fluoroscopy or ultrasound to demonstrate paradoxical movement of the diaphragm with spontaneous inspiration. Additional evaluation with transdiaphragmatic pressure measurements and phrenic nerve conduction studies may be necessary (14). Ventilatory support by pacing of the diaphragm has been developed and used in a number of patients with trauma or infarction of the cervical cord above C2 when it was certain that the lower motor neurons of the phrenic nerve were viable (15).

## Drug Overdoses

There are a variety of sedative and hypnotic drugs that directly depress respiration and result in the need for mechanical ventilation. In addition, tricyclic depressant overdose is a common cause of acute respiratory failure. Cardiopulmonary complications of drug overdose occur commonly and may include hypotension, arrhythmias, and central nervous system dysfunction, including status epilepticus. This section focuses primarily on acute respiratory failure that may occur in drug-overdosed patients.

In general, the patient's history of specific drugs that have been ingested may not be reliable. Medication containers and samples of drugs or substances, if they can be obtained, are very helpful in the emergency room. Gastric contents, urine, and blood may also be collected for toxicologic examination. Initial treatment of drug overdose patients in the emergency room includes attempts to remove any unabsorbed drug with emesis or gastric lavage. Activated charcoal can be used to bind and prevent absorption of some drugs that were not removed by emesis or by lavage, as well

as helping to remove some drugs that undergo intrahepatic recirculation. Further discussion of these issues is available in other texts (16).

Most patients who require intubation and mechanical ventilation from drug overdoses do not develop primary pulmonary complications. Their need for mechanical ventilation is usually related to a depression of central ventilatory drive, which recovers as the drug is removed from the circulation. The decision to intubate and ventilate patients with drug overdose is based on clinical evaluation of the patient, including mental status, hemodynamic stability, and the ability of the patient to protect his or her airway. As a general rule, it is preferable to intubate patients with known drug overdose who have a decrease in mental function, even if their arterial blood gases remain acceptable.

Acute respiratory failure secondary to intrinsic lung disease, however, does occur in some patients following drug overdose and may become the primary clinical problem in the management of the patient (17). For example, gastric aspiration can lead to diffuse and severe lung injury with secondary pulmonary and pleural space infections (18). In addition, some drugs have been specifically implicated as causing acute lung injury even in the absence of gastric aspiration. In patients overdosed on these drugs, pulmonary edema may occur from an increase in lung vascular permeability, resulting in protein-rich edema fluid collecting in the interstitium and air spaces of the lung, even in the absence of elevated pulmonary microvascular pressures. For example, salicylate overdose has been associated with noncardiogenic pulmonary edema in some studies (19). Other drugs that cause noncardiogenic pulmonary edema include heroin, other narcotics, and ethchlorvynol.

## Chest Wall Abnormalities as a Cause of Acute Respiratory Failure

Traumatic injury to the chest wall with subsequent rib fractures is the most frequent cause of acute respiratory failure in this category. Such an injury is usually associated with pain that prevents full lung inflation and results in atelectasis and occasionally alveolar hypoventilation. If multiple ribs are fractured in multiple locations, lung inflation may be limited because of loss of normal chest wall rigidity and a subsequent paradoxical motion of the involved area (flail chest). Underlying injury to the lung contributes to abnormalities of gas exchange. Some patients can be managed without intubation and mechanical ventilation, depending on the severity of the injury and associated pulmonary dysfunction, as indicated by arterial blood gas tensions (see Chapter 24). The primary indications for placement of an endotracheal tube and mechanical ventilation are deteriorating gas exchange, particularly hypoxemia, and a requirement for large doses of narcotic agents to control pain (20).

Chronic deformities of the chest wall or marked pleural disease may also result in acute respiratory failure, although in these situations the pathophysiologic alterations are more complex than in acute injuries to the chest wall because they involve chronic parenchymal and pulmonary vascular abnormalities as well (21). These abnormalities include ventilation-perfusion mismatching due to airway closure when lung volumes are reduced by a deformed thoracic cage, inability to cough, malfunction or an acquired defect of the respiratory center in conjunction with increased work of breathing, and excessive blood volume and fluid retention that aggravate the work of breathing and ventilation-perfusion mismatch.

Table 21.1 includes a list of clinical conditions that can best be described as mechanical causes of respiratory failure. These include scoliosis, severe obesity, fibrothorax, thoracoplasty, and ankylosing spondylitis. The incidence of respiratory failure, its clinical course, and associated problems are indicated in Table 21.1 (21).

Many of the disorders that affect the chest wall are associated with chronic respiratory failure that may be accompanied by chronic alveolar hypoventilation and hypoxemia, which in turn may lead to chronic pulmonary hypertension. Thus, some patients who present with acute respiratory failure may also have associated cor pulmonale with signs and symptoms of right heart failure in association with moderate-to-severe pulmonary hypertension. The pulmonary hypertension may also be related to mechanical compression of portions of the pulmonary circulation. Some data suggest that there is a relationship between pulmonary arterial pressures and the angle of spinal deformity in patients with scoliosis (21).

Treatment for acute respiratory failure in patients with chest wall abnormalities described in Table 21.1 must be directed toward reversing hypoxemia and improving alveolar ventilation. There is some evidence that hyperinflation with positive-pressure breathing devices or incentive spirometers may be useful in improving lung inflation and oxygenation. In many cases, acute respiratory failure occurs because of the development of an associated lung infection (21).

Endotracheal intubation and mechanical ventilation may be necessary to reverse acute deteriorations in blood gases as well as to help clear pulmonary secretions. Mechanical ventilation may also be necessary in patients with the obesity-hypoventilation syndrome in whom central respiratory drive is inadequate to maintain ventilation. Treatment of right heart failure can best be accomplished by improving oxygenation. In general, digitalis has not been shown to be of major benefit in right heart failure alone.

There are other mechanical causes of acute respiratory failure that should be remembered. These include tension pneumothorax, severe ascites, and metabolic disorders such as hypothyroidism. In addition, chest wall or pleural abnormalities may contribute to respiratory failure in patients who have a primary pulmonary etiology for their respiratory distress. For example, patients with acute exacerbations of chronic obstructive lung disease may have their respiratory failure worsened by ascites, obesity, or an endocrine disorder such as hypothyroidism. Similarly, patients with primary chest wall or pleural disease may develop secondary parenchyma abnormalities such as pneumonia or pulmonary edema, which in the presence of their underlying chest wall abnormality leads to acute respiratory failure. Thus, acute respiratory failure can often be attributed to multiple factors.

## UPPER AIRWAY OBSTRUCTION

There are many possible causes of upper airway obstruction that may lead to acute respiratory failure and the need for emergency treatment. In children, croup and epiglottitis are the most common causes of upper airway obstruction. Acute epiglottitis also occurs in adults. In addition, upper airway obstruction may be the result of obstructing tumors in the base of the tongue, the larynx, or in the hypopharynx. Acute upper airway obstruction may also occur from aspirated liquid or food contents or any foreign object that becomes lodged in the airway. In some massively obese patients, obstruction of the upper airway may occur when the patient is supine.

Management of acute upper airway obstruction requires an understanding of the pathogenesis of the disorder. In patients who have severe carbon dioxide retention or apnea, emergency endotracheal intubation must be performed. If oral intubation is not possible, an emergency cricothyroidotomy or tracheostomy must be done. In patients with progressive upper airway obstruction, as may occur in acute epiglottitis, a number of studies have shown that early intubation in a controlled setting with a skilled anesthesiologist present is the best treatment. In some patients with tumors causing upper airway obstruction, temporizing measures such as treatment with helium-oxygen mixtures have been reported to preclude the need for intubation while the patient is receiving radiation therapy, chemotherapy, and corticosteroids to reduce the size of the tumor (22). Pulmonary edema may complicate upper airway obstruction in both children and adults (23). The mechanism for the relationship between upper airway obstruction and pulmonary edema has not been well established.

## CHRONIC OBSTRUCTIVE AIRWAYS DISEASE

As opposed to the disorders that primarily involve alveoli, acute respiratory failure in patients with chronic airways obstruction is characterized by an increase in $PaCO_2$ as well as a decrease in $PaO_2$. The pathogenesis of the hypoxemia depends mainly on mismatching of ventilation and perfusion (24). This is a consequence of the anatomic abnormalities described previously. In addition, superimposed conditions such as pneumonia, atelectasis, or left ventricular failure cause hypoxemia because of intrapulmonary right-to-left shunting of blood.

The mechanisms of impaired $CO_2$ elimination are more complex but also relate in part to mismatching of ventilation to perfusion (24). Unless there is rather severe airways obstruction, reductions in ventilation to some alveoli can be offset by increased ventilation to other alveoli. However, with increasing airways obstruction, this compensatory mechanism is not sufficient to cope with the overall reduction in alveolar ventilation. At least three important factors also play a role in compounding the effects of airways obstruction. First, because of the increased work of breathing in the face of hypoxic conditions, the respiratory muscles may become fatigued and be unable to maintain the necessary level of minute ventilation (25). Second, also related to the increased work of breathing, $CO_2$ production is increased (26). Finally, there may be a decrease in central ventilatory drive, partly genetic (27, 28) and partly acquired (29). Also, the hypercarbia and hypoxemia or both may depress central respiratory drive, leading to further hypoventilation. In patients with acute decompensation, administration of oxygen leads to further hypercapnia. This may be partly due to a decrease in ventilatory drive from the loss of hypoxic stimulus, although recent studies have suggested that an increase in alveolar dead space associated with oxygen therapy may be primarily responsible (30).

Chronic obstructive airways disease is generally regarded as an inexorably, albeit slowly, progressive disorder (31). Patients may have symptoms of cough and sputum production for many years. As the airways obstruction progresses, however, patients become more vulnerable to what in persons with normal lungs would be minor insults. Although acute respiratory failure may be a consequence of severe progressive airways obstruction, first episodes are generally precipitated by some complicating disorder. Most commonly, the precipitating problem is a lower respiratory tract infection, either bronchitis or pneumonia (32). The inflammation resulting from the infection, together with increased mucus production, causes further airways narrowing. If pneumonia is present, the alveolar filling causes shunting of blood and worsens lung mechanics. As a result, a vicious cycle may be initiated in which the acute process superimposed on chronic airways disease results in further increases in airways resistance, worsening of gas exchange with both increases in $PaCO_2$ and decreases in $PaO_2$, and increased work of breathing. As a consequence of increasing demands placed on respiratory muscles at a time when oxygen delivery is reduced, muscle fatigue ensues. The increased work of breathing also increases $CO_2$ production, as does fever if present, thereby presenting the lungs with an increased load of $CO_2$, which they are incapable of eliminating. This results in a progressively increasing $PaCO_2$ and decreasing $PaO_2$ unless the cycle is interrupted.

A number of other processes in addition to infection may also be involved, either alone or in combination, in producing acute respiratory failure. These include left ventricular failure, pneumothorax, pulmonary embolism, and worsening of the airways obstruction in response to inhaled irritants.

As the abnormalities of gas exchange become more severe, the function of other organs, especially the heart and central nervous system, may be affected. With regard to the heart, these effects may be manifested as arrhythmias, ischemia, heart failure, or actual myocardial infarction. Central nervous system effects include alterations in behavior, reduction in level of consciousness, coma, seizures, or myoclonus. Obviously, either cardiovascular or central nervous system effects could have a major adverse influence on the course of respiratory failure and themselves become a part of the progressive downward spiral.

The symptoms associated with respiratory failure in patients with chronic airways obstruction usually represent an accentuation of the baseline symptoms. Most patients with airways obstruction have cough and sputum production. Acute lower respiratory tract infections generally increase these symptoms and are often associated with an increase in the volume of sputum and its being darker and thicker. However, as airways obstruction increases, the ability to clear mucus from the lungs may decrease. Thus, a decrease in sputum production associated with other symptoms may also indicate worsening clinical status.

In some patients, cardiovascular complaints may

predominate. These include palpitations, orthopnea, paroxysmal nocturnal dyspnea, ankle swelling, and chest pain. Complaints related to central nervous system dysfunction may also be prominent. Headache, visual problems, sleep disturbances, memory loss, and behavioral alterations may be reported. In some patients, these may be severe enough to obscure the respiratory symptoms.

Findings on physical examination may be quite helpful and provide an important context in which to evaluate the more objective measurements such as blood gas tensions. Of the physical findings, the general appearance of the patient is very important. A patient who looks reasonably well and is alert and able to cooperate with therapy obviously represents quite a different management problem than the patient who is confused, combative, stuporous, or comatose, even though both patients may have the same blood gas and pH values. Alterations in behavior or level of consciousness may not be caused by the abnormal blood gas tensions per se, but could be related to drugs or other factors; however, the implications for treatment are the same. In addition to providing information concerning the lung disease per se, the physical examination should be targeted to detect disorders that may

have precipitated the acute deterioration, for example, left ventricular failure. At least in the acute setting, the degree of pulsus paradoxus correlates with the severity of airways obstruction. Chest examination may or may not be helpful. Most patients with acute exacerbations of chronic airways obstruction have supraclavicular and intercostal space retractions. The chest is usually hyperinflated and tympanitic with very limited diaphragmatic excursion. Breath sounds commonly are markedly diminished. Wheezing may or may not be heard.

The chest film may simply show the classic changes of longstanding obstructive lung disease (Fig. 21.1). However, there may also be evidence for pneumonia, left ventricular failure, or pneumothorax that was not evident on physical examination. The electrocardiogram is less often helpful, but it is important if it shows right atrial or right ventricular enlargement, an arrhythmia, or evidence of left ventricular disease. Routine blood studies may provide evidence of other processes, but except for the hematocrit, they do not relate to lung disease. Patients who have been hypoxemic for long periods of time, unless other factors supervene, will have secondary polycythemia (33). This

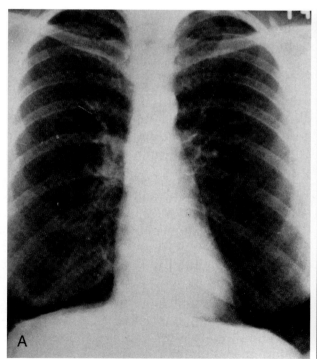
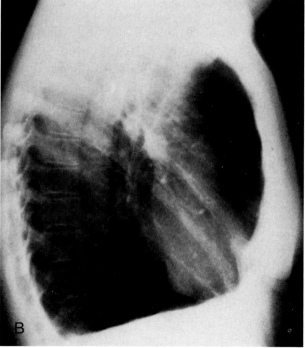

**FIGURE 21.1.** Posterior-anterior (**A**) and lateral (**B**) chest roentgenograms of a 62-year-old woman with advanced chronic obstructive pulmonary disease, mainly emphysema, showing low, flattened diaphragms, large retrosternal airspace, vertically oriented heart, and hyperlucency of peripheral lung fields. (From Hinshaw HC, Murray JF: Chronic bronchitis and emphysema. In Hinshaw HC, Murray JF [eds]: *Diseases of the Chest*. Philadelphia, WB Saunders, 1980, p 578.)

finding gives some indication of the duration of the hypoxemia.

Of all the assessments that can be made, measurements of arterial $P_{O_2}$, $P_{CO_2}$, and pH are the most important. Serial measurements of $Pa_{O_2}$, $Pa_{CO_2}$, and pH are much more helpful than a single determination and can indicate success or failure of initial therapy. Blood gas and pH values taken together with the general status of the patient often determine the necessary intensity of supportive measures, particularly whether or not endotracheal intubation and mechanical ventilation will be necessary. Nearly all patients with chronic airways obstruction will have some degree of hypoxemia, and some will have $CO_2$ retention when they are at their functional baseline. As noted above, chronicity of hypoxemia may be attested to by polycythemia and, in addition, by findings of pulmonary hypertension with or without right ventricular failure. A single measurement of $Pa_{CO_2}$ without a prior baseline value may be very difficult to interpret; hence the clinical context is important. An elevated plasma bicarbonate concentration indicates that an elevated $Pa_{CO_2}$ has been present long enough to allow metabolic compensation.

Direct measurements of air flow are often difficult to obtain in severely ill patients and may not be useful. If feasible, measurements of $FEV_1$ and FVC may, however be helpful in evaluating response to therapy.

Effective management of acute respiratory failure in patients with chronic airways obstruction requires a critical care unit. The approach to treatment should always be directed to providing supportive care while at the same time treating the specific processes such as lower respiratory tract infection that precipitated the acute deterioration.

The major supportive intervention necessary in this setting is provision of supplemental oxygen. Because the pathophysiologic mechanism by which hypoxemia develops is mismatching of ventilation to perfusion, increases in $Pa_{O_2}$ usually are easily achieved by administration of low concentrations of oxygen. The concern with overadministration of oxygen causing an increase in $Pa_{CO_2}$ has been well described and is a potential problem in patients who have a chronically elevated $Pa_{CO_2}$ (30, 34). This concern, however, should not deter oxygen administration. The basic principle should be to administer the lowest amount of oxygen necessary to increase $Pa_{O_2}$ to approximately 60 mm Hg. Frequently, this can be achieved using nasal prongs or cannulae with flows of 1 to 2 liters/minute. Occasionally, higher flows are needed (Fig. 21.2). The $F_{IO_2}$ delivered by devices such as nasal prongs will vary considerably, depending on the patient's minute ventilation. Although this does not usually present a problem, the $F_{IO_2}$ can be controlled more precisely with a mask that

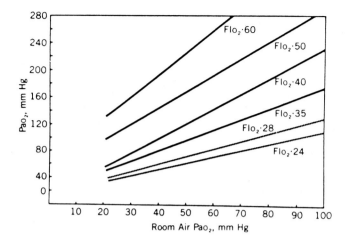

**FIGURE 21.2.** The relationship of $Pa_{O_2}$ to $F_{IO_2}$ administered to patients with COPD. Each line gives the expected arterial oxygen tension for the $F_{IO_2}$ administered. These lines were obtained in a study of patients with acute respiratory failure and stable patients with COPD. (From Bone RC: Treatment of respiratory failure due to advanced chronic obstructive lung disease. *Arch Intern Med* 140:1019, 1980. Copyright 1980, American Medical Association.)

uses a Venturi device to deliver a high flow of oxygen that entrains sufficient room air to produce the desired $F_{IO_2}$. The disadvantages of the Venturi delivery device are that the inspired gas is usually poorly humidified and the mask interferes with talking and eating.

Regardless of the oxygen delivery system, arterial blood gas tension must be measured soon after oxygen therapy is begun. The goal as cited above is to increase the $Pa_{O_2}$ to 60 mm Hg (i.e., 90% hemoglobin saturation) without undue effects on $Pa_{CO_2}$. Blood gas measurements should be made thereafter as frequently as the clinical circumstances dictate. In this situation, because of the concern with the interactions of $Pa_{O_2}$ and $Pa_{CO_2}$, noninvasive oximetric monitoring of oxyhemoglobin saturation alone is not sufficient. Because reductions in $Pa_{O_2}$ below the target value of 60 mm Hg will cause reduction in saturation to less than 90%, monitoring of oxyhemoglobin saturation may complement direct measurements of $Pa_{O_2}$ and $Pa_{CO_2}$.

In most patients, provision of supplemental oxygen is the only supportive therapy needed. Some, however, require endotracheal intubation and mechanical ventilation. Precise criteria for intubation and mechanical ventilation are difficult to define and commonly involve both subjective and objective assessments. Hypoxemia per se is usually not an indication for intubation because of the relative ease with which $Pa_{O_2}$ can be increased with supplemental oxygen provided by external devices. The major indication for ventilatory assistance is a poorly compensated acute respiratory acidosis. This may be apparent at the initial evaluation and dictate prompt institution of mechanical ventilation. Commonly, however, the need for ventilatory assistance is indicated by the the patient failing to improve or worsening with conservative management. This determination is made through careful monitoring of the response to $O_2$ administration as well as an assessment of other variables such as respiratory distress, fatigue, mental status, and ability to cooperate with conservative management.

When necessary, mechanical ventilation should be accomplished using a volume-cycled ventilator and intermittent positive-pressure ventilation (IPPV) rather than intermittent mandatory ventilation (IMV). The use of IPPV enables resting of the respiratory muscles. Respiratory muscle fatigue presumably plays a major role in the need for mechanical ventilation in this setting. Tidal volume should be set to approximately 7 to 10 ml/kg body weight. Assuming the patient is awake, he or she will determine the respiratory rate. Given the tachypnea that is common in such patients, sedation is often necessary to enable an optimum ventilatory pattern. Ideally, the rate should be relatively slow, providing sufficient time for full exhalation of the previous breath to avoid stacking breaths with a consequent further increase in functional residual capacity. A long inspiratory time also is desirable to improve the distribution of inspired gas. Positive end-expiratory pressure (PEEP) should generally not be used. PEEP would further increase the already greatly enlarged functional residual capacity and cause further overdistention of the lungs. In patients with airways obstruction, an auto-PEEP effect may occur because of airway closure prior to full exhalation (35). Because the patient is now being mechanically ventilated, there should no longer be concern with the overadministration of oxygen, and the $F_{IO_2}$ should be sufficient to maintain a $Pa_{O_2}$ over 60 mm Hg.

Within 10 minutes of beginning mechanical ventilation, arterial blood gases should be measured. Because many patients with acute respiratory failure and chronic airways obstruction have had $CO_2$ retention for days, months, or years, metabolic compensation has occurred. This compensation generally is insufficient in the setting of an acute deterioration but is appropriate for the baseline $Pa_{CO_2}$. When mechanical ventilation is applied, the $Pa_{CO_2}$ generally can be decreased very quickly, and if it is reduced well below the patient's baseline to a normal value of 40 mm Hg, the patient will be left with an uncompensated, sometimes profound, metabolic alkalosis. Alkalosis has a

number of potential adverse effects including depressing cardiac output, increasing the risk of both supraventricular and ventricular arrhythmias, depressing the level of consciousness, and causing seizures (36). Because of the concern with alkalosis, the adequacy of mechanical ventilation should be determined not by $Pa_{CO_2}$ but by pH. The $Pa_{CO_2}$ should be maintained at a level that keeps the pH no higher than 7.45 to 7.50, preferably close to 7.40. Also, because of chronic increases in $Pa_{CO_2}$, patients are commonly deficient in potassium and chloride. A reduction in plasma bicarbonate concentration will not occur until sufficient chloride, usually in the form of potassium chloride, has been given (37).

Weaning patients with chronic airways obstruction from mechanical ventilation can present a difficult problem. Implicit in the decision to intubate and ventilate is the assumption that there is a reversible factor contributing to the acute deterioration and that treatment will restore the patient to baseline status. Thus, mechanical ventilation is simply tiding the patient over until specific therapy has had its effect, although resting the muscles of respiration may be of value in itself. Given this assumption, weaning efforts should begin as soon as the reversible component has been improved. In the case of left ventricular failure, for example, this may occur quite rapidly in response to diuresis. On the other hand, if pneumonia caused the acute deterioration, improvement may be slow.

A number of criteria have been developed to predict the ability to be weaned. Unfortunately, these criteria rarely apply to patients with chronic airways obstruction, who may not have been able to perform at the levels indicated by the criteria for many years. For this reason, assessing the ability to be weaned in this setting is more subjective. Measurements such as VC and MIP can be made, but low values should not be assumed to predict failure. The patient should be alert and psychologically prepared for weaning. Serum electrolyte concentrations, especially potassium, phosphate, calcium, and magnesium, should be optimum, and the patient should be hemodynamically stable.

In general, prior to beginning the process of weaning, the $Pa_{O_2}$, $Pa_{CO_2}$, and pH should be maintained approximately at their baseline values, if known. Thus, patients may be mildly hypoxemic, hypercapneic, and acidemic. The technique of weaning is somewhat controversial, with some clinicians favoring spontaneous breathing on a T-piece and others favoring the use of IMV with progressively decreasing ventilatory rates. The use of a T-piece trial offers the advantage of being able to determine fairly quickly if a patient is ready to be extubated, whereas IMV may delay this determination. In addition, because IMV uses both spontaneous and machine-generated breaths, this form of weaning may be associated with increasing respiratory muscle fatigue. If the patient ventilates adequately via a T-piece for 1 or 2 hours without a deterioration in arterial blood gas tension, usually the endotracheal tube can be removed. Longer periods of spontaneous breathing (especially through a small endotracheal tube less than 7 mm in diameter), may cause respiratory muscle fatigue because of the resistance of the tube. Recent studies have indicated that several different approaches to weaning from mechanical ventilation may be equally effective (38).

In managing patients with acute respiratory failure and chronic airways obstruction, important and difficult ethical issues may be raised. As stated previously, in undertaking mechanical ventilatory support it is assumed that the respiratory failure has a reversible component. This may not be the case. The respiratory failure may simply represent the end stage of a disease that is known to be inexorably progressive. Providing mechanical ventilation for a patient who has no reversible component usually means that the patient will not be able to be weaned successfully. Under ideal circumstances the patient and his or her physician will have discussed the outlook for the illness prior to acute deterioration, and the patient can make an informed decision regarding the use of mechanical ventilation. Such a patient may decide that ventilation should be undertaken on the chance that there is a reversible component. If facilities are available, the patient may also chose chronic ventilatory support. Given the multiplicity of disorders commonly present in these sorts of patients, chronic mechanical ventilation is usually a very unattractive option even if available. Patients who are being ventilated mechanically may also elect to have this support discontinued. In the face of previously reviewed difficulties in predicting weanability, abrupt discontinuation of support may not mean death. If mechanical ventilation is not undertaken or is discontinued, vigorous treatment can still be provided, but in addition, particular attention should be paid to the patient's comfort.

Survival rates for acute respiratory failure in patients with chronic airways obstruction have been surprisingly similar in several studies, ranging from 58 to 79%. Not surprisingly, 24-month survival has been much lower, from 35 to 72% (39).

In addition to the supportive care described in this section, treatment of the airways obstruction and the precipitating disorder must be prompt and vigorous. Although the use of bronchodilators in patients with chronic airways obstruction is controversial, a reversible component should always be assumed. Inhaled $\beta_2$-adrenergic agonists such as albuterol, metaproterenol, and terbutaline should be used at intervals of 2 to 4

hours at the beginning of treatment and decreased in frequency if adverse reactions are encountered. They can be administered directly via a nebulizer drive by a compressed gas source or through a mechanical ventilator. With either of these devices, the amount of drug actually delivered is difficult to quantify, and thus the dose given should be limited mainly by side effects. Inhaled ipratropium has also been shown to be useful for bronchodilation and perhaps for reducing the volume of secretions (40). Intravenous theophylline may also be of benefit, albeit less than inhaled $\beta$-agonists. The loading dose of aminophylline in patients who have not been taking the drug is 5 to 6 mg/kg. Maintenance doses in patients with severe airways obstruction, some of whom may have heart failure, should be 0.3 to 0.5 mg/kg/minute (40, 41). After 18 to 24 hours, the serum theophylline concentration should be measured and the infusion rate adjusted appropriately. The concentration should be approximately 15 $\mu$g/ml, with 20 $\mu$g/ml being the usual threshold for toxicity. Theophylline has been shown to increase the strength of respiratory muscles, but in one study, the dose needed to achieve this effect required concentrations that were toxic (42). Also, one recent study suggested that theophylline was of minimal benefit in treating acute respiratory failure in COPD if the patient was already treated with $\beta$-agonists, antibiotics, and corticosteroids (43).

Corticosteroids may also be of benefit (44), although response is not universal. The dose that should be given is not established, but a sufficient amount should be given to ensure an effect (40). Doses of 120 to 240 mg are commonly administered daily early in the course of treatment.

Antimicrobial drugs are given commonly and are of obvious value if there is a bacterial bronchitis or pneumonia (45). The choice of agents should be guided initially by the results of sputum Gram stains. If Gram stains and cultures do not provide guidance, empiric therapy with ampicillin, trimethoprim-sulfamethoxazole, or tetracycline may be used.

## RESPIRATORY FAILURE IN ASTHMA

Asthma mortality is on the rise in the United States and worldwide (46). Most deaths occur in asthmatics from status asthmaticus. Acute airways obstruction in asthma results in increased resistance to air flow during inspiration and especially expiration, and this leads to air trapping and overinflation of the lung (47). Because the air flow obstruction is not uniform, the distribution of inspired air is uneven, causing mismatching of ventilation to perfusion. This results in hypoxemia and an increase in wasted ventilation (48). The hyperinflation serves to maintain airway patency, but as functional residual capacity (FRC) increases and approaches the predicted normal total lung capacity (TLC), a greater change in transpulmonary pressure is required to produce an adequate tidal volume. This, together with the rise in airways resistance, markedly increases the work of breathing. As a consequence of these abnormalities, in severe airways obstruction there is an increased $O_2$ demand caused by the increased work of breathing at the same time that hypoxemia may result from mismatching of ventilation to perfusion. Moreover, the increases in wasted ventilation and in $CO_2$ production require a greater minute ventilation, which can be achieved only by imposing an additional workload on the respiratory muscles. Because of the hyperinflation, the intercostal, accessory, and diaphragmatic muscles are forced to work at a considerable mechanical disadvantage (49). At some point, if the airways obstruction is not corrected, the system fails and $CO_2$ retention occurs. In addition, as the $O_2$ demands of the respiratory muscles begin to outstrip the supply of $O_2$, anaerobic metabolism results, with subsequent metabolic (lactic) acidosis. Because there is no possibility for respiratory compensation, the pH rapidly decreases. Metabolic acidosis in this setting must be dealt with promptly or rapid deterioration will occur.

Assessment of the severity of an asthmatic episode is of obvious importance in determining the approach to management of the patient. Although the vast majority of asthma attacks are treated entirely on an outpatient basis, it is essential that both the patient and medical personnel be aware of when more intensive treatment is needed. Several groups of investigators have identified factors of importance in deciding which patients with asthma require hospital admission (50–52). However, the utility and accuracy of numerical indices derived from such data have been questioned (53, 54). Thus, both objective and subjective individualized patient assessment determines the severity of an asthmatic episode. Factors that should be taken into account in such evaluations are listed in Table 21.2.

The history is of major importance in assessing the severity of a given asthmatic episode and provides information that influences the interpretation of the more objective physiologic data. Patients who have a history of having severe attacks tend to continue to have severe attacks. Thus, information from the patient or from the medical record indicating previously required hospitalization increases concern for the current episode. The duration of the current attack is also important, since the mechanism of airway obstruction changes as the attack persists. Early, it is mainly smooth muscle spasm; later, it is mucous plugging and edema. Spasm can resolve within minutes, but days

**TABLE 21.2**
**IMPORTANT FACTORS IN ASSESSING SEVERITY OF ACUTE ASTHMA**

1. History of prior hospitalization for asthma
2. History of prior or current corticosteroid therapy
3. Patient's subjective sense of severity of attack
4. Failure to respond to usual treatment (i.e., persistent wheezing despite bronchodilator therapy)
5. Duration of attack
6. Patient too distressed to talk
7. Silent chest (i.e., minimal breath sounds)
8. Disturbances in mental status
9. Systemic hypertension, tachycardia >110/min
10. Cardiac arrhythmias
11. Cyanosis
12. Prominent accessory muscle use
13. Pulsus paradoxus >10 mm Hg
14. Mediastinal emphysema, pneumothorax
15. FEV <1.0 liter
16. Acute respiratory acidosis or arterial $Pa_{O_2}$ <60 on room air

may be required to improve obstruction that is caused by edema and plugging.

Patients with acute asthmatic episodes are nearly always tachypneic and tachycardic, either of which correlates well with the degree of airway obstruction. The amount of pulsus paradoxus, however, correlates with greater degrees of obstruction (55). This finding can therefore be used both to indicate severity and to judge response to therapy. The intensity of wheezing cannot be used to infer the amount of airways obstruction, although prolongation of the expiratory phase varies roughly with obstruction. The absence of wheezing in a patient who by all other indicators has asthma is an ominous finding, indicating that air flow is so reduced that there is not sufficient turbulence to cause wheezing. Unilateral absence of wheezing may be the result of a pneumothorax or mucus plug in a large airway and likewise indicates a very serious clinical problem. Although not specific, abnormalities in mental status are important in patients with severe airways obstruction. Such findings may be the result of hypoxia or $CO_2$ retention or be unrelated to the asthma per se but influence management by interfering with patient cooperation.

Although an understanding of the alterations in pulmonary function is necessary to conceptualize the pathophysiology of asthma, in clinical practice the only measurements that can be made routinely are the $FEV_1$, PEF, and FVC. Of these, the PEF is the most easily obtained because it does not require a full forced exhalation but rather a short forced puff similar to a cough after a full inhalation. Severe obstruction is indicated by a peak flow of less than 100 liters/minute. This has been shown to correspond to an $FEV_1$ of less than 0.7 liter (56).

The $FEV_1$ is more difficult to measure because it requires a full inspiration followed by a full forced exhalation, maneuvers that a severe asthmatic may not be able to perform because of dyspnea and that in some patients actually worsen the obstruction (57). Nevertheless, the $FEV_1$ is the most direct measurement of air flow and correlates well with other variables and clinical outcomes. Nowak and associates (56) found that an $FEV_1$ of less than 1 liter or 20% of the predicted value was associated with a poor bronchodilator response, the need for hospitalization, and the likelihood of relapse. Similar findings were reported by Kelsen and coworkers (52). Several investigators have related the $FEV_1$ to $PaO_2$ and $PaCO_2$ (58, 59) and have demonstrated that in general, in acute asthma, $CO_2$ retention begins to occur at an $FEV_1$ of approximately 750 ml or 25% of the predicted value. An increase in $PaCO_2$ is a direct consequence of the airways obstruction with limited ventilatory capability in the face of increased $CO_2$ production. Because mild degrees of acute airways obstruction are usually associated with a lower than normal $PaCO_2$, the finding of a value in the range of 40 mm Hg should be viewed with concern.

Although there is a tendency for the $PaO_2$ to decrease with decreasing values of $FEV_1$, the relationship is not as predictable as with $PaCO_2$ (60). Nearly all patients with any airways obstruction have some arterial hypoxemia. Values below 50 mm Hg are distinctly unusual, however, and suggest that factors in addition to airways obstruction are playing a role.

Acute hypoventilation results in a reduction in arterial pH of about 0.008 pH unit for every 1 mm Hg increase in $PaCO_2$; thus, an increase in $PaCO_2$ from 40 to 60 mm Hg would result in a pH of 7.25. A reduction in pH that is in excess of the change in $PaCO_2$ indicates both metabolic and respiratory acidosis. As discussed previously, metabolic acidosis in this setting is due to an imbalance between the supply and consumption of $O_2$ by the respiratory muscles plus perhaps a reduction in clearance of lactate from blood. The finding of metabolic acidosis in a patient with severe asthma is perhaps the single most ominous finding of all (61).

Chest radiographs should be obtained routinely in patients with severe asthma. The most common finding is overinflation of the lungs, but occasionally pneumonia, pneumomediastinum, pneumothorax, or atelectasis from mucous plugging of larger airways may be found. Electrocardiograms should also be obtained, especially in older patients. The common abnormalities include P-pulmonale, right ventricular strain, and right axis deviation, all of which may be reversible.

Much less commonly, changes indicating ischemia or arrhythmias may be encountered (62). The treatment modalities used in severe asthma are directed toward both support of the patient and reversal of the airways obstruction. Supplemental oxygen is an essential supportive measure that should be instituted in all patients with acute airways obstruction. Because there is no concern with depression of ventilatory drive by oxygen in most patients with asthma, the choice of an oxygen delivery system should mainly be dictated by patient comfort. For example, face masks that fit tightly may not be tolerated, and humidification of the inspired gas mixture, although desirable, may stimulate more bronchoconstriction. Normal saline is less likely to produce this effect than is distilled water. In addition, heated humidification is preferable.

It can be difficult to determine when to institute mechanical ventilation in severe asthma. There are no uniformly applicable criteria that can guide the decision, and as with the general assessment, both subjective and objective criteria should be used (63). Generally, mechanical ventilation should not be undertaken before the patient has been given maximal bronchodilator therapy, even though marked abnormalities of gas exchange may be present. Exceptions to this generalization include the presence of significant mental status changes, life-threatening cardiac arrhythmias, electrocardiographic evidence of myocardial ischemia, or a history of previous severe asthmatic episodes requiring mechanical ventilation (63).

Patients who continue to deteriorate in the face of aggressive, in-hospital management generally require mechanical ventilation. This is indicated by increasing respiratory acidosis often accompanied by metabolic acidosis. Hypoxemia in itself, because it can be managed effectively with supplemental $O_2$, is rarely an indication for mechanical ventilation.

Placement of an endotracheal tube should be done semielectively rather than waiting until the patient is in extremis. A nasotracheal intubation with adequate topical anesthesia may be performed in an awake patient after preoxygenation. Because there are irritant receptors in the larynx and trachea, endotracheal intubation may provoke increased bronchoconstriction. This response is mediated by the parasympathetic nervous system and may be reduced by premedication with atropine or topical lidocaine in the pharynx and larynx. In most patients, orotracheal intubation with sedation and paralysis is necessary.

Once control of the airway is achieved, sedation is generally necessary. Morphine sulfate, 3 to 5 mg given intravenously, is the agent of choice. Although there are theoretical concerns that morphine causes release of histamine and further bronchoconstriction, this has not been clinically significant. Mechanical ventilation should be provided with a volume-cycled ventilator. At least early in the course, the ventilatory mode should be IPPV rather than IMV. This will allow the respiratory muscles to rest completely. Tidal volume should be in the range of 6 to 10 ml/kg body weight. Because the FRC is markedly increased, PEEP, which will further increase the FRC, should not be used, although the auto-PEEP phenomenon is common.

Appropriate adjustment of the ratio of inspiration to expiration is the most difficult aspect of mechanical ventilation in the setting of severe airways obstruction. An interplay of four factors is involved: (*a*) marked slowing of the expiratory flow because of the airways obstruction, (*b*) dyspnea and tachypnea, (*c*) the need for a minute ventilation that will reduce the $PaCO_2$, and (*d*) the desirability of a slow inspiratory time to minimize peak airway pressures and enable optimum distribution of the inspired gas. Because of the reduction in expiratory flow, a relatively long expiratory time is needed. If expiratory time is too short, further air trapping will occur. To avoid this, either the inspiratory time can be shortened or the tidal volume reduced, neither of which is desirable. Thus, it is generally preferable to sedate the patient until apnea is produced so that a slow ventilatory rate can be used, thereby allowing both a slower inspiratory flow and a longer expiratory time. In addition to morphine or diazepam, muscle relaxants may be necessary. Pancuronium or vecuronium are the muscle relaxants of choice because curare, succinylcholine, and atracurium cause release of histamine, but these agents can be associated with prolonged neuromuscular blockade and myopathy, so their use should be minimized (64).

One study reported excellent results with controlled hypoventilation with hyperoxic mixtures in mechanically ventilated patients (65). In this study, the authors did not allow peak airway pressures to exceed 50 cm $H_2O$ and thus allowed the patients to be hypercapnic but well oxygenated. Alveolar hypoventilation was maintained for hours or even up to 4 days until airway obstruction was relieved and the hypercapnia resolved. There were no deaths with this approach, which contrasts with prior studies (Table 21.3).

During the course of mechanical ventilation, in addition to following $PaO_2$, $PaCO_2$, and pH, the peak and mean airway pressures should be noted because they provide a rough indication of the inspiratory flow resistance. With mechanical ventilation, $PaO_2$ and $PaCO_2$ generally can be brought into the normal range quite promptly; however, weaning cannot begin until the airways obstruction remits. This is indicated by a reduction in peak inspiratory pressure, a spontaneous maximum inspiratory force of at least $-30$ cm $H_2O$,

## TABLE 21.3
### Prognosis in Patients Requiring Mechanical Ventilation in Status Asthmaticus

| Study | Year | Episodes (*n*) | Deaths | Mortality (%) |
|---|---|---|---|---|
| Riding and Ambiavagar | 1967 | 26 | 4 | 15 |
| Iisalo et al | 1969 | 29 | 4 | 14 |
| Lissac et al | 1971 | 19 | 4 | 21 |
| Sheehy et al | 1972 | 22 | 2 | 9 |
| Scoggin et al | 1977 | 21 | 8 | 38 |
| Cornil et al | 1977 | 58 | 6 | 10 |
| Westerman et al | 1979 | 42 | 4 | 9.5 |
| Webb et al | 1979 | 20 | 7 | 35 |
| Picado et al | 1983 | 26 | 6 | 23 |
| Darioli et al | 1983 | 34 | 0 | 0 |

From Darioli R, Perrec C: Mechanical controlled hypoventilation in status asthmaticus. *Am Rev Respir Dis* 129:385–387, 1984.

and a vital capacity of at least 15 ml/kg body weight. If these are achieved, weaning can usually proceed using either conventional T-piece trials with spontaneous ventilation or IMV with a progressively decreasing frequency of mechanical breaths.

The principles for the use of bronchodilator agents apply equally in mild, moderate, and severe asthma. As discussed previously, however, one of the clinical features that serves to define severe asthma is a failure to respond promptly to the usual bronchodilators. In spite of the poor early response to bronchodilators in patients with severe asthma, these agents together with corticosteroids remain the keystone of treatment. In severe asthma, the general rule is still to give both theophylline and $\beta$-adrenergic agonists in maximal doses as determined by blood concentrations (theophylline) or toxicity ($\beta$-adrenergic agents and theophylline). In at least two studies, this approach provided more bronchodilation than either agent given alone in maximal doses, although in a third trial, inhaled isoproterenol had as much effect alone as when combined with aminophylline (66). More studies are needed to assess the clinical value of theophylline therapy in severe acute asthma.

$\beta$-Adrenergic agonists may be administered orally, by inhalation, subcutaneously, or intravenously. There is, however, substantial evidence that when given by inhalation there is a much more favorable ratio between benefit and untoward effects (67, 68). Frequently, because of limitation of inspiratory flow, use of a metered dose inhaler is not adequate to deliver the aerosol. Placing a spacer or reservoir between the inhaler and the mouth may enable more effective use of the metered dose inhaler. Of the β-selective agents, only metaproterenol, terbutaline, and albuterol are available in the United States. The usual doses are, for metaproterenol solution, 15 mg (0.3 ml of 5% solution) and, for terbutaline, 1.5 to 2.5 mg. Albuterol is currently available only in metered dose inhalers. Normal saline is added to the drug to make a total volume of 2.5 to 3 ml. Using standard nebulizers, this volume should be completely aerosolized in 10 to 15 minutes. With most compressed gas–driven systems nebulization is continuous, but only the portion of the nebulized drug that is inhaled constitutes an effective dose; thus, the doses listed above are substantially greater than the doses delivered.

Aerosolized agents have an onset of action within minutes and the effect of a single dose peaks at 30 to 60 minutes. The duration of effect is 4 to 6 hours following a single dose. In treating severe episodes of asthma, inhalation of a $\beta_2$-selective agent should be nearly continuous during the first hour unless toxicity develops as indicated by cardiac arrhythmia or intolerable tremor. During the next several hours inhalation can be given at hourly intervals with close monitoring for toxicity. As the airways obstruction improves, the dosing interval can be increased to 4 to 6 hours. In asthmatics who require endotracheal intubation and mechanical ventilation, the drug can be delivered using an in-line nebulizer in the inspiratory limb of the ventilator circuit. Longer-acting β-adrenergic agonists may also prove to be of some value by inhalation, though the delay in the onset of their action may limit their utility in the acute setting (69).

The use of theophylline was discussed in the preceding section on COPD and acute respiratory failure. However, the factors that tend to alter the pharmacokinetics of theophylline (such as pneumonia, heart failure, and severe airways obstruction) are more likely to be present in severe asthma than in milder forms. Because of the severity of the process and perhaps because of coexisting diseases, it is more difficult to determine if a given occurrence (cardiac arrhythmia, seizure) is due to theophylline. For these reasons the use of theophylline in severe asthma must be monitored closely with measurements of serum concentration of the drug.

Treatment with corticosteroids is essential therapy in severe asthma. In patients who do not respond promptly to initial bronchodilator therapy, treatment with a systemic, generally intravenous, corticosteroid should be instituted (70). This does not obligate patients to a long course of corticosteroids nor cause them to be steroid dependent. Because the peak effect occurs no sooner than 4 to 6 hours after intravenous administration, it is best to give the initial dose early in the course of treatment and reevaluate the need for continuation at a later time. There appears to be a dose-response relationship between increasing doses of methylprednisolone (15 mg, 40 mg, and 125 mg all given 3 times a day) and $FEV_1$ (71). Given that the adverse effects of even high doses of corticosteroids are minimal if the duration of administration is short, it is probably better to err on the side of giving too much of the drug than too little. Based on the scant data that are available, a dose of methylprednisolone in the range of 60 to 120 mg given intravenously at 6- to 8-hour intervals for 48 to 72 hours represents a reasonable initial approach to corticosteroid administration in patients with severe asthma. Higher doses should be used in patients who have been taking corticosteroids prior to being seen or who are taking other drugs, such as barbiturates, phenytoin, or rifampin, that accelerate the metabolism of corticosteroids (72). In patients who respond promptly, the dose can be reduced rapidly to maintenance doses given orally or be discontinued altogether.

Aerosols of corticosteroids, although effective in maintenance therapy, have no role in management of the severe attack. However, patients who have asthma and are being mechanically ventilated for other reasons can be given agents such as beclomethasone via the endotracheal tube.

Because both airway smooth muscle and mucociliary function are modulated by the parasympathetic nervous system with stimulation causing both bronchoconstriction and an increase in mucus production, it is logical to assume that antimuscarinic agents such as atropine might be of benefit in asthma. To date, however, there is no evidence that administration of atropine or related compounds results in more bronchodilation than that provided by maximal doses of β-adrenergic agonists.

Antimicrobial agents are of questionable value in the routine management of acute asthmatic episodes (72). However, antimicrobial therapy is clearly indicated in patients who have bacterial pneumonia as seen on chest radiographs and supported by the presence of bacteria and polymorphonuclear leukocytes in a Gram-stained sputum smear. Antimicrobial agents should also be used in patients with severe asthma and bacterial bronchitis. In general, mucolytic agents are of little use in severe asthma. General anesthesia with inhalational agents has been used in the treatment of refractory asthma for a number of years. Halothane, because it possesses inherent bronchodilating properties, is the current agent of choice (73). The drug has been demonstrated to antagonize the effects on smooth muscle of acetylcholine and histamine as well as reducing antigen-induced bronchospasm in dogs. In addition to the pharmacologic effects of the anesthetic agent, general anesthesia may allow more effective mechanical ventilation, although this could also be achieved in the vast majority of instances by proper use of sedatives and muscle relaxants in patients already being ventilated mechanically.

The side effects of halothane must be considered in deciding to administer general anesthesia. These include myocardial depression and arrhythmias, both of which may be potentiated by hypoxia and acid-base disturbance, and worsened hypoxemia caused by a loss of intrapulmonary regulation of blood flow (73).

We gratefully thank Jill Richardson for her assistance in preparing this manuscript.

▼

## REFERENCES

1. Segredo V, Caldwell JE, Matthay MA, Sharma ML, Gruenke LD, Miller RD: Persistent paralysis in critically ill patients after long-term administration of vecuronium. *N Engl J Med* 327:524-528, 1992.
2. Luce JM: Medical management of spinal cord injury. *Crit Care Med* 13:126-131, 1985.
3. Moore P, James O: Guillain-Barré syndrome: incidence, management and outcome of major complications. *Crit Care Med* 9:549-555, 1981.
4. Gracey D, McMichan JC, Divertie MB, Howard JRFM: Respiratory failure in Guillain-Barré syndrome. *Mayo Clin Proc* 57:742-746, 1982.
5. Eisendrath SJ, Matthay MA, Dunkel J, et al: Guillain-Barré syndrome: psychosocial aspects of management. *Psychosomatics* 24:465-475, 1983.
6. Henschel EO: The Guillain-Barré syndrome: a personal experience. *Anesthesiology* 47:228-231, 1977.
7. Guillain-Barré Syndrome Study Group. Plasmapheresis and acute Guillain-Barré syndrome. *Neurology* 35:1096-1104, 1985.
8. Dyck PJ, Kurtzke JF: Plasmapheresis in Guillain-Barré syndrome. *Neurology* 35:1105-1107, 1985.
9. Leventhal SR, Orkin FK, Hirsh RA: Prediction of the need for postoperative mechanical ventilation in myasthenia gravis. *Anesthesiology* 53:26-30, 1980.
10. Grob D: Acute neuromuscular disorders. *Med Clin North Am* 65:189-207, 1981.
11. Dou PL, Lindstrom JM, Cassel LK, et al: Plasmapheresis and immunosuppressive drug therapy in myasthenia gravis. *N Engl J Med* 297:1134-1139, 1977.
12. Keys PA, Blume RP. Therapeutic strategies for myasthenia gravis. *Ann Pharm Therapy* 25:1101-1108, 1991.
13. Mickell JJ, Kook SO, Siewers RD, et al: Clinical implications of postoperative unilateral phrenic nerve paralysis. *J Thorac Cardiovasc Surg* 75:297-304, 1978.
14. Wilcox P, Baile E, Hards J, et al: Phrenic nerve function and its relationship to atelectasis after coronary artery bypass surgery. *Chest* 93:693-698, 1988.
15. Glenn WL, Hogan JF, Loke J, et al: Ventilatory support by pacing of the conditioned diaphragm in quadriplegia. *N Engl J Med* 310:1150-1155,
16. Rippe JM, Irwin RS, Alpert JS, Dalen JE: *Intensive Care Medicine.* Boston, Little, Brown, 1985.
17. Roy TM, Ossorio MA, Cipolla LM, et al: Pulmonary complications after tricyclin antidepressant overdose. *Chest* 96:852-856, 1989.
18. Bynum LJ, Pierce AK: Pulmonary aspiration of gastric contents. *Am Rev Resp Dis* 114:1129-1136, 1976.
19. Heffner JE, Sahn SA: Salicylate-induced pulmonary edema. *Ann Intern Med* 95:405-409, 1981.
20. Schackford SR, Virgilio RW, Peters RM: Selective use of ventilator therapy in flail chest injury. *J Thorac Cardiovasc Surg* 81:194-201, 1981.
21. Bergofsky EH: Respiratory failure in disorders of the thoracic cage. *Am Rev Respir Dis* 119:643-669, 1979.
22. Curtis JL, Mahlmeister M, Fink J, et al: Helium-oxygen gas therapy: use and availability for the emergency treatment of inoperable airway obstruction. *Chest* 90:455-457, 1986.
23. Tami T, Chu F, Wildes T, Kaplan M: Pulmonary edema and acute upper airway obstruction. *Laryngoscope* 96:506-509, 1986.
24. Wagner PD, Dantzker DR, Dueck R, et al: Ventilation-perfusion inequality in chronic obstructive pulmonary disease. *J Clin Invest* 59:203-216, 1977.
25. Roussos C, Moxham J: Respiratory muscle fatigue. In Roussos C, Macklem PT (eds): *The Thorax.* New York, Marcel Dekker, 1985, pp 829-870.
26. Roussos C: Ventilatory failure and respiratory muscle. In Roussos C, Macklem PT (eds): *The Thorax.* New York, Marcel Dekker, 1985, pp 1253-1279.
27. Anthonisen NR, Cherniack RM: Ventilatory control in lung disease. In Roussos C, Macklem PT (eds): *The Thorax.* New York, Marcel Dekker, 1985, pp 965-987.
28. Mountain R, Zwillich C, Weil JV: Hypoventilation in obstructive lung disease. *N Engl J Med* 10:521-525, 1978.
29. Broadovsky D, McDonnell JA, Cherniack RM: The respiratory response to carbon dioxide in health and in emphysema. *J Clin Invest* 39:724-729, 1960.
30. Aubier M, Murciano D, Fournier M, et al: Central respiratory drive in acute respiratory failure of patients with chronic obstructive lung disease. *Am Rev Respir Dis* 122:191-199, 1980.
31. Burrows B, Earle RH: Course and prognosis of chronic obstructive pulmonary disease. *N Engl J Med* 280:397-404, 1969.
32. Gump DW, Phillips CA, Forsyth BR, et al: Role of infection in chronic bronchitis. *Am Rev Respir Dis* 113:465-470, 1976.
33. Murray JF: Classification of polycythemic disorders with comments on the diagnostic value of arterial blood oxygen analysis. *Ann Intern Med* 64:892-903, 1966.
34. Campbell EJM: The management of acute respiratory failure in chronic bronchitis and emphysema. *Am Rev Respir Dis* 95:626-639, 1967.
35. Pepe P, Marini JJ: Occult positive end-expiratory pressure in mechanically ventilated patients with airflow obstruction: the auto-PEEP effect. *Am Rev Respir Dis* 126:166-170, 1982.
36. Kilburn KH: Shock, seizures and coma with alkalosis during mechanical ventilation. *Ann Intern Med* 66:977-984, 1966.
37. Kassires JP, Berkman PM, Lawrence DR, Schwartz WB: The critical role of chloride in the correction of hypokalemic alkalosis in man. *Am J Med* 38:172-189, 1965.
38. Weinberger SE, Weiss JW: Weaning from ventilatory support. *N Engl J Med* 332:388-389, 1995.

39. Martin TR, Lewis S, Albert RK: The prognosis of patients with chronic obstructive pulmonary disease after hospitalization for acute respiratory failure. *Chest* 82:310–314, 1982.

40. Ferguson GT, Cherniack RM. Management of chronic obstructive lung disease. *N Engl J Med* 328:1017–1022, 1993.

41. Weinberger M, Hendeles L, Ahrens R: Pharmacologic management of reversible obstructive lung disease. *Med Clin North Am* 65:579–591, 1980.

42. Dimarco A, Nochomovits M, Dimarco M, et al: Comparative effect of aminophylline on diaphragm and cardiac contractility. *Am Rev Respir Dis* 132:800–805, 1985.

43. Rice K, Leatherman JW, Duane PG, et al: Aminophylline for acute exacerbations of chronic obstructive pulmonary disease. *Ann Intern Med* 107:305–309, 1987.

44. Albert RK, Martin TR, Lewis SW: Controlled clinical trial of methylprednisolone in patients with chronic bronchitis and acute respiratory insufficiency. *Ann Intern Med* 92:753–758, 1980.

45. Towes GB: Use of antibiotics in patients with chronic obstructive pulmonary disease. *Semin Respir Med* 8:165–170, 1986.

46. Barrett TE, Strom BL. Inhaled beta-adrenergic receptor agonists in asthma: more harm than good? *Am J Respir Crit Care Med* 151:574–577, 1995.

47. Woolcock AJ, Read J: Lung volume in exacerbations of asthma. *Am J Med* 41:259–264, 1966.

48. Wagner PD, Dantzker DR, Iacovoni WC, et al: Ventilation perfusion inequality in asymptomatic asthma. *Am Rev Respir Dis* 118:511–524, 1978.

49. Martin J, Powell E, Shore S, et al: The role of respiratory muscles in the hyperinflation of bronchial asthma. *Am Rev Respir Dis* 121:441–447, 1980.

50. Banner AS, Shah RS, Addington WW: Rapid prediction of need for hospitalization in acute asthma. *JAMA* 235:1337–1338, 1976.

51. Fischl MA, Pitchenik A, Gardner LB: An index predicting relapse and need for hospitalization in patients with acute bronchial asthma. *N Engl J Med* 305:783–789, 1981.

52. Kelsen SG, Kelsen DP, Fleezer RF, et al: Emergency room assessment and treatment of patients with acute asthma. *Am J Med* 64:622–628, 1978.

53. Centor RM, Yarbrough B, Wood JP: Inability to predict relapse in bronchial asthma. *N Engl J Med* 310:577–580, 1984.

54. Rose CC, Murphy JG, Schwartz JS: Performance of an index predicting the response of patients with acute bronchial asthma to intensive emergency department treatment. *N Engl J Med* 310:573–577, 1984.

55. Rebuck AS, Pengelly LD: Development of pulsus paradoxus in the presence of airway obstruction. *N Engl J Med* 288:66–69, 1973.

56. Nowak RM, Pensler MJ, Sarkar DD, et al: Comparison of peak expiratory flow and $FEV_1$ admission criteria for acute bronchial asthma. *Ann Emerg Med* 11:64–69, 1982.

57. Nadel JA, Tierney DF, Effect of a previous deep inspiration on airway resistance in man. *J Appl Physiol* 16:401–407, 1961.

58. Rees HA, Millar JS, Wood KW: A study of the clinical course and arterial blood gas tensions of patients in status asthmaticus. *Q J Med* 148:541–561, 1968.

59. Tai E, Read J: Blood gas tensions in bronchial asthma. *Lancet* 1:644–646, 1967.

60. Fanta CH, Rossing TH, McFadden ER Jr: Emergency room treatment of asthma. *Am J Med* 72:416–422, 1982.

61. Appel D, Rubenstein R, Schrager K, et al: Lactic acidosis in severe asthma. *Am J Med* 75:580–584, 1983.

62. Molfino NA, Nannini LJ, Martelli AN, Slutsky AS. Respiratory arrest in near-fatal asthma. *N Engl J Med* 324:285–288, 1991.

63. FitzGerald JM, Hargreave FE. The assessment and management of acute life-threatening asthma. *Chest* 95:4 888–894, 1989.

64. Bellomo R, McLaughlin P, Tai E Parkin G. Asthma requiring mechanical ventilation a low morbidity approach. *Chest* 105:891–896, 1994.

65. Darioli R, Perret C: Mechanical controlled hypoventilation in status asthmaticus. *Am Rev Respir Dis* 129:385–387, 1984.

66. Rossing TH, Fanta CH, McFadden ER Jr, and the Medical Housestaff of the Peter Bent Brigham Hospital: A controlled trial of single versus combined drug therapy in the treatment of acute episodes of asthma. *Am Rev Respir Dis* 123:190–194, 1981.

67. Wolfe JD, Tashkin DP, Calvarese B, et al: Bronchodilator effects of terbutaline and aminophylline alone and in combination in asthmatic patients. *N Engl J Med* 298:363–367, 1978.

68. Larsson S, Svedmyr N: Bronchodilating effect and side effects of β-adrenoceptor stimulants by different routes of administration (tablets, metered aerosol, and combinations thereof). *Am Rev Respir Dis* 116:861–869, 1977.

69. Pearlman DS, Chervinsky P, La Force C, et al: A comparison of salmeterol with albuterol in the treatment of mild to moderate asthma. *N Engl J Med* 327:1420–1425, 1992.

70. King TE, Chang SW: Corticosteroid therapy in the management of asthma. *Semin Respir Med* 8:387–399, 1987.

71. Haskell RJ, Wong BM, Hansen JE: A double-blind, randomized clinical trial of methylprednisolone in status asthmaticus. *Arch Intern Med* 143:1324–1327, 1983.

72. Cook JL: Infection in asthma. *Semin Respir Med* 8:259–263, 1987.

73. O' Rourke PP, Crone PK: Halothane in status asthmaticus. *Crit Care Med* 10:341–343, 1982.

# Chapter 22

# Acute Hypoxemic Respiratory Failure:
## Pulmonary Edema and ARDS

### Michael A. Matthay

---

PHYSIOLOGIC AND STRUCTURAL ASPECTS OF FLUID
    EXCHANGE IN THE LUNG
HIGH-PRESSURE (CARDIOGENIC) PULMONARY
    EDEMA
    Implications for Treatment of High-
      Pressure Cardiogenic Pulmonary
      Edema

INCREASED-PERMEABILITY PULMONARY EDEMA
    (ARDS)
    Implications for Treatment of
      Increased-Permeability Edema and
      ARDS

---

THIS CHAPTER CONSIDERS the causes of acute respiratory failure that are primarily associated with severe hypoxemia. In most patients, the defect in oxygenation is related to disorders that cause filling of the distal air spaces of the lung with edema fluid, blood, or purulent exudate. Microatelectasis often contributes to the hypoxemia in these patients as well. The physiologic basis for the hypoxemia is usually explained by both ventilation to perfusion mismatch as well as frank right-to-left intrapulmonary shunting through fluid-filled or collapsed alveoli. This chapter focuses on cardiogenic and noncardiogenic pulmonary edema, the most common causes of this type of acute respiratory failure.

Two types of pulmonary edema occur in humans: (a) high-pressure edema (usually cardiogenic) and (b) edema secondary to increased permeability of the lung microvascular endothelium or the alveolar epithelium. The correct diagnosis and appropriate treatment of both kinds of pulmonary edema require a good understanding of the normal physiology of fluid exchange in the microcirculation of the lung. In addition, familiarity with the structures that surround the fluid-exchanging vessels is essential to appreciate how and where edema fluid accumulates in the lung.

This discussion of pulmonary edema is divided into

three sections. The first part briefly reviews transvascular fluid and protein movement in the normal lung; it also considers the influence of the lung structure on the distribution and removal of normal and excessive quantities of fluid. The second part of the chapter describes the interstitial and alveolar phases of high-pressure (cardiogenic) pulmonary edema. The chapter concludes with experimental and clinical examples to illustrate the fundamental physiologic abnormalities that characterize increased-permeability edema. This final section also briefly reviews the common clinical disorders that have been associated with increased-permeability edema, also called the adult respiratory distress syndrome (ARDS). Principles of therapy for ARDS are considered in this chapter, although the general principles for the treatment of acute respiratory failure with mechanical ventilation are discussed in Chapter 20, and hemodynamic assessment and management are considered in detail in Chapters 23 and 24.

## PHYSIOLOGIC AND STRUCTURAL ASPECTS OF FLUID EXCHANGE IN THE LUNG

In the normal lung, as in all other organs, there is a net outward movement of fluid from the vascular to the interstitial space. This fluid is removed by lymphatics, which under normal conditions prevent excess fluid from accumulating in the interstitial space of the lung (1). The factors that determine the quantity of fluid that leaves the vascular space are all included in the Starling equation for filtration of fluid across a semipermeable membrane (2). A simplified version of the equation is

$$\dot{Q} = K[(Pmv - Ppmv) - (\pi mv - \pi pmv)]^a$$

where $\dot{Q}$ is the net transvascular flow of fluid, K describes quantitatively the permeability of the membrane, Pmv is the hydrostatic pressure in the lumen of the microvessels, and Ppmv is the hydrostatic pressure in the perimicrovascular interstitial space. The term $\pi mv$ is the plasma protein osmotic pressure in the circulation, and $\pi pmv$ is the protein osmotic pressure in the perimicrovascular compartment. This equation is applicable to the microcirculation of the lung because normal pulmonary capillary permeability allows some water and solutes (electrolytes) to leave the circulation but restricts the movement of larger molecules such as plasma proteins. The net transvascular filtration of fluid ($\dot{Q}$) into the interstitium of the lung depends on the net difference in hydrostatic and protein osmotic pressures, as well as on the permeability of the capillary membrane.

Most of the evidence suggests that under normal circumstances the hydrostatic pressure in the perimicrovascular interstitial space (Ppmv) is close to alveolar pressure, approximately zero, or atmospheric pressure (3). Thus, the main hydrostatic force for fluid filtration in the lung is the hydrostatic pressure within the capillaries (Pmv). The absolute value for hydrostatic pressure in the lung microcirculation must vary from the top to the bottom of the lung (4). Also, hydrostatic pressure in the microvessels varies along the length of the pre- to postcapillary vessels, depending on the resistance of the vessels based on the recent innovative use of direct measurements of lung microvascular pressures with micropuncture (5). Hydrostatic pressure also depends on whether the vessel is in a zone 1, 2, or 3 condition (also see Chapter 2). Clinically, it has generally been assumed that the average value for Pmv in the lung is roughly equal to the left atrial pressure.

However, some investigators have estimated that Pmv is probably closer to left atrial pressure plus about one-half of the difference between mean pulmonary artery pressure and left atrial pressure (6). Thus, "wedge" pressure measurements of left atrial pressure remain the most reliable clinical indicator of hydrostatic pressure in the microcirculation of the lung, but the precapillary or pulmonary arterial pressure will also contribute to fluid filtration under some conditions (7).

Protein osmotic pressure in the circulation ($\pi mv$) is higher than protein osmotic pressure in the perimicrovascular interstitial space ($\pi pmv$). This gradient is maintained because the normal permeability of the endothelial junctions allows only a small quantity of protein to flow out of the circulation into the interstitial space of the lung. Thus, the sum of protein osmotic pressures normally favors fluid absorption into the circulation and thereby partially offsets the net hydrostatic force that causes fluid to leave the vascular space. In Table 22.1 we have estimated a value for each of the Starling forces and then calculated a value for net fluid filtration ($\dot{Q}$) that is consistent with experimental studies of transvascular fluid movement in the normal lung (8).

Most of the available evidence indicates that the major site for fluid exchange in the lung is in the microcirculation of the alveolar vessels (see Chapter 2 for a definition of alveolar versus extraalveolar vessels). Anatomically, the microvessels in humans have no

---

**TABLE 22.1**
**STARLING EQUATION**

$$\dot{Q} = K[(Pmv - Ppmv) - (\pi mv - \pi pmv)]$$

Transvascular fluid flow = permeability fluid flux × [hydrostatic pressure − protein osmotic pressure] Then, substituting estimated values for the variables under normal conditions:

$$\dot{Q} = K[(10 - 0) - (25 - 19)]$$
$$\dot{Q} = K[10 - 6] = K \times 4.$$

1. Net calculated transvascular fluid flow ($\dot{Q}$) is positive from the capillary lumen into the perimicrovascular interstitial space.
2. Note that the protein osmotic pressure gradient normally opposes fluid filtration out of the vessels. If the gradient were abolished, i.e., if protein osmotic pressure were assumed to be equal on both sides of the capillary, then the calculated transvascular fluid flow would more than double.
3. Also, if permeability (K) increases, there are two apparent effects: (a) transvascular fluid flux increases, even at normal hydrostatic pressures, and (b) the protein osmotic pressure difference across the capillary membrane deceases as proteins leak into the interstitium, further increasing transvascular fluid flux.

---

$^a$ The Starling equation in its complete form contains a term $\sigma$, which is the reflection coefficient for the difference in transvascular protein osmotic pressure (1). Also, the term K refers to the endothelial conductance of fluid (filtration coefficient) in the complete version of the equation. The simplified version is used here to focus the reader's attention on the three key variables: hydrostatic pressure, protein osmotic pressure, and the permeability of the endothelial barrier.

media or adventitia, and thus their walls are thinner than those of larger vessels (9). However, a number of experimental studies have shown that some liquid probably also leaks from small arterioles and venules that are located at the corners of alveolar wall junctions (10, 11). Figure 22.1 shows an alveolar vessel (capillary)

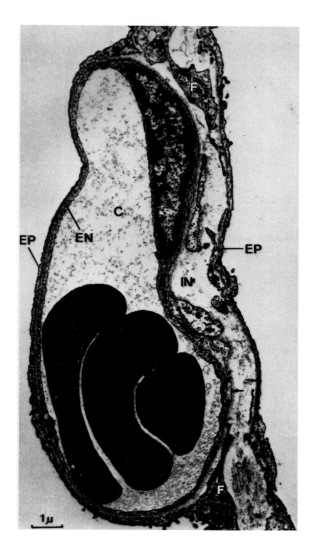

**FIGURE 22.1.** Electron micrograph of an alveolar capillary (C) cross-section from human lung. Blood cells are suspended in the interalveolar septum between two alveolar spaces. The alveolar epithelium (*EP*) is the barrier that separates the air spaces from the interstitium (*IN*). The endothelium (*EN*) separates the vascular space from the interstitium. Fluid and protein exchange probably occurs through small gaps between the endothelial cells in the alveolar capillaries. Connective tissue fibers are found in the interstitium, where the basal laminae (*arrows*) of the epithelium and endothelium are separated. *cf*, fibroblast cell. (From Fishman AP, Renkin E: *Pulmonary Edema.* Bethesda, MD, American Physiological Society, 1979, p 4.)

in the lung, surrounded by an interstitial space. The normal fluid and protein leakage is believed to occur through small gaps between the endothelial cells in the capillary (3, 12).

Fluid that is filtered into the alveolar interstitial space does not enter the alveoli because the normal alveolar epithelium is composed of very tight junctions (Fig. 22.1) that prevent fluid and protein from entering the air spaces (12–14). Once the filtered fluid enters the alveolar interstitial space, it then moves proximally toward the peribronchial and perivascular space in the extraalveolar interstitium (15). Interstitial pressure in the extraalveolar space is negative relative to the alveolar interstitial space. Therefore, the loose connective tissue space can act as a sump to drain fluid from the alveolar wall interstitium (17–19). Under ordinary conditions the lymphatics remove all the filtered fluid and return it to the systemic circulation (Fig. 22.2). It has been estimated that about 10 to 20 ml of fluid per hour is filtered in the lung and removed by the lymphatics in normal humans (20).

Since surface tension in the normal alveolus is low, it is thought that surface tension has a minimal effect on interstitial pressure around alveolar vessels and thus little effect on normal fluid balance in the lung. However, if surface tension were high, then perimicrovascular interstitial hydrostatic pressure ($P_{pmv}$) could become more negative and thereby increase the transvascular pressure gradient for movement of fluid from the alveolar vessels or the extraalveolar corner vessels into the interstitial space (Table 22.1). A deficiency of surfactant could lead to high surface tension and possibly favor the development of pulmonary edema (22, 23). Clinically, abnormal surfactants or inactivated surfactant may contribute to the extent of pulmonary edema in some patients (24).

*In summary*, there is a constant flow of fluid through the interstitium of the lungs. Small amounts of fluid leak from the alveolar and some extraalveolar vessels into the perimicrovascular interstitial space. This fluid does not enter the alveolar space because of the high resistance of the normally tight alveolar epithelium. The filtered fluid moves to the extraalveolar interstitial space, where lymphatics remove it from the lung.

For experimental purposes, lung lymph flow can be collected from some species (sheep, goats, or dogs) to study the normal physiology of fluid and protein balance in the lung as well as to learn how the lung responds to pathologic conditions (8, 15). The quantity of lung lymph flow can be used to estimate the quantity of fluid leaving the vascular space in the lung; the protein concentration of the lymph can be measured to determine the amount of protein leaving the microcirculation and thereby evaluate the permeability of

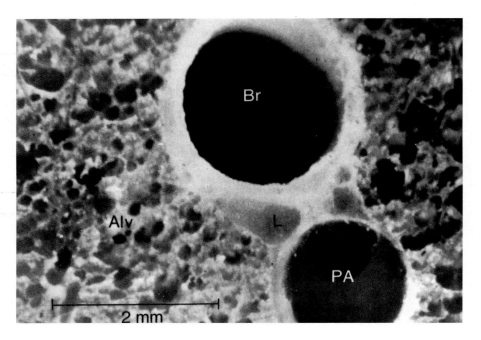

**FIGURE 22.2.** A photomicrograph from a sheep lung frozen at normal inflation pressure. The bronchus (*Br*), lymphatic (*L*), and partially blood-filled pulmonary artery (*PA*) are surrounded by loose connective tissue. This is the extraalveolar interstitial space. The alveolar ducts and alveoli (*Alv*) surround the bronchovascular sheath. The lymphatics drain fluid that is filtered from the capillaries and return this fluid to the systemic circulation.

the pulmonary microvascular barrier (25). In the past decade, a number of investigators have studied lung lymph flow in animal models in an effort to better understand the pathogenesis of the various kinds of pulmonary edema (26–28).

As stated, pulmonary edema is caused by either high pressure, increased permeability, or both. In the next section, high-pressure edema is examined, with an emphasis on correlating the clinical features with the physiologic abnormalities.

## HIGH-PRESSURE (CARDIOGENIC) PULMONARY EDEMA

According to the Starling equation, when hydrostatic pressure increases in the microcirculation, the rate of transvascular fluid filtration rises. The clinical counterpart of this physiologic principle occurs in humans when there is a rise in left atrial pressure, usually secondary to left ventricular failure. This increased left atrial pressure is transmitted to the microcirculation of the lung, resulting in an increase in transvascular fluid flow into the interstitium of the lung. With a small increase in left atrial pressure (14 to 20 mm Hg), most patients experience only a mild degree of dyspnea. The

chest radiograph usually demonstrates prominent interlobular septa (Kerley B lines) consistent with interstitial pulmonary edema alone (Fig. 22.3). Histologically, mild elevations of left atrial pressure leads to interstitial edema in the alveolar septa and in the extraalveolar spaces in the loose connective tissue around the bronchovascular sheath. Figure 22.4 illustrates the prominent perivascular fluid cuffs in this phase of interstitial pulmonary edema.

As left atrial pressure acutely rises above 25 to 30 mm Hg, the pumping ability of the lymphatics and the capacity of the interstitial space in the lung are usually exceeded, and the edema fluid breaks through the alveolar epithelium and begins to flood the alveoli (1). The development of arterial hypoxemia has been shown experimentally to correlate with alveolar flooding (29).

High-pressure, cardiogenic edema has been well studied in experimental animals by using samples of lung lymph to quantify the amount of fluid leaving the vascular space and the protein content of that fluid (8, 15). As left atrial pressure is increased by placing an inflatable balloon in the left atrium, lung lymph flow rises and the concentration of protein declines (Fig. 22.5). This indicates, as the Starling equation predicts, that transvascular flow of water and solutes into the interstitium of the lung is increasing. Since the permeability of the capillary endothelium remains normal,

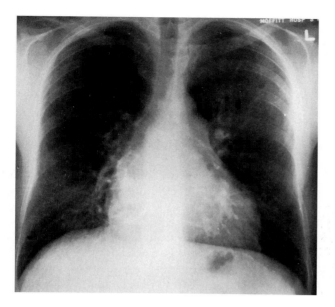

**FIGURE 22.3.** A posterior-anterior chest radiograph from a patient with interstitial pulmonary edema secondary to left ventricular heart failure. Pulmonary capillary wedge pressure was measured as 20 mm Hg. The *arrow* in the left upper lobe indicates prominent vascular markings. The *arrows* in the right lower lobe draw attention to prominent Kerley B lines, which indicate fluid-filled interlobular septa.

the fluid leaving the circulation has a low protein content, resulting in a fall in the lymph:plasma protein ratio.

During the early, interstitial phase of high-pressure pulmonary edema, the lung has at least three safety factors that function to protect against alveolar flooding. First, lung lymph flow increases and helps to clear some of the edema fluid from the lung. Second, the concentration of protein in the perimicrovascular interstitial space falls, since there is an increase in water and solutes entering the interstitial space around the alveolar vessels. The decreasing perimicrovascular concentration of protein leads to an increase in the protein osmotic pressure difference between the plasma and the interstitial fluid. This results in an increased protein osmotic force to absorb fluid into the circulation. It has been estimated that this increased protein osmotic pressure difference offsets about one-half of the rise in transvascular fluid filtration that can occur from a rise in hydrostatic pressure alone (15). It has been shown, in fact, that patients with low plasma protein concentrations are likely to develop clinical pulmonary edema at lower levels of left atrial pressure elevation (30). The third safety factor against alveolar flooding is the capacity of the interstitial space in the lung to contain up to about 500 ml of edema fluid in the bronchovascular cuffs (Fig. 22.4) (15).

When the capacity of the interstitial space is exceeded, the interstitial edema fluid moves through the

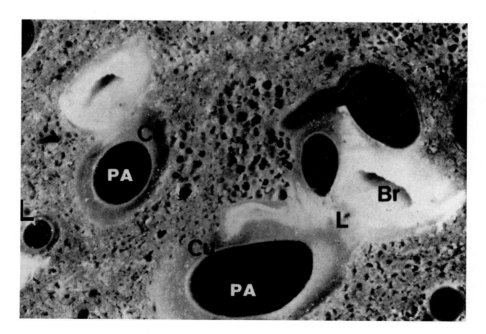

**FIGURE 22.4.** Photograph of a frozen sheep lung. In this experimental study, left atrial pressure was elevated to 20 cm $H_2O$ for 4 hours. The result is interstitial pulmonary edema with perivascular fluid cuffs (*Cu*) around pulmonary arteries (*PA*) and small airways (*Br*). There are some lymphatics (*L*) visible in the fluid cuffs also.

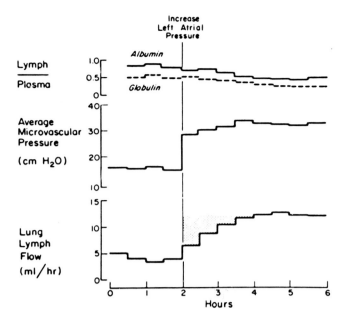

**FIGURE 22.5.** The time course of a sheep experiment in which left atrial pressure was elevated after a 2-hour stable baseline period. Note that with left atrial hypertension, the lung lymph flow rises sharply and the lymph:plasma protein concentrations fall. This is typical of high-pressure pulmonary edema. (From Erdmann AJ III, Vaughn TR, Brigham KL, et al: Effect of increased vascular pressure on lung fluid balance in unanesthetized sheep. *Circ Res* 37:271–284, 1975. By permission of the American Heart Association, Inc.)

visceral pleura and causes pleural effusions (31, 32). These effusions are primarily related to the elevation of left atrial pressure and the magnitude of pulmonary edema as demonstrated by studies in patients with congestive heart failure (33, 34) or in experimental studies of hydrostatic pulmonary edema (35) or increased-permeability pulmonary edema (36).

When the capacity of the interstitial space is exceeded, the edema fluid also breaks through the alveolar epithelium and fills the air spaces by bulk flow. Samples of edema fluid in experimental animals have demonstrated that the initial sample of high-pressure, cardiogenic pulmonary edema flow is low in protein content relative to the plasma protein (about 50%) (25). This can be a useful diagnostic test to separate patients with high-pressure pulmonary edema from those with an increased-permeability edema, since the latter group of patients have an alveolar fluid:plasma protein ratio of 80% or greater, providing the edema fluid is sampled before resolution has occurred and alveolar liquid reabsorption has begun (37–39).

Recently both in vivo and in vitro work has shown that resolution or clearance of edema from the air spaces of the lung depends on active sodium transport across the alveolar epithelial barrier. Alveolar fluid is removed even in the face of a rising alveolar edema protein concentration in excess of the plasma protein concentration (40–42). Also, experimentally, β-adrenergic agonist therapy increases the activity of the sodium transport pump, resulting in a marked increase in the clearance of alveolar liquid in dogs, sheep, rats, and humans (43–47).

Clinically, high-pressure, cardiogenic edema is the most common form of pulmonary edema. Measurement of elevated pulmonary arterial wedge pressures with a pulmonary artery catheter helps to confirm that the pulmonary edema is from high pressure when the cause of the pulmonary edema cannot be established on clinical grounds alone (48–50). Use of noninvasive techniques such as two-dimensional echocardiography to measure left ventricular contractility and ejection fraction can also be helpful. The underlying cause is usually left ventricular failure from ischemic heart disease, aortic or mitral valve disease, or a cardiomyopathy. Occasionally, patients with normal cardiac function develop high-pressure pulmonary edema from fluid overload. In addition, some noncardiogenic causes of pulmonary edema may be complicated by an element of high pressure in the pulmonary circulation (51).

### IMPLICATIONS FOR TREATMENT OF HIGH-PRESSURE CARDIOGENIC PULMONARY EDEMA

Effective therapy for high-pressure pulmonary edema depends on lowering left atrial pressure and thus decreasing the driving force responsible for increased filtration of fluid into the extravascular space. A reduction in left atrial filling pressure (preload) can be accomplished by decreasing venous filling of the heart. Osler's classic method for treatment of cardiogenic pulmonary edema is based on this first principle of decreasing venous return to the heart by sitting the patient upright and using rotating tourniquets on the extremities to impede blood return to the heart (52).

For more than 50 years, morphine sulfate has been known to be effective in treating cardiogenic pulmonary edema. Part of the beneficial effect of morphine depends on a reduction in preload to the heart, because it causes systemic venodilation (53). More potent agents such as sodium nitroprusside can rapidly decrease venous return (54). Nitroprusside also reduces systemic blood pressure, reducing the afterload (resistance) on the left ventricle, which may result in better cardiac function with a subsequent lowering of left atrial filling pressures (55). Potent diuretics such as furosemide lower left atrial filling pressure by decreasing systemic venous tone (when given intravenously) and inducing diuresis of the expanded extracellular volume (56).

Finally, agents that improve myocardial contractility can lower cardiac filling pressures. Acutely, this can be accomplished with inotropic vasopressors such as dopamine or dobutamine given in low doses (57, 58). In patients with chronic congestive heart failure and pulmonary congestion, digitalis augments myocardial contractility and thereby decreases left atrial and left ventricular filling pressures (59).

Patients with acute cardiogenic pulmonary edema and severe respiratory distress often generate very negative pleural pressures in an effort to maintain adequate alveolar ventilation. These negative pleural pressures may increase left ventricular transmural pressure and thus increase left ventricular afterload (60). Patients with acute pulmonary edema also have a reduced cardiac output and are more susceptible to respiratory muscle fatigue (61, 62).

It is not surprising, therefore, that some patients with acute cardiogenic pulmonary edema develop refractory hypoxemia and hypercapnia, even with adequate supplemental oxygen and appropriate pharmacologic therapy. These more seriously ill patients usually require intubation and positive pressure mechanical ventilation to achieve adequate arterial oxygenation and adequate alveolar ventilation. Institution of positive pressure mechanical ventilation in patients with acute cardiogenic pulmonary edema usually results in prompt improvement in oxygenation and sometimes in cardiac output as well. The improved oxygenation is secondary to better lung inflation with improved matching of ventilation and perfusion. An improvement in left ventricular function may occur because of at least four possible factors: (a) improved arterial oxygen saturation, and hence better myocardial oxygen supply; (b) reduction in the extreme pleural pressure swings present with spontaneous ventilation, and hence reduction in afterload on the left ventricle; (c) less workload on the failing heart because the work of breathing (and the oxygen needed to perform it) have been assumed by a mechanical ventilator; and (d) reduction in atrial filling pressure (preload) because positive pressure ventilation decreases venous return.

## INCREASED-PERMEABILITY PULMONARY EDEMA (ARDS)

The Starling equation predicts that a change in permeability of the microvascular membrane will result in a marked increase in the amount of fluid and protein leaving the vascular space. Pulmonary edema of this type should have a high protein content because the vascular membrane does not have a normal capacity to restrict the outward movement of larger molecules such as plasma proteins. Results of clinical and experimental studies demonstrate that this is exactly what happens in most types of noncardiogenic pulmonary edema (26, 27, 42, 63).

When increased-permeability pulmonary edema develops, a syndrome of mild, moderate, or severe acute lung injury may develop. The severe lung injury is associated with very poor oxygenation, dense pulmonary infiltrates, decreased lung compliance, and usually a need for mechanical ventilation. The severe form of acute lung injury was described by Petty and associates and termed the adult respiratory distress syndrome (ARDS) (64), but recent proposals for more specific definition require quantitative scoring of the physiologic and radiographic abnormalities to determine whether the acute lung injury is mild, moderate, or severe ARDS (65). This new scoring system also takes into account the presence of absence of other organ failure besides the lung and the associated clinical disorders, since prognosis depends on all these nonpulmonary factors as well as the extent of acute lung injury (66, 67). There are estimated to be about 150,000 cases of ARDS in the United States annually (68, 69).

The principal clinical manifestations of ARDS are similar, regardless of what the associated clinical condition may be. The typical findings are (a) severe hypoxemia, unresponsive to low-flow oxygen and due to intrapulmonary right-to-left shunting of blood through fluid-filled and atelectatic alveoli; (b) bilateral, fluffy infiltrates on the chest radiograph (Fig. 22.6); and (c) a decrease in the static lung compliance. Clinically, this change in the mechanical properties of the lungs is manifested by the high ventilatory pressures that are required to deliver an adequate tidal volume.

Recently, a consensus conference of North American and European investigators recommended that the definition of acute lung injury and ARDS be standardized and simplified (70). The inclusion criteria for acute lung injury are (a) bilateral infiltrates on the chest radiograph and (b) a $PaO_2 : FiO_2$ ratio below 300. The main exclusion criterion is clinical evidence of left atrial hypertension from intravascular volume overload or left heart failure. If clinically indicated, a pulmonary arterial catheter can be inserted to establish that the pulmonary arterial wedge pressure is less than 18 mm Hg. ARDS is defined with the same criteria as acute lung injury except that the $PaO_2 : FiO_2$ ratio needs to be below 200, thus indicating a more severe oxygenation defect (70).

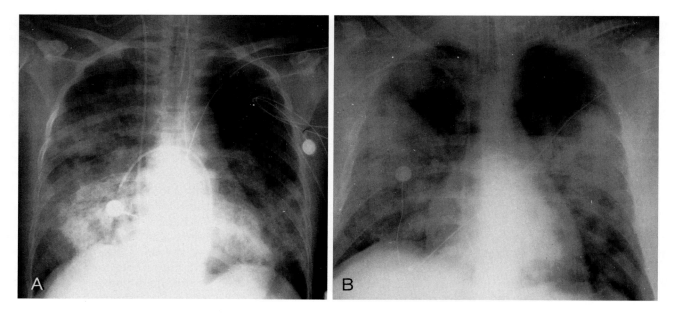

**Figure 22.6.** **A,** Anterior-posterior chest radiograph from a 40-year-old man with acute respiratory failure from gastric aspiration. Note that the endotracheal tube is in good position. The pulmonary artery line, inserted through the right internal jugular vein, passes through the superior vena cava, right atrium, right ventricle, and main pulmonary artery and terminates in a branch of pulmonary artery in the right lower lobe. The wedge pressure was 2 mm Hg. The radiographic pattern indicates a typical location for pulmonary aspiration into dependent segments of the left lower lobe, right lower lobe, and right upper lobe. Before tracheal intubation, this patient's $PaO_2$ was 55 mm Hg on an $FiO_2$ of 0.9. The fluffy bilateral infiltrates progressed to involve all lung zones within 3 days. However, the patient ultimately recovered after 2 weeks of treatment with antibiotics and mechanical ventilation with PEEP. **B,** Anterior-posterior chest radiograph from a 55-year-old man who developed non-cardiogenic pulmonary edema from Gram-negative sepsis. The pulmonary artery line was inserted through the right subclavian vein and terminated in a posterior branch (visible on a lateral chest film) of the right pulmonary artery. The cardiac silhouette appears slightly enlarged, but the wedge pressure was 4 mm Hg, and the cardiac output was high (consistent with sepsis). The $PaO_2$ was 45 mm Hg on an $FiO_2$ of 0.90 prior to ventilation with positive pressure. The patient's acute respiratory failure and sepsis were successfully treated, and the $FiO_2$ was lowered to 0.50 with 15 cm $H_2O$ of PEEP within 2 days. Subsequently the patient did not improve, and he ultimately developed recurrent sepsis and died with severe ARDS.

The terms acute lung injury and ARDS do not designate a specific cause for the acute respiratory failure. In fact, the list of clinical disorders associated with the development of ARDS is impressively long (Table 22.2) (71, 72). The acute lung injury can occur via either the blood (sepsis, fat embolism), the airways (liquid aspiration, pulmonary infections), or perhaps by neural mechanisms (neurogenic pulmonary edema with increased intracranial pressure). In some clinical disorders, such as drug overdose or acute pancreatitis, the route of lung injury is not known. Overall mortality in ARDS remains high, from 50 to 70%, partly because of associated multiorgan failure as well as uncontrolled or recurrent infection (67). Some patients with ARDS have a lower mortality, perhaps because the function of the alveolar epithelial barrier is more preserved and perhaps because of the absence of severe nonpulmonary organ dysfunction (42).

An in-depth discussion of each of the associated causes of ARDS is not possible in this chapter. However, the two most common clinical disorders associated with the development of ARDS, gastric aspiration and sepsis, are considered below.

The acute respiratory failure that can follow gastric aspiration is a good example of ARDS resulting from direct injury to the alveolar epithelium and air spaces of the lung (Fig. 22.6**A**). Aspiration of gastric contents injures the lung if the pH is less than 2.5, even if the volume of aspirated fluid is as small as 50 ml (73). The aspirated, acidic fluid acutely causes an increase in the permeability of the alveolar epithelium and the rapid development of pulmonary edema. The severe hypoxemia that occurs after massive gastric aspiration has been attributed to a combination of pulmonary edema and the atelectasis resulting from alterations of surfactant activity and subsequent closure of small airways

**TABLE 22.2**
**CLINICAL DISORDERS ASSOCIATED WITH ARDS**

Sepsis
Trauma
    Fat emboli
    Lung contusion
    Nonthoracic trauma
Liquid aspiration
    Gastric contents
    Fresh and salt water (drowning)
    Hydrocarbon fluids
Drug-associated
    Heroin
    Methadone
    Propoxyphene
    Barbiturates
    Colchicine
    Ethchlorvynol
    Aspirin
    Hydrochlorothiazide
Inhaled toxins
    Smoke
    Oxygen (high concentration)
    Corrosive chemicals
    ($NO_2$, $Cl_2$, $NH_3$, phosgene)
Shock of any etiology
Hematologic disorders
    Massive blood transfusion
    Disseminated intravascular coagulation
Metabolic
    Acute pancreatitis
    Uremia
Miscellaneous
    Lymphangiography
    Reexpansion pulmonary edema
    Increased intracranial pressure
    Postcardiopulmonary bypass
    Eclampsia
    Air emboli
    Amniotic fluid embolism
    Ascent to high altitude
Primary pneumonias
    Viral
    Bacterial
    Mycobacterium
    Tuberculosis
    Fungal
    *Pneumocystis carinii*

(74). In fact, mortality in patients with ARDS secondary to gastric aspiration can be predicted in part by the severity of the arterial hypoxemia in relation to the alveolar oxygen tension (the $Pa_{O_2}:PA_{O_2}$ ratio). If the $Pa_{O_2}:PA_{O_2}$ is less than 0.50 immediately after gastric aspiration, the mortality rate is 50%, compared with 14% in patients with a ratio above 0.50 (75). The ultimate outcome in patients with ARDS from gastric aspiration is also influenced by the delayed development of secondary bacterial lung infections with aerobic and anaerobic bacteria (76). Recent experimental studies suggest that anti-interleukin-β therapy may be effective in preventing the severe pulmonary injury following acid aspiration, providing that the neutralizing antibody is given within 1 hour of the aspiration (77).

While massive gastric aspiration is a good illustration of acute respiratory failure from direct injury to the alveolar epithelium, systemic sepsis is an example of ARDS that develops from injury to the endothelium of the pulmonary microcirculation (Fig. 22.6**B**). Clinical studies have shown that acute lung injury develops in about 60% of patients with sepsis syndrome, and about 25 to 35% of these patients develop severe acute lung injury (ARDS) (78, 79). The mortality from ARDS secondary to sepsis ranges from 60 to 90% (66, 79, 80).

Studies in experimental animals have provided important information regarding the early phase of acute lung injury from sepsis. Brigham and associates (26, 81, 82) demonstrated that when sheep are given either *Pseudomonas* organisms or *Escherichia coli* endotoxin intravenously, lung lymph flow increases markedly. In these studies, the increase in lymph flow is associated with a high lymph:plasma protein ratio and a dramatic rise in lymph protein transport (Fig. 22.7). The increased lung lymph flow cannot be accounted for exclusively by a change in hydrostatic or protein osmotic pressures in the microcirculation of the lung and therefore must be partly due to an increase in lung vascular permeability. Histologic examination of the sheep lungs in this early phase shows interstitial edema with perivascular fluid cuffs, as seen in the interstitial phase of high-pressure pulmonary edema (Fig. 22.4). The next phase of pulmonary edema is for the edema fluid to flood into the air spaces, although recent experimental studies have shown that the alveolar epithelium is more resistant than the lung endothelium to the injurious effects of *E. coli* endotoxin (83).

Clinically, the early phase of increased-permeability pulmonary edema from sepsis with interstitial edema is often not recognized (84). This is partly due to the lack of sensitive clinical indicators of a mild increase in extravascular lung water. The chest radiograph, for example, may not show edema until there is a 30% increase in lung water content (85, 86). Also, major arterial blood gas abnormalities do not usually develop until edema fluid enters the air spaces, when there is a dramatic decrease in arterial oxygenation secondary to both ventilation-perfusion mismatch and right-to-left shunting of blood through fluid-filled alveoli (29, 70).

Clinical studies of patients with permeability pulmonary edema from sepsis have shown that the pulmonary edema fluid has a high protein concentration (80 to 100%) compared with the plasma protein level

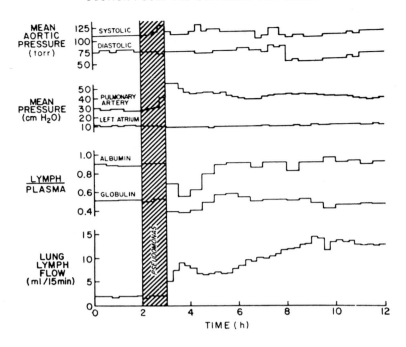

**Figure 22.7.** Effects of infusion of *Pseudomonas aeruginosa* on lung vascular pressures, lymph flow, and lymph:plasma protein concentration in an unanesthetized sheep. Note that the lymph flow rises steeply several hours after the infusion of *Pseudomonas* organism, indicating that the capillary leak of protein-rich fluid occurs a few hours after the septic insult. (Reproduced from Brigham KL, Woolverton WC, Blake LH, et al: Increased sheep lung vascular permeability caused by *Pseudomonas* bactemeria. *J Clin Invest* 54:792–804, 1974 by copyright permission of the American Society for Clinical Investigation.)

(37, 38, 42). In addition, measurements of cardiac filling pressures with a pulmonary artery catheter usually demonstrate normal or even low pressures (63). Both these findings add further support to the concept that pulmonary edema from sepsis occurs because of an increase in permeability of the vascular endothelium and perhaps the alveolar epithelium as well.

In the acute phase of permeability pulmonary edema and respiratory failure, the densities on the chest radiograph result from a combination of interstitial and alveolar edema in addition to a variable degree of atelectasis. Typically, the lung volumes are reduced because of a change in the mechanical properties of the lung. A reduction in vital capacity and functional residual capacity and an increase in lung compliance occur for three main reasons: (*a*) edema fluid in the air spaces displaces air, decreasing gas volumes; (*b*) edema in peribronchovascular interstitial spaces causes airways to narrow or close, which results in atelectasis (Fig. 22.4); and (*c*) there may be a reduction in surfactant (secondary to alveolar epithelial injury), which could increase surface tension and thereby decrease lung compliance (87–89).

Histologically, in this acute phase of lung injury there is widespread interstitial and alveolar edema, with an abundance of polymorphonuclear leukocytes, erythrocytes, macrophages, cell debris, plasma proteins, and strands of fibrin. Electron microscopy studies have shown injury to the capillary endothelium and denuding of the alveolar epithelium (Fig. 22.8) (90). If the patient survives the acute phase of the lung injury, the pulmonary edema may resolve, and the patient may completely recover normal lung function over a few months (91, 92).

However, some patients with ARDS progress from the acute lung injury to a subacute phase over 7 to 14 days, during which time they still require mechanical ventilation with high airway pressures, high fractions of inspired oxygen, and pulmonary hypertension (Fig. 22.9) (93). These patients develop fibrosis and capillary obliteration in the lungs (90, 94). Although barotrauma with pneumothorax occurs in 10 to 15% of patients with acute lung injury, the barotrauma appears to be primarily associated with the severity of lung injury (94). It is not clear why some patients successfully repair their injured lungs and recover, whereas recurrent pneumothoraces progressive fibrosis and even bullae develop in the lungs of others (Fig. 22.10). The role of

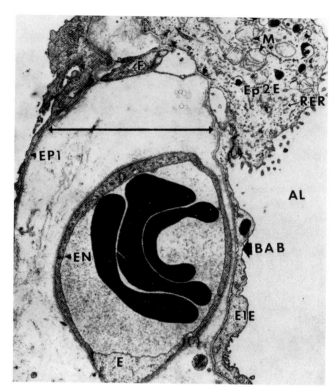

**FIGURE 22.8.** Electron micrograph of an alveolar capillary in the interalveolar septum between alveolar spaces (*AL*) from a patient with ARDS. The interstitial space is widened by edema fluid (*arrows*), and the capillary endothelium has normal areas (*EN*) and swollen, abnormal areas (*E*). Some of the alveolar epithelium is normal (*EP1*), whereas other type 1 and 2 cells are swollen (*E1E* and *Ep2E*). The damaged type 2 cell shows degenerative features with swollen mitochondria (*M*) and degranulating rough endoplasmic reticulum (*RER*). There is a fibrocyte (*F*) that anchors the epithelial basement membrane. (From Fishman AP, Renkin E: *Pulmonary Edema*. Bethesda, MD, American Physiological Society, 1979, p 103.)

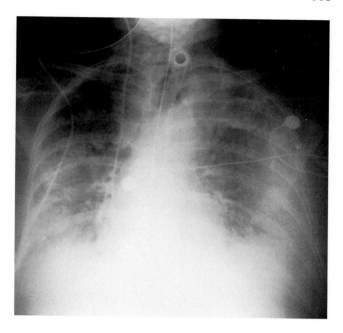

**FIGURE 22.9.** Anterior-posterior chest radiograph of a 42-year-old woman being ventilated through a cuffed tracheostomy tube. Her respiratory failure had begun 3 weeks previously when she developed ARDS from severe acute pancreatitis. Note the diffuse ground-glass appearance of the lung fields. At this point in her clinical course she had noncompliant lungs that required very high airway pressures to provide an adequate tidal volume. She died of persistent respiratory failure 1 week after this chest radiograph was taken. Postmortem examination of the lungs revealed extensive interstitial fibrosis and hyaline membranes.

secondary lung injury from oxygen toxicity has been difficult to quantify experimentally or even to estimate clinically (95,96).

Numerous experimental and clinical studies have been done during the last 10 years to determine the mechanisms of acute lung injury in noncardiogenic pulmonary edema. Since many disorders are associated with ARDS, the cause of the increased-permeability edema may depend on the specific associated etiology. For example, neutrophils have been implicated as a major factor in lung injury from sepsis and microembolism (97). Complement activation in sepsis may play a role in activating white blood cells to release toxic enzymes (e.g., neutral proteases) that could increase endothelial permeability in the lung (98). One study

showed that neutrophil elastolytic activity in air spaces is very high in half of ARDS patients (99). However, some investigators have shown that neither white blood cells nor complement is necessary for some kinds of permeability pulmonary edema (100, 101). Also, other investigators have implicated the fibrinogen and coagulation system in the pathogenesis of acute lung injury (102, 103). The possible role of cytokines, such as tumor necrosis factor or interleukin-8, in mediating pulmonary and systemic lung injury from sepsis, has been studied in experimental and clinical studies (104, 105).

Some cases of noncardiogenic pulmonary edema may be mediated by neural mechanisms that could increase lung vascular permeability. This mechanism has been demonstrated in one animal model of neurogenic pulmonary edema in which an α-adrenergic blocker, phentolamine, prevented the increased pulmonary vascular permeability that occurred with intracranial hypertension in dogs (106). Also, some investigators have shown that in the presence of increased vascular

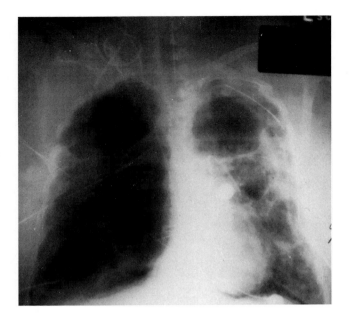

**Figure 22.10.** Anteroposterior chest radiograph of a 36-year-old woman who had developed ARDS from Gram-negative sepsis 6 weeks prior to this chest film. Her clinical course was characterized by persistent respiratory failure and ventilator dependence. Her chest radiograph initially showed noncardiogenic pulmonary edema with fluffy infiltrates (as in Fig. 22.6**B**). About 2 weeks following the development of ARDS from sepsis, her chest radiograph showed a diffuse ground-glass appearance (as in Fig. 22.6), and her lungs became very noncompliant. Finally, 5 weeks following the onset of ARDS she developed bilateral bullae in the upper and lower lung zones and required multiple chest tubes to drain recurrent pneumothoraces. She died 2 days after this chest film was taken. At postmortem examination her lungs showed large bullae with extensive loss of lung tissue. She had no prior history of smoking, and her chest film was normal prior to the onset of sepsis and ARDS.

permeability in the lung, there may be an element of high pressure from constriction of pulmonary veins that may compound the degree of pulmonary edema that develops (107).

There are several reviews which summarize much of the progress that has been made in unraveling the mechanisms of acute lung injury (108,109). Further research in the next few years probably will yield more specific information about the basic causes of acute lung injury.

Although the lung appears to be the primary target organ for failure in ARDS, a number of studies have shown that mortality in ARDS is closely related to multiorgan failure, uncontrolled infection, and chronic medical diseases that are associated with ARDS (65–67, 110). In fact, mortality is directly caused by

respiratory failure alone in less than 20% of ARDS cases, although most patients die with severe respiratory failure (67). Sepsis appears to be the most important cause of both early and late mortality (67, 110).

### Implications for Treatment of Increased-Permeability Edema and ARDS

Ideal treatment for patients with increased-permeability edema would be an agent that could restore the abnormal vascular permeability of the pulmonary microcirculation to its normal state. This would prevent additional leakage of protein-rich fluid into the interstitium and alveoli of the lung. Unfortunately, no such agent is available at present. Although corticosteroids and antioxidant agents (superoxide dismutase) have been shown to be effective experimentally in modestly ameliorating the acute lung injury if they are given before or immediately after the injury occurs, clinical studies have demonstrated no benefit of glucocorticoids for treatment of septic-induced ARDS (111).

At present, the best approach to therapy of ARDS is to identify and treat, if possible, the precipitating cause of the acute respiratory failure. The most treatable causes of ARDS are sepsis, respiratory infections, and shock. In many cases, such as smoke inhalation, trauma, and gastric aspiration, the injury has already occurred when the patient is first seen. In other cases, such as acute pancreatitis, viral pneumonia, or neurogenic pulmonary edema from increased intracranial pressure, the cause of the ARDS cannot be easily controlled.

The diagnosis of noncardiogenic pulmonary edema may need to be confirmed by measuring the vascular filling pressures in the pulmonary circulation to be certain that the pulmonary edema is not of cardiogenic origin (49). A pulmonary arterial catheter can be passed percutaneously into the pulmonary artery via the antecubital, internal jugular, subclavian, or femoral vein. As described in Chapters 2 and 23, a wedge pressure usually reflects the left atrial filling pressure. Normal or low pressures (less than 12 mm Hg) indicate that the pulmonary edema is from a noncardiogenic cause. Occasionally, patients with pulmonary edema primarily from increased vascular permeability also have an element of fluid overload with mildly elevated wedge pressures (112). As the Starling equation predicts, an increase in hydrostatic pressure (Pmv) in the face of increased vascular permeability (K) will result in an exponential rise in transvascular fluid flux (20, 112–114). These patients may benefit from treatment (diuretics) that decreases left atrial filling pressures to a normal range.

Since most patients with ARDS have severe pulmonary edema and poorly compliant lungs, they usually experience respiratory muscle fatigue from the hypoxemia and the increased work of breathing. Mechanical ventilation with positive pressure is usually necessary to improve oxygenation and stabilize alveolar ventilation in patients with ARDS. Positive end-expiratory pressure (PEEP) in the range of 5 to 15 cm $H_2O$ improves oxygenation further by inflating poorly ventilated alveoli and thereby decreasing the amount of venous admixture (or intrapulmonary shunting) in the lung (112). PEEP usually permits the fraction of inspired oxygen to be lowered, thus reducing the risk of superimposed oxygen toxicity to the lungs.

PEEP does not, however, alter the course of the primary lung injury. It does not, for example, reduce extravascular lung water content in pulmonary edema (115, 116). High levels of PEEP (above 10 cm $H_2O$) usually cause a reduction in cardiac output (112), which may result in an even higher arterial $Pao_2$. This improved oxygenation with a declining cardiac output results from either decreased blood flow to poorly ventilated lung regions or a longer time for oxygen diffusion in edematous lung units when pulmonary blood flow is reduced. Clinically, a reduction in cardiac output from PEEP may interfere with overall oxygen transport even if the arterial oxygen tension is adequate. Careful monitoring of the effects of PEEP on cardiac output and perfusion to vital organs (brain, kidney) may be helpful in patients with ARDS and a low-output syndrome (112).

In the future, other modalities of therapy for ARDS may be helpful, including surfactant replacement (117) and monoclonal antibody treatment for sepsis (118), although recent experience with both of these approaches has not been encouraging (119). New ventilatory strategies have been considered, though none have yet been shown to alter mortality or the duration of mechanical ventilation (119). It is possible that efforts directed at accelerating recovery from acute lung injury may offer more long-term promise for effective therapy (120–122).

▼

## REFERENCES

1. Staub NC: Pulmonary edema. *Physiol Rev* 54:678–811, 1974.
2. Starling EH: On the absorption of fluids from the connective tissue spaces. *J Physiol* 19:312–326, 1986.
3. Staub NC: The pathogenesis of pulmonary edema. *Prog Cardiovasc Dis* 23:53–80, 1980.
4. Blake LH, Staub NC: Pulmonary vascular transport in sheep. A mathematical model. *Microvasc Res* 12:197–220, 1976.
5. Blattacharya J, Staub NC: Direct measurement of microvascular pressure in the isolated, perfused dog lung. *Microvasc Res* 17 (Part 2):586, 1979.
6. Gaar KA, Taylor AE, Owens LJ: Pulmonary capillary pressure and filtration coefficient in the isolated perfused lung. *Am J Physiol* 213:910–914, 1967.
7. Brigham KL: Mechanisms of acute lung injury. *Clin Chest Med* 3:9–24, 1982.
8. Erdmann JA, Vaughn TR Jr, Brigham KL, et al: Effect of increased vascular pressure on lung fluid balance in unanesthetized sheep. *Circ Res* 37:271–284, 1975.
9. Reid l, Meyrick B: Microcirculation: definition and organization at tissue level. *Ann NY Acad Sci* 384:3–20, 1982.
10. Bo G, Hauge A, Nicolaysen G: Alveolar pressure and lung volume as determinants of net transvascular fluid filtration. *J Appl Physiol* 42:476–482, 1977.
11. Albert RK, Lakshminarayan S, Kirk W, Butler J: Lung inflation can cause pulmonary edema in zone I of in situ dog lungs. *J Appl Physiol* 49:815–819, 1980.
12. Schneeberger-Keeley EE, Karnovsky MJ: The ultrastructural basis of alveolar capillary membrane permeability to peroxidase used as a tracer. *J Cell Biol* 37:781–793, 1968.
13. Gorin AB, Stewart PA: Differential permeability of endothelial and epithelial barriers to albumin flux. *J Appl Physiol* 47:1315–1324, 1979.
14. Taylor AE, Gaar KA Jr: Estimation of equivalent pore radii of pulmonary capillary and alveolar membranes. *Am J Physiol* 218:1133–1140, 1970.
15. Gee MH, Havil AM: The relationship between pulmonary perivascular cuff fluid and lung lymph in dogs with edema. *Microvasc Res* 19:209–216, 1978.
16. Bhattacharya J, Gropper M, Staub NC: Interstitial fluid pressure gradient measured by micropuncture in excised dog lung. *J Appl Physiol* 56:271–277, 1984.
17. Howell JBL, Permutt S, Proctor DF, Riley RL: Effect of inflation of the lung on different parts of the pulmonary vascular bed. *J Appl Physiol* 16:71, 1961.
18. Gee MH, William DO: Effect of lung inflation on perivascular cuff fluid volume in isolated dog lung lobes. *Microvasc Res* 17:192–201, 1979.
19. Goshy M, Lai-Fook SJ, Hyatt RE: Perivascular pressure measurements by wick-catheter technique in isolated dog lobes. *J Appl Physiol* 46:950–955, 1979.
20. Staub NC: Pulmonary edema. Physiologic approaches to management. *Chest* 74:559–564, 1978.
21. Clements JA: Pulmonary edema and permeability of alveolar membranes. *Arch Environ Health* 2:280–283, 1961.
22. Albert RK, Lakshminarayan S, Hildebrandt J, et al: Increased surface tension favors pulmonary edema formation in anesthetized dogs' lungs. *J Clin Invest* 63:1015, 1979.
23. Raj U: Alveolar liquid pressure measured by micropuncture in isolated lungs of mature and immature fetal rabbits. *J Clin Invest* 79:1579–1588, 1987.
24. Gregory TJ. Surfactant chemical composition and biophysical activity in acute respiratory distress syndrome. *J Clin Invest* 88:1976–1981, 1991.
25. Vreim CE, Snashall PD, Demling RH, Staub NC: Lung lymph and free interstitial fluid protein composition in sheep with edema. *Am J Physiol* 230:1650–1653, 1976.
26. Brigham KL, Woolverton WC, Blake LH, et al: Increased

sheep lung vascular permeability caused by *Pseudomonas* bacteremia. *J Clin Invest* 54:792–804, 1974.

27. Ohkuda K, Nakahara K, Weidner WJ, et al: Lung fluid exchange after uneven pulmonary artery obstruction in sheep. *Circ Res* 43:152–161, 1978.

28. Jayr C, and Matthay MA: Alveolar and lung liquid clearance in the absence of pulmonary blood flow in sheep. *J Appl Physiol* 71(5):1679–1687, 1991.

29. Bongard F, Matthay MA, Mackeasie RC, Lewis FR: Morphologic and physiologic correlates of increased extravascular lung water. *Surgery* 96:395–403, 1984.

30. DaLuz PL, Shubia H, Weil MH: Pulmonary edema related to changes in colloid osmotic and pulmonary artery pressure in patients after acute myocardial infarction. *Circulation* 51:350–357, 1975.

31. Aberle DR, Wiener-Kronish JP, Webb RW, Matthay MA: Hydrostatic versus increased permeability pulmonary edema: diagnosis based on radiographic criteria in critically ill patients. *Radiology* 168:73–79, 1988.

32. Wiener-Kronish JP, Matthay MA: Pleural effusions associated with hydrostatic and increased permeability pulmonary edema. *Chest* 93:852–858, 1988.

33. Wiener-Kronish JP, Matthay MA, Collen PW, et al: Relationship of pulmonary hemodynamics to pleural effusions in patients with heart failure. *Am Rev Respir Dis* 132:1253–1256, 1985.

34. Wiener-Kronish JP, Goldstein R, Matthay RA, et al: Chronic pulmonary arterial and right atrial hypertension are not associated with pleural effusions. *Chest* 92:967–970, 1987.

35. Broaddus VC, Wiener-Kronish JP, Staub NC: Removal of pleural liquid and protein by lymphatics in awake sheep. *J Appl Physiol* 64:384–390, 1990.

36. Wiener-Kronish JP, Broaddus VC, Albertine K, et al: The relationship of pleural effusions to increased permeability pulmonary edema in anesthetized sheep. *J Clin Invest* 82:1422–1429, 1988.

37. Fein A, Grossman RF, Jones JG, et al: The value of edema fluid protein measurements in patients with pulmonary edema. *Am J Med* 67:32–38, 1979.

38. Matthay MA, Eschenbacher WL, Goetzl E: Elevated concentration of leukotriene $D_4$ in the pulmonary edema fluid of patients with the adult respiratory distress syndrome. *J Clin Immunol* 4:479–483, 1984.

39. Matthay MA, Landolt CC, Staub NC: Differential liquid and protein clearance from the alveoli of anesthetized sheep. *J Appl Physiol* 53:96–104, 1982.

40. Matthay MA, Berthiaume Y, Staub NC: Long-term clearance of liquid and protein from the lungs of unanesthetized sheep. *J Appl Physiol* 59:928–934, 1985.

41. Goodman BE, Brown JE, Crandall EP: Regulation of transport across pulmonary alveolar epithelial cell monolayers. *J Appl Physiol* 57:703–710, 1984.

42. Matthay MA, Wiener-Kronish JP: Intact epithelial barrier function is critical for the resolution of alveolar edema in humans. *Am Rev Respir Dis* 142:1250–1257, 1990.

43. Berthiaume Y, Staub NC, Matthay MA: β-Adrenergic agonists increase lung liquid clearance in anesthetized sheep. *J Clin Invest* 79:335–343, 1987.

44. Berthiaume Y, Broadus VC, Gropper MA, et al: Alveolar liquid and protein clearance from normal dog lungs. *J Appl Physiol* 65:585–593, 1988.

45. Crandall SD, Heming TA, Palombo RL, Goodman BE: Effects of terbutaline on sodium transport in isolated perfused rat lungs. *J Appl Physiol* 60:289–294, 1986.

46. Jayr C, Garat C, Meignan M, Pittet JF, Zelter M, Matthay MA: Alveolar liquid and protein clearance in anesthetized ventilated rats. *J Appl Physiol* 76(6):2636–2642, 1994.

47. Sakuma OG, Nakada T, Nishimura T, Fujimura S, Matthay MA: Alveolar fluid clearance in the resected human lung. *Am J Respir Crit Care Med* 150:305–310, 1994.

48. Swan HJC, Ganz W, Forrester J, et al: Catheterization of the heart in man with use of a flow directed balloon-tipped catheter. *N Engl J Med* 283:447–451, 1970.

49. Conners AF, McCaffree RD, Gray BA: Evaluation of right heart catheterization in the critically ill patient without acute myocardial infarction. *N Engl J Med* 308:263–267, 1983.

50. Matthay MA, Chatterjee K: Bedside catheterization of the pulmonary artery: risks versus benefits. *Ann Intern Med* 109:826–834, 1988.

51. Unger KM, Shibel EM, Moser KM: Detection of left ventricular failure in patients with the adult respiratory distress syndrome. *Chest* 67:8–13, 1975.

52. Osler W, McCrae T: *The Principles and Practice of Medicine*, 10th ed. New York, D. Appleton, 1927.

53. Lee G, De Maria A, Amsterdam EA, et al: Comparative effects of morphine, meperidine, and pentazocine on cardiocirculatory dynamics in patients with acute myocardial infarction. *Am J Med* 60:949–955, 1976.

54. Packer M: Do vasodilators prolong life in heart failure: *N Engl J Med* 316:1471–1473, 1987.

55. Cohn JN: Physiologic basis for vasodilator therapy for heart failure. *Am J Med* 71:135–139, 1981.

56. Biddle TL, Ju PN: Effect of furosemide on hemodynamics and lung water in acute pulmonary edema secondary to myocardial infarction. *Am J Cardiol* 43:86–90, 1979.

57. Goldstein RA, Passamani ER, Roberts R: A comparison of digoxin and dobutamine in patients with acute infarction and cardiac failure. *N Engl J Med* 303:846–850, 1980.

58. Gray R, Shah PK, Singh B, et al: Low cardiac output states after open heart surgery. *Chest* 80:16–22, 1981.

59. Arnold SB, Byrd RC, Meister W: Long-term digitalis therapy improves left ventricular function in heart failure. *N Engl J Med* 303:1443–1448, 1980.

60. Buda AJ, Pinsky MR, Ingels NB Jr, et al: Effect of intrathoracic pressure on left ventricular performance. *N Engl J Med* 301:453–459, 1979.

61. Macklem PT: Respiratory muscles: the vital pump. *Chest* 78:753–758, 1980.

62. Aubier M, Trippenback T, Roussos C: Respiratory muscle fatigue during cardiogenic shock. *J Appl Physiol* 51:499–508, 1981.

63. Anderson RR, Holliday RL, Driedger AA: Documentation of pulmonary capillary permeability in the adult respiratory distress syndrome accompanying human sepsis. *Am Rev Respir Dis* 119:869–877, 1979.

64. Petty TL, Ashbaugh DG: The adult respiratory distress syndrome. *Chest* 60:233–239, 1971.

65. Murray JF, Matthay MA, Luce JM, Flick MR: An expanded definition of the adult respiratory distress syndrome. *Am Rev Respir Dis* 138:720–723, 1988.

66. Rubin DB, Wiener-Kronish JP, Murray JF, Turner J, Luce JM, et al: Elevated von-Willebrand factor antigen is an

early plasma predictor of impending acute lung injury and death in non-pulmonary sepsis syndrome. *J Clin Invest* 86:474–480, 1990.

67. Montgomery AB, Stager MA, Carrico CJ, Hudson LH: Causes of mortality in patients with the adult respiratory distress syndrome. *Am Rev Respir Dis* 132:485–489, 1985.

68. Murray JF: Mechanisms of acute respiratory failure. *Am Rev Respir Dis* 115:1071–1078, 1977.

69. Villar J, Slutsky AS; The incidence of the adult respiratory distress syndrome. *Am Rev Resp Dis* 140:814–816, 1989.

70. Bernard GR, Artigas A, Brigham RL, et al: The American-European consensus conference on ARDS: definitions, mechanisms, relevant outcomes, and clinical trial coordination. *Am J Respir Crit Care Med* 149:818–824, 1994.

71. Pepe PE, Potkin RT, Reus DH, et al: Clinical predictors of the adult respiratory distress syndrome. *Am J Surg* 144:124–130, 1982.

72. Fowler AA, Hamman RF, Good JT, Petty TL: Adult respiratory distress syndrome: risks with common predispositions. *Ann Intern Med* 98:593–597, 1983.

73. Cameron JL, Zuidema GD: Aspiration pneumonia. Magnitude and frequency of the problem. *JAMA* 219:1194–1196, 1972.

74. Wynne JW, Modell JH: Respiratory aspiration of stomach contents. *Ann Intern Med* 87:466–474, 1977.

75. Bynum LJ, Pierce AK: Pulmonary aspiration of gastric contents. *Am Rev Respir Dis* 114:1129–1136, 1976.

76. Bartlett JG, Gorback SL, Finegold SM: The bacteriology of aspiration pneumonia. *Am J Med* 56:202–207, 1974.

77. Folkesson HG, Hebert C, Broaddus VC, Matthay MA: Acid aspiration-induced acute lung injury is mediated by interleukin-β dependent mechanisms. *Clin Res* 43:143A, 1995.

78. Kaplan RL, Sahn SA, Petty TL: Incidence and outcome of the respiratory distress syndrome in Gram-negative sepsis. *Arch Intern Med* 139:867–869, 1979.

79. Weinberg PF, Matthay MA, Webster RO, et al: Biologically active products of complement and acute lung injury in patients with the sepsis syndrome. *Am Rev Respir Dis* 130:791–796, 1984.

80. Hechtman HB, Lonergan EA, Shepro D: Platelet and leukocyte lung interactions in patients with respiratory failure. *Surgery* 83:155–163, 1978.

81. Brigham KL, Meyrick B: Endotoxin and lung injury. *Am Rev Resp Dis* 133:913–927, 1986.

82. Brigham KL, Bowers RE, Haynes J: Increased lung vascular permeability caused by *E. coli* endotoxin. *Circ Res* 45:292–297, 1979.

83. Wiener-Kronish JP, Albertine KH, Matthay MA: Differential responses of the endothelial and epithelial barrier of the lung in sheep to *E. coli* endotoxin. *J Clin Invest* 88:864–875, 1991.

84. Staub NC: Conference report on a workshop on the measurement of lung water. *Crit Care Med* 8:752–759, 1980.

85. Pistolesi M, Guintini C: Assessment of extravascular lung water. *Radiol Clin North Am* 16:551–574, 1978.

86. Noble WH, Kay JC, Obdrzalek J: Lung mechanics in hypervolemic pulmonary edema. *J Appl Physiol* 38:681–687, 1975.

87. Said SI, Avery ME, Davis RK, et al: Pulmonary surface activity in induced pulmonary edema. *J Clin Invest* 44:458–464, 1965.

88. Hallman M, Spragg R, Harrell JH, et al: Evidence of lung surfactant abnormality in respiratory failure—a study of bronchoalveolar lavage phospholipids, surface activity, phospholipase activity, and plasma myoinositol. *J Clin Invest* 70:673–683, 1982.

89. Gregory TJ, Longmore WJ, Moxley MA, Whitsett JA, Reed CR, Fowler AA III, Hudson LD, Maunder RJ, Crim C, Hyers TM: Surfactant chemical composition and biophysical activity in acute respiratory distress syndrome. *J Clin Invest* 88:1976–1981, 1991.

90. Bachofen M, Weibel ER: Alterations of the gas exchange apparatus in adult respiratory insufficiency associated with septicemia. *Am Rev Respir Dis* 116:589–615, 1977.

91. Elliott CG, Morris AH, Cengiz M: Pulmonary function and exercise gas exchange in survivors of adult respiratory distress syndrome. *Am Rev Respir Dis* 123:492–495, 1981.

92. Lakshminarayan S, Stanford RE, Petty TL: Prognosis after recovery from adult respiratory distress syndrome. *Am Rev Respir Dis* 113:7–16, 1976.

93. Zapol WM, Snider MT: Pulmonary hypertension in severe acute respiratory failure. *N Engl J Med* 296:476–480, 1977.

94. Schnapp LM, Chin DP, Szaflarshi N, Matthay MA: Frequency and importance of barotrauma in 100 patients with acute lung injury. *Crit Care Med* 23:272–278, 1995.

95. Pratt PC, Vollmer RT, Shelburne JD, Crapo JD: Pulmonary morphology in a multihospital collaborative extracorporeal membrane oxygenation project. I. Light microscopy. *Am J Pathol* 85:210–228, 1979.

96. Witschi HR, Haschek WM, Klein-Szanto AJR, Hakkinen PJ: Potentiation of diffuse lung damage by oxygen: determining variables. *Am Rev Respir Dis* 123:98, 1981.

97. Rinaldo J: Mediation of ARDS by leukocytes. *Chest* 89:590–593, 1986.

98. Stevens JH, O'Hanley P, Shapiro JM, Raffin T: Effects of anti-C5a antibodies on the adult respiratory distress syndrome in septic primates. *J Clin Invest* 77:1812–1816, 1986.

99. Lee CT, Fein AM, Lippmann M, et al: Elastolytic activity in pulmonary lavage fluid from patients with adult respiratory distress syndrome. *N Engl J Med* 304:192–196, 1981.

100. Maunder RJ, Hackman RC, Riff E, et al: Occurrence of the adult respiratory distress syndrome in neutropenic patients. *Am Rev Respir Dis* 133:313–316, 1986.

101. Rinaldo JE, Borovetz H: Deterioration of oxygenation and abnormal lung microvascular permeability during resolution of leukopenia in patients with diffuse lung injury. *Am Rev Respir Dis* 131:579–583, 1985.

102. Haynes JB, Hyers TM, Giclas PC, et al: Elevated fibrinogen degradation products in the adult respiratory distress syndrome. *Am Rev Respir Dis* 122:841–847, 1980.

103. Malik AB, Vander Zee H: Mechanism of pulmonary edema induced by microembolism in dogs. *Circ Res* 42:72–79, 1978.

104. Tracey KJ, Fong Y, Hesse DG, et al: Anti-cachetin/TNF monoclonal antibodies prevent septic shock during lethal bacteremia. *Nature* 330:662–664, 1987.

105. Miller EJ, Cohen AB, Nagao S, Griffith D, Maunder RJ, et al: Elevated levels of NAP-1/interleukin-8 are present in the airspaces of patients with the adult respiratory

distress syndrome and are associated with increased mortality. *Am Rev Resp Dis* 146:427–432, 1992.

106. Vander Zee H, Malik AB, Lee BC, Hakim TS: Lung fluid and protein exchange during intracranial hypertension and the role of sympathetic mechanisms. *J Appl Physiol* 48:273, 1980.

107. Dauber IM, Hofmeister S, Weil JV: Preventing sympathetically mediated pulmonary venoconstriction decreases permeability pulmonary edema. *Clin Res* 29:67A, 1981.

108. Rinaldo JE, Rogers RM: Adult respiratory distress syndrome: changing concepts of lung injury and repair. *N Engl J Med* 306:901–908, 1982.

109. Wiedemann H, Matthay RA, Matthay MA (eds): *Acute Lung Injury. Critical Care Clinics.* Philadelphia, WB Saunders, 1986.

110. Bell RC, Coalson J, Smith JD, et al: Multiple organ failure and infection in the adult respiratory distress syndrome. *Ann Intern Med* 99:293–298, 1983.

111. Luce JM, Montgomery AB, Marks JD, Turner J, Metz CA, Murray JF: Ineffectiveness of high-dose methylprednisolone in preventing parenchymal lung injury and improving mortality in patients with septic shock. *Am Rev Respir Dis* 138:62–68, 1988.

112. Matthay MA, Broaddus VL: Fluid and hemodynamic management in acute lung injury. *Semin Respir Crit Care Med* 15:271–288, 1994.

113. Ohkuda K, Nakahara K, Binder A, Staub NC: Venous air emboli in sheep: reversible increase in lung microvascular permeability. *J Appl Physiol* 51:887–894, 1981.

114. Prewitt RM, McCarthy J, Wood LDH: Treatment of acute low pressure pulmonary edema in dogs. *J Clin Invest* 67:409–418, 1981.

115. Demling RH, Staub NC, Edmunds LH Jr: Effect of end-expiratory airway pressure on accumulation of extravascular lung water. *J Appl Physiol* 38:907–912, 1975.

116. Hopewell PC, Murray JF: Effects of continuous positive pressure ventilation in experimental pulmonary edema. *J Appl Physiol* 40:568–574, 1976.

117. Merritt TA, Hallman M, Bloom BT, et al: Prophylactic treatment of very premature infants with human surfactant. *N Engl J Med* 315:785–789, 1986.

118. Baumgartner JD, McCutchan JA, Melle GV, et al: Prevention of Gram-negative, shock and death in surgical patients by antibody to core glycolipid. *Lancet* 2:59–63, 1985.

119. Kollef M, Schuster DP: The acute respiratory distress syndrome. *N Engl J Med* 332:27–37, 1995.

120. Matthay MA: Function of the alveolar epithelial barrier under pathologic conditions. *Chest* 105(Suppl):67S–74S, 1994.

121. Wortel CH, Doerschuk CM. Neutrophils and neutrophil-endothelial cell adhesion in adult respiratory distress syndrome. *New Horizons* 1:631–637, 1993.

122. Matthay MA: Fibrosing alveolitis in the adult respiratory distress syndrome. *Ann Intern Med* 122:65–66, 1995.

# Chapter 23

# Principles of Managing the Patient with Hemodynamic Insufficiency and Shock

## Michael A. Matthay

| | |
|---|---|
| CARDIORESPIRATORY MONITORING | Acute Noncardiogenic Pulmonary |
|   **Systemic Arterial Catheterization** |   **Edema** |
|   **Pulmonary Artery Catheterization** | **Shock** |
| CLINICAL INDICATIONS FOR PULMONARY ARTERY | **Management of Patients after Cardiac** |
|   CATHETERIZATION |   **and Major Vascular Surgery** |
|   **Acute Cardiogenic Pulmonary Edema** | HOW TO DETERMINE THE PHYSIOLOGIC BASIS FOR |
| |   SHOCK |

THIS CHAPTER FOCUSES primarily on (*a*) the methods available for the diagnosis and monitoring of hemodynamic insufficiency in critically ill patients, (*b*) the indications for invasive hemodynamic monitoring in critically ill patients, and (*c*) the basic principles of determining the etiology of shock. A more detailed discussion of sepsis and multiple organ failure is provided in Chapter 24.

## CARDIORESPIRATORY MONITORING

In this section, techniques for monitoring the hemodynamic and respiratory status of critically ill patients with respiratory failure are discussed. In the last three decades many invasive techniques for monitoring the systemic and pulmonary circulation have been developed. More recently, however, there has been increasing interest in developing noninvasive methods for monitoring important physiologic variables with the goal of reducing the risk and expense of invasive measurements whenever possible.

### SYSTEMIC ARTERIAL CATHETERIZATION

Systemic arterial catheters are widely used in a variety of critically ill patients. They are most useful for monitoring systemic arterial blood pressure in patients who are hemodynamically unstable, including patients with severe, uncontrolled hypertension as well as patients with hypotension and clinical shock. In addition, systemic arterial catheters are useful as a means of obtaining repeated blood samples from patients, thus obviating the need for repeated percutaneous venous or arterial puncture. In general, systemic arterial catheters are well tolerated, although there are a few important concerns regarding insertion technique and complications that need to be remembered.

### Insertion Techniques for Systemic Arterial Catheters

Peripheral arterial cannulation is accomplished most frequently by percutaneous insertion of an 18- or 20-gauge catheter using sterile technique. When percutaneous insertion is not possible, a surgical cutdown may be necessary. The radial artery is usually chosen because of its accessibility and because there is generally good collateral circulation via the ulnar artery. Prior to insertion, the status of this collateral circulation should be assessed with an Allen's test. With this test, both the ulnar and radial arteries are occluded by pressure at the wrist; after the hand becomes pale and cool, releasing only the ulnar artery occlusion should restore adequate circulation within 5 seconds. The femoral, dorsales pedis, and brachial arteries may be cannulated also. Femoral arterial catheterization has not been associated with any increased risk of complication compared with that of the radial artery, providing that the catheters are inserted with sterile technique percutaneously (1).

### Complications of Systemic Arterial Catheters

Infection and ischemia are the most important major complications that may occur from systemic arterial catheterization. Ischemia may occur secondary to either thrombosis with local occlusion or distal embolization. One large prospective study found a 4% incidence of catheter-related septicemia and an 18% incidence of local infection (defined by semiquantitative culture of the catheter tip) (2). The risk factors favoring infection include insertion by surgical cutdown rather than percutaneously, duration of cannulation exceeding 4 days, and inflammation at the catheter site (2). Infection may originate in the transducer or fluid-delivery apparatus. One prospective study indicated that catheter-related infection can be decreased markedly if a continuous flush device is located immediately distal to the transducer apparatus rather than close to the insertion site (3). This eliminates a long proximal static fluid column between the transducer and flush intake. With this design and careful sterile precautions at the blood-sampling stopcock, the incidence of catheter-related septicemia was reduced to less than 1%.

Clinically significant thrombosis or embolism is rare. In over 12,000 consecutive placements of arterial lines (including radial, brachial, and/or dorsalis pedis arteries), necrosis of the fingers or toes occurred in only 15 (0.2%) (4). Similarly, in another study, only 3 (0.6%) of 531 patients required emergency thrombectomies for distal ischemia (5). The clinical risk factors for acute distal ischemia include systemic hypotension, severe peripheral vascular disease, and the use of vasopressor drugs. Even though clinically important ischemia is rare, reversible subclinical arterial occlusion or reduced flow is common, with up to 24% of arteries still occluded 1 week after catheter removal (6). The risk factors for such occlusion include larger catheter size (18- versus 20-gauge), smaller wrist size (women and

children), repeated attempts before successful cannulation, and duration of cannulation (risk increases after 3 to 4 days). Ulnar refill time determined by the Allen's test prior to insertion is also of some predictive value. As mentioned, a palmar blush caused by filling via the ulnar artery should appear within 5 seconds. If 15 seconds is used as an acceptable upper limit, then distal ischemia is more frequent (approximately 10%) (7).

Once the catheter is placed, distal perfusion should be assessed at least daily by noting any changes in skin color, temperature, or capillary refill time. If the arterial pressure tracing becomes persistently dampened, or if blood drawing is difficult, thrombosis formation on the catheter tip is likely and the catheters should be removed, since the risk of occlusion is high (8).

### PULMONARY ARTERY CATHETERIZATION

The availability of bedside pulmonary artery catheterization has had a major impact on the management of critically ill patients. There are numerous clinical conditions for which pulmonary artery catheterization has been accepted as useful (1). These include shock associated with acute myocardial infarction, sepsis or major trauma, acute respiratory failure from cardiogenic or noncardiogenic pulmonary edema, and management of patients following cardiac or major vascular surgery. However, there has been increasing concern that clinicians need to be better informed regarding the risk and potential benefits of systemic and pulmonary artery catheterization (9–11). The clinical literature contains numerous examples of how incorrect information may be conveyed from pulmonary arterial pressure measurements when physicians are not sufficiently skilled at interpreting pressure and waveform tracings (1, 12, 13).

### Insertion Techniques

The pulmonary circulation can be monitored by percutaneous insertion of a balloon-tipped pulmonary artery catheter via the subclavian, internal jugular, external jugular, femoral, or antecubital vein. Catheterization can be done at the patient's bedside with only pressure waveform and amplitude and electrocardiographic monitoring. Fluoroscopy is not necessary, although the prescribed waveform must be displayed on the bedside oscilloscope. The pulmonary artery catheter used most frequently has four lumina plus a small thermistor near the tip for thermodilution cardiac output measurements. One lumen is used to inflate the balloon on the tip of the catheter. After the catheter is advanced into the thorax, the balloon is inflated. The flow-directed catheter then usually passes easily from the right atrium across the tricuspid valve

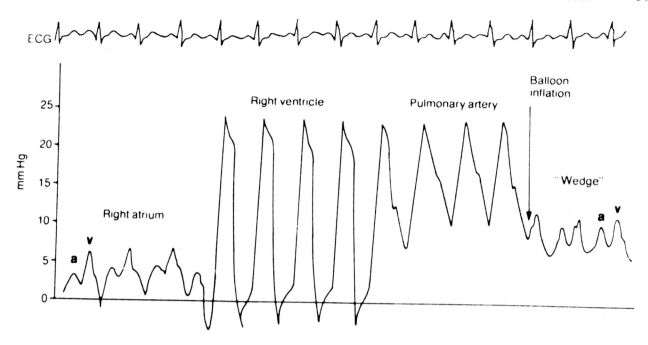

**FIGURE 23.1.** Representative recording of pressures as a Swan-Ganz catheter is inserted through an internal jugular vein through the right side of the heart into the pulmonary artery. The first recorded wave form is a right atrial tracing with characteristic a and v waves. In the right ventricle, note that end-diastolic pressure is zero. In the pulmonary artery, a normal pressure wave form is recorded. The catheter is then advanced to the wedge position with the balloon inflated. The wedge pressure tracing shows a and v waves transmitted from the left atrium. The wedge tracing is not always this clear, but it should not be overly damped. The pressures shown here are normal. (From Matthay MA: Invasive hemodynamic monitoring in critically ill patients. *Clin Chest Med* 4(2), 1983, with permission.)

through the right ventricle and into the pulmonary artery (Fig. 23.1). If the catheter is advanced further with the balloon inflated, it will wedge in the pulmonary artery and occlude blood flow. The distal lumen, which opens at the tip of the catheter, will then record the downstream vascular pressure, the pulmonary arterial wedge pressure (Fig. 23.1). When the balloon is deflated, the distal lumen records the phasic pulmonary arterial pressure. The proximal lumen, located 30 cm from the tip of the catheter, will then be positioned in the right atrium to measure central venous pressure when the tip of the catheter is in the pulmonary artery. This proximal lumen is also used to inject a bolus of indicator (10 ml of 5% dextrose) to determine cardiac output by thermodilution. The bolus is injected through the lumen in the right atrium so that the thermistor near the tip of the catheter in the pulmonary artery can sense the change in temperature as the bolus flows into the pulmonary artery. A small bedside computer then integrates the time-temperature curve and prints out the cardiac output. The fourth lumen, located 31 cm from the tip of the catheter, is used for infusion of intravenous solutions. An introducer sheath that has an additional lumen is also available for the intravenous infusion of fluids.

### Obtaining Reliable Pressure Measurements

Once the catheter is in place, the pressure is transmitted via the catheter through the fluid-filled tubing to the diaphragm of a transducer and then converted to an electronic signal. The signal is amplified, the pressure waveform is shown on an oscilloscope, and the pressure is shown on a digital display (Fig. 23.1). Correct pressure measurements depend on accurately calibrated transducers, a fluid-filled catheter system without blood clots or air bubbles, and a monitor that displays the pressure tracing in an appropriate size to demonstrate the waveforms clearly. The pulmonary arterial and wedge pressure tracing in Figure 23.1 fulfills these requirements. Note that there is a single major pulmonary arterial pressure wave for each spike on the electrocardiogram. Correct amplitude settings are needed to display the waveform correctly. In general, amplitudes in the range of 0 to 30 or 0 to 60 mm Hg are appropriate for the pulmonary circulation. In addition, the contour of the tracing is important. Figure

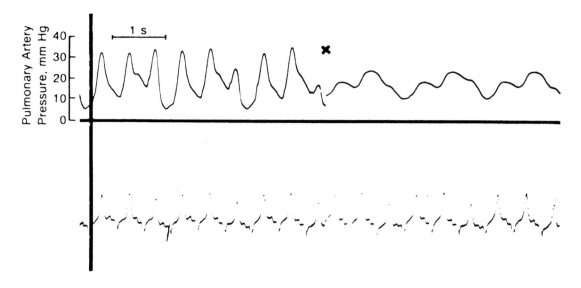

**FIGURE 23.2.** Pulmonary artery tracing after introduction of 0.5 cm³ of air into the connecting tubing at X, with the electrocardiogram recorded below. The phasic contour of the pulmonary artery tracing is damped out by the air bubble; the same pattern can be produced by clots in the catheter or on the catheter tip. (From Quinn K, Quebbeman EJ: Pulmonary artery pressure monitoring in the surgical intensive care unit. *Arch Surg* 116: 872–876, 1981, with permission.)

23.2 illustrates the dampening effect of a small air bubble in the catheter system. The dampening of the tracing also can be caused by a clot on the end of the catheter.

Calibration of the transducer is important because transducers may not be linear over a wide range. Thus, the transducer for the pulmonary artery catheter must be calibrated for the lower pressures of the pulmonary circulation (0 to 40 mm Hg) rather than for the higher pressure range of the systemic circulation (1, 13). Another common pitfall is improper location of the zero reference point, particularly because patients are moving from side to side or the head of the bed is raised or lowered. In general, the proper zero reference is the midchest position.

Perhaps the most common source of error in making intrathoracic pressure measurements is failure to take into account the effects of respiration on these pressure measurements (1, 12, 14). Pleural pressure becomes negative during spontaneous inspiration and positive during the inspiratory cycle of mechanical ventilation (IPPV). Consequently, the pressure readout and the waveform on the oscilloscope will change, depending on the phase of respiration. In Figure 23.3, the recording of pulmonary arterial wedge pressure is interrupted by deep troughs in the tracing produced by the patient's spontaneous inspiratory efforts. During these troughs, the pressure reading was zero. Thus, the problem is how to obtain a reliable transmural pressure measurement when the reference pressure (pleural pressure) is changing. To minimize the effects of changing pleural pressure, pulmonary arterial pressures should be measured at end-expiration when pleural pressures will be close to zero. In Figure 23.3, end-expiration can be clearly seen in both the pulmonary arterial pressure and the wedge pressure tracing. This approach enables the clinician to consider the measured pressure at end-expiration as a very close approximation of the true transmural pressure. This approach can be complicated if the patient is breathing so rapidly that the end-expiratory phase is very brief (Fig. 23.4). In most circumstances, the best approach for obtaining a reliable pressure tracing is to obtain a printout of the actual pressure tracing, ideally on a strip-chart recorder, but alternatively on the oscilloscopy electrocardiographic monitor paper. First, the calibration lines for the pressure range are recorded on the paper, then the actual pressure tracing is recorded, and then the end-expiratory period can be noted on the paper. The pressure at end-expiration can then be measured from the tracing on the paper. When the patient's respiratory rate is rapid, the digital readout will not be accurate because the frequency response of the electronic system is usually too slow to detect the brief period of end-expiration.

Accurate measurements of pulmonary arterial pressures can be particularly difficult in patients with acute, severe airways obstruction. To overcome the high airway resistance, patients generate very positive intrathoracic pressures throughout expiration, and this

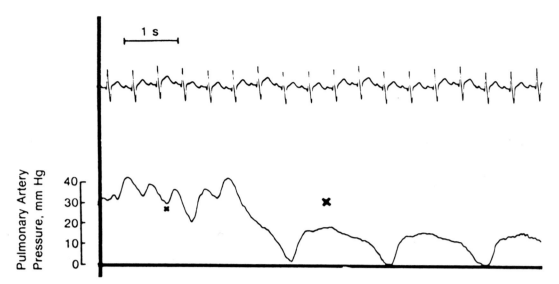

**FIGURE 23.3.** Continuous monitoring of the electrocardiogram and the phasic pulmonary artery pressure plus a segment of a pulmonary artery wedge tracing. Note that the troughs in the pulmonary artery and in the wedge tracings occur when the patient takes a spontaneous breath and pleural pressure becomes negative, thus causing a downward deflection in the tracing. The *X marks* indicate end-expiration in the respiratory cycle. At end-expiration, pleural pressure is zero; therefore, the measured in-traluminal pressure should be close to the real transmural pressure. Wedge pressure is about 15 mm Hg below the pulmonary artery end-diastolic pressure; the patient had pulmonary hypertension from acute pulmonary embolism, which accounts for the gradient between the end-diastolic and the wedge pressures. (From Quinn K, Quebbeman EJ: Pulmonary artery pressure monitoring in the surgical intensive care unit. *Arch Surg* 116: 872–876, 1981, with permission.)

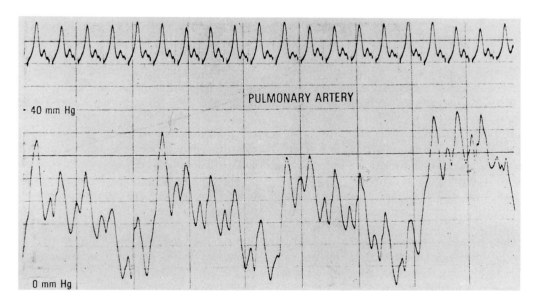

**FIGURE 23.4.** Example of how rapid labored respirations can result in rapid oscillations of the pulmonary artery pressure tracing and highly variable pressure measurements. The patient's respiratory rate was 40, and the peak pulmonary artery pressure varied from 35–40 to 18 mm Hg. A brief period of end-expiration could be identified, but the electronic digital readout could not reflect that brief end-expiratory period alone. So the pulmonary artery tracing was recorded on calibrated paper, and the pressures read off the paper at the point of end-expiration. (From Matthay MA. Invasive hemodynamic monitoring in critically ill patients. *Clin Chest Med* 4:233–250, 1983, with permission.)

leads to an elevated pulmonary arterial pressure or an elevated wedge pressure. During inspiration, the patient's pleural pressure may be markedly negative, and there will be a wide swing in the pulmonary arterial pressure tracing in the opposite direction. The problems posed by measuring pressures in patients on positive end-expiratory pressure (PEEP) are considered in the next section after discussion of the relationship of wedge pressure to left atrial pressure.

### Relation of Wedge Pressure to Left Arterial Pressure

The pulmonary arterial wedge pressure is used widely as an index of left atrial filling pressure. In general, most studies have demonstrated that the correlation between wedge pressure and left atrial pressure in patients is very good (1, 14). The correlation of left atrial pressure to left ventricular end-diastolic pressure likewise is good, provided there is no mitral valve disease. The pulmonary arterial end-diastolic pressure provides an accurate indication of the pulmonary arterial wedge pressure except when there is an increase in pulmonary vascular resistance, in which case the end-diastolic pressure will be higher than the wedge pressure. Pulmonary vascular resistance is elevated in several clinical conditions associated with acute or chronic pulmonary hypertension (see Chapters 10, 11, 13, and 22).

### Effect of PEEP on Wedge Pressure Measurements

Accurate transmural arterial and wedge pressure measurements may be more difficult to obtain in patients on PEEP in excess of 10 cm $H_2O$. PEEP may interfere with accurate measurements in two ways. First, it may result in an undetermined increase in pleural pressure. Second, the airway pressure generated by PEEP may be transmitted to the pulmonary microcirculation (14). Because PEEP prevents transpulmonary pressure from falling to zero at the end of expiration, this means the pleural pressure remains positive at the end of expiration; thus, the reference pressure for the pulmonary arterial pressure measurement is not zero. Hence, the recorded intraluminal pressure (central venous pressure, pulmonary arterial pressure, or wedge pressure) may be higher than the actual transmural pressure. One way to solve this problem is to measure esophageal pressure as an indicator of pleural pressure to obtain a more accurate reference pressure. However, reliable esophageal pressure measurements are difficult to obtain, especially in a supine patient in a critical care unit. The best working solution to the problem, in general, is to make an estimate of pleural pressure and subtract this value from the measured wedge pressure. In clinical studies in which pleural pressure was

measured in patients with the adult respiratory distress syndrome (ARDS), pleural pressure does not usually become significantly positive with levels of PEEP below 10 cm $H_2O$ (15, 16). With levels of PEEP above 10 cm $H_2O$, pleural pressure usually will be approximately 2 to 3 cm $H_2O$ positive for every 5 cm $H_2O$ increase in PEEP above 10 cm $H_2O$ (15, 16).

The other potential difficulty with levels of PEEP above 10 cm $H_2O$ is that if alveolar pressure exceeds the pulmonary arterial pressure, the catheter tip may reflect airway pressure rather than vascular pressures. Theoretically, the wedge pressure will reflect left atrial pressure if the wedged catheter tip is located in a portion of the lung where pulmonary arterial and pulmonary venous pressures exceed the alveolar pressure (zone 3) (1, 14). If the catheter tip is in an area where alveolar pressure exceeds venous pressure when pulmonary arterial flow is occluded with balloon inflation, the recorded pressure will be airway pressure rather than pulmonary artery pressure. If the catheter is located in zone 3, the wedge catheter can look through the pulmonary vasculature to sense left atrial pressure. Thus, to have an accurate indication of left atrial pressure, the pulmonary artery catheter must be in a zone 3 area.

Usually, the flow-directed pulmonary artery catheter migrates to zone 3, and the wedge pressure accurately reflects left atrial pressure (1). If PEEP is increased, it is possible that the zone 3 area, where the catheter was initially placed, may become a zone 2 area, where alveolar pressure exceeds venous pressure. Although this does not happen very often, it has been shown experimentally that if the tip of the pulmonary artery catheter is at or below the left atrium, the mean wedge pressure at end-expiration still reflects left atrial pressure, even with levels of PEEP up to 30 cm $H_2O$ (17). Therefore, it is reasonable to confirm the position of the catheter tip with an anteroposterior portable chest roentgenogram and, if necessary, a lateral chest radiograph (1). When a question arises concerning the location of the catheter tip, there are a few maneuvers that can be done to verify zone 3 conditions (Table 23.1). (18) For wedge pressure tracings outside zone 3, the wedge contour appears unusually smooth and the pulmonary artery end-diastolic pressure tends to be lower than the balloon-occlusion pressure. In zones 1 and 2, changes in the wedge pressure tend to follow alveolar rather than left atrial pressure. Thus, the swings in the wedge pressure during ventilation with positive pressure are unusually wide because only half or less of the change in static airway pressure (peak greater than pressure) transmits to the pleural spaces, left atrium, and intrathoracic vessels. For the same reason, a trial of PEEP reduction causes a fall in

**TABLE 23.1**
**CHECKLIST FOR VERIFYING POSITION OF PULMONARY ARTERIAL CATHETER**[a]

| Condition | Zone 3 | Zone 1 or 2 |
|---|---|---|
| Respiratory variation of PW | $\frac{1}{2}$ $\Delta$ Palv | $> \frac{1}{2}$ $\Delta$ Palv |
| PW contour | Cardiac ripple | Unnaturally smooth |
| Catheter tip location | LA level or below | Above LA level |
| Decrease PEEP trial | $\Delta$PW 1.2 PEEP | $\Delta$PW $> \frac{1}{2}$ $\Delta$PEEP |
| PPAD vs. PW | PPAD $>$ PW | PPAD  PW |

From Marini JJ: Obtaining meaningful data from the Swan-Ganz catheter. *Respir Care* 30:572, 1985.
[a] PW, wedge pressure; Palv, static airway pressure; LA, left atrium; PEEP, positive end-expiratory pressure; PPAD, pulmonary artery diastolic pressure.

the wedge pressure of unexpected magnitude (more than half the PEEP decrement) when the catheter tip is in zone 1 or 2 (Table 23.1) (18).

## CLINICAL INDICATIONS FOR PULMONARY ARTERY CATHETERIZATION

The most common clinical conditions for which pulmonary artery catheterization is used in intensive care units include acute pulmonary edema, shock, and management of patients after cardiac or major vascular surgery (1, 9).

### ACUTE CARDIOGENIC PULMONARY EDEMA

In general, acute cardiogenic pulmonary edema is accompanied by either systemic hypertension or hypotension. Indications for pulmonary artery catheterization depend mainly on the patient's systemic blood pressure. The diagnosis of cardiogenic pulmonary edema in the setting of systemic hypertension is nearly always accompanied by physical findings that point to left ventricular failure as the cause of the pulmonary edema (11). Treatment of the heart failure almost always results in prompt improvement, making it unnecessary to insert a pulmonary artery catheter for diagnosis or management. In fact, the pulmonary arterial wedge pressure may return to the normal range before the pulmonary artery catheter can be inserted (19). Treatment of the acute pulmonary edema does not require pulmonary artery catheterization in these patients unless hemodynamic instability develops (11).

In contrast, patients with acute pulmonary edema in association with systemic hypotension secondary to

an acute myocardial infarction present more difficult problems. A number of studies have documented that the hemodynamic profiles of patients within this group may vary considerably. Some patients will have markedly elevated left ventricular end-diastolic pressures in association with a very low cardiac output, while others may have a much more moderate elevation in the pulmonary arterial wedge pressure and better ventricular function (11, 20). Occasionally, patients thought to have left ventricular failure will be found to have noncardiogenic pulmonary edema. Rational decisions regarding the use of vasopressors, vasodilators, and volume replacement can best be made with knowledge of the left ventricular filling pressure and systemic vascular resistance (9, 11)

### ACUTE NONCARDIOGENIC PULMONARY EDEMA

There are a number of reasons why pulmonary arterial catheterization may be indicated in most patients with suspected noncardiogenic pulmonary edema. First, differentiation of cardiogenic from noncardiogenic pulmonary edema can be difficult both radiographically (21) and clinically. In one study, the clinical diagnosis of noncardiogenic pulmonary edema was substantiated on pulmonary artery catheterization in only 56% of patients (22). In addition, some patients who have primary lung injury also may have a mild elevation in the pulmonary arterial wedge pressure that contributes to the pulmonary edema (23). Therefore, in many patients with pulmonary edema that appears to be of a noncardiac origin, it is reasonable to obtain pulmonary hemodynamic measurements to be certain that the diagnosis is correct.

The management of certain patients with noncardiogenic pulmonary edema is facilitated by hemodynamic measurements (23). This is particularly true in patients with sepsis in whom systemic hypotension and acute respiratory failure occur together. In this setting, the goals of management are to produce optimal cardiac output and systemic perfusion with as little increase as possible in the pulmonary arterial wedge pressure. This balance can be achieved with the use of invasive hemodynamic monitoring, although there is no definite proof that measurement of these physiologic variables ultimately results in an improved patient outcome (9).

Most patients with ARDS should have their pulmonary artery catheters removed within 3 to 4 days to reduce the risk of secondary infection and to convert the central line to a triple-lumen catheter that can be used for the administration of fluids, antibiotics, and hyperalimentation. There are some patients with ARDS who are very stable hemodynamically and in whom the oxygenation defect is not very severe. Some of these patients can be managed without pulmonary arterial catheterization (24, 25).

## SHOCK

One of the original justifications for pulmonary artery catheterization rests on the evidence that some patients with acute myocardial infarction may have a normal central venous pressure in the presence of an elevated pulmonary arterial wedge pressure (26). Also, some patients with an acute myocardial infarction and shock are found to have low left ventricular filling pressures that can be best treated with volume expansion to increase preload. Thus, the argument has been that pulmonary arterial catheterization helps provide information that cannot be obtained by clinical examination alone. In fact, one study confirmed that clinical assessment of hemodynamic variables in patients with shock prior to insertion of a pulmonary artery catheter was poor (22). In patients with pulmonary arterial wedge pressures greater than 18 mm Hg, the wedge pressure was predicted correctly only 35% of the time. Similarly, in the same group of patients with a measured cardiac index of less than 2.2 liters/minute/m$^2$, the cardiac index was predicted correctly only 55% of the time.

### MANAGEMENT OF PATIENTS AFTER CARDIAC AND MAJOR VASCULAR SURGERY

The indications for pulmonary artery catheterization in patients who have had cardiac surgery are controversial (9). In some institutions, for example, clinicians insert pulmonary artery catheters in all patients who undergo cardiac surgery; in other institutions, even cardiac transplant patients do not have routine pulmonary artery pressure monitoring. However, available data regarding risks versus benefits of pulmonary artery catheterization after cardiac surgery support a more selective approach, reserving pulmonary artery catheterization for patients with a reduced left ventricular ejection fraction (9). Moreover, one study demonstrated that the pulmonary arterial wedge pressure was not a reliable indicator of left ventricular preload in the immediate period following coronary artery bypass surgery (27).

Patients who have undergone major vascular surgery often have coexistent cardiac and renal disease that places them at high risk for postoperative hemodynamic instability. In addition, it is common for these patients to have large collections of peritoneal fluid and a diffuse systemic capillary leak following cross-clamping of the aorta, so they have major fluid shifts postoperatively. Because these patients are at high risk of postoperative heart failure, volume overload respiratory failure, and renal failure, they may benefit from pulmonary artery catheterization, although the decision should be made on a case-by-case basis (9).

## HOW TO DETERMINE THE PHYSIOLOGIC BASIS FOR SHOCK

Shock is present if evidence of multisystem organ hypoperfusion is apparent. Evidence of hypoperfusion obtained during the rapid initial clinical evaluation of a patient in shock may include tachycardia, a low mean blood pressure, an altered mental status, and a decreased urine output. There are several causes of shock that need to be differentiated as early as possible in the patient's clinical course.

A systemic approach to determining the etiology of shock is helpful in the initial diagnosis and management of the hypotensive patient. This approach acknowledges that shock is identified in most patients by systemic hypotension and that mean arterial blood pressure is the product of cardiac output and the systemic vascular resistance (28). Accordingly, hypotension may be due to reduced cardiac output or reduced systemic vascular resistance. Initial examination of the hypotensive patient seeks to determine if cardiac output is reduced or not. High cardiac output hypotension is most often signaled by a large pulse pressure, a low diastolic pressure, warm extremities, fever (or hypothermia), and leukocytosis (or leukopenia); these clinical findings strongly suggest a working diagnosis of septic shock, the initial treatment for which is antimicrobial therapy combined with adequate, but not excessive, expansion of the vascular volume (Table 23.2).

By contrast, a low cardiac output is indicated by a small pulse pressure and cool extremities with poor nail bed return. In this case, the clinical need is to determine if the heart is too full or not. A heart that is too full in a hypotensive patient is signaled by elevated jugular venous pressure (JVP), peripheral edema, crepitations on lung auscultation, a large heart with extra heart sounds (S$_3$, S$_4$), chest pain, ischemic changes on the electrocardiogram (ECG), and a chest radiograph showing a large heart with dilated upper lobe vessels and pulmonary edema. These findings suggest cardiogenic shock, most often due to ischemic heart disease, and are generally absent when the low cardiac output is due to hypovolemia (Table 23.2). Then, clinical examination reveals manifestations of blood loss (hematemesis, tarry stools, abdominal distention, reduced hematocrit, trauma, or manifestations of dehydration (reduced tissue turgor, vomiting or diarrhea, negative fluid balance). This distinction between cardiogenic

## TABLE 23.2
### CHARACTERISTICS OF SEPTIC, CARDIOGENIC, AND HYPOVOLEMIC SHOCK

| Abnormalities in Shock | Septic | Cardiogenic | Hypovolemic |
|---|---|---|---|
| Blood pressure | ↓ | ↓ | ↓ |
| Heart rate | ↑ | ↑ | ↑ |
| Respiratory rate | ↑ | ↑ | ↑ |
| Mentation | ↓ | ↓ | ↓ |
| Urine output | ↓ | ↓ | ↓ |
| Arterial pH | ↓ | ↓ | ↓ |
| **Is cardiac output reduced?** | | | |
| Pulse pressure | ↑ | ↓ | ↓ |
| Diastolic pressure | ↓↓↓ | ↓ | ↓ |
| Extremities/digits | Warm | Cool | Cool |
| Temperature | ↑ or ↓ | ↔ | ↔ |
| White cell count | ↑ or ↓ | ↔ | ↔ |
| Site of infection | + + | − | − |
| **Is the heart too full?** | No | Yes | No |
| Symptoms/clinical context | Sepsis/liver failure | Ischemia/infarction | Hemorrhage/dehydration |
| Jugular venous pressure | ↓ | ↑ | ↓ |
| $S_3$, $S_4$, gallop rhythm | − | + + + | − |
| Chest radiograph | Normal (early in course) | Large heart<br>↑ upper lobe flow<br>Pulmonary edema | Normal |

**What does not fit?**
Overlapping etiologies (septic + cardiogenic, septic + hypovolemic, cardiogenic + hypovolemic)

| Short list of other etiologies | *High-output hypotension* | *High right atrial pressure hypotension* | *Nonresponsive hypovolemia* |
|---|---|---|---|
| | Thyroid storm<br>Arteriovenous fistula<br>Paget's disease | Cardiac tamponade<br>Right ventricular infarction<br>Pulmonary hypertension | Adrenal insufficiency<br>Anapylaxis<br>Spinal shock |
| Obtain more information | Echocardiography, right heart catheterization | | |

From Hall JB, Schmidt GA, Wood LDH (eds): *Principles of Critical Care*, New York, McGraw-Hill, 1992, pp 1393–1395.

and hypovolemic shock allows initial therapy to focus on vasoactive drugs or on volume infusions, respectively (Table 23.2).

Whenever the clinical formulation is not obvious, it helpful to determine what does not fit. Most often, the answer is that the hypotension is due to two or more causes of shock: septic shock complicated by myocardial ischemia or hypovolemia, cardiogenic shock complicated by hypovolemia or sepsis, and hypovolemic shock masking sepsis or ischemia heart disease. At this time, more data are frequently needed, especially aided by echocardiography and and pulmonary arterial catheterization. Interpretation of the data and response to initial therapy frequently confirm the multiple causes or lead to a broader differential diagnosis of the causes of shock (Table 23.2).

### REFERENCES

1. Wiedemann HP, Matthay MA, Matthay RA: Cardiovascular-pulmonary monitoring in the intensive care unit. *Chest* 85:537–549 (pt I), 656–668 (pt II), 1984.
2. Band JD, Maki DG: Infections caused by arterial catheters used for hemodynamic monitoring *Am J Med* 67:735–741, 1979.
3. Shinozaki T, et al: Bacterial contamination of arterial lines: a prospective study. *JAMA* 249:223–227, 1983.
4. Shapiro BA: Monitoring gas exchange in acute respiratory failure. *Respir Care* 28:605–607, 1983.
5. Gardner RM: Percutaneous indwelling radial-artery catheters for monitoring cardiovascular function. *N Engl J Med* 290:1227–1231, 1974.
6. Bedford RF: Long-term radial artery cannulation: effects

on subsequent vessel function. *Crit Care Med* 6:64–67, 1978.

7. Bedford RF: Radial arterial function following percutaneous cannulation with 18- and 20-gauge catheters. *Anesthesiology* 47:37–39, 1977.

8. Davis FM, Stewart JM: Radial artery cannulation. *Br J Anaesth* 52:41–47, 1980.

9. Matthay MA, Chatterjee K: Bedside catheterization of the pulmonary artery: risks compared with benefits. *Ann Intern Med* 109:826–834, 1988.

10. Robin ED: The cult of the Swan-Ganz catheter: overuse and abuse of pulmonary flow catheters. *Ann Intern Med* 103:445–449, 1985.

11. Shaver JA: Hemodynamic monitoring in the critically ill patient (editorial). *N Engl J Med* 308:277–278, 1983.

12. Matthay MA: Invasive hemodynamic monitoring. *Clin Chest Med* 4:233–249, 1983.

13. Quinn K, Quebbeman EJ: Pulmonary artery pressure: monitoring in the surgical intensive care unit. *Arch Surg* 116:872–876, 1981.

14. O'Quinn R, Marini JJ: Pulmonary artery occlusion pressure: clinical physiology measurement, and interpretation. *Am Rev Respir Dis* 128:319–326, 1983.

15. Dhainault JF, Devaux J, Monsallier J: Mechanisms of decreased left ventricular preload during continuous positive pressure ventilation in ARDS. *Chest* 90:74–80, 1986.

16. Jardin F, Farcot JC, Boisante L, et al: Influence of positive end-expiratory pressure on left ventricular performance. *N Engl J Med* 304:387–392, 1981.

17. Tooker J, Huseby J, Butler J: The effect of Swan-Ganz catheter height on the wedge pressure relationship in edema during positive pressure ventilation. *Am Rev Respir Dis* 117:721–725, 1978.

18. Marini JJ: Obtaining meaningful data from the Swan-Ganz catheter. *Respir Care* 30:572–578, 1985.

19. Fein A, Goldberg S, Walhenstein M, Gershaw B, Braitman L, Liddmann M, et al: Is pulmonary artery catheterization necessary for the diagnosis of pulmonary edema? *Am Rev Respir Dis* 129:1006–1009, 1984.

20. Chatterjee K, Swan HJ, Kaushik VS, et al: Effects of vasodilator therapy for severe pump failure in acute myocardial infarction on short-term and late prognosis. *Circulation* 53:797–802, 1976.

21. Aberle DR: Hydrostatic versus increased permeability pulmonary edema: diagnosis based on radiographic criteria in critically ill patients. *Radiology* 168:73–79, 1988.

22. Connors AF Jr, McCaffree DR, Gray BA: Evaluation of right-heart catheterization in the critically ill patient without acute myocardial infarction. *N Engl J Med* 308:263–267, 1983.

23. Matthay MA, Broaddus VC: Fluid and hemodynamic management in acute lung injury. *Sem Respir Crit Care Med* 15:271–288, 1994.

24. Matthay MA, Eschenbacher WL, Goetzl EJ: Elevated concentrations of leukotriene $D_4$ in pulmonary edema fluid of patients with the ARDS. *J Clin Immunol* 4:479–483, 1984.

25. Rinaldo JE: Indicators of risk, course, and prognosis in ARDS. *Annu Rev Respir Dis* 133:343–346, 1986.

26. Swan HJ, Ganz TW, Forrester J, et al: Catheterization of the heart in man with the use of a flow-directed balloon-tipped catheter. *N Engl J Med* 283:447–451, 1970.

27. Hansen RM, Viquerat CE, Matthay MA, et al: Poor correlation between pulmonary arterial wedge pressure and left ventricular end-diastolic volume after coronary artery bypass surgery. *Anesthesiology* 64:764–770, 1986.

28. Hall JB, Schmidt GA, Wood LDH (eds): *Principles of Critical Care*. New York, McGraw-Hill, 1992, pp 1393–1395.

Chapter **24**

# Sepsis and Multiple Organ Failure

**Michael A. Matthay**
**Paul M. Dorinsky**

THIS CHAPTER FOCUSES on multiple organ failure (MOF) in critically ill patients (1). Since sepsis is a major cause of MOF, the importance of infection in these patients is discussed as well. One of the earliest descriptions of MOF was written by Baue in 1975:

> The sequence of events often begins with a period of shock or circulatory failure at some point during the initial injury, accompanied sooner or later by failure of ventilation and the need for ventilatory support. This may be followed by renal failure, hepatic failure (jaundice and decreasing albumin levels), gastrointestinal failure (stress ulcers and gastrointestinal bleeding), and metabolic failure (decrease in lean body mass and weakness due to progressive catabolism). Our ability to support a single system that has failed, transiently at least, is reasonably good. The support of two or more failed units, however, stresses our knowledge and capability. Survivors of multiple systems failure are infrequent (2).

Since this description, a number of medical and surgical studies have reported a high mortality rate associated with MOF in critically ill patients. Sepsis syndrome is clearly the most frequently encountered clinical problem associated with the development of MOF (2). Some patients who have MOF, however, do not seem to have a clear-cut infectious etiology. For example, patients who have been treated with interleukin-2 for malignant disorders frequently develop renal failure, gastrointestinal failure, neurologic disturbances, and sometimes even acute respiratory failure. These observations suggest that release of potent endogenous humoral factors during noninfectious disorders (e.g., severe hypovolemic shock) may produce the clinical features of the sepsis syndrome without necessarily being related to infection. Finally, it is also possible that primary lung injury itself can lead to the development of nonpulmonary organ failure (1, 2). In any case, sepsis often complicates MOF, even if sepsis is not the initial clinical disorder (3, 4).

In this chapter, the definition and epidemiology of MOF is discussed, with an emphasis on specific guidelines for defining the failure or dysfunction of the respiratory, cardiovascular, renal, hepatic, central nervous, and hematologic systems. In the second part of the chapter, the pathogenesis of MOF is considered. In the third section, guidelines are provided for the management of patients with MOF, with an emphasis on guidelines for therapy with fluids, colloid, blood, and vasoactive agents, as well as antiinflammatory agents. In the final section, the prevention and early recognition of MOF and sepsis syndrome are reviewed.

## DEFINITION AND EPIDEMIOLOGY

MOF is often a major complication in patients with shock from sepsis, major trauma, severe pancreatitis, drug overdose, or thermal injury (1–6). The extent to which an individual organ is likely to be damaged in these clinical settings depends on numerous factors, including age, preexisting medical illnesses, severity of illness on admission to the intensive care unit, and the specific precipitating event (1, 4, 5). The clinical features of organ dysfunction in this patient group also vary and have been defined by different criteria. Specifically, organ dysfunction in critically ill patients ranges from minor biochemical abnormalities to irreversible organ failure. Nonetheless, the incidence of renal, gastrointestinal, hepatic, central nervous, and hematologic failure has been studied, especially in patients with acute respiratory failure. The definition and incidence of acute respiratory failure are discussed after considering criteria for failure of the nonpulmonary organ systems.

### CARDIOVASCULAR FAILURE

The incidence of cardiovascular failure among critically ill patients varies from 10 to 23% (1). Although a uniform definition in critically ill patients has yet to be established, most clinicians agree that cardiovascular failure exists when one or more of the following are present: (*a*) mean arterial pressure less than or equal to 60 mm Hg, (*b*) cardiac index of 2 liters/minute/m$^2$ or less, or (*c*) reversible ventricular fibrillation or asystole. This definition could include a patient with an acute myocardial infarction and severe pump failure. It could also include a patient with septic shock who has a high cardiac output, a low systemic vascular resistance, and a low mean arterial blood pressure.

Cardiovascular failure, therefore, includes those disturbances that cause a major decrease in myocardial function as well as those clinical disorders associated with abnormalities in the peripheral circulation.

Although human septic shock is usually characterized by elevated cardiac output and reduced systemic vascular resistance, it may also be associated with a decrease in the left ventricular ejection fraction. In addition, studies have shown that septic patients have increased left ventricular ejection fraction, increased end-systolic and end-diastolic volumes, normal or decreased stroke work, and decreased right ventricular ejection fraction. Among patients who survive, these cardiovascular parameters normalize (7).

The mechanism of myocardial dysfunction during sepsis is not entirely known (7, 8). Nonetheless, serum obtained from patients with septic shock has been shown to depress myocardial cell contractility in vitro. Moreover, evidence suggests that tumor necrosis factor (TNF), an important humoral mediator of sepsis, is capable of depressing myocardial cell contractility. It is likely that one or more of these myocardial depressant substances are responsible for the reduction in ejection fracture and the ventricular volume changes that occur during sepsis.

Two other important features of sepsis syndrome are the abnormal vasodilation of the systemic circulation and the abnormalities of peripheral oxygen uptake. These issues are discussed in the section on pathogenesis.

### RENAL FAILURE

Renal dysfunction is a frequent complication in critically ill patients (40 to 55% incidence) and is manifested by reductions in urine output and a rise in the serum urea and creatinine values (1, 8). Specifically, renal failure may be defined in this patient group as a serum creatinine value above 2 mg/dl and a urine output below 600 ml/24 hours (4).

The three most important risk factors for the development of renal failure in critically ill patients are hypotension, sepsis, and nephrotoxic drugs (9). Acute nonoliguric renal failure associated primarily with nephrotoxic drugs has a better prognosis than acute oliguric renal failure that occurs with septic shock or after major cardiovascular surgery.

### GASTROINTESTINAL FAILURE

Alterations in gastrointestinal tract function are estimated to occur in 30% of critically ill patients (1, 8). The pathologic basis for gastrointestinal dysfunction appears to be both an alteration in microvascular permeability and mucosal ischemia. For example, TNF causes necrosis of intestinal villi when infused into experimental animals. These morphologic observations suggest a pathologic basis for the functional abnormalities of the gastrointestinal tract that occur in critically ill patients (10).

The clinical features of gastrointestinal tract dysfunction vary and include hemorrhage, ileus, malabsorption (e.g., inability to tolerate enteral feedings), and, occasionally, acalculous cholecystitis or pancreatitis. Among these complications, gastrointestinal bleeding is common, but it is difficult to quantify. Gastrointestinal blood loss in excess of 1 g/dL of hemoglobin per 24 hours is generally accepted to be clinically significant, however (11).

An intact gastrointestinal tract mucosa provides an essential barrier to the entry of bacteria into the systemic circulation. Since this mucosal integrity is frequently impaired in critically ill patients, bacteria may translocate or migrate from the bowel lumen into the peritoneal cavity or to regional gastrointestinal lymph nodes and to the portosystemic circulation. To the extent that this occurs, bacterial translocation may propagate septic shock and result in further organ dysfunction.

## HEPATIC FAILURE

Fulminant hepatic failure as a feature of organ failure in critically ill patients is uncommon and occurs in less than 10% of critically ill patients (1, 8). By contrast, reversible elevations in serum transaminases and elevations in serum bilirubin or clotting parameters are common and may be found in as many as 95% of critically ill patients. Criteria for hepatic failure in critically ill patients are evolving. Nonetheless, elevations in serum bilirubin that exceed 4 to 5 mg/dl, a prothrombin time of more than 1.5 times control, and a serum albumin level below 2 g/dl indicate significant hepatic dysfunction (4, 12).

As a complication of septic shock or other critical illnesses, hepatic dysfunction is of more than academic interest. The liver is an important reticuloendothelial organ whose function is also altered when the liver is damaged. For example, fibronectin, an opsonin that is important in the maintenance of host defense, is frequently decreased in critically ill patients. Mortality data indicate the importance of intact hepatic function to the outcome of critically ill patients. Mortality from septic shock approaches 100% in patients with severe hepatic damage. Also, when hepatic failure occurs in the setting of acute respiratory failure, the prognosis for recovery from the acute lung injury is poor (12). Thus, evidence is accumulating to suggest that the various systemic organs are not merely targets of damage during critical illnesses. Rather, once these organs are damaged, their dysfunction has a substantial impact on host defense and the propagation of the underlying injury.

## CENTRAL NERVOUS SYSTEM FAILURE

Abnormalities of central nervous system (CNS) function have been frequently described in critically ill patients (5, 8, 13). For example, CNS dysfunction, including disorientation, confusion, agitation, obtundation, and seizures, occurs commonly in septic patients. One study reported a 9% incidence of CNS dysfunction, defined as an inability to follow simple commands, in 106 patients with intraabdominal sepsis. By contrast, another study, using an altered sensorium as the criterion for CNS dysfunction, reported a 33% incidence of CNS abnormalities in sepsis (1).

Use of the Glasgow Coma Scale helps to provide a more uniform, standard approach to defining CNS function (13). This scale provides a measurement of visual, motor, and verbal (e.g., orientation) responsiveness (Table 24.1). The Glasgow Coma Scale can be used in intubated patients and is considered abnormal in critically ill patients with a score of less than 6 to 8 (maximal score = 15). Using this criterion, abnormalities of CNS function have been found to occur in 7 to 30% of critically ill patients. The factors that underlie CNS dysfunction in this patient population are unclear

**TABLE 24.1**
**GLASGOW COMA SCALE**

| Parameter | Score |
|---|---|
| Eye opening | |
| Spontaneous | 4 |
| To speech | 3 |
| To pain | 2 |
| None | 1 |
| Motor response | |
| Obeys verbal commands | 6 |
| Responds appropriately to painful stimuli (localizes pain) | 5 |
| Withdraws to pain leg, flexion withdrawal | 4 |
| Decorticate posturing | 3 |
| Decerebrate posturing | 2 |
| No response | 1 |
| Verbal responses | |
| Oriented and conversant | 5 |
| Disoriented but conversant | 4 |
| Inappropriate response | 3 |
| Incomprehensible sounds | 2 |
| No response | 1 |

but may include the production of false neurotransmitters, direct microvascular injury, and brain ischemia from global or regional reductions in cerebral blood flow (13).

## HEMATOLOGIC FAILURE

Hematologic abnormalities occur with a frequency that ranges from 0 to 26% among critically ill patients (1, 8). There is little clinical consensus regarding the definition of hematologic failure in this patient group. A number of parameters including the platelet count, the white blood cell count, fibrinogen levels, and coagulation parameters have been used to assess the adequacy of the hematologic system in these patients. Despite some differences, most clinical studies use criteria that include a platelet count of 50,000 cells/$\mu$liter or less, a white blood cell count of 1000 cells/$\mu$liter or less, and a fibrinogen level below 100 mg/dl to define hematologic failure. Obviously, severe neutropenia decreases host resistance to infection while thrombocytopenia increases the risk of bleeding and the need for transfusion of blood products. Disseminated intravascular coagulation is sometimes associated with acute lung injury (14).

## ACUTE RESPIRATORY FAILURE

The incidence of acute respiratory failure in critically ill patients varies considerably depending on the criteria used to define failure of the respiratory system. Although the term adult respiratory distress syndrome (ARDS) has been useful for designating the clinical syndrome, a more quantitative definition has been needed. A quantitative scoring system for assessing acute lung injury was proposed and has been used in several studies (Table 24.2) (15). This system is based on the severity of hypoxemia and the extent of infiltrates on the chest radiograph. If the patient is mechanically ventilated, abnormalities in the compliance of the lungs and the level of positive end-expiratory pressure are also scored. With the use of these criteria patients can be classified as having mild, moderate, or severe lung injury (15).

## SPECIAL CONSIDERATIONS

Although not unique to any particular organ system, a number of serious problems exist with respect to the MOF syndrome. Since there is a general lack of consensus regarding the criteria for individual organ system failure, the incidence of organ failure varies among different study centers and contributes to the general confusion in this area. Until uniform criteria

### TABLE 24.2
#### COMPONENTS OF THE ACUTE LUNG INJURY SCORE

| | Value |
|---|---|
| **Chest radiograph score** | |
| No alveolar consolidation | 0 |
| Alveolar consolidation in 1 quadrant | 1 |
| Alveolar consolidations in 2 quadrants | 2 |
| Alveolar consolidation in 3 quadrants | 3 |
| Alveolar consolidation in all quadrants | 4 |
| **Hypoxemia score** | |
| $Pao_2/Fio_2$ 300 | 0 |
| $Pao_2/Fio_2$ 225–299 | 1 |
| $Pao_2/Fio_2$ 175–224 | 2 |
| $Pao_2/Fio_2$ 100–174 | 3 |
| $Pao_2/Fio_2$ <100 | 4 |
| **Respiratory system compliance score** (when ventilated) | |
| Compliance 80 ml/cm $H_2O$ | 0 |
| Compliance 60–79 ml/cm $H_2O$ | 1 |
| Compliance 40–59 ml/cm $H_2O$ | 2 |
| Compliance 20–39 ml/cm $H_2O$ | 3 |
| Compliance 19 ml/cm $H_2O$ | 4 |
| **Positive end-expiratory pressure (PEEP)** score (when ventilated) | |
| PEEP 5 cm $H_2O$ | 0 |
| PEEP 6–8 cm $H_2O$ | 1 |
| PEEP 9–11 cm $H_2O$ | 2 |
| PEEP 12–14 cm $H_2O$ | 3 |
| PEEP 15 cm $H_2O$ | 4 |

The final value is obtained by dividing the aggregate sum by the number of components that were used.

| | Score |
|---|---|
| No lung injury | 0 |
| Mild to modern lung injury | 0.1–2.5 |
| Severe lung injury (ARDS) | >2.5 |

From Murray JF, Matthay MA, Luce J, Flick MR: An expanded definition of the adult respiratory distress syndrome. *Am Rev Respir Dis* 138:720, 1988.

are established, the true incidence and natural history of MOF will remain unclear. These problems are further compounded by the lack of uniform diagnostic criteria for the definition of septic shock and acute lung injury. The net effect of this diagnostic imprecision is that patients with dissimilar critical illnesses are often inappropriately grouped together. However, a number of recent cooperative efforts have been undertaken to reach consensus on this issue and more precisely define the criteria for organ system failure in this patient group (16).

Despite the current uncertainties, a number of important issues regarding MOF among critically ill patients have been resolved. First, the number of involved organ systems has a significant impact on patient mortality (5). Mortality for a single organ failure ranges from 15 to 30% and from 45 to 55% for failure of two organ systems. By contrast, mortality exceeds 80% when three or more organ systems have failed and reaches 100% if the MOF persists beyond 4 hospital days (5). Second, certain organ systems (e.g., heart, kidney, lung, and liver) are involved more frequently than other organ systems. Third, although individual organs may be preferentially injured in specific situations (e.g., renal failure and respiratory failure in septic shock), MOF may occur after acute cardiorespiratory failure of any etiology. Finally, early detection and treatment of the underlying cause of the MOF may offer the best hope for treatment of this potentially fatal disorder (10, 17, 18).

## PATHOGENESIS

The MOF syndrome occurs in a variety of clinical settings including infection, severe hypotension, and multiple trauma. Prototypic among the risk factors for MOF is septic shock. Although a scientific consensus has yet to be reached, evidence is accumulating to suggest that MOF during sepsis, and perhaps other critical illnesses, is due to widespread organ injury that is caused by activated inflammatory cells and a variety of humoral mediators (8, 10, 19). Any theory regarding the pathogenesis of MOF during sepsis or other acute catastrophic illnesses must take into account the abnormalities in systemic gas exchange that occur in these disorders and that are manifested as an abnormal relationship between oxygen uptake and oxygen delivery ($\dot{Q}O_2$).

As illustrated in Figure 24.1, whole-body oxygen uptake is normally maintained at a constant level over wide ranges of oxygen delivery (20). This is accomplished by means of local compensatory mechanisms, which include increases in oxygen extraction and increases in recruitable capillary reserves (e.g., the cross-sectional area of perfused capillaries within an individual organ). Once these mechanisms for the preservation of a constant oxygen uptake are exhausted, $\dot{V}O_2$ falls in a manner that is directly related to the reductions in oxygen delivery. The level of oxygen delivery below which oxygen uptake begins to fall is termed $\dot{Q}O_{2c}$ (i.e., critical threshold for oxygen delivery), and it signifies the level of $\dot{Q}O_2$ below which oxygen supply-demand imbalances exist (20). Some recent data indicate that this imbalance in oxygen supply and demand may sometimes occur because the methods for measur-

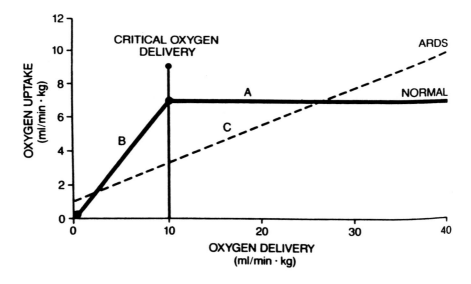

**FIGURE 24.1.** Oxygen uptake and oxygen delivery ($\dot{V}O_2$ and $\dot{Q}O_2$) relationships in normal subjects and in patients with ARDS. $\dot{V}O_2$ is regulated by whole body metabolic demand and is normally constant over a wide range of $\dot{Q}O_2$. This is accomplished by local compensatory mechanisms, including increases in oxygen extraction and increases in the cross-sectional density of perfused capillaries. Once these compensatory mechanisms are exhausted, further reductions in $\dot{Q}O_2$ are accompanied by reduc- tions in $\dot{V}O_2$ (*line B*). The $\dot{Q}O_2$ below which $\dot{V}O_2$ begins to decrease is termed the critical threshold for $\dot{Q}O_2$ ($\dot{Q}O_{2c}$) In contrast to the normal situation, $\dot{V}O_2$ is dependent on $\dot{Q}O_2$ at nearly all levels of $\dot{Q}O_2$ in ARDS. This finding indicates that an oxygen supply-demand imbalance may exist at all levels of $\dot{Q}O_2$ in ARDS patients. (From Dorinsky PM, Gadek JE: Mechanisms of multiple nonpulmonary organ failure in ARDS. *Chest* 96:885, 1989.)

ing the $\dot{V}_{O_2}$ and $\dot{Q}_{O_2}$ in the intensive care unit may not always be accurate (21).

In contrast to the situation described above for the normal $\dot{V}_{O_2}/\dot{Q}_{O_2}$ relationship, the relationship between $\dot{V}_{O_2}$ and $\dot{Q}_{O_2}$ in critically ill patients is often markedly altered (22, 23). For example, in many critically ill patients, $\dot{V}_{O_2}$ depends on $\dot{Q}_{O_2}$ at nearly all levels of oxygen delivery, including levels that would normally be more than adequate to meet tissue metabolic demands. These abnormalities indicate that oxygen supply-demand imbalances exist at all levels of $\dot{Q}_{O_2}$ in these patients.

There are a number of mechanisms that may explain both the nonpulmonary organ failure and the $\dot{V}_{O_2}/\dot{Q}_{O_2}$ abnormalities that occur in this patient population. These may be divided into two broad categories (a) altered blood flow distribution and (b) endothelial or parenchymal injury (8).

### ALTERED BLOOD FLOW DISTRIBUTION

Oxygenated blood that bypasses nutrient capillary beds could alter $\dot{V}_{O_2}/\dot{Q}_{O_2}$ relationships and cause organ damage. This sequence of events may result from (a) a redistribution of cardiac output to organs with inherently low oxygen extraction fractions (e.g., skeletal muscle); (b) an increase in the fraction of cardiac output that bypasses nutrient capillaries through anatomic, precapillary arteriovenous channels (e.g., shunt flow); or (c) a reduction in recruitable capillary reserves that would prevent effective compensation for reductions in oxygen supply (23).

### ENDOTHELIAL OR PARENCHYMAL INJURY

Endothelial injury may be accompanied by local edema formation with subsequent increases in diffusion distances for oxygen and reductions in capillary surface area (e.g., reduced recruitable capillary reserves). Alternatively, direct parenchymal cell injury may impair the ability of individual organs to utilize oxygen by interfering with cellular oxidative metabolism.

Little direct experimental evidence exists to support the idea that either MOF or the systemic $\dot{V}_{O_2}/\dot{Q}_{O_2}$ alterations associated with ARDS, septic shock, and other critical illnesses are caused by primary alterations in the distribution of cardiac output (e.g., increased anatomic shunt flow or increased blood flow to organs with low oxygen extraction). However, there is evidence to indicate that nonpulmonary organs are damaged both structurally and functionally during critical illness, and this damage often includes alterations in individual organ $\dot{V}_{O_2}/\dot{Q}_{O_2}$ matching (20–23).

### POSSIBLE MECHANISMS OF INJURY

The best-studied experimental model for MOF has been septic shock that is produced either by live bacterial organisms or by endotoxin. In this context, structural studies of endothelial monolayers exposed to endotoxin show that these cells undergo contraction, become pyknotic, and finally die. Likewise, it is known that endotoxin or live bacteria can induce the release of various mediators, each of which can cause cell injury (24). Considerable experimental evidence indicates that both cyclooxygenase and lipoxygenase products of arachidonic acid metabolism participate in the hemodynamic, pathologic, and metabolic derangements that occur during sepsis. Also, complement is activated in sepsis, and some evidence indicates that the elevated levels of a C5a derivative correlate with the severity of hypotension and metabolic acidosis during sepsis. There has also been considerable interest in the possible role of cytokines (e.g., TNF) in mediating systemic organ injury during sepsis (10, 25). In this regard, antibodies to TNF can prevent the development of endotoxin-mediated hypotension, fibrin deposition, and death in animals. Likewise, anti-TNF antibody prevented shock and death in baboons given live *Escherichia coli* organisms, but only if they were given 2 hours before the bacteremia (26).

Finally, many studies (but not all) suggest a central role for neutrophils in mediating both systemic and pulmonary injury from bacteria or endotoxin (10). Along this line, monoclonal antibodies to the adherence-promoting leukocyte glycoprotein complex (i.e., CD18) reduce systemic organ injury and improve survival from hemorrhagic shock in many species of animals. Although many schemes have been proposed to explain the mechanism by which neutrophils cause tissue injury, recent work suggests that there may be important interactions between elastases and toxic oxygen radicals elaborated by neutrophils (10, 27). Thus, in septic shock, endotoxin and bacteria may directly damage endothelial cells, promote the activation of polymorphonuclear leukocytes and mononuclear cells, as well as mediate the release of numerous proinflammatory agents (e.g., kinins, prostaglandins, complement, and monokines). Acting in concert, these events culminate in widespread organ injury (10).

### MANAGEMENT OF THE PATIENT WITH MULTIPLE ORGAN FAILURE

Critically ill patients at risk for developing MOF generally present with one or more of the following clinical problems: shock (hypovolemic, cardiac, or septic), acute respiratory failure, or major alterations in mental status. These clinical problems initially require a prompt therapeutic response to stabilize the patient. In general, initial management is directed toward maintaining an adequate blood pressure and supporting gas exchange (28). For example, patients with hypovolemic shock, either from trauma or from gastrointestinal bleeding, require rapid intravascular volume expansion with blood. Likewise, patients who have severe alterations in mental status with failure to protect the airway and/or progressive respiratory failure require prompt endotracheal intubation and mechanical ventilation. The physician caring for critically ill patients must recognize that the initial priority must be to stabilize the patient's circulatory and respiratory status. For example, the decision to insert a pulmonary arterial catheter should not take precedence over initial management of the hypotension and respiratory failure (28, 29). Once the patient is stabilized and appropriate support has been given to the circulatory and respiratory systems, a careful assessment of the likely cause of the patient's condition should be undertaken.

A logical starting point in the evaluation of critically ill patients is to search for the usual causes of shock, which include sepsis, cardiac failure (especially acute myocardial infarction), gastrointestinal bleeding, acute pancreatitis, drug overdose, and occult bleeding from recent trauma. However, one must always maintain a high index of suspicion of septicemia. There should be a low threshold for obtaining blood cultures and appropriate cultures of other possible sources of infection. In addition, patients with even presumptive evidence for infection should be promptly given broad-spectrum antibiotics. Given these general supportive measures, the remainder of this section is devoted to a discussion of specific issues related to support of the circulatory system.

## GUIDELINES FOR FLUID THERAPY

With the exception of patients with acute blood loss, for whom there is a need to transfuse blood to maintain the hematocrit between 25 and 35%, most patients also need crystalloid or colloid therapy (28). Most medical and surgical centers favor the use of crystalloid in preference to colloid for volume expansion. This preference is based, in part, on the fact that crystalloid, unlike colloid, can restore both the intravascular and the interstitial component of the extracellular fluid space. Some physicians do administer colloid in an attempt to maintain circulating plasma protein osmotic pressure, but large volumes of colloid are often needed to achieve this objective, and the clearance of infused protein from the intravascular space is usually quite rapid (28). Despite the advantages of crystalloid over colloid, red

blood cells remain the ideal volume expander because they have the advantage of both increasing oxygen transport to the tissues as well as maintaining intravascular volume (28).

The appropriate guidelines for fluid therapy depend on the cause of the patient's shock. For the patient with an acute myocardial infarction, fluid replacement should be titrated to maintain the pulmonary arterial wedge pressure between 15 and 20 mm Hg. By contrast, for patients with hypovolemic shock, traumatic shock, or septic shock, an increase in the central venous pressure or pulmonary arterial wedge pressure to 15 to 20 mm Hg may not be optimal. For example, in one study that examined volume resuscitation in patients with septic shock, the investigators found that increases in pulmonary arterial wedge pressure beyond 11 to 12 mm Hg did not result in a higher cardiac output (28).

Ideally, optimal fluid resuscitation in any form of shock should include the restoration of euvolemia. Euvolemia is often difficult to define in critically ill patients. In addition, the adjustment of fluid therapy will depend on the use of vasoactive agents (28). Finally, although invasive hemodynamic monitoring with a pulmonary arterial catheter is frequently used to assist in the management of patients with septic shock, no evidence suggests that this kind of monitoring changes outcome (29). Given these uncertainties, the best indices for evaluating fluid replacement therapy are the patient's acid-base status, mental status, skin perfusion, and, perhaps most importantly, urine flow and renal function. Please see Chapter 23 for further discussion of these issues.

## VASOACTIVE AGENTS

The most useful vasopressor for treating patients with septic shock is dopamine (28). Dopamine improves cardiac output through a positive chronotropic effect, an increase in preload to the heart, and an increase in contractility. This agent is particularly efficacious in septic shock because it both increases cardiac output and improves blood flow to the kidneys, when given at doses below 10 $\mu$g/kg/minute. Moreover, dopamine, in contrast to fluid replacement therapy, has the additional advantage of being able to increase cardiac output with a minimal increase in the pulmonary arterial wedge pressure (28). Finally, dopamine, unlike dobutamine, does not cause vasodilation, thus making it preferable in treatment of shock caused by factors other than primary cardiac failure.

In some patients, septic shock will be unresponsive to even high doses of dopamine. In these patients, norepinephrine can be added to increase systemic arterial pressure. Epinephrine is another catecholamine that can be used for blood pressure support in severe septic shock. In doses above 1-2 $\mu$g/minute, epinephrine causes primarily $\alpha$-stimulation. High doses of any of these potent vasopressors will cause vasoconstriction that may maintain systemic blood pressure, but blood flow to the kidneys, the splanchnic bed, muscles, and skin may be markedly reduced.

It is often difficult to determine the level of mean arterial pressure or cardiac output that is optimal in septic shock. In general, it is best to try to adjust the mean arterial pressure and cardiac output to a level that stabilizes the metabolic acidosis associated with sepsis and improves tissue perfusion, particularly as indicated by urine flow. Some patients with severe septic shock will require high doses of dopamine, norepinephrine, or epinephrine to maintain even a barely adequate blood pressure. In most patients, vasodilator therapy is not appropriate in the setting of septic shock. In a minority of cases, patients with primary cardiac disease may present with hypotension and an elevation of systemic vascular resistance associated with septicemia. These patients may benefit from dobutamine and occasionally from low doses of afterload reduction with a vasodilator such as nitroprusside or nitroglycerin. With the exception of these patients, the use of vasodilators in the setting of MOF and septic shock remains experimental.

## ANTIINFLAMMATORY AGENTS

A large number of experimental animal model studies have demonstrated the potential value of various antiinflammatory agents for the treatment of septic shock. In many studies, however, the pharmacologic agents were effective only as prevention, not as treatment. In this regard, no antiinflammatory agents are clinically proven to decrease morbidity or improve mortality in patients with septicemia and MOF (10, 28).

Corticosteroids had been used for a number of years in the management of patients with septicemia and ARDS, based largely on the unproven clinical impression that they might be beneficial. In the past few years, however, a number of prospective, well-controlled studies have demonstrated that corticosteroids are of no therapeutic value in patients with either septic shock or ARDS (24). Specifically, these clinical studies demonstrate that corticosteroids do not prevent the development of ARDS in patients with sepsis, nor do they prevent MOF, and they have no favorable effect on mortality (see Chapter 22). Several agents are being evaluated in clinical trials currently, though none have yet been shown to be of clinical value (10, 30).

## ANTIBIOTICS

Selection of appropriate antibiotics for patients with septic shock and MOF is important. In general, a careful search for the likely source of sepsis should be undertaken and then appropriate broad-spectrum antibiotics administered. The antibiotic spectrum should include Gram-negative, enteric bacteria as well as $\beta$-lactamase producers. Effects of the agents on renal function should be considered and monitored.

## NUTRITIONAL SUPPORT

Nutritional and metabolic support is an essential part of the management of patients with MOF. Hypermetabolism develops early in the syndrome, and severe malnutrition can become a prominent feature within days after the onset of illness. The characteristics of the hypermetabolic state include (a) increases in resting energy expenditure and oxygen consumption; (b) increased use of carbohydrate, fat, and amino acids as energy substrates; and (c) increased loss of nitrogen in the urine. The hypermetabolic state results in profound protein catabolism, which is associated with a decrease in total-body protein synthesis. The mechanism for the alteration of metabolism observed in patients with MOF appears to be related to the inflammatory mediators and the hormonal response to injury. Unfortunately, these fundamental alterations in metabolism do not appear to be readily altered by therapy. However, if adequate nutritional support is not provided, then it is likely that organ dysfunction will be accelerated.

The goal of nutritional support in patients with or at risk for MOF is to prevent substrate-limited metabolism and to support, rather than attempt to alter, the hypermetabolism (see Chapter 26 for detailed discussion of nutritional support). In general, nutrition should be provided by the enteral route whenever possible. Enteral feeding eliminates cholestasis and reduces the risk of acalculous cholecystitis. Enteral alimentation may also offer some protection against gastrointestinal hemorrhage in mechanically ventilated patients.

## ETHICAL SUPPORT

It is important for physicians to assess carefully the likelihood of meaningful recovery in each critically ill patient with MOF. This assessment will depend on the natural history of the patient's underlying disease, as well as on the extent and severity of their organ failure. There is a growing awareness among the medical community that reasonable limits should be exercised by physicians and patient's families in supporting patients with critical illnesses and MOF. Studies have demonstrated that some patient groups have a particularly poor prognosis for recovery. For example, patients with ARDS following bone marrow transplantation have a less than 10% chance for recovery, while patients with a combination of hepatic failure and acute lung injury have a nearly 100% mortality. In addition, one study in two intensive care units at the University of California Medical Center has shown that withdrawal of life support was the mechanism for death in more than 50% of patients in the intensive care unit setting (31). As more information becomes available regarding prognostic indices for specific disease processes, it may help guide decisions to discontinue life support in patients who do not have a reasonable chance for meaningful recovery.

## EARLY RECOGNITION AND PREVENTION OF MULTIPLE ORGAN FAILURE

### EARLY RECOGNITION

A number of studies have identified patients who are at the highest risk for developing MOF. Patients with multiple trauma and hypotension who require emergency surgery and multiple transfusions are one common group of patients at high risk. Other patients considered to be at high risk for the development of MOF include patients with septic shock, patients with advanced chronic diseases (e.g., chronic liver disease or chronic renal failure) who are hospitalized for cardiac failure or a primary infection, and patients with the acquired immunodeficiency syndrome. Finally, patients who are immunosuppressed because of an underlying malignancy or its treatment may be at particularly high risk for MOF, both from the toxic effects of the chemotherapy as well as the increased susceptibility to septicemia.

Some investigators have evaluated clinical factors as well as easily measurable plasma factors that might predict which patients with nonpulmonary sepsis syndrome would progress to develop acute lung injury. One study investigated the possible value of a product of endothelial cells for predicting acute lung injury (4). This study was based on the premise that endothelial cell injury is a ubiquitous, early event in the pathogenesis of sepsis. In this regard, a variety of in vitro and in vivo studies have shown that both pulmonary and systemic endothelial cell injury occurs during endotoxemia and septicemia. The investigators measured plasma levels of von Willebrand factor-antigen (VWF-Ag) because VWF-Ag has been shown to be released from endothelial cells in vitro when they are injured

and because two prior clinical studies demonstrated that plasma VWF-Ag levels are markedly elevated in patients with established acute respiratory failure. In this study, plasma VWF-Ag levels were increased two-fold in patients with nonpulmonary sepsis who subsequently developed acute lung injury, compared with patients with nonpulmonary sepsis who did not progress to develop acute lung injury. Moreover, of the 15 patients who developed acute lung injury from sepsis, 14 patients died (93% mortality). An elevated VWF-Ag level above 450 (percentage of control) was predictive of the development of acute lung injury (87% sensitivity, 77% specificity) and had a positive predictive value of 80% for identifying septic patients who were not likely to survive.

More studies are needed to combine clinical factors and readily measurable plasma factors to identify those patients with sepsis syndrome who have the greatest risk of developing acute lung injury and not surviving. These patients would be reasonable candidates for early treatment with immunotherapy, antiinflammatory agents, and other new treatments that may become available in the near future.

### PREVENTION

There has been a growing interest in various approaches to reducing the risk of MOF, particularly because the outcome is so poor once a patient develops MOF. Although specific treatment approaches have yet to be established, a number of general supportive measures are available. Perhaps the most important supportive measure is prevention of infection. Nosocomial infection can be reduced by good hand washing, removal of unnecessary intravascular and urinary catheters, and the prevention of skin ulcers. Moreover, it is important to change central venous catheters in a timely manner (e.g., every 3 to 4 days) and to remain diligent to detect surgically treatable infections.

▼

### REFERENCES

1. Dorinsky PM, Matthay MA: Management of the critically ill patient with multiple organ failure. In Kelley WN (ed): *Textbook of Internal Medicine*, 2nd ed. Philadelphia, JB Lippincott, 1992, pp 1850–1856.
2. Baue AE: Multiple, progressive, or sequential systems failure. *Arch Surg* 110:779–781, 1975.
3. Bell RC, Coalson J, Smith JD, Johanson WG: Multiple organ failure and infection in adult respiratory distress syndrome. *Ann Intern Med* 99:293–298, 1983.
4. Rubin DB, Wiener-Kronish JP, Murray JF, et al: Elevated

von Willebrand factor antigen is an early plasma predictor of impending acute lung injury and death in non-pulmonary sepsis syndrome. *J Clin Invest* 86:474–480, 1990.

5. Knaus WA, Wagner DP: Multiple systems organ failure: epidemiology and prognosis. *Crit Care Clin* 5(2):221–232, 1989.

6. Montgomery AB, Stager MA, Carrico CJ, Hudson LD: Causes of mortality in patients with the adult respiratory distress syndrome. *Am Rev Respir Dis* 132:485–489, 1985.

7. Parillo JE, Parker MM, Natanson C, Suffredini AF, Danner RL, Cunnion RE, et al: Septic shock in humans. *Ann Intern Med* 113:227–242, 1990.

8. Dorinsky PM, Gadek JE: Mechanisms of multiple non-pulmonary organ failure in ARDS. *Chest* 96:885–892, 1989.

9. Kramar S, Khan F, Patel S, Seriff N: Renal failure in the respiratory intensive care unit. *Crit Care Med* 7:263–266, 1979.

10. St John RC, Dorinsky PM: Immunologic therapy for ARDS, septic shock and multiple organ failure. *Chest* 103:932–943, 1993.

11. Cook DJ, Fuller HD, Gordon MD, et al: Risk factors for gastrointestinal bleeding in critically ill patients. *N Engl J Med* 330:377–381, 1994.

12. Schwartz DB, Bone RC, Balk RA, Szidon JP: Hepatic dysfunction in the adult respiratory distress syndrome. *Chest* 95:871–875, 1989.

13. Prough DS: Neurologic critical care. *Critl Care Clin* 5, 1989.

14. Bone RC, Francis PB, Pierce AK: Intravascular coagulation associated with the adult respiratory distress syndrome. *Am J Med* 61:585–589, 1976.

15. Murray JF, Matthay MA, Luce J, Flick MR: An expanded definition of the adult respiratory distress syndrome. *Am Rev Respir Dis* l38:720–723, 1988.

16. Bone RC, Balk RA, Cerraf B, Dellinger RP, Fein AM, Knaus WA, Schein RM, Sibbaid WJ: Definitions for sepsis and organ failure and guidelines for the use of innovative therapies in sepsis. *Chest* 101:1644–1655, 1992.

17. Macho JR, Luce JM: Rational approach to the management of multiple systems organ failure. *Crit Care Clin* 5: 379–392, 1989.

18. Pinsky MR, Matuschak GM (eds): Multiple systems organ failure. *Crit Care Clin* 5: 1989.

19. Goris RJA, Boekhorst TPA, Nuytinck JKS, Gimbrere JSF: Multiple-organ failure: generalized autodestructive inflammation? *Arch Surg* 120:1109–1115, 1985.

20. Cain SM: Assessment of tissue oxygenation. *Crit Care Clin* 2:537–550, 1986.

21. Ronco JJ, Fenwick JC, Tweeddale MG, et al: Identification of the critical oxygen delivery for anaerobic metabolism in critically ill septic and nonseptic humans. *JAMA* 270: 1724–1728, 1993.

22. Danek SJ, Lynch JP, Weg JG, Dantzker DR: The dependence of oxygen uptake on oxygen delivery in the adult respiratory distress syndrome. *Am Rev Respir Dis* 122: 387–395, 1980.

23. Dorinsky PM, Costello JL, Gadek JE: Oxygen uptake–oxygen delivery relationship in non-ARDS respiratory failure. *Chest* 93:103–111, 1988.

24. Baumgartner JD, Glauser MP, McCutchan JA, et al: Prevention of Gram-negative shock and death in surgical patients by antibody to endotoxin core glycolipid. *Lancet* 2:59–63, 1985.

25. Tracey KJ, Beutler B, Lowry SF, Merryweather J, Wolpe S, Milsark JW, et al: Shock and tissue injury induced by recombinant human cachectin. *Science* 234:470–474, 1986.

26. Tracey KJ, Fong Y, Hesse DG, Manogue KR, Lee AT, Kuo GC, et al: Anti-cachectin/TNF monoclonal antibodies prevent septic shock during lethal bacteraemia. *Nature* 330:662–664, 1987.

27. Weiss SJ: Tissue destruction by neutrophils. *N Engl J Med* 320:365–376, 1989.

28. Matthay MA, Broaddus VC: Fluid and hemodynamic management in acute lung injury. *Sem Resp Crit Care Med* 15:271–288, 1994.

29. Matthay MA, Chatterjee K: Bedside catheterization of the pulmonary artery: risks compared with benefits. *Ann Intern Med* 109:826–834, 1988.

30. Bernard GR: Sepsis trials intersection of investigation, regulation, funding, and practice. *Am J Resp Crit Care Med* (*in press*, 1995).

31. Smedira N, Evans B, Grais L, et al: Withholding and withdrawing of life support from the critically ill. *N Engl J Med* 332:309–315, 1990.

Chapter **25**

# Thoracic Trauma, Surgery, and Perioperative Management

**Steven A Conrad**
**Christian Jayr**
**Eric A. Peper**

SURGICAL PROCEDURES, BOTH thoracic and extrathoracic, and thoracic trauma can adversely affect pulmonary function and result in significant morbidity and mortality. This chapter first discusses the changes in pulmonary function with general anesthesia and surgery, and the preoperative assessment and management of elective surgical patients. The common postoperative pulmonary complications seen in surgical patients are reviewed, with emphasis on identifying those groups at risk for these complications and

629

on their prevention. The chapter then focuses on the pathophysiology, diagnosis, and treatment of traumatic thoracic and pulmonary disease.

## Respiratory Effects of Anesthesia and Surgery

Postoperative pulmonary complications may be related to preoperative lung disease, effects of anesthesia on lung function, or the effects of surgery itself on lung function. A number of mechanisms account for these complications (Table 25.1).

### General Anesthesia—Related

Anesthetic agents affect several aspects of pulmonary physiology, including lung volumes, diaphragm function, pulmonary vasomotor tone, ventilation-perfusion matching, mucociliary function, and respiratory control. The effects of general anesthesia have implications not only for intraoperative patient management but also for postoperative management.

Pulmonary gas exchange is impaired during general anesthesia and may result in intraoperative and postoperative hypoxemia. A 20% reduction in functional residual capacity (FRC) typically occurs when a patient assumes the supine position, independent of muscular paralysis (1). This response is exaggerated in obese subjects and may be as large as 60%. The introduction of general anesthesia, muscle relaxation, and mechanical ventilation results in a further reduction in FRC of about 15% (2). The shape and motion of the chest wall changes after induction of general anesthesia, with a decrease in anteroposterior diameter of both the thorax and abdomen and an increase in the lateral diameter (3). These changes are attributed to loss of muscle tone

and increase in chest wall deformability. Although thoracic cross-sectional area remains unchanged, thoracic volume is reduced, from a cephalad diaphragmatic shift that occurs almost immediately upon induction of general anesthesia (4). Recent work suggests that this may be due to the effect of general anesthesia on central nervous system innervation of diaphragmatic tone (5). It is possible that this cephalad diaphragmatic shift is responsible, at least in part, for the observed decrease in FRC and that persistent pulmonary arterial perfusion of these unventilated alveoli results in shunt and hypoxemia. Closing capacity decreases in parallel with the decrease in FRC. Patients with pulmonary diseases with elevated closing capacities are predisposed to increased airway closure following induction of anesthesia. These changes in lung volume promote the development of atelectasis, which can occur in up to 95% of patients (6). The degree of atelectasis averages 4% of thoracic cross-sectional area (7) and can be decreased with the application of positive end-expiratory pressure (PEEP) (8).

Inhalational anesthetics may inhibit the hypoxic pulmonary arterial vasoconstrictive response, allowing perfusion to continue to poorly ventilated regions of the lung (9). The clinical consequences of this effect are controversial, however, and some investigators have shown that concentrations of agents used clinically have little effect (10, 11).

The net result of these changes during general anesthesia is to increase intrapulmonary shunt, widening the alveolar to arterial oxygen difference ($P_{AO_2}$ − $Pa_{O_2}$). Nunn (12) has estimated the intraoperative $Pa_{O_2}$ to be approximately one-half the inspired oxygen tension, which is equivalent to an intrapulmonary shunt of 10 to 15%. Measurements in healthy volunteers under halothane—nitrous oxide anesthesia with paralysis have shown the shunt to be $13.9 \pm 5.3\%$. This is in

**Table 25.1**
**Effects of Anesthesia and Surgery on Pulmonary Function**

| Effect | Pathologic Mechanism | Result |
|---|---|---|
| General anesthesia–related | | |
| Reduction in FRC[a] | Shunt | Hypoxemia |
| Atelectasis | Shunt | Hypoxemia |
| Abnormal distribution of ventilation | $\dot{V}/\dot{Q}$ mismatch | Hypoxemia, hypercapnia |
| Loss of hypoxic pulmonary vasoconstriction | $\dot{V}/\dot{Q}$ mismatch | Hypoxemia |
| Reduced ventilatory drive | Hypoventilation | Hypercapnia |
| Surgery-related | | |
| Upper abdominal surgery, diaphragmatic dysfunction | Shunt, decreased FRC | Hypoxemia |
| Thoracotomy, nonresectional, lung contusion | Shunt | Hypoxemia |
| Coronary bypass surgery, phrenic nerve palsy | Shunt, decreased FRC, hypoventilation | Hypoxemia, hypercapnia |

[a] FRC, functional residual capacity.

contrast to the awake normal volunteer or to a person anesthetized with pentobarbital and paralysis, in whom the shunt is approximately 1%.

Dead space increases with the induction of general anesthesia and positive pressure ventilation. Ventilation is increased to the nondependent areas of the lungs, which have a lesser blood flow. The use of positive pressure compounds the problem further by causing pulmonary microvascular compression, with further reduction in blood flow, resulting in an increase in dead space. In practice this is of little clinical consequence, since it can be compensated for by increasing overall minute ventilation.

Ventilatory drive is also abnormal during general anesthesia. General anesthetics depress respiration centrally and result in a decreased ventilatory response to both hypercarbia and hypoxia. The depression of ventilation may be aggravated by mechanical loading such as added external resistance from increased airway resistance due to a small-bore endotracheal tube or bronchospasm or from added abdominal mass due to obesity or ascites. This may explain in part why obese patients or patients with chronic obstructive pulmonary disease (COPD) hypoventilate more while under general anesthesia than do normal patients. The depression of the hypoxic and hypercapnic ventilatory drive extends into the immediate postoperative period and is further aggravated by the administration of narcotic analgesia, especially in the elderly.

Some studies have suggested that epidural analgesia may improve postoperative respiratory mechanics, compared with parenteral opioid analgesia (13, 14). However, these results have not been confirmed by other investigators (15, 16). Diaphragmatic dysfunction, a major cause of respiratory complications after upper abdominal surgery, is not modified by the administration of opioids in the epidural space (17). Using clinical, radiologic, spirometric, and oxygenation criteria, some authors have reported a similar incidence of pulmonary complications in a large prospective study of patients who received either parenteral or epidural morphine after major abdominal surgery (16). In contrast, the administration of epidural local anesthetics and opioids may improve postoperative diaphragmatic function and gas exchange (18). However, some studies have reported fewer complications with epidural bupivacaine than with parenteral morphine (19). Others found no difference in postoperative respiratory complications between these two analgesic regimens. Postoperative epidural analgesia with a local anesthetic and an opioid provides good pain relief but does not seem to reduce postoperative respiratory morbidity (20). However, the benefits of epidural analgesia during and after anesthesia must be balanced against possible adverse effects. Respiratory depression can occur with epidural morphine. Epidural analgesia with local anesthetics may be associated with a bilateral sympathetic and motor blockade, resulting in hypotension and paralysis in a small percentage of patients.

## SURGERY-RELATED

Postoperative pulmonary complications depend on the type and location of operation performed. Upper abdominal operations are more frequently associated with pulmonary function defects than are operations involving the lower abdomen or extremities (21). Pulmonary function after upper abdominal surgery is characterized as a restrictive defect with up to 55% decrease in forced vital capacity (FVC) and 30% reduction in FRC, but no change in the ratio of the forced expiratory volume in 1 second to the forced vital capacity, $FEV_1/FVC$. Measurements of FRC during the postoperative period in groups at high risk for postoperative hypoxemia and atelectasis (Table 25.2) demonstrate that FRC continues to decrease postoperatively, reaching a nadir at 24 to 48 hours, followed by a delayed return to normal values over the next 5 days; full recovery may require 2 weeks. In contrast, FRC and alveolar-arterial oxygen differences following surgery on the extremities return to normal within 24 hours (22).

The pathogenesis of surgery-induced abnormalities in pulmonary function is not entirely clear. Originally, it was proposed that stimulation of nociceptive abdominal or parietal receptors resulted in postoperative pain and splinting, with resultant shallow respirations. However, as already discussed, excellent analgesia with epidural narcotics fails to improve pulmonary function (23). It is unlikely that pulmonary abnormalities result from persistent anesthesia and analgesia

**TABLE 25.2**
**POSTOPERATIVE RISK FACTORS FOR ATELECTASIS**

Upper abdominal surgery
Thoracotomy
Bypass surgery with external cardiac hypothermia
Smoking
Chronic obstructive pulmonary disease
Restrictive pulmonary disease
Obesity
Age >70
Postoperative immobility

postoperatively, because these abnormalities are uncommon following lower abdominal and extremity surgery using similar anesthetic agents.

Postoperative changes in pulmonary function after upper abdominal surgery resemble those that occur in patients with unilateral diaphragmatic paralysis (24). Diaphragmatic dysfunction has been demonstrated in these patients (25), although diaphragmatic contractility in response to phrenic nerve stimulation is unchanged postoperatively. Diaphragmatic dysfunction may result from a reflex reduction in central phrenic nerve output secondary to vagal, splanchnic, or sympathetic afferent receptors. Stimulation of gallbladder afferent receptors results in the immediate cessation of diaphragmatic electrical activity (26). Diaphragmatic function improves following upper abdominal surgery with administration of aminophylline, a drug that increases central phrenic nerve output (27). It is not known if pulmonary function improves with augmented diaphragmatic function in this setting.

Like surgery in the upper abdomen, thoracic procedures even without pulmonary resection have a high incidence of intraoperative and postoperative pulmonary function abnormalities (28). Hypoxemia can occur intraoperatively in the lateral decubitus position from venous admixture, with blood flowing preferentially to the dependent lung, and ventilation distributing preferentially to the nondependent lung. In cases in which the upper lung is temporarily collapsed to aid surgical exposure, perfusion of the completely unventilated lung results in even more intrapulmonary shunt. Although lung volumes are reduced by resection of pulmonary parenchyma, thoracic surgical procedures without lung resection are more likely to lead to postoperative arterial hypoxemia. This has been attributed to the better matching of perfusion and ventilation in the unresected lung following pneumonectomy.

In contrast to the situation with upper abdominal surgery, phrenic nerve function after thoracotomy has not been well defined. Diaphragmatic dysfunction after thoracic procedures, however, has been documented. Following cardiopulmonary bypass, diaphragmatic dysfunction can occur and may be due to hypothermic damage to the phrenic nerve during external cardiac cooling. When liberal external cardiac cooling was used in addition to intracoronary cold cardioplegia, phrenic nerve palsy (diagnosed by left hemidiaphragm elevation) occurred in 70% of one group of patients, with 14% of the patients developing life-threatening respiratory complications (29). Use of an insulating pad in the pericardial sac reduced the incidence significantly (30). Nerve paralysis usually lasts 2 to 3 weeks but may take as long as 2 months to resolve.

## RISKS FOR POSTOPERATIVE PULMONARY COMPLICATIONS

Several preexisting conditions serve to increase the risk of postoperative pulmonary complications. The risk factors that may be modified preoperatively, at least to some extent, include smoking, air flow limitation from COPD or asthma, nutritional status, and cardiovascular disease. Factors over which we have little or no control include the age of the patient, the type of operation, and the location of its incision. It is important to assess these risk factors in the preoperative evaluation of any patient scheduled to undergo an operation. The time taken to improve any potentially reversible factor and its potential for later complications should be weighed against the potential for harm caused by delay of the operation.

### SMOKING

Cigarette smoking is known to increase the risk of postoperative pulmonary complications and increase perioperative mortality two- to threefold. Morton, in 1944 (31), found a sixfold increase in postoperative respiratory morbidity in patients smoking more than 10 cigarettes per day. Wightman subsequently demonstrated that smokers had more postoperative fever, sputum production, and abnormal chest physical findings after elective surgery than did nonsmokers (32). Other findings include an increased frequency of abnormal chest radiographs and an increased risk of postoperative pneumonia in smokers. In a study of younger smokers most of whom had normal pulmonary function tests, however, these findings were not prominent (33). Thus, the older patient who has smoked longer and has established abnormal pulmonary function is probably at the highest risk for postoperative respiratory complication.

Smoking exerts its deleterious effects primarily on the cardiovascular and pulmonary systems (Table 25.3). Nicotine is a direct adrenergic agonist that increases heart rate, systemic vascular resistance, and blood pressure (34, 35). Smoking directly increases coronary vascular resistance, especially at sites of atherosclerotic plaques and stenoses (36). Inhaled cigarette smoke also exerts a negative inotropic effect on the myocardium, possibly due to the binding of carbon monoxide to cytochrome oxidase and myoglobin, resulting in increased myocardial oxygen consumption and decreased oxygen delivery. Carbon monoxide has

**TABLE 25.3**
**CARDIORESPIRATORY EFFECTS OF SMOKING**

Cardiovascular effects
  Increased myocardial oxygen consumption
    Increased heart rate and systemic vascular resistance
      from $\beta_2$-adrenergic stimulation
    Decreased myocardial inotropic activity
  Decreased myocardial oxygen supply
    Carboxyhemoglobin reduction in available hemo-
      globin
    Coronary artery vasospasm
    Leftward shift of oxyhemoglobin dissociation curve
Respiratory effects
  Decreased mucociliary clearance
  Decreased circulating immunoglobulin levels
  Decreased neutrophil chemotaxis
  Decreased pulmonary macrophage count and adher-
    ence
  Altered T lymphocyte immunoregulatory activity
  Decreased natural killer lymphocyte activity

a binding affinity for the hemoglobin molecule 250 times greater than that of oxygen. In heavy smokers, as much as 15% of circulating hemoglobin may be bound to carbon monoxide, reducing the oxygen-carrying capacity of the blood. In addition, carbon monoxide shifts the oxyhemoglobin dissociation curve to the left, inhibiting the release of oxygen. The half-life of the carboxyhemoglobin complex is 4 hours when breathing room air; therefore, patients should abstain from smoking for a minimum of 12 hours before an operation.

The effects of smoking on the respiratory system are diverse. Smoking is known to disrupt mucociliary function and its ability to clear particles from the peripheral airways before any abnormality in pulmonary function is measured. This impairment in mucociliary clearance can be partially reversed by inhalation of $\beta_2$ agonists (37). In mice exposed to cigarette smoke, mucociliary anatomy is disrupted following the subsequent inhalation of halothane (38). The effect of inhalational agents on mucociliary clearance in humans who smoke remains to be determined. The time course for resolution of mucociliary dysfunction with the cessation of smoking is not certain, but anecdotal evidence from smoking cessation clinics suggests that sputum volume declines over a 6-week period.

Smoking also alters pulmonary immune defense mechanisms by depressing neutrophil chemotaxis, decreasing immunoglobulin levels, reducing natural killer lymphocyte activity, decreasing macrophage adherence, and altering immunoregulatory T lymphocyte activity (39). The full contribution of these effects

to the pathogenesis of postoperative pulmonary complications is unknown. However, based on the measured time of recovery of T lymphocyte immunoregulatory activity, smokers should abstain from smoking for a minimum of 6 weeks prior to operation to reduce the risk of pulmonary complications.

Theoretically, ceasing smoking should provide immediate benefit in the perioperative period through decreased irritation of mucosa, improved mucociliary function, decreased sputum production, and lower carboxyhemoglobin levels. Unfortunately, a study of patients undergoing coronary artery bypass did not bear this out (40). Current smokers had a postoperative pulmonary complication rate of 33%, exsmokers who had stopped smoking for up to 8 weeks had a complication rate of 57%, and exsmokers of more than 8 weeks duration had a 15% rate of complications.

### CHRONIC OBSTRUCTIVE PULMONARY DISEASE

Patients with COPD are at increased risk for postoperative pulmonary complications of atelectasis, exacerbation of bronchitis, pneumonia, and prolonged mechanical ventilation (41). Among patients with a history of smoking and abnormal pulmonary function tests, 50 to 70% can expect to suffer one or more of these complications. In contrast, there is only a 3 to 6% incidence of these complications in nonsmokers with normal pulmonary function tests. Multiple studies confirm that pulmonary function tests can only identify a group of patients at risk for these postoperative pulmonary complications, but no test or group of tests can predict which patients ultimately will develop these complications.

The risk of postoperative pulmonary complications in patients with COPD can be reduced approximately two- or threefold with a preoperative pulmonary preparation consisting of cessation of smoking, treatment with inhaled bronchodilators, and oral antibiotics if sputum is purulent (42). In spite of the risk reduction, however, changes in measured preoperative pulmonary function after therapy are frequently not evident. It is not clear whether preoperative pulmonary preparation administered with the patient hospitalized is superior to that obtained with maximal outpatient therapy. The incidence of postoperative pneumonia appears to increase with the length of preoperative hospital stay. Nonetheless, some preoperative pulmonary therapy, whether administered in an inpatient or an outpatient setting, is reasonable in patients with moderate to severe COPD.

### ASTHMA

Until recently, it had not been demonstrated that asthma was a risk factor for postoperative pulmonary complications in the absence of acute bronchospasm. Tyler and coworkers (43) reported that the two greatest risk factors for postoperative hypoxemia in low-risk anesthetic patients, American Society of Anesthesiology (ASA) class I or II, were obesity and a medical history of asthma. Several anesthetic maneuvers may precipitate bronchospasm in the asthmatic and therefore require close attention. These maneuvers include (a) direct airway irritation by tracheal intubation, (b) the inhalation of cool, dry gases (in which bronchospasm is triggered by transmucosal heat loss), and (c) the administration of intravenous agents that can cause histamine release. For these reasons, regional anesthesia should be considered in asthmatic patients whenever possible, and warm, humidified gas should be administered intraoperatively. The inhalational agents used in anesthesia are themselves excellent bronchodilators (44) and have been used to treat status asthmaticus (45). Classically, halothane has been described as the agent of choice; however, its arrhythmogenic effects are more pronounced when catecholamines and toxic levels of aminophylline are present than when other inhalational agents are used, such as enflurane and isoflurane (46). Agents that are known to release histamine, such as morphine and atracurium, have the potential to induce bronchospasm. These agents should be used with caution in patients with asthma.

A recent upper respiratory infection (URI) is a common clinical history in patients who develop an increase in the severity of bronchospasm. Even patients without underlying bronchospasm may develop increased airway reactivity following such infections (47), so it is not surprising that asthma can be aggravated. Although definitive evidence on when it is safest to proceed with elective surgery does not exist, it seems prudent to wait 2 to 3 weeks after clinical recovery from a URI in asthmatics, even if clinical symptoms are not present. Evidence supporting this in children comes from investigators who found that respiratory complications increased 11-fold, even in normal children with a preoperative URI (48).

Recognition of the fundamental role of inflammation has led several prominent chest physicians to advocate inhaled corticosteroids as the first therapeutic agent used in patients with moderate asthma (49). Ideally, the bronchospastic patient will have been treated with one of the several topical inhaled therapy. While topical steroids need to be administered for a period of several days or more before major benefit is seen, the action of systemic steroids is generally much quicker. In humans, clinical benefit is achieved in less than 12 hours (50). In an animal study on asthmatic dogs, Parker et al (51) demonstrated that the airway resistance response to a citric aerosol challenge was markedly diminished by 24 hours after a single subcutaneous dose of 2 mg/kg of methylprednisolone. Oral administration is cheaper than, and just as efficacious as, intravenous administration.

While there is increasing use of inhaled corticosteroids as the first-line maintenance drug for asthmatics, $\beta$-agonists remain a mainstay of treatment, both chronically and acutely, in the patient with mild to moderate reactive airways. While many question whether that association is real, the drugs currently available are extremely safe. $\beta$-Agonists lead to an increase in the intracellular concentration of cyclic AMP in bronchial smooth muscle, relaxing the muscle and decreasing airway resistance. They may also have a secondary action in inhibiting the release of mediators from mast cells (52). Rather than treating the patient with an inhaled $\beta$-adrenergic agonist prior to arrival in the operating room, the patient should be treated with a metered dose inhaler (MDI) on arrival in the preanesthetic preparation area. This approach serves several purposes. First, the anesthesiologist can ensure that treatment is actually given. Second, it ensures proper timing. Most of these agents have peak effects in the first 10 to 30 minutes, with efficacy waning in about 3 hours. Thus, the peak can be reached prior to induction with sustained effect throughout the course of anesthesia.

The use of theophylline in the therapy of bronchospasm appears to be declining. It is a relatively weak bronchodilator that adds little other than toxicity to the therapeutic effect of inhaled $\beta_2$-agonists (53). In addition, it does not treat the underlying inflammation (54). In the preoperative preparation of the patient, theophylline has the added disadvantage of increasing arrhythmias during halothane administration (55). Although it does not increase arrhythmogenicity during isoflurane or enflurane administration, many anesthesiologists prefer to use halothane for the asthmatic because of the lower incidence of coughing during mask induction (56). Despite its disadvantages, the clinician will still encounter many patients taking theophylline. For some, it provides a nighttime baseline of bronchodilation that is not achievable with existing inhaled $\beta_2$-adrenergic agonists because of their short duration of action. Patients receiving theophylline should be continued on their preoperative regimen if it appears adequate and nontoxic.

Anticholinergic agents block smooth muscle muscarinic receptors, interfering with vagal cholinergic tone and blocking cholinergic reflex bronchoconstriction. They appear to be more effective in patients with chronic obstructive lung disease than in asthmatics. The advent of ipratropium bromide, a poorly absorbed inhaled anticholinergic, has made this class of drug an important adjunctive therapy. Because of the low systemic absorption, there is virtually no toxicity.

## OBESITY

Patients whose body weight is more than 30% above their ideal weight are defined as "morbidly" obese. Obesity is associated with increased morbidity and mortality from pulmonary and cardiovascular dysfunction. Because of the added resistive load of adipose tissue to the chest wall, obese patients have a decrease in chest wall compliance, which increases their work of breathing and reduces lung volumes, including total lung capacity (TLC), vital capacity (VC), and FRC. FRC falls below the closing volume and early airway closure ensues, resulting in an increase in intrapulmonary shunt and a widened alveolar-arterial oxygen gradient.

The cardiovascular system is also involved. Morbidly obese patients have an increased circulating blood volume and increased metabolic demand and may have elevated systemic arterial, pulmonary arterial, and pulmonary artery occlusion pressures. These factors increase myocardial oxygen consumption. An increased incidence of coronary atherosclerotic disease in obese patients results in a potentially tenuous balance of myocardial oxygen demand and supply, so that even minor increases in myocardial oxygen consumption can have devastating consequences.

These cardiopulmonary risk factors combined with the increased risk of postoperative hypoxemia, atelectasis, aspiration pneumonitis, postoperative pneumonia, and pulmonary embolism all require added vigilance and aggressive supportive pulmonary care of obese patients throughout all phases of the hospital course.

## MALNUTRITION

Few studies have evaluated the incidence of postoperative pulmonary complications in patients who are malnourished. Wightman found that 9% of all patients who developed postoperative pulmonary complications weighed less than 95% of ideal body weight, compared with an overall incidence of 6.2% (32). Arora and Rochester demonstrated that malnourished patients without superimposed chronic pulmonary disease did indeed have a significant decrease in respiratory muscle endurance as measured by the maximal mandatory ventilation maneuver (57). Furthermore, protein calorie malnutrition decreases the response of ventilatory drive to hypoxemia (58) and also reduces secretory IgA levels (59). These studies suggest that malnutrition may result in an increased risk of postoperative pulmonary complications, such as atelectasis and pneumonia.

An increased risk for postoperative pneumonia has been found in patients whose serum albumin levels were below 3 g/100 ml (60).

## CARDIOVASCULAR DISEASE

The presence of significant cardiac disease was not found to correlate with an increased incidence of postoperative *pulmonary* complications in one study, although pulmonary edema was not identified as a pulmonary complication (32). However, in a large, prospective study, Goldman and coworkers identified nine clinical factors associated with an increased incidence of perioperative *cardiac* morbidity and mortality in patients undergoing nonthoracic surgery; one of these cardiac complications was pulmonary edema (Table 25.4) (61).

## OPERATIVE SITE

The increased incidence of postoperative pulmonary complications associated with upper abdominal and thoracic procedures is discussed in detail earlier in this chapter. Fewer postoperative pulmonary complications and improved pulmonary function following abdominal surgery have been reported when transverse incisions are used in place of vertical-midline incisions (62, 63), but this is not a universal finding. The retroperitoneal approach for operation on the abdominal aorta results in fewer postoperative pulmonary complications and a shorter hospital stay (64). Median sternotomy is better tolerated than a lateral thoracotomy for pulmonary resection, with improved patient comfort and fewer postoperative pulmonary

**TABLE 25.4**

**PREOPERATIVE FACTORS RELATED TO POSTOPERATIVE CARDIAC COMPLICATIONS**[a,b]

| |
|---|
| $S_3$ gallop or jugular venous distention |
| Myocardial infarction within past 6 months |
| Rhythm other than sinus |
| More than 5 documented premature contractions per minute |
| Intraperitoneal, intrathoracic, or aortic operation |
| Age >70 years |
| Important aortic stenosis |
| Emergency operation |
| Poor general medical condition |

[a] Multivariate analysis, in order of decreasing significance.
[b] Adapted from information appearing in Goldman L, Cadera DL, Nussbaum SR, et al: Multifactorial index of cardiac risk in noncardiac surgical procedures. *N Engl J Med* 297:845–850, 1977.

complications (65). The median sternotomy incision is the preferred approach for exposure of the heart and great vessels; however, it may also be used for bilateral pulmonary wedge resections and pulmonary resections not involving the left lower lobe, or extension to the posterior chest wall. For reasons of exposure, lateral thoracotomy incisions for thoracic exploration are usually preferred in obese patients, patients with cardiomegaly or an elevated hemidiaphragm, and patients with superior sulcus carcinomas.

Laparoscopy cholecystectomy is said to have many advantages, compared with the open operation; the major one is a shorter hospital stay (66, 67). There are also fewer respiratory complications than with a laparotomy. Further studies have to confirm that this new type of surgical approach to abdominal operations can decrease the incidence of postoperative pulmonary complications in patients with COPD.

## AGE

Surgical risk is increased in the elderly population. However, perioperative mortality for major operations in patients over age 70 has decreased from more than 20% to between 4 and 10% since the 1960s (68). This has resulted from advances in anesthetic, surgical, and postoperative care techniques. Nonetheless, elderly patients have an estimated four- to eightfold increase in surgical mortality compared with younger patients undergoing comparable major operations (69). This age-related risk probably represents a risk due to age itself, as much as it represents the increased incidence of cardiovascular, pulmonary, and renal pathology with advancing age.

Half of the postoperative deaths occurring in elderly postoperative patients may be ultimately related to myocardial dysfunction (70). Age greater than 70 years is associated with an increased incidence of postoperative cardiac morbidity and mortality in patients undergoing nonthoracic surgical procedures.

Respiratory complications are second only to cardiac complications in being responsible for perioperative death in the elderly. Normal physiologic effects of aging include decreases in lung compliance, TLC, and VC and increases in dead space and closing volumes. FRC appears to remain unaffected; however, closing volume may rise above FRC, resulting in early airway closure and shunt. In addition, ventilatory drive in elderly patients in response to hypoxia and hypercapnia is decreased, while sensitivity to the respiratory depressant effects of sedatives and narcotics is increased. All of these changes place the elderly at risk for atelectasis, lobar pneumonia, and aspiration pneumonia (71).

In summary, the safest operations in the elderly appear to be those that are elective, are away from the diaphragm, do not involve suppurative disease, and allow minimal postoperative analgesia and sedation and early ambulation. Surgical therapy should certainly not be denied to a patient on the basis of age alone. A person who is 70 years of age may have 10 to 15 years or more of life remaining. However the elderly are at a higher risk for postoperative cardiopulmonary complications and thus require appropriate preoperative evaluation and therapy.

## PULMONARY ASSESSMENT OF THE THORACIC SURGERY PATIENT

The high morbidity and mortality of patients with limited pulmonary reserve undergoing thoracic surgery, particularly lung resection, has been known for decades (72). Most patients with neoplastic disease who are candidates for resection have coexisting COPD because of the common association of these two diseases with smoking. Despite this risk, surgery currently remains the only chance for long-term survival or cure in patients with non–oat cell carcinoma of the lung. The determination of operability is crucial in the preoperative evaluation of lung cancer patients, for it is desirable to give patients a chance for curative resection when possible and avoid surgery on those patients who would not survive resection.

The causes of perioperative pulmonary complications are multifactorial, and it is not possible to predict outcome on the basis of any single abnormality in cardiopulmonary function. The goals of assessment are twofold: (*a*) to determine operability for pulmonary resection and (*b*) to determine the risk of cardiopulmonary complications following upper abdominal and resectional and nonresectional thoracic surgery.

### DETERMINATION OF OPERABILITY FOR RESECTION

Preoperative assessment of the candidate for pulmonary resection begins with screening pulmonary function tests to measure VC, air flow limitation, and ventilatory reserve. $FEV_1$, FVC, and maximal voluntary ventilation (MVV) test greater than 50% of the predicted value are considered sufficient for pneumonectomy or lobectomy on the basis of residual pulmonary function. Lower values of $FEV_1$ or FVC indicate a high risk for postoperative respiratory failure because of inability to maintain alveolar ventilation. The MVV is perhaps a more sensitive indicator of flow-dependent pulmonary complications because it also assesses ventilatory reserve. A patient who does not meet one or more of these criteria should undergo split function studies.

Split function studies are intended to estimate residual pulmonary function following lung resection and include bronchospirometry, the lateral position test, and quantitative radionuclide scanning. *Bronchospirometry* entails differential bronchial intubation and gas exchange measurements, but it has been replaced by the more current radionuclide techniques and in general is no longer performed. The *lateral position test* attempts to measure the relative contribution of each lung to total minute ventilation measuring tidal volume while the subject is positioned on each side, but it has significant variability. It too has been largely replaced by quantitative radionuclide techniques but remains an option should radionuclide tests be unavailable.

The preferred method at present for estimating residual pulmonary function following pneumonectomy is *quantitative ventilation or perfusion scanning*. Microaggregate perfusion scanning correlates well with ventilation scanning and is perhaps simpler to perform. Scintillation counts are obtained for each lung individually, and residual $FEV_1$ is calculated as follows:

$$FEV_1 \text{ (postop)} = FEV_1 \text{ (preop)} \times \frac{\text{counts in nonresected lung}}{\text{total counts in both lungs}}$$

A predicted postoperative $FEV_1$ of 0.8 to 1.0 liter has traditionally been used as the lower limit of operability (73), based on the observations of activity and $CO_2$ retention of patients with similar degrees of impairment (74). More recently, Gass and Olsen (75) suggested use of a cutoff value of 30% of the predicted normal to take into account patient size, but this approach is not universally used, and the value of 30% may be subject to refinement.

Not infrequently a potential candidate will fall into the borderline category in which the predicted $FEV_1$ is in the range of 0.8 to 1.0 liter. Two additional testing methods may prove useful in making the decision of operability in these patients. Fee and coworkers (76) demonstrated that vascular compliance correlates with survival. A pulmonary vascular resistance (PVR) during exercise of under $190 \text{ dyn·cm·s}^{-5}$ predicts a good outcome following pneumonectomy or lobectomy, while a value above this is associated with a high mortality. Measurement of PVR during exercise goes beyond assessment of ventilation and tests the cardiopulmonary response to stress, which may better assess the postoperative condition. However, this test is invasive, requiring pulmonary artery catheterization, and is infrequently performed. Another test that has fallen into

disuse because of a high technical failure rate is temporary unilateral occlusion of the pulmonary artery, in which the presence of pulmonary hypertension or hypoxemia during occlusion of blood flow to the diseased lung indicates inoperability.

Noninvasive cardiopulmonary exercise testing for preoperative evaluation has recently been described and appears to assess the cardiopulmonary stress response as does measurement of PVR. Smith and coworkers (77) have shown that a $\dot{V}O_2max$ over 20 ml/min/kg was associated with a low complication rate after resectional surgery even when screening pulmonary function tests were nearly "unacceptable." A $\dot{V}O_2max$ under 15 ml/min/kg predicted a high rate of complications. Bechard and Wetstein (78) have confirmed these results in a larger study, noting that a $\dot{V}O_2max$ above 20 ml/min/kg was associated with no complications in their series. In addition, they recommend a lower threshold of 10 ml/min/kg, since most patients between 10 and 20 ml/min/kg had no complications. The role of cardiopulmonary exercise testing is not fully elucidated, but it appears to be useful in arriving at a decision when quantitative lung scanning does not provide a clear answer.

The workup of the patient for lung resectional surgery should therefore follow a stepwise approach such as that depicted in Figure 25.1. This workup should be undertaken in the absence of any intercurrent illness that may transiently impair pulmonary function. However there are no proven or universally accepted guidelines for preoperative evaluation (79). The patient who fails a staged evaluation using noninvasive testing may be considered for invasive testing of pulmonary vascular and right heart function if the lesion is potentially curable (80).

## Risk of Complications in Nonresectional Surgery

Except for lung resection surgery, there is little evidence of benefit of pulmonary function testing as a routine screening technique in the absence of clinical symptoms (81). Spirometry, the most commonly obtained pulmonary function test, provides the information of most concern to the anesthesiologist, the presence or absence of obstructive disease. When obstruction is present, pulmonary function laboratories generally administer a bronchodilator and then retest the patient. Although evidence of acute reversibility is encouraging, its absence should not prevent the clinician from initiating a trial of bronchodilators and then retesting the patient at a later time. In a review of 135 articles, it was concluded that abnormal preoperative spirometry was not predictive of postoperative

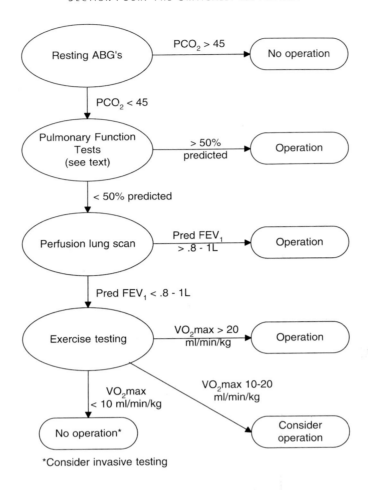

**FIGURE 25.1.** Preoperative assessment for pulmonary resection.

pulmonary complications (81). Although many investigators have found that patients with chronic obstructive disease have an increased incidence of postoperative pulmonary complications after abdominal surgery, none of these studies addressed why and how often these patients required prolonged mechanical ventilation.

Zilbrach contended that patient populations that have been studied using preoperative pulmonary function tests have not been homogenous (82).

A recent prospective study evaluated an homogenous group of elderly smokers who underwent abdominal vascular surgery, to determine the incidence and causes of postoperative respiratory failure (83). A longer history of cigarette smoking and preoperative hypoxemia, as well as intraoperative blood loss, were all associated with the need for more than 24 hours of postoperative ventilation. Preoperative abnormalities of spirometry did not identify patients who were destined to require postoperative ventilation.

In summary, patients who smoke or have chronic obstructive lung disease appear to be at increased risk for postoperative pulmonary complications, but predicting these complications is difficult, except for those undergoing lung resection.

The decision to delay surgery is complex and depends on the severity of the underlying disease, the extent of reversible disease, and the site of surgery. In an older study of 1500 surgical patients, the incidence of respiratory complications averaged 63% after upper abdominal and thoracic procedures versus only 9% for lower abdominal procedures. The likelihood of complications following peripheral procedures is even lower (84). Thus, postponing surgery is more important for procedures in the upper abdomen than for other procedures. Although emergent surgery cannot be postponed, urgent cases may be worth postponing for hours or days to permit better preparation of the patient.

For patients undergoing upper abdominal or thoracic procedures, incentive spirometry can reduce postoperative complications and hospital stay. This therapy is inexpensive and cost effective and consequently is used routinely, although the cost:benefit ratio is most favorable for those with the most severe disease. The technique should be taught preoperatively, when the patient is most alert and cooperative.

## POSTOPERATIVE PULMONARY COMPLICATIONS

Given the common occurrence of intraoperative pulmonary abnormalities and the incidence of preoperative risk factors in patients, it is not surprising that the most frequent postoperative complications are related to the pulmonary system. The more common postoperative pulmonary complications are discussed in further detail in this section.

### HYPOXEMIA

Hypoxemia occurring in the postoperative period has long been recognized as one of the earliest of the postoperative complications (85). It is seen in its most severe form in the obese, the elderly, patients with preoperative cardiac or pulmonary insufficiency, and patients who have had operations on the thorax and upper abdomen. Its true prevalence is becoming more apparent with more frequent intraoperative and postoperative monitoring of saturation by pulse oximetry. A prospective study of 95 ASA class I and II patients on room air revealed a 35% incidence of arterial hemoglobin saturation of 90% or less (a $Pa_{O_2}$ under about 58 mm Hg) and 12% incidence of arterial saturation less than 85% (a $Pa_{O_2}$ under about 50 mm Hg). Arterial desaturation did not correlate with the anesthetic agent (inhalational versus intravenous), duration of operation, or level of consciousness but was associated with obesity and a history of asthma.

The causes of immediate postoperative hypoxemia are not clear. The dilution of alveolar gases by the release of nitrous oxide from body stores is one possibility but is inconsistent with the finding that inhalation of 100% oxygen fails to correct the alveolar-arterial oxygen difference. A more likely explanation is intraoperative decrease of FRC below closing volume, resulting in microatelectasis with increased intrapulmonary shunting. This is consistent with the finding that the degree of hypoxemia is related to the severity of the reduction in FRC and an increased incidence of intraoperative and postoperative abnormalities in FRC in patients who are obese or elderly, in those with COPD, and in those undergoing upper abdominal operations.

Therapeutic interventions to prevent postoperative hypoxemia have included the use of periodic hyperinflation, use of larger tidal volumes (10 to 15 ml/kg), and prophylactic PEEP or continuous positive airway pressure (CPAP). While improvements in arterial oxygenation intraoperatively have been reported with all of these interventions, they have not consistently demonstrated postoperative prevention of this complication. Epidural anesthesia has the potential to reduce postoperative hypoxemia through its ability to permit maintenance of more normal spontaneous ventilatory function. This form of anesthesia has been shown to be useful in preventing postoperative pulmonary complications, with the exception of deep venous thrombosis, in the obese patient. This improvement is attributed to the superior pain control of epidural narcotics over intramuscular narcotics, resulting in earlier ambulation (86, 87). Given the prevalence and unpredictable occurrence of hypoxemia in the immediate postoperative period, supplemental oxygen should be used routinely when transporting patients who have been given a general anesthetic to the recovery room and should be continued in the early postoperative period.

### ATELECTASIS

Atelectasis is the most common postoperative pulmonary complication. Risk factors for its development are listed in Table 25.2. Atelectasis appears most frequently following upper abdominal and thoracic procedures, with rates up to 80%. Possible mechanisms with respect to diaphragmatic dysfunction have been reviewed earlier in this chapter. In a study of eight patients without preexisting cardiopulmonary disease undergoing CT scanning during anesthetic induction and up to 24 hours postoperatively, all patients developed plaque-like densities in the most dependent portions of their lungs from the time of induction (88). These densities did not increase in size when muscular paralysis and mechanical ventilation were started, suggesting they were caused by the anesthetic agent and not by muscular paralysis. Furthermore, these densities persisted for at least 24 hours in up to 50% of the patients. It is tempting to speculate that the observed CT scan abnormalities seen in this study represent the precursors to postoperative atelectasis.

Most postoperative atelectasis is subclinical and resolves spontaneously within 24 to 48 hours. There is currently no evidence that atelectasis actually predisposes to pneumonia. This assumption is often made, since retrospective data support the conclusion in that the patients at risk for postoperative pneumonia are those at risk for atelectasis. Atelectasis theoretically can alter production of alveolar surfactant through local effects of hypoxia, thus making reexpansion difficult.

Clinically significant atelectasis that persists requires therapy. The standard methods of improving pulmonary function postoperatively are incentive spirometry, deep breathing, intermittent positive-pressure breathing, and CPAP. All are equally superior to no treatment at all in reducing the incidence of postoperative atelectasis in patients undergoing upper abdominal surgery (33). Of these treatments, CPAP by mask appears to be superior to the others in producing measurable differences in pulmonary function by increasing FRC (89). The treatment of persistent atelectasis by bronchoscopic removal of mucus plugs appears to offer little or no advantage over conventional aggressive chest physiotherapy in most patients (90).

### PNEUMONIA AND ASPIRATION

Nosocomial pneumonias occur most frequently in surgical patients and are the third most frequent type of nosocomial infection and the most common cause of postoperative mortality due to nosocomial infections (91). Only urinary tract infections and wound infections occur more frequently. The occurrence rate is 1.3% of all postoperative patients and ranges from 12 to 20% of patients following upper abdominal surgery. Postoperative nosocomial pneumonia has a mortality rate that approaches 50%. Several factors increase the risk of postoperative pneumonia (Table 25.5). Increasing the length of preoperative stay increases the risk of postoperative pneumonia, possibly by increasing oropharyngeal colonization with virulent, hospital-acquired, Gram-negative bacilli (92). The role of atelectasis in the development of postoperative pneumonia remains unclear, although a retrospective study found that 41% of the patients who developed postoperative pneumonia had preceding radiographic evidence of atelectasis (93).

The most prevalent organisms in postoperative pneumonias are Gram-negative aerobic rods, in particular *Pseudomonas, Klebsiella,* and *Escherichia coli,* while

**TABLE 25.5**
**RISK FACTORS FOR POSTOPERATIVE PNEUMONIA**

Severe underlying illness—peritonitis, sepsis, burn
Emergency operation
Prolonged operation
History of smoking or abnormal pulmonary function tests
Malnutrition
Thoracic or upper abdominal procedures
History of aspiration
Obesity
? Atelectasis

**TABLE 25.6**
**RISK FACTORS FOR ASPIRATION PNEUMONIA**

Decreased gastroesophageal tone
  Anesthetics
  Narcotics, sedatives
  Alkaline gastric pH
Incompetent gastroesophageal junction
  Nasogastric or enteral feeding tubes
  Hiatal hernia
  Esophageal motility disorders
  Elderly
Elevated intragastric pressure or volume
  Gastric outlet obstruction
  Small bowel obstruction
  Diabetes (functional gastric outlet obstruction)
  Pregnancy, ascites, intraabdominal mass
Abnormal glottic closure
  Anesthetic induction or postanesthetic recovery
  Neurologic disorders (central or peripheral)
  Sedatives, narcotics
  Intubation or tracheostomy
  Postextubation

the most prevalent Gram-positive organism is *Staphylococcus aureus.* Postoperative pneumonias may result from subclinical aspiration of oropharyngeal secretions containing hospital-acquired bacteria combined with a diminution of host defenses. Prevention of postoperative pneumonia begins by early identification of the groups at risk. Severely ill patients should have prompt, aggressive treatment of underlying pathology followed by the early institution of nutritional support; smokers should abstain from smoking 6 weeks prior to elective operation; sedation and narcotics should be titrated carefully in the elderly and those with COPD; prophylactic antibiotics should be discontinued within 24 to 48 hours postoperatively to minimize the risk of bacterial colonization; and postoperative pulmonary toilet should be aggressive, especially in patients prone to atelectasis.

Aspiration of gastric contents, or Mendelson's syndrome (94), is a dreaded complication in the postoperative patient and is more often suspected than confirmed. The syndrome results from the breakdown of one or more physiologic defense mechanisms: (*a*) a competent gastroesophageal junction, (*b*) coordinated glottic closure, and (*c*) intact pulmonary mucociliary clearance and macrophage phagocytosis (Table 25.6).

The gastroesophageal junction in its tonically contracted, resting state exerts a constant pressure of 25 to 30 cm $H_2O$. Only when intragastric pressure exceeds this resting pressure or when the gastroesophageal junction is rendered incompetent does reflux of gastric contents occur. Gastroesophageal sphincter tone is reduced by such agents as narcotics, benzodiazepines, alcohol, and alkaline gastric pH, while its competency is violated by such devices as nasogastric or enteral feeding tubes. Even small 7F silastic nasogastric feeding tubes place the patient at increased risk for postoperative pneumonia and aspiration pneumonia, although this risk decreases slightly when the tube is advanced beyond the pylorus. Pathologic processes that increase the risk of gastric reflux include hiatal hernias (sliding variety only) and esophageal motility disorders. Intragastric pressures are elevated in pregnant patients and patients with massive ascites or morbid obesity. Patients with gastric outlet obstruction or small bowel obstruction have increased gastric volumes, which may increase intragastric pressure. Elderly patients have a higher incidence of sliding hiatal hernia, loss of gastroesophageal sphincter tone, and delayed gastric emptying, all of which put them at an increased risk of gastric reflux (95).

Patients may not recover normal glottic closure for up to 8 hours after extubation, even after short periods of intubation (96). Almost half of normal subjects aspirate oropharyngeal secretions while sleeping, but the low-volume, alkaline pH, and nonparticulate nature of the secretions of the oropharynx do not cause alveolar injury (97). With colonization of the oropharynx by more virulent bacteria, however, these "minor" aspiration events could play an important role in the pathogenesis of postoperative pneumonia in patients whose clearing mechanisms are abnormal or overwhelmed. Even while intubated with low-pressure, high-volume cuffs, one-third of patients will aspirate oropharyngeal contents (98).

The pathogenesis and significance of an aspiration event are directly related to the pH, volume, and particulate nature of the aspirate. An aspirate with pH less than 2.5, a volume over 0.4 ml/kg (about 25 ml), and with larger particulate content has the worst prognosis. Aspiration of alkaline contents, on the other hand, is not a benign process either, raising concern about the preoperative administration of antacids, especially particulate antacid suspensions, to patients at high risk for aspiration (99). Antacids have the further disadvantages of increasing gastric volume and gastric pH, reducing gastroesophageal sphincter tone.

Mortality from a significant gastric aspiration event ranges from 10 to 30%. Death usually occurs within the first 48 hours (100, 101). Treatment after aspiration pneumonia is supportive. No apparent benefit has been found from the use of corticosteroids, bronchoalveolar lavage, or prophylactic antibiotics (101, 102). Bronchoscopy may be of benefit in the removal of large food particles blocking major or segmental bronchi.

The greater risk of gastric aspiration in surgical patients occurs at the time of anesthetic induction. Patients undergoing intubation for emergent operation or those at risk for aspiration should have manual pressure applied on the cricoid cartilage (Sellick maneuver) (103). This maneuver should be maintained until the endotracheal tube is confirmed to be in the trachea and the cuff is inflated. An intraesophageal pressure exceeding 60 to 100 cm $H_2O$ is required to overcome properly applied cricoid pressure (104). Esophageal rupture from forced emesis during cricoid pressure is uncommon and should not deter one from continuing to apply cricoid pressure if emesis should occur.

Elective surgical patients are not allowed to eat or drink anything 8 to 12 hours prior to operation, to reduce the risk of aspiration on induction. Fasting will cause a progressive decrease in gastric volume and an increase in gastric pH in most patients. However, despite a 12-hour fast, up to 76% of patients without gastrointestinal pathology undergoing elective operation will have a gastric pH below 2.5, and up to 35% will have a gastric volume exceeding 0.4 ml/kg (95). These findings are more prevalent in the pediatric and geriatric age groups. The current trend is to use $H_2$-antagonists such as cimetidine or ranitidine to increase gastric pH and decrease gastric volume. The use of two doses of one of these agents in the 12 hours preceding elective operation, optionally in combination with metoclopramide (an agent known to increase gastroesophageal sphincter tone and increase antral motility and gastric emptying), has been demonstrated to decrease gastric volume and increase gastric pH.

These precautions should be combined with other preventive measures in patients at high risk for aspiration, including elevation of the head of the bed in unsupervised patients; early discontinuation or less frequent use of nasogastric tubes; careful titration of pain medication and sedation, especially in the elderly; and close observation of obtunded patients.

## PULMONARY EMBOLISM

Pulmonary embolism is discussed in detail in Chapter 13. Without prophylaxis, fatal postoperative pulmonary embolism varies in frequency from 0.1 to 0.8% following elective general surgery, 0.3 to 1.7% following elective hip surgery, and 4 to 7% in patients undergoing emergency hip surgery. Two-thirds of patients who die from pulmonary embolism do so within 30 minutes after the acute event, before thrombolytic or anticoagulant therapy can ever be effectively instituted. It is therefore not surprising that a major emphasis has been placed on the identification of the groups of patients at risk for pulmonary embolus and their prophylaxis.

Although venous thromboembolism is an elusive,

life-threatening disease whose natural history still remains unclear, groups at risk for this disease can be identified. There are now multiple modalities available for the prevention of venous thromboembolism, including low-dose subcutaneous or adjusted-dose heparin, leg exercises, and external pneumatic compression, with no single method currently showing clear superiority in all patient groups. Combined therapy shows promise in helping to improve the results of prophylaxis. Consequently, until more definitive regimens have been studied prospectively, the choice of a prophylactic regimen to use in a given patient will remain a complex and difficult decision.

## THORACIC TRAUMA

Thoracic injuries are directly responsible for 25% of all civilian traumatic deaths, with 50% of these patients succumbing prior to arrival at a medical facility. Furthermore, thoracic injuries contribute to another 25 to 50% of civilian trauma deaths (105). Only 5 to 15% of all thoracic injuries require a thoracotomy for treatment; the remainder are adequately treated by basic resuscitation, intubation, or tube thoracostomy (105, 106).

The patient with thoracic trauma is frequently the victim of multiple trauma, with coexisting extrathoacic injuries. With rare exception, however, the thoracic components of the injuries are the ones that pose the greatest threat to survival in the first few hours. As with any critically ill patient, the initial management of the trauma victim is directed toward the ABCs (airway, breathing, and circulation) of resuscitation and the identification and treatment of *immediately* life-threatening injuries (Table 25.7). This rapid initial evaluation and treatment is termed the primary survey. *Potentially*

life-threatening injuries are identified shortly thereafter in a detailed head-to-toe physical examination known as the secondary survey. Thus, the quick establishment of an airway with adequate ventilation and oxygenation takes priority over all other injuries.

For purposes of this chapter, however, we will concentrate on thoracic and pulmonary trauma, dividing thoracic trauma into injuries that involve the thoracic cage itself (rib fractures and flail chest), and those that are intrathoracic. Intrathoracic injuries include pleural injuries (e.g., pneumothorax or hemothorax), pulmonary injuries (e.g., pulmonary contusion, pulmonary hematoma, or adult respiratory distress syndrome (ARDS)), tracheal injuries, and diaphragmatic injuries.

### DIAGNOSTIC AND THERAPEUTIC MODALITIES

#### Tube Thoracostomy

Drainage of the pleural space is a mainstay in the management of pneumothorax and hemothorax in blunt and penetrating thoracic trauma. It is frequently the only measure necessary for management of pneumothorax and for hemothorax due to lung parenchymal injury. Indications for tube thoracostomy are given in Table 25.8.

#### Thoracotomy

Thoracotomy is required in only a minority of thoracic trauma patients, because tube thoracostomy provides effective therapy in most thoracic trauma victims. Large or persistent hemorrhage requires thoracotomy. Specific indications for thoracotomy are given in Table 25.9.

Emergency department thoracotomy, while once commonly performed in trauma centers, has shown survival benefit only in patients with penetrating thoracic trauma who have signs of life at the scene but have a trauma arrest either en route to the emergency department or in the emergency department (107). Blunt trauma victims who have no signs of life before

---

**TABLE 25.7**
**INITIAL SURVEY OF THORACIC INJURIES**

Primary survey of immediately life-threatening injuries
    Airway obstruction
    Tension pneumothorax
    Open pneumothorax
    Massive hemothorax
    Flail chest
    Cardiac tamponade
Secondary survey of potentially life-threatening injuries
    Pulmonary contusion
    Aortic rupture
    Tracheobronchial disruption
    Esophageal disruption
    Traumatic diaphragmatic hernia
    Myocardial contusion

---

**TABLE 25.8**
**INDICATIONS FOR TUBE THORACOSTOMY IN THORACIC TRAUMA**

Pneumothorax above minimal size
Pneumothorax increasing in size
Pneumothorax in intubated, ventilated patient
Tension pneumothorax
Pneumothorax in any unstable patient
Hemothorax or hemopneumothorax
Bilateral pneumothorax

**TABLE 25.9**

**INDICATIONS FOR THORACOTOMY IN THORACIC TRAUMA**

Operating room thoracotomy
  Persistent hemorrhage >500 ml/hour
  Initial thoracostomy tube drainage >1–1.5 liters
  Failure of tube thoracostomy with enlarging hemo-
    thorax
  Hemodynamic instability despite adequate resuscitation
Emergency department thoracotomy
  Penetrating injury with trauma arrest enroute to or in
    emergency department

**TABLE 25.10**

**APPLICATIONS OF THORACOSCOPY IN THORACIC TRAUMA**

Diagnostic evaluation
  Persistent hemorrhage
  Diaphragmatic injuries
  Mediastinal (tracheal, esophageal) injuries
  Continued air leak
Therapeutic applications
Stapling of lung parenchymal injury
Ligation of isolated bleeding vessels
Evacuation of hemothoraces
Evacuation of posttraumatic empyema

arrival in the emergency department are not considered candidates for emergency department thoracotomy.

## Thoracoscopy

Although most victims of thoracic trauma do not
require thoracotomy, a significant number of delayed
deaths occur in this group as a result of complications
of trauma that may not be identified at the time of
injury. Thoracoscopy is a minimally invasive technique that has an expanding role in the diagnosis and
management of thoracic injuries (108) (Table 25.10). Diagnostic applications have been reported in penetrating trauma (109), diaphragmatic injuries (110, 111), and
pleural evacuation (112). Diagnostic applications often
result in identification of problems amenable to thoracoscopic therapy, such as ligation of bleeding vessels,
stapling of pulmonary lacerations, or evacuation of
clotted hemithoraces, thereby avoiding thoracotomy.

## Bronchoscopy

Diagnostic flexible fiberoptic bronchoscopy may be
invaluable in the evaluation of the thoracic trauma patient in the emergency department or the operating
room. The identification of tracheobronchial injuries
and localization of airway foreign bodies are the most

common uses. The evaluation and localization of massive hemoptysis prior to thoracotomy, however, is best
performed with the rigid bronchoscope in the operating room.

### RIB FRACTURES

The most frequent thoracic injuries causing respiratory embarrassment are rib fractures. Simple rib fractures (i.e., without associated injuries) are reported in
up to 36% of cases of blunt thoracic trauma and most
commonly involve the fifth through the ninth ribs.
These ribs are fixed anteriorly to the costochondral
junction and posteriorly to the spine, as opposed to the
floating or vertebral ribs (11th and 12th), and are more
directly exposed to the kinetic energy of the traumatic
insult. In comparison, ribs 1 through 4 are afforded
protection by the clavicle, upper extremity, pectoral
muscles, and scapulae, and are much less frequently
injured.

The diagnosis of rib fractures is often elusive with
nonspecific physical findings, unreliable clinical
impressions, and chest radiographs that frequently do
not show the lesion on initial examination. Since therapy of simple rib fractures is symptomatic and not influenced by the radiographic presence or absence of an
identifiable fracture, spot films of the point of maximal
tenderness are unwarranted (113). Indeed, the posteroanterior chest film more frequently detects the presence of suspected rib fractures than spot rib films and,
more importantly, detects the potentially serious complications of rib fractures, such as pneumothorax and
hemothorax, which require additional therapy.

The pain associated with rib fractures causes the patient to take shallow, splinted breaths with low tidal
volumes. The potential consequences are decreases in
FRC, ventilation-perfusion ($\dot{V}/\dot{Q}$) mismatching, hypoxemia, atelectasis, and pneumonia (114). Certain patients are at greater risk for these complications, including patients with multiple rib fractures, those over the
age of 50, or those with underlying chronic cardiac or
pulmonary disease. Patients in these high-risk groups
are probably best served by admission to the hospital
for observation, pain control, and aggressive pulmonary toilet. Patients not in these risk groups and who
have a normal posteroanterior chest radiograph usually tolerate rib fractures well and require only oral
analgesics for treatment. It is important to remember,
however, that patients with seven or more rib fractures
have a 50% incidence of an intrathoracic injury and a
15% incidence of intraabdominal injury and therefore
require close observation (115). Patients at risk should
be observed by serial measurements of VC. When expired volumes fall below 15 ml/kg body weight, there

**TABLE 25.11**
**INDICATIONS FOR ARTERIOGRAPHY IN HIGH THORACIC INJURIES**

Evidence of distal vascular insufficiency

Evidence of hemorrhage (hemothorax or extrapleural hematoma)

Concomitant brachial plexus injury

Marked displacement of the rib fragments

Subclavian groove (anterior one-third) fracture of the first rib

Fractures of the scapula, vertebrae, or sternum

Presence of a widened mediastinum

Left apical capping

Downward displacement of the left mainstem bronchus

---

is a high likelihood of ventilatory failure, and early intervention is indicated.

Treatment of rib fractures by strapping the chest wall with tape or elastic belts is not recommended because it further limits chest wall excursion, possibly leading to atelectasis and pneumonia. Intercostal nerve block of the neurovascular bundle of the involved rib can provide analgesia in the surrounding dermatomes for periods of 3 to 15 hours. Epidural anesthesia has the capability of providing continuous relief and is being used with increasing preference over other forms of analgesia. Both therapies improve maximal inspiratory force (MIF) and VC in patients with rib fractures, presumably through pain relief (116, 117).

Special mention needs to be made of fractures of the first and second ribs. These ribs are well protected from trauma. Fractures of these ribs are uncommon and usually indicate a high-kinetic-energy injury. The physician should be aware of the possibility of serious thoracic injury, such as disruption of the subclavian artery or thoracic aorta (up to 15%), as well as serious intraabdominal or neurologic injury (over 50%). Patients with a first rib fracture combined with other rib fractures have a significantly higher morbidity (70%) and mortality (15%) resulting from more severe extrathoracic injuries than those patients with an isolated first rib fracture, whose morbidity and mortality are 15% and 1.5%, respectively (118). All patients with a first or second rib fracture require close observation. Routine arteriography in these patients, however, discloses surprisingly few thoracic arterial injuries and is generally indicated only in selected situations (Table 25.11).

## FLAIL CHEST

The unilateral fracture of multiple (usually four or five) ribs both anteriorly and posteriorly or the bilateral fracture of multiple costochondral junctions anteriorly results in a free-floating segment of ribs known as flail chest. In the spontaneously breathing patient whose pain is well controlled, this segment can be identified by its paradoxical respiratory motion in which the flail segment moves in with the negative intrapleural pressure created during inspiration and out during expiration. However, pain may cause patients to splint their respiratory efforts so that the paradoxical excursion of the flail segment is subtle and may be missed on the initial physical examination. Patients who are ventilated in controlled modes with continuously positive intrapleural pressures will also not demonstrate the paradoxical motion of their flail segments until spontaneous ventilation is allowed during weaning attempts.

Pulmonary function abnormalities seen in flail chest include decreases in VC, total static lung compliance, MIF, FRC, and arterial oxygenation and increases in airway resistance and work of breathing (119). Several processes appear to be operating simultaneously. Pain associated with breathing can result in splinting and diminished regional ventilation as well as an inability to generate adequate tidal volumes. In addition to the abnormal motion of the flail segment, there is often some degree of pulmonary contusion. The hypoxemia seen in flail chest is in large part due to shunt through the fluid-filled alveoli of the underlying contused lung and not due to motion of the flail segment (120).

Therapy for flail chest has changed considerably over the past several decades. Originally, it was considered important to stabilize the flail segment to reverse the pulmonary abnormalities. Stabilization methods included use of a towel clamp to grasp a central rib of the flail segment and suspend it with a weight. With the advent of volume-controlled ventilation, Avery, Morch, and Benson in 1956 advanced the concept of "internal pneumatic stabilization" (121). Although the mortality rate from flail chest was lowered with this approach, there was a subsequent rise in morbidity from an increase in the incidence of tracheostomy complications and nosocomial pulmonary infections (122). Shackford and coworkers (123) and Richardson and coworkers (124) showed that successful management could be done without mechanical ventilation, by providing excellent analgesia and aggressive pulmonary toilet. With this approach, morbidity was reduced and hospital stays were shorter than with the use of mechanical ventilation. The concept of selective management of flail chest injuries by mechanical ventilation has since become commonplace, with ventilatory support instituted only for specific indications, including tachypnea (respiratory rate over 40), progressive decrease in VC to less than 10 to 15 ml/kg body weight, hypoxemia (PaO$_2$ below 60 mm Hg with FIO$_2$ at least 50%), or hypercapnia (PaCO$_2$ over 50 mm Hg in patients with chronic pulmonary disease). Other major indications for intubation in patients with flail chest are the presence of central nervous system trauma, shock, and the need for operation associated with abdominal and thoracic injuries.

In these selected cases, mechanical ventilation for periods as long as 2 to 4 weeks may be required in 50 to 75% of all patients with flail chest. Criteria for extubation are similar to the standard weaning criteria. In flail chest, however, VC should *exceed* 15 ml/kg and the maximal inspiratory force should exceed $-40$ cm $H_2O$. These values help ensure a stable chest wall. In contrast, patients without flail chest can usually be extubated with a VC of 10 to 15 ml/kg and an MIF above $-25$ cm $H_2O$.

Another treatment option in selected patients with flail chest is operative stabilization. It is most commonly required when chest wall injury has been severe, in particular with sternal fractures or massive disruption of lateral portions of the chest wall (more than eight ribs) and marked displacement of the fracture fragments. In these circumstances in which prolonged mechanical ventilation is probable, in patients with tracheal or bronchial injuries or persistent air leaks, or when other intrathoracic injuries require a thoracotomy, operative stabilization should be considered. Potential advantages of this form of therapy over mechanical ventilation are a shortened duration of ventilation (usually less than 7 days), improved pain control, and perhaps improved anatomic healing resulting in improved pulmonary function (125).

Long-term pulmonary disability in patients with flail chest, with or without associated intrathoracic injuries, is significant. As many as 60% of these patients continue to have complaints of chest wall pain, marked chest wall deformity, or dyspnea on exertion for months to years after the injury. Measurements of pulmonary function reveal an overall decrease in the MVV as well as mild restrictive pulmonary disease (126, 127). Mortality from flail chest continues to remain high, up to 35%, despite recent advances in knowledge and treatment of this injury. Mortality is usually related to extrathoracic injuries (especially central nervous system trauma) and appears to be independent of the degree of underlying pulmonary and other intrathoracic injuries (128). Flail chest is thus an important indicator that the patient has sustained a major traumatic insult and demands that the physician maintain a close vigilance for associated life-threatening injuries.

## PNEUMOTHORAX

Traumatic pneumothorax, defined as the entry of air into the pleural cavity, occurs after both penetrating and nonpenetrating thoracic trauma. An *open* pneumothorax occurs when air in the pleural cavity communicates freely with the environment. Free communication occurs when the size of the chest wall defect is at least two-thirds of the cross-sectional area of the trachea. It is most frequently seen in combat victims and in civilians who have suffered a close-range shotgun blast injury. An open pneumothorax results in an inability of the patient to maintain intrapleural pressures between the two hemithoraces. It precludes the generation of an effective negative intrathoracic pressure in both the unaffected and the affected hemithorax, resulting in respiratory embarrassment.

When the egress of pleural air to the external environment is prevented, intrapleural pressure on the affected side rapidly increases, resulting in the development of a *tension pneumothorax*. This causes a shift of the mediastinum away from the affected side, a progressive decrease in venous return, hypotension, and shock. The exact mechanism for the decrease in venous return is still unclear. "Kinking" of the great vessels by a mediastinal shift does not appear to be responsible for the decrease in venous return (129, 130). Furthermore, as long as the negative intrathoracic pressure swing occurs with inspiration, as in the spontaneously ventilating animal, cardiac output is maintained. This remains true even with an intrapleural pressure of $+20$ cm $H_2O$ caused by a unilateral tension pneumothorax. However, when spontaneous ventilation is abolished and the negative intrathoracic pressure swing abates, cardiac output may decrease significantly. A bellows mechanism of spontaneous breathing may contribute to the maintenance of venous return. Hypoxemia often develops with a tension pneumothorax from both increased shunt and worsened ventilation-perfusion mismatch in both the collapsed lung and the uninvolved lung. The uninvolved lung may develop a 40% decrease in FRC (131).

The diagnosis of an open pneumothorax is based on the findings of respiratory distress in combination with an open, sucking chest wound and decreased breath sounds on the side of the affected hemithorax. Pulmonary collapse can be confirmed with a chest radiograph. The diagnosis of a tension pneumothorax is also clinical and identified by the presence of respiratory distress, the unilateral absence of breath sounds, and the presence of hypertympanic percussion note. Late signs include tracheal deviation and distended neck veins. Distended neck veins are also found in cardiac tamponade, but this can usually be distinguished from a tension pneumothorax by the lack of tracheal deviation and hypertympany to percussion.

Treatment of an open pneumothorax is directed at ventilatory support, when needed, combined with the prompt reexpansion of the collapsed lung. The latter is accomplished by occlusion of the open, sucking chest wound with an airtight, sterile dressing, followed by the immediate placement of a large-bore, straight chest tube (size 36 French or greater) into the fourth or fifth intercostal space in the midaxillary line. Suction is applied at $-15$ to $-20$ cm $H_2O$ pressure. Large-bore chest tubes placed posterolaterally are preferred in the treatment of a traumatic pneumothorax (instead of small-bore anteriorly placed chest tubes) to provide better drainage for blood from an associated hemothorax. As much as 300 ml of blood may be hidden in the pleural cavity of a patient, and an upright posteroanterior chest radiograph may be interpreted as "pneumothorax only." In a supine chest radiograph, 1000 ml of blood may appear as nothing more than a mild increase in density over the affected hemithorax.

The life-threatening nature of a tension pneumothorax demands immediate relief of the increased intrapleural pressure. In the hypotensive patient who is suspected of having a tension pneumothorax, this is most rapidly accomplished by inserting an uncapped 14- or 16-gauge 2-inch plastic intravenous catheter into the second intercostal space in the midclavicular line. Care must be taken to insert the needle over the superior edge of the third rib to avoid the intercostal vessels, which run along the inferior margin of adjacent superior rib. Only the pleural cavity is entered, the catheter is left in place and the needle removed while arrangements are made for the immediate placement of a large-bore chest tube as described above. Even if no rush of air out of the pleural cavity occurs with the placement of the needle thoracostomy, one is then committed to inserting a chest tube into the pleural space. A chest radiograph should be obtained after insertion of the chest tube, to ensure that the evacuation of air has been complete and that lung reexpansion is full.

At times the complete evacuation of air from the pleural space can be difficult. New or multiple additional chest tubes and increased suction may be required. In patients who have suffered recent thoracic trauma, a persistent pneumothorax and air leak should alert one to the possibility of a bronchial or tracheal disruption (see below). In the chronically ventilated patient with ARDS, incomplete evacuation of a pneumothorax may be due to loculations that form within the pleural cavity, making accurate chest tube placement into these pockets mandatory.

### HEMOTHORAX

One of the most common injuries of both penetrating and blunt thoracic trauma is hemothorax, occurring in approximately 70% of both of these forms of trauma. A "massive hemothorax," defined as the presence of 1500 ml or more of blood in the pleural cavity, is an uncommon occurrence accounting for less than 20% of all hemothoraces. A massive hemothorax often represents an injury to the heart, great vessels, or other major systemic artery, rather than an injury to the pulmonary parenchyma, which is perfused at low blood pressures. A massive hemothorax causes hypotension on the basis of intravascular volume loss but can also cause hypoxemia as a result of ventilation-perfusion mismatching and shunting of blood through the compressed lung. Tension hemothorax does not occur, because the blood volumes required to produce significant increases in intrathoracic pressure are so massive that they inevitably first cause hypotension from volume loss.

The diagnosis of a massive hemothorax should rarely be missed, since shock will be the major presenting feature. Physical examination reveals diminished breath sounds and dullness to percussion. As noted above, 1 liter of blood can occupy a hemithorax, and the only finding on the supine chest radiograph will be a subtle increase in the density of the overlying affected hemithorax. This underscores the necessity for obtaining an upright or decubitus film in all cases of blunt or penetrating thoracic trauma. Even the upright posteroanterior chest radiograph can hide 300 ml of blood. The initial treatment of any hemothorax is the evacuation of the pleural cavity with a large-bore (size 36 French or greater) chest tube placed into the fifth or sixth intercostal space in the midaxillary line and directed superiorly and posteriorly. Needle thoracentesis other than for diagnostic purposes is inadequate and risky therapy of a hemothorax, because of an inability to monitor blood loss and the risk of incomplete evacuation of blood from the pleural space (see below). After insertion, the chest tube is connected to a suction of $-15$ to $-20$ cm $H_2O$ pressure.

Autotransfusion devices are becoming commonplace in many emergency departments in the United States; if one is readily available, it should be set up in the presence of a suspected massive hemothorax to expedite the important restoration of blood volume. Up to 5 liters of blood may be retransfused in this fashion without any ill effects. Monitoring of the initial and subsequent blood volume output via the tube thoracostomy will help determine the need for a thoracotomy. An initial output of 1500 ml of blood immediately following the insertion of the chest tube or the persistence of bleeding at a rate of greater than 150 to 200 ml/hour for 3 hours or longer are rough guidelines for the need for an exploratory thoracotomy (131, 132).

After the placement of the chest tube, a chest radiograph is obtained immediately to evaluate the adequacy of evacuation of blood from the pleural cavity and the degree of pulmonary reexpansion. If any residual blood remains in the pleural space, the tube, if malpositioned, should be removed and a new tube inserted. However, if the chest tube is properly positioned, an additional chest tube should be placed into the residual collection. Failure to evacuate a hemothorax may place the patient at increased risk for the formation of a restrictive pleural rind, which limits lung expansion, resulting in restrictive pulmonary function abnormalities and an increased risk of atelectatic and pneumonic complications (133).

### POSTTRAUMATIC EMPYEMA

Bacterial contamination of the pleural space results in posttraumatic empyema in about 5% of patients with penetrating or blunt thoracic injury (134). Gram-positive organisms, especially *Staphylococcus* and *Streptococcus* species occur most frequently. In patients with associated intraabdominal injury or in those who require laparotomy, Gram-negative aerobic organisms, including *E. coli, Klebsiella,* and *Pseudomonas,* are the most common (135).

Effective treatment of posttraumatic empyema requires evacuation of infected material from the pleural space and reexpansion of the lung. This frequently requires thoracotomy and removal of all clot and organized material, although multiple chest tubes may be tried initially.

### PULMONARY CONTUSION

Pulmonary contusion is most commonly caused by blunt chest trauma, in which the lung impacts directly against the chest wall. This trauma results in the local disruption of the alveolar microvasculature, allowing red blood cells and plasma to exude and flood the alveoli. It is radiographically distinct from ARDS in that it involves a focal area of lung, it appears immediately after the traumatic insult, and it resolves within 72 hours. The filling of alveoli with blood and plasma results in decreases in pulmonary compliance, TLC, and FRC and an increase in shunt, with consequent decreases in arterial oxygenation. Oppenheimer and coworkers have shown in animal models that overall perfusion to the contused lung segments is reduced, thus somewhat limiting the oxygenation defect (136). The severity of hypoxemia is proportional to the amount of lung involved by the contusion.

The diagnosis of pulmonary contusion is made by the combination of clinical history along with early chest radiographs showing focal infiltrates occurring in a nonsegmental or nonlobar distribution. Treatment is supportive, with mechanical ventilation for refractory hypoxemia.

There are currently three areas of controversy in the treatment of pulmonary contusion. The first is the use of volume restriction and diuresis. There is no evidence to support the use of either of these therapies (137). Most agree that volume overloading and creation of pulmonary edema is to be avoided in any patient, including those with pulmonary contusion; however, it is unlikely that patients with pulmonary contusion would benefit from volume restriction and diuresis. A reasonable clinical approach is the judicious administration of volume as necessary to maintain adequate perfusion of vital organs, balanced by an awareness of the problem of maintaining oxygenation. Volume restriction and diuretics should be reserved for patients with evidence of volume overload as evidenced by physical examination and elevated central pressures.

The second controversy in the treatment of pulmonary contusion is whether volume resuscitation using colloid instead of crystalloid improves respiratory parameters and outcome. The essence of this argument is that colloid solution resuscitation will remain intravascular, thus maintaining colloid osmotic pressure, and decrease the tendency toward pulmonary edema, while crystalloid solution resuscitation will lower the plasma colloid osmotic pressure, increasing filtration in vascular beds. Dodek and coworkers (138) studied the effects of plasmapheresis and hypoproteinemia on lung lymph flow and lung microvascular conductance in unanesthetized sheep and found that although there was a transient decrease in the lymph:serum protein concentration and a transient increase in lung microvascular conductance, there was a simultaneous increase in lung lymph flow. Furthermore, all these changes resolved within 4 hours. There is currently no evidence to support the conclusion that crystalloid resuscitation, in comparison to colloid resuscitation, causes a greater net accumulation of pulmonary fluid, results in fewer pulmonary complications, or improves outcome in patients with pulmonary contusion.

The third area of debate involves the use of corticosteroids in pulmonary contusion. There is experimental evidence in animals supporting the use of corticosteroids in the treatment of pulmonary contusion (139). However, Lucas and Ledgerwood (140) found that massive doses of corticosteroids in humans neither prevented nor ameliorated pulmonary failure after shock and indeed may have aggravated it. Richardson and coworkers (141) found that bacterial clearance in contused animal lungs was decreased only when associated with hypovolemia or steroid administration and not in pulmonary contusion alone. There are currently no data from humans to support the use of corticosteroids in the treatment of pulmonary contusion.

Mortality rates of patients with pulmonary contusion appear to depend on the severity of associated injuries (with Glasgow Coma Score less than 7, Injury Severity Score over 25, and more than three units of blood transfused reflecting poorer outcome) and possibly the degree of hypoxemia ($PaO_2/FIO_2$ 300). Bongard and Lewis (142), however, found no difference in the ratio $PaO_2/FIO_2$ between survivors and nonsurvivors with pulmonary contusions in their retrospective study. They did, however, find that an initial respiratory acidosis due to ventilatory impairment correlated with a high mortality. Another major influence on mortality rates in patients with pulmonary contusion is the development of major pulmonary complications in the involved lung segment. For example, 50 to 70% of patients with pulmonary contusion will develop pneumonia in the contused segment, and another 35% of these will proceed to develop an empyema. This emphasizes the importance of the ability to clear bacteria from contused lung segments in the presence of hypovolemia, as well as the possible importance of aggressive pulmonary toilet in these patients.

### ADULT RESPIRATORY DISTRESS SYNDROME

ARDS is a pathologic entity characterized by increased permeability of the pulmonary microvasculature. The syndrome most commonly occurs in the setting of sepsis or trauma (75 to 90% of the cases). The pathophysiologic mechanism responsible for the abnormal pulmonary microvascular permeability is currently an area of intense scientific investigation and debate. There seem to be initial pathogenic differences between ARDS induced by sepsis and that induced by trauma, probably followed by a final common pathway of cellular disruption via the production of oxygen free radicals. Trauma-induced ARDS appears to involve the clotting cascade, with a tendency toward a hypercoagulable state and the collection of platelet microemboli in pulmonary microvasculature (143). The secretory products of platelets and neutrophils enhance each other's activity (144). Activated neutrophils are able to attract platelets and cause them to release their vasoactive substances; on the other hand, serotonin released by the platelets is known to increase the adhesion of neutrophils to endothelial membranes and increase their cytotoxic effect on those membranes. The syndrome is more fully discussed in Chapter 23.

### FAT EMBOLISM SYNDROME

The fat embolism syndrome (FES) is an uncommon but serious clinical syndrome seen primarily in patients with traumatic injuries that can result in pulmonary insufficiency and neurological dysfunction. The

**TABLE 25.12**
**CRITERIA FOR DIAGNOSIS OF FAT EMBOLISM SYNDROME (FES)**

Major criteria
  Hypoxemia ($PO_2$ <60 on $FIO_2$ on 0.40)
  Pulmonary edema
  CNS depression or dysfunction
  Axillary or conjunctival petechiae
Minor criteria
  Tachycardia (HR >110)
  Fever above 38.5 C
  Decrease in hematocrit or platelet count
  Retinal emboli on fundoscopic examination
  Fat globules in sputum
  Lipuria

first description of FES was by von Bergman in 1873 (145), in a patient who sustained a fractured femur followed by respiratory insufficiency, coma, and death. The classic triad includes respiratory distress, neurologic dysfunction, and petechiae, although all three findings may not be present. Gurd has provided major and minor criteria that have gained widespread acceptance (146). Diagnosis of the syndrome requires the presence of at least one major criterion and four minor criteria (Table 25.12).

The clinical syndrome usually develops between 12 to 72 hours following fractures of the long bones or pelvis. There is widespread variation in incidence among various studies, but historically the incidence in multiple trauma patients is 5 to 10% (147, 148). A recent study of isolated fractures in skiers found a 23% incidence, suggesting that features of the syndrome may be mild and may have been masked by other injuries in multiple trauma patients and not identified unless the symptoms were more severe (149).

The pathogenesis of the pulmonary injury has not been fully elucidated. Fat globules from bone marrow embolize to pulmonary vessels, causing obstruction. Lipases are thought to hydrolyze the neutral fat, releasing free fatty acids with resulting inflammation, endothelial injury, and other pathways leading to acute lung injury. The syndrome has been described in critically ill patients without trauma, in which case agglutinated intravascular chylomicrons may be the source of the emboli and free fatty acids. The pathogenesis in other organs such as the CNS may result from similar mechanisms. The presence of lipid emboli in the lung microvessels, however, does not necessarily result in FES, since fat emboli have been found in over 90% of major trauma patients (150).

The clinical presentation of FES typically begins with pulmonary signs of dyspnea, tachypnea, and respiratory distress as early as 4 hours following an inciting event such as trauma or orthopaedic surgery. CNS disturbances occur about this time and range from mild disorientation to seizures and coma. Focal neurological findings are less common. The development of petechiae is typically delayed by hours and found on the chest, axillae, groin, or conjunctivae. Laboratory abnormalities are present by this time. The chest radiograph, while it may be normal initially, demonstrates diffuse bilateral interstitial or alveolar infiltrates consistent with an acute lung injury. Patients with multiple trauma may have other injuries to which these findings may be attributed, so a high index of suspicion is warranted.

Identification of neutral fat droplets in pulmonary capillary (151, 152) and bronchoalveolar washings (153) has been reported as a potential means of more definitive diagnosis. The presence of fat in the pulmonary microcirculation does not always result in FES or lung injury and may occur in other conditions (154, 155). It may also occur from biochemical changes following trauma and be a result, not a cause, of pulmonary injury (156). The usefulness of these methods remains to be established.

Treatment is both preventive and supportive. Definitive fracture management may lessen the incidence of FES (157, 158), as may aggressive trauma resuscitation and rapid reversal of shock. Once the syndrome becomes established, supportive treatment follows that for ARDS. Prophylactic corticosteroids have been evaluated in clinical trials and consistently found to reduce the incidence of FES in dosages of 7.5 to 10 mg/kg/dose (159, 160) and more recently at lower doses of 1.5 mg/kg/dose (161). The role of corticosteroids is still controversial because the safety of their use is not completely established.

## PULMONARY HEMATOMA

Pulmonary hematomas most commonly result from blunt chest trauma through the generation of shear forces, resulting in pulmonary laceration. Blood quickly fills the space created by the parenchymal disruption, initially creating an indistinct infiltrate on the chest radiograph. Over a period of several days, there is improved radiographic delineation on the border of the lesion, leaving a typical "coin lesion" in the pulmonary parenchyma. If an adjacent segmental bronchus is disrupted simultaneously with the vessel, air in addition to blood will fill and expand the cavity, creating a traumatic pneumatocele. These lesions are most often asymptomatic. The natural history of pulmonary hematomas and traumatic pneumatoceles is one of spontaneous resolution within 3 to 4 weeks. Most surgeons favor a conservative regimen of observation unless continued hemorrhage, air leak, or infection supervenes. If, on the other hand, the lesion has not resolved within 4 to 6 weeks and there are no prior films available for comparison, the lesion should be excised and examined pathologically.

## PULMONARY LACERATION AND AIR EMBOLIZATION

Pulmonary lacerations may be caused by both penetrating and blunt trauma, although the vast majority are caused by penetrating injuries. In blunt chest trauma, they occur most commonly by direct piercing or tearing of the lung by the jagged edges of broken ribs and less commonly through shear forces generated by abrupt thoracic compression and rebound decompression. The most common presentation of a pulmonary laceration is either hemothorax or pneumothorax or a combination of the two. Because the bleeding is from the lung parenchyma, which is perfused at relatively low pressures, bleeding tends not to be profuse, and less than 4% of these patients require thoracotomy to control either the continued bleeding or a persistent air leak (162).

One of the most dreaded complications resulting from penetrating or blunt thoracic trauma is air embolism through a traumatic fistula created between a bronchus and either the pulmonary artery or pulmonary vein (163, 164). Once an airway-circulatory fistula exists, a pressure gradient is needed to drive the air into the circulation. Peak airway pressures during emergent resuscitation of an intubated patient who is being hand ventilated can be as high as 100 mm Hg, thus explaining one common presentation of an air embolus as the immediate onset of shock and cardiac arrest in a patient with thoracic trauma who has just been intubated (164, 165). The fistulous connection of the pulmonary venous circulation to an airway is the major cause of air entry into the systemic circulation following trauma. There is good evidence that air may also enter the right side of the heart through a lacerated intercostal or bronchial vein, while air may also enter the left side of the heart through a cardiac anomaly connecting the right and left circulation; for example, a traumatic ventricular septal defect (VSD) or a patent foramen ovale (probe patency of the foramen ovale occurs in 15 to 25% of the general population) (166).

A subtle clinical sign serving as the harbinger to a potential air embolus is hemoptysis. A relatively large volume of air (5 to 8 ml/kg body weight) can be tolerated into the right side of the circulation (right ventricle and pulmonary artery), while as little as 0.5 ml of air can be lethal when entered into the left side of the circulation (pulmonary vein, left ventricle, and systemic circulation) (167). The clinical presentation of right-sided air embolism results from the blockade of the right ventricle or pulmonary circulation by air, with consequent signs and symptoms of shock or electromechanical dissociation (EMD). Clinically, left-sided air embolism is evident through its effects on the coronary circulation, as evidenced by arrhythmias (especially ventricular ectopy, asystole, or EMD), or effects on the cerebral circulation, as evidenced by feelings of dizziness or light-headedness, progressing in severity to loss of consciousness, seizures, blindness, and paresis. Once the diagnosis is suspected, the patient should immediately be placed in the head-down position to minimize the risk of further cerebral air emboli and with the affected hemithorax in the dependent position, to increase the pulmonary venous pressure and decrease the airway-circulatory pressure differential. In addition, high peak airway pressures from positive-pressure ventilation should be avoided. Immediate thoracotomy is indicated to allow cross-clamping of the hilum of the affected lung, if that is the probable source of the air emboli, and venting of the aortic root with a large-bore needle, as well as the aspiration of air from the left and right ventricles with a needle.

## TRACHEAL AND BRONCHIAL DISRUPTION

Disruption of the tracheobronchial tree can occur with both blunt and penetrating trauma, but blunt trauma accounts for the larger portion of tracheobronchial injuries in the civilian population. The exact mechanism responsible for tracheobronchial disruption is unknown but may involve shearing forces produced by the rapid deceleration of mobile lungs against a fixed cricoid cartilage and carina or may involve the sudden increase in intraluminal airway pressure with a resultant tracheobronchial "blowout" as the external decelerating force is applied to the chest wall while the glottis is closed (168). The most common site of tracheobronchial injury due to blunt chest trauma is within 2.5 cm of the carina (168–170). The tracheal lacerations usually occur at the junction of the membranous trachea with the cartilaginous trachea and are vertical and posterior where the cartilage is deficient. The bronchial injuries usually occur at the takeoff of the main or upper lobe bronchus and are often transverse (171).

The diagnosis of tracheobronchial disruption can be difficult to make. Collins and coworkers found that 68% of the injuries were not diagnosed until atelectasis or sepsis had arisen (172). The clinical presentation of tracheobronchial injury occurs in one of two ways, depending on whether the disruption does or does not communicate with the pleural cavity. In the first group, when the tracheobronchial disruption communicates

with the pleural cavity, the predominant finding will be of a large pneumothorax. When a chest tube is placed into the pleural space, a persistent and large air leak is encountered, the pneumothorax persists, and the lung fails to reexpand. These patients are dyspneic and have increasing subcutaneous emphysema along the chest wall and the mediastinum. Hypoxemia resulting from shunt through the collapsed lung may be severe, causing the patient to be cyanotic. Hemoptysis from rupture of a bronchial vessel occurs in less than 20% of injuries. In the second group, when the tracheobronchial disruption fails to communicate with the pleural space, air escapes into the surrounding tissues and dissects into the mediastinum, not into the pleural cavity. Uncommonly, a small pneumothorax is present secondary to slight extension of the airway disruption into the pleural space, which is then quickly sealed off by fibrin or clot. The resultant small pneumothorax is easily treated with a tube thoracostomy, does not recur, and does not persist in leaking air. Hemoptysis is uncommon. Mediastinal emphysema may be slight and not extend into the deep cervical tissues, making this type of tracheobronchial disruption extremely difficult to diagnose. The most sensitive test in this case is detection of the pneumomediastinum or deep cervical emphysema on the chest x-ray.

Frequently, the diagnosis of tracheobronchial disruption is missed only to become evident 3 to 4 weeks later when the fibrous ridge of scar tissue created by the healing of the disrupted airway leads to a partial or complete occlusion of the airway, with resultant atelectasis of the lung distal to the disrupted airway. Other important radiologic clues aiding in the early diagnosis of tracheobronchial disruption include abrupt cutoff of the course of an air-filled bronchus and rib fractures limited to the upper thorax (ribs 1 through 4). Most important of all, however, is maintenance of a high index of clinical suspicion for the diagnosis of tracheobronchial disruption in all patients who have suffered severe thoracic trauma.

Once the diagnosis of tracheobronchial disruption is suspected, it is best confirmed in the acute situation by bronchoscopy. This should be performed in an operating room with provisions ready for an emergency thoracotomy. In cases in which there may be a cervical spine injury, a fiberoptic bronchoscope can be used instead of a rigid bronchoscope. Bronchography is usually contraindicated as a diagnostic technique in the acute evaluation of tracheobronchial disruption because of the patient's unstable condition. Once the diagnosis of a tracheobronchial disruption is made, early surgical repair is indicated. An exception is made for lesions meeting all three of the following criteria: (*a*) bronchial tears involve less than one-third of the circumference of the bronchus; (b) a chest tube thoracostomy successfully treats any associated pneumothorax; and (c) an air leak does not persist after tube thoracostomy (173). When required, repair is performed by debridement of the divided airway edges and a primary, delicate anastomosis using interrupted nonabsorbable sutures. When the diagnosis of a tracheobronchial disruption is not entertained until several weeks or more after the injury has occurred, bronchography is very useful in delineating the extent and site of the injury, and surgical reconstruction should still be pursued unless there is distal suppuration, in which case lobectomy is indicated.

The overall mortality of tracheobronchial disruption is approximately 30% and is related to the location of the disruption (proximal lesions being more fatal than distal lesions), the severity of the complications associated with the injury, and the severity of other extrathoracic injuries (174). This number probably underestimates the true mortality rate because it does not include patients who die at the scene of the accident or prior to their arrival at the hospital. The results of patients undergoing early repair are excellent, with more than 90% of the patients having no residual deficits.

Tracheoesophageal fistulas are rarely due to thoracic trauma alone and are more commonly seen as the result of pressure applied on the tracheal and esophageal walls by the simultaneous placement of endotracheal and nasogastric tubes. The lesion solely due to thoracic trauma is created in a manner similar to that described earlier in this section for tracheal disruption; however, in this case the disruptive process extends to include the esophagus. Later the damaged segment of esophageal wall breaks down, after it becomes adherent to the adjacently damaged trachea. A fistula is thus formed between the two structures with minimal, if any, mediastinal contamination. The tracheal lesion is usually located within 2.5 cm of the carina, in the weak posterior portion of the trachea where cartilage is deficient. The diagnosis is made when the patient shows signs of aspiration pneumonia, usually 3 to 5 days after the injury. If the patient is intubated, gastric contents are found in the bronchial secretions, and ventilation is heard to fill the stomach with each breath. Immediate management consists of endotracheal intubation below the site of the fistula to protect the lungs against further aspiration. Early operative repair with debridement of the wound edges and primary anastomosis is the treatment of choice (175).

### DIAPHRAGMATIC TRAUMA

Diaphragmatic disruption may result from both penetrating and blunt trauma. Diaphragmatic defects due to penetrating trauma are usually less than 4 cm in diameter, and their location is determined by the point of entry and direction of entry of the missile. Left-sided lesions predominate in penetrating diaphragmatic injuries, probably because of the predominance of right-handed assailants. In the spontaneously ventilating patient, the dome of the diaphragm can reach as high as the fourth intercostal space, and penetrating thoracic injuries as high as the level of the nipples anteriorly or the tip of the scapula posteriorly may involve the diaphragm. Small right-sided diaphragmatic defects are effectively plugged by the liver and therefore often remain clinically shut and difficult to detect. Diaphragmatic defects due to blunt trauma tend to be large, over 6 cm, peripherally located, and predominantly left-sided. This left-sided predominance is hypothesized to be due to the lack of visceral support by the liver. In both blunt and penetrating diaphragmatic trauma, the peritoneum and parietal pleura (and more rarely the pericardium) are disrupted, thus explaining the free communication of the contents of each cavity with one another and the anatomic fact that diaphragmatic hernias lack a hernia sac. Diaphragmatic defects are important pathologically in that they allow abdominal viscera to herniate into the thoracic cavity. Organs that tend to herniate are, in decreasing order of frequency, colon, stomach, spleen, omentum, liver, and ileum. Herniation of these organs into the thoracic cavity may result in nothing more than compression of the adjacent lung parenchyma and atelectasis or may be complicated by strangulation and infarction (most commonly the colon), displacement of both lung and mediastinum, or massive bleeding (most commonly spleen or liver).

The preoperative diagnosis of a traumatic defect in the diaphragm is often difficult to make, because these patients usually have multiple injuries that often mask the subtle findings of the diaphragmatic injury. Clinical signs and symptoms are abdominal, cardiovascular, or pulmonary and are insensitive and nonspecific. They include vague abdominal pain, peritonitis, intestinal obstruction, ventricular ectopy, tachypnea, cough, chest pain, and hypotension. Pain referred to the shoulder or bowel sounds in the thoracic cavity are infrequently found. Chest radiographs are normal in up to 40% of the patients with penetrating diaphragmatic trauma, with another 50% showing only a nonspecific hemothorax or pneumothorax. Chest radiographs in blunt diaphragmatic disruption show a herniated viscus in up to 30% of cases, with 60% showing a nonspecific hemothorax or pneumothorax. The presence of a nasogastric tube curled in the stomach in a supradiaphragmatic position is a rare but useful finding. Computed tomography is also of value in the rapid diagnosis of this injury in the acute setting. Thoracoscopy is a highly sensitive diagnostic method when performed within the first 24 hours of the injury (111). Diagnostic pneumoperitoneum with the infusion of 300 to 500 ml of nitrous oxide into the left lower quadrant creates a diagnostic pneumothorax when open communication exists between the peritoneal and pleural cavities. The optimum time for this open communication is in the first 24 hours, prior to the formation of an adherent clot or tight herniation of an abdominal viscus at the site of diaphragmatic disruption. The infusion of gas into the peritoneal cavity, however, can cause or worsen abdominal pain, thus making its use in the acute setting less desirable. Other reported, but less useful, diagnostic modalities include hepatic and splenic radioisotopic scanning and celiac angiography.

Most frequently the diagnosis of a traumatic rent in the diaphragm is made at the time of operative exploration for another major injury. In one series of diaphragmatic disruption due to blunt trauma, 100% of the patients had an associated intraabdominal major injury, most frequently a ruptured spleen (176). In the case of penetrating diaphragmatic injuries, 30 to 70% had associated intraabdominal injuries (177). Many advocate abdominal exploration of all penetrating wounds below the nipple, including those on the flank. Even at the time of operation, 2 to 10% of diaphragmatic injuries will be missed because attention is directed toward an associated major injury, thus emphasizing the need for careful exploration of the entire abdominal or thoracic cavity once the major injury has been treated. Delayed diagnosis, later than 24 hours, occurs in roughly 10 to 15% of cases, which most frequently present as acute intestinal obstruction or acute respiratory distress.

Once the diagnosis is made, urgent operation is indicated, even if the patient is asymptomatic. In the acute situation, this is done via an exploratory laparotomy. When the diagnosis is made late and intrathoracic adhesions have formed, it is not clear whether a thoracic or an abdominal approach is best. Careful inspection for associated injuries is required. Although diaphragmatic dysfunction in these patients is not understood, the possibility exists for dysfunction at least as severe as that associated with operations near the diaphragm.

In the acute setting, mortality rates in patients with diaphragmatic defects range from 10 to 20% and reflect the severity of associated injuries (lower for penetrating trauma than for blunt trauma) (178). Patients rarely die from their diaphragmatic defects (less than 1%); however, once a viscus becomes strangulated and infarcted, mortality rates increase to 25 to 66% (179).

## ESOPHAGEAL PERFORATION

Perforation or rupture of the esophagus can occur spontaneously or following trauma, instrumentation, or foreign body ingestion (180). The diagnosis of perforation is frequently difficult, and a high index of suspicion in appropriate settings is required. The most common cause is iatrogenic perforation during esophageal endoscopic or dilatory procedures, with a rate of about 0.13% (181). The region of the cricopharyngeus muscle is the narrowest portion of the esophagus and the most common site of iatrogenic perforation. Perforations occur with nearly equal frequency in flexible and rigid endoscopies (182). Procedures performed in the presence of esophageal disease are more likely to result in perforation. Traumatic attempts at endotracheal intubation can result in perforation, which is often not recognized at the time of the procedure.

Penetrating trauma is more common in the cervical esophagus because of the protection afforded by the chest wall, but thoracic injuries have a fourfold higher mortality. Blunt trauma to the abdomen or chest is an uncommon cause of perforation. Foreign bodies can result in traumatic perforation from direct injury, attempts at removal, or subsequent pressure necrosis.

Spontaneous perforation can occur with forceful emesis (Boerhaave's syndrome) as well as other abrupt increases in intraabdominal pressure, such as blunt trauma or heavy lifting. The mechanism is not clear, but an increased intraluminal pressure in the presence of a functional obstruction is felt to be responsible. Preexisting esophageal disease predisposes to traumatic rupture.

The complications of perforation include mediastinitis and mediastinal sepsis, which may extend to include the pleural and abdominal cavities.

The diagnosis of perforation can be difficult, because symptoms may initially be absent. Examination may reveal subcutaneous emphysema. A mediastinal crunch may be heard on auscultation. Hematemesis may be the only sign. On plain radiographs, a prevertebral shadow, a widened mediastinum, and cervical or mediastinal emphysema are helpful signs. If these signs are present or suspicion is high, esophagography with a water-soluble contrast agent is the most helpful test. Penetrating wounds to the cervical area should be explored if the wound extends through the platysma, even in the absence of other findings.

The approaches to treatment have traditionally been operative, but nonoperative treatment in selected circumstances may result in lower morbidity and may be a therapeutic option. Nonoperative management should be considered if the perforation appears to be localized, without significant symptoms, and without sepsis and if the involved area can drain to the esophagus. The mainstays of medical therapy include discontinuation of oral intake, intravenous hydration, antibiotic therapy, and parenteral nutritional support.

Operative management is indicated in the presence of sepsis, respiratory failure, communication with the pleural or peritoneal cavities, extension from the site by the presence of mediastinal emphysema, or obstruction. The operative procedure depends on the site and extent of involvement but ranges from drainage procedures to closure with a local tissue flap. Drainage gastrostomy may be performed simultaneously. Occasionally, esophageal resection or exclusion is required.

▼

## REFERENCES

1. Marsh HM, Southorn PA, Rehder K: Anesthesia, sedation, and the chest wall. *Int Anesthesiol Clin* 22:1–12, 1984.
2. Dueck R, Prutow RJ, Davies NJ, Clausen JL, Davidson TM: The lung volume at which shunting occurs with inhalational anesthesia. *Anesthesiology* 69:854–861, 1988.
3. Schmid ER, Rehder K: General anesthesia and the chest wall. *Anesthesiology* 55:668–675, 1981.
4. Froese AB, Bryan AC: Effects of anesthesia and paralysis on diaphragmatic mechanics in men. *Anesthesiology* 41:242–255, 1974.
5. Covino B, Fozzard H, Rehder K, Strichartz G: *Effects of Anesthesia.* Bethesda, MD, American Physiological Society, 1985.
6. Hedenstierna G, Tokics L, Strandberg A, Lundquist H, Brismar B: Correlation of gas exchange impairment to development of atelectasis during anaesthesia and muscle paralysis. *Acta Anaesthesiol Scand* 30:183–191, 1986.
7. Hedenstierna G: New aspects on atelectasis formation and gas exchange impairment during anaesthesia. *Clin Physiol* 9:407–417, 1989.
8. Brismar B, Hedenstierna G, Lundquist H, et al: Pulmonary densities during anesthesia with muscular relaxation—a proposal of atelectasis. *Anesthesiology* 62:422–428, 1985.
9. Duek R: Gas exchange. *Int Anesthesiol Clin* 22:13, 1984.
10. Eisenkraft JB: Effects of anaesthetics on the pulmonary circulation. *Br J Anaesth* 65:63–78, 1990.
11. Carlsson J, Hedenstierna G, Bindsley L: Hypoxia-induced vasoconstriction in human lung exposed to enflurane anaesthesia. *Acta Anaesthesiol Scand* 31:57–62, 1987.
12. Nunn JF: *Applied Respiratory Physiology,* ed 2. London, Butterworth, 1977.
13. Rybro L, Schurizek BA, Petersen TK, Wernberg M: Postoperative analgesia and lung function a comparison of intramuscular with epidural morphine. *Acta Anaesthesiol Scand* 26:514–518, 1982.
14. Rawal N, Sjöstrand U, Christoffersson E, et al: Comparison of intramuscular and epidural morphine for postoperative analgesia in the grossly obese: influence on postoperative ambulation and pulmonary function. *Anesth Analg* 63:583–592, 1984.
15. Bonnet F, Blery C, Zatan M, Simonet O, Brage D, Guady J: Effect of epidural morphine on postoperative pulmonary dysfunction. *Acta Anaesthesiol Scand* 28:147–151, 1984.
16. Jayr C, Mollie A, Bourgain JL, Alarcon J, Masselot J, Lasser P, Denjean A, Trauffa-Bachi J: Postoperative pulmonary complications: general anesthesia with postoperative parenteral morphine compared with epidural analgesia. *Surgery* 104:57–63, 1989.
17. Simmoneau G, Vivien A, Sartene R, Kunstlinger F, Samii K, Noviant Y, Duroux P: Diaphragmatic dysfunction induced by upper abdominal surgery: role of postoperative pain. *Am Rev Respir Dis* 128:899–903, 1983.
18. Mankikian B, Cantineau JP, Bertrand M, Kieffer E, Sartene R, Viars P: Improvement of diaphragmatic function by a thoracic extradural block after upper abdominal surgery. *Anesthesiology* 68:379–386, 1988.
19. Cushieri RJ, Morran CG, Howie JC, McArdle CS: Postoperative pain and pulmonary complications. Comparison of three analgesic regimens. *Br J Surg* 72:495–498, 1985.
20. Jayr C, Thomas H, Rey A, Farhat F, Lasser PH, Bourgain JL: Postoperative pulmonary complications: epidural analgesia using bupivacaine and opioids versus parenteral opioids. *Anesthesiology* 78:666–676, 1993.
21. Craig DB: Postoperative recovery of pulmonary function. *Anesth Analg* 60:46–52, 1981.
22. Alexander JI, Spence AA, Parikh RK, Stuart B: The role of airway closure in postoperative hypoxaemia. *Br J Anaesth* 45:34–40, 1973.
23. Wahba WM, Don HF, Craig DB: Post-operative epidural analgesia: effects on lung volumes. *Can Anaesth Soc J* 22:519–527, 1975.
24. Ford GT, Whitelaw WA, Rosenal TW, Cruse PJ, Guenter CA: Diaphragm function after upper abdominal surgery in humans. *Am Rev Respir Dis* 127:431–436, 1983.
25. Tahir AH, George RB, Weill H, Adriani J: Effects of abdominal surgery upon diaphragmatic function and regional ventilation. *Int Surg* 58:337–340, 1973.
26. Ford GT, Rideout KS, Bozdech LK, et al: Inhibition of breathing arising from gallbladder in dogs. *Physiologist* 26:20–28, 1983.
27. Dureuil B, Desmonts JM, Mankikian B, Prokocimer P: Effects of aminophylline on diaphragmatic dysfunction after upper abdominal surgery. *Anesthesiology* 62:242–246, 1985.
28. Gothard JW, Branthwaite MA: The effects of thoracic surgery. *Int Anesthesiol Clin* 22:45–57, 1984.
29. Esposito RA, Spencer FC: The effect of pericardial insulation on hypothermic phrenic nerve injury during open-heart surgery. *Ann Thorac Surg* 43:303–308, 1987.
30. Wheeler WE, Rubis LJ, Jones CW, Harrah JD: Etiology and prevention of topical cardiac hypothermia-induced phrenic nerve injury and left lower lobe atelectasis during cardiac surgery. *Chest* 88:680–683, 1985.
31. Morton HJV: Tobacco smoking and pulmonary complications after operation. *Lancet* 1:368–370, 1944.
32. Wightman JA: A prospective survey of the incidence of postoperative pulmonary complications. *Br J Surg* 55:85–91, 1968.
33. Celli BR, Rodriguez KS, Snider GL: A controlled trial of intermittent positive pressure breathing, incentive spirometry, and deep breathing exercises in preventing

pulmonary complications after abdominal surgery. *Am Rev Respir Dis* 130:12–15, 1984.

34. Aronow WS, Cassidy J, Vangrow JS, et al: Effect of cigarette smoking and breathing carbon monoxide on cardiovascular hemodynamics in anginal patients. *Circulation* 50:340–347, 1974.

35. Turino GM: Effect of carbon monoxide on the cardiorespiratory system. Carbon monoxide toxicity: physiology and biochemistry. *Circulation* 63:253A–259A, 1981.

36. Klein LW, Ambrose J, Pichard A, et al: Acute coronary hemodynamic response to cigarette smoking in patients with coronary artery disease. *J Am Coll Cardiol* 3:879–886, 1984.

37. Foster WM, Langenback EG, Bergofsky EH: Disassociation in the mucociliary function of central and peripheral airways of asymptomatic smokers. *Am Rev Respir Dis* 132:633–639, 1985.

38. Hegab ES, Matulionis DH: Pulmonary macrophage mobilization in cigarette smoke–exposed mice after halothane anesthesia. *Anesth Analg* 65:37–45, 1986.

39. McLeod R, Mack DG, McLeod EG, et al: Alveolar macrophage function and inflammatory stimuli in smokers with and without obstructive lung disease. *Am Rev Respir Dis* 131:377–384, 1985.

40. Warner MA, Divertie MB, Tinker JH: Preoperative cessation of smoking and pulmonary complications in coronary artery bypass patients. *Anesthesiology* 60:380–383, 1984.

41. Stein M, Koota GM, Simon M, Frank HA: Pulmonary evaluation of surgical patients. *JAMA* 181:765–770, 1962.

42. Gracey DR, Divertie MB, Didier EP: Preoperative pulmonary preparation of patients with chronic obstructive pulmonary disease: a prospective study. *Chest* 76:123–129, 1979.

43. Tyler IL, Tantisira B, Winter PM, Motoyama EK: Continuous monitoring of arterial oxygen saturation with pulse oximetry during transfer to the recovery room. *Anesth Analg* 64:1108–1112, 1985.

44. Hirshman CA, Edelstein G, Peetz S, et al: Mechanism of action of inhalational anesthesia on airways. *Anesthesiology* 56:107–111, 1982.

45. Rosseel P, Lauwers LF, Baute L: Halothane treatment in life-threatening asthma. *Intensive Care Med* 11:241–246, 1985.

46. Johnston RR, Eger EI II, Wilson C: A comparative interaction of epinephrine with enflurane, isoflurane, and halothane in man. *Anesth Analg* 55:709–712, 1976.

47. Empey DW, Laitinen LA, Jacobs L, Gold WM, Nadel JA: Mechanisms of bronchial hyperactivity in normal subjects after upper respiratory tract infections. *Am Rev Respir Dis* 113:131–139, 1976.

48. Cohen MM, Cameron CB: Should you cancel the operation when a child has an upper respiratory tract infection? *Anesth Analg* 72:282–288, 1991.

49. Barnes PJ: A new approach to the treatment of asthma. *N Engl J Med* 321(22):1517–1527, 1989.

50. Fanta CH, Rossing TH, McFadden ER: Glucocorticoids in acute asthma: a critical controlled trial. *Am J Med* 74:845–851, 1983.

51. Parker SD, Brown RH, Darowski MJ, Hirschman CA: Time related decrease in airway reactivity by corticosteroids. *Anesthesiology* 71:A1077, 1989.

52. Howarth PH, Durham SR, Lee TH, Kay AB, Church MK, Holgate ST: Influence of albuterol, cromolyn sodium and ipratopium bromide on the airway and circulating mediator responses to allergen bronchial provocation in asthma. *Am Rev Respir Dis* 132:86–92, 1985.

53. Chieb J, Beecher N, Rees PJ: Maximum achievable bronchodilation in asthma. *Respiratory Med* 83:97–102, 1989.

54. Hargreave FE, O'Byrne PM, Ramsdale EH: Mediators, airway responsiveness and asthma. *J Allergy Clin Immunol* 76:272–276, 1985.

55. Stirt JA, Berger JM, Roe SD, Ricker SM, Sullivan SF: Halothane-induced cardiac arrhythmias following administration of aminophylline in experimental animals. *Anesth Analg* 60:517–520, 1981.

56. Stirt JA, Berger JM, Roe SD, Ricker SM, Sullivan SF: Safety of enflurane following administration of aminophylline to experimental animals. *Anesth Analg* 60:871–873, 1981.

57. Arora NS, Rochester DF: Respiratory muscle strength and maximal voluntary ventilation in undernourished patients. *Am Rev Respir Dis* 126:5–8, 1982.

58. Doekel RC Jr, Zwillich CW, Scoggin CH, et al: Clinical semistarvation: depression of hypoxic ventilatory response. *N Engl J Med* 295:358–361, 1976.

59. Sirisinha S, Suskind R, Edelman R, et al: Secretory and serum IgA in children with protein-calorie malnutrition. *Pediatrics* 55:166–170, 1975.

60. Garibaldi RA, Britt MR, Coleman ML, et al: Risk factors for postoperative pneumonia. *Am J Med* 70:677–680, 1981.

61. Goldman L, Caldera DL, Nussbaum SR, et al: Multifactorial index of cardiac risk in noncardiac surgical procedures. *N Engl J Med* 297:845–850, 1977.

62. Vaughan RW, Wise L: Choice of abdominal operative incision in the obese patient: a study using blood gas measurements. *Ann Surg* 181:829–835, 1975.

63. Halasz NA: Vertical vs horizontal laparotomies. *Arch Surg* 46:911, 1964.

64. Peck JJ, McReynolds DG, Baker DH, Eastman AB: Extraperitoneal approach for aortoiliac reconstruction of the abdominal aorta. *Am J Surg* 151:620–623, 1986.

65. Urschel HC Jr, Razzuk MA: Median sternotomy as a standard approach for pulmonary resection. *Ann Thorac Surg* 41:130–134, 1986.

66. Grace PA, Quereshi A, Colenian J, Keane R, McEntee G, et al: Reduced postoperative hospitalization after laparoscopic cholecystectomy. *Br J Surg* 78:160–162, 1991.

67. Frazee R, Roberts J, Okeson G, Symmonds R, Snyder S, Hendricks J, Smith R: Open versus laparoscopic cholecystectomy: a comparison of postoperative pulmonary function. *Ann Surg* 213:651–653, 1991.

68. Mohr DN: Estimation of surgical risk in the elderly: a correlative review. *J Am Geriatr Soc* 31:99–102, 1983.

69. Siegel JH, Fabian M, Lankau C, et al: Clinical and experimental use of thoracic impedance plethysmography in quantifying myocardial contractility. *Surgery* 67:907–917, 1970.

70. Cole WH: Prediction of operative reserve in the elderly patient, (editorial). *Ann Surg* 168:310, 1968.

71. Grodsinsky C, Brush BE, Ponka JL: Postoperative pulmonary complications in the geriatric age group. *J Am Geriatr Soc* 22:407–412, 1974.

72. Gaensler EA, Cugell DW, Lindgren I, et al: The role of pulmonary insufficiency in mortality and invalidism

following surgery for pulmonary tuberculosis. *J Thorac Surg* 29:163–185, 1955.

73. Olsen GN, Block AJ, Swenson EW, et al: Pulmonary function evaluation of the lung resection candidate: a prospective study. *Am Rev Respir Dis* 111:379–387, 1975.

74. Segall JJ, Butterworth BA: Ventilatory capacity in chronic bronchitis in relation to carbon dioxide reduction. *Scand J Respir Dis* 47:215–224, 1966.

75. Gass GD, Olsen GN: Preoperative pulmonary function testing to predict postoperative morbidity and mortality. *Chest* 89:127–135, 1986.

76. Fee HJ, Holmes EC, Gewirtz HS, et al: Role of pulmonary vascular resistance measurements in preoperative evaluation of candidates for pulmonary resection. *J Thorac Cardiovasc Surg* 75:519–524, 1978.

77. Smith TP, Kinasewitz GT, Tucker WY, et al: Exercise capacity as a predictor of post-thoracotomy morbidity. *Am Rev Respir Dis* 129:730–734, 1984.

78. Bechard D, Wetstein L: Assessment of exercise oxygen consumption as preoperative criterion for lung resection. *Ann Thorac Surg* 44:344–349, 1987.

79. Reilly JJ, Mentzer SJ, Sugarbaker DJ: Preoperative assessment of patients undergoing pulmonary resection. *Chest* 103:342S–345S, 1993.

80. Crapo RO: Pulmonary function testing. *N Engl J Med* 331:25–30, 1994.

81. Lawrence VA, Page CP, Harris GD: Preoperative spirometry before abdominal operations. A critical appraisal of its predictive value. *Arch Intern Med* 149:280–285, 1989.

82. Zibrak JD, O'Donell CR, Marton K: Indications for pulmonary function testing. *Ann Intern Med* 112:763–771, 1990.

83. Jayr C, Matthay MA, Goldstone J, Gold WM, Wiener-Kronish JP: Preoperative and intraoperative factors associated with prolonged mechanical ventilation following major abdominal vascular surgery. *Chest* 103:1231–1236, 1993.

84. Anderson WH, Dosett BE Jr, Hamilton GE: Prevention of postoperative pulmonary complications. *JAMA* 186:763–766, 1963.

85. Fairley HB: Oxygen therapy for surgical patients. *Am Rev Respir Dis* 122:37–44, 1980.

86. Buckley FP, Robinson NB, Simonwitz DA, Dellinger EP: Anesthesia in the morbidly obese. *Anesthesia* 38:840, 1983.

87. Rawal N, Sjostrand U, Christoffersson E, et al: Comparison of intramuscular and epidural morphine for postoperative analgesia in the grossly obese: influence on postoperative ambulation and pulmonary function. *Anesth Analg* 63:583–592, 1984.

88. Strandberg A, Tokics L, Brismar B, et al: Atelectasis during anesthesia and in the postoperative period. *Acta Anaesthesiol Scand* 30:154–158, 1986.

89. Ricksten SE, Bengtsson A, Soderberg C, et al: Effects of periodic positive airway pressure by mask on postoperative pulmonary function. *Chest* 89:774–781, 1986.

90. Marini JJ, Pierson DJ, Hudson LD: Acute lobar atelectasis: a prospective comparison of fiberoptic bronchoscopy and respiratory therapy. *Am Rev Respir Dis* 119:971–978, 1979.

91. Eickhoff TC: Pulmonary infections in surgical patients. *Surg Clin North Am* 60:175–183, 1980.

92. Valenti WM, Trudell RG, Bentley DW: Factors predisposing to oropharyngeal colonization with Gram-negative bacilli in the aged. *N Engl J Med* 298:1108–1111, 1978.

93. Martin LF, Asher EF, Casey JM, Fry DE: Postoperative pneumonia. Determinants of mortality. *Arch Surg* 119:379–383, 1984.

94. Mendelson CL: The aspiration of stomach contents into the lungs during obstetric anesthesia. *Am J Obstet Gynecol* 52:191–205, 1946.

95. Manchikanti L, Colliver JA, Marrero TC, Roush JR: Assessment of age-related acid aspiration risk factors in pediatric, adult, and geriatric patients. *Anesth Analg* 64:11–17, 1985. [published erratum appears in *Anesth Analg* 65:210, 1986].

96. Burgess GE, Cooper LR Jr, Marino RJ, et al: Laryngeal competence after tracheal extubation. *Anesthesiology* 51:73–77, 1979.

97. Huxley EJ, Viroslav J, Gray WR, Pierce AK: Pharyngeal aspiration in normal adults and patients with depressed consciousness. *Am J Med* 64:564–568, 1978.

98. Spray SB, Zuidema GD, Cameron JL: Aspiration pneumonia; incidence of aspiration with endotracheal tubes. *Am J Surg* 131:701–703, 1976.

99. Schwartz DJ, Wynne JW, Gibbs CP, et al: The pulmonary consequences of aspiration of gastric contents at pH values greater than 2.5. *Am Rev Respir Dis* 121:119–126, 1980.

100. Bynum LJ, Pierce AK: Pulmonary aspiration of gastric contents. *Am Rev Respir Dis* 114:1129–1136, 1976.

101. LeFrock JL, Clark TS, Davies B, Klainer AS: Aspiration pneumonia: a ten-year review. *Am Surg* 45:305–313, 1979.

102. Toung TJ, Bordos D, Benson DW, et al: Aspiration pneumonia: experimental evaluation of albumin and steroid therapy. *Ann Surg* 183:179–184, 1976.

103. Sellick BA: Cricoid pressure to control regurgitation of stomach contents during induction of anesthesia. *Lancet* 2:404–406, 1961.

104. Fanning GL: The efficacy of cricoid pressure in preventing regurgitation of gastric contents. *Anesthesiology* 32:553–555, 1970.

105. Trunkey DD, Lewis FR: Chest trauma. *Surg Clin North Am* 60:1541–1549, 1980.

106. Zuidema GD, Rutherford RB: *The Management of Trauma*. Philadelphia, WB Saunders, 1979.

107. Cogbill TH, Moore EE, Millikan JS, Cleveland HC, et al: Rationale for selective application of emergency department thoracotomy in trauma. *J Trauma* 23:453, 1983.

108. Graeber GM, Jones DR: The role of thoracoscopy in thoracic trauma. *Ann Thorac Surg* 56:646–648, 1993.

109. Jones JW, Kitahama A, Webb WR, McSwain N: Emergency thoracoscopy: a logical approach to chest trauma management. *J Trauma* 21:280–284, 1981.

110. Feliciano DV: The diagnostic and therapeutic approach to chest trauma. *Semin Thorac Cardiovasc Surg* 4:156–162, 1992.

111. Adamthwaite DN: Traumatic diaphragmatic hernia. *Surg Annu* 15:73–97, 1983.

112. Wakabayashi A: Expanded applications of diagnostic and therapeutic thoracoscopy. *J Thorac Cardiovasc Surg* 102:721–723, 1991.

113. Thompson BM, Finger W, Tonsfeldt D, et al: Rib radiographs for trauma: useful or wasteful? *Ann Emerg Med* 15:261–265, 1986.

114. Little RA, Yates DW, Atkins RE, et al: The effects of minor and moderately severe accidental chest injuries on pulmonary function in man. *Arch Emerg Med* 1: 29–38, 1984.

115. Wilson RF, Murray C, Antonenko DR: Nonpenetrating thoracic injuries. *Surg Clin North Am* 57:17–36, 1977.

116. Pedersen VM, Schulze S, Hier-Madsen K, Halkier E: Air-flow meter assessment of the effect of intercostal nerve blockade on respiratory function in rib fractures. *Acta Chir Scand* 149:119–120, 1983.

117. Abouhatem R, Hendrickx P, Titeca M, Guerisse P: Thoracic epidural analgesia in the treatment of rib fractures. *Acta Anaesthesiol Belg* 35:271–275, 1984.

118. Yee ES, Thomas AN, Goodman PC: Isolated first rib fracture: clinical significance after blunt chest trauma. *Ann Thorac Surg* 32:278–283, 1981.

119. Garzon AA, Seltzer B, Karlson KE: Physiopathology of crushed chest injuries. *Ann Surg* 168:128–136, 1968.

120. Craven KD, Oppenheimer L, Wood LD: Effects of contusion and flail chest on pulmonary perfusion and oxygen exchange. *J Appl Physiol* 47:729–737, 1979.

121. Avery EE, Morch ET, Benson DW: Critically crushed chests. A new method of treatment with continuous mechanical hyperventilation to produce alkalotic apnea and internal pneumatic stabilization. *J Thorac Surg* 32: 291–311, 1956.

122. Relihan M, Litwin MS: Morbidity and mortality associated with flail chest injury: a review of 85 cases. *J Trauma* 13:663–671, 1973.

123. Shackford SR, Virgilio RW, Peters RM: Selective use of ventilator therapy in flail chest injury. *J Thorac Cardiovasc Surg* 81:194–201, 1981.

124. Richardson JD, Adams L, Flint LM: Selective management of flail chest and pulmonary contusion. *Ann Surg* 196:481–487, 1982.

125. Thomas AN, Blaisdell FW, Lewis FR Jr, Schlobohm RM: Operative stabilization for flail chest after blunt trauma. *J Thorac Cardiovasc Surg* 75:793–801, 1978.

126. Landercasper J, Cogbill TH, Lindesmith LA: Long-term disability after flail chest injury. *J Trauma* 24:410–414, 1984.

127. Beal SL, Oreskovich MR: Long-term disability associated with flail chest injury. *Am J Surg* 150:324–326, 1985.

128. Schaal MA, Fischer RP, Perry JF: The unchanged mortality of flail chest injuries. *J Trauma* 19:492–496, 1979.

129. Rutherford RB, Hurt HH Jr, Brickman RD, Tubb JM: The pathophysiology of progressive, tension pneumothorax. *J Trauma* 8:212–227, 1968.

130. Gustman P, Yerger L, Wanner A: Immediate cardiovascular effects of tension pneumothorax. *Am Rev Respir Dis* 127:171–174, 1983.

131. Kish G, Kozloff L, Joseph WL, Adkins PC: Indications for early thoracotomy in the management of chest trauma. *Ann Thorac Surg* 22:23–28, 1976.

132. Richardson JD: Indications for thoracotomy in thoracic trauma. *Curr Surg* 42:361–364, 1985.

133. Coselli JS, Mattox KL, Beall AC Jr: Reevaluation of early evacuation of clotted hemothorax. *Am J Surg* 148: 786–790, 1984.

134. Arom KV, Grover FL, Richardson JD, et al: Posttraumatic empyema *Ann Thorac Surg* 23:254–258, 1977.

135. Caplan ES, Hoyt NJ, Rodriguez A, Cowley RA: Empyema occurring in the multiple traumatized patient. *J Trauma* 24:785–789, 1984.

136. Oppenheimer L, Craven KD, Forkert L, Wood LD: Pathophysiology of pulmonary contusion in dogs. *J Appl Physiol* 47:718–728, 1979.

137. Johnson JA, Cogbill TH, Winga ER: Determinants of outcome after pulmonary contusion. *J Trauma* 26: 695–697, 1986.

138. Dodek PM, Rice TW, Bonsignore MR, et al: Effects of plasmapheresis and hypoproteinemia on lung liquid conductance in awake sheep. *Circ Res* 58:269–280, 1986.

139. Franz JL, Richardson JD, Grover FL, Trinkle JK: Effect of methylprednisolone sodium succinate on experimental pulmonary contusion. *J Thorac Cardiovasc Surg* 68: 842–844, 1974.

140. Lucas CE, Ledgerwood AM: Pulmonary response of massive steroids in seriously injured patients. *Ann Surg* 194:256–261, 1981.

141. Richardson JD, Woods D, Johanson WG Jr, Trinkle JK: Lung bacterial clearance following pulmonary contusion. *Surgery* 86:730–735, 1979.

142. Bongard FS, Lewis FR: Crystalloid resuscitation of patients with pulmonary contusion. *Am J Surg* 148: 145–151, 1984.

143. Demling RH: The pathogenesis of respiratory failure after trauma and sepsis. *Surg Clin North Am* 60: 1373–1390, 1980.

144. Jacob HS, Moldow CF, Flynn PJ, et al: Therapeutic ramifications of the interaction of complement, granulocytes, and platelets in the production of acute lung injury. In Malik AB, Staub NC (eds): *Mechanisms of Lung Microvascular Injury*. New York, New York Academy of Sciences, 1982, pp 489–495.

145. von Bergman E: Ein Fall tödlicher Fettembolie. *Berl Klin Wochenschr* 10:385, 1873.

146. Gurd AR: Fat embolism: an aid to diagnosis. *J Bone Joint Surg* 52B:732, 1970.

147. Peltier LF, Collins JA, Evarts CM et al: Fat embolism. *Arch Surg* 109:12–16, 1974.

148. Fabian TC, Hoots AV, Stanford DS, Patterson CR, Mangiante EC: Fat embolism syndrome: prospective evaluation in 92 fracture patients. *Crit Care Med* 18:42–46, 1990.

149. Ganong RB: Fat emboli syndrome in isolated fractures of the tibia and femur. *Clin Orthop* 291:208–214, 1993.

150. Palmovic V, McCarroll JR: Fat embolism in trauma. *Arch Pathol* 80:630, 1965.

151. Masson R, Ruggieri J: Pulmonary microvascular cytology: a new diagnostic application of the pulmonary artery catheter. *Chest* 88:908–914, 1985.

152. Castella X, Valles J, Cabezuelo MA, Fernandez R, Artigas A: Fat embolism syndrome and pulmonary microvascular cytology. *Chest* 101:1710–1711, 1992.

153. Chastre J, Fagon J-Y, Soler P, Fichelle A, Dombret M-C, et al: Bronchoalveolar lavage for rapid diagnosis of the fat embolism syndrome in trauma patients. *Ann Intern Med* 113:583–588, 1990.

154. Gitin TA, Seidel T, Cera PJ, Glidewell OJ, Smith JL: Pulmonary microvascular fat: the significance? *Crit Care Med* 21:673–677, 1993.

155. Vedrinne JM, Guillaume C, Gagnieu MC, Gratadour P, Fleuret C, Motin J: Bronchoalveolar lavage in trauma patients for diagnosis of fat embolism syndrome. *Chest* 102:1323–1327, 1992.

156. Bone RC: Pulmonary microvascular fat in lung injury: an epiphenomenon? *Crit Care Med* 21:644, 1993.

157. Johnson KD, Cadambi A, Seibert GB et al: Incidence of adult respiratory distress syndrome in patients with multiple musculoskeletal injuries: effect of early operative stabilization of fractures. *J Trauma* 25:375, 1985.

158. Berhman SW, Fabian TC, Kudsk KA, et al: Improved outcome with femur fractures: early vs. delayed fixation. *J Trauma* 30:792, 1990.

159. Alho A, Saikku K, Eerola P, Koskinen M, Hämäläinen M: Corticosteroids in patients with a high risk of fat embolism syndrome. *Surg Gynecol Obstet* 147:358–362, 1978.

160. Schonfeld SA, Ploysongsang Y, DiLisio R, Crissman JD, Miller E, et al: Fat embolism prophylaxis with corticosteroids. *Ann Intern Med* 99:438–443, 1983.

161. Kallenbach J, Lewis M, Zaltzman M, Feldman C, Orford A, Zwi S: "Low dose" corticosteroid prophylaxis against fat embolism. *J Trauma* 27:1173–1176, 1987.

162. Hankins JR, McAslan TC, Shin B, et al: Extensive pulmonary laceration caused by blunt trauma. *J Thorac Cardiovasc Surg* 74:519–527, 1977.

163. Thomas AN, Roe BB: Air embolism following penetrating lung injuries. *J Thorac Cardiovasc Surg* 66:533–540, 1973.

164. Graham JM, Beall AC Jr, Mattox KL, Vaughan GD: Systemic air embolism following penetrating trauma to the lung. *Chest* 72:449–454, 1977.

165. Yee ES, Verrier ED, Thomas AN: Management of air embolism in blunt and penetrating thoracic trauma. *J Thorac Cardiovasc Surg* 85:661–668, 1983.

166. Thomas AN, Stephens BG: Air embolism: a cause of morbidity and death after penetrating chest trauma. *J Trauma* 14:633–638, 1974.

167. Durant TM, Oppenheimer MJ, Webster MR, Long J: Arterial air embolism. *Am Heart J* 38:481–500, 1949.

168. Kirsh MM, Orringer MB, Behrendt DM, Sloan H: Management of tracheobronchial disruption secondary to nonpenetrating trauma. *Ann Thorac Surg* 22:93–101, 1976.

169. Amauchi W, Birolini D, Branco PD, Oliveira MR: Injuries to the tracheobronchial tree in closed trauma. *Thorax* 38:923–928, 1983.

170. Guest JL Jr, Anderson JN: Major airway injury in closed chest trauma. *Chest* 72:63–66, 1977.

171. Halttunen PE, Kostiainen SA, Meurala HG: Bronchial rupture caused by blunt chest trauma. *Scand J Thorac Cardiovasc Surg* 18:141–144, 1984.

172. Collins JP, Ketharanathan V, McConchie I: Rupture of major bronchi resulting from closed chest injuries. *Thorax* 28:371–375, 1973.

173. Grover FL, Ellestad C, Arom KV, et al: Diagnosis and management of major tracheobronchial injuries. *Ann Thorac Surg* 28:384–391, 1979.

174. Chesterman JT, Satsangi PN: Rupture of the trachea and bronchi by closed injury. *Thorax* 21:21–27, 1966.

175. Gerwat J, Bryce DP: Management of traumatic tracheo-esophageal fistula. *Arch Otolaryngol* 101:67–70, 1975.

176. Ward RE, Flynn TC, Clark WP: Diaphragmatic disruption secondary to blunt abdominal trauma. *J Trauma* 21:35–38, 1981.

177. Miller L, Bennett EV Jr, Root HD, et al: Management of penetrating and blunt diaphragmatic injury. *J Trauma* 24:403–409, 1984.

178. Wise L, Connors J, Hwang YH, Anderson C: Traumatic injuries to the diaphragm. *J Trauma* 13:946–950, 1973.

179. Grimes OF: Traumatic injuries of the diaphragm. Diaphragmatic hernia. *Am J Surg* 128:175–181, 1974.

180. Michel L, Grillo HC, Malt RA: Esophageal perforation. *Ann Thorac Surg* 33:203–210, 1982.

181. Silvis SE, Nebel O, Rogers G, et al: Endoscopic complications. Results of the 1974 American Society for Gastrointestinal Endoscopy Survey. *JAMA* 235:928–930, 1976.

182. Katz D: Morbidity and mortality in standard and flexible gastrointestinal endoscopy. *Gastrointest Endosc* 15:134–141, 1969.

# Chapter 26

# Metabolism, Nutrition, and Respiration in Critically Ill Patients

## C. Kees Mahutte

A HYPERMETABOLIC HYPERCATABOLIC state commonly occurs early in critical illnesses caused by burns, sepsis, or trauma. This stress response is mediated primarily via the release of counterregulatory hormones (glucagon, cortisol, and catecholamines). Gluconeogenesis, lipolysis, and hyperglycemia result. In addition, protein breakdown occurs, and a negative nitrogen balance that may be difficult to correct ensues. If the hypermetabolic hypercatabolic state is coupled with inadequate nutritional support, malnutrition may develop rapidly. Malnutrition adversely affects organ function, morbidity, and mortality. Specifically, immune function is depressed, wound healing is impaired, and lean body mass is decreased. Malnutrition also deleteriously affects gut integrity and results in increased bacterial translocation. In the patient with respiratory failure, the adverse effects of malnutrition include decreased respiratory muscle strength, decreased ventilatory drive, and impaired lung defenses.

It is thought that early nutritional support in the critically ill patient may mitigate the adverse consequences associated with malnutrition. Specifically, there is evidence that optimal early nutritional support will decrease infection rates, improve wound healing, and improve patient outcome. In addition, specific nutrients may maintain gut integrity, decrease bacterial translocation, modulate the inflammatory response, and enhance the body's immune function. It is therefore important to perform a proper nutritional assessment in the critically ill patient. It is also vital to estimate the patient's energy requirements and to establish the required protein and caloric needs. There is increasing evidence that enteral feeding is preferable to parenteral nutrition. Alimentation via the enteral route has particularly salutary effects on the bowel, since it preserves mucosal integrity together with immune function and thereby decreases bacterial translocation.

In patients with or prone to respiratory failure, overfeeding will increase carbon dioxide production and compromise the respiratory system. In these patients, judicious selection of total calories with an appropriate fat-to-carbohydrate ratio may prevent the development of respiratory failure and/or facilitate weaning.

It is incumbent upon the intensivist to monitor nutritional therapy carefully to minimize the development of malnutrition and to optimize patient outcome.

## FUEL UTILIZATION DURING CRITICAL ILLNESS

Injury caused by burns, trauma, or sepsis evokes increases in both metabolic and catabolic rates. Even in the presence of inadequate intake, these hormone-mediated responses ensure the delivery of abundant glucose, obtained primarily via gluconeogenesis from endogenous proteins, to the sites of injury. Teleologically one might therefore argue that these metabolic and catabolic responses enhance survival. Both afferent nerve signals and cytokines (interleukin-1 (IL-1), tumor necrosis factor (TNF), and others) originating at the site of injury act on the hypothalamus, which in turn activates the sympathetic nervous system and pituitary gland (1). Consequent increases in norepinephrine, epinephrine, cortisol, glucagon, and insulin ensue. Infusion of cortisol, glucagon, and epinephrine into normal subjects elicits the same metabolic stress responses as are seen in critical illness, including the increased levels of insulin (2). The overriding influence of the counterregulatory hormones—cortisol, glucagon and epinephrine—stimulates gluconeogenesis,

glycogenolysis, lipolysis, and proteolysis. As a result, circulating levels of glucose are increased. Substrate cycling (turnover) of carbohydrates, proteins, and fats all increase (Fig. 26.1).

To better understand the changes that occur during the hypermetabolic hypercatabolic state of stress, the hypometabolic catabolic state of nonstressed starvation is first discussed (Table 26.1).

### NONSTRESSED STARVATION

The normal body contains substantial caloric reserves (3). Of these reserves, the oxidative metabolism of fat yields considerably more energy than that of protein or glucose (Table 26.2). During the initial phase of

**TABLE 26.1**
**NONSTRESSED STARVATION AND THE HYPERMETABOLIC HYPERCATABOLIC STRESS RESPONSE**

|  | Starvation | Stress |
|---|---|---|
| Metabolic rate | ↓ | ↑ |
| Urinary nitrogen losses | ↓ | ↑ |
| Insulin | ↓ | ↑ (resistance) |
| Counterregulatory hormones[a] | Normal | ↑ |
| Ketones | ↑ | Absent |
| Glucose | Normal | ↑ |
| Gluconeogenesis | Present | ↑ |
| Glycogenolysis | ↑ | ↑ |
| Lipolysis | ↑ | ↑ |
| Proteolysis | ↓ | ↑ |
| Primary fuel sources | Fat | Fat |

[a] Glucagon, cortisol, catecholamines.

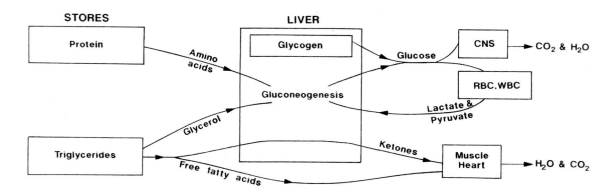

**FIGURE 26.1.** Major metabolic pathways. During stress, amino acids are used to produce glucose, and fats are used for energy, but the elevated glucose level suppresses ketone production.

During nonstressed starvation, ketones are present and supply a substantial portion of the brain's energy.

TABLE 26.2
NORMAL CALORIC STORES IN A 70-KG MAN

| Fuel | kg | kcal/g[a] | Calories (kcal) |
|---|---|---|---|
| Fat | 15 | 9.3 | 140,000 |
| Muscle protein | 6 | 4.4 | 26,000 |
| Glycogen | 0.26 | 4.2 | 1,000 |
| Total | | | 167,000 |

[a] Energy from the body's oxidative metabolism of fat, protein, and carbohydrates (3.7 kcal/g for glucose).

nonstressed starvation (lasting a few days), glycogen stores are broken down to provide the glucose necessary for the brain, erythrocytes, white blood cells, and renal medulla. Glycogen stores are soon depleted, since they are small (containing about 1000 kcal), and the brain alone requires 100 to 150 g of glucose per day, and in addition, the blood cells require about 40 g/day (3). Insulin levels are low to facilitate mobilization of carbohydrate, fat, and protein for energy. As glycogen is depleted within 48 to 72 hours, fat gradually becomes the major caloric source, providing about 85% of the total required calories from free fatty acids or ketones (produced in the liver). The remaining 15% of calories, required by the glucose-dependent tissues (brain, blood cells, and renal medulla) is obtained from glucose. Most of this glucose is derived from gluconeogenesis of amino acids, and only a small portion of the glucose is derived from gluconeogenesis of glycerol. Within a few days the brain adapts to the utilization of ketone bodies, which thereafter may supply 50 to 80% of the brain's energy needs. Brain utilization of ketones spares the breakdown of protein that would otherwise be required for gluconeogenesis. In addition, the metabolic rate may also decrease by 20 to 40% below basal levels. Thus, urinary nitrogen excretion (indicating protein breakdown), which increases from about 10 g/day in the equilibrium state prior to the fast to about 12 g/day in the initial days of the fast, may with prolonged fasting decrease to about 3 g/day. Despite these adaptive processes and total potential energy stores in a 70-kg man of approximately 170,000 kcal (Table 26.2), death typically occurs in about 2 months.

## GLUCOSE METABOLISM DURING STRESS

During the stressed state of critical illness, carbohydrate metabolism is characterized by hyperglycemia, which in turn induces a relative hyperinsulinemia. However, because of the predominance of the counter-regulatory hormones (glucagon, cortisol, catecholamines), the glucose levels are higher than expected for a given insulin level, leading to the so-called insulin resistance of critical illness. The high glucose levels fuel the cells involved in the reparative processes. These cells are the white blood cells, macrophages, and fibroblasts, all of which require glucose to generate energy via the glycolytic pathway. Since the hyperglycemia of critical illness may therefore be beneficial, it is usually recommended that glucose not be tightly controlled with insulin, even though there is some evidence that insulin infusion can decrease protein catabolism (4). The necessity for frequent glucose sampling (to monitor for hypoglycemia) and the risk of causing lipogenesis (with consequent increases in carbon dioxide production) temper the enthusiasm for insulin administration. Consequently, glucose values of 200 to 250 mg/ml are generally tolerated during critical illness.

During very severe stresses such as those induced by burns, glucose utilization and turnover increase (from a normal value of less than 2 mg/kg/minute) and maximally may reach 5 to 7 mg/kg/minute (5). Since the body's glycogen stores are small and rapidly depleted, these quantities of glucose are primarily obtained from gluconeogenesis, which occurs in the liver (typically more than 75%) and kidney (less than 25%). The major gluconeogenic precursors are lactate, pyruvate, glycerol, and some amino acids, such as alanine and glutamine. Lactate and pyruvate, resulting from glycolysis of glucose by the red blood and phagocytic cells, are used as substrates for gluconeogenesis in the liver. The newly produced glucose is then again transferred to the peripheral tissues where it is needed, and where it is incompletely oxidized via glycolysis to lactate (Cori cycle). Increased rates of lactate cycling via the Cori cycle (Fig. 26.2) occur in trauma, sepsis, and burns (6). Glycerol, derived from fat, may also be metabolized to glucose. Whereas during nonstressed starvation glycerol accounts for only a small portion of total glucose production (about 3%), during sepsis the amount of glucose produced from glycerol may reach 20% (7). However, most of the glucose derived from gluconeogenesis originates from degradation of muscle protein. Alanine is the major amino acid precursor in this pathway (Fig. 26.3). The alanine used for gluconeogenesis is derived from two sources: direct release of alanine from muscle and conversion of glutamine (released from muscle) to alanine in the gastrointestinal tract. Alanine and pyruvate (from glycolysis and protein breakdown) are then again converted to glucose via the glucose-alanine cycle. In the stressed patient, the exogenous infusion of glucose (up to 6 mg/kg/minute) only partially suppresses gluconeogenesis, and a portion of the infused glucose is metabolized to glycogen and fat (8). Glucose infusions exceeding 6

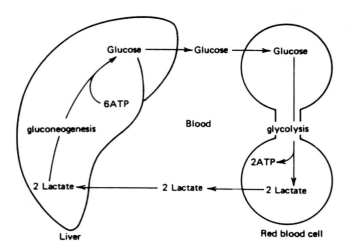

**FIGURE 26.2.** The Cori cycle. Glucose carbons shuttle potential energy between the liver and anaerobically metabolizing cells. Energy ultimately derives from lipid. (From Devlin T (ed): *Textbook of Biochemistry*. New York, John Wiley & Sons, 1982; with permission.)

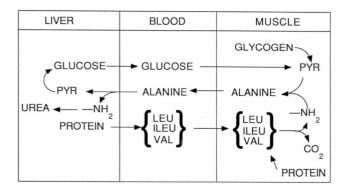

**FIGURE 26.3.** The glucose-alanine cycle. (From Felig P, Wahren J: Amino acid metabolism in exercising man. *J Clin Invest* 50: 2703–2714, 1971; with permission.)

mg/kg/minute result in a respiratory quotient above 1, indicating net lipogenesis (9). Since these amounts of glucose (6 mg/kg/minute) also do not suppress protein breakdown, glucose alone cannot meet the nutritional requirements in critically ill patients. The overriding stimulation for glucose production appears to derive from several factors: a decreased level of pyruvate dehydrogenase activity (10), an increase in the glucagon-to-insulin ratio, and an elevation of plasma catecholamine levels.

In summary, during stress, hyperglycemia satisfies the increased peripheral glucose demands. The hyperglycemia is the result of incomplete glucose oxidation

(glycolysis in phagocytic cells and insulin resistance in other tissues) and increased glucose synthesis. The latter uses amino acid, pyruvate, and lactate substrates.

## FAT METABOLISM DURING STRESS

Fat becomes the preferred oxidative fuel in the hypermetabolic patient (1, 11). This shift from glucose to fat oxidation decreases the muscle proteolysis that would otherwise occur. In contrast to the situation during nonstressed starvation, the increased turnover of fat persists even when exogenous glucose is infused (7, 11). Despite this increase in lipolysis, the concentration of free fatty acids is generally not significantly increased, whereas the triglyceride and glycerol concentrations are increased (1, 11). Oxidation of free fatty acids may provide 70 to 90% of the total energy needs. However, in septic or injured patients, the elevated glucose levels suppress the conversion of free fatty acids to ketones in proportion to the severity of the insult (12). Thus, in contrast to prolonged nonstressed starvation, during the stressed state ketone production is inadequate to meet the energy needs of the brain. Therefore, the brain's energy requirements (about 100 to 150 g of glucose per day) must be satisfied via gluconeogenesis fueled (in part) by protein degradation (it takes about 200 g of protein to make 100 g of glucose).

In summary, in the stressed patient, fat becomes the preferred oxidative fuel. Ketone production is decreased and is insufficient to meet the brain's energy demands (necessitating proteolysis to provide glucose).

## PROTEIN METABOLISM DURING STRESS

Under normal equilibrium conditions, protein degradation is balanced by protein synthesis. After a few days of starvation in normal man, the initial catabolic response diminishes and protein sparing occurs. In contrast, with burns, trauma, or sepsis, protein catabolism far exceeds synthesis. In addition, in contrast to nonstressed starvation, during stress the administration of glucose alone does not suppress the proteolysis that occurs (8). Similarly, administration of fat alone does not suppress proteolysis. Protein sparing is optimal when either a combination of carbohydrate and protein (13) or fat and protein (14) is administered. Protein requirements range from 1 to 1.5 g/kg/day (15), and excessive protein administration (more than 2 g/kg/day) neither prevents endogenous protein catabolism nor leads to enhanced protein synthesis. During the stress response, only about 20% of the muscle protein that is broken down is used directly for energy generation. The remainder enters the liver and is used for gluconeogenesis or synthesis of acute-phase reactant proteins (C-reactive protein, fibrinogen, $\alpha_1$-antitrypsin). As mentioned, glucose is required by the brain and phagocytic cells involved in the reparative processes. The synthesis of acute-phase reactant proteins enhances immune function, coagulation, and antiprotease activity and thereby may enhance survival. The muscle proteolysis occurs because of an increase in stress hormones (catecholamines, glucagon, and cortisol) as well as cytokines, including IL-1 (16). In the liver, the amino acids not used directly in gluconeogenesis or acute-phase reactant protein production are deaminated to yield pyruvate (used in gluconeogenesis) and an amino group. The latter is eventually excreted as urea, resulting in increased urinary nitrogen excretion. In the critically ill patient, muscle mass and protein losses may be substantial (Fig. 26.4). To appreciate the magnitude of these losses, 30 g of muscle mass contains 6.25 g of protein, which when fully catabolized leads to 1 g of urinary nitrogen excretion. Daily urinary nitrogen excretion may range from 20 to 40 g with burns and 20 to 30 g with trauma or sepsis. Therefore, a loss of 30 g of urinary nitrogen each day corresponds to a loss of 0.9 kg of muscle per day. Such a loss will lead to severe life-threatening protein malnutrition within 1 to 2 weeks.

In summary, during critical illness increased proteolysis of skeletal muscle occurs. The resultant amino acids are used to produce glucose (via gluconeogenesis) and acute-phase reactant proteins. Massive protein losses (measured by urinary nitrogen excretion) may be incurred rapidly, with catastrophic consequences.

## NUTRITIONAL ASSESSMENT

Traditionally, the nutritional assessment of a patient involves a history, physical examination, anthropometric measurements, and a number of laboratory tests (Tables 26.3 and 26.4). Because the traditional objective measurements and tests have wide confidence limits and because they can be affected by various underlying disease states, no single test or measurement can be relied upon in an individual patient. Indeed, it has been shown in stable patients that simple clinical judg-

**TABLE 26.3**
**NUTRITIONAL ASSESSMENT**

| Procedure | Emphasis |
| --- | --- |
| History | ↓ weight<br>↓ intake<br>↓ absorption (surgery, vomiting, diarrhea)<br>↑ requirements (burns, sepsis)<br>Catabolic drugs<br>Chronic disease |
| Physical examination | Muscle wasting (protein/calorie)<br>Fat loss (protein/calorie)<br>Edema (protein)<br>Pluckable hair (protein)<br>Dry skin (essential fatty acids)<br>Bleeding (vitamin K)<br>Glossitis (B vitamins)<br>Cheilosis (riboflavin, niacin) |
| Most useful | ↓ weight, fat, muscle, and albumin |

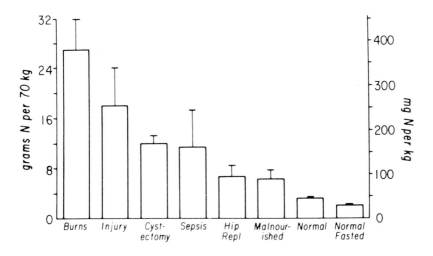

**FIGURE 26.4.** Total nitrogen excretion during 5% dextrose infusion in injured, septic, burned, or malnourished patients and normal subjects. Mean + SD. (From Elwyn DH: Protein metabolism and requirements in the critically ill patient. *Crit Care Clin* 3:57–69, 1987; with permission.)

**TABLE 26.4**
**ROUTINE NUTRITIONAL STATUS LABORATORY TESTS**

| Test | Comments |
|---|---|
| Serum albumin | Half-life ≈20 days; a value <2.4 g/dl suggests severe protein deficiency; may be normal (despite presence of malnutrition) in dehydration or if whole blood, fresh frozen plasma, or albumin is infused; may be decreased (despite absence of malnutrition) in fluid overload, congestive heart failure, liver failure, or stress (sepsis, trauma, surgery, burns); stress alters vascular permeability, with consequent leakage of protein to the extravascular compartment |
| Prealbumin | Half-life ≈1 to 2 days; a value <5 mg/ml suggests severe protein deficiency; may be normal (despite presence of malnutrition) in dehydration or renal disease; may be decreased (despite absence of malnutrition) in fluid overload or stress (sepsis, trauma, surgery, burns); increasing level over several days suggests improving nitrogen balance |
| Retinol-binding protein | Half-life ≈10 hours; changes rapidly with stress; may be normal (despite presence of malnutrition) in dehydration or renal disease; may be decreased (despite absence of malnutrition) in stress |
| Transferrin | Half-life ≈9 days; calculated usually from total iron-binding capacity (TIBC) as 0.8 TIBC − 43 mg/dl; may be normal (despite presence of malnutrition) in iron deficiency; may be decreased (despite absence of malnutrition) in iron overload, fluid overload, and stress |
| Cutaneous reactivity | Poor measure of nutritional status or immune system, affected by sepsis, fever, steroids, malignancy, drugs (immunosuppressants) |
| Total lymphocyte count | <1500/mm$^3$ may indicate malnutrition; not useful in acute situation since fluctuates rapidly and is affected by infection, stress, or malignancy |
| Nitrogen balance | Useful for assessing the degree of catabolism; may be useful to estimate and follow metabolic needs |

ment (termed *subjective global assessment*), consisting merely of a nutritionally oriented history and physical examination, is reproducible between observers and is as valid in assessing nutritional status as the objective traditional measurements (17).

The history and physical examination are helpful in identifying malnourished patients or patients at risk for the development of malnutrition. Obvious factors to look for in the history include weight loss, decreased food intake, nutrient losses (e.g., malabsorption, diarrhea, vomiting, bowel surgery), chronic diseases (e.g., alcoholism, cancer), catabolic drugs (e.g., steroids, antineoplastic agents), and metabolic needs (e.g. sepsis, burns). The physical examination should focus on muscle wasting, edema, subcutaneous fat, jaundice, easily pluckable hair, dry skin, glossitis, and cheilosis (dry ulcerated lips indicating vitamin deficiency).

The traditional objective indicators are even less reliable when they are applied to unstable critically ill patients. Specifically, they do not identify patients whose energy requirements exceed their intake or those who are at risk for the development of malnutrition. Anthropometric measures have limited usefulness because they can not detect acute changes. Visceral proteins (Table 26.4) such as albumin, transferrin, and prealbumin change too slowly to either indicate current nutritional status or acute changes in nutritional status with changes in therapy. Retinol-binding

protein has a short half-life of 10 hours but changes rapidly with minor stress. The preceding visceral proteins are all affected by the metabolic stress response, which is characterized by an increase in acute-phase protein synthesis at the expense of visceral protein synthesis. Furthermore, with the stress response, vascular permeability can change rapidly, leading to extravasation of proteins with consequent substantial acute decreases in measured serum proteins. Thus, all of the visceral proteins (Table 26.4) are affected by any kind of stress as well as such other conditions as chronic illness, renal disease, or fluid status (18). For the preceding reasons, serial collection of visceral proteins cannot be used to adjust the delivered nutritional support in real time. On the other hand, a recent study in infants concluded that if prealbumin increases over several days, the provided nutrition is adequate and that if such an increase in prealbumin occurs, it may correlate with survival (19). Thus, if albumin and/or prealbumin levels increase over relatively long time periods (one to several weeks), the stress response is resolving and/or nutritional repletion has been adequate.

The above difficulties with the nutritional assessment make it particularly important to match the administered nutrition with the energy requirements of the patient.

## Energy Requirements

Severely stressed patients typically are both hypermetabolic and hypercatabolic. Resting energy expenditure may be doubled, and nitrogen losses can be substantial. On the other hand, starvation itself is commonly encountered in critically ill patients, and this decreases the metabolic rate. Thus, it is not surprising that the energy expenditures in critically ill patients may vary widely (20). Energy expenditure may be estimated or measured. In practice, a patient's caloric and protein needs are usually estimated, and the adequacy of the administered nutrition is followed by the clinical response and serial changes in albumin, prealbumin, or nitrogen balance.

### Estimation of Caloric Requirements

The basal resting energy expenditure (REE) in kcal/day may be estimated from the Harris-Benedict equations. The REE depends on the patient's sex, weight (W in kg), height (H in cm), and age (A in years). The equations are

$$\text{Males REE} = 66 + 13.7W + 5H - 6.8A$$

$$\text{Females REE} = 655 + 9.6W + 1.8H - 4.7A.$$

Whereas these equations may yield approximately a 10% error in normal individuals, in stressed patients the errors may be substantially larger. Consequently, in patient populations, special correction factors have been found that correct for the degree of stress. For mild, moderate, and severe stress, the REE may typically be multiplied by the factors 1.2 (surgery or trauma), 1.4 to 1.6 (sepsis), 1.5 to 2.0 (burns), and 0.8 (starvation). These correction factors are valid in patient populations and when applied will correct the differences between estimated and measured REE in most individuals to within about 20%. However in some patients the differences between estimated and measured REE may remain substantial and reach 30 to 50% (20, 21).

Alternatively, it has been suggested (22) that the required daily calories in critically ill patients may be estimated simply as follows:

$$\text{REE} = 25 \times \text{weight (kg)}$$

This rule of thumb probably estimates the REE as accurately as the Harris-Benedict equations with correction factors. The above formula provides a "ballpark" caloric goal for the initiation of feeding and is adequate for the clinical management of most ICU patients.

### Measurement of Caloric Requirements

A patient's energy expenditure may also be measured. Theoretically, this energy expenditure may be obtained from direct measurement of a patient's heat loss (termed direct calorimetry). This procedure is obviously impractical in critically ill patients. Measurement of a patient's oxygen consumption ($\dot{V}O_2$) and carbon dioxide production ($\dot{V}CO_2$) together with nitrogen excretion may also be used to estimate energy expenditure. This method is referred to as indirect calorimetry. The method is based on the assumption that the energy liberated by the body from the utilization of each food source is a constant for each fuel and is identical to the complete combustion of each fuel (carbohydrate, fat, protein) in a bomb calorimeter (23). The latter assumption is valid for carbohydrate and fat but not protein, since oxidation of protein in a bomb calorimeter yields 5.7 kcal/g whereas oxidation in the body yields 4.4 kcal/g. Thus indirect calorimetry cannot provide the "gold standard" for measurement of energy expenditure. In the body, complete oxidation of 1 g of carbohydrate yields 4.2 kcal; 1 g of fat yields 9.3 kcal; and 1 g of protein yields 4.4 kcal (Table 26.5). From the chemical mass balance equations for carbohydrate, fat, and protein combustion, the quantities of oxygen utilized and carbon dioxide produced by combustion of each of these fuels are known (Table 26.5). Consequently, the equations for $\dot{V}O_2$, $\dot{V}CO_2$, and energy expenditure (EE) may be written in terms of the (unknown and to be solved for) quantities of carbohydrate, protein, and fat that are metabolized. In addition, the urinary nitrogen (UN) yields the protein metabolized. The preceding equations may then be solved (23) to yield the energy expenditure per minute:

$$\text{EE (kcal)} = 3.59\dot{V}O_2 + 1.44\dot{V}CO_2 - 1.2\text{UN}$$

where the $\dot{V}O_2$ and $\dot{V}CO_2$ are in liters/minute and UN is in g/minute. The urinary nitrogen excretion is usually neglected in the EE calculation since it makes a relatively small contribution. However, the urinary nitrogen is essential to estimate protein breakdown and requirements (see below). Neglecting the UN, the daily resting energy expenditure (REE in kcal/day) then becomes

$$\text{REE} = 5.2\dot{V}O_2 + 2.1\dot{V}CO_2$$

**TABLE 26.5**
**Oxidation of Carbohydrate, Fat, and Protein in the Body**

|  | Carbohydrate | Fat | Protein |
|---|---|---|---|
| $\dot{V}O_2$ (liters/g) | 0.83 | 2.0 | 0.97 |
| $\dot{V}CO_2$ (liters/g) | 0.83 | 1.4 | 0.78 |
| Respiratory quotient | 1.0 | 0.7 | 0.8 |
| Energy (kcal/g) | 4.2 | 9.3 | 4.4 |

where the measured $\dot{V}O_2$ and $\dot{V}CO_2$ are expressed in ml/minute (obtained by multiplying the preceding EE by 1.44 [24 hours $\times$ 60 minutes/1000 ml]). The $\dot{V}O_2$ and $\dot{V}CO_2$ can be measured on-line at the patient's bedside with a metabolic gas monitor. Numerous such devices are commercially available. Resting measurements of $\dot{V}O_2$ and $\dot{V}CO_2$ are usually made over 15- to 30-minute periods several times a day (24). Since there is considerable variation in energy expenditure from day to day, these measurements have to be performed daily (25). In addition, since metabolic rate can vary substantially (10 to 20%) over time (26) or with minimal activities, the measured resting (and presumed basal) energy expenditure may be multiplied by 1.1 or 1.2 to account for these activities and to estimate daily caloric needs.

The respiratory quotient (RQ), defined as the ratio of carbon dioxide produced to oxygen uptake (RQ = $\dot{V}CO_2/\dot{V}O_2$) can also provide important information. The RQ associated with carbohydrate metabolism is 1.0, with fat metabolism it is 0.7, and with protein metabolism it is 0.8 (Table 26.5). A mixed balanced diet then results in an overall RQ of 0.85. If too much carbohydrate is administered, lipogenesis results. The RQ of net lipogenesis is 8.0! Thus, if a patient has a measured RQ above 1.0, net lipogenesis is taking place and too much carbohydrate is being administered. Similarly, if the overall RQ is 0.7, the patient is primarily burning fat, and if the RQ is less than 0.7, ketosis is likely. On the other hand, an RQ of 0.8 could be either due to balanced metabolism of carbohydrate, fat, and protein or solely due to protein metabolism.

Indirect calorimetry provides the most accurate clinically available estimate of daily caloric requirements. However, in patients with a fractional inspired oxygen above 0.5, the $\dot{V}O_2$ measurement becomes unreliable. In addition, accurate measurements require a stable state, and therefore indirect calorimetry may be most useful in assessing difficult patients who require long-term support. It is also difficult and time consuming to obtain accurate measurements; a competent dedicated technician is required. The equipment is expensive and therefore not universally available. Finally, the use of this equipment has not yet been shown to alter patient outcome.

In patients with a right heart catheter in situ, the oxygen uptake ($\dot{V}O_2$ in milliliters per minute) may also be calculated from the Fick equation. Accordingly,

$$\dot{V}O_2 \text{ (Fick)} = 10 \dot{Q}_{th} (CaO_2 - CvO_2)$$

where $\dot{Q}_{th}$ (liters/minute) is the thermodilution cardiac output and $CaO_2$ and $CvO_2$ are the arterial ($a$) and venous ($v$) oxygen contents (ml/dl) calculated from the formula $CxO_2 = 1.34Hb \, SxO_2 + 0.003 \, PxO_2$; where Hb

is the hemoglobin; where $SO_2$ and $PO_2$ refer to the oxygen saturation and partial pressure, respectively, and $x$ refers to $a$ (arterial) or $v$ (venous). Measurement errors in thermodilution cardiac output, hemoglobin, and saturation will all affect the error in calculated $\dot{V}O_2$. The Fick calculated $\dot{V}O_2$ also does not include the $\dot{V}O_2$ used by the lung nor does it account for the bronchial blood supply, most of which empties into the pulmonary veins. The Fick calculated $\dot{V}O_2$ is typically 5 to 10% less than the directly measured $\dot{V}O_2$ (27). If one further assumes that the patient is consuming a normal mixed fuel source with a respiratory quotient of 0.85, the $\dot{V}CO_2$ (= 0.85 $\dot{V}O_2$) may be eliminated from the above energy expenditure equation, EE = $3.59\dot{V}O_2$ + $1.44\dot{V}CO_2$, to obtain EE (kcal/minute) = $4.81\dot{V}O_2$. Daily caloric needs are obtained by multiplication by 1.44 to yield the Fick estimated REE (kcal/day) simply as

$$\text{REE} \simeq 7\dot{V}O_2 \text{ (Fick)}$$

where the $\dot{V}O_2$ in milliliters per minute is calculated from the Fick equation. This formula will give a reasonable approximation to the daily caloric requirements (27).

## NITROGEN REQUIREMENTS

Nutritional supplementation should contain sufficient protein to maintain the patient's lean body mass. Protein breakdown may be quite variable in ICU patients. Whereas the normal recommended intake is 0.8 g/kg/day, in catabolic patients an intake typically ranging from 1.0 to 1.5 g/kg/day or even higher may be required to maintain nitrogen balance.

Nitrogen is excreted via the kidneys, skin, and gut. The 24-hour urinary nitrogen (UN) represents the renal nitrogen excretion. Each gram of urinary nitrogen results from the breakdown of 6.25 g of protein (equivalent to 30 g of muscle mass). When renal function is stable, the urinary nitrogen level is an estimate of the breakdown of the body's protein. Thus 10 g of urinary nitrogen in 24 hours would imply that 62.5 g of protein is broken down and would need to be ingested to maintain balance. In critically ill patients, values of up to 40 g urine nitrogen may be encountered (Fig. 26.4). Fecal and skin nitrogen losses are typically estimated at 2 g each, for a total of 4 g. However, in patients with diarrhea, gastrointestinal bleeding, or protein-losing enteropathy, gut nitrogen losses alone may reach 4 g. Taking account of protein intake as well as renal and gastrointestinal nitrogen losses, the nitrogen balance equation then becomes

$$\text{Nitrogen balance (g)} = \text{(Protein intake/6.25)}$$
$$- \text{(UN + 4)}$$

In patients with unstable renal function, the urinary nitrogen will not equal the protein breakdown. In this case, the change (Δ) in total body BUN (g) has to be included, so the nitrogen balance equation becomes

$$\text{Nitrogen balance (g)} = (\text{Protein intake}/6.25) - (\text{UN} + 4 + \Delta\text{BUN})$$

The change in total body BUN (g) is the product of the change in blood urea nitrogen (mg/dl) and total body water (TBW [liters] = 0.6 weight [kg]) divided by 100.

A negative nitrogen balance implies net protein loss. With feeding, one then aims to achieve and maintain a positive nitrogen balance. It is important to realize that if excessive protein (more than 2 to 3 g/kg/day) is administered, it may contribute to ureagenesis, thereby creating a futile cycle. In this situation an improving nitrogen balance does not necessarily imply increased net protein synthesis. In the hormone-mediated catabolic state of stress, net protein anabolism may not occur whatever the protein intake and whatever the nitrogen balance. Provided the protein intake is adequate (1.5 g/kg/day), the nitrogen balance may be most useful in assessing the severity of the catabolic state. Evidence that the nitrogen balance is an effective predictor of outcome is lacking.

## THE ROLE OF THE GUT

In the critically ill patient, hypo- and hypermotility problems frequently interfere with the delivery of enteral nutrition. In addition, the gut's mucosal barrier is often compromised, allowing bacteria and/or their products to cross this barrier (28). It has been postulated that gut barrier dysfunction may play an important role in the multiple organ dysfunction syndrome

**TABLE 26.6**
**NUTRIENTS WITH POTENTIAL BENEFITS**[a]

| | |
|---|---|
| Glutamine | Fuel for enterocyte; maintains gut barrier integrity; decreases bacterial translocation |
| Fiber | Needed by colonocyte; decreases bacterial translocation; may decrease enteral feeding-induced diarrhea |
| Arginine | Improves nitrogen retention; improves wound healing; enhances immunity |
| Growth hormones | Improves nitrogen retention; maintains muscle mass |
| Nucleic acids | May improve immune function |
| ω-3 Fatty acids | May improve wound healing and immune function |

[a] See text.

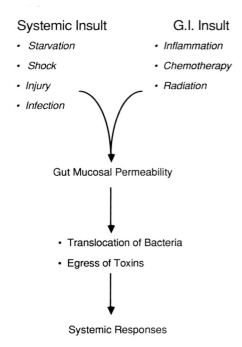

**FIGURE 26.5.** The gut hypothesis. A variety of insults increase bowel permeability, which allows the egress of bacteria or their toxins or both to initiate systemic responses. (From Wilmore DW, Smith RJ, O'Dwyer ST, et al: The gut: a central organ after surgical stress. *Surgery* 104:917–923, 1988; with permission.)

seen so frequently in these patients (Fig. 26.5). Early initiation of enteral feeding has beneficial effects on gut mucosa, its integrity and permeability (29). Administration of specific nutrients, such as glutamine and others (Table 26.6), which once were not considered essential, may have marked salutary effects on the immune and barrier function of the gut. Finally, administration of specific nutrients may also affect wound healing, systemic immunity, and the systemic inflammatory response.

## GUT MOTILITY

Motility disorders are particularly common in patients with ventilatory failure. Hypomotility disorders may present with altered bowel sounds, abdominal distention and pain, increased gastric residuals, vomiting, or aspiration. Abdominal distention decreases functional residual capacity and causes atelectasis, both of which deleteriously affect gas exchange. Distention, with its increased intraabdominal pressure, also increases the pressure the diaphragm must generate with each breath. This in turn increases the work of breathing. Common causes of hypomotility include drugs (narcotics), respiratory failure, intraabdominal processes, electrolyte abnormalities, shock, sepsis, and trauma. Hypomotility will of course interfere with or interrupt the administration of enteral nutrition. Small bowel function commonly remains intact even in the presence of gastric atony. Consequently, if increased gastric residuals are present, placing the feeding tube into the small bowel may bypass the atonic area and allow continuation of enteral alimentation. Metoclopramide may also be tried and can be especially useful in diabetic patients. However, an ileus or colonic obstruction requires cessation of feeding and decompression.

Diarrhea also often interferes with the administration of enteral nutrition. Causes include drugs (magnesium-containing antacids, $H_2$-receptor antagonists, metoclopramide, antibiotics, sorbitol-containing theophylline elixirs, etc.), lactose intolerance, bacterial overgrowth, mediator release (IL-1, TNF), protein calorie malnutrition, decreased plasma oncotic pressure (low albumin), and intolerance to enteral feeding (particularly common with gastric feeding). When one is faced with a patient with diarrhea, any medications that could cause the diarrhea should be stopped. Stool samples should be cultured for *Clostridium difficile*. Furthermore, if possible, isotonic feeding solutions should be used. If enteral feeding causes the diarrhea, the feeding rate should be decreased by 50% and then gradually increased again over the next few days. Adding a fermentable fiber (e.g., Kaopectate, 30 ml t.i.d.), which increases the cecal concentrations of short-chain fatty acids (see below) may also be useful (30). There is also some, albeit controversial, evidence that albumin infusion may decrease diarrhea due to dietary intolerance (by decreasing villus edema) in hypoalbuminemic patients (31). Lastly, narcotic agents that decrease bowel motility should be used cautiously, since they may not be helpful and can cause an ileus.

## GUT BARRIER DYSFUNCTION

The normal gut effectively prevents bacteria and their products from reaching the systemic circulation by the utilization of several defense mechanisms. Competitive bacterial antagonistic actions by normal bowel flora protects against overgrowth by potential pathogens. In addition, gastrointestinal mucus combined with continuous epithelial desquamation and peristalsis limits the intimate contact between gut and bacteria. Secretory immunoglobulins (IgA) also curtail the attachment of bacteria to epithelial cells. Finally, the lymphocytes in the gut-associated lymphoid tissue (GALT) provide a formidable defense barrier.

The enterocyte primarily uses glutamine (normally considered a nonessential amino acid) as its energy source. Whereas glucose is also used by the enterocyte and metabolized via glycolysis to lactate, during times of stress the glucose is needed elsewhere, i.e., at the sites of injury. Consequently, during stress, glutamine uptake by the mucosal cells and GALT increases markedly (32). The glutamine is derived from (and therefore contributes to) endogenous protein catabolism. Unless adequate glutamine is provided, mucosal atrophy and bacterial translocation occur (Fig. 26.6). Soluble fiber has similar trophic effects on the colonocyte (33). One of the metabolic products of soluble fiber is the short-chain fatty acid butyrate, which serves as a fuel for the colonocyte. The lack of both glutamine and soluble fiber may therefore contribute to decreased bowel mass, increased intestinal permeability, and increased bacterial translocation. Once in the systemic circulation, these bacteria and their products contribute to the inflammatory response, and this may play a role in the pathogenesis of the multiple organ dysfunction syndrome (Fig. 26.5).

## NUTRIENTS OF SPECIAL SIGNIFICANCE

Initiation of prompt enteral alimentation after injury as well as alimentation with specific nutrients (glutamine, arginine, and others) may have direct salutary effects on bowel integrity and immunity as well as on the systemic inflammatory response (Table 26.6).

Initiation of enteral nutrition promptly after injury decreases the hypermetabolic hypercatabolic response to burns (34, 35). In addition, early enteral feeding after injury may prevent bacterial translocation. In experimental animal models, initiation of enteral feeding immediately after injury prevents mucosal sloughing and decreases the hypermetabolic response otherwise seen after injury (29). Thus, there is some evidence to suggest that after injury, enteral alimentation should be started as soon as possible, since this may protect the gut as well as decrease the systemic inflammatory response to injury.

The addition of glutamine to the diet preserves gut mass and decreases bacterial translocation in experimental animals with injury induced by chemotherapy or radiation (36). In man, glutamine uptake by the gut increases markedly after injury (37). Furthermore, since glutamine is also a fuel for the GALT, the decreases in plasma glutamine concentration that occur with stress have been implicated in causing immunosuppression (38). Recent studies in man have shown that the addition of glutamine to parenteral nutrition solutions improves nitrogen balance after major surgery (39). Addition of glutamine to parenteral nutrition

## GUT-GLUTAMINE CYCLE

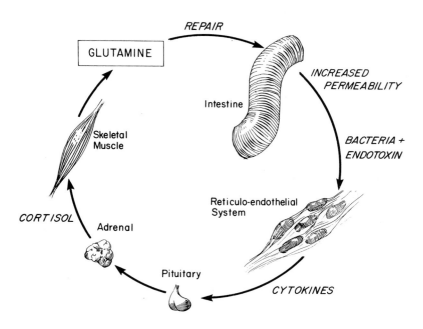

**FIGURE 26.6.**   The gut-glutamine cycle. If bowel permeability is increased (see Figure 26.5), bacteria and/or their toxins invade the host and cause release of cytokines, which stimulate the pituitary-adrenal axis. The elaboration of cortisol mediates skeletal muscle proteolysis, releasing glutamine for gut repair. If the factors that initiated the increased gut permeability persist or if the patient is unable to take enteral feeding and remains glutamine deficient, the cycle continues and results in a prolonged hypercatabolic state. (From Wilmore DW, Smith RJ, O'Dwyer ST, et al: The gut: a central organ after surgical stress. *Surgery* 104:917–923, 1988; with permission.)

solutions also prevents the deterioration in gut permeability and mucosal structure that would otherwise occur with parenteral nutrition (40). Thus, glutamine plays a major role in the maintenance of a healthy gut.

Besides glutamine, various other nutrients (arginine, growth hormone, nucleotides, ω-3 fatty acids) alone or in combination show considerable promise in minimizing proteolysis and enhancing immunologic function. In animal studies, addition of arginine to the diet has beneficial effects on systemic immunity and survival (41). Other studies demonstrate improved nitrogen retention, wound healing, and immune function when arginine is added to the diet (42). To achieve some of these actions, arginine may act in part via the hypothalamic pituitary axis to stimulate secretion of various hormones (glucagon, insulin, growth hormone, and catecholamines). Human growth hormone given postoperatively preserves muscle glutamine and promotes nitrogen retention (43). The combination of glutamine and epidermal growth factor in a septic rat model improves nitrogen balance and preserves gut mass (44). Fish oils and ω-3 polyunsaturated fatty acids

also appear to enhance the immune system and to have antiinflammatory properties (45). Nucleotides, essential for the formation of various coenzymes (e.g. ATP, NAD), may also have beneficial effects on immune function (46). A recent study in postoperative patients showed that the combination of arginine, RNA, and ω-3 fatty acids improves nitrogen retention and wound healing and decreases hospital stay (47). Finally, supplementation with zinc (220 mg twice daily) and vitamin C (1 g daily) in patients deficient in the latter accelerates wound healing.

## ADMINISTRATION OF NUTRITION

The goal of nutritional therapy in the ICU patient is to aid in the patient's recovery and to minimize losses in lean body mass. If malnutrition is present in patients admitted for medical or surgical illness, subsequent morbidity and mortality are increased. The required hospital stay is prolonged, and in fact, infectious complications (pneumonia, wound infections) are increased (48). However, data from prospective randomized trials to support the thesis that well-nourished patients who develop a brief critical illness benefit from nutritional support are less clear-cut (49). Thus, there are no easy or hard answers to the questions of "who" should be fed; when "who" should be fed; how much "who" should be fed; or with what "who" should be fed. Data cited above suggest that early enteral feeding maintains gut integrity and protects against bacterial translocation (29, 34, 35). Early feeding may also increase wound healing (50), decrease infectious complications (51), and decrease the inflammatory response (34, 35). Finally, in selected patient groups, nutritional supplementation improves outcome and decreases the morbidity, mortality, rate of infection, and the duration of hospitalization (47, 52–54). Current data therefore suggest that nutritional supplementation should generally be started as soon as possible. Even though initially it may be difficult to match nutrition to energy expenditure (see below), there may be substantial benefits associated with even partial enteral feeding in preserving gut integrity.

There is increasing evidence that enteral alimentation, if feasible, is preferable to parenteral alimentation (55). Enteral nutrition contains important nutrients (complex carbohydrates, fiber, glutamine) not contained in parenteral solutions. Enteral nutrition is also cheaper, less invasive, and easier to administer (56). Enteral alimentation preserves the structural and functional integrity of the gut. In particular, when compared with parenteral alimentation, enteral alimentation is associated with decreased gastrointestinal mucosal atrophy (56), decreased bacterial translocation through the gastrointestinal barrier (57), and decreased septic morbidity (58). Furthermore, enteral nutrition maintains the immune function of the gut (59, 60). The preceding nonnutritive effects may well be as important as the caloric benefits obtained from enteral nutrition. Therefore, whenever feasible, nutrition should be administered via the enteral route.

## NUTRIENTS ADMINISTERED

Nutritional supplements need to contain sufficient protein to maintain the patient's protein stores and sufficient carbohydrates and lipids to satisfy the caloric requirements (Table 26.7). If the administered carbohydrate and lipid calories are insufficient, additional endogenous protein will be catabolized to serve as a caloric source (15). As previously mentioned, critically ill patients may be very catabolic (Fig. 26.4). Administration of either carbohydrate and protein or fat and protein will result in protein sparing (13–15). The brain, blood cells, and fibroblasts (at the site of injury)

**TABLE 26.7**
**INITIAL NUTRITIONAL SUPPLEMENTATION IN STRESSED PATIENTS**

| | |
|---|---|
| Protein | 1.0 to 1.5 mg/kg/day |
| Calories (30 to 50% lipid, remainder carbohydrate) | 25 kcal/kg/day |

together may utilize approximately 200 to 250 g of glucose daily, so that administration of even such small amounts of glucose will have protein-sparing effects (as long as the glucose is infused together with some protein [13]). However, regardless of the protein intake, one may not be able to achieve a positive nitrogen balance in severely stressed patients (1, 15, 61). The optimal amount of protein that preserves lean tissue mass after severe injury is not established. Even though up to 2 to 3 g/kg/day of protein are sometimes given after severe burns, this may not induce net protein synthesis. An important study (15) in catabolic septic patients suggested that increasing protein infusion rates above 1.5 g/kg/day had no further effect on net protein synthesis. In view of these data, it is commonly recommended to start protein supplementation at a rate of 1.0 to 1.5 g/kg/day. Subsequent changes in rate may be guided by clinical response and by serial changes in nitrogen balance, albumin, or prealbumin. If malnutrition is absent prior to the systemic insult, a negative nitrogen balance up to 5 g/day can usually be well tolerated for a few weeks, whereas losses of 30 g/day (corresponding to 0.9 kg/day of muscle) lead to life-threatening protein malnutrition within a few weeks.

If metabolic measurements are not available, a reasonable clinical approach consists of starting calories at an initial rate equal to 25 kcal/kg/day. The optimal ratio of carbohydrates to fats is a matter of debate and choice that may be tailored to the individual patient's needs. Carbohydrates and fats spare protein equally well (13, 14). There are data to suggest that the protein-sparing effect of carbohydrates levels off when the caloric value of infused dextrose reached 1.2 times the daily resting energy expenditure (62). During stress, maximal glucose utilization rates of 5 to 7 mg/kg/minute (corresponding to infusion of 7 to 10 g/kg/day of glucose) have also been demonstrated (5). Exceeding these rates led to no further increases in glucose oxidation or protein synthesis (9). Since oxidation of glucose releases 3.7 kcal/g (Table 26.2), these maximal rates correspond to infusion of glucose calories equal to 26 to 37 kcal/kg/day. Generally, it is therefore recommended that the administered glucose calories should not exceed these rates of administration (5 to 7 mg/

**TABLE 26.8**
**ADVERSE EFFECTS OF OVERFEEDING**

| | |
|---|---|
| Carbohydrate | ↑ Lipogenesis |
| | ↑ Hepatic steatosis |
| | ↑ $CO_2$ production |
| | ↑ Glucose |
| Lipids | ↓ Arterial $Po_2$ |
| | ↓ Immune function |
| General | ↑ Infections |
| | ↑ Mortality |

kg/minute) or 1.2 times the daily resting energy expenditure. However, after severe burns, up to 100 kcal/kg/day is sometimes required, necessitating a substantial percentage of fat calories to meet caloric requirements.

Since neither carbohydrate nor fat have major advantages as a caloric fuel, typically 30 to 50% of the calories are provided as lipids and the remainder as carbohydrates. However, administration of excess carbohydrates or fats can be hazardous (Table 26.8). Excessive administration of carbohydrates (characterized by an RQ above 1.0) may lead to hyperglycemia, increased $CO_2$ production, decreased mobilization of fatty acids from endogenous fat stores (because of insulin release), and hepatic steatosis (characterized by increasing alkaline phosphatase and bilirubin levels). Similarly, excessive lipid administration may cause immune suppression (63) or a decrease in arterial $Po_2$ by altering ventilation-perfusion matching via interference with prostaglandin production (64). In addition, there is evidence from animal studies that overfeeding may lead to increased infectious complications and increased mortality (65, 66). Thus the catabolic stress response may well have survival advantages, and overfeeding should be avoided. Remember that it is better to be a thin survivor than a fat corpse.

After starting with 25 kcal/kg/day, subsequent changes in calories are guided by clinical response, measurements via indirect calorimetry, and appearance of any side effects (Table 26.8).

### ENTERAL NUTRITION

Enteral nutrition is typically administered via small-bore (6–8 French), flexible, weighted tubes made of polyurethane or silicone that may be inserted with stylets, from the nose into the stomach, duodenum, or jejunum. These smaller tubes are more comfortable to the patient and reduce the risk of reflux and aspiration compared with the large feeding tubes (14–16 French) that were in use a few years ago. Placement of feeding tubes can result in a pneumothorax, hydrothorax, or

esophageal perforation (67). To reduce these placement complications, the stylet should be removed after the nasopharynx is passed. A chest x-ray is needed prior to initiation of feeding to ensure correct placement. A PA chest film alone may not definitively locate the feeding tube in the stomach, since the tube can be located behind the dome of the diaphragm in the costophrenic sulcus. Insufflation of air into the tube while listening for gurgling noises over the left upper quadrant can be helpful (although not definitive) for tube localization in the stomach. Aspiration of stomach contents showing an acidic pH (if the flexible tube allows aspiration and does not collapse) is also helpful.

It is generally believed that postpyloric enteral alimentation is associated with fewer infectious complications due to aspiration than is gastric feeding. The evidence for this tenet is rather weak (68, 69). However, if gastric residuals are substantial, aspiration can ensue. In addition, if gastric paresis is present, as is frequently the case, it will contribute to decreased caloric intake. Compared with gastric feeding, small bowel feedings have been shown to allow increased caloric intake (68). Peristalsis in the small bowel may precede the return of gastric motility, so that if gastric paresis is present, consideration needs to be given to placing the feeding tube in the small bowel. About one-third of weighted feeding tubes pass spontaneously into the small bowel within 24 hours. One bedside procedure reported a 92% success rate for feeding tube placement in the small bowel by manipulation and corkscrew rotation of the tube with a stylet to pass the pylorus (70). If the latter procedure is not successful, fluoroscopic- or endoscopic-assisted small bowel placement may be required.

Gastric feeding is commonly started with an initial dilute (half-strength formula or 5% D/W) infusion equal to the anticipated hourly infusion rate. The tube is then clamped for 30 minutes and the residual is aspirated. If the returned volume is less than 50% of the infused volume, feeding can start (71). If the used formula is isotonic, feeding may immediately start at full strength. There is little advantage to starting with a dilute formula at slow infusion rates (25 to 50 ml/hour), unless the patient has had prolonged bowel rest or has substantial gastric residuals. Gastric residuals should be checked every 4 hours. Gastric residuals should be less than the hourly infusion rate and maximally should not exceed 150 to 200 ml. With duodenal or jejunal feeding, regimens consisting of slow (25 ml/hr) initial infusions of dilute (one-quarter strength) isotonic formula, are commonly used. The flow rate is then gradually increased until the desired rate is achieved, and this is then followed by subsequent increases in concentration. Duodenal or jejunal feeding should be stopped if there is evidence of reflux into the stomach.

Numerous enteral feeding formulas (more than 80) are currently available with a variety of osmolalities (120 to 1200 mOsm/kg), calories (0.5 to 2 kcal/ml), and percentages of calories as protein (4 to 32%), carbohydrate (27 to 91%), or fat (1 to 55%). Polymeric formulas, useful if gut absorption is normal, contain complex proteins, carbohydrates, and fats. Elemental formulas, intended for small bowel feeding, contain little fat, simple amino acids, and oligosaccharides. Enteral formulas also differ in the amounts of fiber, glutamine, arginine, nucleic acids, lactose, vitamins, and trace elements that they contain. A detailed discussion of these formulas as well as a patient's vitamin and trace element requirements is beyond the scope of this review, and the reader is referred elsewhere (72).

Common complications of enteral nutrition are aspiration, diarrhea, and tube obstruction. Aspiration occurs in up to 44% of patients. Simple elevation of the head of the bed may reduce the occurrence of this problem. Similar to histamine $H_2$-receptor antagonists, enteral feedings also increase gastric colonization with Gram-negative bacteria. Acidification of enteral feedings has been shown to decrease this gastric microbial growth (73). As mentioned, jejunal feeding may be associated with fewer pulmonary infections, compared with gastric feeding (68). Diarrhea also occurs commonly (10 to 20% of cases) with enteral feeding. If this occurs with gastric feeding, use of isotonic solutions, reduction in the rate of administration, and/or addition of fiber may alleviate the problem. Agents that decrease gastrointestinal motility should be avoided, since they can lead to an ileus. Finally, small feeding tubes can easily become clogged. Flushing with warm water, crushed pancrelipase tablets, diet sodas, or papain can be tried to clear the obstruction (74).

## PARENTERAL NUTRITION

Increasing acknowledgment that enteral alimentation is possible with most conditions as well as recognition of the benefits associated with enteral alimentation (see above) have led to a decrease in the use of total parenteral nutrition (TPN). Consequently, our discussion of TPN will be limited, and the reader is referred elsewhere for details (75).

Inability of the gut to tolerate or digest an adequate amount of nutrients for an extended period is the indication for TPN. Common indications for TPN thus include bowel obstruction, ileus, bowel ischemia, short bowel syndrome, severe pancreatitis, and severe inflammatory bowel disease. TPN is provided with various solutions of dextrose (10 to 70%), amino acids (5

to 10%), and lipids (10 to 20%). The dextrose (at 3.4 kcal/g) is mixed with an equal amount of amino acids to yield the final solution. Fat emulsions, obtained from soybean or safflower oil, are infused separately or via a Y-connector with the amino acid–dextrose solution. Fats are primarily given to prevent essential fatty acid deficiency (500 ml twice a week suffices) or to provide extra calories (not to exceed 60% of total), as when carbohydrate calories are poorly tolerated. Electrolytes, vitamins, and trace elements (zinc, copper, manganese, chromium, selenium) are added to the dextrose–amino acid solution. If TPN is given via a peripheral vein, the osmolality of the solution has to be reduced to minimize the commonly associated phlebitis (117). Thus peripheral TPN requires the administration of large, dilute (5–15% D/W) volumes of dextrose to administer adequate calories. These large volumes limit the use of peripheral TPN to providing only partial or interim nutritional support. To minimize initial glucose intolerance, central TPN is started with a low dextrose concentration (2 mg/kg/minute) that is increased within a day to full strength (about 4 mg/kg/minute). Insulin may be added if persistent hyperglycemia (above 250 mg/dl) occurs. Insulin administration should be minimized because it inhibits lipoprotein lipase, the enzyme necessary for endogenous fat mobilization from adipose tissue. Initiation of TPN can also lead to hypophosphatemia and consequent muscle weakness (including the respiratory muscles). Similarly, excess glucose can lead to increased $CO_2$ production with associated nutritionally induced hypercapnia and difficulty in weaning patients from mechanical ventilation. Fatty liver due to excessive carbohydrate calories or lipid administration as well as hyperlipidemia, thrombocytopenia, and electrolyte abnormalities may also develop. Finally, TPN does not prevent the development of mucosal atrophy and the consequent bacterial barrier dysfunction of the gut (28) unless glutamine is added to the solution (40).

## RESPIRATION AND NUTRITION

In the patient with respiratory failure, the pulmonary consequences of malnutrition (decreased respiratory muscle strength, decreased ventilatory drive, and impaired lung defenses) can be particularly detrimental. Malnutrition is a risk factor for the development of respiratory failure and may also develop rapidly in these patients because their energy demands (work of breathing) are increased. Whereas nutritional supplementation will eventually improve respiratory muscle strength and facilitate weaning, feedings initially cause an increased ventilatory demand. Furthermore, overfeeding is to be avoided because it leads to increased $CO_2$ production and may result in hypercapnic ventilatory failure. Respiratory muscle weakness may be caused by electrolyte abnormalities (hypophosphatemia, hypokalemia, hypomagnesemia) commonly associated with refeeding. Finally, feeding is an invasive support modality that may be withheld or withdrawn under certain conditions.

### EFFECT OF MALNUTRITION ON LUNG FUNCTION

Malnutrition has major adverse effects on the respiratory muscles, lung defenses, and ventilatory drive. With starvation, loss of respiratory muscle mass and weakness in the remaining fibers occur (76). As a result of the decreased respiratory muscle strength, the maximal voluntary ventilation (an index of endurance) and the vital capacity are decreased (76). In rats, starvation induces emphysema-like morphologic changes in the lung parenchyma (77). Protein restriction also results in reductions in alveolar macrophages in rats. Secretory IgA and complement levels are reduced in malnourished children (78). These abnormalities in the immune system could contribute to the incidence and severity of pulmonary infections commonly seen in malnourished critically ill patients. Finally, semistarvation is accompanied by decreases in both basal oxygen consumption and hypoxic drive (79). The implementation of early nutritional support might mitigate the development of the preceding respiratory complications, which are particularly detrimental to ICU patients with respiratory failure.

### NUTRITION AND RESPIRATORY FAILURE

Malnutrition has been reported to occur in up to 50% of patients with acute respiratory failure (80) and is also common in patients with emphysema or cystic fibrosis (81). In malnourished critically ill patients, major causes of death are respiratory failure, pneumonia, and sepsis (82). If malnutrition is present in patients with chronic obstructive pulmonary disease (COPD), it is a risk factor for the development of respiratory failure as well as death. Progressive malnutrition develops commonly in ventilator-dependent patients (83). The increased metabolic needs associated with respiratory failure (and critical illness) can be substantial. Increased work of breathing leads to increased oxygen demand by the respiratory muscles, which may demand up to 50% of the resting $O_2$ (84). Unless nutritional supplementation is adequate to balance the increased caloric expenditures, malnutrition will develop particularly rapidly in these patients. Although there are no, and are unlikely to be any, randomized prospective controlled trials to determine which patients require nutritional support during mechanical ventilation, it is generally felt that patients who are fed do better than those who are not. However, most data in this area come from anecdotal reports of poorly malnourished ventilator-dependent patients improving after nutrition is added to their therapy (85).

### NUTRITION AND WEANING

The sequelae of malnutrition (viz., decreased muscle strength and decreased respiratory drive) may contribute to failure in weaning patients from ventilatory support. A number of studies suggest that nutritional repletion will improve respiratory muscle strength within several weeks (86). However, the immediate effects of initiation of feeding are an increase in metabolic rate (which may be restored to normal within 4 hours) with a concomitant increase in carbon dioxide production and an increase in respiratory drive (87). Proteins and amino acid solutions may especially increase respiratory drive (88). The increased ventilation resulting from the increase in drive and the added carbon dioxide load (from the increased metabolic rate) may both initially hinder weaning patients with limited pulmonary reserve.

Ventilation also has to increase if total (or carbohydrate) calories provided exceed the energy requirements of the patient. In that case, lipogenesis ensues and the $CO_2$ production increases (89). The increased $CO_2$ production in turn demands an increase in ventilation to keep the arterial $P_{CO_2}$ constant. The amount of $CO_2$ produced depends primarily on the total calories provided and secondarily on the nutritional composition (carbohydrate vs. fat). Although glucose (RQ = 1.0) is associated with a higher carbon dioxide production than fat (RQ = 0.7), only a 20 to 25% increase in $CO_2$ production occurs when an all-fat fuel source is switched to an all-carbohydrate source. On the other hand, excess glucose calories result in net lipogenesis with an associated respiratory quotient of 8.0. Increasing the calories provided by a fixed 60% carbohydrate: 20% fat mixture from estimated resting energy expenditure (REE) to 2 times REE resulted in a far greater increase in $CO_2$ production than did changing the fat: carbohydrate compositions of an isocaloric regimen (89). Since the total calories provided has a far greater effect on the $CO_2$ production than the fat: carbohydrate ratio, overfeeding has to be avoided to prevent increases in $CO_2$ production and ventilation. A number of years ago it was reported that high carbohydrate loads impaired successful weaning of COPD patients from mechanical ventilation, and it was suggested that utilization of formulae high in fat and low in carbohydrate might facilitate weaning. This was supported by data that suggested that high-carbohydrate diets resulted in hypercapnic respiratory failure in patients with compromised ventilatory function (e.g., caused by weak respiratory muscles) (90). However, the more recent evidence cited above suggests that the increased $CO_2$ production is primarily related to the total calories administered rather than to the specific carbohydrate: fat calorie ratio (89). Thus a moderate caloric intake appears to be more important in avoiding nutritionally induced hypercapnia than a low carbohydrate:high fat ratio.

## RESPIRATORY COMPLICATIONS OF NUTRITIONAL SUPPORT

A variety of respiratory complications (Table 26.9) can occur when refeeding is initiated in malnourished patients (91). As described above, overfeeding or administration of excessive carbohydrate calories will result in increased $CO_2$ production and consequent increased ventilatory demands. Overfeeding can also lead to hyperglycemia with consequent impaired resistance to infection as well as hyperosmolar nonketotic coma. Chronically malnourished patients, patients with alcoholism, diabetes, or stressed patients who have not been fed for a few days are also prone to the development of electrolyte abnormalities (hypophosphatemia, hypokalemia, hypomagnesemia). Severe hypophosphatemia (serum phosphorus levels below 1.5

mg/dl [0.5 mmol/liter]) may be precipitated by parenteral or enteral alimentation, phosphate-binding antacids, diuretics, and steroids as well as sepsis. Hypophosphatemia may also occur with the institution of mechanical ventilation in COPD patients secondary to the correction of respiratory acidosis (92). Hypophosphatemia reduces diaphragmatic contractility (93) and may therefore precipitate respiratory failure or be a cause for failure to wean (94).

Refeeding shifts potassium into cells, and hypokalemia can result. Hypokalemia causes muscle weakness, and this weakness can include the respiratory muscles. Common factors that may precipitate hypokalemia include vomiting, diarrhea, diuretics, amphotericin B, nasogastric suctioning, and hypomagnesemia. There is a high incidence (20 to 60%) of often unsuspected hypomagnesemia in critically ill patients (95). Causes include decreased gastrointestinal absorption, renal losses, or intracellular shifts. Hypomagnesemia should be especially suspected in patients with alcoholism and in patients on diuretics, digoxin, or aminoglycosides. Hypomagnesemia decreases respiratory muscle strength and can contribute to hypoventilation (96). Correction of the hypomagnesemia improves respiratory muscle strength.

Finally, the initiation of nutrition is associated with rapid increases in metabolic rate within 30 to 60 minutes. The associated increased carbon dioxide load requires an increase in ventilation to maintain a normal arterial $P_{CO_2}$.

## TABLE 26.9
### RESPIRATORY COMPLICATIONS ASSOCIATED WITH REFEEDING

| Consequences | Cause |
| --- | --- |
| ↑ Ventilation | Feeding increases metabolic rate and drive to breathe; may hinder weaning |
| ↑ $CO_2$ production | Excessive calories or carbohydrate administration; may lead to hypercapnic respiratory failure in patients with little or no respiratory reserve |
| ↓ Phosphate | Feeding causes shifts to intracellular space, common in alcoholics or diabetics; causes muscle weakness and may lead to respiratory failure |
| ↓ Potassium | Vomiting, diuretics, steroids, ↓ magnesium, amphotericin B; causes muscle weakness |
| ↓ Magnesium | Suspect in alcoholics or patients on diuretics or aminoglycosides; causes muscle weakness |

## ETHICAL CONSIDERATIONS OF NUTRITIONAL SUPPORT

The conditions under which it is acceptable to withhold or withdraw nutritional support currently remain controversial. The provision of hydration and nutrition has substantial symbolic and/or religious significance for some health care personnel, patients, or their families. Nevertheless, enteral and parenteral nutrition are generally considered invasive support modalities from clinical (97), ethical (98), and legal (99) points of view. According to ethical guidelines developed by the Hastings Center (98), any treatment modality that imposes an undue burden or that provides no benefit may be withheld or withdrawn. If, as is often the case, the prognosis and benefits to be derived by a patient from nutritional support are uncertain, nutrition should be provided. If, on the other hand, it is deemed that there is no benefit to be derived or that the therapy provided is futile, the support may be withdrawn. This withdrawal of nutritional support should only occur after careful deliberation involving the patient or a surrogate as well as the family. The decision process must consider the ethical principles of beneficence (that benefits must outweigh the burdens), autonomy (that patients have the right to make their own decisions including refusal of treatment), and justice (that individuals have equal access to health care and that treatment decisions should not be based on cost alone). In the Nancy Cruzan case, the U.S. Supreme Court upheld the principle that nutrition and hydration may be stopped in individuals (even once they become incompetent) as long as they had expressed a desire for such an action when they were still competent. Ethical guidelines for withholding and withdrawing life-sustaining therapy are discussed in detail in various professional society position articles (100, 101). Increasing acceptance by patients and health care personnel of the inevitability of death in certain circumstances as well as recognition of the limits of what medical science can reasonably accomplish will both influence the future role of nutritional supplementation. The economic burdens associated with prolonging the dying process will inevitably have a major influence on this evolution.

▼

## References

1. Goldstein SA, Elwyn DH: The effects of injury and sepsis on fuel utilization. *Annu Rev Nutr* 9:445–473, 1989.
2. Bessey PQ, Watters J, Aoki TT, Wilmore DW: Combined hormone infusion stimulates the metabolic response to injury. *Ann Surg* 200:264–281, 1984.
3. Cahill GF Jr: Starvation in man. *N Engl J Med* 282:668–675, 1970.
4. Woolfson AMJ, Heatly RV, Allison SP: Insulin to inhibit protein catabolism after injury. *N Engl J Med* 300:14–17, 1979.
5. Wolfe RR, Herndon DN, Jahoor F, et al: Effect of severe burn injury on substrate cycling by glucose and fatty acids. *N Engl J Med* 317:403–408, 1987.
6. Clowes GHA, Randall HT, Cha JC: Amino acid and energy metabolism in septic and traumatized patients. *JPEN* 4:195–205, 1980.
7. Jeevanadam M, Grote-Holman AE, Chikenji T, et al: Effects of glucose on fuel utilization and turnover in normal and injured man. *Crit Care Med* 18:125–135, 1990.
8. Long CL, Kinney JM, Geiger JW: Nonsuppressibility of gluconeogenesis by glucose in septic patients. *Metabolism* 25:193–201, 1976.
9. Burke JF, Wolfe RR, Mullany CJ, et al: Glucose requirements following burn injury: parameters of optimal glucose infusion and possible hepatic and respiratory abnormalities following excessive glucose intake. *Ann Surg* 190:274–285, 1979.
10. Vary TC, Siegel JH, Nakatani T, et al: Regulation of glucose metabolism by altered pyruvate dehydrogenase activity in sepsis. *JPEN* 10:351–355, 1986.
11. Nordenstrom J, Carpentier YA, Askanazi IE, et al: Free fatty acid mobilization and oxidation during total parenteral nutrition in trauma and infection. *Ann Surg* 198:725–735, 1983.
12. Birkhahn RH, Long CL, Fitkin DL, et al: A comparison of the effects of skeletal trauma and surgery on ketosis of starvation in man. *J Trauma* 21:513–518, 1981.
13. Elwyn DH, Gump FE, Iles M, et al: Protein and energy sparing of glucose added in hypocaloric amounts to peripheral infusions of amino acids. *Metabolism* 27:325–331, 1978.
14. Yamazaki K, Maiz A, Sobrado J, et al: Hypocaloric lipid emulsions and amino acid metabolism in injured rats. *JPEN* 8:360–366, 1984.
15. Shaw JHF, Wildbore M, Wolfe RR: An integrated analysis of glucose, fat, and protein metabolism in severely traumatized patients: studies in the basal state and the response to total parenteral nutrition. *Ann Surg* 209:66–72, 1987.
16. Baracos V, Rodemann HP, Dinarello, et al: Stimulation of muscle protein degradation and prostaglandin E$_2$ release by leukocyte pyrogen (interleukin-1). *N Engl J Med* 308:553–558, 1983.
17. Detsky AS, McLaughlin JR, Baker JP, et al: What is subjective global assessment of nutritional status? *JPEN* 11:8–13, 1987.
18. Gianino S, St John RE: Nutritional assessment of the patient in the intensive care unit. *Crit Care Nurs Clin* 5:1–16, 1993.
19. Chwals WJ, Fernandez ME, Jamie AC, et al: Relationship of metabolic indexes to postoperative mortality in surgical infants. *J Pediatr Surg* 28:819–822, 1993.
20. Weissman C, Kemper M, Askanazi J, et al: Resting metabolic rate of the critically ill patient: Measured versus predicted. *Anesthesiology* 64:673–676, 1986.
21. van Landschot JJB, Feenstra BWA, Vermeij CG, et al: Calculation versus measurement of total energy expenditure. *Crit Care Med* 14:981–985, 1986.
22. Daley BJ, Bistrian BR: Nutritional assessment. In Zaloga GP (ed): *Nutrition in Critical Care*. St Louis, Mosby, 1994, pp 9–33.
23. Burzstein S, Elwyn DH, Askanazi J, et al: The theoretical framework of indirect calorimetry and energy balance. In Bursztein S, Elwyn DH, Askanazi J, Kinney JM (eds): *Energy Metabolism, Indirect Calorimetry and Nutrition*. Baltimore, Williams & Wilkins, 1989, pp 27–80.
24. van Landschot JJB, Feenstra BW, Vermeij CG, et al: Accuracy of intermittent metabolic gas exchange recordings extrapolated for diurnal variation. *Crit Care Med* 16:737–742, 1988.
25. Vermeij CG, Feenstra BW, van Landschot JJB, et al: Day-to-day variability of energy expenditure in critically ill surgical patients. *Crit Care Med* 17:623–626, 1989.
26. Mahutte CK, Jaffe MB, Sasse SA, et al: Relationship of thermodilution cardiac output to metabolic measurements and mixed venous oxygen saturation. *Chest* 104:1236–1242, 1993.
27. Brandi LS, Grana M, Mazzanti T, et al: Energy expenditure and gas exchange measurements in postoperative patients: thermodilution versus indirect calorimetry. *Crit Care Med* 20:1273–1283, 1992.
28. Wilmore DW, Smith RJ, O'Dwyer ST, et al: The gut: a central organ after surgical stress. *Surgery* 104:917–923, 1988.
29. Lo CW, Walker WA: Changes in the gastrointestinal

tract during enteral or parenteral feeding. *Nutr Rev* 47: 193–198, 1989.

30. Bowling TE, Raimundo AH, Grimble GK, et al: Reversal by short-chain fatty acids of colonic fluid secretion induced by enteral feeding. *Lancet* 342:1266–1268, 1993.

31. Mowatt-Larssen CA, Brown RO, Wojtysiak SL, et al: Comparison of tolerance and nutritional outcome between a peptide and a standard enteral formula in critically ill, hypoalbuminemic patients. *JPEN* 16:20–24, 1992.

32. Souba WW, Klimberg VS, Plumley DA, et al: The role of glutamine in maintaining a healthy gut and supporting the metabolic response to injury and infection. *J Surg Res* 48:383–391, 1990.

33. Kripke SA, Fox AD, Berman JM, et al: Stimulation of intestinal mucosal growth with intracolonic infusion of short chain fatty acids. *JPEN* 13:109–116, 1989.

34. Mochizuki H, Trocki O, Dominioni L, et al: Mechanism of prevention of postburn hypermetabolism and catabolism by early enteral feeding. *Ann Surg* 200:297–310, 1984.

35. Barber AE, Jones WG, Minei JP, et al: Glutamine or fiber supplementation of a defined formula diet: impact on bacterial translocation, tissue composition and response to endotoxin. *JPEN* 14:335–343, 1990.

36. Fox A, Kripke S, Berman J, et al: Reduction of severity of enterocolitis by glutamine supplemented enteral diets. *Surg Forum* 38:43–44, 1987.

37. McAnena OJ, Moore FA, Moore EE, et al: Selective uptake of glutamine in the gastrointestinal tract: confirmation in a human study. *Br J Surg* 78:480–482, 1991.

38. Parry-Billings M, Evans J, Calder PC, et al: Does glutamine contribute to immunosuppression after major burns. *Lancet* 336:523–525, 1990.

39. Stehle P, Zander J, Mertes N, et al: Effect of parenteral glutamine peptide supplementation on muscle glutamine loss and nitrogen balance after major surgery. *Lancet* 1:231–233, 1989.

40. Van der Hulst RRWJ, Van Kreel BK, Von Meyenfeldt MF, et al: Glutamine and the preservation of gut integrity. *Lancet* 341:1363–1365, 1993.

41. Kirk S, Barbul A: Role of arginine in trauma, sepsis and immunity. *JPEN* 14:226S–229S, 1990.

42. Daly JM, Reynolds J, Thom A, et al: Immune and metabolic effects of arginine in the surgical patient. *Ann Surg* 208:512–523, 1988.

43. Hammarqvist F, Stromberg C, von der Decken A, et al: Biosynthetic human growth hormone preserves both muscle protein synthesis and the decrease in muscle-free glutamine, and improves whole-body nitrogen economy after operation. *Ann Surg* 216: 184–191, 1992.

44. Ardawi MSM: Effects of epidermal growth factor and glutamine supplemented parenteral nutrition on the small bowel of septic rats. *Clin Sci* 82:573–580, 1992.

45. Katz DP, Kvetan V, Askanazi J: Enteral nutrition: potential role in regulating immune function. *Curr Opin Gastroenterol* 6:199–203, 1990.

46. Van Buren C: Nucleotides. In Zaloga GP (ed): *Nutrition in Critical Care*. St Louis, CV Mosby, 1994, pp 205–214.

47. Daly J, Lieberman M, Goldfine J, et al: Enteral nutrition with supplemental arginine, RNA and omega-3 fatty acids: immunologic metabolic and clinical outcome. *Surgery* 112:56–67, 1992.

48. Hill GL: Body composition research—implications for the practice of clinical nutrition. *JPEN* 16:197–218, 1992.

49. Koretz RL: Feeding controversies. In Zaloga GP (ed): *Nutrition in Critical Care*. St Louis, Mosby, 1994, pp 283–296.

50. Zaloga GP, Bortenschlager L, Black KW, et al: Immediate postoperative enteral feeding decreases weight loss and improves wound healing after abdominal surgery in rats. *Crit Care Med* 20:115–118, 1992.

51. Chiarelli A, Enzi G, Casadei A, et al: Very early nutrition supplementation in burned patients. *Am J Clin Nutr* 51: 1035–1039, 1990.

52. Mullen JL, Buzby GP, Matthews DC, et al: Reduction of operative morbidity and mortality by combined preoperative and postoperative nutritional support. *Ann Surg* 192:604–613, 1981.

53. Askanazi J, Hensle TW, Starker PA, et al: Effect of immediate postoperative nutritional support on lengths of hospitalization. *Ann Surg* 203:236–239, 1986.

54. Grahm TW, Zadrozny DB, Harrington T, et al: The benefits of early jejunal hyperalimentation in the head-injured patient. *Neurosurg* 25:729–735, 1989.

55. Zaloga GP: Timing and route of nutritional support. In Zaloga GP (ed): *Nutrition in Critical Care*. St Louis, Mosby, 1994, pp 283–330.

56. Heymsfeld SB, Bethel RA, Ansley JD, et al: Enteral alimentation: an alternative to central venous hyperalimentation. *Ann Intern Med* 90:63–71, 1979.

57. Alverdy JC, Aoys E, Moss GS: Total parenteral nutrition promotes bacterial translocation from the gut. *Surgery* 104:185–190, 1988.

58. Kudsk KA, Croce MA, Fabian TC, et al: Enteral versus parenteral feeding: effects on septic morbidity after blunt and penetrating abdominal trauma. *Ann Surg* 215: 503–513, 1992.

59. Kaminski MV, Blumeyer TJ: Metabolic and nutritional support of the intensive care unit patient. *Crit Care Clin* 9:363–376, 1993.

60. Manous MR, Deitch EA: The gut barrier. In Zaloga GP (ed): *Nutrition in Critical Care*. St Louis, Mosby, 1994, pp 557–568.

61. Bursztein S, Elwyn DH: Nitrogen balance. In Bursztein S, Elwyn DH, Askanazi J, Kinney JM (eds): *Energy Metabolism, Indirect Calorimetry and Nutrition*. Baltimore, Williams & Wilkins, 1989, pp 85–118.

62. Iapichino G, Gattinoni L, Solca M, et al: Protein sparing and protein replacement in acutely injured patients during TPN with and without amino acid supply. *Intensive Care Med* 8:25–31, 1982.

63. Seidner DL, Mascioli EA, Istfan NW, et al: Effects of long-chain triglyceride emulsions on reticuloendothelial system function in humans. *JPEN* 13:614–619, 1989.

64. McKeen CR, Brigham KL, Bowers RE, et al: Pulmonary vascular effects of fat emulsion infusion in sheep. Prevention by indomethacin. *J Clin Invest* 61:1291–1297.

65. Alexander JW, Gonce SJ, Miskell PW, et al: A new model for studying nutrition in peritonitis. *Ann Surg* 209: 334–340, 1989.

66. Dominioni L, Trocki O, Fang CH, et al: Enteral feeding in burn metabolism: nutritional and metabolic effects of different levels of calorie and protein intake. *JPEN* 9: 269–279, 1985.

67. McWey RE, Curry NS, Schabel SI, et al: Complications

of nasoenteric feeding tubes. *Am J Surg* 155:253–257, 1988.

68. Montecalvo MA, Steger KA, Farber HW, et al: Nutritional outcome and pneumonia in critical care patients randomized to gastric versus jejunal tube feedings. *Crit Care Med* 20:1377–1387, 1992.

69. Strong RM, Condom SC, Solinger MR, et al: Equal aspiration rates from post pylorus and intragastric-placed small bore nasoenteric feeding tubes. A randomized prospective study. *JPEN* 16:59–63, 1992.

70. Zaloga GP: Bedside method for placing small bowel feeding tubes in critically ill patients: a prospective study. *Chest* 100:1643–1646, 1991.

71. Rombeau JL, Caldwell MD, Forlaw L, Guenter PA (eds): *Atlas of Nutritional Support Techniques.* Boston: Little, Brown & Co, pp 77–106, 1989.

72. Zaloga GP (ed): *Nutrition in Critical Care.* St Louis, Mosby, 1994.

73. Heyland D, Bradley C, Mandell LA: Effect of acidified enteral feedings on gastric colonization in the critically ill patient. *Crit Care Med* 20:1388–1394, 1992.

74. Marqard CP, Segall KL, Trogdon S: Clearing obstructed feeding tubes. *JPEN* 12:469–472, 1988; 13:81–83, 1989.

75. Rombeau JL, Caldwell MD (eds): *Parenteral Nutrition.* Philadelphia: Lea & Febiger, 1986.

76. Rochester DF, Esau SA: Malnutrition and the respiratory system. *Chest* 85:411–415, 1984.

77. Kerr JS, Riley DJ, Lanza-Jacobi S, et al: Nutritional emphysema in the rat: influence of protein depletion and impaired lung growth. *Am Rev Respir Dis* 131:644–650, 1984.

78. Stiehm ER: Humoral immunity in malnutrition. *Fed Proc* 39:3093–3097, 1980.

79. Doekel RC Jr, Zwillich CW, Scoggin CH, et al: Clinical semistarvation: depression of hypoxic ventilatory response. *N Engl J Med* 295:358–361, 1976.

80. Pingleton SK: Nutritional management in acute respiratory failure. *JAMA* 22:3094–3097, 1987.

81. Wilson DO, Rogers RM, Hoffman RM: Nutrition and chronic lung disease. *Am Rev Respir Dis* 132:1347–1365, 1985.

82. Askanazi J, Weissman C, Rosenbaum SH, et al: Nutrition and the respiratory system. *Chest* 10:163–172, 1982.

83. Driver AG, LeBrun M: Iatrogenic malnutrition in patients receiving ventilatory support. *JAMA* 244: 2195–2196, 1980.

84. Field S, Kelly SM, Macklem PT: The oxygen cost of breathing in patients with cardiorespiratory disease. *Am Rev Respir Dis* 126:9–13, 1982.

85. Larca L, Greenbaum DM: Effectiveness of intensive nutritional regimes in patients who fail to wean from mechanical ventilation. *Crit Care Med* 10:297–300, 1982.

86. Whittaker JS, Ryan CF, Buckley PA, et al: The effects of refeeding on peripheral and respiratory muscle function in malnourished chronic obstructive pulmonary disease. *Am Rev Respir Dis* 142:283–288, 1990.

87. Weissman C, Askanazi J, Rosenbaum S, et al: Amino acids and respiration. *Ann Intern Med* 98:41–44, 1983.

88. Takala J, Askanazi J, Weissman C, et al: Changes in respiratory control induced by amino acid infusion. *Crit Care Med* 16:465–469, 1988.

89. Talpers SS, Romberger DJ, Bunce SB, et al: Nutritionally associated increased carbon dioxide production: excess total calories vs high proportion of carbohydrate calories. *Chest* 102:551–555, 1992.

90. Herve P, Simonneau G, Girard P, et al: Hypercapnic acidosis induced by nutrition in mechanically ventilated patients: glucose versus fat. *Crit Care Med* 13: 537–540, 1985.

91. Solomon SM, Kirby DF: The refeeding syndrome: a review. *JPEN* 14:90–97, 1990.

92. Laaban JP, Grateau G, Psychoyos I, et al: Hypophosphatemia induced by mechanical ventilation in patients with chronic obstructive pulmonary disease. *Crit Care Med* 17:1115–1120, 1989.

93. Aubier M, Murciano D, Lecocguic Y, et al: Effect of hypophosphatemia on diaphragmatic contractility in patients with acute respiratory failure. *N Engl J Med* 313: 420–424, 1985.

94. Agusti AGN, Torres A, Estopa R, et al: Hypophosphatemia as a cause of failed weaning: the importance of metabolic factors. *Crit Care Med* 12:142–144, 1984.

95. Ryzen E, Wagers PW, Singer FR, et al: Magnesium deficiency in a medical ICU population. *Crit Care Med* 13: 19–21, 1985.

96. Fiaccadori E, DelCanale S, Coffrini E, et al: Muscle and serum magnesium in pulmonary intensive care unit patients. *Crit Care Med* 16:751–760, 1988.

97. American Medical Association Council on Ethical and Judicial Affairs: *Withholding or Withdrawing Life-Prolonging Medical Treatment.* Chicago, American Medical Association, 1989.

98. Hastings Center: *Guidelines in the Termination of Life-Sustaining Treatment and the Care of the Dying.* Briarcliff Manor, NY, Hastings Center, 1987.

99. Paris JJ, Reardon JD: Court responses to withholding or withdrawing artificial nutrition and fluids. *JAMA* 253: 2243–2245, 1985.

100. An ACCP/SCCM consensus panel: Ethical and moral guidelines for the initiation, continuation, and withdrawal of intensive care. *Chest* 97:949–958, 1990.

101. American Thoracic Society: Withholding and withdrawing life-sustaining therapy. *Am Rev Respir Dis* 144: 726–731, 1991.

# Index

Page numbers followed by *f* denote figures; those followed by *t* denote tables.

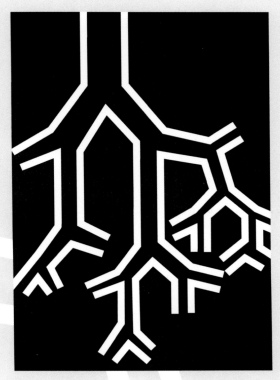

# Pulmonary Care Resources

From Williams & Wilkins

## Try them for 30 days...
## There's No Risk To You—

You can preview these books for a full month.  If you're not completely satisfied, return them to us within 30 days at no further obligation (US only).  There's never any risk to you.

## To order CALL:

Toll Free    1-800-638-0672
Refer to #A4 436 I when you order
FAX          1-800-447-8438
INTERNET
E-mail: wwbooks@access.digex.net
Electronic Newstand (Mini-Catalog): gopher enews.com

---

# Please Send Me:

_____ Feinsilver: **A Textbook of Bronchoscopy** May 1995/about 800 pages/3107-4/$125.00
_____ Light: **Pleural Diseases, 3rd edition** May 1995/5017-6/$75.00
_____ George: **Chest Medicine, 3rd edition** May 1995/608 pages/230 illustrations/3458-8/$77.00
_____ Perel: **Handbook of Mechanical Ventilatory Support**
_____ Marino: **The ICU Book** 1991/1306-3/$49.50
_____ **Stedman's Medical Dictionary, 25th ed.** 1990/7916-6/$43.00

**Try them for 30 days...There's No Risk To You—**
You can preview these books for a full month.  If you're not completely satisfied, return them to us within 30 days at no further obligation (US only).  There's never any risk to you.

## To order CALL:
## Toll Free   1-800-638-0672
Refer to #A4 436 I when you order
FAX 1-800-447-8438
INTERNET
E-mail: wwbooks@access.digex.net
Electronic Newstand (Mini-Catalog): gopher enews.com

## Payment Options:

☐ Check enclosed (plus $4.00 handling)
☐ Bill me (plus  postage and handling)
☐ Charge my credit card (plus postage &handling)

___ Mastercard  ___Visa  ___ American Express

card #

exp. date

signature or p.o.#
(        )
your telephone #
CA, IL, MD, and PA residents please add state sales tax.
Prices subject to change without notice.

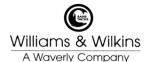
Williams & Wilkins
A Waverly Company

Printed in US  11  94
GEORGBI      A4 436 I

---

# Please Send Me:

_____ Feinsilver: **A Textbook of Bronchoscopy** May 1995/about 800 pages/3107-4/$125.00
_____ Light: **Pleural Diseases, 3rd edition** May 1995/5017-6/$75.00
_____ George: **Chest Medicine, 3rd edition** May 1995/608 pages/230 illustrations/3458-8/$77.00
_____ Perel: **Handbook of Mechanical Ventilatory Support**
_____ Marino: **The ICU Book** 1991/1306-3/$49.50
_____ **Stedman's Medical Dictionary, 25th ed.** 1990/7916-6/$43.00

**Try them for 30 days...There's No Risk To You—**
You can preview these books for a full month.  If you're not completely satisfied, return them to us within 30 days at no further obligation (US only).  There's never any risk to you.

## To order CALL:
## Toll Free   1-800-638-0672
Refer to #A4 436 I when you order
FAX 1-800-447-8438
INTERNET
E-mail: wwbooks@access.digex.net
Electronic Newstand (Mini-Catalog): gopher enews.com

## Payment Options:

☐ Check enclosed (plus $4.00 handling)
☐ Bill me (plus  postage and handling)
☐ Charge my credit card (plus postage &handling)

___ Mastercard  ___Visa  ___ American Express

card #

exp. date

signature or p.o.#
(        )
your telephone #
CA, IL, MD, and PA residents please add state sales tax.
Prices subject to change without notice.

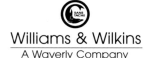
Williams & Wilkins
A Waverly Company

Printed in US  11  94
GEORGBI      A4 436 I

**BUSINESS REPLY MAIL**

FIRST CLASS    PERMIT NO. 724    BALTIMORE, MD.

POSTAGE WILL BE PAID BY ADDRESSEE

**Williams & Wilkins**
P.O. Box 1496
Baltimore, Maryland 21298-9724

NO POSTAGE
NECESSARY
IF MAILED
IN THE
UNITED STATES

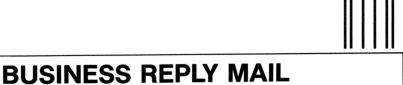

**BUSINESS REPLY MAIL**

FIRST CLASS    PERMIT NO. 724    BALTIMORE, MD.

POSTAGE WILL BE PAID BY ADDRESSEE

**Williams & Wilkins**
P.O. Box 1496
Baltimore, Maryland 21298-9724

NO POSTAGE
NECESSARY
IF MAILED
IN THE
UNITED STATES

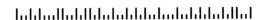